PDR FOR HERBAL MEDICINES

FIRST EDITION

PDR®

for Herbal Medicines

MEDICAL ECONOMICS COMPANY

MONTVALE, NEW JERSEY

PDR®

for Herbal Medicines

ISBN: 1-56363-292-6

Contents

Foreword

Almost overnight, herbal remedies have become a major factor in American health care. Botanicals with names like Ginseng, St. John's Wort, and Ma Huang have suddenly become household words throughout the U.S. Sales of herbal remedies are doubling every four years. And as herbs move out of the health food stores and into mainstream supermarkets and drugstores, the trend towards self-medication with "natural" supplements seems certain to accelerate.

The majority of today's herbal remedies exhibit varying degrees of therapeutic value. Some—such as ginkgo, valerian, and saw palmetto—seem genuinely useful, while others—such as ephedra, tansy, and nightshade—can actually be dangerous. As the use of unfamiliar botanicals spreads, the need to steer patients towards the few truly useful preparations—and warn them away from ineffective and dangerous alternatives—is becoming an increasingly significant priority.

Which herbals should be taken seriously and which dismissed? In the free-wheeling dietary-supplement segment of the health care marketplace, reliable information has been very hard to come by. Spared the rigors of FDA review, suppliers are free to make controversial claims based on limited or anecdotal evidence, and no standard, generally accepted compendium of scientific information has been available to contradict them.

To rectify this situation, *Physicians' Desk Reference®* is pleased to bring you the closest available analog to FDA-approved labeling—the findings of the German Regulatory Authority's herbal watchdog agency, commonly called "Commission E." This agency has conducted an intensive assessment of the peer-reviewed literature on some 300 common botanicals, weighing the quality of the clinical evidence and identifying the uses for which the herb can reasonably be considered effective. Its conclusions represent the best expert consensus on medicinal herbs currently to be found.

For those herbs not considered by Commission E, *Physicians' Desk Reference* has augmented this compendium with the results of an exhaustive literature review conducted by the respected PhytoPharm U.S. Institute of Phytopharmaceuticals under the direction of noted botanist, Dr. Joerg Gruenwald. These additional monographs, some 300 in number, provide a detailed introduction to an array of exotic botanicals that you'll be hard pressed to find in any other source.

To make the information in the monographs as useful and accessible as possible, *PDR* has echoed the structure of standard U.S. product labeling. Each monograph contains up to nine standard sections, covering considerations ranging from description to dosage. Here's a closer look at what you will find:

- **Names:** Each monograph begins with the herb's scientific name, followed by its most widely accepted common name. In addition, all monographs are cross-referenced by the accepted common name.
- **Description:** This section provides a detailed botanical overview of the herb, including information on its medicinal parts; flower and fruit; leaves, stem and root; unique characteristics, habitat, production, related plants, and additional common names and synonyms.
- **Actions and Pharmacology:** Here you'll find data on the active compounds or heterogeneous mixtures found in the plant, followed by a summary of the herb's clinical effects. If various parts of the plant possess different pharmacological activity, the parts are discussed individually, here and throughout the remainder of the monograph.
- **Indications and Usage:** Uses for which the herb has been judged effective by Commission E are presented here in list fashion. Provisos regarding route and form of administration for each indication are appended as necessary. Unsubstantiated uses found in folk medicine, Asian medicine, and homeopathic practice are also enumerated.
- **Contraindications:** Although most natural remedies can be used under all medical circumstances, a few pharmacologically potent herbs must be avoided in certain patient populations and in the presence of certain medical conditions. If any such contraindications exist, they are summarized here.
- **Precautions and Adverse Reactions:** Found in this section are any cautions or special considerations regarding safe use of the herb, including any restrictions on use in pregnancy or childhood. Although most herbal remedies are notably free of known side effects, any reported in the available literature are noted here.
- **Overdosage:** As we all know, "natural" is not synonymous with "benign," and an overdose of many "healing" herbs can have serious—even fatal—consequences. Whenever adverse effects of overdose have been found in the literature, they are reported here, along with the appropriate medical interventions to be undertaken when an overdose occurs.
- **Dosage:** Listed here are common modes of administration and representative dosage recommendations drawn from the literature. Note, however, that this information can be used only as a general guide, and that it is often applicable only to the natural herb. The potency of individual preparations and extracts is subject to substantial variation, so the manufacturer's directions should be consulted whenever available.
- **Literature:** This section provides you with a unique bibliography of the technical literature. Because German researchers have been particularly active in the herbal arena, you will find an unusual number of German-language citations. However, work in the English literature is included as well.

To assist you in quickly locating the information you require, the monographs have been indexed by name, therapeutic category, indications, and side effects. Here's an overview of what each index provides:

- **Scientific and Common Name Index:** This index presents a list of all plant names and their page numbers, with scientific and common names intermingled alphabetically. For quick reference, each herb's common names are repeated under its scientific name.
- **Indications Index:** This index lists the herbal products and their page numbers, alphabetically by scientific name, under their various indications. Herbs deemed effective for an indication are shown in Roman type. If the indication is tentative or controversial, the herb appears in italics. For your convenience, the most widely accepted common name is appended to each entry. To help you quickly identify conventional alternatives, the indication headings match those found in *PDR's* Indications Index, which appears in the *PDR® Companion Guide*™ and the *PDR® Electronic Library CD-ROM.*
- **Therapeutic Category Index:** This index lists the monographs and their page numbers, alphabetically by scientific name, under appropriate therapeutic category headings. As in the Indications Index, the most widely accepted common name is appended to each entry. To facilitate comparison with prescription and nonprescription drugs, *PDR's* standard therapeutic categories are used throughout.
- **Side Effects Index:** In this index, you'll find a list of all herbs associated with a given adverse reaction. As in the other indices, the herbs are listed alphabetically by scientific name, with the common name and page number appended. Nomenclature employed in the side effect headings matches that used in *PDR's* Side Effects Index, another feature of the *PDR®*

Companion Guide™ and the *PDR*® *Electronic Library CD-ROM.*

In addition to these convenient indices, you will also find a brief guide to drug/herb interactions. In this section, each potential interaction is listed under both the name of the drug and the name of the interacting herb. Each entry includes a brief description of the interaction's effect.

Following the indices, just as in *PDR* itself, you'll find an extensive full-color identification guide encompassing nearly 400 of the most widely used herbs—a truly unique reference unmatched in any other printed resource. We've also included a brief glossary of the unfamiliar terms found in the monographs.

PDR for Herbal Medicines is the product of one of the most thorough and inclusive examinations of the herbal literature ever undertaken. Nevertheless, it's important to remember that it merely summarizes and synthesizes key data from the underlying research reports, and of necessity includes neither every published report nor every recorded fact.

As in all scientific investigation, conclusions regarding the effectiveness of the herbs discussed in this compendium are based on the preponderance of current evidence and cannot be considered firm or final. The publisher does not warrant that any herb will unfailingly and uniformly exhibit the properties ascribed to it in these pages. Likewise, the publisher does not guarantee that every possible hazard, adverse effect, contraindication, precaution, or consequence of overdose is included in the summaries presented here. The publisher has performed no independent verification of the data reported herein, and expressly disclaims responsibility for any error, whether inherent in the underlying literature or resulting from erroneous translation, transcription, or typography.

Although the publisher has endeavored to provide the most extensive possible coverage of currently available botanical preparations, not all medicinal herbs can be found herein. As review of the literature continues, additional herbs will be included in future editions. Inclusion of an herb in the current editions does not signify an endorsement by the publisher; absence of an herb does not imply its rejection.

It should be understood that by making this material available, the publisher is not advocating the use of any substance described herein. Please remember that in the United States, herbal products must be in compliance with the Dietary Supplement Health and Education Act of 1994, which stipulates that they may not be marketed for the diagnosis, treatment, cure, or prevention of any disease. The monographs in *PDR for Herbal Medicines* do not discuss claims made for any proprietary herbal preparation. They merely report general findings on generic botanicals and their extracts.

When patients approach you—as they surely will—for advice on the latest herbal "discovery" to hit the nightly news, we hope that *PDR for Herbal Medicines* will provide you with all the facts you need to offer sound, rational guidance firmly grounded in fact. Certainly such counseling is the aim of every dedicated health care professional. And at PDR, we fully share that goal.

Scientific and Common Name Index

In this index, all botanicals profiled in the Herbal Monographs section are listed alphabetically by both their scientific and common names. The scientific name appears in bold type, common names are shown in standard type. Under each scientific name, all associated common names are repeated in italic type. If an entry lists two page numbers, the first refers to a photograph of the plant in the Herb Identification Guide, the second to the herbal monograph.

Indications Index

Entries in this index are organized by specific indication, enabling you to quickly review the botanical alternatives for a particular diagnosis. For ease of comparison with prescription and over-the-counter medications, the index employs the same nomenclature found in the Indications Index of the PDR Companion Guide™. Under each heading, herbs are listed alphabetically by scientific name, with the leading common name shown in parentheses. Botanicals deemed effective by the German Regulatory Authority's "Commission E" appear in standard type. Those which have not received the commission's imprimatur are shown in italics. If an entry lists two page numbers, the first refers to a photograph of the plant in the Herb Identification Guide, the second to the herbal monograph. For more information on both proven and traditional remedies, be sure to check the appropriate underlying monograph.

Passiflora Incarnata (Passion Flower) **517, 1015**
Strychnos Nux Vomica (Nux Vomica) **522, 1161**
Syzygium Cumini (Jambolan) **1168**

DERMATITIS, ECZEMATOID

Calendula Officinalis (Marigold) **505, 704**

DERMATITIS, SEBORRHEIC

Arachis Hypogaea (Peanuts) **655**
Avena Sativa (Oats) **504, 680**
Betula Species (Birch) **504, 691**
Daphne Mezereum (Mezereon) **508, 800**
Lawsonia Inermis (Henna) ... **513, 930**
Mahonia Aquifolium (Mountain Grape) **515, 953**
Quillaja Saponaria (Soap Bark) **519, 1079**
Urtica Dioica (Nettle) **523, 1197**
Viola Tricolor (Heartsease) **1218**

DERMATITIS, UNSPECIFIED

Carlina Acaulis (Carline Thistle) **505, 719**
Drimys Winteri (Winter's Bark) .. **813**
Vaccinium Myrtillus (Bilberry) **524, 1201**

DIABETES

Allium Cepa (Onion) **502, 624**
Allium Sativum (Garlic) **502, 626**
Aloe Barbadensis (Aloe) **502, 630**
Avena Sativa (Oats) **504, 680**
Caesalpinia Bonducella (Divi-Divi) **703**
Carex Arenaria (German Sarsaparilla) **717**
Centaurium Umbellatum (Centaury) **505, 728**
Elymus Repens (Couch Grass) **509, 825**
Eucalyptus Globulus (Eucalyptus) **509, 836**
Galega Officinalis (Goat's Rue) **510, 857**
Medicago Sativa (Alfalfa) ... **515, 963**
Phaseolus Vulgaris (Bean) .. **518, 1027**
Phragmites Communis (Reed Herb) **1028**
Solidago Species (Golden Rod) **522, 1148**
Sorbus Aucuparia (Mountain Ash Berry) **522, 1151**
Sorbus Torminalis (Ash) **1153**
Syzygium Cumini (Jambolan) **1168**
Taraxacum Officinale (Dandelion) **1174**
Theobroma Cacao (Cocoa) . **523, 1179**
Urtica Dioica (Nettle) **523, 1197**

DIABETES MELLITUS

Helianthus Annuus (Sunflower) **511, 891**
Senecio Nemorensis (Life Root) .. **1134**
Vaccinium Myrtillus (Bilberry) **524, 1201**

DIARRHEA

Acacia Senegal (Acacia) **603**
Castanea Sativa (Chestnut) **724**
Centella Asiatica (Hydrocotyle) **505, 729**
Ceratonia Siliqua (Carob) ... **506, 732**
Lysimachia Vulgaris (Loosestrife) **514, 951**
Lythrum Salicaria (Purple Loosestrife) **514, 952**
Maranta Arundinaceae (Arrowroot) **958**
Marrubium Vulgare (White Horehound) **515, 959**
Mentha Aquatica (Wild Mint) **515, 969**
Sanguisorba Officinalis (Great Burnet) **521, 1118**
Teucrium Scordium (Water Germander) **1178**
Ulmus Minor (Elm Bark) **1196**

DIARRHEA, BLOODY, SYMPTOMATIC RELIEF OF

Cumimum Cyminum (Cumin) . **508, 785**

DIARRHEA, CHRONIC

Ailanthus Altissima (Tree of Heaven) **501, 618**
Cornus Florida (Dogwood) .. **507, 777**
Nymphaea Odorata (American White Pond Lily) **516,994**

DIARRHEA, SYMPTOMATIC RELIEF OF

Acacia Arabica (Acacia) **601**
Achillea Millefolium (Yarrow) **501, 604**
Achillea Ptarmica (Sneezewort) ... **606**
Aegle Marmelos (Bael) **612**
Aethusa Cynapium (Fool's Parsley) **501, 616**
Agrimonia Eupatoria (Agrimony) **501, 617**
Ailanthus Altissima (Tree of Heaven) **501, 618**
Alchemilla Vulgaris (Lady's Mantle) **501, 621**
Alkanna Tinctoria (Alkanna) . **502, 623**
Alstonia Constricta (Fever Bark) . **635**
Althaea Officinalis (Marshmallow) **635**
Amaranthus Hypochondriacus (Amaranth) **502, 638**
Avena Sativa (Oats) **504, 680**
Bellis Perennis (Wild Daisy) . **504, 687**
Berberis Vulgaris (Barberry) . **504, 688**
Betonica Officinalis (Wood Betony) **504, 690**
Calluna Vulgaris (Heather) .. **505, 706**
Camellia Sinensis (Green Tea) **505, 710**
Capsicum Annuum (Cayenne) **505, 715**
Chondrus Crispus (Carrageen) ... **742**
Cinnamomum Aromaticum (Chinese Cinnamon) **749**
Cinnamomum Verum (Cinnamon) **506, 752**
Coffea Arabica (Coffee) **507, 763**
Croton Eleuteria (Cascarilla) **782**
Curcuma Domestica (Turmeric) ... **786**
Cydonia Oblongata (Quince) **791**
Cynoglossum Officinale (Hound's Tongue) **794**
Cypripedium Calceolus (Nerve Root) **796**
Daemonorops Draco (Dragon's Blood) **800**
Erigeron Canadensis (Canadian Fleabane) **509, 831**
Eugenia Chequen (Cheken) **839**
Euphorbia Cyparissias (Cypress Spurge) **510, 843**
Fragaria Vesca (Strawberry Leaf) **510, 852**
Galipea Officinalis (Angostura) ... **858**
Geranium Robertianum (Herb Robert) **511, 867**
Geum Rivale (Water Avens) .. **511, 869**
Geum Urbanum (Bennet's Root) **511, 869**
Glechoma Hederacea (Ground Ivy) **511, 873**
Gossypium Herbaceum (Cotton) **511, 880**
Haematoxylon Campechianum (Logwood) **884**
Hamamelis Virginiana (Witch Hazel) **511, 885**

DIGESTIVE DISORDERS, SYMPTOMATIC RELIEF OF

DIGESTIVE INSUFFICIENCIES, SYMPTOMATIC RELIEF OF

DROPSY

(*See under* Edema, Idiopathic)

DYSENTERY

DYSMENORRHEA, UNSPECIFIED, SYMPTOMATIC RELIEF OF

RHEUMATIC DISORDERS, UNSPECIFIED

URINARY TRACT PAIN, RELIEF OF

(*See under* Pain, Urinary Tract)

UTERINE ATONY, POSTPARTUM

UTERINE BLEEDING

UTERINE SPASTICITY

VAGINAL ITCHING

VAGINAL PROLAPSE

VAGINAL SECRETIONS

VENEREAL DISEASE

VENOUS CONDITIONS

Therapeutic Category Index

Entries in this index are organized by prescribing category, enabling you to quickly identify botanicals with similar properties. Please note that this index reflects not only scientifically verified applications, but also uninvestigated folk uses with varying degrees of promise. For an assessment of the herb's precise clinical status, please check the underlying monograph.

Within each category, herbs are listed alphabetically by scientific name, with the leading common name shown in parentheses. If an entry lists two page numbers, the first refers to a photograph of the plant in the Herb Identification Guide, the second to the herbal monograph. The index lists herbs by general category only. To locate botanicals considered appropriate for a specific indication, please consult the Indications Index.

ANTACID PREPARATIONS

ANTHELMINTICS

ANTIANXIETY AGENTS

ANTIARRHYTHMICS

ANTICONVULSANTS

ANTIDEPRESSANTS

ANTIDIABETIC AGENTS

ANTIDIARRHEALS

ANTIEMETICS

ANTIFLATULENTS

ANTIFUNGALS

ANTIHISTAMINES & COMBINATIONS

ANTI-INFECTIVES

ANTI-INFLAMMATORY AGENTS

ANTILIPEMIC AGENTS

ANTIMALARIAL AGENTS

ANTIPANIC AGENTS

ANTIPRURITICS

ANTIPSORIATIC AGENTS

ANTIRHEUMATIC AGENTS

ANTISEBORRHEIC AGENTS

ANTISPASMODICS

ANTITHYROID AGENTS

ANTITUBERCULOSIS AGENTS

ANTIVIRALS

APPETITE STIMULANTS

APPETITE SUPPRESSANTS

BENIGN PROSTATIC HYPERPLASIA (BPH) THERAPY

BOWEL EVACUANTS

BURN PREPARATIONS

CALCIUM OXALATE STONE PREVENTION

CARDIOVASCULAR AGENTS

CENTRAL NERVOUS SYSTEM STIMULANTS

COLD & COUGH PRODUCTS WITH ANALGESICS

COUGH & COLD PRODUCTS

DECONGESTANTS & COMBINATIONS

DECONGESTANTS, EXPECTORANTS & COMBINATIONS

DENTAL PREPARATIONS

DEODORANTS

DEPIGMENTING AGENTS

DIGESTIVE AIDS

DIGESTIVE ENZYMES

DIURETIC AGENTS

EMOLLIENTS & MOISTURIZERS

ENURESIS MANAGEMENT

ERECTILE DYSFUNCTION THERAPY

LOCAL ANESTHETICS

MIGRAINE PREPARATIONS

MOTION SICKNESS PRODUCTS

MOUTH & THROAT PRODUCTS

NARCOTIC ANTITUSSIVES & COMBINATIONS

NARCOTICS & COMBINATIONS

NON-NARCOTIC ANTITUSSIVES & COMBINATIONS

SMOKING CESSATION AIDS

SMOOTH MUSCLE RELAXANTS

STIMULANT LAXATIVES & COMBINATIONS

SUNBURN PREPARATIONS

TEETHING REMEDIES

TREMOR PREPARATIONS

URINARY ANTI-INFECTIVES & COMBINATIONS

URINARY TRACT AGENTS

VAGINAL PREPARATIONS

VENOUS INSUFFICIENCY PRODUCTS

VERTIGO AGENTS

VITAMIN C & COMBINATIONS

WART PREPARATIONS

WOUND CARE PRODUCTS

Side Effects Index

Presented here is an alphabetical list of every side effect cited in the herbal monographs. Under each heading, herbs associated with the reaction are listed alphabetically by scientific name, with the leading common name shown in parentheses. For ease of comparison with prescription and over-the-counter medications, the index employs the same nomenclature found in the Side Effects Index of the PDR Companion Guide.™ If an entry lists two page numbers, the first refers to a photograph of the plant in the Herb Identification Guide, the second to the herbal monograph.

Drug/Herb Interactions Guide

This section catalogs potentially adverse drug/herb combinations by both the generic name of the drug and the scientific name of the herb. Under each bold-face drug entry you'll find a list of the herbs with which the agent may interact. Likewise, under a bold-face herb entry you'll find a list of potentially interactive drugs. A description of the interaction's effect follows each item in the list. Further information on each drug can be found in Physicians' Desk Reference®. Information on each herb appears in the Herbal Monographs section of this book.

ADONIS
(*See under* Adonis Vernalis)

ADONIS VERNALIS
Calcium
(*Increases action of Adonis*)
Glucocorticoids
(*Increases action of Adonis*)
Laxatives
(*Increases action of Adonis*)
Quinidine
(*Increases action of Adonis*)
Saluretics
(*Increases action of Adonis*)

ALCOHOL
Rauwolfia Serpentina
(*Increases impairment of motor skills*)

ALKALINE DRUGS
Quercus Robur
(*Absorption of alkaline drugs may be reduced or inhibited*)

ALKALOIDS
Quercus Robur
(*Absorption of alkaloids may be reduced or inhibited*)

ALOE
(*See under* Aloe Barbadensis)

ALOE BARBADENSIS
Antiarrhythmics
(*Effect not specified*)
Cardiac Glycosides
(*Increases effect of cardiac glycosides*)
Corticosteroids
(*Increased potassium loss*)
Licorice
(*Increased potassium loss*)
Thiazide Diuretics
(*Increased potassium loss*)

ALPINE CRANBERRY
(*See under* Vaccinium Vitis-Idaea)

AMANTADINE HYDROCHLORIDE
Atropa Belladonna
(*Increases anticholinergic effect of herb*)
Hyoscyamus Niger
(*Increased anticholinergic action*)
Scopolia Carniolica
(*Increased effect when given simultaneously with herb*)

ANTIARRHYTHMICS
Aloe Barbadensis
(*Effect not specified*)
Rhamnus Cathartica
(*Increased effect due to potassium loss with chronic use of herb*)
Rhamnus Purshianus
(*Effect unspecified*)

ANTIHISTAMINES
Hyoscyamus Niger
(*Increased anticholinergic action*)

ANTITHROMBOLYTIC DRUGS
Ginkgo Biloba
(*Increases effect of antithrombolytic drugs*)

ARCTOSTAPHYLOS UVA-URSI
Medication and Food that Increase Uric Acid Levels
(*Decreases effect of herb*)

ASPIRIN
Tanacetum Parthenium
(*Increased antithrombotic effect*)

ATROPA BELLADONNA
Amantadine Hydrochloride
(*Increases anticholinergic effect of herb*)
Quinidine
(*Increases anticholinergic effect of herb*)
Tricyclic Antidepressants
(*Increases anticholinergic effect of herb*)

BARBITURATES
Rauwolfia Serpentina
(*Synergistic effect*)

BELLADONNA
(*See under* Atropa Belladonna)

BREWER'S YEAST
(*See under* Saccharomyces Cerevisiae)

BROOM
(*See under* Cytisus Scoparius)

BUCKTHORN
(*See under* Rhamnus Cathartica)

BUCKTHORN BARK
(*See under* Rhamnus Frangula)

BUGLEWEED
(*See under* Lycopus Virginicus)

CALCIUM

Adonis Vernalis
(Increases action of Adonis)
Convallaria Majalis
(Increases the effect of Convallaria)
Drimia Maritima
(Increases effectiveness and side effects of herb)

CALCIUM SALTS

Nerium Odoratum
(Increased efficacy and side effects when given simultaneously with herb)
Strophanthus Species
(Simultaneous administration with herb enhance both effects and side effects)

CARDIAC GLYCOSIDES

Aloe Barbadensis
(Increases effect of cardiac glycosides)
Ephedra Sinica
(Disturbance of heart rhythm)
Rhamnus Cathartica
(Increased effect due to potassium loss with chronic use of herb)
Rhamnus Frangula
(Increased effect due to potassium loss with chronic use of herb)
Rhamnus Purshianus
(Increased effect due to potassium loss with chronic use of herb)
Rheum Palmatum
(Increased effect due to potassium loss with chronic use of herb)

CARDIOACTIVE STEROIDS

Ricinus Communis
(Increased effect due to potassium loss with chronic use of herb)

CARICA PAPAYA

Warfarin Sodium
(Increased INR levels)

CASCARA SAGRADA

(See under Rhamnus Purshianus)

CASTOR OIL PLANT

(See under Ricinus Communis)

CHASTE TREE

(See under Vitex Agnus-Castus)

CINCHONA

(See under Cinchona Pubescens)

CINCHONA PUBESCENS

Drugs that Cause Thrombocytopenia
(Herb increases risk of thrombocytopenia)

COFFEA ARABICA

Drugs, unspecified
(Herb can hinder (or decrease) resorption of other drugs)

COFFEE

(See under Coffea Arabica)

CONVALLARIA MAJALIS

Calcium
(Increases the effect of Convallaria)
Glucocorticoids
(Increases the effect of Convallaria)
Laxatives
(Increases the effect of Convallaria)
Quinidine
(Increases the effect of Convallaria)
Saluretics
(Increases the effect of Convallaria)

CORTICOSTEROIDS

Aloe Barbadensis
(Increased potassium loss)
Rhamnus Cathartica
(Increases hypokalemic effects)
Rhamnus Purshianus
(Increases hypokalemic effect)

CYTISUS SCOPARIUS

MAO Inhibitors
(Increased risk of hypertensive crisis)

DIAGNOSTIC PROCEDURES USING RADIOACTIVE ISOTOPES

Lycopus Virginicus
(Lycopus interferes with these isotopes)

DIGITALIS GLYCOSIDE PREPARATIONS

Rauwolfia Serpentina
(Severe bradycardia when used in combination with digitalis glycosides)

DIGITALIS PURPUREA

Methylxanthines
(Increases risk of cardiac arrhythmias)
Phosphodiesterase Inhibitors
(Increases risk of cardiac arrhythmias)
Quinidine
(Increases risk of cardiac arrhythmias)
Sympathomimetic Agents
(Increases risk of cardiac arrhythmias)

DOPAMINE ANTAGONISTS

Vitex Agnus-Castus
(Decreased dopaminergic effect of herb)

DRIMIA MARITIMA

Calcium
(Increases effectiveness and side effects of herb)
Glucocorticoids
(Increases effectiveness and side effects of herb)
Laxatives
(Increases effectiveness and side effects of herb)
Methylxanthines
(Increases risk of cardiac arrhythmias)
Phosphodiesterase Inhibitors
(Increases risk of cardiac arrhythmias)
Quinidine
(Increases risk of cardiac arrhythmias; increases effectiveness and side effects of herb)
Saluretics
(Increases effectiveness and side effects of herb)
Sympathomimetic Agents
(Increases risk of cardiac arrhythmias)

DRUGS THAT CAUSE THROMBOCYTOPENIA

Cinchona Pubescens
(Herb increases risk of thrombocytopenia)

DRUGS, UNSPECIFIED

Coffea Arabica
(Herb can hinder (or decrease) resorption of other drugs)
Linum Usitatissimum
(Absorption of other drugs may be delayed when taken simultaneously)
Melaleucea Viridiflora
(Co-administration may result in decreased effect of drugs that undergo liver metabolism)
Plantago Afra
(Absorption of other drugs may be decreased if taken simultaneously with herb)

Plantago Isphagula
(*Absorption of other drugs may be delayed when taken simultaneously*)

EPHEDRA SINICA

Cardiac Glycosides
(*Disturbance of heart rhythm*)
Guanethidine
(*Increased sympathomimetic effects*)
Halothane
(*Disturbance of heart rhythm*)
MAO Inhibitors
(*Increases sympathomimetic effects of ephedrine*)
Oxytocin
(*Development of high blood pressure*)

FEVERFEW

(*See under* Tanacetum Parthenium)

FLAXSEED

(*See under* Linum Usitatissimum)

FOXGLOVE

(*See under* Digitalis Purpurea)

GINKGO

(*See under* Ginkgo Biloba)

GINKGO BILOBA

Antithrombolytic Drugs
(*Increases effect of antithrombolytic drugs*)

GLUCOCORTICOIDS

Adonis Vernalis
(*Increases action of Adonis*)
Convallaria Majalis
(*Increases the effect of Convallaria*)
Drimia Maritima
(*Increases effectiveness and side effects of herb*)
Nerium Odoratum
(*Increased efficacy and side effects when given simultaneously with herb*)
Strophanthus Species
(*Simultaneous administration with herb enhance both effects and side effects*)

GUANETHIDINE

Ephedra Sinica
(*Increased sympathomimetic effects*)

HALOTHANE

Ephedra Sinica
(*Disturbance of heart rhythm*)

HENBANE

(*See under* Hyoscyamus Niger)

HYOSCYAMUS NIGER

Amantadine Hydrochloride
(*Increased anticholinergic action*)
Antihistamines
(*Increased anticholinergic action*)
Phenothiazines
(*Increased anticholinergic action*)
Procainamide
(*Increased anticholinergic action*)
Quinidine
(*Increased anticholinergic action*)
Tricyclic Antidepressants
(*Increased anticholinergic action*)

INSULIN

Plantago Isphagula
(*Effect unspecified; insulin dose should be decreased*)

LAXATIVES

Adonis Vernalis
(*Increases action of Adonis*)
Convallaria Majalis
(*Increases the effect of Convallaria*)
Drimia Maritima
(*Increases effectiveness and side effects of herb*)
Nerium Odoratum
(*Increased efficacy and side effects when given simultaneously with herb*)
Strophanthus Species
(*Simultaneous administration with herb enhance both effects and side effects*)

LEVODOPA

Rauwolfia Serpentina
(*Decreased effect; increases in extra-pyramidal symptoms*)

LICORICE

Aloe Barbadensis
(*Increased potassium loss*)

LICORICE ROOT

Rhamnus Cathartica
(*Increases hypokalemic effects*)

LILY-OF-THE-VALLEY

(*See under* Convallaria Majalis)

LINUM USITATISSIMUM

Drugs, unspecified
(*Absorption of other drugs may be delayed when taken simultaneously*)

LYCOPUS VIRGINICUS

Diagnostic Procedures Using Radioactive Isotopes
(*Lycopus interferes with these isotopes*)
Thyroid Preparations
(*Effect not specified*)

MA-HUANG

(*See under* Ephedra Sinica)

MAO INHIBITORS

Cytisus Scoparius
(*Increased risk of hypertensive crisis*)
Ephedra Sinica
(*Increases sympathomimetic effects of ephedrine*)
Saccharomyces Cerevisiae
(*Increase in blood pressure*)

MEDICATION AND FOOD THAT INCREASE URIC ACID LEVELS

Arctostaphylos Uva-Ursi
(*Decreases effect of herb*)
Vaccinium Vitis-Idaea
(*Decreases effect of Vaccinium*)

MELALEUCEA VIRIDIFLORA

Drugs, unspecified
(*Co-administration may result in decreased effect of drugs that undergo liver metabolism*)

METHYLXANTHINES

Digitalis Purpurea
(*Increases risk of cardiac arrhythmias*)
Drimia Maritima
(*Increases risk of cardiac arrhythmias*)

NERIUM ODORATUM

Calcium Salts
(*Increased efficacy and side effects when given simultaneously with herb*)
Glucocorticoids
(*Increased efficacy and side effects when given simultaneously with herb*)
Laxatives
(*Increased efficacy and side effects when given simultaneously with herb*)
Quinidine
(*Increased efficacy and side effects when given simultaneously with herb*)

Saluretics
(*Increased efficacy and side effects when given simultaneously with herb*)

NEUROLEPTICS
Rauwolfia Serpentina
(*Synergistic effect*)

NIAULI
(*See under* Melaleucea Viridiflora)

NON-STEROIDAL ANTI-INFLAMMATORY DRUGS
Salix Species
(*Use with caution; effect not specified*)

OAK BARK
(*See under* Quercus Robur)

OLEANDER LEAF
(*See under* Nerium Odoratum)

OXYTOCIN
Ephedra Sinica
(*Development of high blood pressure*)

PAPAYA
(*See under* Carica Papaya)

PHENOTHIAZINES
Hyoscyamus Niger
(*Increased anticholinergic action*)

PHOSPHODIESTERASE INHIBITORS
Digitalis Purpurea
(*Increases risk of cardiac arrhythmias*)
Drimia Maritima
(*Increases risk of cardiac arrhythmias*)

PLANTAGO AFRA
Drugs, unspecified
(*Absorption of other drugs may be decreased if taken simultaneously with herb*)

PLANTAGO ISPHAGULA
Drugs, unspecified
(*Absorption of other drugs may be delayed when taken simultaneously*)
Insulin
(*Effect unspecified; insulin dose should be decreased*)

PROCAINAMIDE
Hyoscyamus Niger
(*Increased anticholinergic action*)

PSYLLIUM
(*See under* Plantago Isphagula)

PSYLLIUM SEED
(*See under* Plantago Afra)

QUERCUS ROBUR
Alkaline Drugs
(*Absorption of alkaline drugs may be reduced or inhibited*)
Alkaloids
(*Absorption of alkaloids may be reduced or inhibited*)

QUINIDINE
Adonis Vernalis
(*Increases action of Adonis*)
Atropa Belladonna
(*Increases anticholinergic effect of herb*)
Convallaria Majalis
(*Increases the effect of Convallaria*)
Digitalis Purpurea
(*Increases risk of cardiac arrhythmias*)
Drimia Maritima
(*Increases risk of cardiac arrhythmias; increases effectiveness and side effects of herb*)
Hyoscyamus Niger
(*Increased anticholinergic action*)
Nerium Odoratum
(*Increased efficacy and side effects when given simultaneously with herb*)
Scopolia Carniolica
(*Increased effect when given simultaneously with herb*)
Strophanthus Species
(*Simultaneous administration with herb enhance both effects and side effects*)

RAUWOLFIA
(*See under* Rauwolfia Serpentina)

RAUWOLFIA SERPENTINA
Alcohol
(*Increases impairment of motor skills*)
Barbiturates
(*Synergistic effect*)
Digitalis Glycoside Preparations
(*Severe bradycardia when used in combination with digitalis glycosides*)
Levodopa
(*Decreased effect; increases in extra-pyramidal symptoms*)
Neuroleptics
(*Synergistic effect*)
Sympathomimetic Agents
(*Increases blood pressure*)

RHAMNUS CATHARTICA
Antiarrhythmics
(*Increased effect due to potassium loss with chronic use of herb*)
Cardiac Glycosides
(*Increased effect due to potassium loss with chronic use of herb*)
Corticosteroids
(*Increases hypokalemic effects*)
Licorice Root
(*Increases hypokalemic effects*)
Thiazide Diuretics
(*Increases hypokalemic effects*)

RHAMNUS FRANGULA
Cardiac Glycosides
(*Increased effect due to potassium loss with chronic use of herb*)

RHAMNUS PURSHIANUS
Antiarrhythmics
(*Effect unspecified*)
Cardiac Glycosides
(*Increased effect due to potassium loss with chronic use of herb*)
Corticosteroids
(*Increases hypokalemic effect*)
Thiazide Diuretics
(*Increases hypokalemic effect*)

RHEUM PALMATUM
Cardiac Glycosides
(*Increased effect due to potassium loss with chronic use of herb*)

RHUBARB
(*See under* Rheum Palmatum)

RICINUS COMMUNIS
Cardioactive Steroids
(*Increased effect due to potassium loss with chronic use of herb*)

SACCHAROMYCES CEREVISIAE
MAO Inhibitors
(*Increase in blood pressure*)

SALICYLATES
Salix Species
(*Use with caution; effect not specified*)

SALIX SPECIES

Non-Steroidal Anti-Inflammatory Drugs
(Use with caution; effect not specified)

Salicylates
(Use with caution; effect not specified)

SALURETICS

Adonis Vernalis
(Increases action of Adonis)

Convallaria Majalis
(Increases the effect of Convallaria)

Drimia Maritima
(Increases effectiveness and side effects of herb)

Nerium Odoratum
(Increased efficacy and side effects when given simultaneously with herb)

Strophanthus Species
(Simultaneous administration with herb enhance both effects and side effects)

SCOPOLIA

(*See under* Scopolia Carniolica)

SCOPOLIA CARNIOLICA

Amantadine Hydrochloride
(Increased effect when given simultaneously with herb)

Quinidine
(Increased effect when given simultaneously with herb)

Tricyclic Antidepressants
(Increased effect when given simultaneously with herb)

SQUILL

(*See under* Drimia Maritima)

STROPHANTHUS

(*See under* Strophanthus Species)

STROPHANTHUS SPECIES

Calcium Salts
(Simultaneous administration with herb enhance both effects and side effects)

Glucocorticoids
(Simultaneous administration with herb enhance both effects and side effects)

Laxatives
(Simultaneous administration with herb enhance both effects and side effects)

Quinidine
(Simultaneous administration with herb enhance both effects and side effects)

Saluretics
(Simultaneous administration with herb enhance both effects and side effects)

SYMPATHOMIMETIC AGENTS

Digitalis Purpurea
(Increases risk of cardiac arrhythmias)

Drimia Maritima
(Increases risk of cardiac arrhythmias)

Rauwolfia Serpentina
(Increases blood pressure)

TANACETUM PARTHENIUM

Aspirin
(Increased antithrombotic effect)

Warfarin Sodium
(Increased antithrombotic effect)

THIAZIDE DIURETICS

Aloe Barbadensis
(Increased potassium loss)

Rhamnus Cathartica
(Increases hypokalemic effects)

Rhamnus Purshianus
(Increases hypokalemic effect)

THYROID PREPARATIONS

Lycopus Virginicus
(Effect not specified)

TRICYCLIC ANTIDEPRESSANTS

Atropa Belladonna
(Increases anticholinergic effect of herb)

Hyoscyamus Niger
(Increased anticholinergic action)

Scopolia Carniolica
(Increased effect when given simultaneously with herb)

UVA-URSI

(*See under* Arctostaphylos Uva-Ursi)

VACCINIUM VITIS-IDAEA

Medication and Food that Increase Uric Acid Levels
(Decreases effect of Vaccinium)

VITEX AGNUS-CASTUS

Dopamine Antagonists
(Decreased dopaminergic effect of herb)

WARFARIN SODIUM

Carica Papaya
(Increased INR levels)

WARFARIN SODIUM

Tanacetum Parthenium
(Increased antithrombotic effect)

WHITE WILLOW

(*See under* Salix Species)

Herb Identification Guide

Shown on the following pages are full-color photographs of over 380 common medicinal herbs. Each plant is labeled with its scientific name immediately above the photo, and its accepted common name immediately below. The photos are arranged alphabetically by the scientific name.

To locate a photo by its common name, please check the Scientific and Common Name Index at the front of the book. If a photo of the herb is available, its page number will be found immediately after the alphabetical entry for the herb's common name.

Please note that the plants are not reproduced in actual size, and that the scale of the photos varies. For the average dimensions of the plant and its component structures, please check the Description section of corresponding herbal monograph.

ACER RUBRUM

Red Maple

ADONIS VERNALIS

Adonis

AFRAMOMUM MELEGUETA

Grains of Paradise

AJUGA REPTANS

Bugle

ACHILLEA MILLEFOLIUM

Yarrow

AEGOPODIUM PODAGRARIA

Goutweed

AGRIMONIA EUPATORIA

Agrimony

ALCEA ROSEA

Hollyhock

ACONITUM NAPELLUS

Monkshood

AESCULUS HIPPOCASTANUM

Horse Chestnut

AILANTHUS ALTISSIMA

Tree of Heaven

ALCHEMILLA VULGARIS

Lady's Mantle

ACORUS CALAMUS

Calamus

AETHUSA CYNAPIUM

Fool's Parsley

AJUGA CHAMAEPITYS

Ground Pine

ALISMA PLANTAGO-AQUATICA

Water Plantain

ALKANNA TINCTORIA

Alkanna

ALNUS GLUTINOSA

Black Alder

AMMI VISNAGA

Bishop's Weed

ANGELICA ARCHANGELICA

Angelica

ALLIUM CEPA

Onion

ALOE SPECIES

Aloe

ANACARDIUM OCCIDENTALE

Cashew

ANTENNARIA DIOICA

Cat's Foot

ALLIUM SATIVUM

Garlic

AMANITA MUSCARIA

Aga

ANAGALLIS ARVENSIS

Scarlet Pimpernel

ANTHOXANTHUM ODORATUM

Sweet Vernal Grass

ALLIUM SCHOENOPRASUM

Chive

AMARANTHUS SPECIES

Amaranth

ANETHUM GRAVEOLENS

Dill

ANTHYLLIS VULNERARIA

Woundwort

APIUM GRAVEOLENS

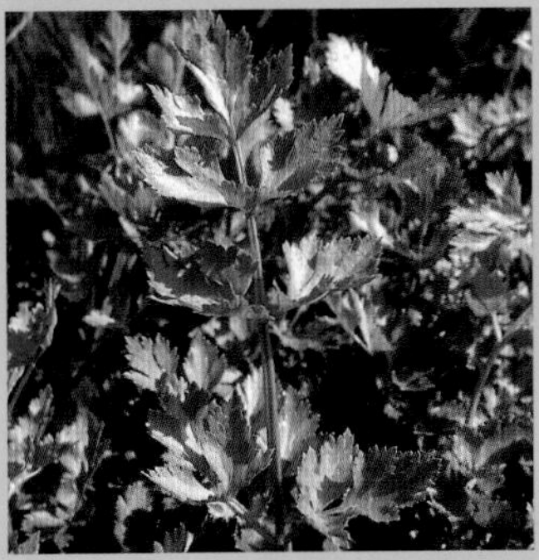

Celery

AQUILEGIA VULGARIS

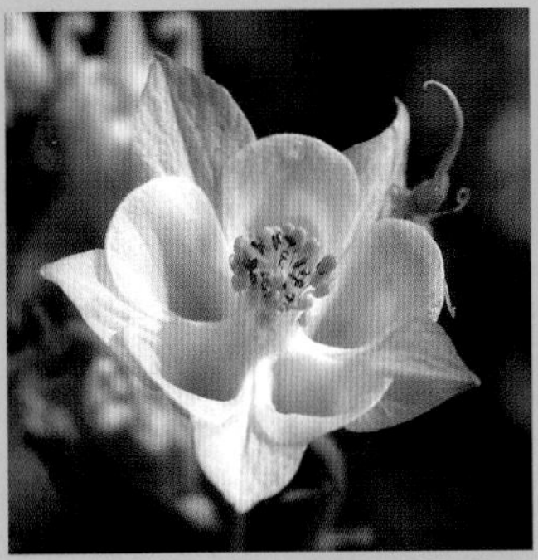

Columbine

ARALIA RACEMOSA

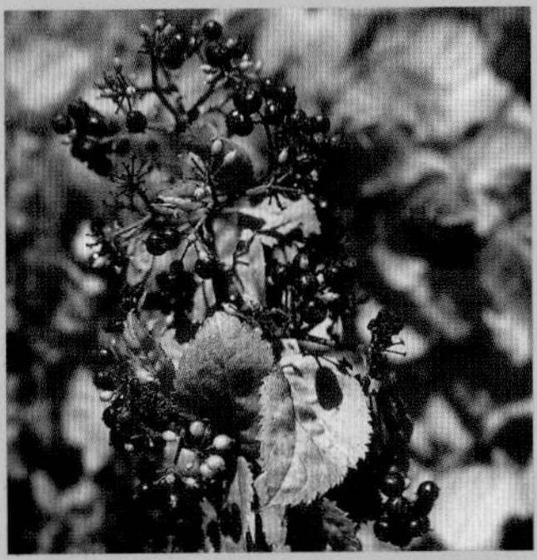

Spikenard

ARCTIUM LAPPA

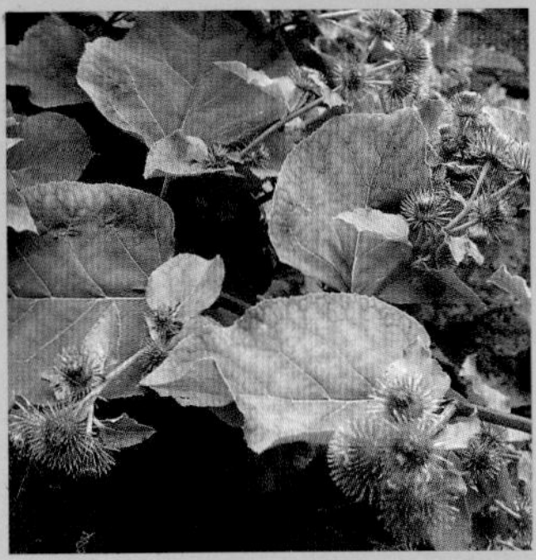

Burdock

ARCTOSTAPHYLOS UVA-URSI

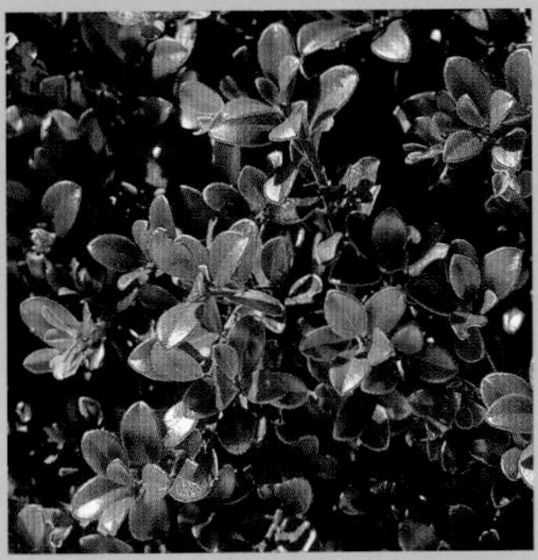

Uva-Ursi

ARECA CATECHU

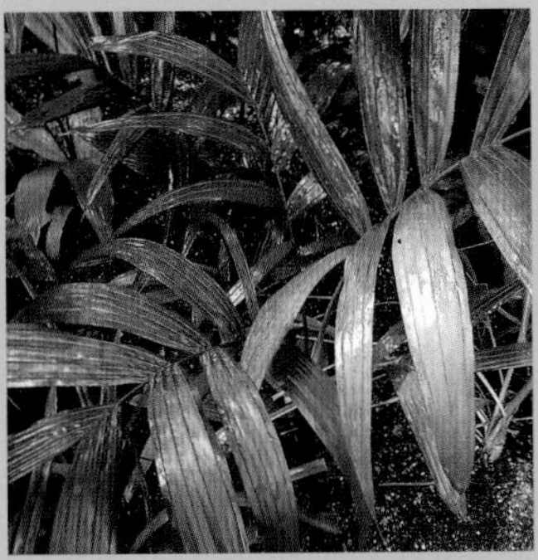

Areca Nut

ARISTOLOCHIA CLEMATITIS

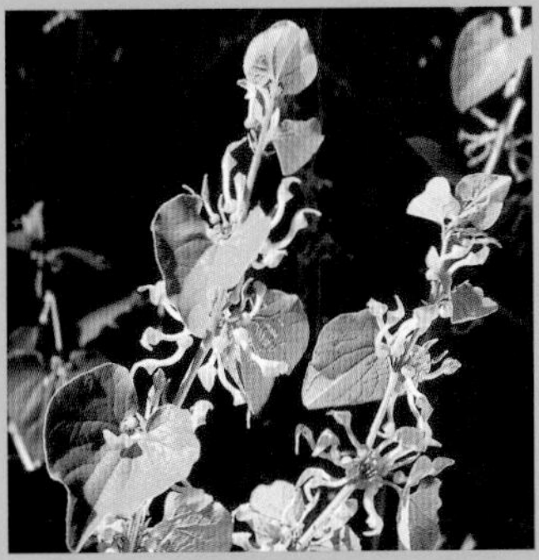

Birthwort

ARMORACIA RUSTICANA

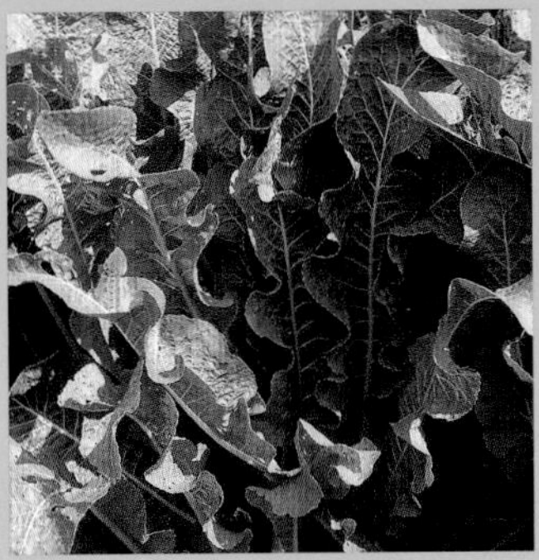

Horseradish

ARTEMISIA ABSINTHIUM

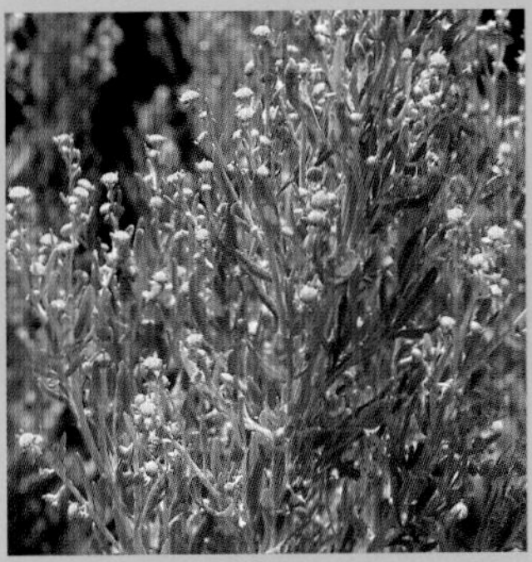

Wormwood

ARTEMISIA DRACUNCULUS

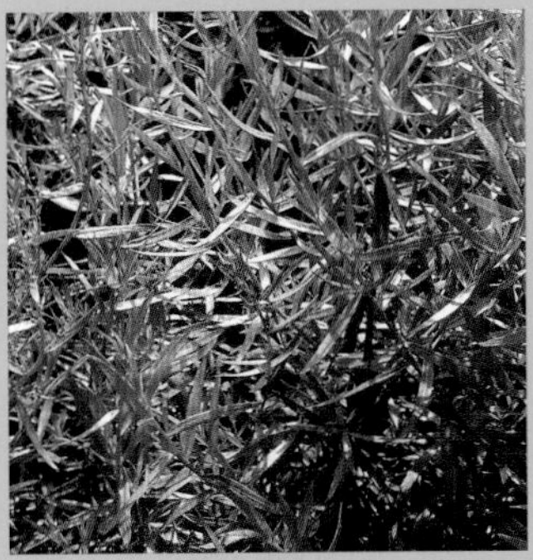

Tarragon

ARTEMISIA VULGARIS

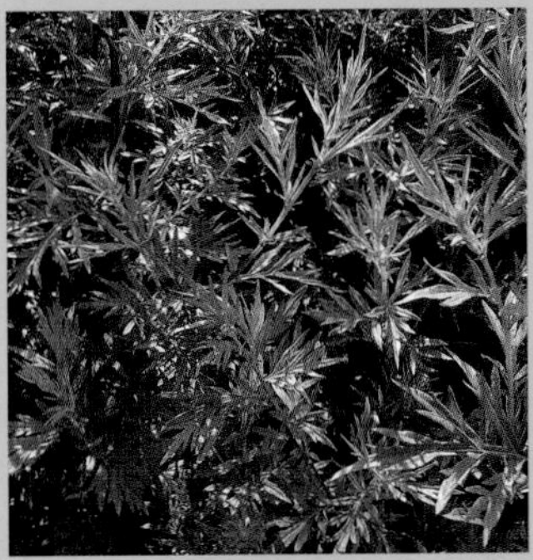

Mugwort

ARUNDINARIA JAPONICA

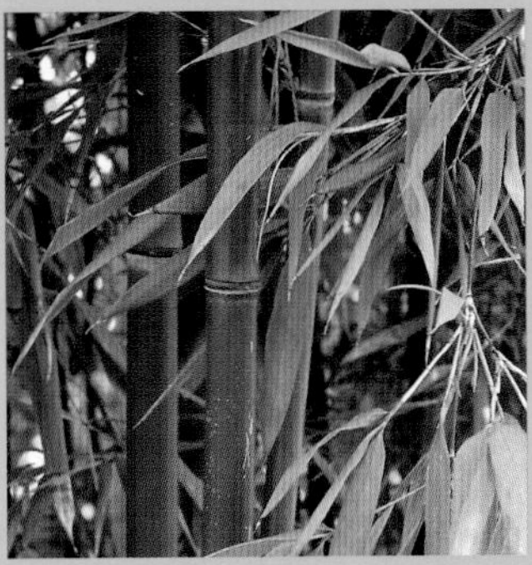

Bamboo

ASARUM EUROPAEUM

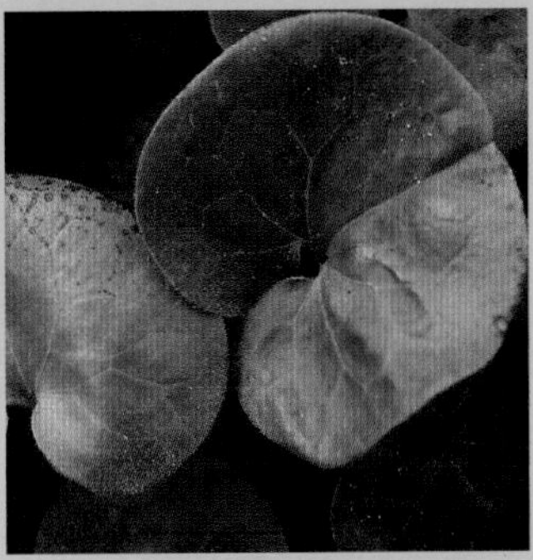

Asarum

ASCLEPIAS INCARNATA

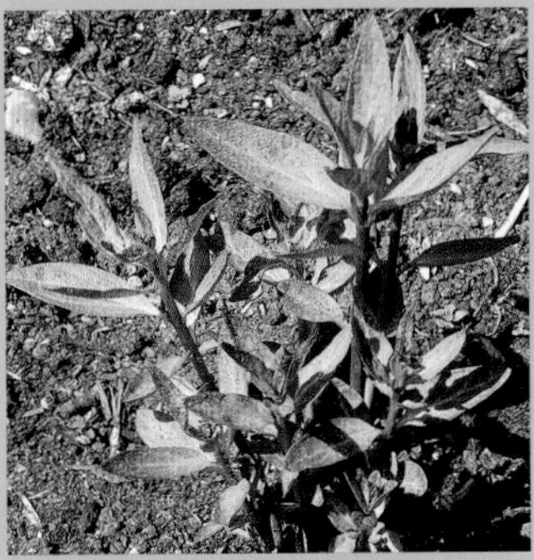

Swamp Milkweed

ASCLEPIAS TUBEROSA

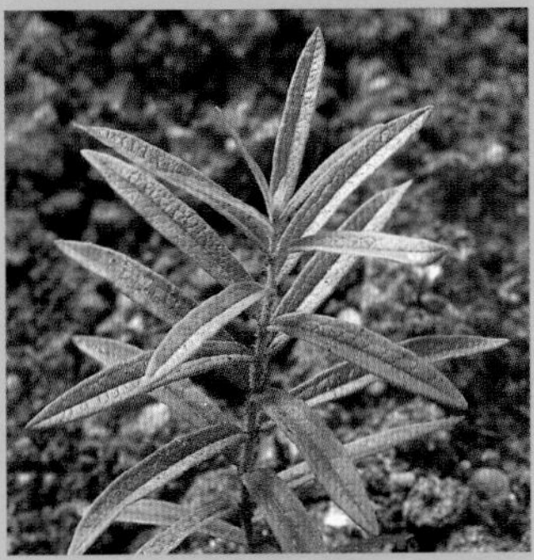

Pleurisy Root

ASPARAGUS OFFICINALIS

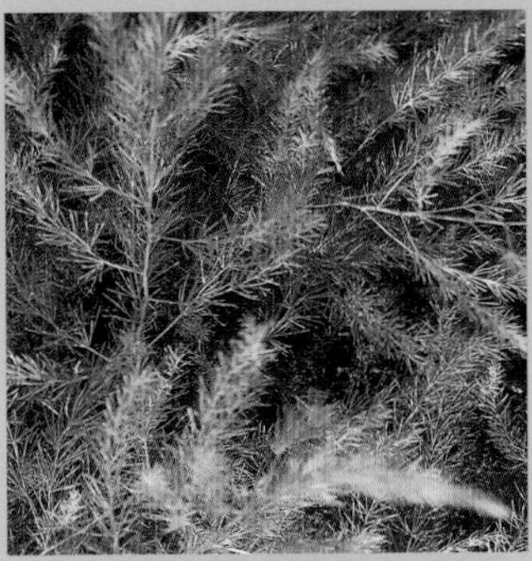

Asparagus

ATHYRIUM FILIX-FEMINA

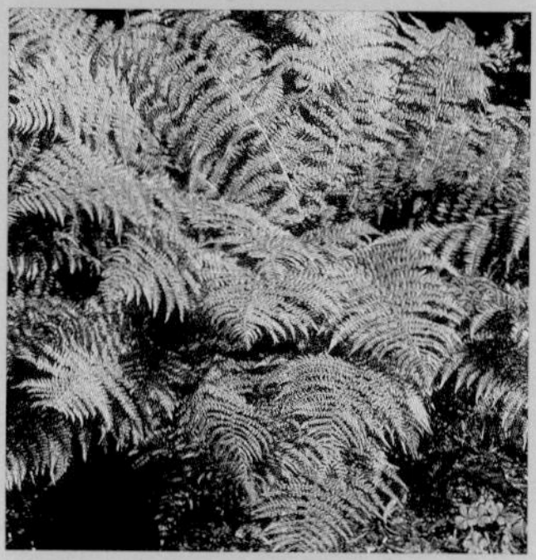

Lady Fern

ATROPA BELLADONNA

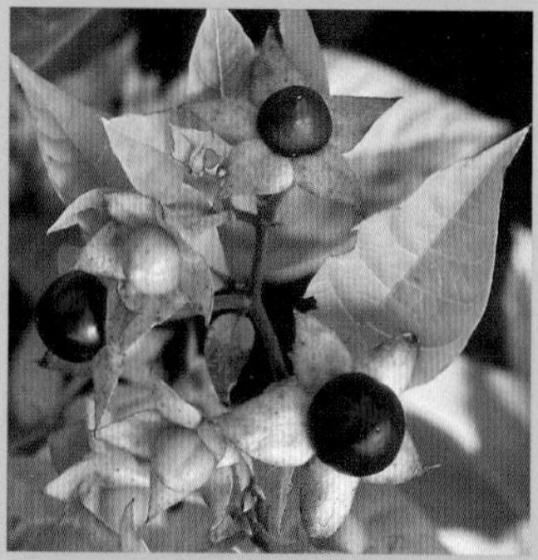

Belladonna

AVENA SATIVA

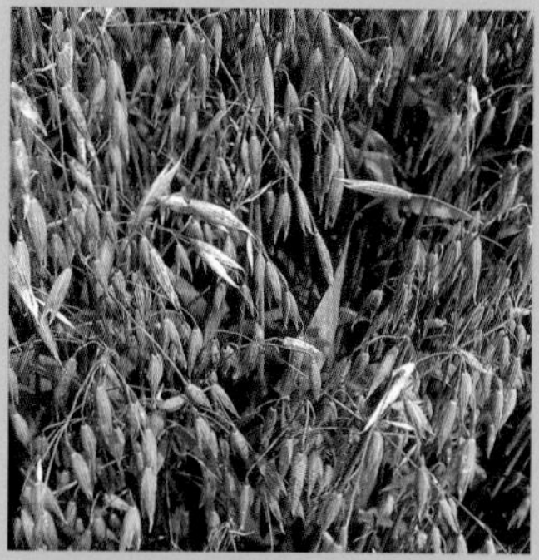

Oats

AZADIRACHTA INDICA

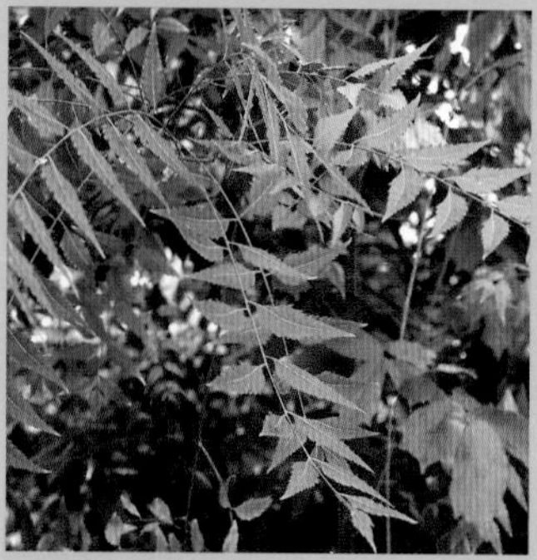

Azedarach

BALLOTA NIGRA

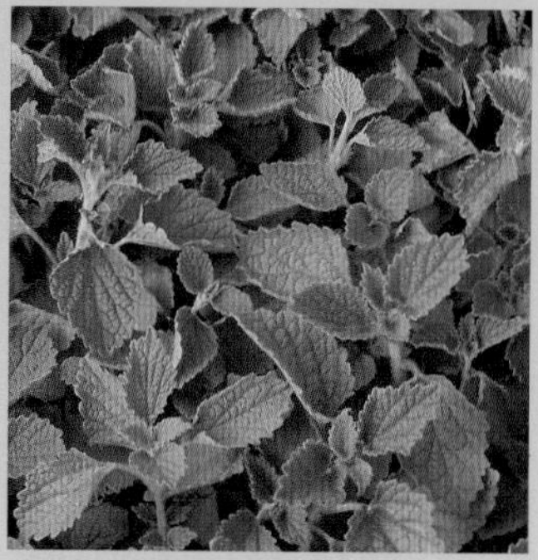

Horehound

BAPTISIA TINCTORIA

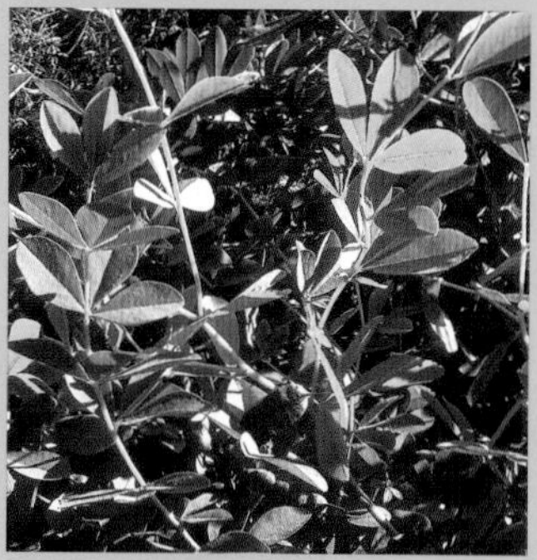

Wild Indigo

BELLIS PERENNIS

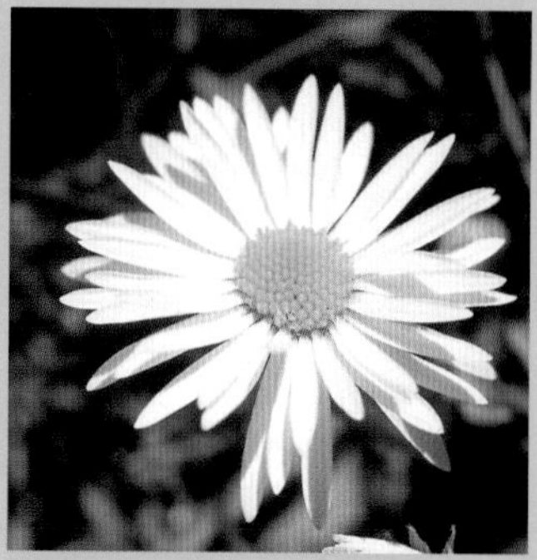

Wild Daisy

BERBERIS VULGARIS

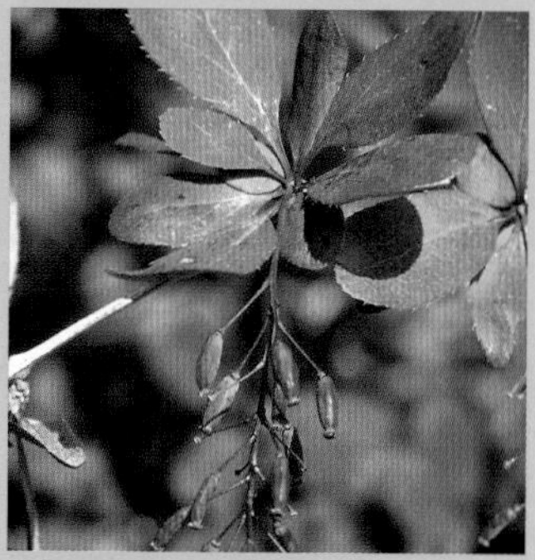

Barberry

BETA VULGARIS

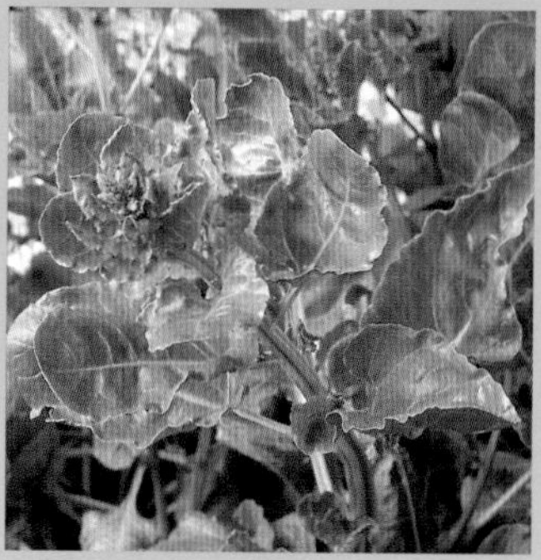

Beet

BETONICA OFFICINALIS

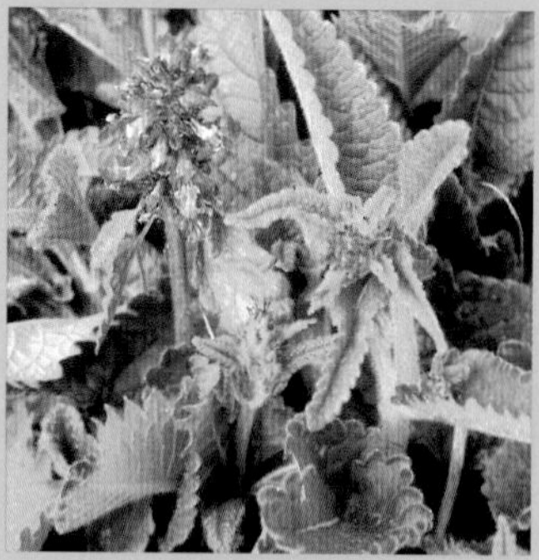

Wood Betony

BETULA SPECIES

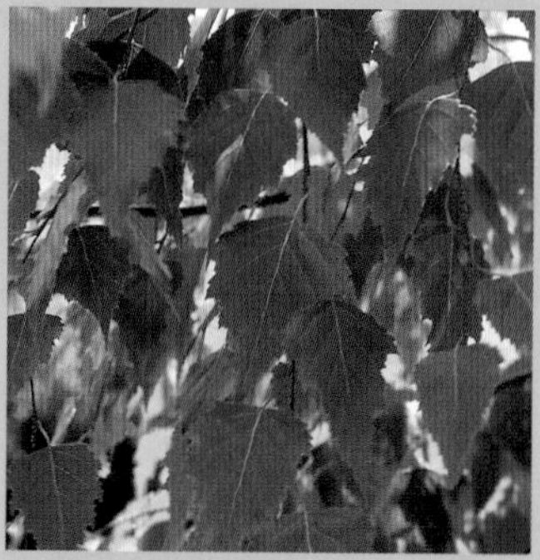

Birch

BIDENS TRIPARTITA

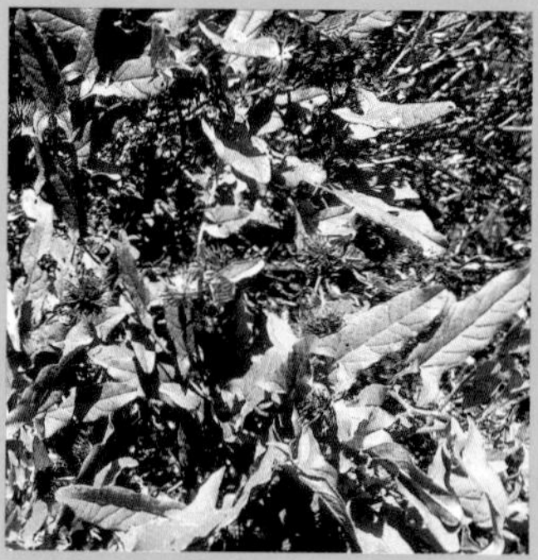

Burr Marigold

BORAGO OFFICINALIS

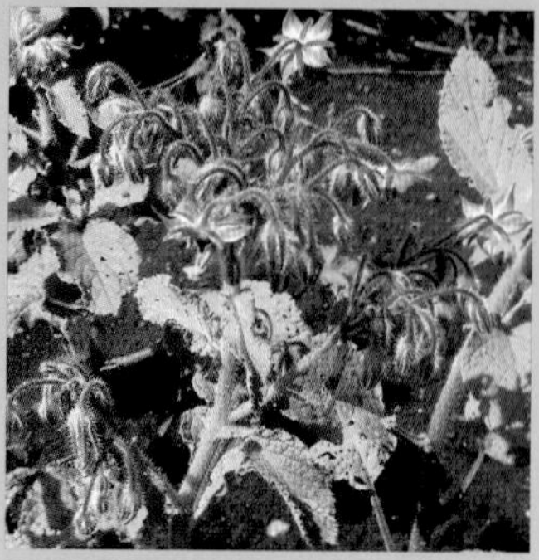

Borage

BRASSICA NIGRA

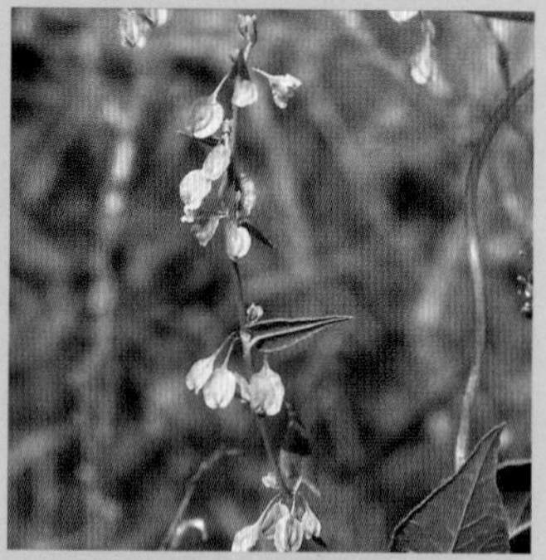

Black Mustard

BRASSICA OLERACEA VAR. CAPITATA

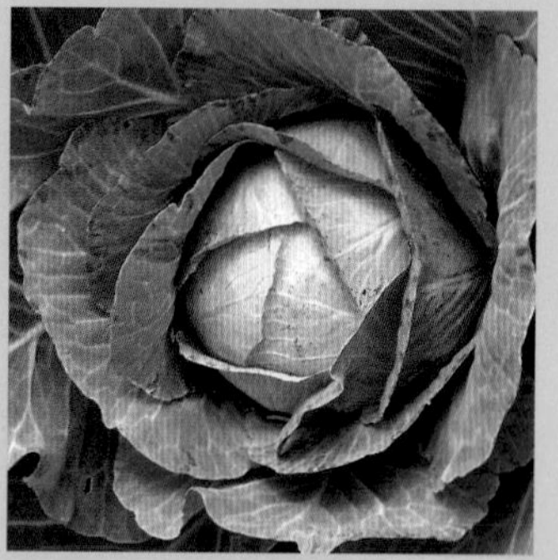

Cabbage

BRYONIA ALBA

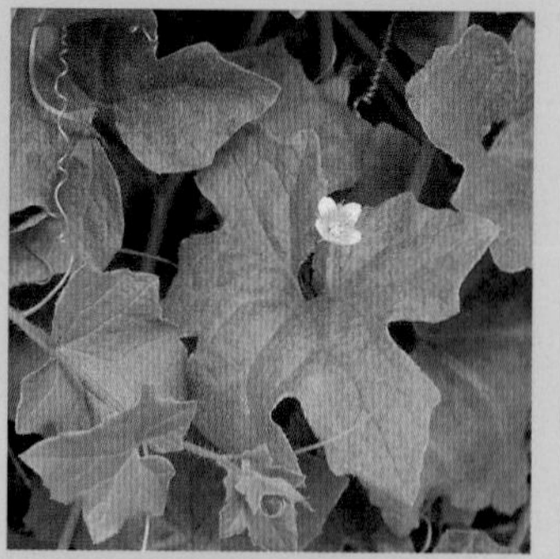

White Bryony

BUXUS SEMPERVIRENS

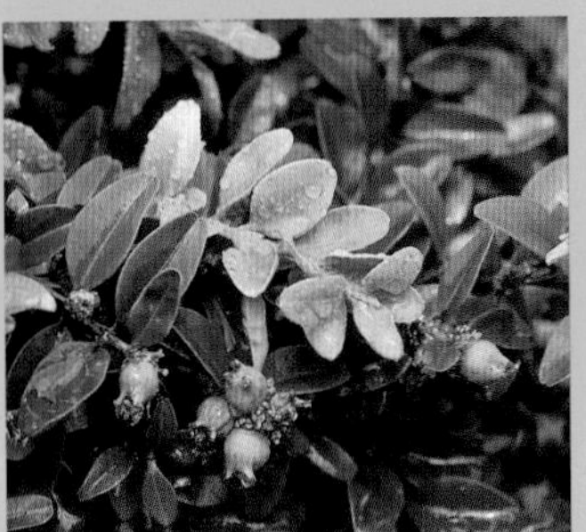

Boxwood

CALENDULA OFFICINALIS

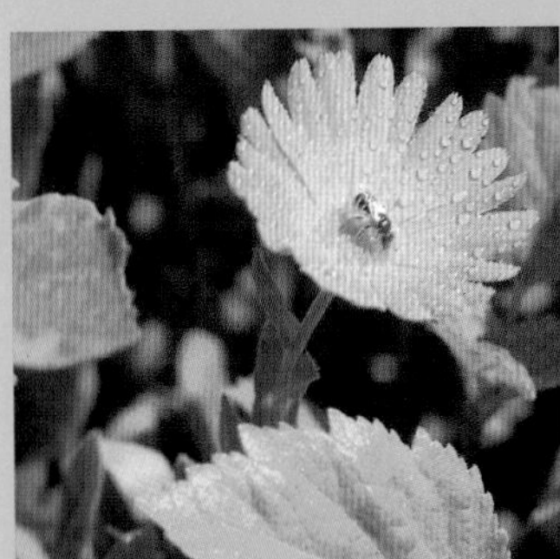

Marigold

CALLUNA VULGARIS

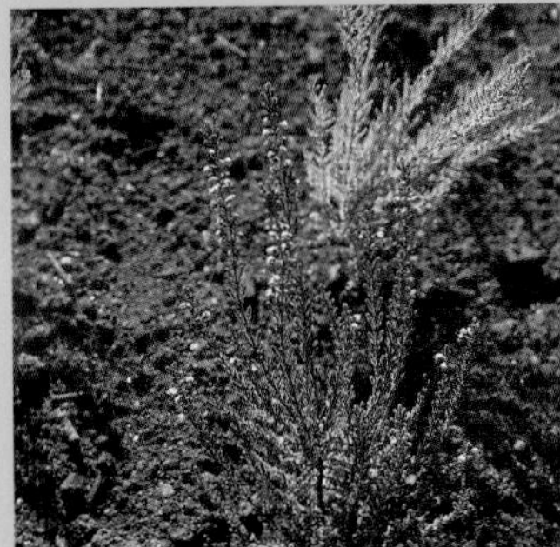

Heather

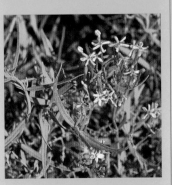

CALTHA PALUSTRIS

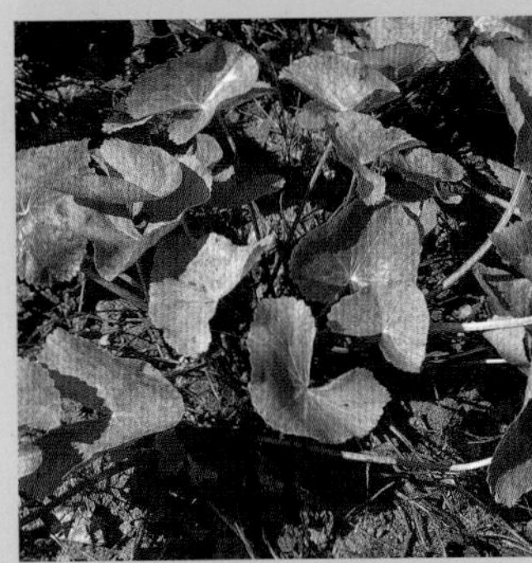

Marsh Marigold

CALYSTEGIA SEPIUM

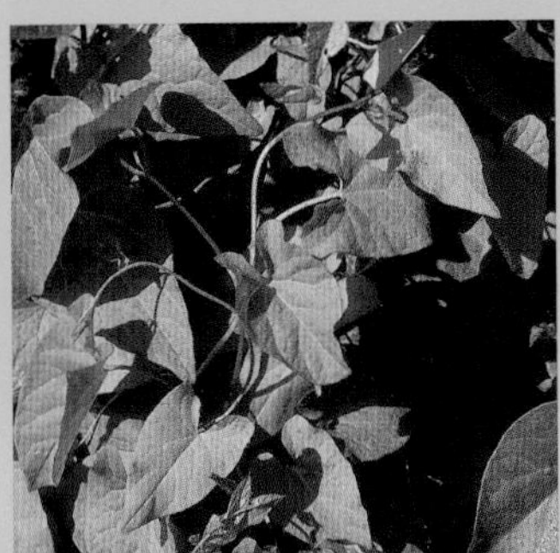

Greater Bindweed

CAMELLIA SINENSIS

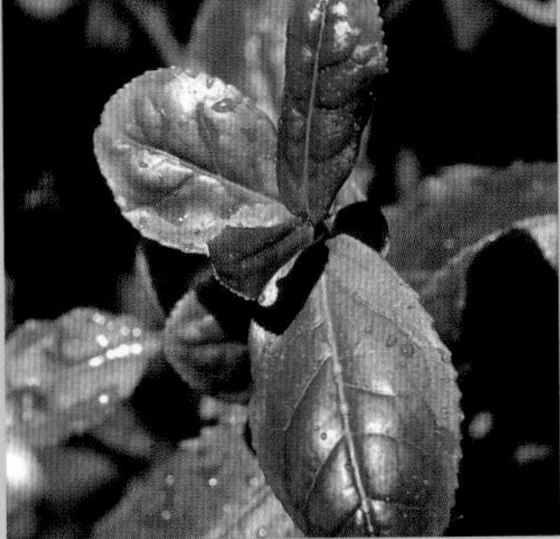

Green Tea

CANNABIS SATIVA

Marijuana

CAPSICUM ANNUUM

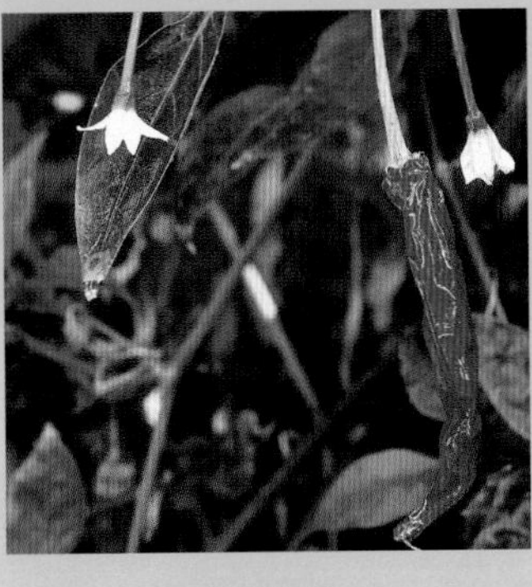

Cayenne

CARICA PAPAYA

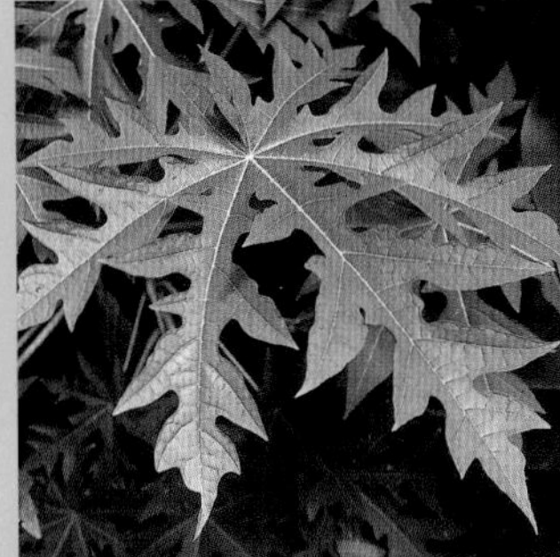

Papaya

CARLINA ACAULIS

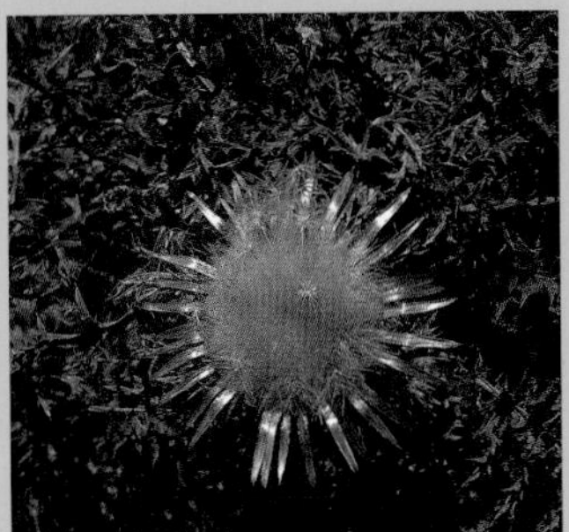

Carline Thistle

CARUM CARVI

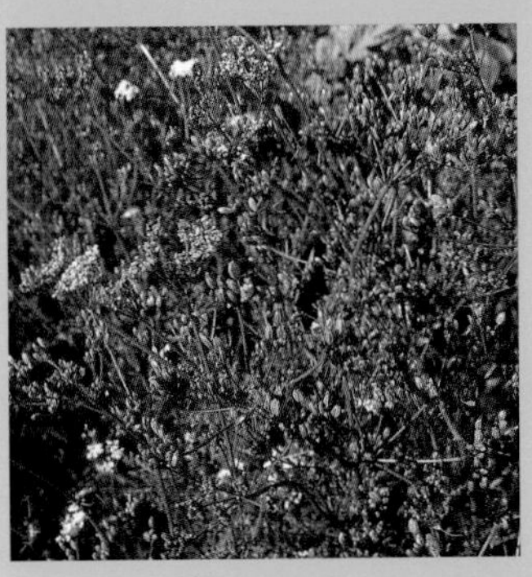

Caraway

CASSIA ALEXANDRINA

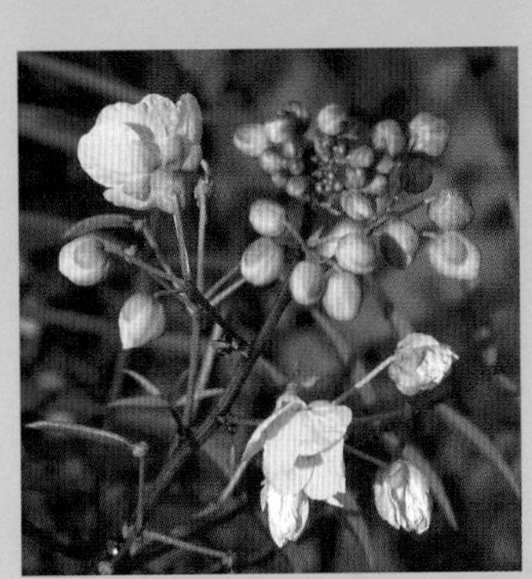

Senna

CENTAUREA CYANUS

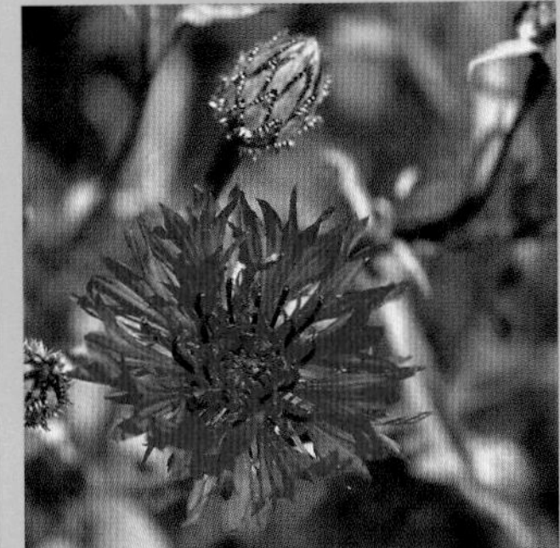

Cornflower

CENTAURIUM SPECIES

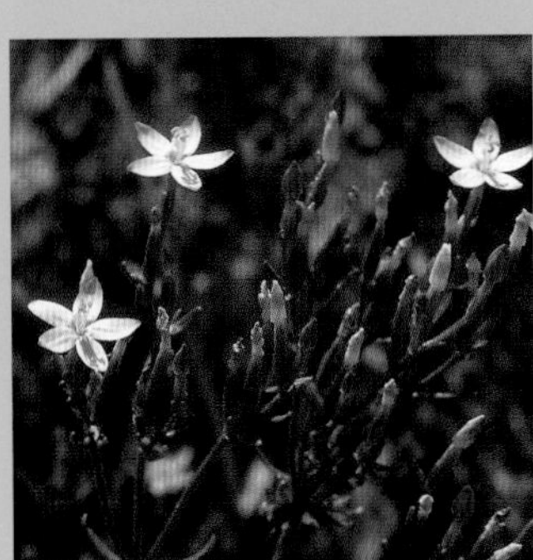

Centaury

CENTELLA ASIATICA

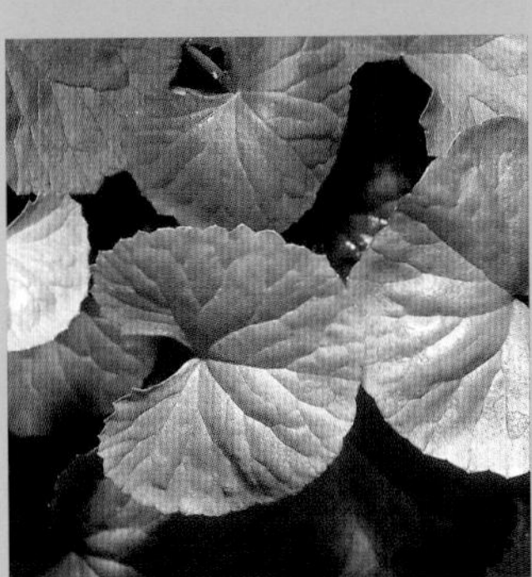

Hydrocotyle

CENTRANTHUS SPECIES

Red-Spur Valerian

CERATONIA SILIQUA

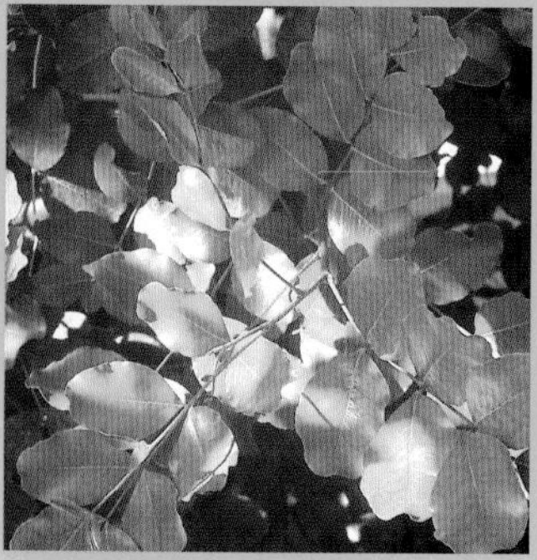

Carob

CHAMAEMELUM NOBILE

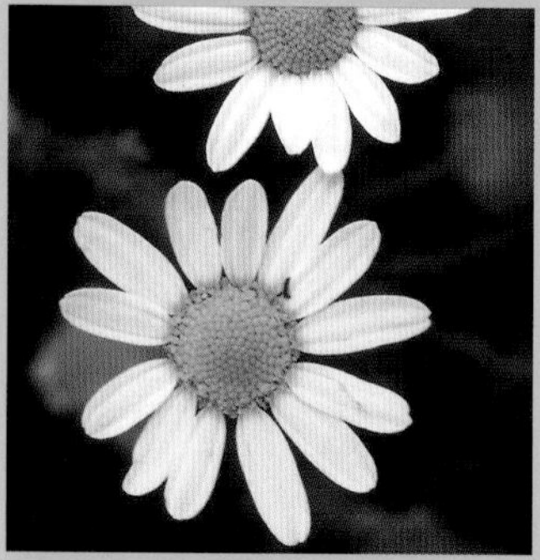

Roman Chamomile

CHEIRANTHUS CHEIRI

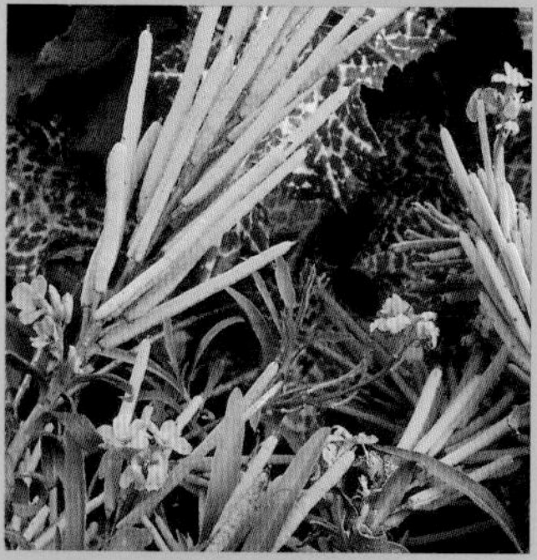

Wallflower

CHELIDONIUM MAJUS

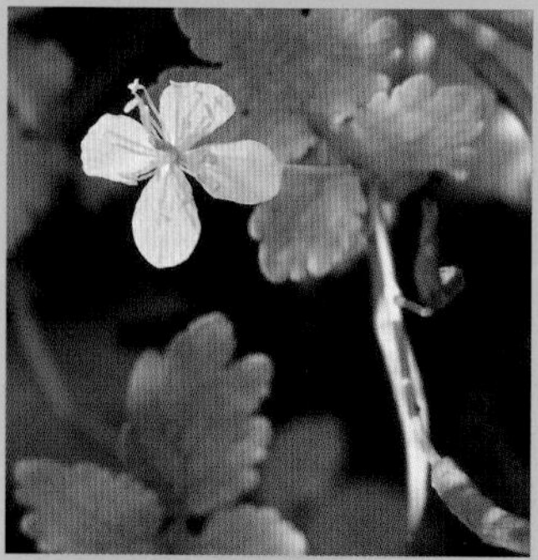

Celandine

CHELONE GLABRA

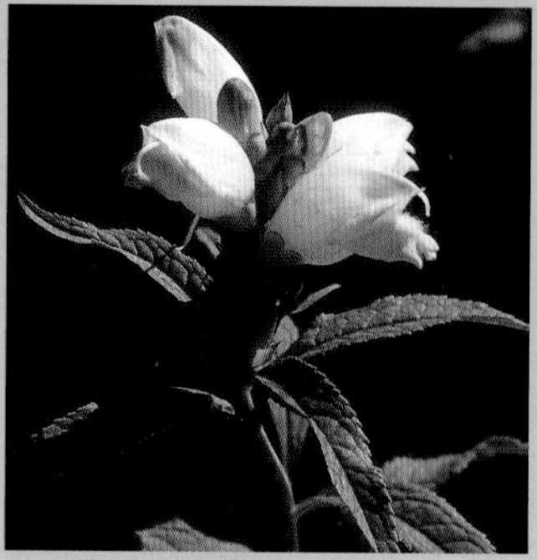

Turtle Head

CHENOPODIUM AMBROSIOIDES

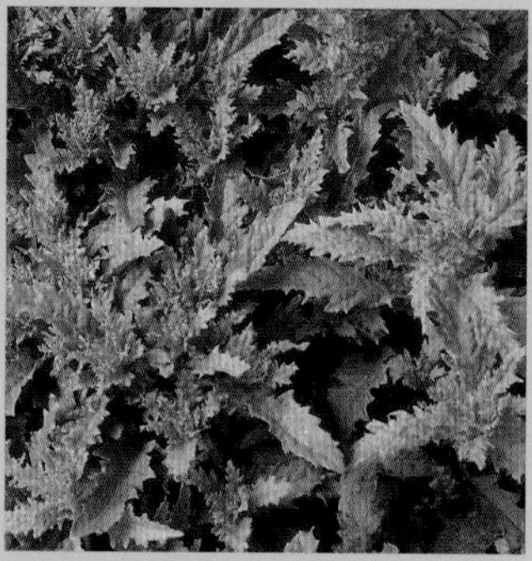

Wormseed Oil

CHIONANTHUS VIRGINICUS

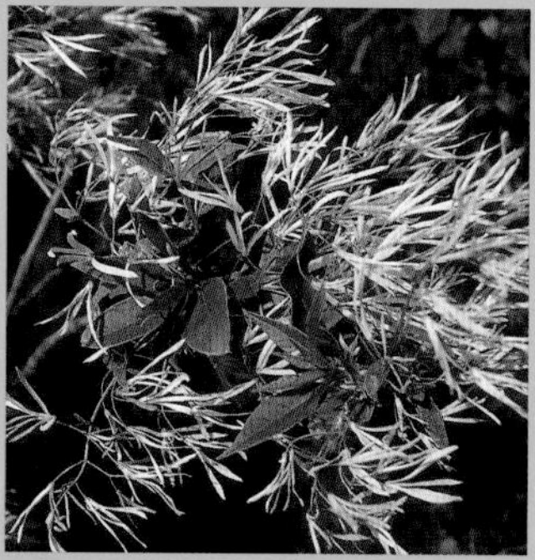

Fringetree

CICHORIUM INTYBUS

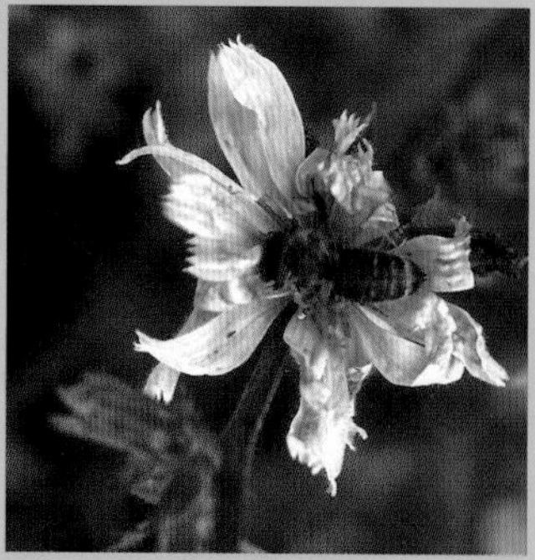

Chicory

CICUTA VIROSA

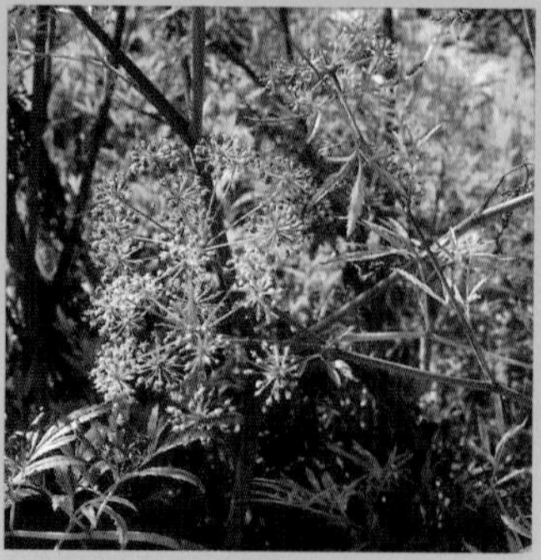

European Water Hemlock

CIMICIFUGA RACEMOSA

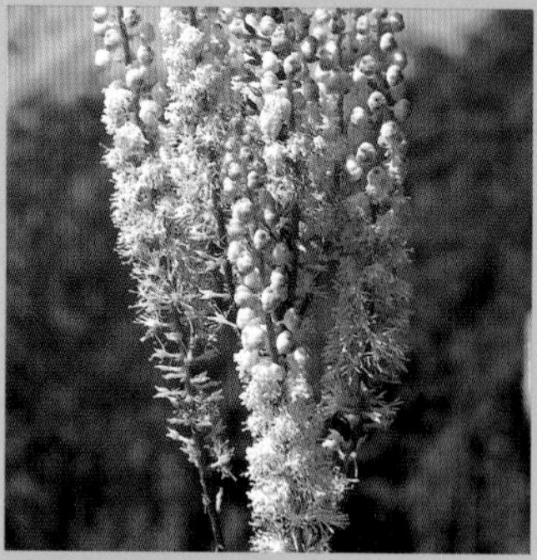

Black Cohosh

CINCHONA PUBESCENS

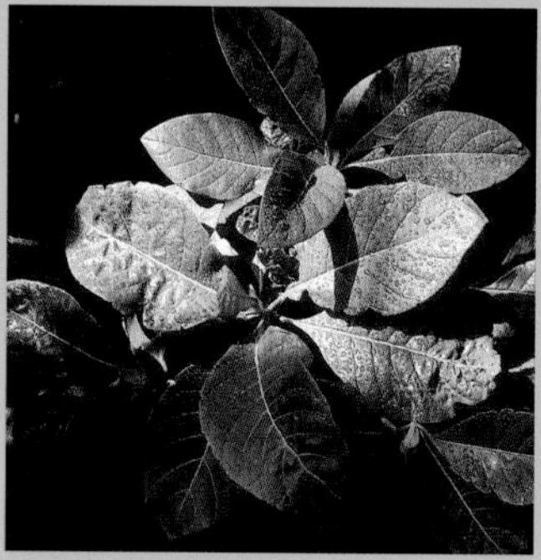

Cinchona

CINNAMOMUM CAMPHORA

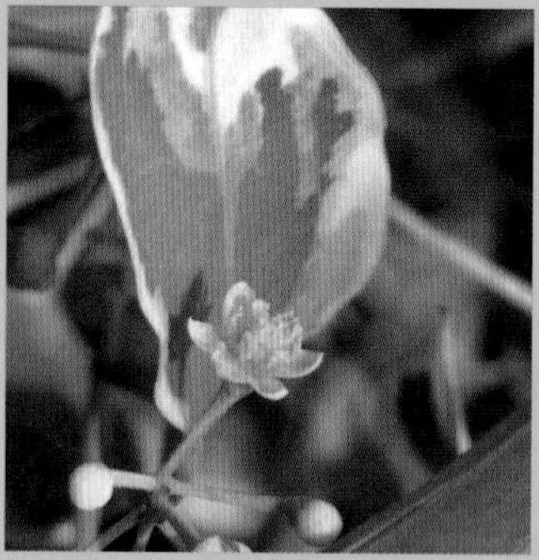

Camphor Tree

CINNAMOMUM VERUM

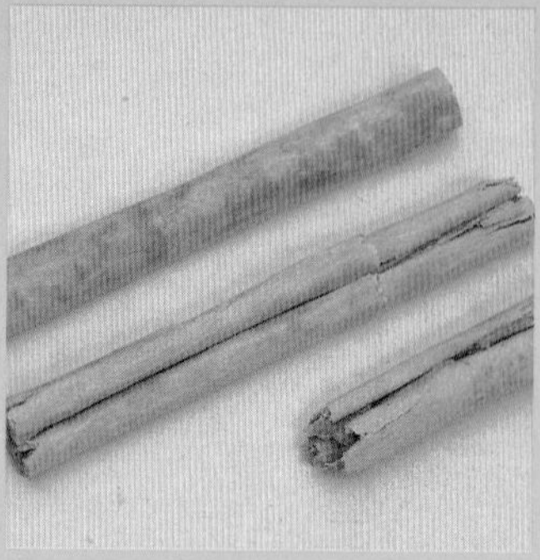

Cinnamon

CITRULLUS COLOCYNTHIS

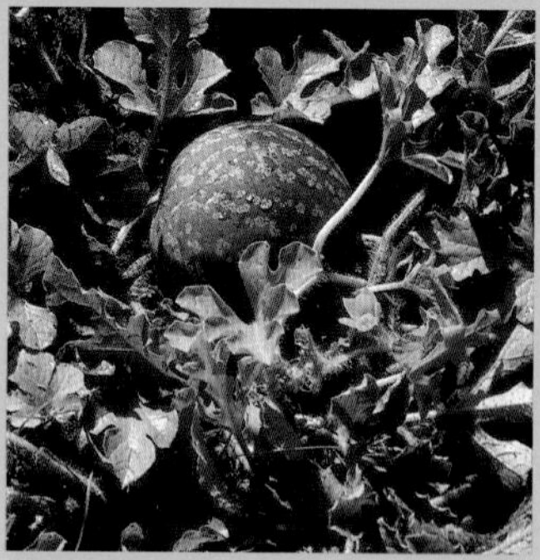

Bitter Apple

CITRUS AURANTIFOLIA

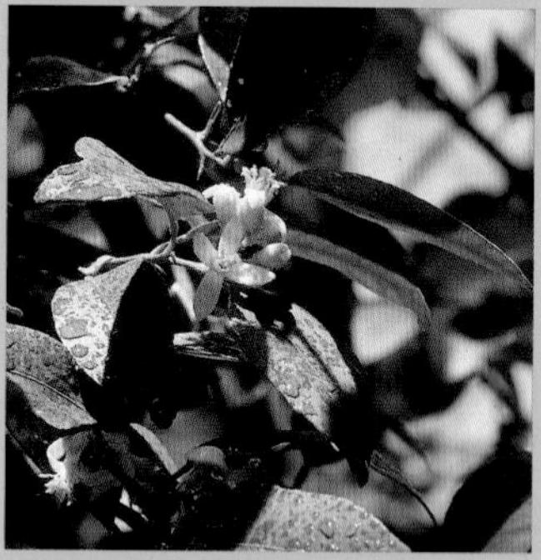

Lime

CITRUS AURANTIUM

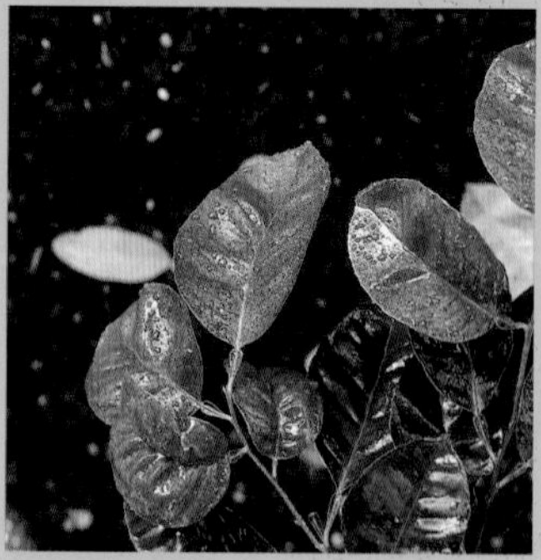

Bitter Orange

CITRUS LIMON

Lemon

CNICUS BENEDICTUS

St. Benedict Thistle

COLLINSONIA CANADENSIS

Stone Root

CORIANDRUM SATIVUM

Coriander

CITRUS SINENSIS

Sweet Orange

COCHLEARIA OFFICINALIS

Scurvy Grass

COMMIPHORA MOLMOL

Myrrh

CORNUS FLORIDA

Dogwood

CLEMATIS RECTA

Clematis

COFFEA ARABICA

Coffee

CONIUM MACULATUM

Hemlock

CRATAEGUS SPECIES

Hawthorn

CLEMATIS VITALBA

Traveller's Joy

COLCHICUM AUTUMNALE

Colchicum

CONVALLARIA MAJALIS

Lily-Of-The-Valley

CROCUS SATIVUS

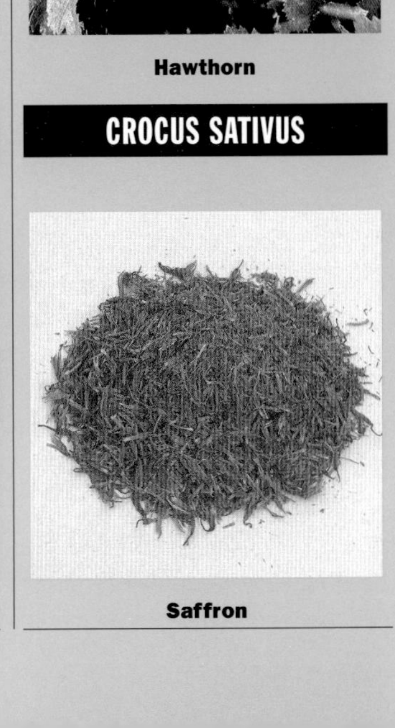

Saffron

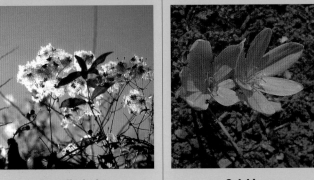

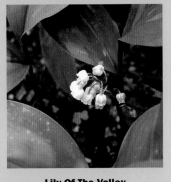

CUCURBITA PEPO
Pumpkin

CURCUMA ZEDOARIA
Zedoary

CYPERUS SPECIES
Adrue

DAUCUS CAROTA
Carrot

CUMIMUM CYMINUM
Cumin

CUSCUTA SPECIES
Dodder

CYTISUS SCOPARIUS
Broom

DELPHINIUM SPECIES
Larkspur

CUPRESSUS SEMPERVIRENS
Cypress

CYMBOPOGON CITRATUS
Citronella

DAPHNE MEZEREUM
Mezereon

DICTAMNUS ALBUS
Burning Bush

CURCUMA XANTHORRHIZIA
Curcuma

CYNARA SCOLYMUS
Artichoke

DATURA STRAMONIUM
Jimson Weed

DIGITALIS PURPUREA
Foxglove

DIOSCOREA VILLOSA

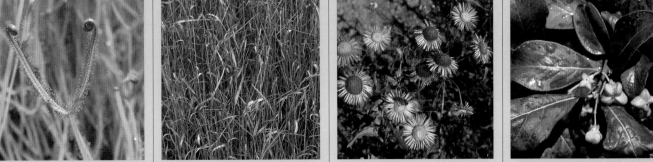

Wild Yam

DIPSACUS SILVESTRIS

Teazle

DRIMIA MARITIMA

Squill

DROSERA SPECIES

Sundew

DRYOPTERIS FILIX-MAS

Male Fern

ECHINACEA PURPUREA

Purple Coneflower

ELETTARIA CARDAMOMUM

Cardamom

ELYMUS REPENS

Couch Grass

EPHEDRA SINICA

Ma-Huang

EPILOBIUM HIRSUTUM

Willow Herb

EQUISETUM ARVENSE

Horsetail

ERIGERON SPECIES

Canadian Fleabane

ERYNGIUM CAMPESTRE

Eryngo

ESCHSCHOLTZIA CALIFORNICA

California Poppy

EUCALYPTUS GLOBULUS

Eucalyptus

EUONYMUS ATROPURPUREUS

Wahoo Root Bark

EUPATORIUM CANNABINUM

Hemp Agrimony

FERULA SPECIES

Ferula

FRAGARIA VESCA

Strawberry Leaf

GALEGA OFFICINALIS

Goat's Rue

EUPATORIUM PERFOLIATUM

Boneset

FICUS CARICA

Figs

FRAXINUS EXCELSIOR

Ash

GALEOPSIS SEGETUM

Hempnettle

EUPHORBIA CYPARISSIAS

Cypress Spurge

FILIPENDULA ULMARIA

Meadowsweet

FRAXINUS ORNUS

Manna

GALIUM ODORATA

Woodruff

FAGOPYRUM ESCULENTUM

Buckwheat

FOENICULUM VULGARE

Fennel

FUMARIA OFFICINALIS

Fumitory

GALIUM VERUM

Lady's Beadstraw

GARCINIA SPECIES

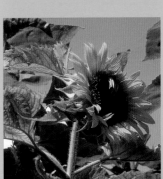

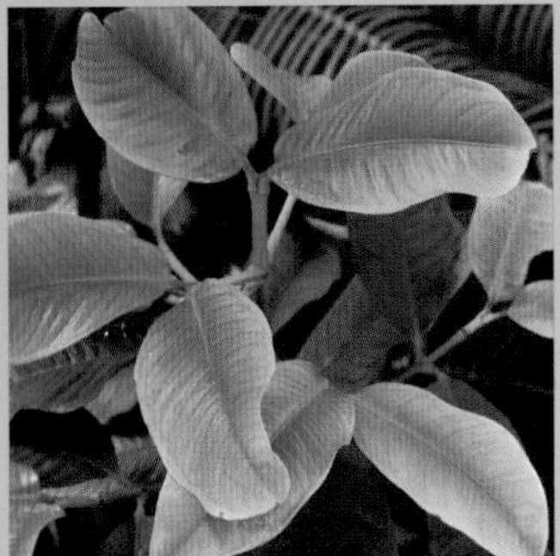

Gamboge

GENISTA TINCTORIA

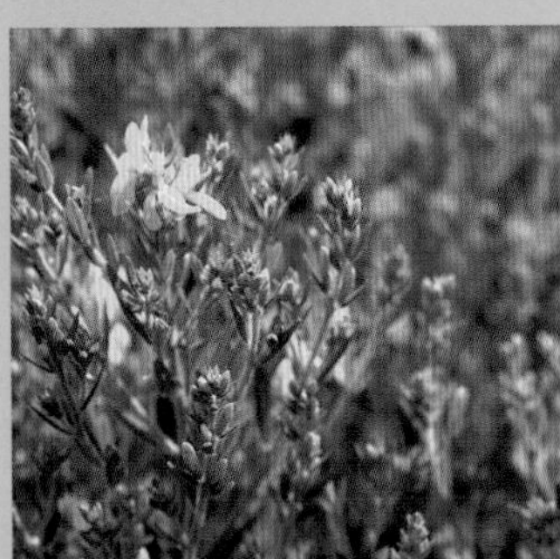

Dyer's Broom

GERANIUM ROBERTIANUM

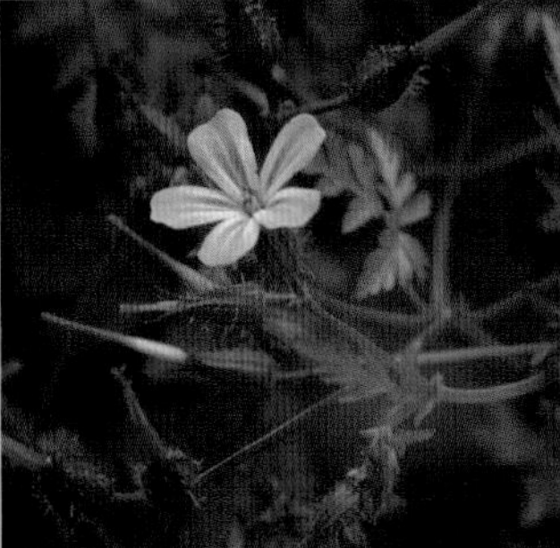

Herb Robert

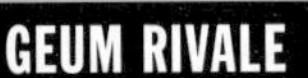

GEUM RIVALE

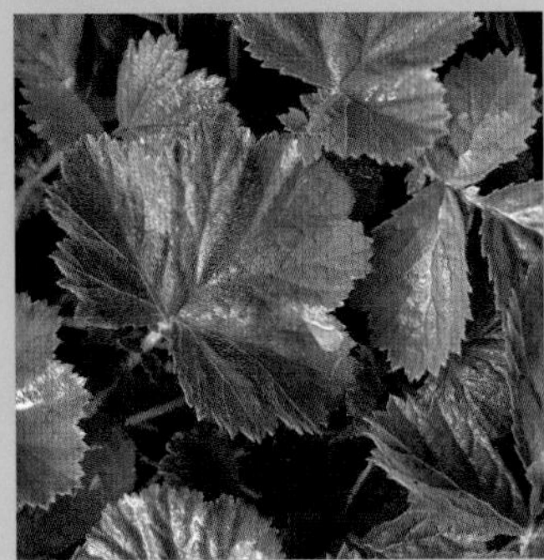

Water Avens

GEUM URBANUM

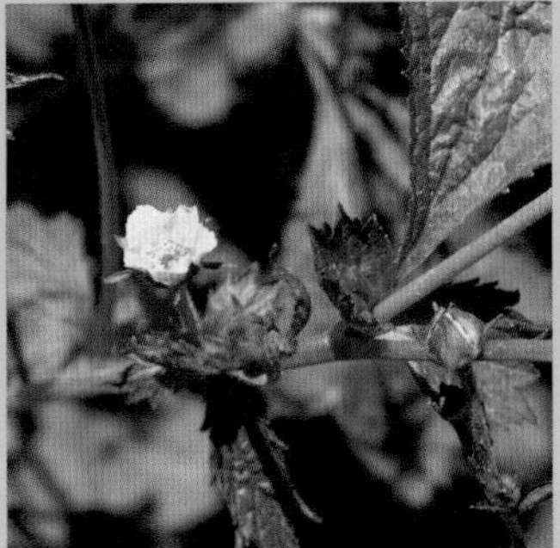

Bennet's Root

GINKGO BILOBA

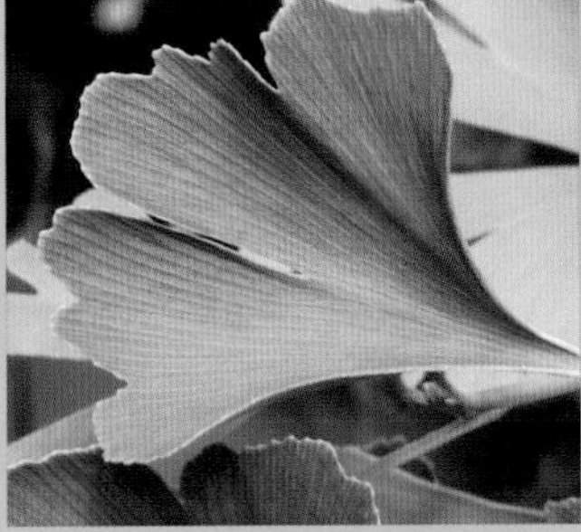

Ginkgo

GLECHOMA HEDERACEA

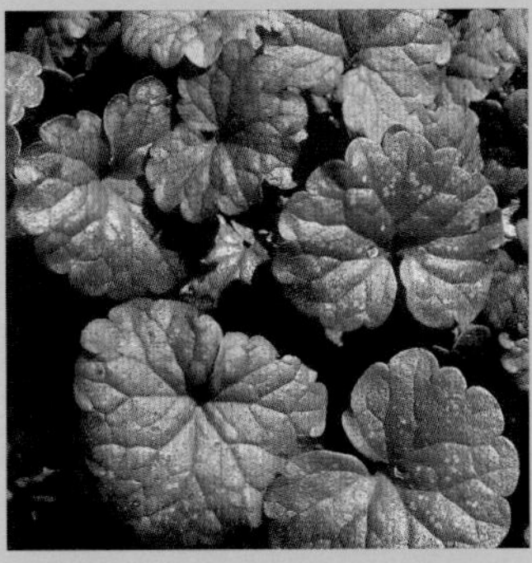

Ground Ivy

GLYCINE SOJA

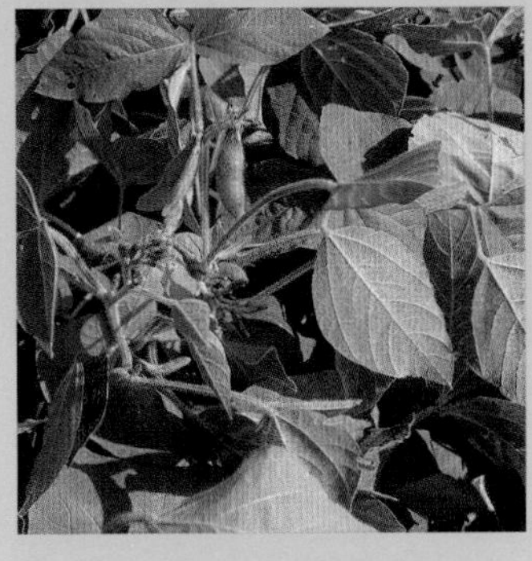

Soybean

GLYCYRRHIZA GLABRA

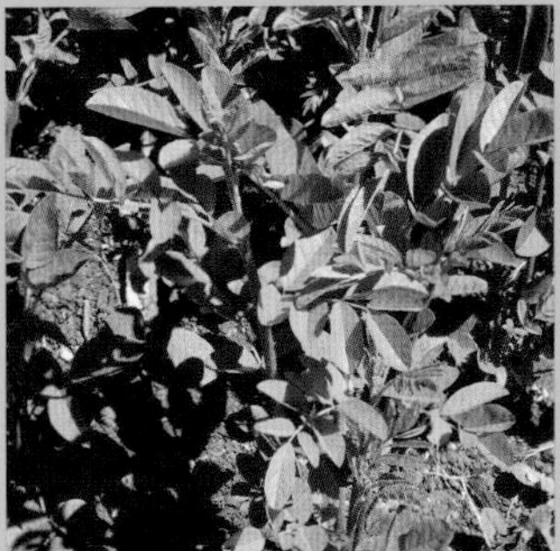

Licorice

GOSSYPIUM HERBACEUM

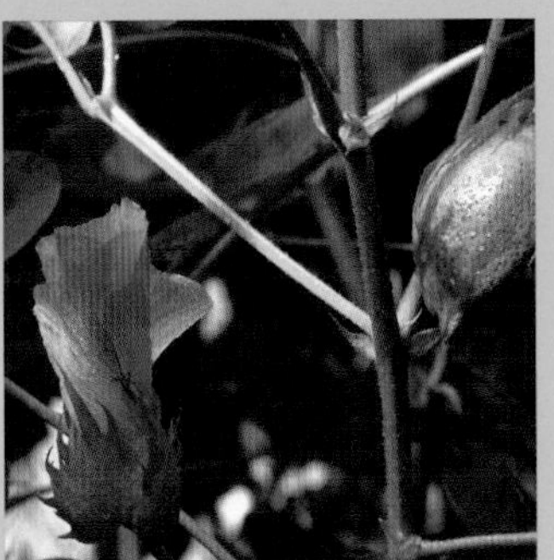

Cotton

GRATIOLA OFFICINALIS

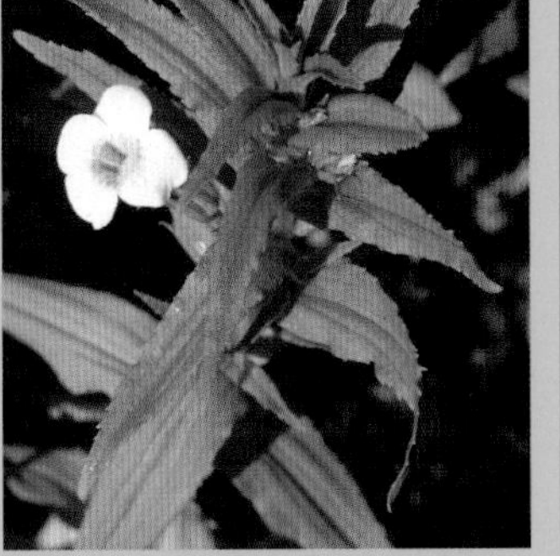

Hedge-Hyssop

HAMAMELIS VIRGINIANA

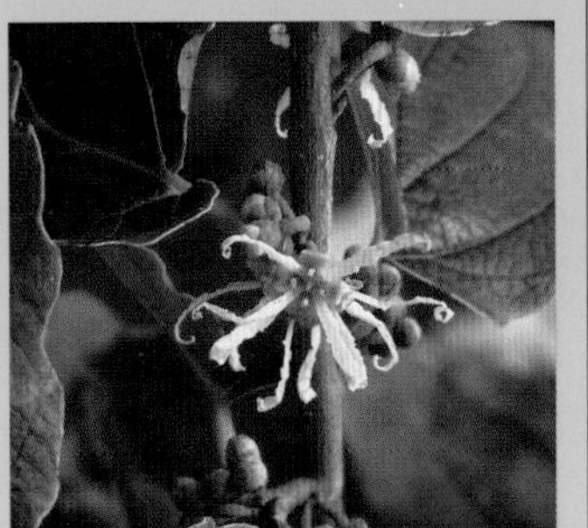

Witch Hazel

HEDERA HELIX

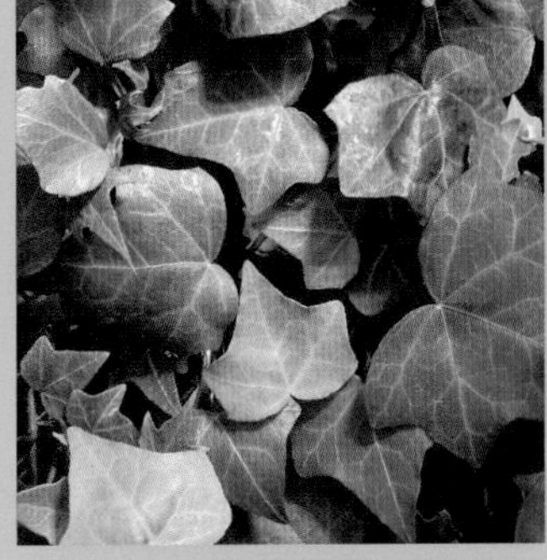

English Ivy

HELIANTHEMUM CANADENSE

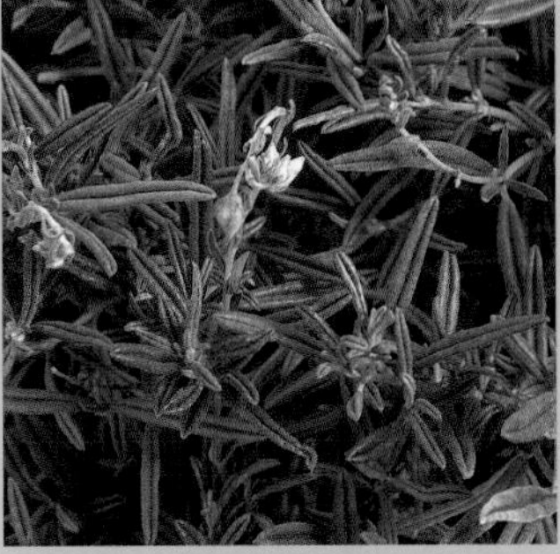

Frostwort

HELIANTHUS ANNUUS

Sunflower

HELICHRYSUM ARENARIUM

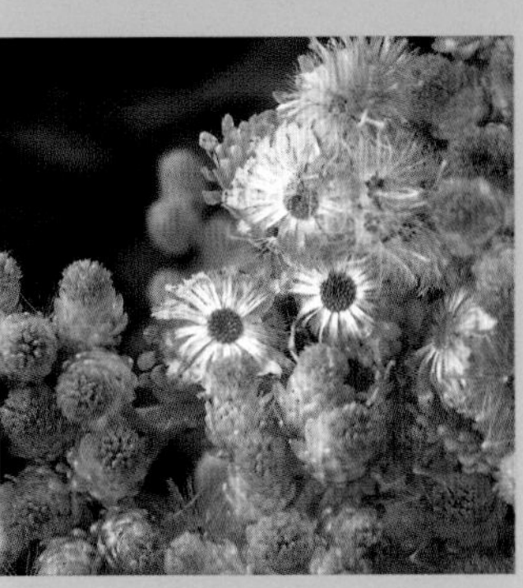

Immortelle

HELLEBORUS NIGER

Black Hellebore

HERACLEUM SPHONDYLIUM

Masterwort

HERNIARIA GLABRA

Rupturewort

HIBISCUS SPECIES

Hibiscus

HIPPOPHAË RHAMNOIDES

Sea Buckthorn

HORDEUM SPECIES

Barley

HUMULUS LUPULUS

Hops

HYDRANGEA SPECIES

Hydrangea

HYDRASTIS CANADENSIS

Golden Seal

HYOSCYAMUS NIGER

Henbane

HYPERICUM PERFORATUM

St. John's Wort

HYSSOPUS OFFICINALIS

Hyssop

ILEX AQUIFOLIUM

Holly

ILEX PARAGUARIENSIS

Mate

ILLICIUM VERUM

Star Anise

INULA HELENIUM

Elecampane

IPOMOEA SPECIES

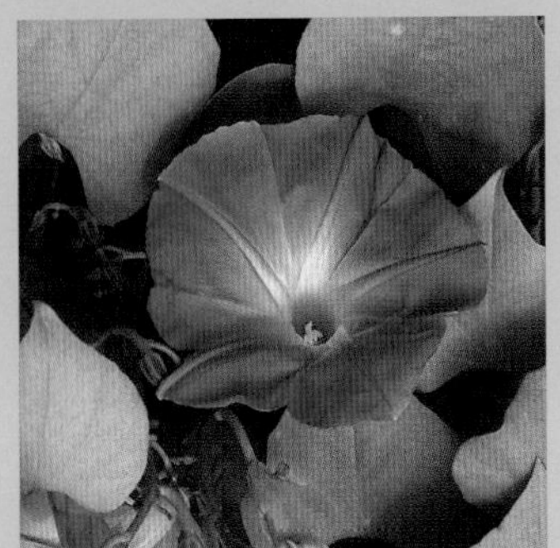

Jalap

IRIS SPECIES

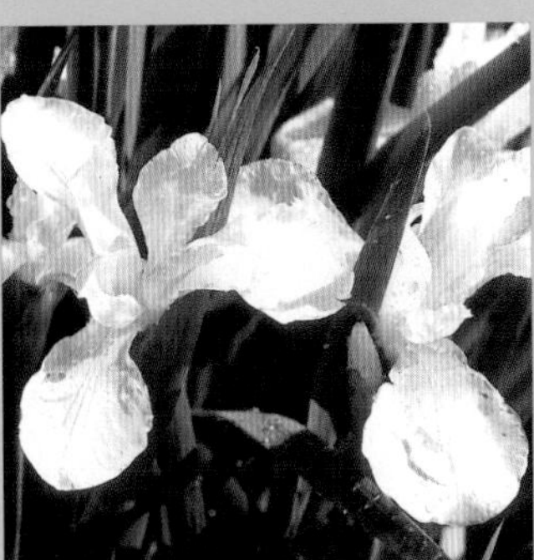

Orris Root

JUGLANS REGIA

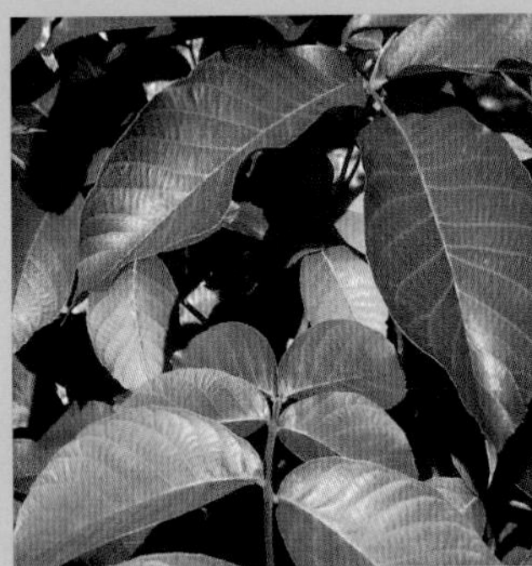

Walnut

JUNIPERUS COMMUNIS

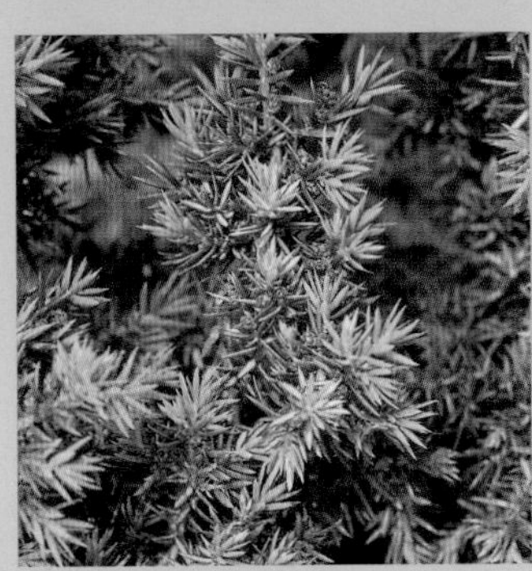

Juniper

JUNIPERUS SABINA

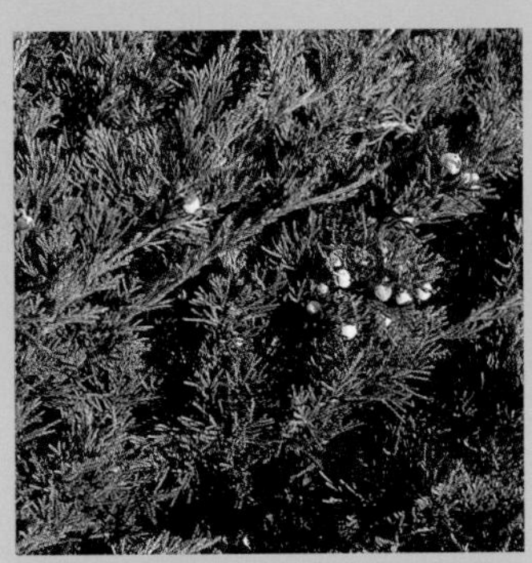

Savin Tops

JUSTICIA ADHATODA

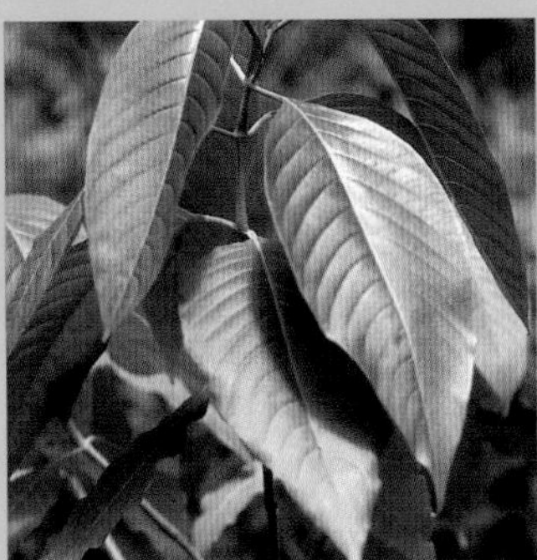

Malabar Nut

KALMIA LATIFOLIA

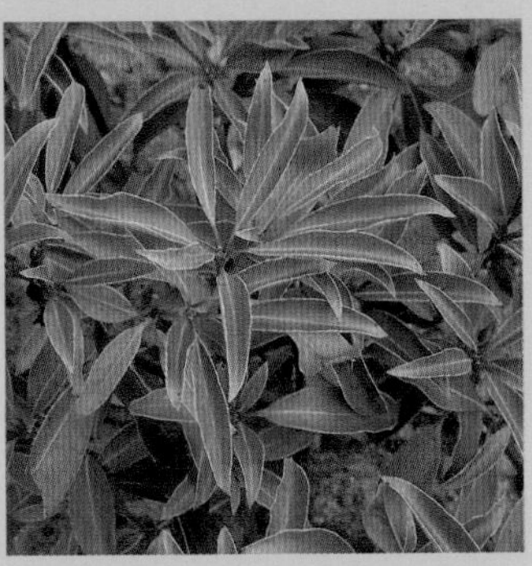

Mountain Laurel

KNAUTIA ARVENSIS

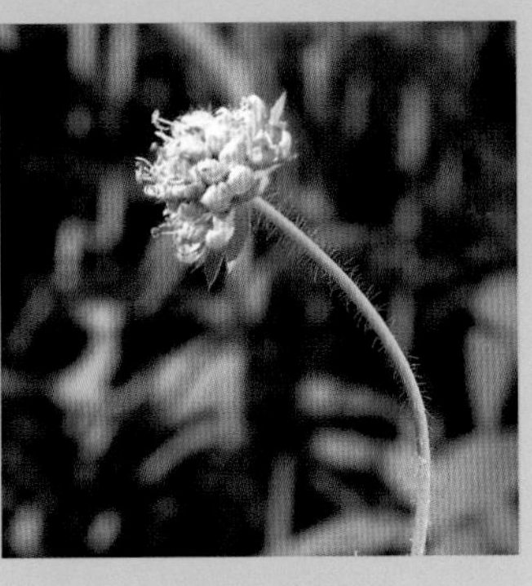

Field Scabious

LACTUCA VIROSA

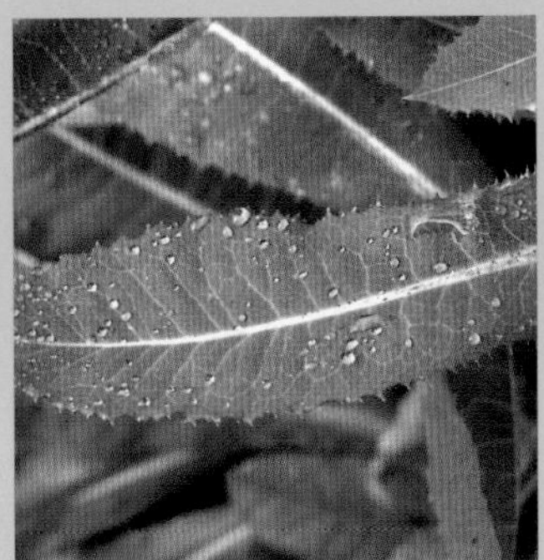

Wild Lettuce

LAMIUM ALBUM

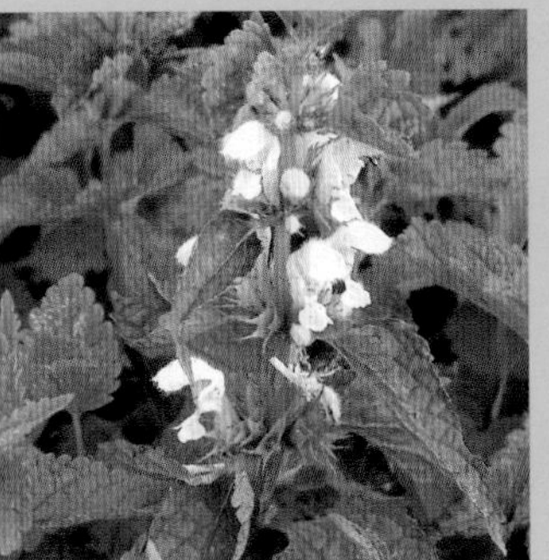

White Dead Nettle

LARIX DECIDUA

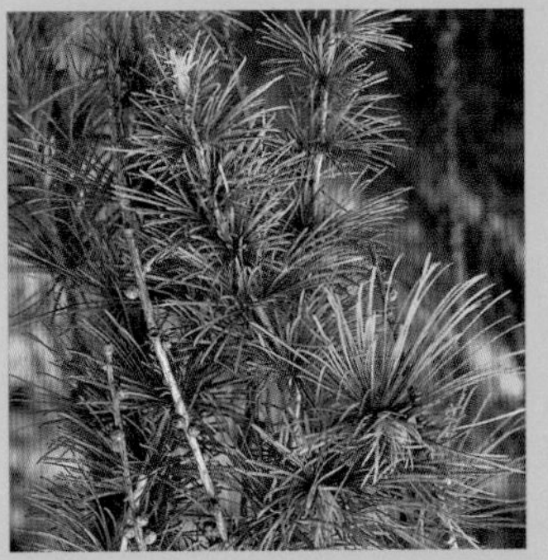

Larch

LAURUS NOBILIS

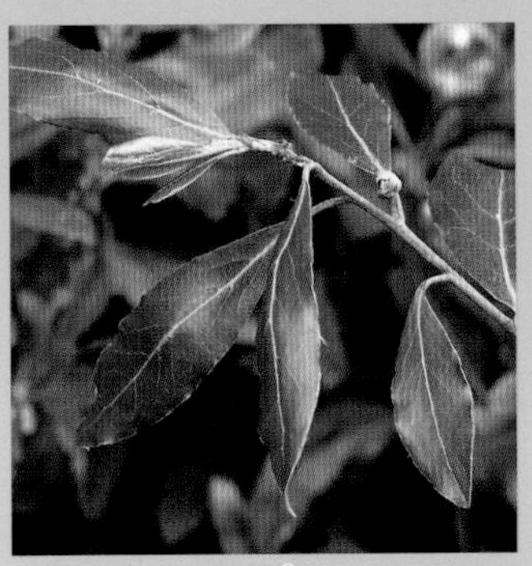

Laurel

LAVANDULA ANGUSTIFOLIA

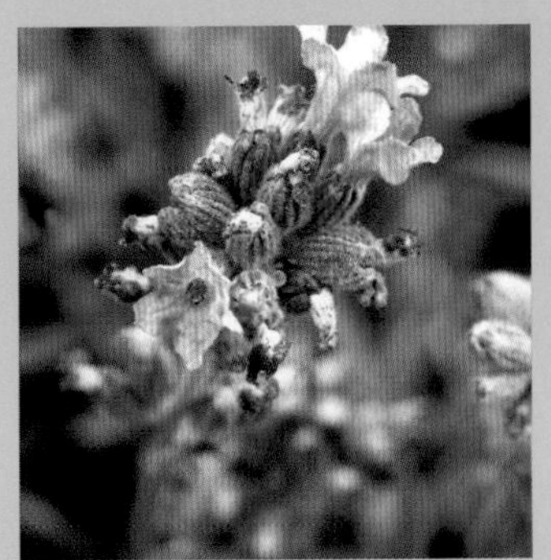

Lavender

LAWSONIA INERMIS

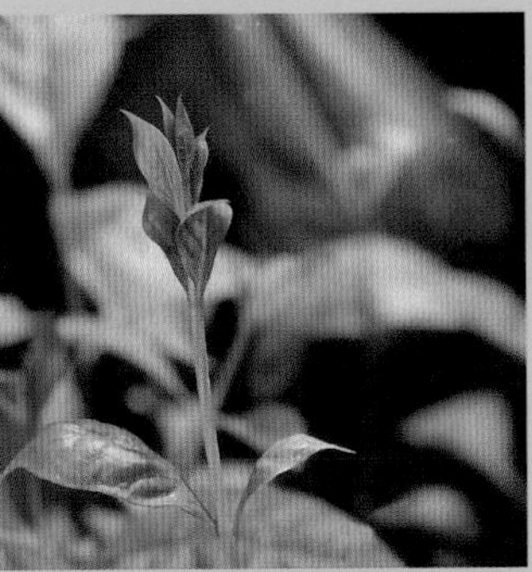

Henna

LEMNA MINOR

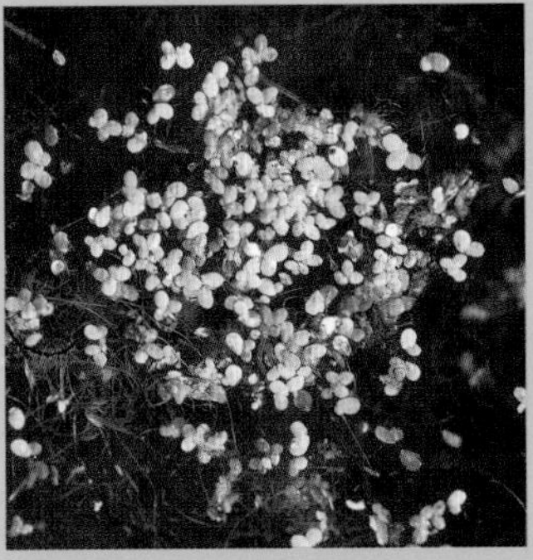

Duckweed

LEONURUS CARDIACA

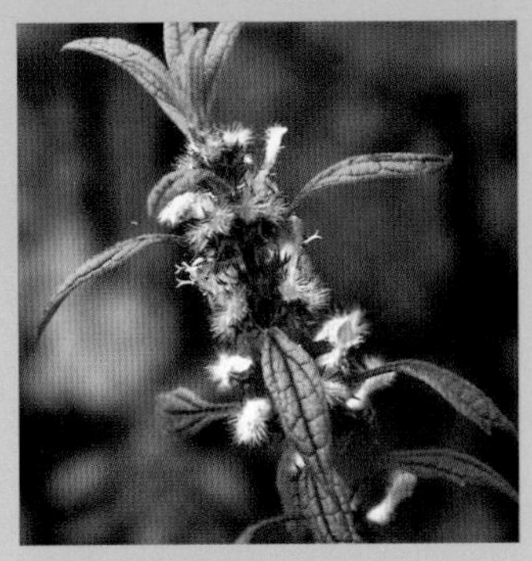

Motherwort

LEPIDIUM SATIVUM

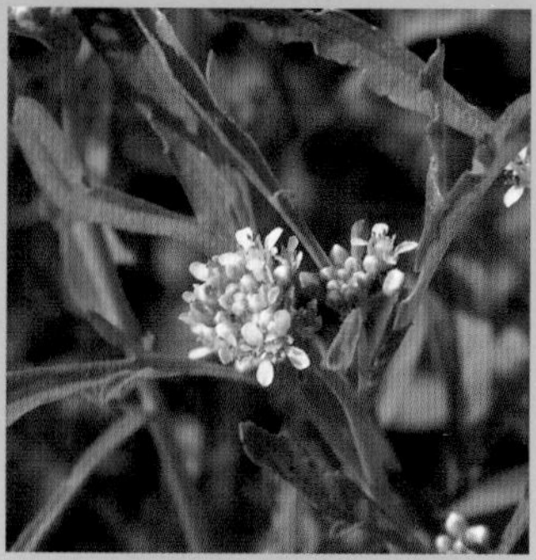

Garden Cress

LEVISTICUM OFFICINALE

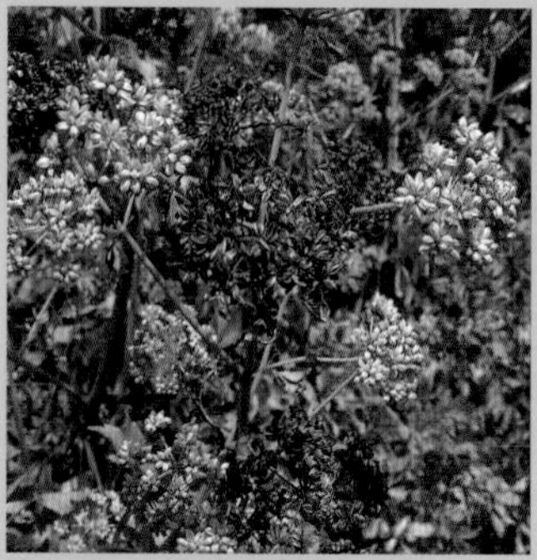

Lovage

LIATRIS SPICATA

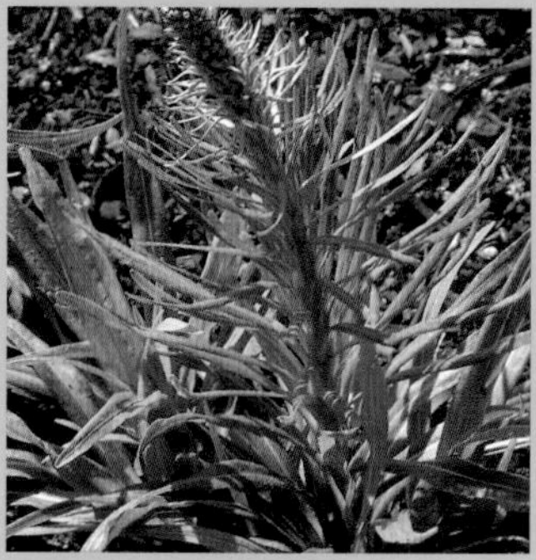

Marsh Blazing Star

LINARIA VULGARIS

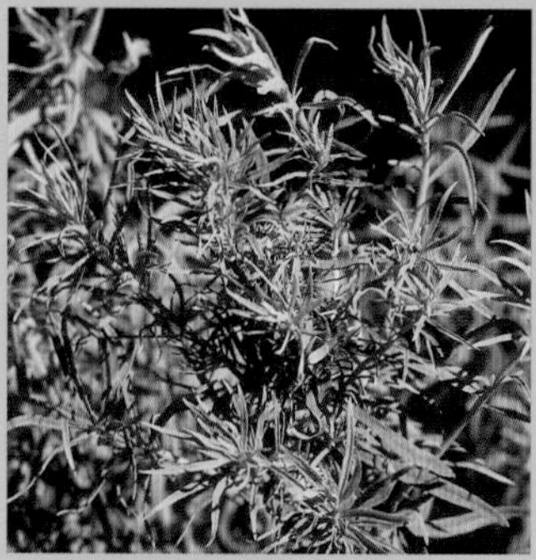

Yellow Toadflax

LINUM USITATISSIMUM

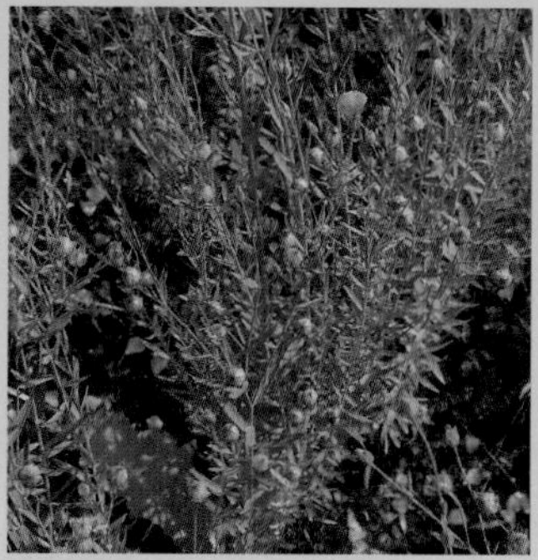

Flaxseed

LIQUIDAMBAR ORIENTALIS

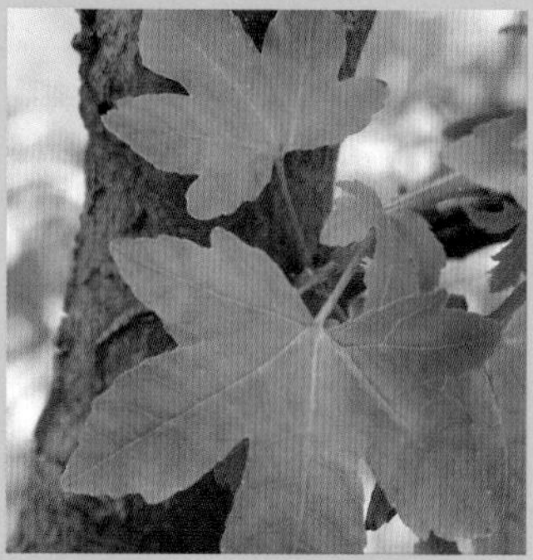

Storax

LOBELIA INFLATA

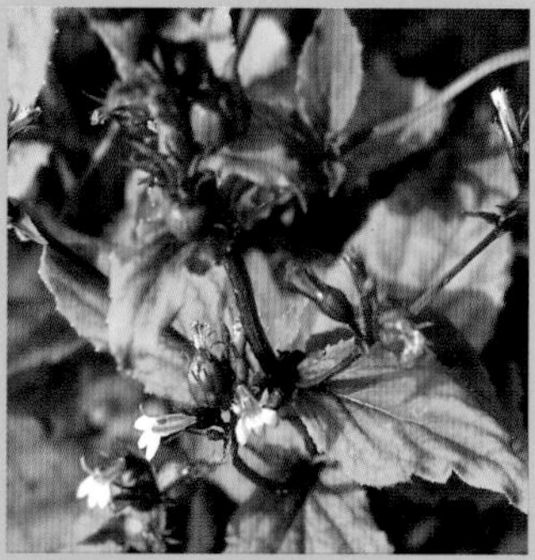

Lobelia

LOLIUM TEMULENTUM

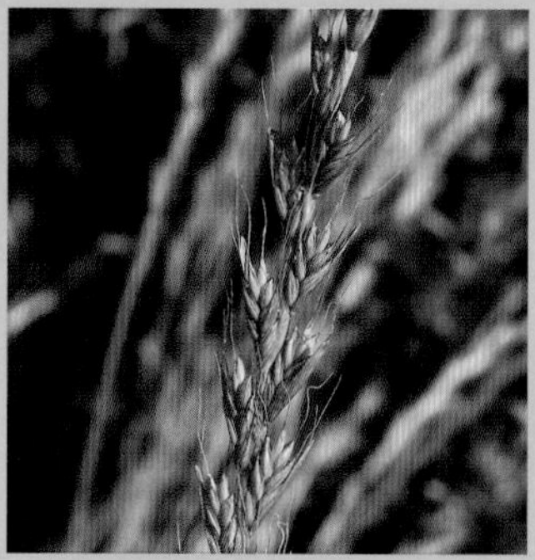

Taumelloolch

LOPHOPHORA WILLIAMSII

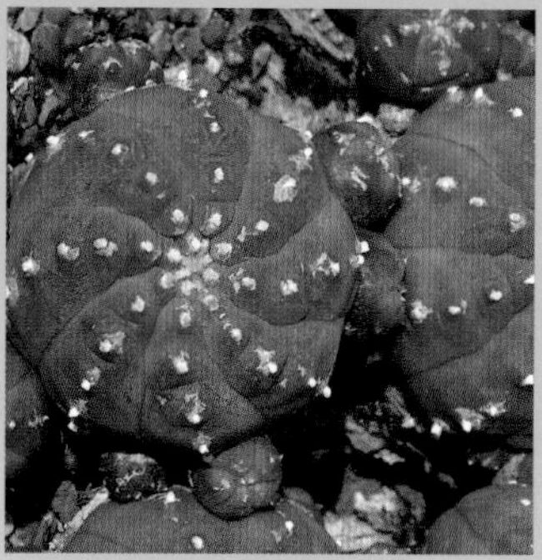

Peyote

LUFFA SPECIES

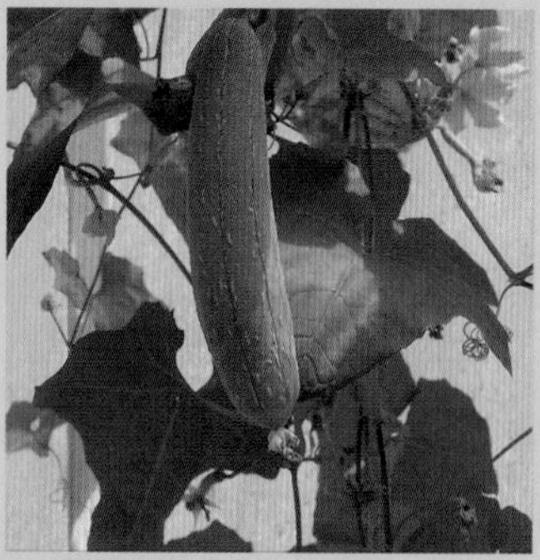

Luffa

LUPINUS LUTEUS

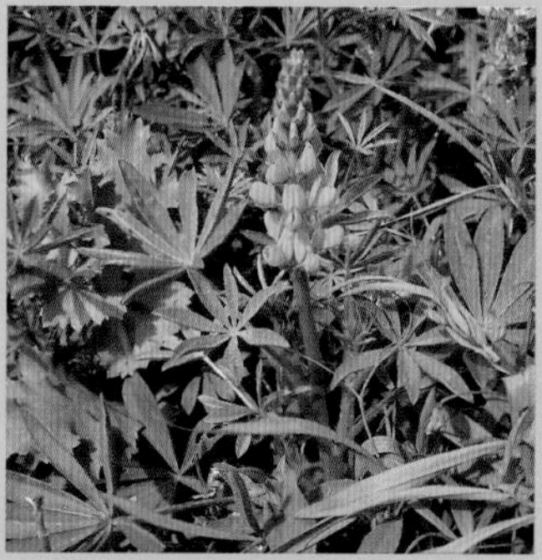

Yellow Lupin

LYCOPERSICON ESCULENTUM

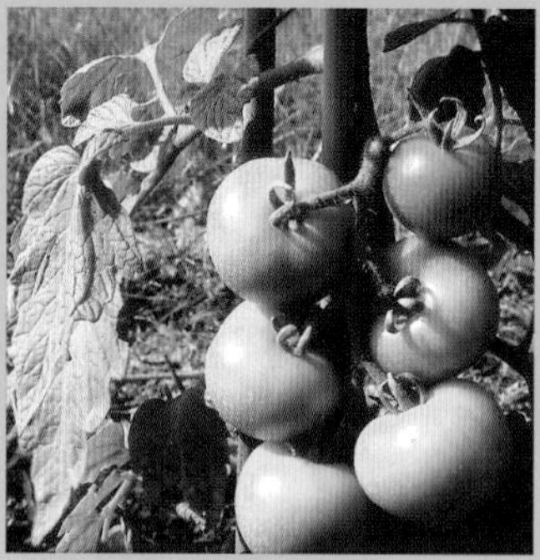

Tomato

LYCOPUS VIRGINICUS

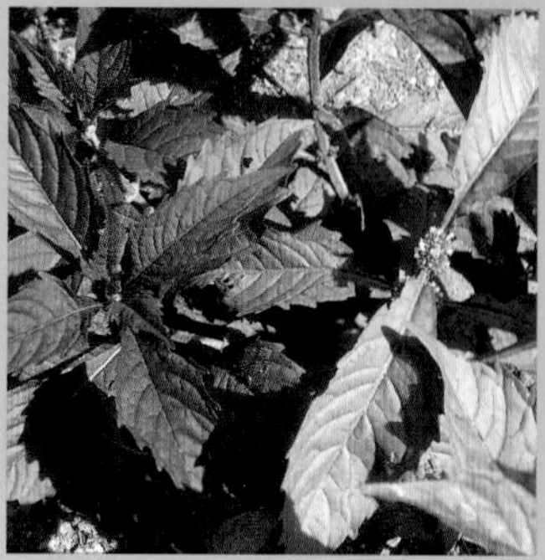

Bugleweed

LYSIMACHIA NUMMULARIA

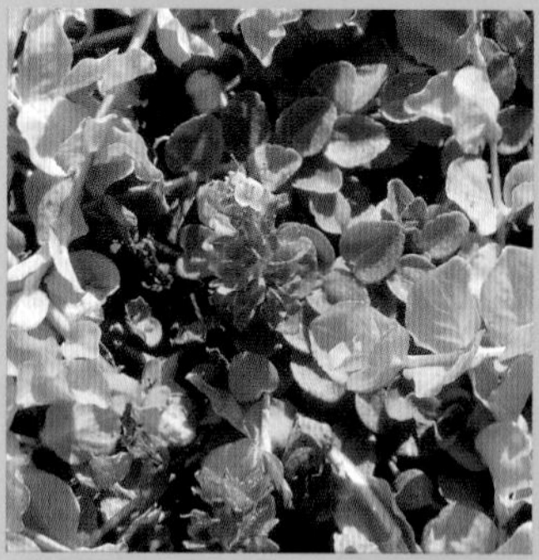

Moneywort

LYSIMACHIA VULGARIS

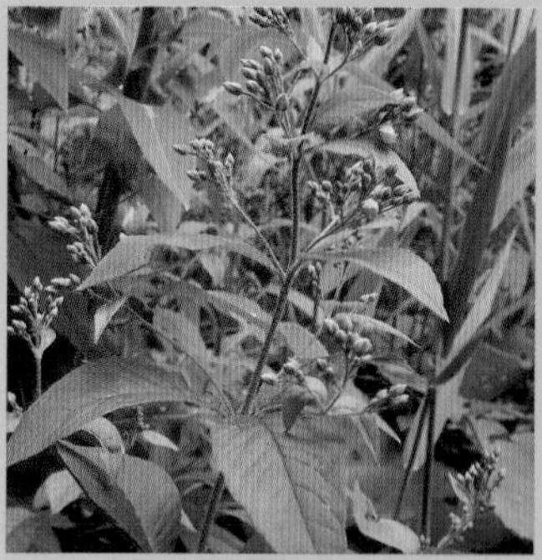

Loosestrife

LYTHRUM SALICARIA

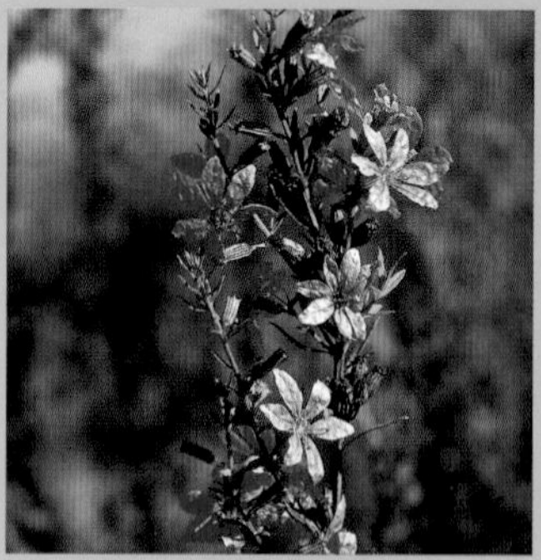

Purple Loosestrife

MAHONIA AQUIFOLIUM

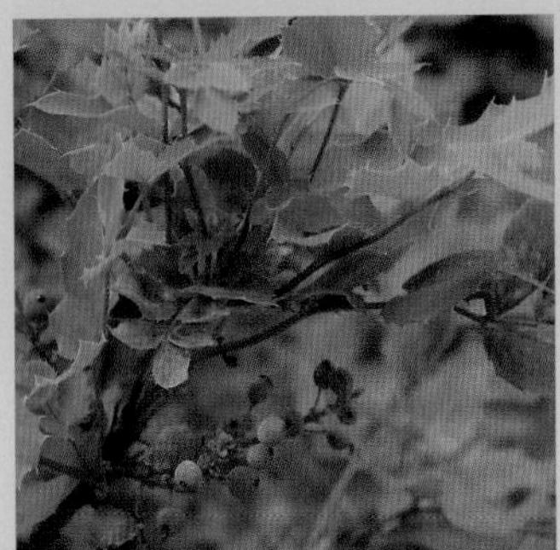

Mountain Grape

MALUS DOMESTICA

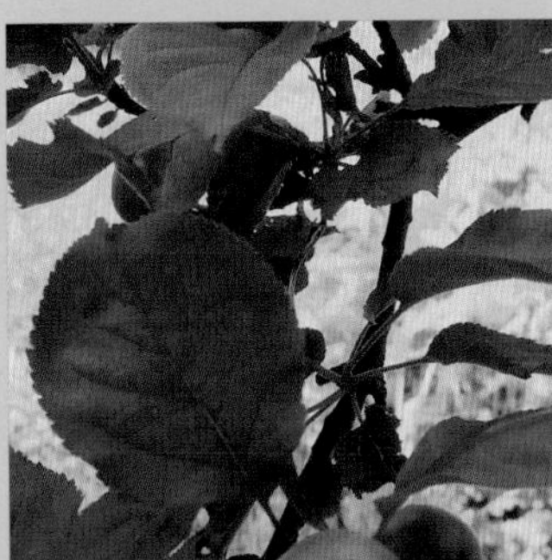

Apple Tree

MALVA SYLVESTRIS

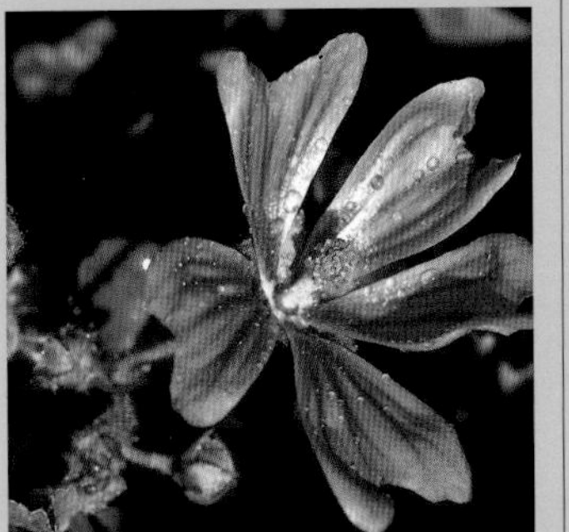

Mallow

MANDRAGORA SPECIES

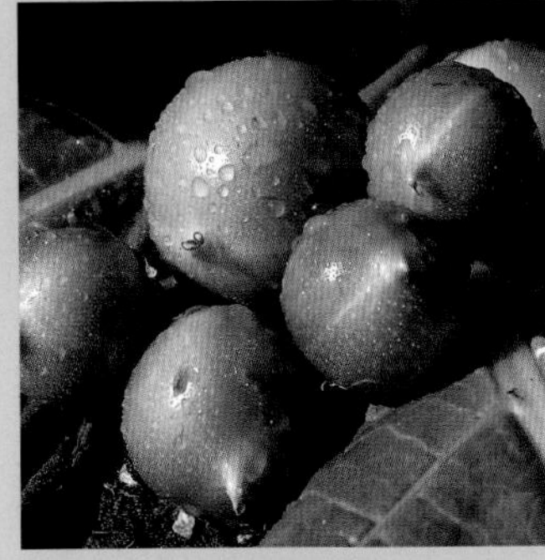

Mandrake

MARRUBIUM VULGARE

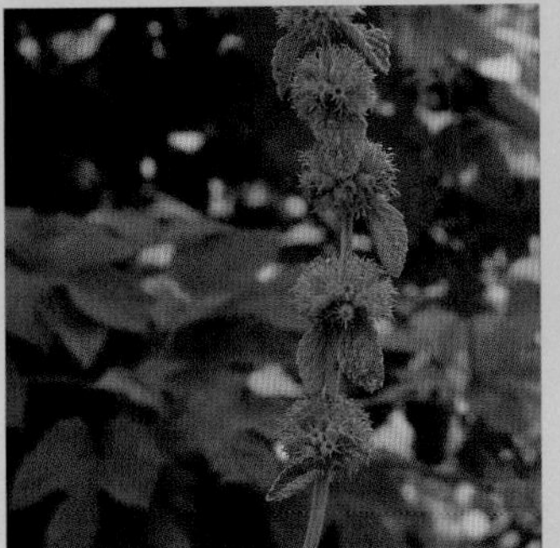

White Horsehound

MATRICARIA CHAMOMILLA

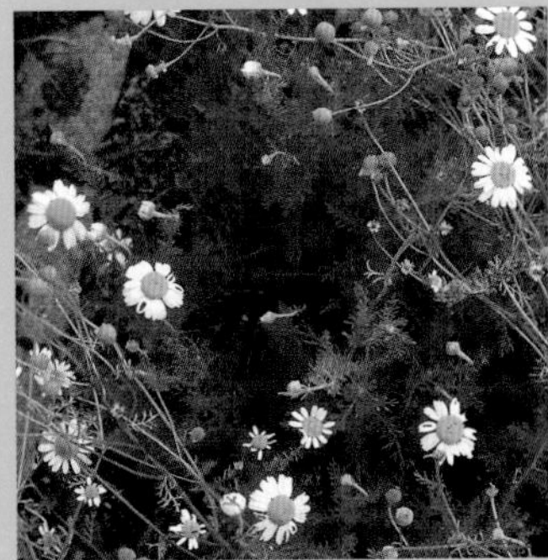

Chamomile

MEDICAGO SATIVA

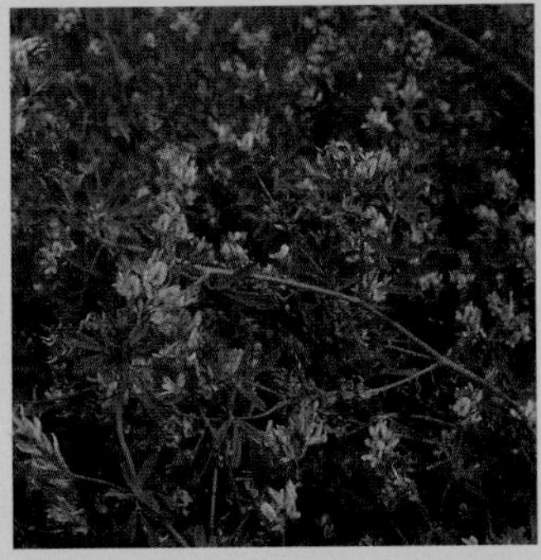

Alfalfa

MELALEUCA SPECIES

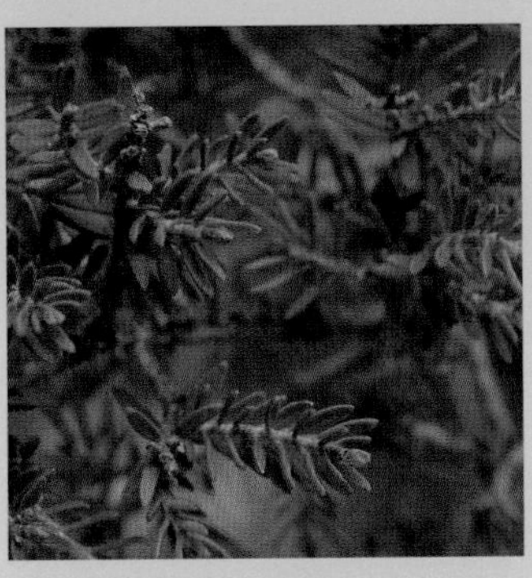

Cajuput

MELILOTUS OFFICINALIS

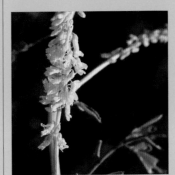

Sweet Clover

MELISSA OFFICINALIS

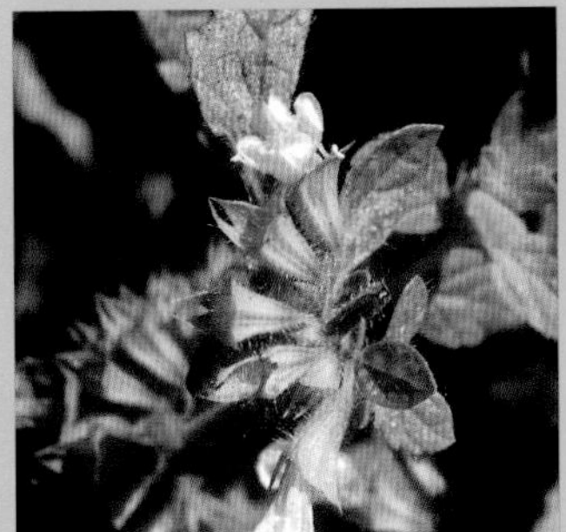

Lemon Balm

MENTHA AQUATICA

Wild Mint

MENTHA LONGIFOLIA

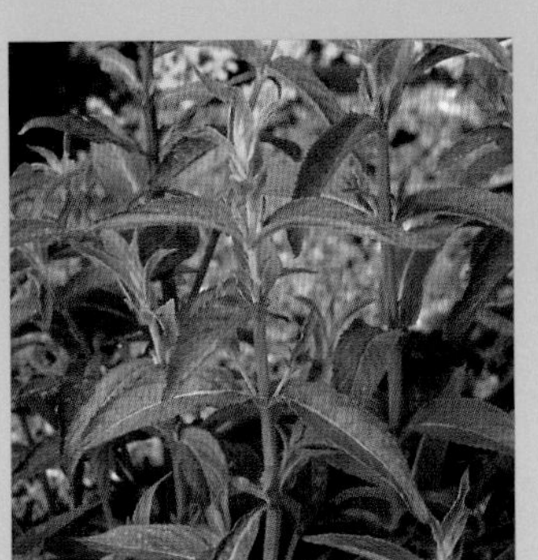

English Horsemint

MENTHA PIPERITA

Peppermint

MENTHA SPICATA

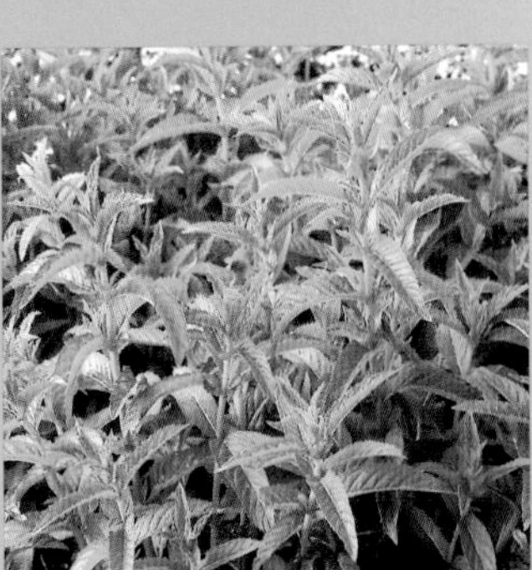

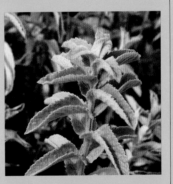

Spearmint

MENYANTHES TRIFOLIATA

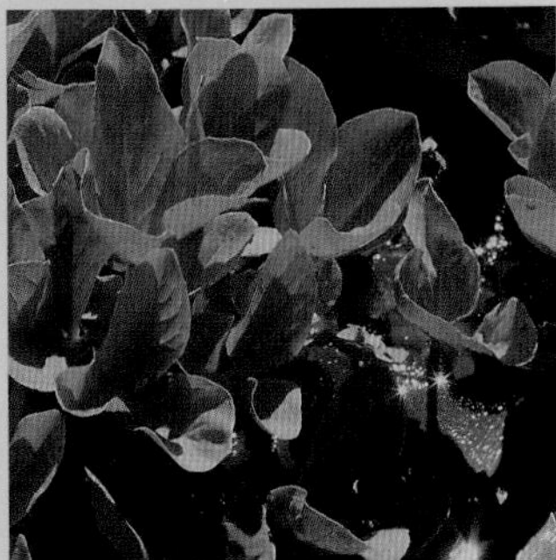

Buck Bean

MERCURIALIS ANNUA

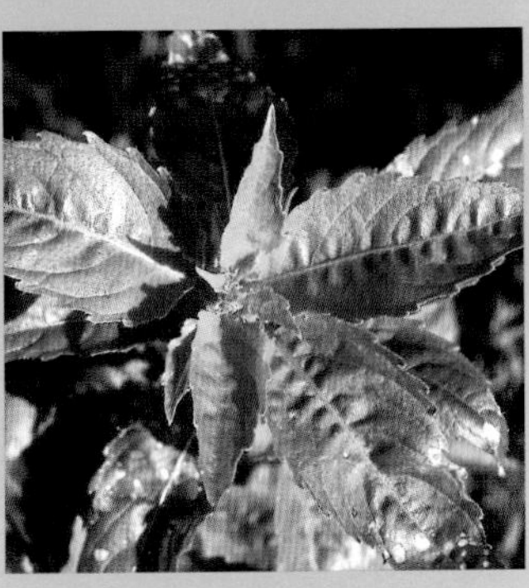

Mercury Herb

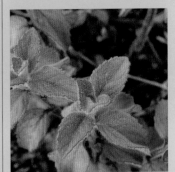

MYOSOTIS ARVENSIS

Forget-Me-Not

MYROXYLON BALSAMUM

Peruvian Balsam

NEPETA CATARIA

Catnip

OCIMUM BASILICUM

Basil

MYRICA CERIFERA

Wax Myrtle

MYRRHIS ODORATA

Sweet Cicely

NERIUM OLEANDER

Oleander Leaf

OENANTHE AQUATICA

Water Fennel

MYRICA GALE

Sweet Gale

MYRTUS COMMUNIS

Myrtle

NICOTIANA TABACUM

Tobacco

OENOTHERA BIENNIS

Evening Primrose

MYRISTICA FRAGRANS

Nutmeg

NELUMBO NUCIFERA

Lotus

NYMPHAEA ODORATA

American White Pond Lily

OLEA EUROPAEA

Olive

ONONIS SPINOSA

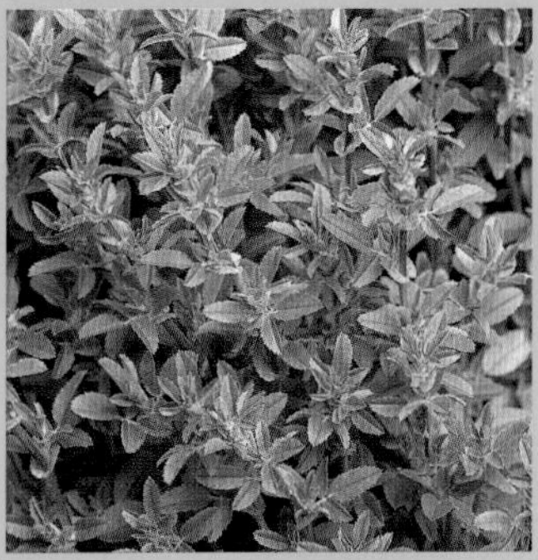

Spiny Rest Harrow

ONOPORDUM ACANTHIUM

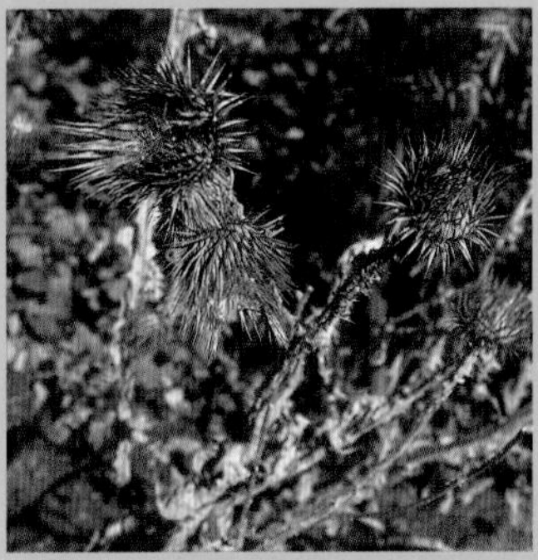

Scotch Thistle

ORIGANUM MAJORANA

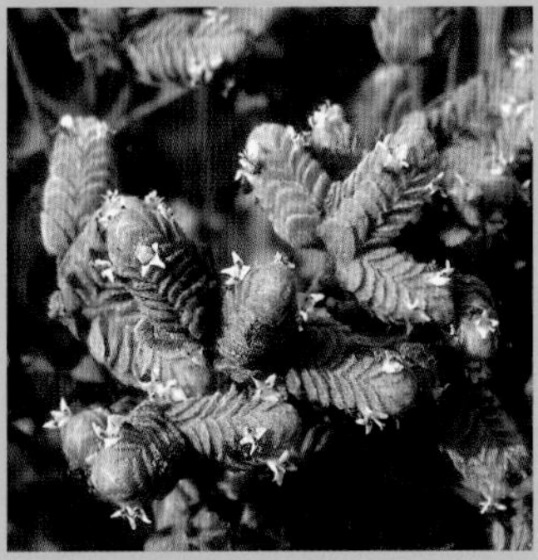

Marjoram

ORIGANUM VULGARE

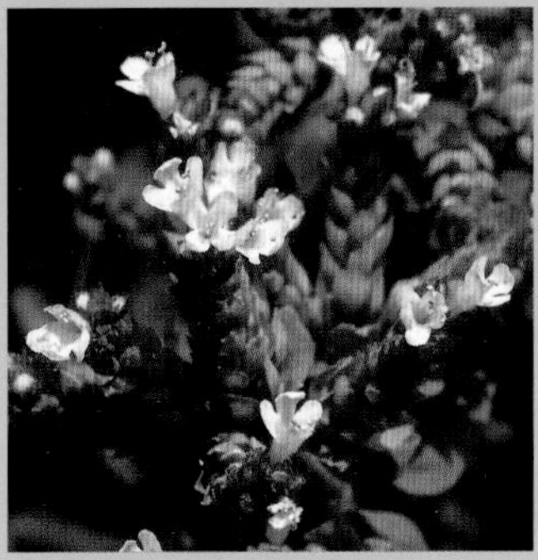

Oregano

ORYZA SATIVA

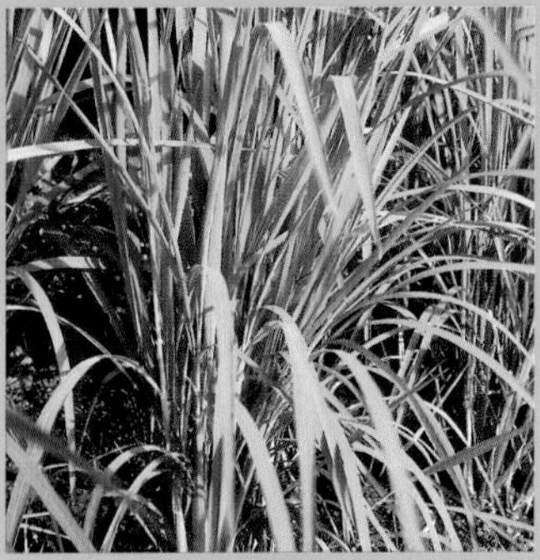

Rice

PAEONIA OFFICINALIS

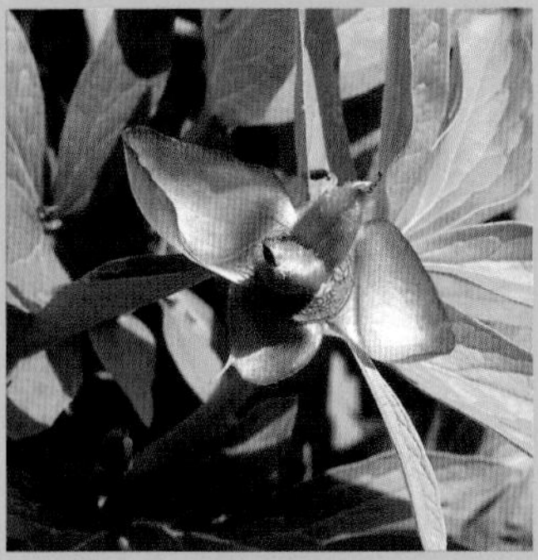

Peony

PAPAVER RHOEAS

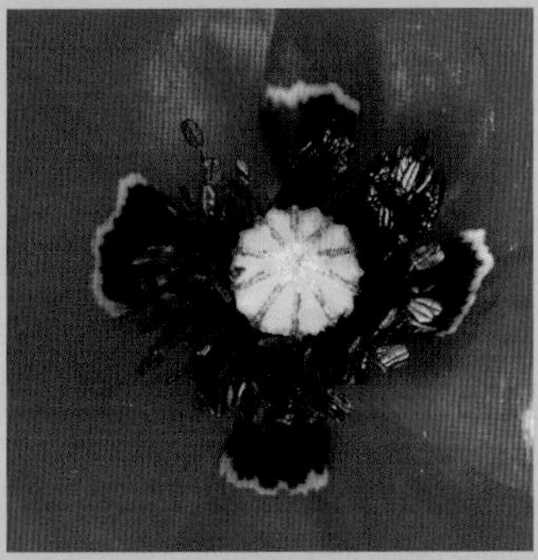

Corn Poppy

PAPAVER SOMNIFERUM

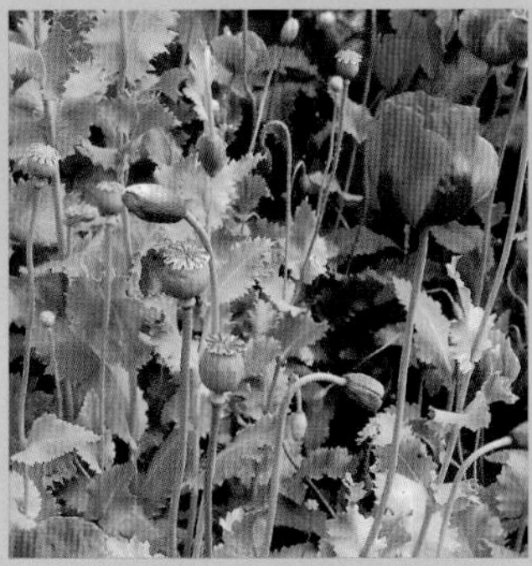

Poppy

PARIS QUADRIFOLIA

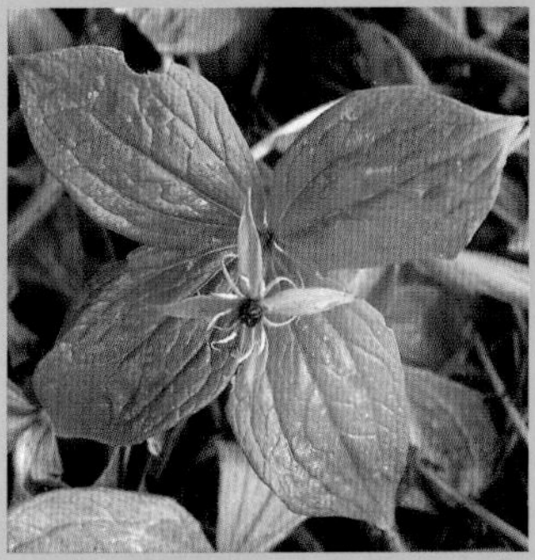

Herb Paris

PARTHENOCISSUS SPECIES

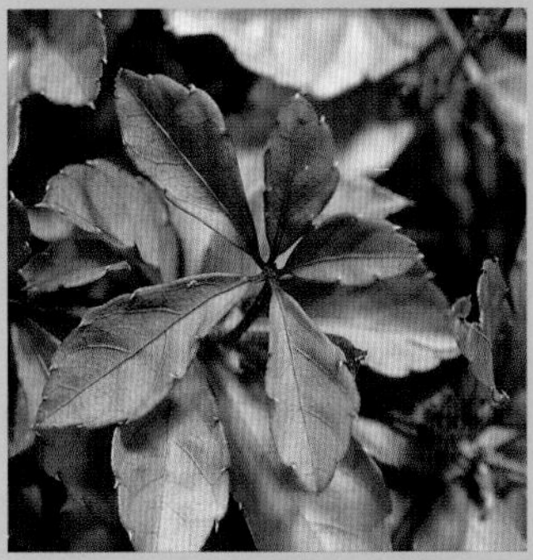

American Ivy

PASSIFLORA INCARNATA

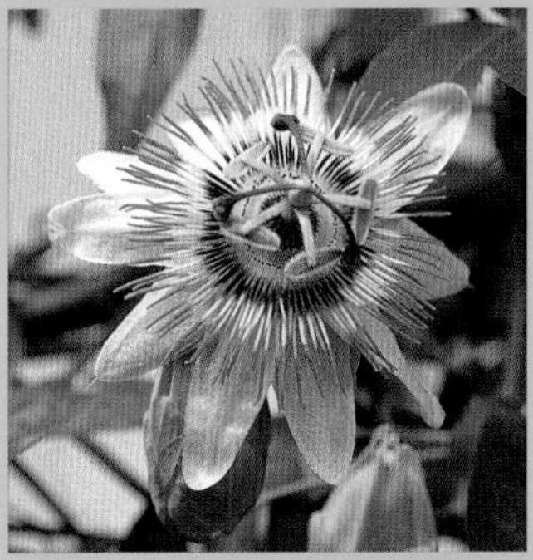

Passion Flower

PASTINACA SATIVA

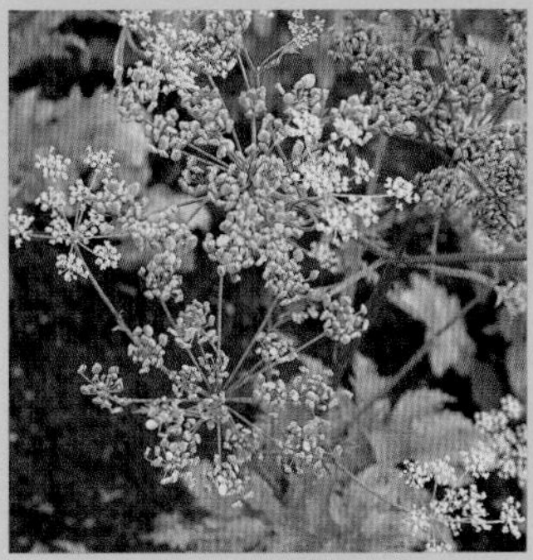

Parsnip

PERSEA AMERICANA

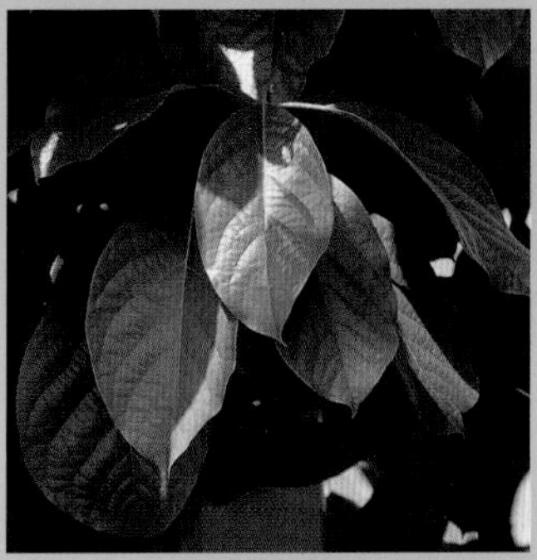

Avocado

PETASITES HYBRIDUS

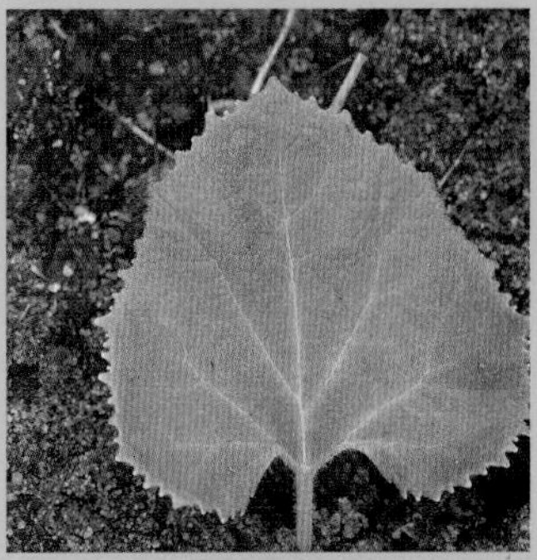

Petasites

PETROSELINUM CRISPUM

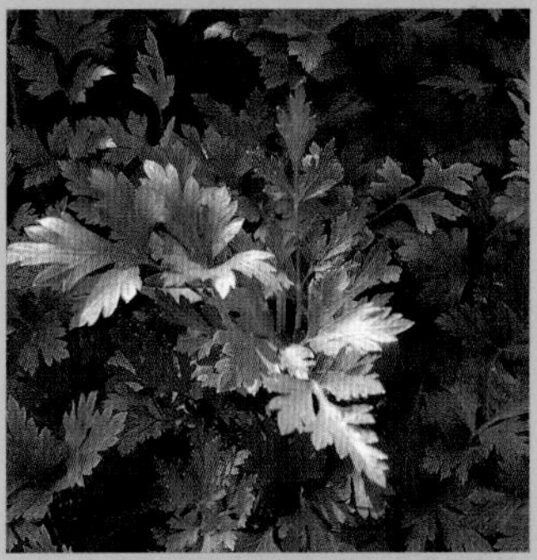

Parsley

PEUMUS BOLDO

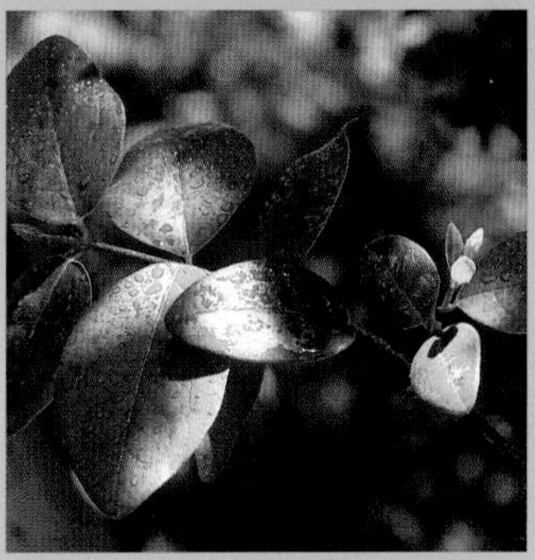

Boldo

PHASEOLUS VULGARIS

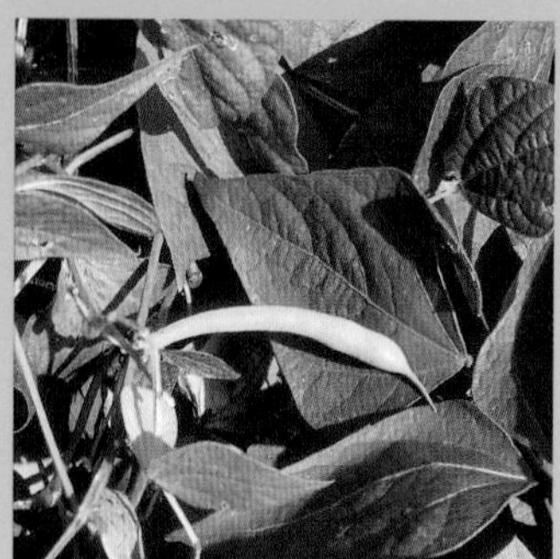

Bean

PHOENIX DACTYLIFERA

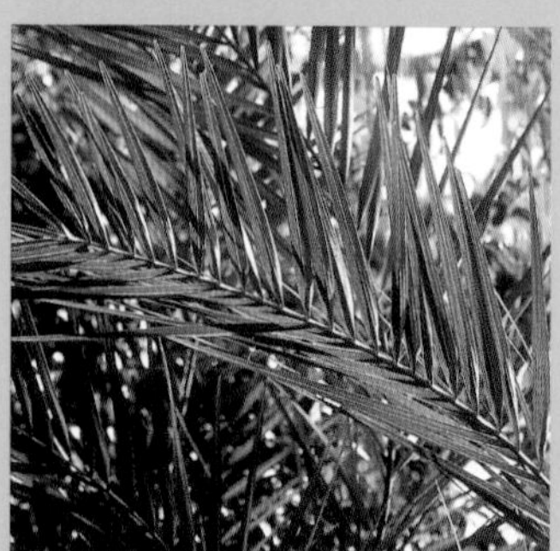

Date Palm

PHYSALIS ALKEKENGI

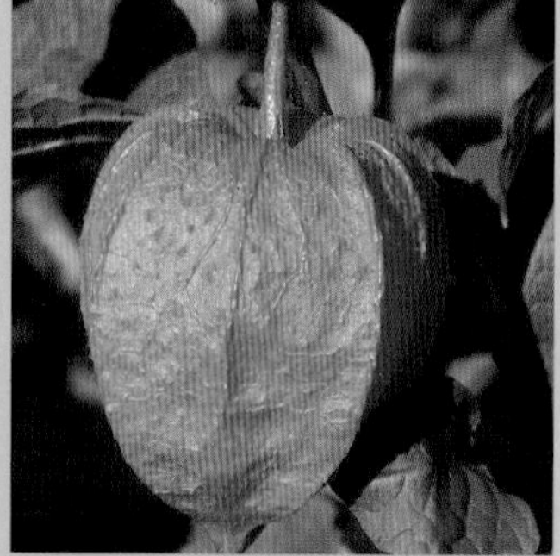

Winter Cherry

PHYTOLACCA AMERICANA

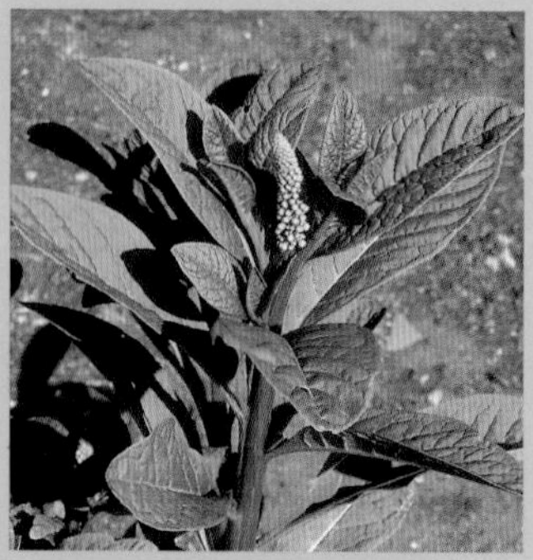

Poke Root

PILOCARPUS SPECIES

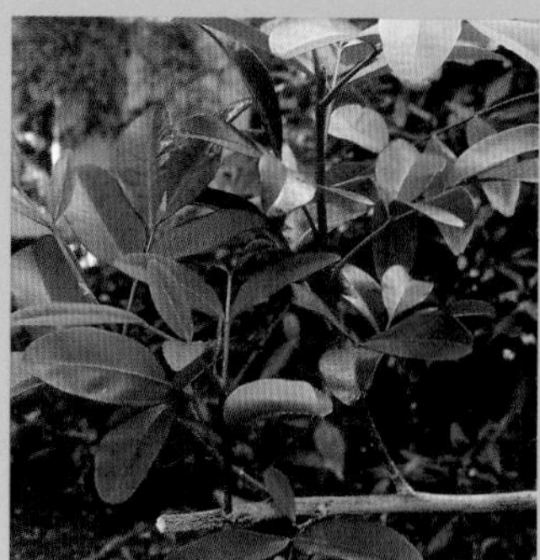

Jaborandi

PIMPINELLA ANISUM

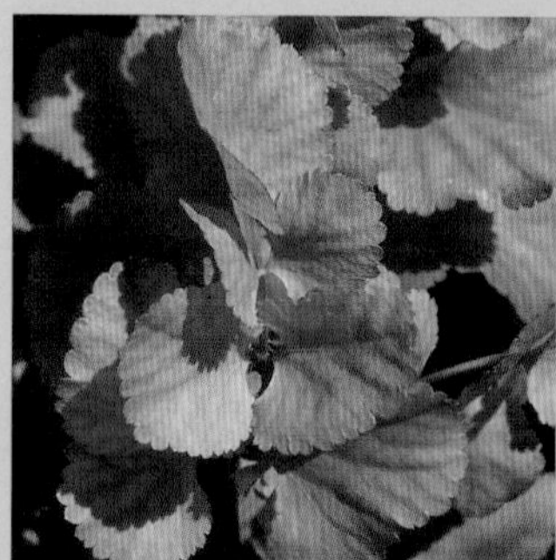

Anise

PIMPINELLA MAJOR

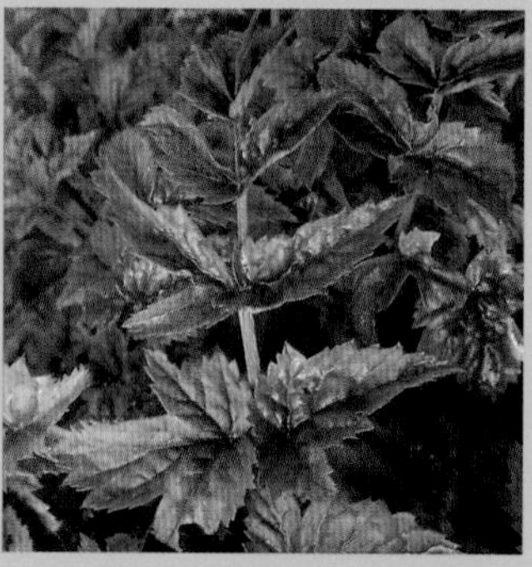

Burnet Saxifrage

PINUS SYLVESTRIS

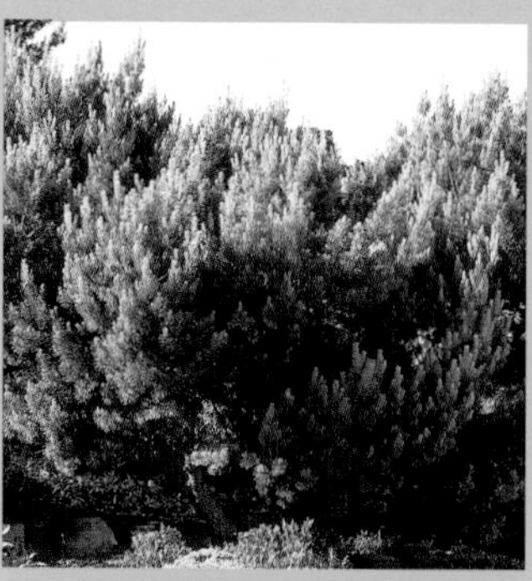

Scotch Pine

PIPER METHYSTICUM

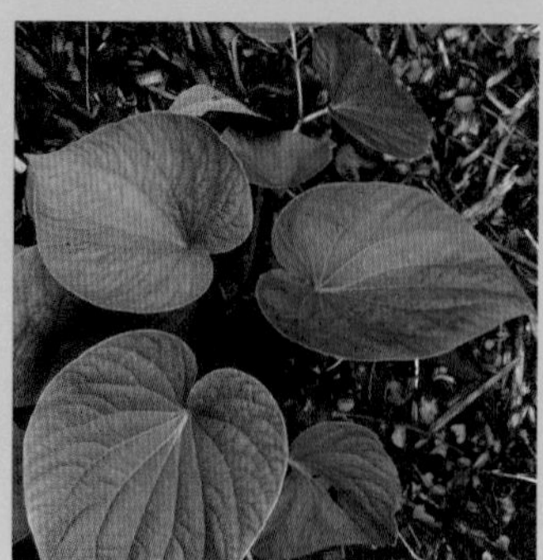

Kava-Kava

PIPER NIGRUM

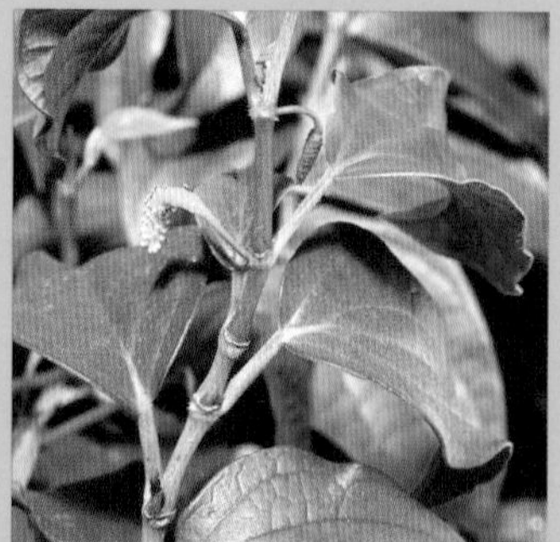

Black Pepper

PISTACIA LENTISCUS

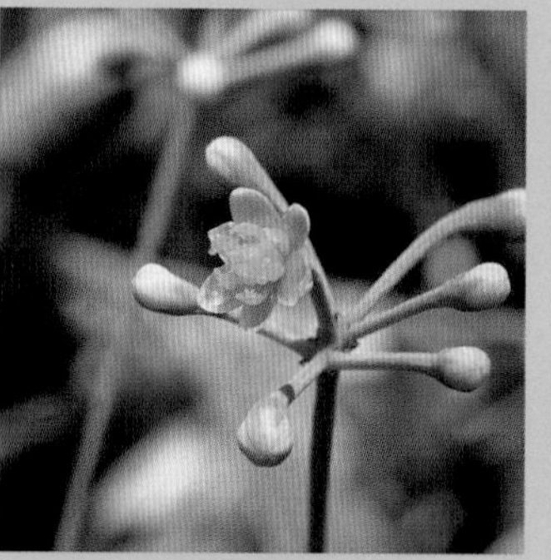

Mastic Tree

PLANTAGO AFRA

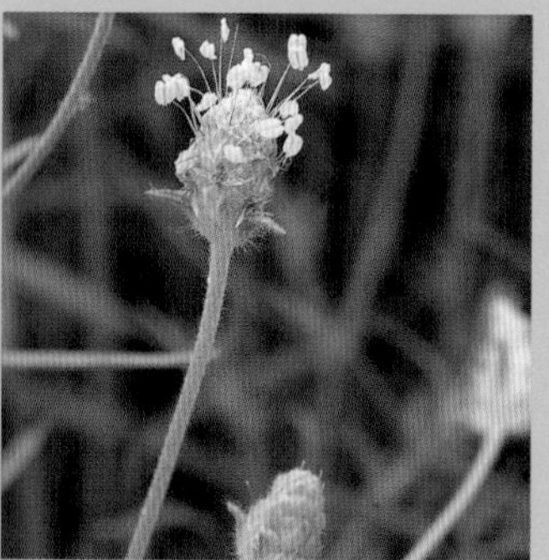

Psyllium Seed

PLANTAGO LANCEOLATA

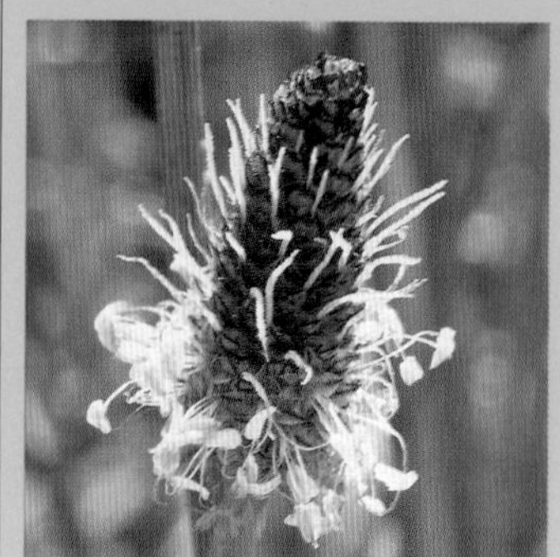

Plantain

POGOSTEMON CABLIN

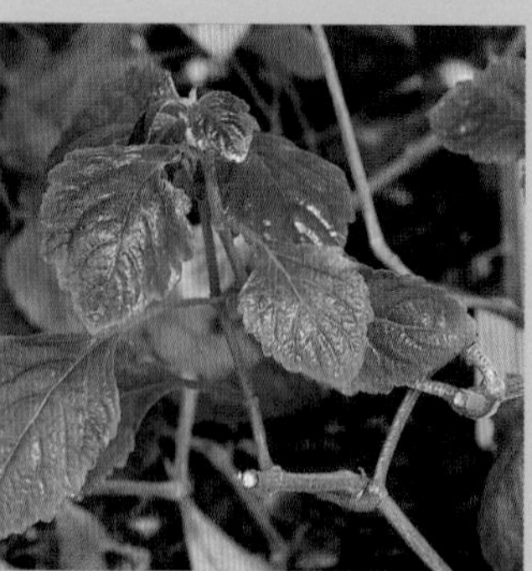

Patchouli

POLEMONIUM COERULEUM

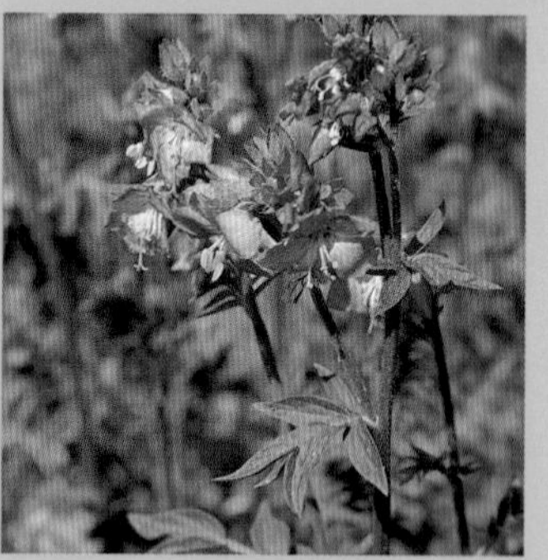

Jacob's Ladder

POLEMONIUM REPTANS

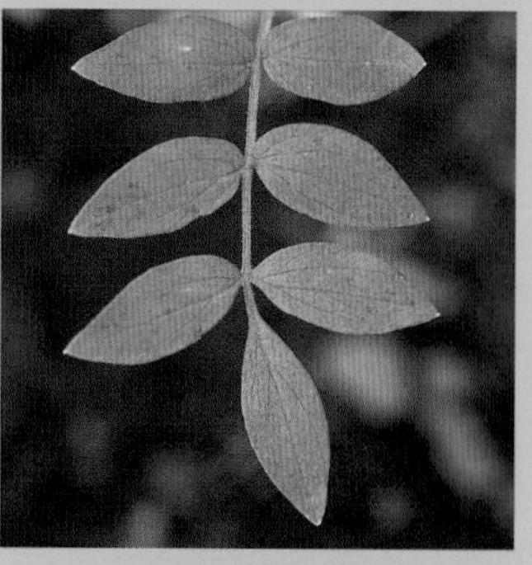

Abscess Root

POLYGONATUM MULTIFLORUM

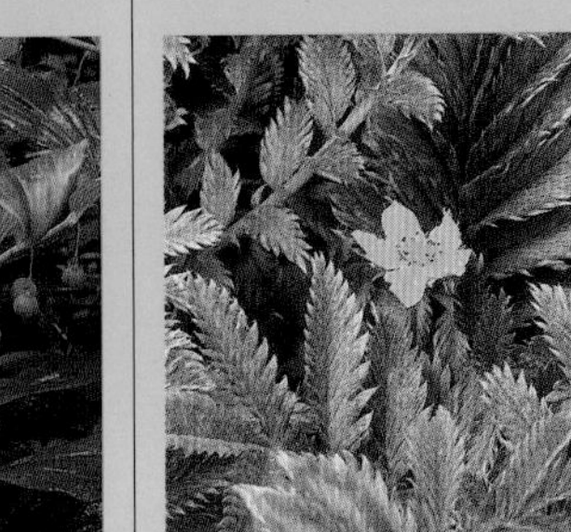

Solomon's Seal

POLYGONUM AVICULARE

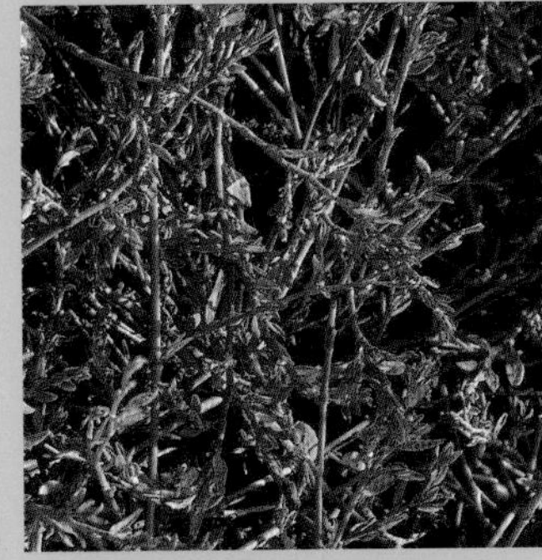

Knotweed

POLYGONUM BISTORTA

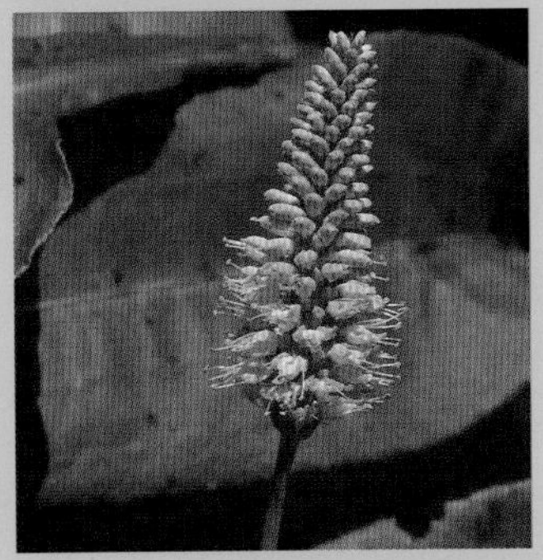

Bistort

POPULUS SPECIES

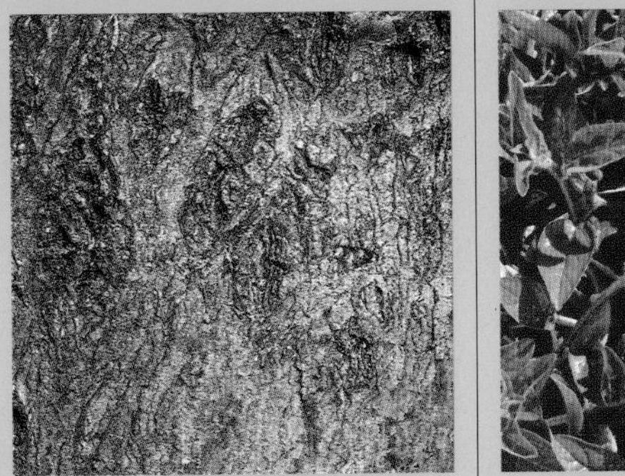

Poplar Bark

POTENTILLA ANSERINA

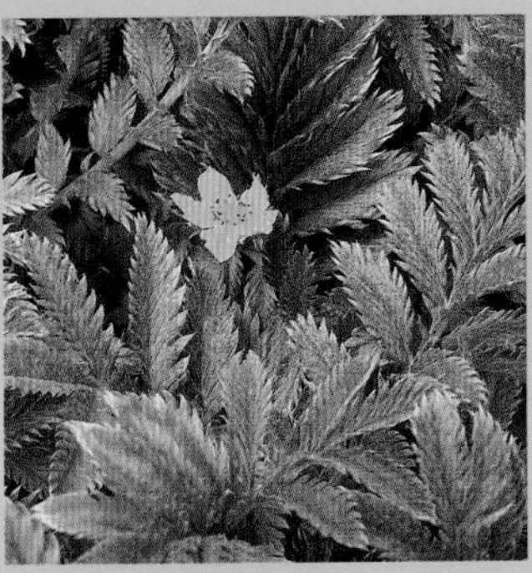

Potentilla

POTENTILLA ERECTA

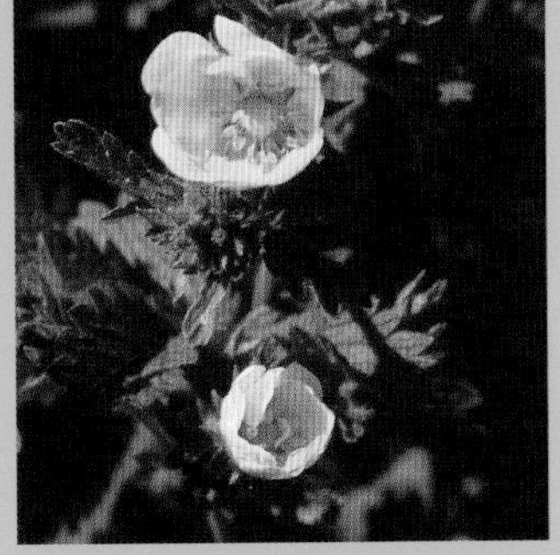

Tormentil Root

POTENTILLA REPTANS

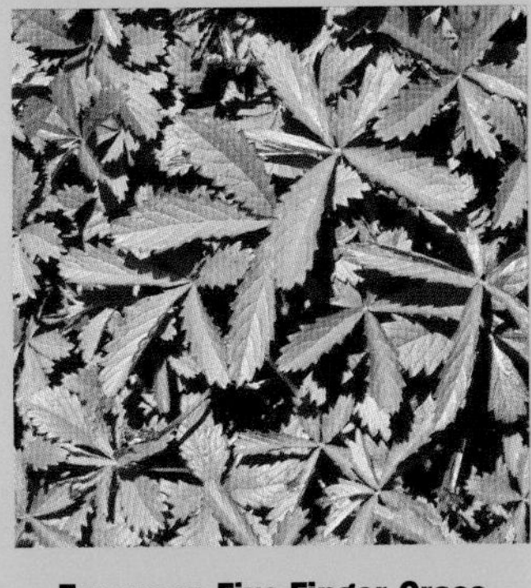

European Five-Finger Grass

PRUNELLA VULGARIS

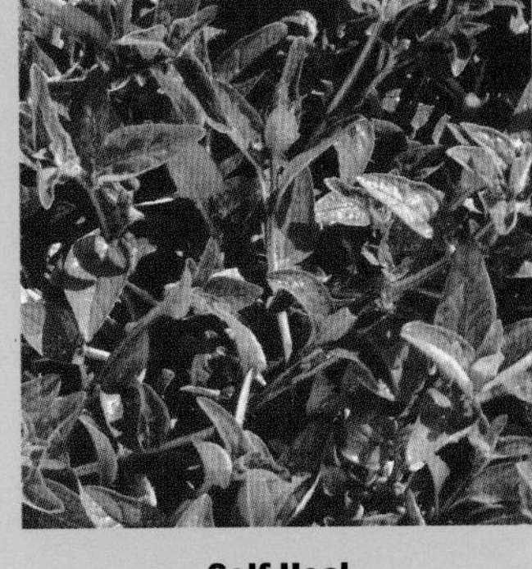

Self-Heal

PRUNUS LAUROCERASUS

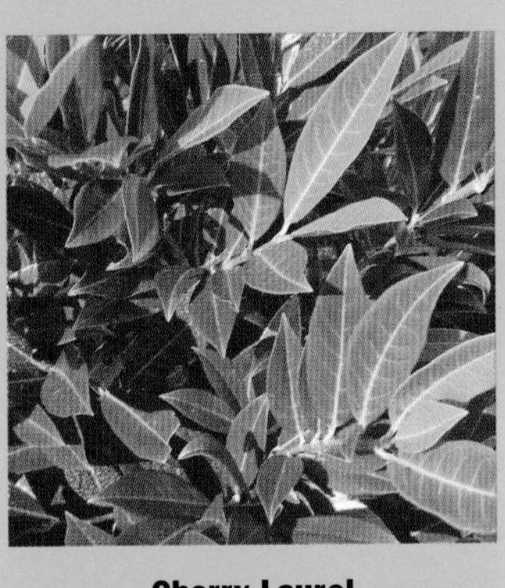

Cherry Laurel

PRUNUS SPINOSA

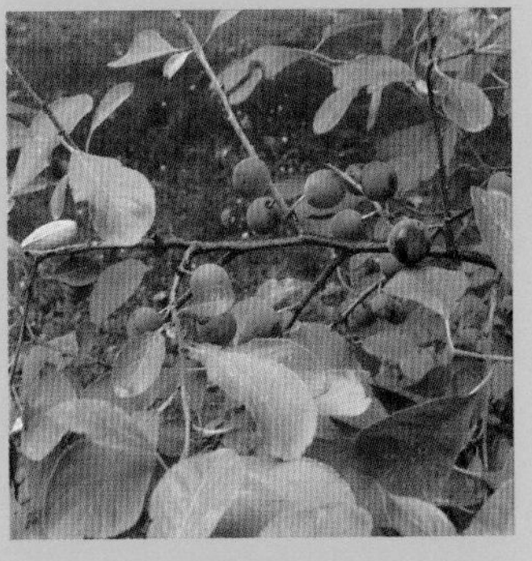

Blackthorn

PULMONARIA OFFICINALIS

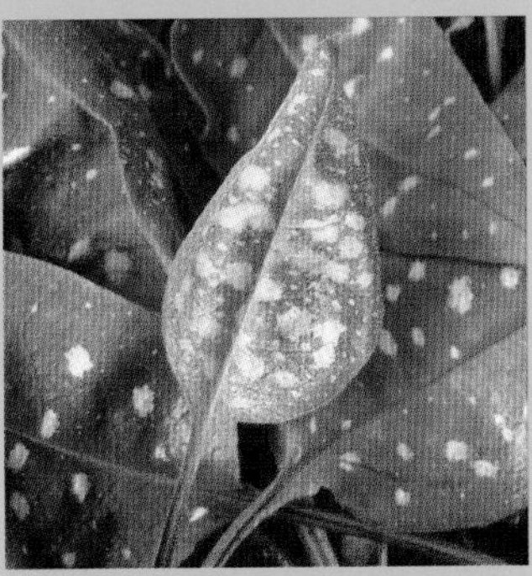

Lungwort

PUNICA GRANATUM

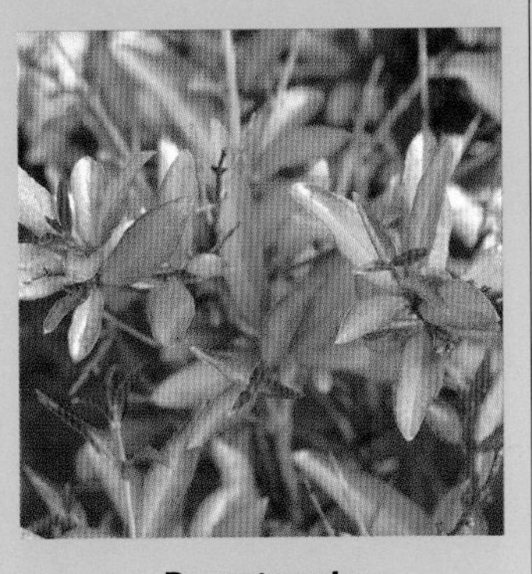

Pomegranate

QUASSIA AMARA

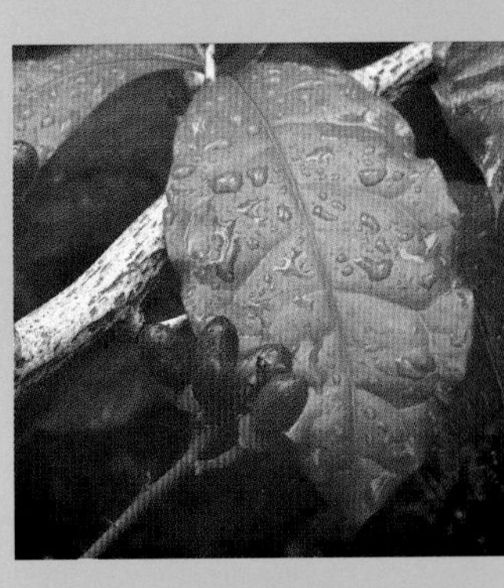

Bitter Wood

QUERCUS ROBUR

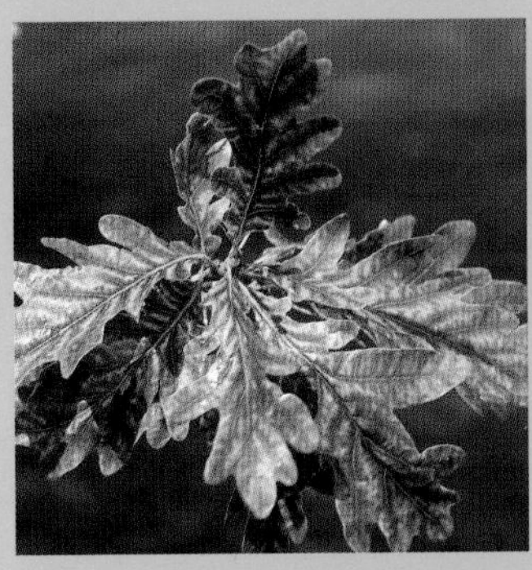

Oak Barn

QUILLAJA SAPONARIA

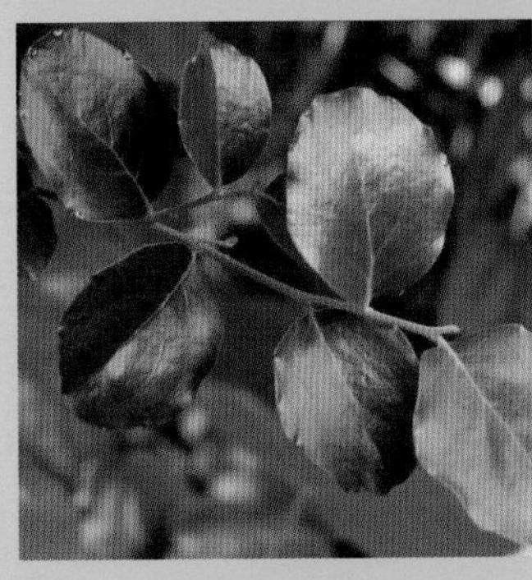

Soap Bark

RANUNCULUS SCELERATUS

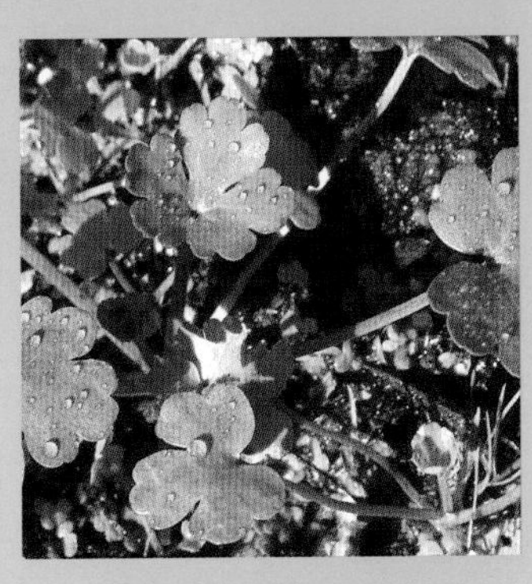

Poisonous Buttercup

RAPHANUS RAPHANISTRUM

Wild Radish

RHAMNUS PURSHIANUS

Cascara Sagrada

ROSA CENTIFOLIA

Rose

RUBUS IDAEUS

Raspberry

RAPHANUS SATIVUS

Radish

RHEUM PALMATUM

Rhubarb

ROSMARINUS OFFICINALIS

Rosemary

RUSCUS ACULEATUS

Butcher's Broom

RHAMNUS CATHARTICA

Buckthorn

RICINUS COMMUNIS

Castor Oil Plant

RUBIA TINCTORUM

Madder

RUTA GRAVEOLENS

Rue

RHAMNUS FRANGULA

Buckthorn Bark

ROSA CANINA

Rose Hip

RUBUS FRUTICOSUS

Blackberry

SALIX SPECIES

White Willow

SALVIA OFFICINALIS

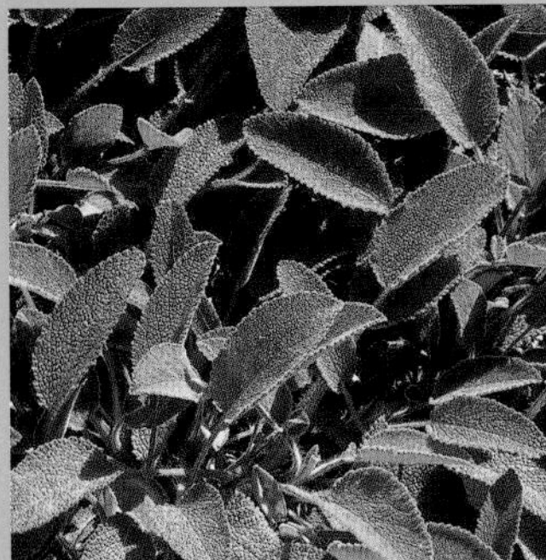

Sage

SAMBUCUS NIGRA

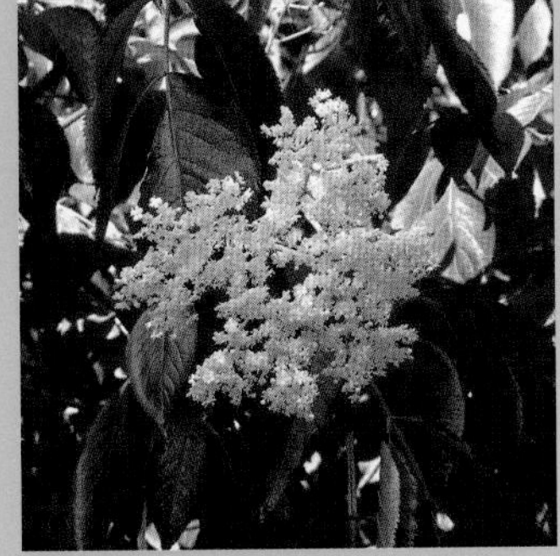

Black Elder

SANGUISORBA OFFICINALIS

Great Burnet

SANTOLINA CHAMAECYPARISSIAS

Lavender Cotton

SAPONARIA OFFICINALIS

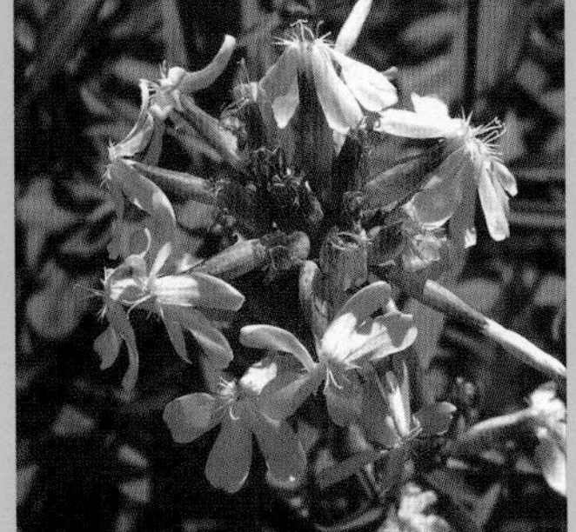

Soapwort

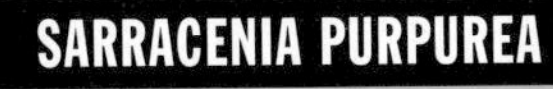

SARRACENIA PURPUREA

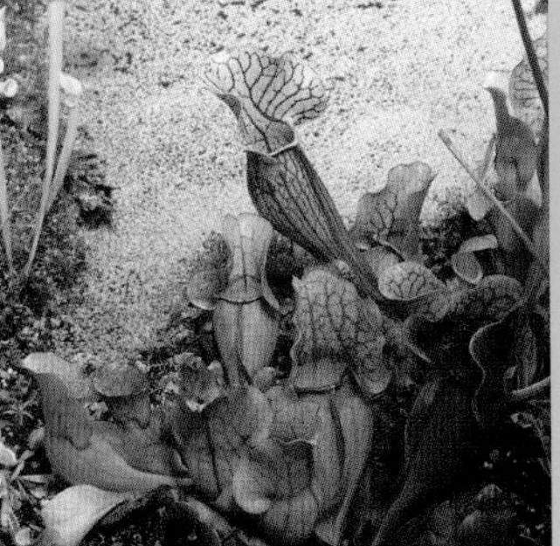

Pitcher Plant

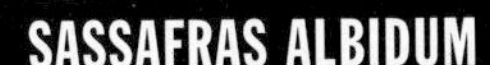

SASSAFRAS ALBIDUM

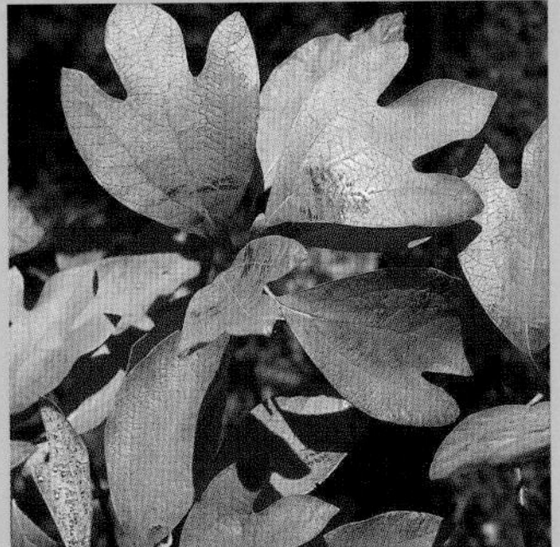

Sassafras

SATUREJA SPECIES

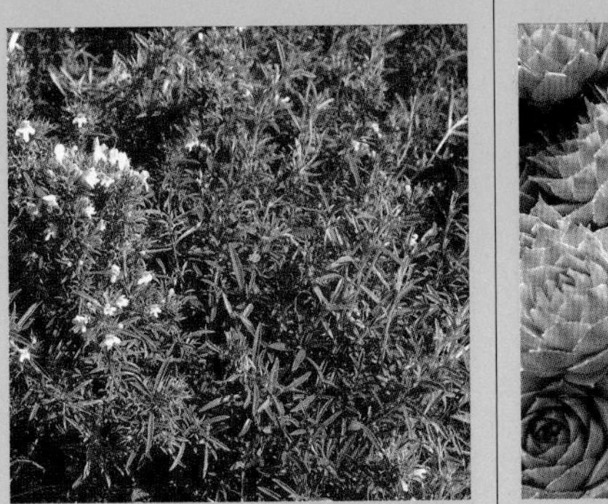

Savory

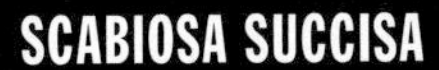

SCABIOSA SUCCISA

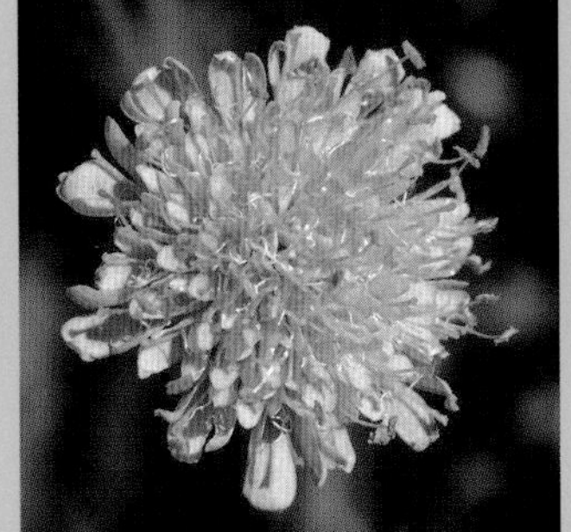

Premorse

SCROPHULARIA NODOSA

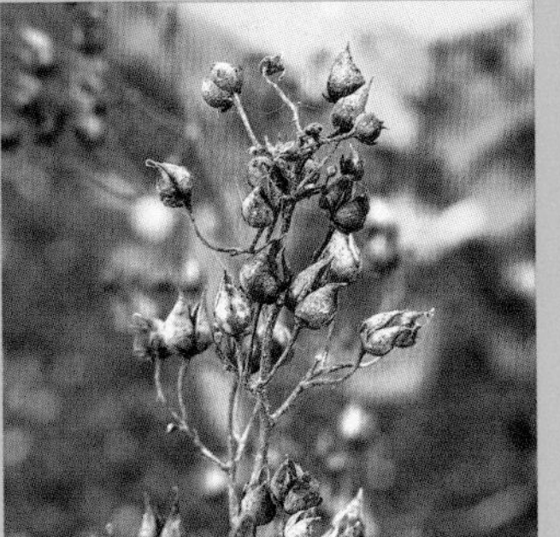

Figwort

SCUTELLARIA LATERIFLORA

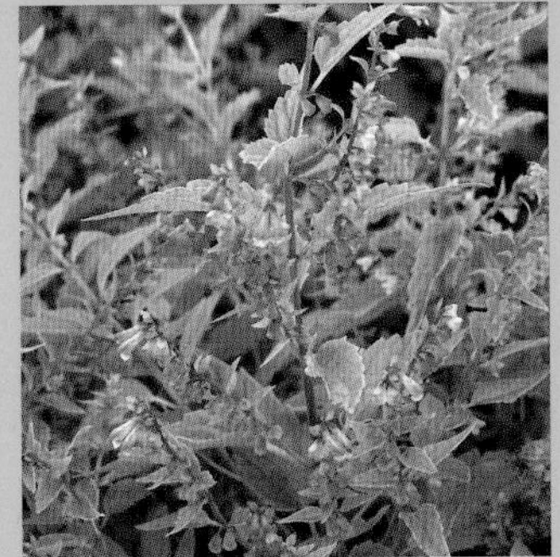

Scullcap

SEMPERVIVUM TECTORUM

Houseleek

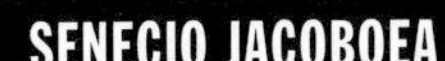

SENECIO JACOBOEA

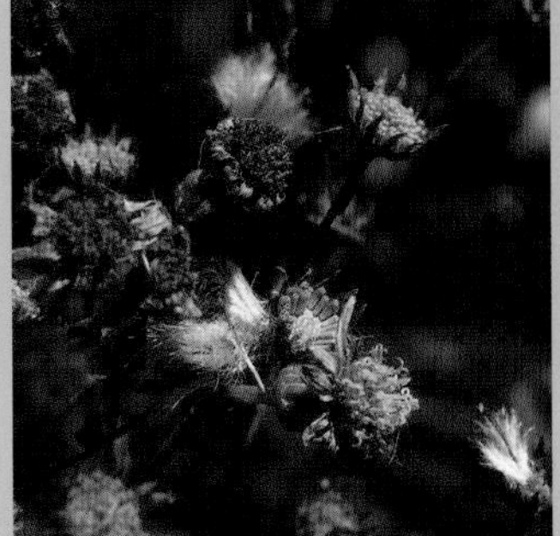

Ragwort

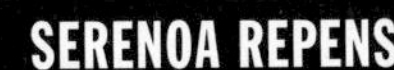

SERENOA REPENS

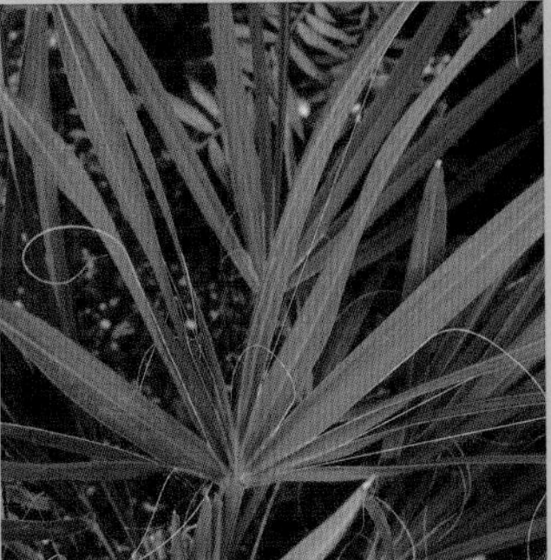

Saw Palmetto

SILPHIUM LACINIATUM

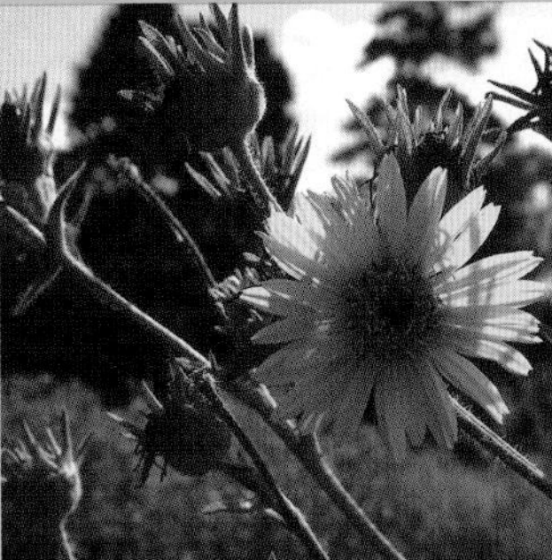

Rosinweed

SILPHIUM PERFOLIATUM

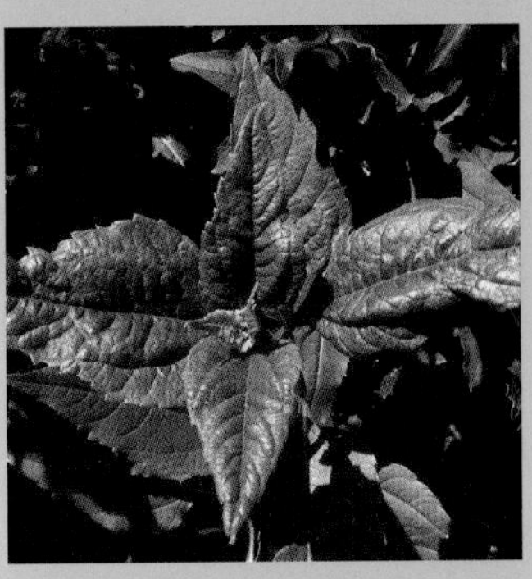

Cup Plant

SIMMONDSIA CHINESIS

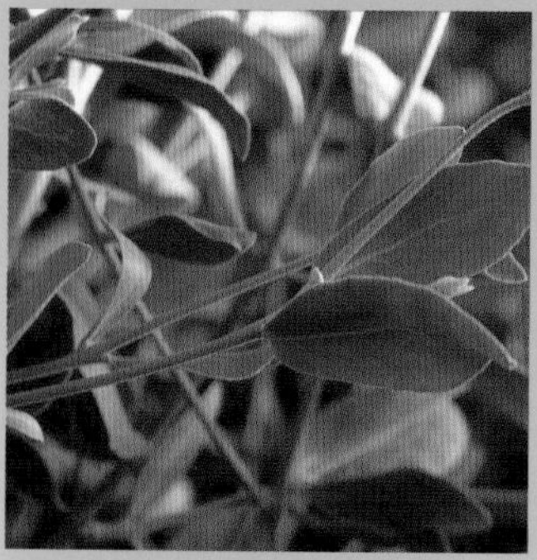

Jojoba

SOLANUM DULCAMARA

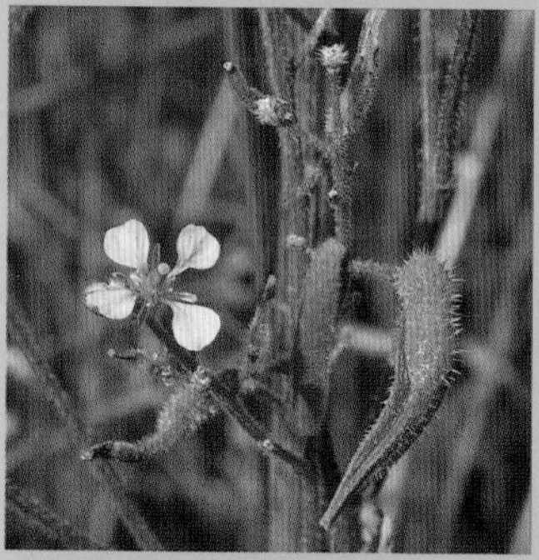

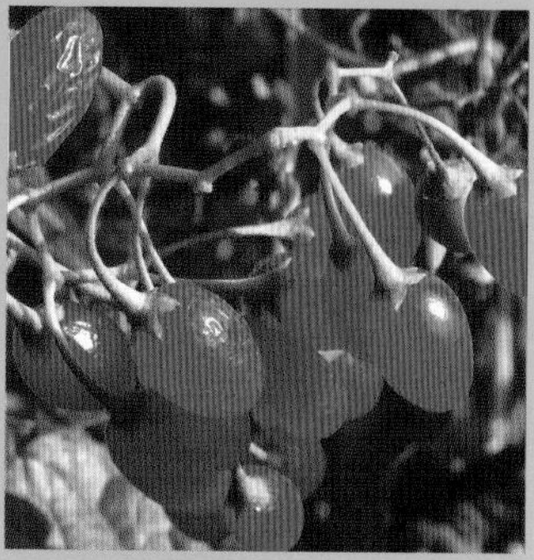

Bittersweet Nightshade

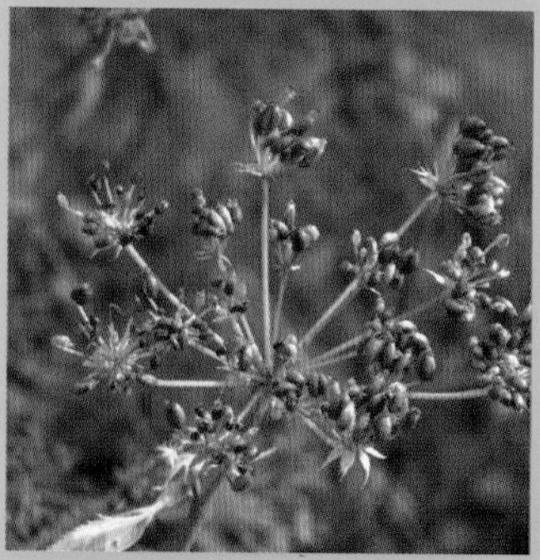

SPINACIA OLERACEA

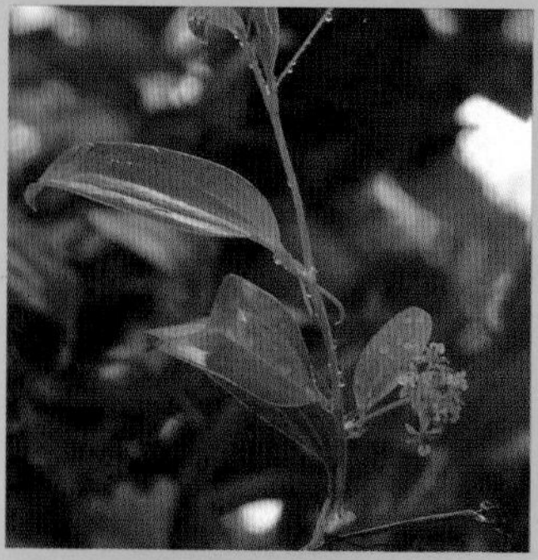

Spinach

SYZYGIUM AROMATICUM

Clove

SINAPIS ALBA

Mustard

SOLANUM NIGRUM

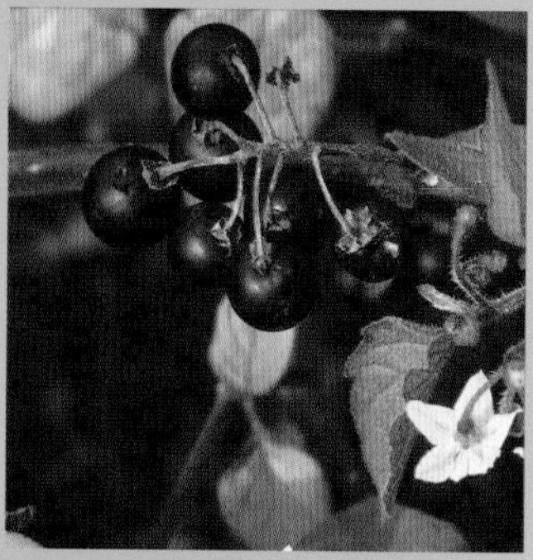

Black Nightshade

STACHYS PALUSTRIS

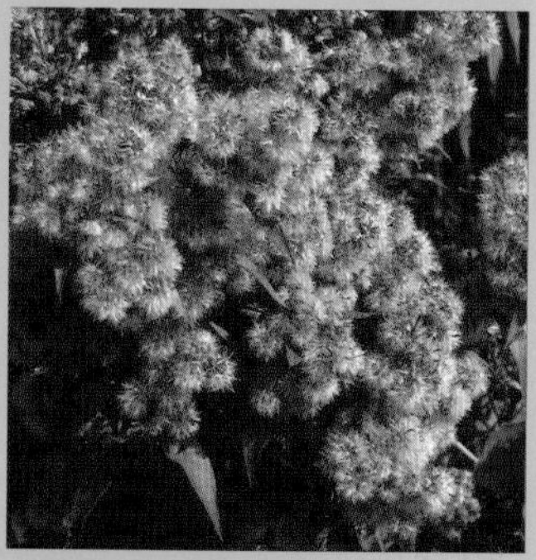

Woundwort

TAMUS COMMUNIS

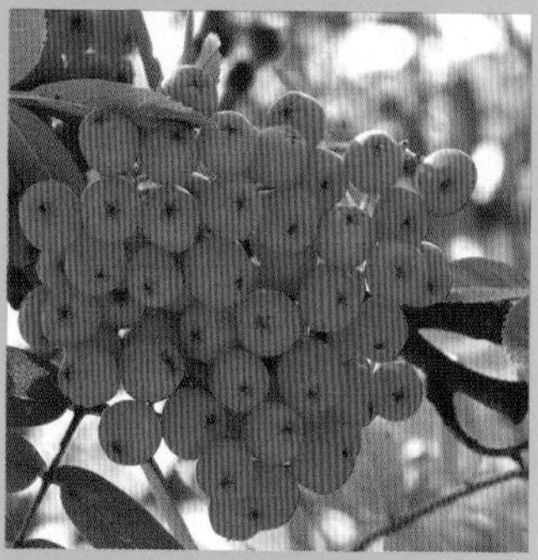

Black Bryony

SIUM SISARUM

Skirret

SOLIDAGO VIRGAUREA

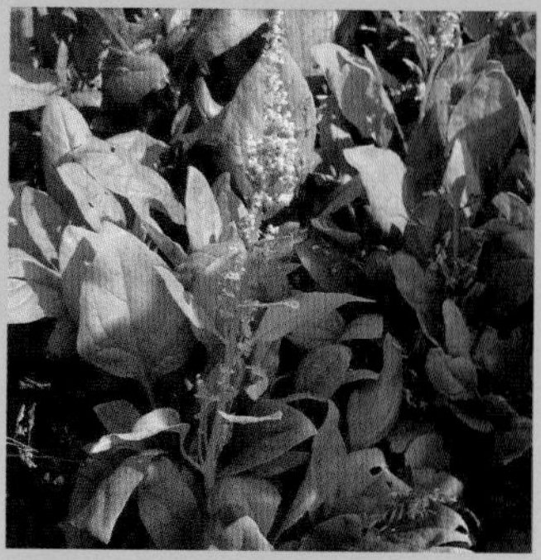

Golden Rod

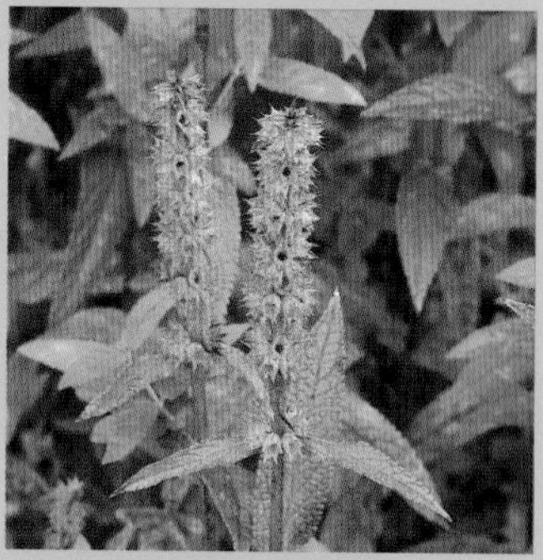

STRYCHNOS NUX VOMICA

Nux Vomica

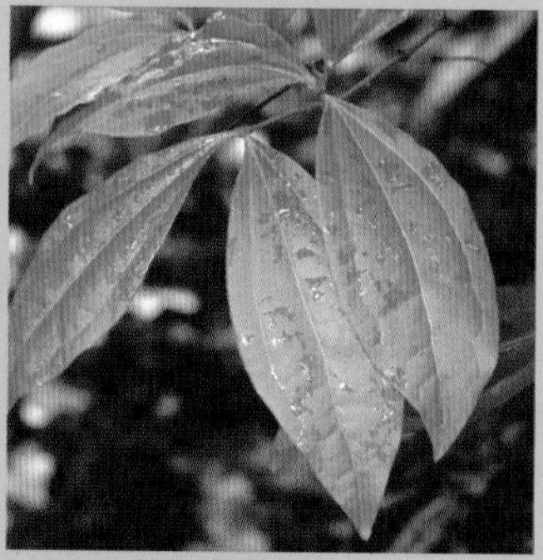

TANACETUM VULGARE

Tansy

SMILAX SPECIES

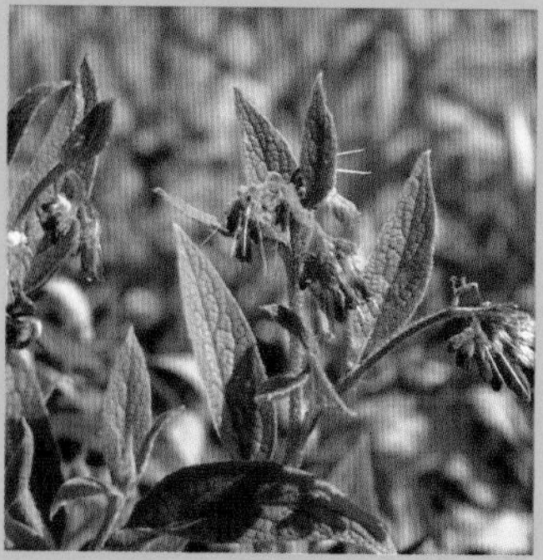

Sarsaparilla

SORBUS AUCUPARIA

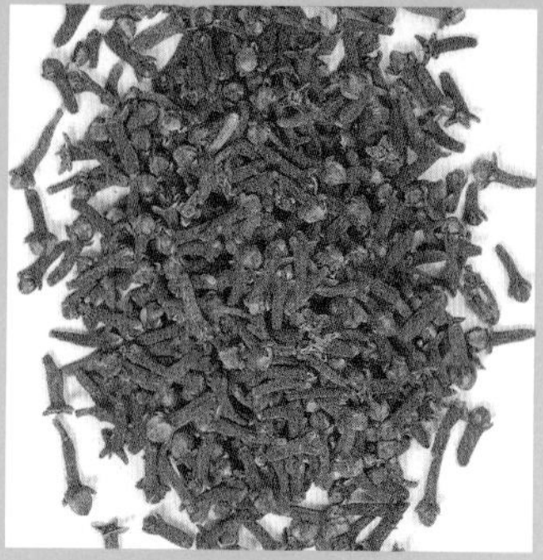

Mountain Ash Berry

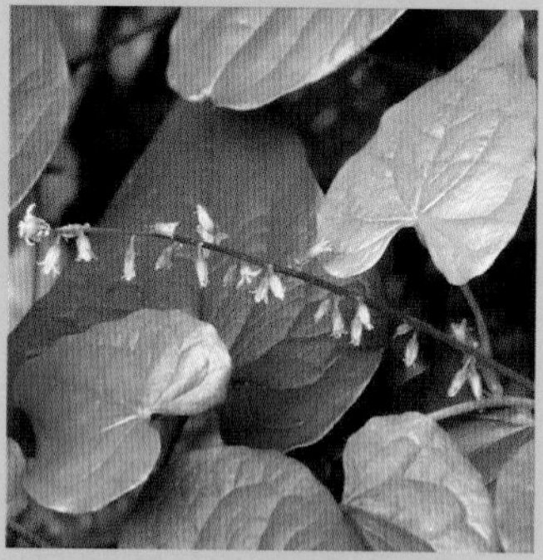

SYMPHYTUM OFFICINALE

Comfrey

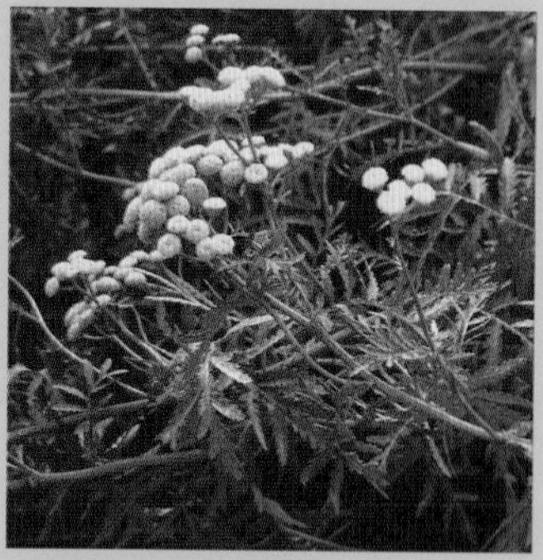

TAXUS BACCATA

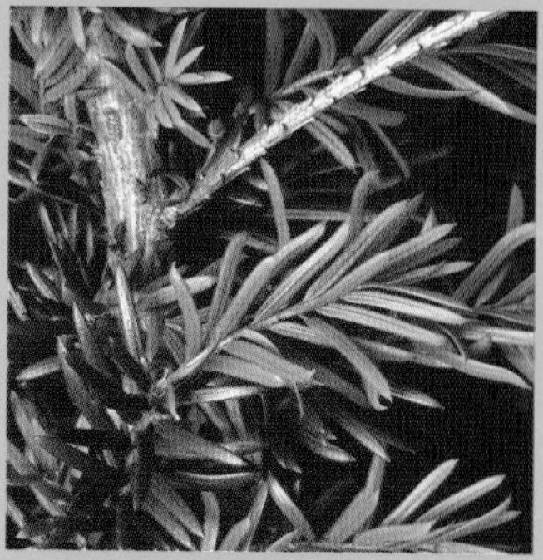

Yew

TEUCRIUM CHAMAEDRYS

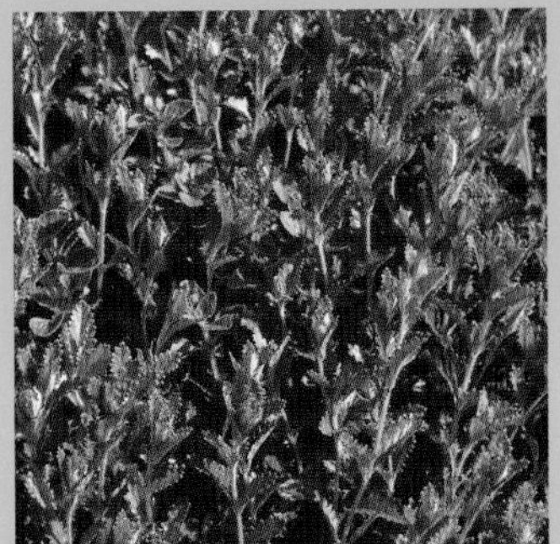

Germander

THYMUS SERPYLLUM

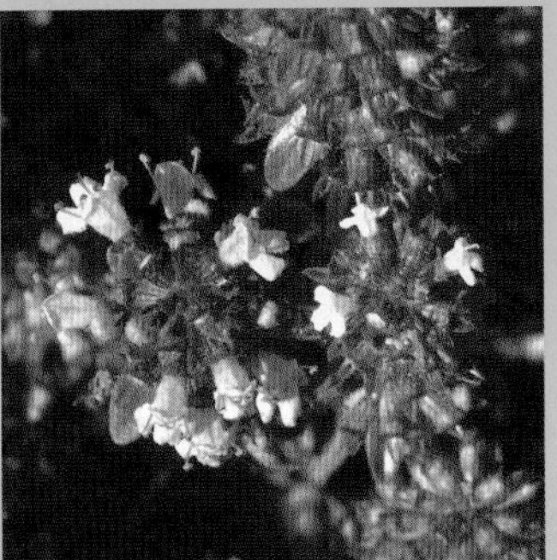

Wild Thyme

TRIFOLIUM PRATENSE

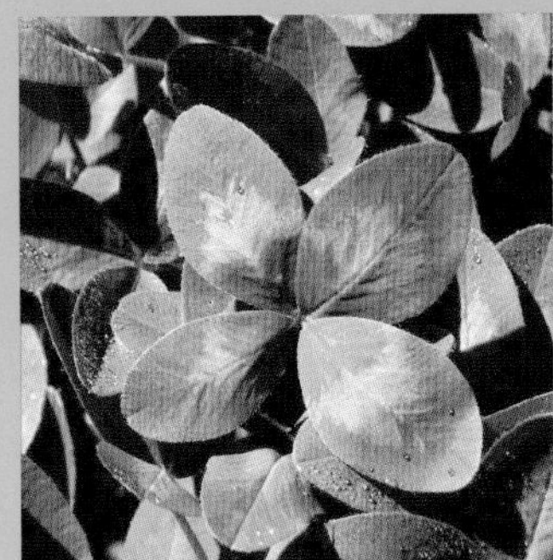

Red Clover

TROPAEOLUM MAJUS

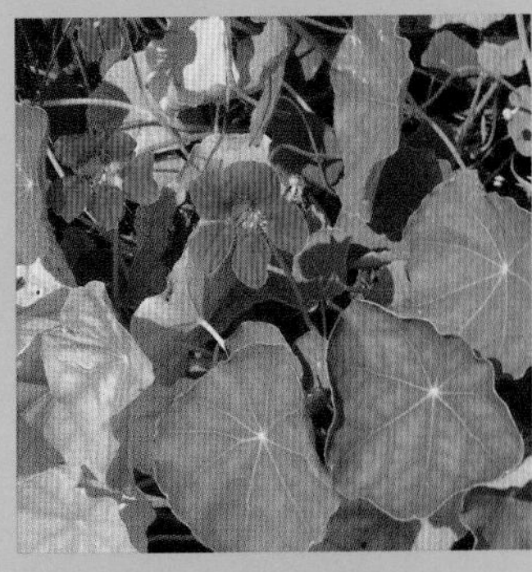

Nasturtium

TEUCRIUM SCORODONIA

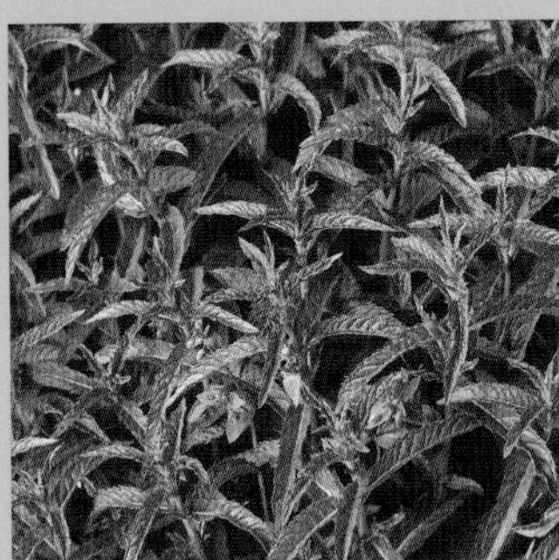

Wood Sage

THYMUS VULGARIS

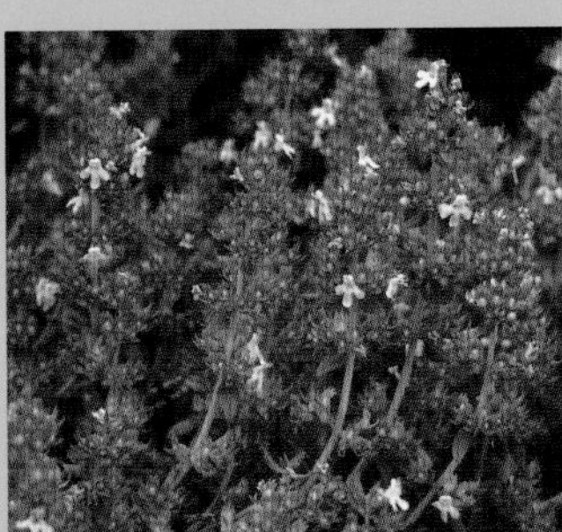

Thyme

TRIGONELLA FOENUM-GRAECUM

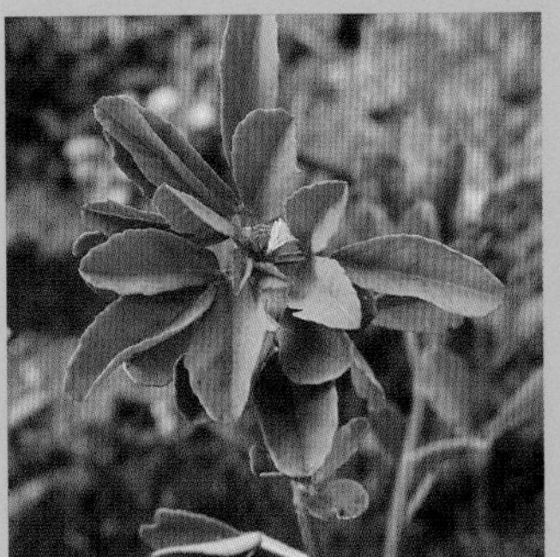

Fenugreek

TSUGA CANADENSIS

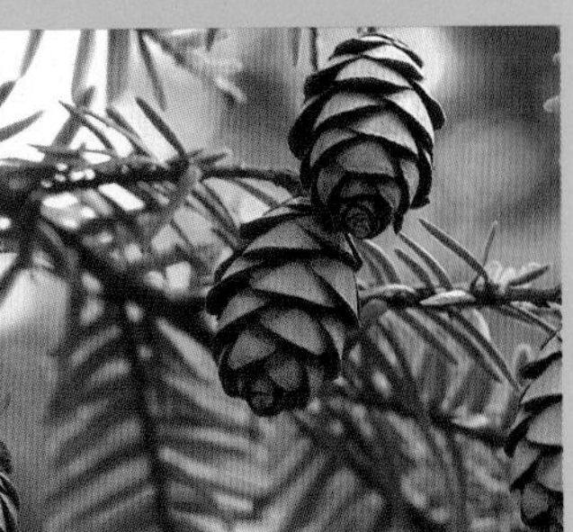

Pinus Bark

THEOBROMA CACAO

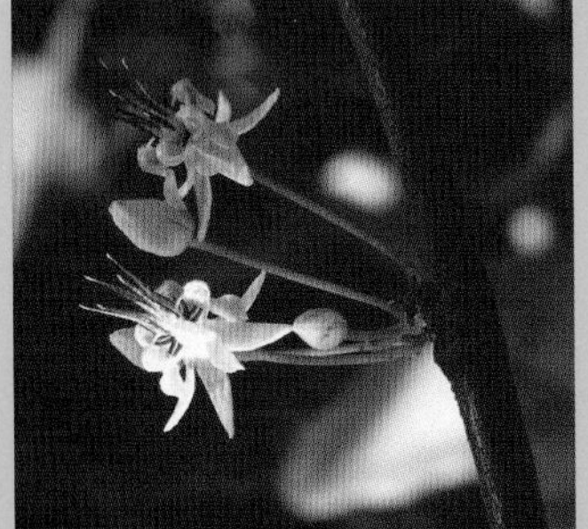

Cocoa

TIARELLA CORDIFOLIA

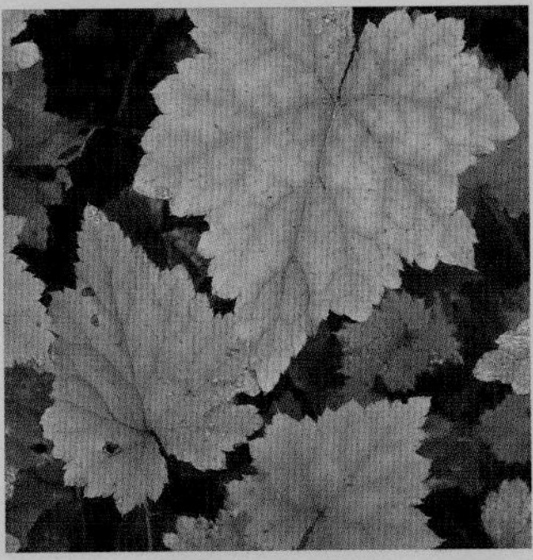

Coolwort

TRILLIUM ERECTUM

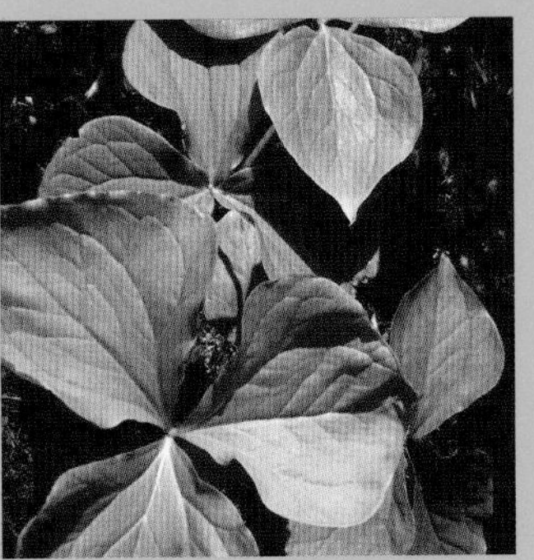

Beth Root

TUSSILAGO FARFARA

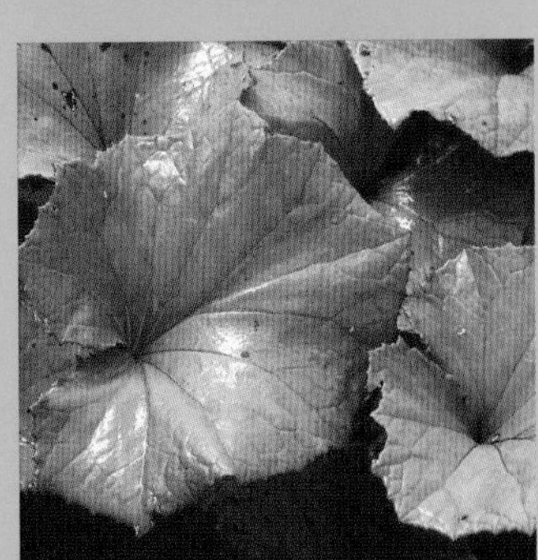

Colt's Foot

THUJA OCCIDENTALIS

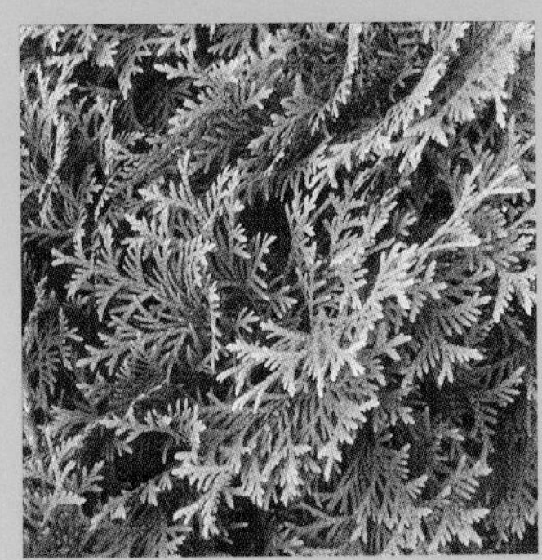

Thuja

TILIA SPECIES

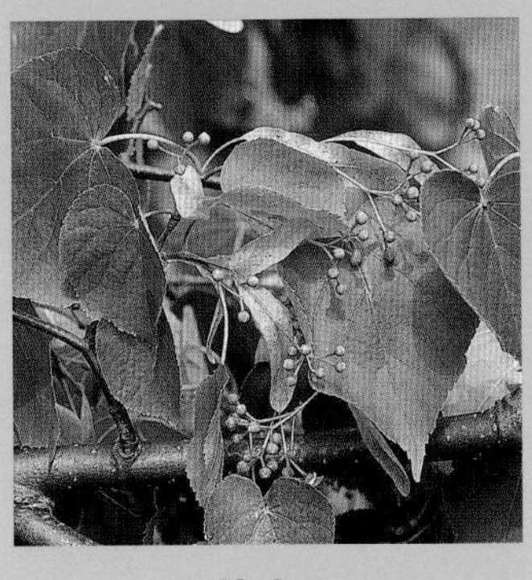

Linden

TROLLIUS EUROPAEUS

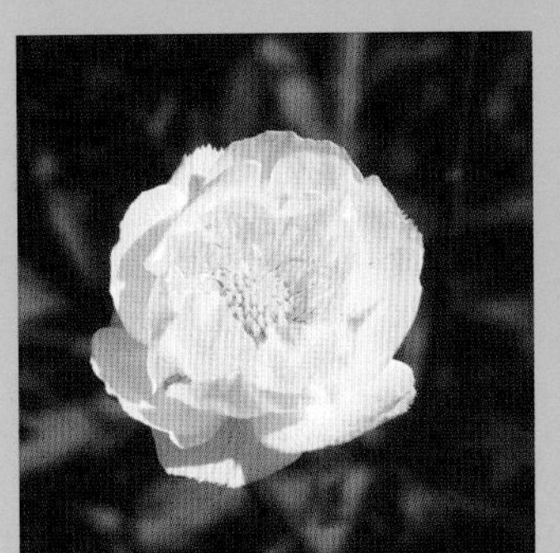

Globe Flower

URTICA DIOICA

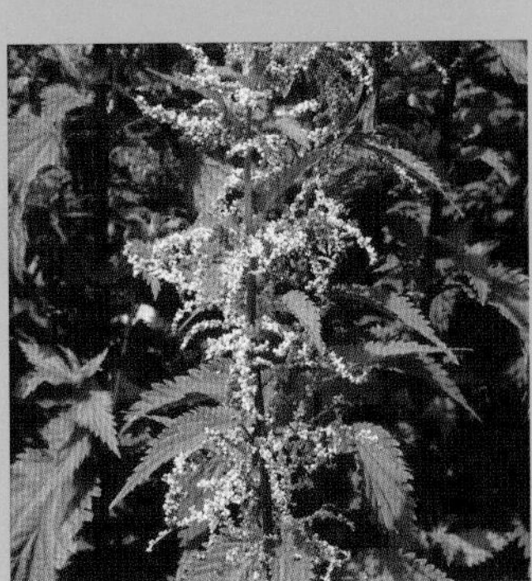

Nettle

UTRICULARIA VULGARIS

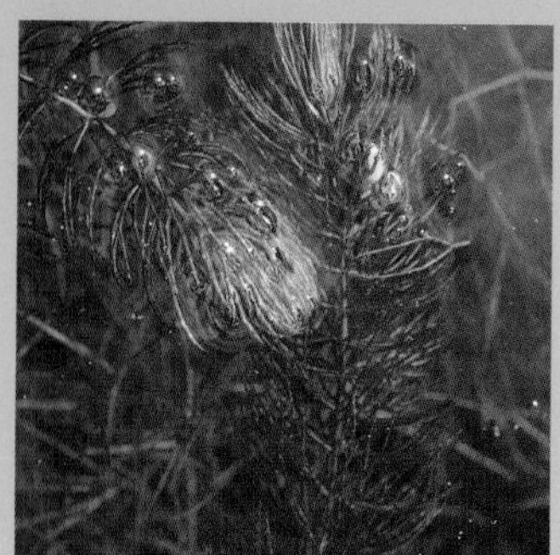

Bladderwort

VACCINIUM MYRTILLUS

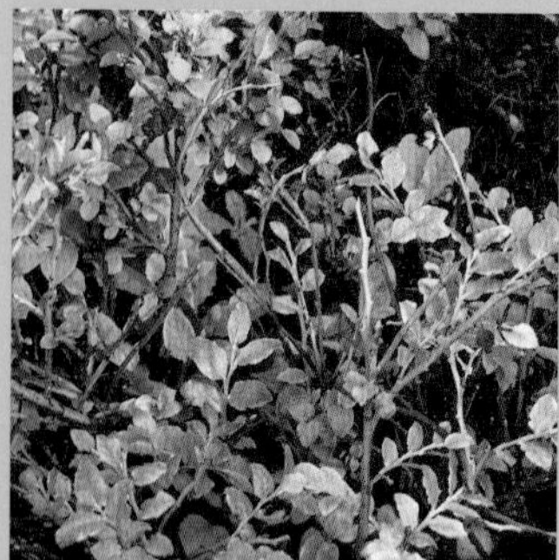

Bilberry

VACCINIUM ULIGINOSUM

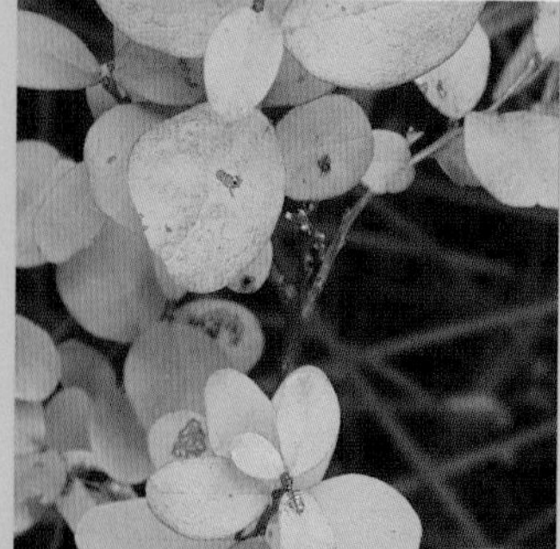

Bog Bilberry

VACCINIUM VITIS-IDAEA

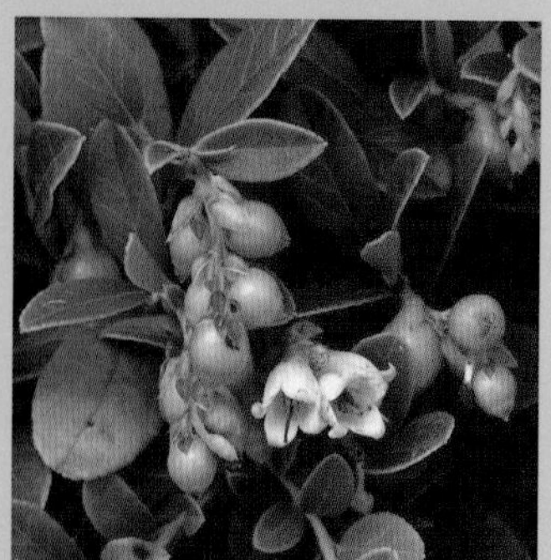

Alpine Cranberry

VALERIANA OFFICINALIS

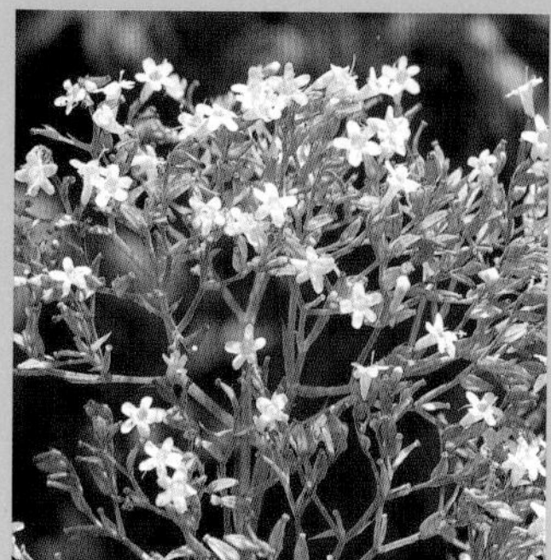

Valerian

VERATRUM ALBUM

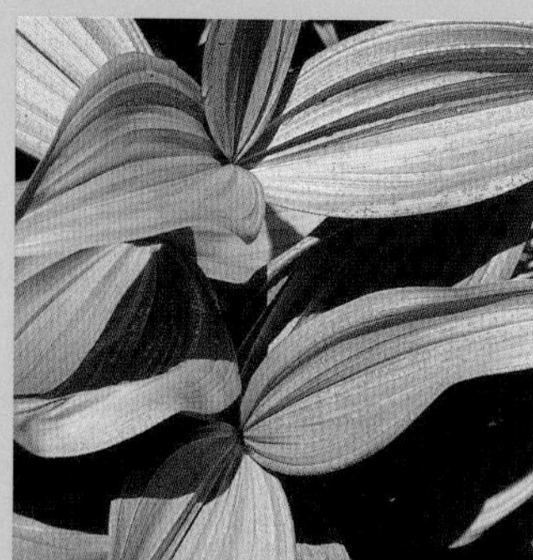

White Hellebore

VERBASCUM DENSIFLORUM

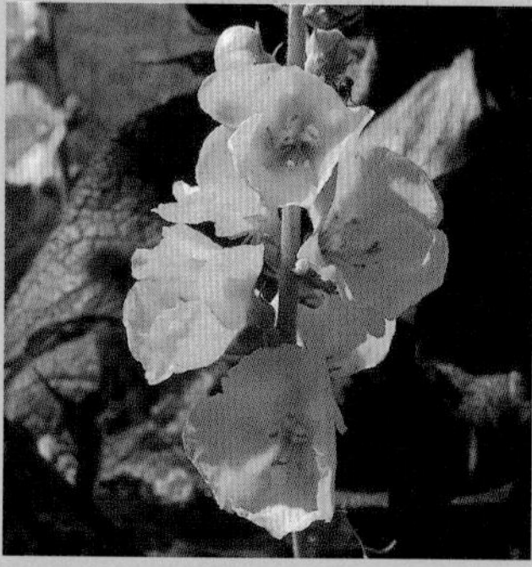

Mullein

VERBENA OFFICINALIS

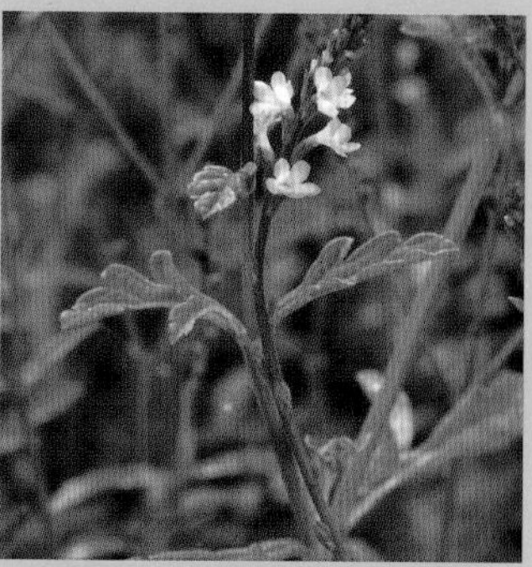

Vervain

VERONICA BECCABUNGA

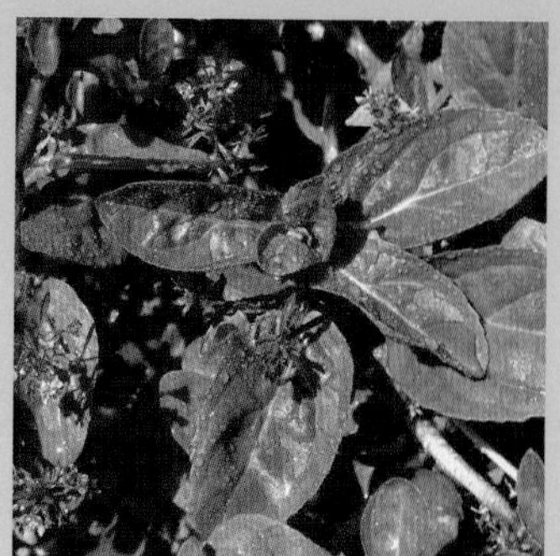

Brooklime

VERONICA OFFICINALIS

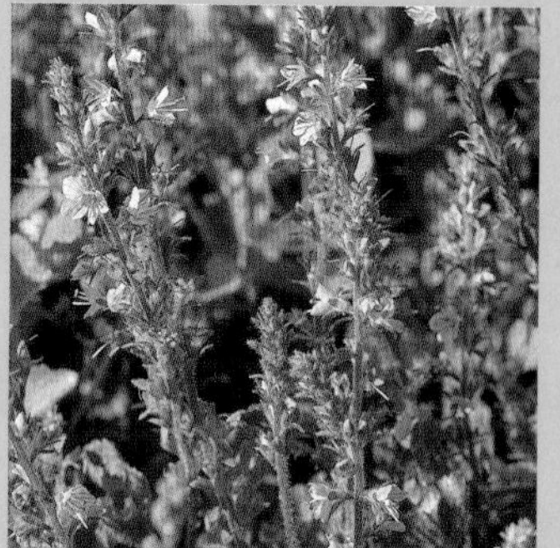

Speedwell

VIBURNUM PRUNIFOLIUM

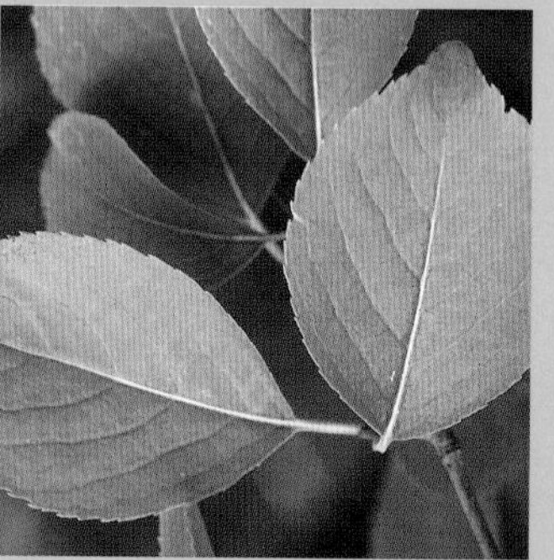

Black Haw

VIOLA ODORATA

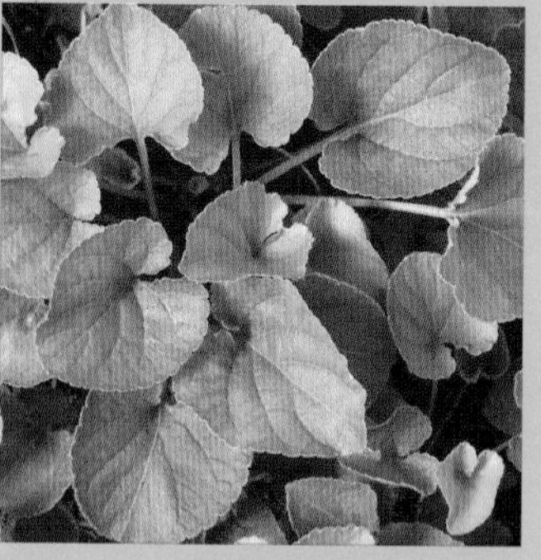

Garden Violet

VISCUM ALBUM

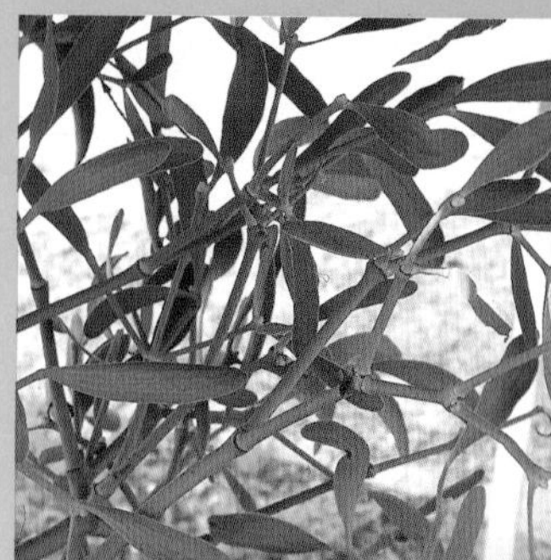

Mistletoe

VITEX AGNUS-CASTUS

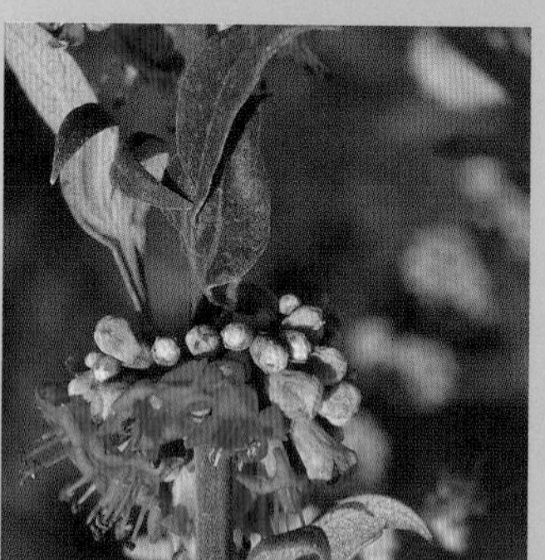

Chaste Tree

VITIS VINIFERA

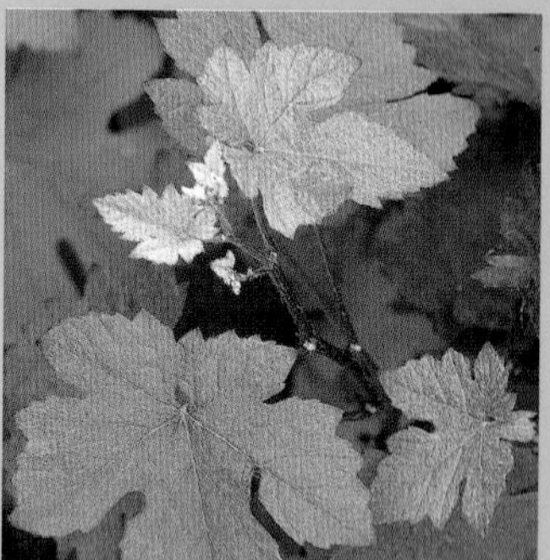

Grape

ZINGIBER OFFICINALE

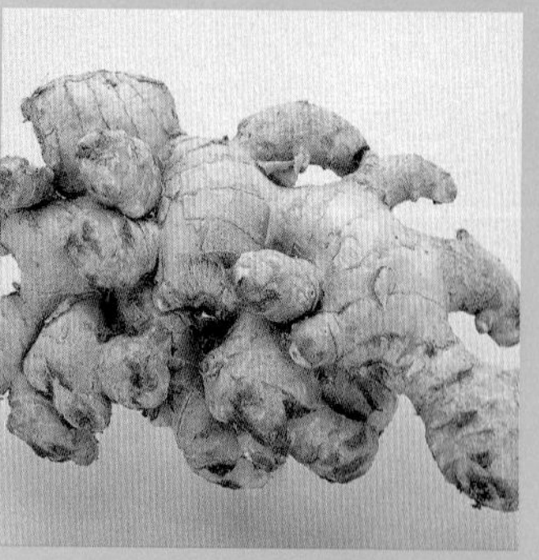

Ginger

Herbal Monographs

This section contains comprehensive profiles of over 600 medicinal herbs, including the findings of the German Regulatory Authority's herbal watchdog agency, commonly called "Commission E." This agency has conducted an intensive assessment of the peer-reviewed literature on some 300 common botanicals, weighing the quality of the clinical evidence and identifying the uses for which the herb can reasonably be considered effective. Its conclusions represent the best expert consensus on medicinal herbs currently to be found.

For those herbs not considered by Commission E, Physicians' Desk Reference has augmented this section with the results of an exhaustive literature review conducted by the respected PhytoPharm U.S. Institute of Phytopharmaceuticals under the direction of noted botanist, Dr. Joerg Gruenwald. These monographs, some 300 in number, provide a detailed introduction to an array of exotic botanicals that you'll be hard pressed to find in any other source.

To make the information in the monographs as useful and accessible as possible, PDR has echoed the structure of standard U.S. product labeling. Each monograph contains up to nine standard sections, covering considerations ranging from description to dosage. Specifically, here's what you will find:

- **Names:** Each monograph begins with the herb's scientific name, followed by its most widely accepted common name. In addition, all monographs are cross-referenced by the accepted common name.

- **Description:** This section provides a detailed botanical overview of the herb, including information on its medicinal parts; flower and fruit; leaves, stem and root; unique characteristics, habitat, production, related plants, and additional common names and synonyms.

- **Actions and Pharmacology:** Here you'll find data on the active compounds or heterogeneous mixtures found in the plant, followed by a summary of the herb's clinical effects. If various parts of the plant possess different pharmacological activity, the parts are discussed individually, here and throughout the remainder of the monograph.

- **Indications and Usage:** Uses for which the herb has been judged effective by Commission E are presented here in list fashion. Provisos regarding route and form of administration for each indication are appended as necessary. Unsubstantiated uses found in folk medicine, Asian medicine, and homeopathic practice are also enumerated.

■ **Contraindications:** Although most natural remedies can be used under all medical circumstances, a few pharmacological potent herbs must be avoided in the presence of certain medical conditions. If any such contraindications exist, they are summarized here.

■ **Precautions and Adverse Reactions:** Found in this section are any cautions or special considerations regarding safe use of the herb, including any restrictions on use in pregnancy or childhood. Although most herbal remedies are notably free of known side effects, any reported in the available literature are noted here.

■ **Overdosage:** As we all know, "natural" is not synonymous with "benign," and an overdose of many "healing" herbs can have serious—even fatal—consequences. Whenever adverse effects of overdose have been found in the literature, they are reported here, along with the appropriate medical interventions to be undertaken when an overdose occurs.

■ **Dosage:** Listed here are common modes of administration and representative dosage recommendations drawn from the literature. Note, however, that this information can be used only as a general guide, and that it is often applicable only to the natural herb. The potency of individual preparations and extracts is subject to substantial variation, so the manufacturer's directions should be consulted whenever available.

■ **Literature:** This section provides you with a unique bibliography of the technical literature. Because German researchers have been particularly active in the herbal arena, you will find an unusual number of German-language citations. However, work in the English literature is included as well.

PDR for Herbal Medicines is the product of one of the most thorough and inclusive examinations of the herbal literature ever undertaken. Nevertheless, it's important to remember that it merely summarizes and synthesizes key data from the underlying research reports, and of necessity includes neither every published report nor every recorded fact.

As in all scientific investigation, conclusions regarding the effectiveness of the herbs discussed in this compendium are based on the preponderance of current evidence and cannot be considered firm or final. The publisher does not warrant that any herb will unfailingly and uniformly exhibit the properties ascribed to it in these pages. Likewise, the publisher does not guarantee that every possible hazard, adverse effect, contraindication, precaution, or consequence of overdose is included in the summaries presented here. The publisher has performed no independent verification of the data reported herein, and expressly disclaims responsibility for any error, whether inherent in the underlying literature or resulting from erroneous translation, transcription, or typography.

Although the publisher has endeavored to provide the most extensive possible coverage of currently available botanical preparations, not all medicinal herbs can be found herein. As review of the literature continues, additional herbs will be included in future editions. Inclusion of an herb in the current editions does not signify an endorsement by the publisher; absence of an herb does not imply its rejection.

It should be understood that by making this material available, the publisher is not advocating the use of any substance described herein. Please remember that in the United States, herbal products must be in compliance with the Dietary Supplement Health and Education Act of 1994, which stipulates that they may not be marketed for the diagnosis, treatment, cure, or prevention of any disease. The monographs in PDR for Herbal Medicines do not discuss claims made for any proprietary herbal preparation. They merely report general findings on generic botanicals and their extracts.

Abrus Precatorius

Jequirity

DESCRIPTION

Medicinal Parts: The medicinal parts are the leaves, roots, and seeds.

Flower and Fruit: The flowers are racemes of pink blossoms. The fruit is a pod with oval seeds which are rounded at the ends. They are about 3 mm in diameter, hard, red and glossy, with a large black dot at one end. One variety has white seeds.

Leaves, Stem and Root: This deciduous climbing plant with compound leaves grows to about 4 m.

Characteristics: The plant is a protected species in some countries.

Habitat: The plant originated in India and is found today in all tropical regions of the world.

Other Names: Indian Liquorice, Wild Liquorice, Prayer Beads, Crab's Eyes, Gunga, Goonteh, Rati

ACTIONS AND PHARMACOLOGY

COMPOUNDS

Toxic lectins: abrine and isotoxins

EFFECTS

Jequirity is an irritant and abortifacient.

INDICATIONS AND USAGE

The drug was used for chronic conjunctivitis and as a contraceptive in folk medicine, but is no longer used.

PRECAUTIONS AND ADVERSE REACTIONS

The drug is very poisonous because it contains the toxic lectin abrine and isolectins.

OVERDOSAGE

Severe poisonings among adults following the intake of one half to two seeds, as well as cases of death among children following the consumption of two seeds, have been recorded. Counter-measures include, besides gastrointestinal emptying, administration of large amounts of fluid, monitoring of the circulatory system, administration of anti-epileptic drugs and possibly artificial respiration.

LITERATURE

Desai VB, Rupawala EN, (1966) Ind J Pharm 29:235.

Desai VB, Sirsi M, (1966) Ind J Pharmac 28:340.

Dupaigne P, (1974) Plantes Med Phytother 8:104.

Karawya MS et al., (1981) Fitoterapia 4:175.

Ku SC et al., (1995) Planta Med 61:307.

Lin JY, Liu SV, (1986) Toxikon 24:757.

Lin JY et al., (1981) Toxikon 19:41.

Murray DR, Vairinhos F, (1982) Z Pflanzenphysiol 108:471.

Further information in:

Frohne D, Pfänder HJ, Giftpflanzen - Ein Handbuch für Apotheker, Toxikologen und Biologen, 4. Aufl., Wiss. Verlags-Ges Stuttgart 1997.

Kern W, List PH, Hörhammer L (Herausg.), Hagers Handbuch der Pharmazeutischen Praxis, 4. Aufl., Springer Verlag Berlin, Heidelberg, New York, 1969.

Roth L, Daunderer M., Kormann K, Giftpflanzen, Pflanzengifte - Vorkommen, Wirkung, Therapie, allergische Reaktionen, 3. Aufl., ecomed 1988.

Teuscher E, Lindequist U, Biogene Gifte - Biologie, Chemie, Pharmakologie, 2. Aufl., Fischer Verlag Stuttgart 1994.

Abscess Root

See Polemonium Reptans

Acacia

See Acacia Arabica; Acacia Senegal

Acacia Arabica

Acacia

DESCRIPTION

Medicinal Parts: The medicinal parts are the bark, the gum, and the fruit of the plant.

Flower and Fruit: The flowers are yellow and sweetly scented. Two to 6 inflorescence peduncles with capitula-like inflorescences grow from the axils of the upper leaflets. The flowers have short calyces with numerous overlapping sepals and the completely fused petals are almost twice as large as the sepals. The fruit is a 12 to 16 cm long and 1.5 cm wide pod, which is straight or lightly curved, flat to convex, and pinched in to create segments. It is matte-black to dark-red. The seeds are 7 x 6 mm and the same color as the pod.

Leaves, Stem and Root: Acacia arabica is a 6 m high tree with a compact, round to flat crown. Older branches are bare, younger ones measuring 15 to 20 mm in diameter are covered in hairy down. The bark is black and fissured; the coloring in the fissure changes to red-brown. There are stipule thorns at the nodes. The leaflets of the double-pinnate leaves are in 3 to 12 pairs on the bare to downy petiole which is covered with glands. The leaflets are oblong, blunt, and bare or thinly ciliate.

Habitat: The plant is indigenous to the Nile area, Ethiopia, East Africa, Angola, Mozambique, South Africa, Arabia, Iran, Afghanistan, and India.

Production: The bark is collected from plants that are at least 7 years old and then left to mature for a year.

Not To Be Confused With: The bark of the Australian species Acacia decurrens; commercially available under the same name.

Other Names: Acacia Bark, Babul Bark, Wattle Bark, Indian Gum, Black Wattle

ACTIONS AND PHARMACOLOGY

COMPOUNDS

Tannins

EFFECTS

The drug has an astringent effect.

INDICATIONS AND USAGE

The drug is used as a decoction for gum disease and inflammations of the mucous membrane of the mouth and throat (rarely used today).

In Indian medicine, Acacia is also used as a decoction in the treatment of diarrhea, vaginal secretions, and as an enema for hemorrhoids.

Efficacy has not been proven.

PRECAUTIONS AND ADVERSE REACTIONS

Large doses taken internally can lead to indigestion and constipation.

LITERATURE

Berger F, Handbuch der Drogenkunde, W Maudrich Verlag Wien 1964.

Hänsel R, Keller K, Rimpler H, Schneider G (Hrsg.), Hagers Handbuch der Pharmazeutischen Praxis, 5. Aufl., Bde 4-6 (Drogen), Springer Verlag Berlin, Heidelberg, New York, 1992-1994.

Trease GE, Evans WC (Eds.), Pharmacognosy, 12th Ed., Bailliere Tindall 1983.

Acacia Catechu

Catechu

DESCRIPTION

Medicinal Parts: Black catechu is extracted from the heartwood in a process of distillation and is used in a variety of preparations.

Flower and Fruit: The flowers grow in closely sitting spikes from the leaf axils. The calyx is about 1 to 2 mm and covered in gray hairs. The corolla is yellow. The pod is about 10 to 15 cm long, dark brown, and veined with 6 to 8 seeds.

Leaves, Stem and Root: Acacia catechu is a medium-sized tree with brown bark and downy-haired branches. The leaf stems of the double-pinnate leaves are about 15 cm long and have glands at the base and between the upper 5 to 7 cm long fronds. The leaflets are sessile, close, pale green, and smaller than 1 cm. There are a few short thorns in pairs.

Habitat: The plant is indigenous to India and Burma.

Production: The heartwood is ground and boiled in water for 12 hours. The wood residue is removed and the extract is steamed to the consistency of a syrup. The syrup is stirred and cooled in moulds. The dried mass is broken up into irregular pieces.

Not To Be Confused With: Haematoxylon campechium and the seeds of Areca catechu, tar products and admixtures of earth, alumen, iron carbonate and sand.

Other Names: Cutch

ACTIONS AND PHARMACOLOGY

COMPOUNDS

Catechins (2-12%): (+)- and (-)-catechin, (+)- and (-)-epicatechin

Catechin tannins (20-60%)

EFFECTS

Catechu is an astringent and antiseptic.

INDICATIONS AND USAGE

Internally, catechu is used for chronic catarrh of the mucous membranes, dysentery, and bleeding.

Externally, catechu is a constituent of tooth tinctures, mouth washes, and gargles. It is used externally in hemostatic powders, dressing solutions, and injection solutions. It is also used for colitis mucosa, gingivitis, stomatitis, and pharyngitis.

In Hindu medicine, it is a constituent of preparations for mouth ulcers, throat infections, and toothache.

In Chinese medicine, it is used for poorly healing ulcers, weeping skin diseases, oral ulcers with bleeding and traumatic injuries.

Sufficient material on the above indications is unavailable. Efficacy has not been proven.

PRECAUTIONS AND ADVERSE REACTIONS

No health hazards or side effects are known in conjunction with the proper administration of designated therapeutic dosages.

DOSAGE

Mode of Administration: Catechu tincture to be painted on mucous membranes and for mouth washes. The drug is used internally.

Preparation: Catechu tincture.

Daily Dosage: The average daily dose of the drug is 0.3 to 2 gm to be taken orally, 3 times daily; single dose is 0.5 gm.

Twenty drops in a glass of lukewarm water or to be applied with a brush in undiluted form.

LITERATURE

Sham JSK et al., (1984) Planta Med 2:177.

Further information in:

Hänsel R, Keller K, Rimpler H, Schneider G (Hrsg.), Hagers Handbuch der Pharmazeutischen Praxis, 5. Aufl., Bde 4-6 (Drogen), Springer Verlag Berlin, Heidelberg, New York, 1992-1994.

Leung AY, Encyclopedia of Common Natural Ingredients Used in Food Drugs and Cosmetics, John Wiley & Sons Inc., New York 1980.

Acacia Senegal

Acacia

DESCRIPTION

Medicinal Parts: The latex from the trunk and branches is the medicinal part of the plant.

Flower and Fruit: The inflorescences, which grow from the leaf axils, are up to 10 cm long. The flowers are white and grow in cylindrical, dense spikes. The calyx is cup-shaped with 5 sepals. The 5 petals are lanceolate. The numerous stamens are long and fused at the base. The pods are about 10 cm long and contain 5 to 6 shiny brown seeds.

Leaves, Stem and Root: Acacia senegal is up to 6 m tall with a 12 to 25 cm thick, slightly leaning trunk, which has knotty branches and a thin crown. The sapwood is white and the heart wood black. The bark is fibrous, gray on the outside, and rust-colored on the inside. The leaves are double abruptly-pinnate. The leaflets are in 10 to 15 pairs, narrow, gray-green, up to 5 mm long, opposite, and very short-petioled. There are 2 to 3 stipules, which have formed into thorns, and are covered on the upper surface with yellow fleshy glands.

Habitat: Found in the tropical Savannah belt of Africa, in the southern Sahara (Senegal, Gambia), in Arabia, Beludschistan and in Sind. Grown in forest-like conditions in the western and southwestern Sahara region (Senegal, Gambia, Ivory Coast, northern Dahomey, and northern Nigeria).

Production: Acacia gummi, the latex, is the result of a wound infection of the tree, which has occurred naturally or has been induced. The incised bark is removed in strips of approximately 4 cm by 60 cm. The liquid discharge dries to form a hard, glazed substance, which is collected on a weekly basis. The latex is harvested from trees, ranging from 3 to 12 years old.

Not To Be Confused With: According to DAB 10 (EUR), USP XXII, only latex from Acacia senegal or other African varieties are officially recognized. In other words, Asian, Australian, and American latex is not official.

Other Names: Cape Gum, Egyptian Thorn, Gum Acacia, Gum Arabic, Gum Senegal

ACTIONS AND PHARMACOLOGY

COMPOUNDS

Colloidally soluble polysaccharides: especially Arabic acid (acidic arabinogalactan)

Glycoproteins

EFFECTS

No information is available.

INDICATIONS AND USAGE

Acacia gummi is used in the preparation of emulsions. The drug is used as a mild stimulant and to impede absorption. It is also used for the treatment of catarrh and diarrhea. Acacia is often a constituent of cough drops.

PRECAUTIONS AND ADVERSE REACTIONS

No health hazards or side effects are known in conjunction with the proper administration of designated therapeutic dosages.

DOSAGE

Mode of Administration: Acacia is used as a pharmaceutical aid and is also administered internally in combination preparations.

Storage: The drug should be stored in tightly closed containers.

LITERATURE

Beuscher N, Bodinet C, Willigmann I, Harnischfeger G, Biological activity of Baptisia tinctoria extracts. In: Inst. für Angew. Botanik der Univ. Hamburg, Angewandte Botanik, Berichte 6, 46-61. 1997.

Randall RC, Phillips GO, Williams PA, Food Hydrocolloids 3:65-75. 1989.

Further information in:

Berger F, Handbuch der Drogenkunde, W Maudrich Verlag Wien 1964.

Hänsel R, Keller K, Rimpler H, Schneider G (Hrsg.), Hagers Handbuch der Pharmazeutischen Praxis, 5. Aufl., Bde 4-6

(Drogen): Springer Verlag Berlin, Heidelberg, New York, 1992-1994.

Steinegger E, Hänsel R, Pharmakognosie, 5. Aufl., Springer Verlag Heidelberg 1992.

Teuscher E, Biogene Arzneimittel, 5. Aufl., Wiss. Verlagsges. Stuttgart 1997.

Acer Rubrum

Red Maple

DESCRIPTION

Medicinal Parts: The medicinal part is the bark.

Flower and Fruit: The flowers are red, aromatic and form round bunches. The ovary is formed from 2 simple carpels pressed together at the sides, which are also present in the male flowers in rudimentary form. Each section contains 2 ovules. The fruit is a schizocarp with 2 one-sided or many-sided, often heavily-veined wings. There is usually only one seed in each section.

Leaves, Stem and Root: The Red Maple tree grows to a height of up to 36 m. The leaves are crossed-opposite, petiolate and partially 3-lobed.

Habitat: Canada and the U.S., introduced into England and Europe around 1650.

Production: Red Acorn bark is the trunk bark of Acer rubrum.

Other Names: Swamp Maple, Bird's Eye Maple, Sugar Maple

ACTIONS AND PHARMACOLOGY

COMPOUNDS

Tannins

Triterpenoid saponins

Allantoins

EFFECTS

Astringent.

INDICATIONS AND USAGE

Red Maple is used for eye conditions (folk medicine of the North American Indians).

This product should not be used otherwise.

PRECAUTIONS AND ADVERSE REACTIONS

No health hazards or side effects are known in conjunction with the proper administration of designated therapeutic dosages.

DOSAGE

Mode of Administration: Comminuted drug.

LITERATURE

No literature references are available.

Achillea Millefolium

Yarrow

DESCRIPTION

Medicinal Parts: The yarrow flowers (dried inflorescences), and aerial parts of the herb, which are collected during flowering and dried, are the medicinal plant parts.

Flower and Fruit: The plant has white, pink or purple composite flowers in dense cymes with small capitula. The bracts are imbricate and long. There are 5 white female linguiform florets. The disc florets are tubular, yellowish-white and androgynous. The bracts are lanceolate and thorn-tipped. The fruit is a 1.5 to 2 mm long hairless achaen.

Leaves, Stem and Root: Achillea millefolium are 0.1 to 1.5 m high plants with hardy, horizontal rhizomes, which grow from underground runners. The stem is simple, erect and hairy. The leaves are lanceolate and multi-pinnate with short acute tips.

Habitat: The numerous subspecies of the Achillea millefolium group are found in various regions. The most important regions are eastern, southeastern and central Europe as well as on the southern edge of the Alps from Switzerland to the Balkans.

Production: Yarrow herb consists of the fresh or dried, above-ground parts of Achillea millefolium, harvested at flowering season. Yarrow flower consists of the dried inflorescence of Achillea milleefolium.

Other Names: Band Man's Plaything, Bloodwort, Carpenter's Weed, Devil's Nettle, Devil's Plaything, Milfoil, Nose Bleed, Old Man's Pepper, Sanguinary, Soldier's Woundwort, Staunchweed, Thousand Weed

ACTIONS AND PHARMACOLOGY

COMPOUNDS

Volatile oil (0.2-1.0%): chief components are chamazulene (blue, 6-19%, maximum 40%), camphor (up to 20%), beta-pinene (up to 23%), 1,8-cineole (up to 10%), caryophyllene (up to 10%), alpha-pinene (ca. 5%), isoartemisiaketon (up to 8%). The composition depends greatly upon the strain; the volatile oil of some strains is free of chamazulene

Sesquiterpene lactones (chiefly guaianolides): including, among others, achillicin, 8-alpha-angeloyloxy-10-epi-artabsin, 2,3-dihydro-desacetoxy-matricin, alpha-peroxyachifolide. Some sesquiterpenes are transformed through steam distillation into chamazulene (proazulenes)

Polyynes: including, among others, ponticaepoxide

Alkamids: including, among others, tetradeca-4,6-diin-10,12-dien acetyl isobutylamides

Flavonoids: including, among others, apigenine-7-O-glucoside, luteolin-7-O-glucoside, rutin

Betaine: including, among others, L-stachydrine

EFFECTS

Yarrow is a cholagogue, an antibacterial, an astringent, and an antispasmodic. The effect probably results from the interplay of various structured connections (chamazulen, flavonoids), in a similar fashion to camomile flowers, as their components are partially identical.

INDICATIONS AND USAGE

- Loss of appetite
- Dyspeptic complaints
- Liver and gallbladder complaints

Internally, Yarrow is used as Amarum aromaticum for loss of appetite and dyspeptic ailments such as mild, spastic discomforts of the gastrointestinal tract, including inflammation, diarrhea, bloating and cramps. Externally, it is used as a partial bath for painful, cramp-like conditions of psychosomatic origin in the lower part of the female pelvis, liver disorders, and the healing of wounds. Applications in folk medicine include use as a hemostyptic for conditions such as bleeding hemorrhoids, for menstrual complaints, and as a bath for the removal of perspiration.

CONTRAINDICATIONS

Contraindications include allergy to Yarrow and other composites.

PRECAUTIONS AND ADVERSE REACTIONS

No health hazards or side effects are known in conjunction with the proper administration of designated therapeutic dosages. The drug possesses a weak to medium-severe potential for sensitization.

DOSAGE

Mode of Administration: As a comminuted drug for teas and other galenic preparations for internal use and for hip baths. The pressed juice of fresh plants is used internally. The drug is contained in standardized preparations of cholagogic and gallbladder therapeutics and as an adjunct in many other preparations, such as laxatives, antitussives, gynecological products, cardiac remedies and preparations for varicose veins.

Preparation: To make a tea, place 2 gm of finely cut drug in boiling water, cover, steep for 10 to 15 minutes, and strain. For partial baths, use 100 gm Yarrow per 20 liter of water.

Daily Dosage: The daily dosage is 4.5 gm Yarrow herb or 3 gm Yarrow flowers.

Storage: The drug must be protected from light and moisture. The essential oil should not be stored in synthetic containers.

LITERATURE

Chandler RF et al., (1982) Econ Bot 36 (2): 203.

Cuong BN et al., (1979) Phytochemistry 18: 331.

Czygan FC, Das ätherische Öl der Schafgarbe. In: DAZ 134(3):228. 1994.

Czygan FC, Schafgarbe: Alte Heilpflanze neu untersucht. In: PZ 139(6):439. 1994.

Falk AJ et al., (1974) Lloydia 37: 598.

Falk AJ et al., (1975) J Pharm Sci 64: 1838.

Kastner U et al., Anti-edematous activity of sesquiterepene lactones from different taxa of the Achillea millefolium group. In: PM 59(7):A669. 1993.

Kastner U, Glasl S, Jurenitsch J, Achillea millefolium - ein Gallentherapeuticum. In: ZPT 16(1):34-36. 1995.

Kastner U, Glasl S, Jurentisch J, Kubelka W, Isolation and structure elucidation of the main proazulenes of the cultivar Achillea collina ''Proa''. In: PM 58(7):A718. 1992.

Kastner U, Jurenitsch J, Lehner S, Baumann A, Robien W, Kubelka W, The major proazulenes from Achillea collina BECKER: a revision of structure. In: Pharm Pharmacol Letters 1(1):27. 1991.

Müller-Jakic B et al., In vitro inhibition of cyclooxygenase and 5-lipoxygenase by alkamides from Echinacea and Achillea species. In: PM 60:37. 1994.

Ochir G, Budesinsky M, Motl O, 3-Oxa-guaianolides from Achillea-millefolium. In: PH 30(12):4163. 1991.

Orth M Berg T van den, Czygan FC, Die Schafgarbe - Achillea millefolium L. In: ZPT 15(3):176-182. 1994.

Schmidt M, Phytotherapie: Pflanzliche Gallenwegstherapeutika. In: DAZ 135(8):680-682. 1995.

Smolenski SJ et al., (1967) Lloydia 30: 144.

Verzár-Petri G et al., (1979) Herba Hung. 18 (2): 83.

Further information in:

Hänsel R, Keller K, Rimpler H, Schneider G (Hrsg.), Hagers Handbuch der Pharmazeutischen Praxis, 5. Aufl., Bde 4-6 (Drogen), Springer Verlag Berlin, Heidelberg, New York, 1992-1994.

Hausen B, Allergiepflanzen, Pflanzenallergene, ecomed Verlagsgesellsch. mbH, Landsberg 1988.

Madaus G, Lehrbuch der Biologischen Arzneimittel, Bde 1-3, Nachdruck, Georg Olms Verlag Hildesheim 1979.

Schulz R, Hänsel R, Rationale Phytotherapie, Springer Verlag Heidelberg 1996.

Steinegger E, Hänsel R, Pharmakognosie, 5. Aufl., Springer Verlag Heidelberg 1992.

Teuscher E, Lindequist U, Biogene Gifte - Biologie, Chemie, Pharmakologie, 2. Aufl., Fischer Verlag Stuttgart 1994.

Teuscher E, Biogene Arzneimittel, 5. Aufl., Wiss. Verlagsges. Stuttgart 1997.

Wagner H, Wiesenauer M, Phytotherapie. Phytopharmaka und pflanzliche Homöopathika, Fischer-Verlag, Stuttgart, Jena, New York 1995.

Wichtl M (Hrsg.), Teedrogen, 4. Aufl., Wiss. Verlagsges. Stuttgart 1997.

Achillea Ptarmica

Sneezewort

DESCRIPTION

Medicinal Parts: The medicinal part is the dried root.

Flower and Fruit: The flowers are white, composite and in cymes at the tip of the stem. The bracts are lanceolate and short-haired. The ray florets are linguiform and female. The disc florets are tubular and androgynous. The chaff scales are lanceolate and hairy tipped. The fruit is hairless.

Leaves, Stem and Root: The plant grows from 30 to 80 cm high. The rhizome is creeping, and the stem is upright and glabrous. The leaves are glabrous, alternate, simple, lanceolate, acute, sessile and finely serrated. They are slightly glossy and dark green.

Habitat: The plant is indigenous to northern and central Europe.

Production: The rhizome is dug up in the autumn of its second year of baring fruit, washed, freed of any green areas and dried in the shade at a temperature of 35°C.

ACTIONS AND PHARMACOLOGY

COMPOUNDS

Volatile oil

Polyynes

Alkamides: including trans-dehydro matricaria acid isobutylamide

EFFECTS

No information is available.

INDICATIONS AND USAGE

In folk medicine, the drug was used as a remedy for tiredness, loss of appetite and urinary tract complaints. Sneezewort is also used for rheumatic and painful disorders, nausea, vomiting, and diarrhea. The drug helps to relieve problems with excretion, flatulence, toothache, and regulates the stool.

PRECAUTIONS AND ADVERSE REACTIONS

No health hazards or side effects are known in conjunction with the proper administration of designated therapeutic dosages, although persons with compound allergies should avoid salves prepared from the drug.

DOSAGE

Mode of Administration: Topically and in alcoholic extracts.

Preparation: To prepare an infusion, use 2 teaspoonfuls of the cut drug to 2 cups of water.

Daily Dosage: A daily infusion is administered or the fresh root can be chewed.

LITERATURE

Kuropka G, Neugebauer M, Glombitza KW, Essential oils of Achillea ptarmica. In: PM 57:492. 1991.

Rücker G et al., trans-Pinocarveylhydroxid aus Achillea ptarmica. In: PM 60(2):194. 1994.

Aconitum Napellus

Monkshood

DESCRIPTION

Medicinal Parts: Deadly poison.

Flower and Fruit: The flowers are 50 to 160 cm and form violet, bluish or reddish upright racemes. The calyx has 5 petal-like sepals. The upper sepal is convex and helmet-shaped. There are 2 petals with nectar releasing spurs under the upper sepal. There are numerous glabrous or ciliate stamens. There are 3 glabrous ovaries with 10 to 14 ovules. The fruit is a 16 to 20 mm long by 5 mm thick follicle. The seeds are glossy black and triangular with narrow wings on the edges.

Leaves, Stem and Root: A. napellus is a 0.5 to 1.5 m high shrub with a tuberous, thickened, fleshy root and an erect, rigid, undivided stem. The racem axis and petioles are glabrous or hairy. The leaves are dark green, glossy above and lighter beneath. They are palmate and 5 to 7-pinnatasect. The sections of the leaf are rhomboid in outline and deeply indented with oblong tips.

Characteristics: Extremely poisonous.

Habitat: A. napellus is common to the Alps and the Carpathians and is to be found in all the mountainous regions of Europe. The plant is found as far as Sweden in the north, as far as England and Portugal in the west, as far as the Pyrenees in the south and as far as the Carpatians in the east.

Production: Monkshood tuber consists of the fresh or dried tubers and roots of Aconitum napellus harvested in autumn after flowering. Monkshood herb consists of the dried herb of Aconitum napellus collected at the beginning of the flowering season. The collected roots are quickly dried at approx. 40°C.

Not To Be Confused With: Other blue-flowering Aconitum species. The yellow-flowering species may be mixed with falsifications.

Other names: Aconite, Wolfsbane, Blue Rocket, Friar's Cap, Mousebane

ACTIONS AND PHARMACOLOGY

COMPOUNDS

Nor-diterpene alkaloids: including aconitine, mesaconitine, hypaconitine, N-desethyl aconitine, oxoaconitine

EFFECTS

The efficacy of the drug is based on the di-ester alkaloids aconitin, mesaconitin, and hypaconitin. Aconitin raises membrane permeability for sodium ions, and retards repolarization. Aconitin is initially stimulating, and then causes paralysis in the motor and sensitive nerve ends, and in the CNS. The other di-ester alkaloids function in a similar fashion. Hypaconitin works more intensely. Aconitin applied in small doses triggers bradycardia and hypotension; in higher doses it has, at first, a positive inotropic effect, followed by tachycardia, cardiac arrhythmia, and cardiac arrest. Di-ester alkaloids were shown to be analgesic in animal experiments. Applied topically in humans, the drug is initially stimulating, in the form of itchiness or burning, and then anaesthetizing. In people with fever, the drug causes outbreaks of sweat and has an anti-febrile effect. Therapeutic doses influence the heart minimally; the heart rate may increase slightly. Given orally, the drug is active after a few minutes.

INDICATIONS AND USAGE

The drug is at most still used popularly to reduce pain from neuralgia, particularly with trigeminus and intercostal neuralgia. It is also used for myalgia, muscular and articular rheumatism, serous skin inflammation, and migraine. Effectiveness is unproven.

Preparations of blue monkshood are used for pain, facial paralyses, ailments of the joints, arthritis, gout, rheumatic complaints, inflammation, pleurisy, pericarditis sicca, fever, skin and mucosal diseases, as well as for disinfecting and wound treatment.

In experimental pharmacology, aconitin is used due to its ability to trigger cardiac arrhythmia.

PRECAUTIONS AND ADVERSE REACTIONS

The drug is highly toxic. Signs of poisoning can appear even with the administration of therapeutic dosages. The first sign of poisoning is a tingling of the mouth as well as of the fingers and toes, that then spreads over the entire body surface and changes into a furry sensation. Body temperature falls heavily. Queasiness, vomiting, diarrhea and urination occur.

OVERDOSAGE

With fatal doses, breathing becomes irregular and the heartbeat slows down and becomes arrythmic. Intense pains are characteristic. Death usually follows within 6 hours due to heart failure or asphyxiation. For adults, the estimated fatal dosage lies between 1 to 2 g. Countermeasures include gastrointestinal emptying, keeping the patient warm, cardiovascular and pulmonary support, magnesium and calcium infusions, administration of atropine to fight bradycardia, lidocaine for relieving the arrythmias, possibly artificial respiration, pain relief (no opiates).

DOSAGE

Mode of Administration: Administration of the drug is prohibited.

The use of the drug is nowadays judged to be too risky and inadvisable, especially as the active agent is available. Externally: Aconiti tinctura applied with a brush. Used in homeopathy.

Preparation: Aconiti tinctura: 1:1

Daily Dose: Drug: Administration is prohibited.

Aconiti tinktura: average dose 0.1g; maximum dose 0.2g; maximum daily dose 0.6g; standardized preparations are advisable.

Storage: The herb must be kept in a dry place, and be protected from light and insects.

LITERATURE

Bugatti C, Colombo ML, Tomé F, Extraction and purification of lipoalkaloids from Aconitum napellus Roots and leaves. In: PM 58(7):A695. 1992.

Hikino H et al., J Pharm Dyn 2:78-83. 1979.

Honerjäger P, Meissner A, Naunyn-Schmiedeberg's Arch Pharmacol 322:49-58. 1983.

Katz A, Rudin HP, Staehlin E, Pharm Acta Helv 62: 216-220. 1987.

Katz A, Staehlin E, Pharm Acta Helv 54:253-265. 1979.

Kimura M et al., Japan J Pharmacol 48:290-299. 1988.

Liu H, Katz A, Norditerpenoid alkaloids from Aconitum napellus ssp. neomontanum. In: PM 62(2):190-191. 1997.

Rao MR, (1966) Acta Pharm Sinica 3, 195.

Further information in:

Chan H, But P (Eds.), Pharmacology and Applications of Chinese Materia Medica, Vol 1, Ed. World Scientific Singapore 1986.

Frohne D, Pfänder HJ, Giftpflanzen - Ein Handbuch für Apotheker, Toxikologen und Biologen, 4. Aufl., Wiss. Verlags-Ges Stuttgart 1997.

Hänsel R, Keller K, Rimpler H, Schneider G (Hrsg.), Hagers Handbuch der Pharmazeutischen Praxis, 5. Aufl., Bde 4-6 (Drogen), Springer Verlag Berlin, Heidelberg, New York, 1992-1994.

Lewin L, Gifte und Vergiftungen, 6. Aufl., Nachdruck, Haug Verlag, Heidelberg 1992.

Madaus G, Lehrbuch der Biologischen Arzneimittel, Bde 1-3, Nachdruck, Georg Olms Verlag Hildesheim 1979.

Roth L, Daunderer M, Kormann K, Giftpflanzen, Pflanzengifte, 4. Aufl., Ecomed Fachverlag Landsberg Lech 1993.

Steinegger E, Hänsel R, Pharmakognosie, 5. Aufl., Springer Verlag Heidelberg 1992.

Teuscher E, Lindequist U, Biogene Gifte - Biologie, Chemie, Pharmakologie, 2. Aufl., Fischer Verlag Stuttgart 1994.

Teuscher E, Biogene Arzneimittel, 5. Aufl., Wiss. Verlagsges. Stuttgart 1997.

Wagner H, Wiesenauer M, Phytotherapie. Phytopharmaka und pflanzliche Homöopathika, Fischer-Verlag, Stuttgart, Jena, New York 1995.

Acorus Calamus

Calamus

DESCRIPTION

Medicinal Parts: The medicinal part is the rhizome after the removal of all other material.

Flower and Fruit: Green flowers, like small dice, form a tightly packed, slim, conical spadix. The plant is non-fruit-bearing and propagates from the rhizome.

Leaves, Stem and Root: The plant grows from 60 to 100 cm tall. The stem is triangular and sprouts from a horizontal, round root-stock, which has the thickness of a thumb. The upper shoot forms a grooved flower sheath. The leaves are oblong, sword-shaped and arranged in two rows. The leaves have no stems.

Characteristics: The rhizome has an intensely aromatic fragrance and a tangy, pungent and bitter taste. The leaves often undulate on the margins.

Habitat: Today Calamus is found all over the world. It probably originated in India and North America.

Production: Calamus root-stock is the dried, coarsely ground and mostly peeled, root-stock of Acorus calamus. Calamus oil is extracted from the same plant.

Other Names: Sweet Flag, Sweet Sedge, Grass Myrtle, Myrtle Flag, Sweet Grass, Sweet Myrtle, Sweet Rush, Sweet Root, Sweet Cane, Gladdon, Myrtle Sedge, Cinnamon Sedge

ACTION AND PHARMACOLOGY

COMPOUNDS

Volatile oil: chief constituents are heavily dependent upon the chemical strain (di-, tri-, tetraploid); beta-asarone (cis-isoasarone), alpha- and gamma-asarone, beta- gurjuns, acorone (bitter), ZZ-Deca-4,7-dienal (odor-determining)

EFFECTS

Calamus is an aromatic, bitter stomachic, which stimulates appetite and digestion and is a stomach tonic. It has spasmolytic, carminative and sedative effects, in addition to being externally hyperemic.

INDICATIONS AND USAGE

The drug is used in the form of teas for dyspeptic disorders, gastritis, and ulcers. It is used externally for rheumatism, gum disease, and angina.

PRECAUTIONS AND ADVERSE REACTIONS

No health hazards or side effects are known in conjunction with the proper administration of designated therapeutic dosages of European origin (triploid strain, up to 15% beta-asarone in volatile oil). Long-term use of this drug should be avoided. Malignant tumors appeared in rats that received Indian Kalmus oils over an extended period (tetraploid strain, over 80% β-asarone in volatile oil).

DOSAGE

Mode of Administration: Calamus preparations are for internal and external use.

Preparation: Steep with hot water to make a tea. For use in a bath, add 250 to 500 g of the drug to the bath water.

Storage: Store for a maximum of 18 months, however if in powder form, do not keep for more than 24 hours.

LITERATURE

Iguchi M et al., (1973) Tetrahedron Letters 29:2759.

Keller K et al., (1985) Planta Med 51(1):6.

Keller K, Stahl E, Composition of the essential oil from beta-asarone free calamus. In: PM 47(2):71. 1983.

Keller K, Stahl E, Kalmus: Inhalsstoffe und β-Asarongehalt bei verschiedenen Herkünften. In: DAZ 122(48):2463-2466. 1982.

Mazza G, Gas chromatographic and mass spectrometric studies of the constituents of the rhizome of calamus. In: J Chromatogr 328:179-206. 1985.

Rohr M, Naegeli P, (1979) Phytochemistry 18(2):279 and 328.

Saxena DB, Phenyl indane from Acorus calamus. In: PH 25(2):553. 1986.

Schneider K, Jurenitsch J, Kalmus als Arzneidroge: Nutzen oder Risiko. In: Pharmazie 47(2):79-85. 1992.

Stahl E, Keller K, Classification of typical commercial Calamus drugs. In: PM 43(2):128-140. 1981.

Taylor JM et al., Toxicity of oli of calamus (Jammu variety). In: Toxicol Appl Pharmacol 10:405 (Abstract). 1967.

Further information in:

Chan, EH et al. (Eds.), Advances in Chinese Medicinal Materials Research, World Scientific Pub. Co. Singapore 1985.

Kern W, List PH, Hörhammer L (Hrsg.), Hagers Handbuch der Pharmazeutischen Praxis, 4. Aufl., Bde 1-8, Springer Verlag Berlin, Heidelberg, New York, 1969.

Leung AY, Encyclopedia of Common Natural Ingredients Used in Food Drugs and Cosmetics, John Wiley & Sons Inc., New York 1980.

Madaus G, Lehrbuch der Biologischen Arzneimittel, Bde 1-3, Nachdruck, Georg Olms Verlag Hildesheim 1979.

Roth L, Daunderer M, Kormann K, Giftpflanzen, Pflanzengifte, 4. Aufl., Ecomed Fachverlag Landsberg Lech 1993.

Steinegger E, Hänsel R, Pharmakognosie, 5. Aufl., Springer Verlag Heidelberg 1992.

Teuscher E, Lindequist U, Biogene Gifte - Biologie, Chemie, Pharmakologie, 2. Aufl., Fischer Verlag Stuttgart 1994.

Teuscher E, Biogene Arzneimittel, 5. Aufl., Wiss. Verlagsges. Stuttgart 1997.

Wagner H, Wiesenauer M, Phytotherapie. Phytopharmaka und pflanzliche Homöopathika, Fischer-Verlag, Stuttgart, Jena, New York 1995.

Wichtl M (Hrsg.), Teedrogen, 4. Aufl., Wiss. Verlagsges. Stuttgart. 1997.

Actaea Spicata

Baneberry

DESCRIPTION

Medicinal Parts: The medicinal part is the root.

Flower and Fruit: The white flowers are in ovate racemes. They have 4 to 6 bracts, white stamens and 1 ovary. The fruit is a black, many-seeded berry.

Leaves, Stem and Root: The plant grows 30 to 60 cm tall. It is large, long-petioled, trifoliate and pinnate. The leaflets are pinnatisect and serrate. The stem is erect and glabrous.

Characteristics: Baneberry is poisonous, as are several other plants with similar qualities.

Habitat: The plant grows worldwide.

Production: Baneberry or Herb Christopher root is the root of Actaea spicata.

Not To Be Confused With: Helleborus niger is occasionally used as a substitute by mistake.

Other Names: Bugbane, Herb Christopher, Toadroot

ACTIONS AND PHARMACOLOGY

COMPOUNDS

Triterpene glycosides: including actein

Trans-aconitic acid

EFFECTS

No information is available.

INDICATIONS AND USAGE

Baneberry is used as an emetic and purgative in folk medicine.

PRECAUTIONS AND ADVERSE REACTIONS

No health hazards or side effects are known in conjunction with the proper administration of designated therapeutic dosages.

DOSAGE

Mode of Administration: There is no information available to evaluate its use in folk medicine. In homeopathy, Baneberry is available as dilutions of the mother tincture.

LITERATURE

Fardella G, Corsano St, Preliminary study on actein biosynthesis. In: Ann Chim(Rom)63:333-337. 1973.

Nikonow GK, Syrkina SA, Chemische Untersuchungen der aktiven Prinzipien von Actaea spicata L. In: Pharm Zentralhalle 103(8):601. 1964.

Further information in:

Frohne D, Pfänder HJ, Giftpflanzen - Ein Handbuch für Apotheker, Toxikologen und Biologen, 4. Aufl., Wiss. Verlags-Ges Stuttgart 1997.

Kern W, List PH, Hörhammer L (Hrsg.), Hagers Handbuch der Pharmazeutischen Praxis, 4. Aufl., Bde. 1-8, Springer Verlag Berlin, Heidelberg, New York, 1969.

Madaus G, Lehrbuch der Biologischen Arzneimittel, Bde 1-3, Nachdruck, Georg Olms Verlag Hildesheim 1979.

Adam's Needle

See Yucca Filamentosa

Adiantum Capillus-veneris

Maidenhair

DESCRIPTION

Medicinal Parts: The fronds and rhizomes were once made into ''syrup de capillaire'' and used in France to cure pulmonary catarrhs. The dried fronds (Maiden Hair) are used as a drug as well the dried herb with rhizome and roots (Maiden Hair with roots).

Flower and Fruit: There are lumps of sporangia without a veil on the underside of the lateral lobes, these sporangia are square to reniform and later, dark brown.

Leaves, Stem and Root: Maidenhair is a hardy, up to 35 cm high plant with an aromatic lily fragrance. It has a creeping rhizome. The leaves are double-rowed, tender, glabrous and up to 50 cm long. They have a glossy black petiole and are covered with hairs at the base. The leaf-blade is ovate to oblong-ovate. The leaflets are light green periolate. The pinnules have hair-like petioles. The veins of the sterile pinna terminate in teeth at the edge of the leaf.

Habitat: Southern Europe, Atlantic coast as far as Ireland, from the south to the southern Alpine valleys (Tessin, southern Tyrol).

Production: Maidenhair fern, which is gathered in June and dried, is the frond of Adiantum capillus-veneris.

Not To Be Confused With: It has sometimes been observed that the drug has been made impure by an addition of bracken leaf fronds (Pteridium aquilinum).

Other Names: Venus Hair, Rock Fern, Hair of Venus, Five-finger fern, Maiden fern

ACTION AND PHARMACOLOGY

COMPOUNDS

Flavonoids

Proanthocyanidins

Hydroxycinnamic acid ester

EFFECTS

The drug is an expectorant, beneficial in bringing up phlegm, and a demulcent.

INDICATIONS AND USAGE

In the middle ages, the drug was used for various illnesses of the respiratory tract, in the form of so-called pectoral teas and as a syrup for severe coughs. Because of its similarity to maiden hair, the drug was used to treat a lack of hair growth and to promote dark hair color.

It is still taken as an infusion in Spain, Belgium and the Canary Islands to treat bronchitis, coughs and whooping cough, and also for painful and excessive menstruation. Efficacy has not been proven.

PRECAUTIONS AND ADVERSE REACTIONS

No health hazards or side effects are known in conjunction with the proper administration of designated therapeutic dosages.

DOSAGE

Mode of Administration: The drug is taken internally as a tea prepared from the ground or powdered drug.

Daily Dosage: The standard single dose is 1.5 g of the drug to 1 cup of liquid per dose.

Storage: Protect from light.

LITERATURE

Berti G et al., Tetrahedron Lett: 1-5. 1964.

Cooper-Driver G, Swain T, Bot J Linn Soc 74:1-21. 1977.

Imperato F, PH 21:2158-2159. 1982.

Imperator F, (1982) Phytochemistry 21(8):2158.

Jain SR, Sharma SN, (1967) Planta Med(4):439.

Twaij HAA et al., (1985) Indian J Pharmacol 17(1):73.

Adonis Vernalis

Adonis

DESCRIPTION

Medicinal Parts: The medicinal part is derived from the aerial parts of the herb which are collected during the flowering season and dried.

Flower and Fruit: The erect, solitary, terminal flower is 4 to 7 cm in diameter and the 5 broad-ovate, downy sepals are half as long as the petals. The 10 to 20 petals are narrow, wedge-shaped, simple or finely serrated at the tip. They are 20 to 40 mm long and lemon yellow, splayed, glossy, reddish on the outside or greenish-tinged. There are numerous stamens and carpels. The small fruit forms a globose capitulum. The fruit is tomentose, wrinkled, laterally veined and keeled with a sideways-facing hook-shaped beak. They are arranged on the spindle-shaped, oblong receptacle.

Leaves, Stem and Root: The plant is 10 to 40 cm high with a sturdy, black-brown rhizome. The stem is erect, undivided, covered with scales at the base, vertically grooved and succulent. There are few branches. The leaves have many slits and a curved, glabrous or sparsely-haired tip. The middle leaves are half clasping.

Characteristics: Adonis is a poisonous plant; heavily protected in Germany.

Habitat: This Siberian/East European plant is found in the north as far as the central Urals and south-west Sweden. In central Europe is limited to the basins of the Weichsel and the Oder as far as the Main and Rhine.

Production: The drug is gathered in forests and should be dried quickly.

Not To Be Confused With: Other Adonis species may be added to Adonidis herba.

Other Names: False Hellebore, Yellow Pheasant's Eye, Ox-eye, Sweet Vernal, Pheasant's Eye, Red Morocco, Rose-a-rubie

ACTIONS AND PHARMACOLOGY

COMPOUNDS

Cardioactive steroid gylcosides (cardenolids): including adonitoxin, k-strophanthoside, k-strophanthoside-β and cymarin

Flavonoids: including vitexin and luteolin

EFFECTS

Adonis has a positive inotropic effect. Animal tests showed a tonic effect on the veins. The adonitoxin component is slightly more toxic than coumarin.

The drug is insufficiently documented.

INDICATIONS AND USAGE

- Arrhythmia
- Cardiac insufficiency (NYHA I and II)
- Nervous heart complaints

The drug is used for mild impairment of heart functions (NYHA I and II), especially when accompanied by nervous symptoms.

In Russian folk medicine, the drug is used for dehydration, cramps, fever, and menstrual disorders, but efficacy is unproven.

CONTRAINDICATIONS

Adonis is contraindicated with digitalis glycoside therapy and also in potassium deficiency.

PRECAUTIONS AND ADVERSE REACTIONS

General: Despite the strong efficacy of the drug's cardioactive steroid gylcosides in parenteral application, serious poisoning in the course of per oral administration is hardly to be expected due to the low resorption rate.

Drug Interactions: Enhancement of efficacy, and thus also of side effects, with simultaneous administration of quinidine, calcium, saluretics, laxatives, and extended therapy with glucocorticoids.

OVERDOSAGE

For possible symptoms of overdose and treatment of poisonings see *Digitalis folium.*

DOSAGE

Mode of Administration: Comminuted herb and preparations thereof for internal use.

Daily Dosage: The average daily dose is 0.5 gm of standardized Adonis powder. The maximum single dose is 1.0 gm; maximum daily dose is 3.0 gm.

Storage: Adonis herb and powder should be stored carefully. Adonis powder should be kept away from light in tightly sealed containers.

LITERATURE

Brevoort P, Der Heilpflanzenmarkt der USA - Ein Überblick. In: ZPT 18(3):155-162. 1997.

ESCOP-Monographs. In: ESCOP-Monographs Fascicule I and II. 1996.

Hiller KO, Rahlfs V, Therapeutische Äquivalenz eines hochdosierten Phytopharmakons mit Amytriptylin bei ängstlich-depressiven Versimmungen - Reanalyse einer randomisierten Studie unter besonderer Beachtung biometrischer und klinischer Aspekte. In: Forsch.

Karrer W (1950) Helv Chim Acta 33:433.

Lee MK et al., Antihepatotoxic activity of Icariin, a major constutent of Epimedium koreanum. In: PM 61(6):523-526. 1995.

Loew, Buch. In: Loew D, Rietbrock N: Phytopharmaka II: Forschung und klinische Anwendung, Steinkopff Verlag, Darmstadt, 1996.

Loew DA, Loew AD, Pharmakokinetik von herzglykosidhaltigen Pflanzenextrakten. In: ZPT 15(4):197-202. 1994.

Loew D, Phytotherapie bei Herzinsuffizienz. In: ZPT 18(2):92-96. 1997.

Martinez-Vazquez M, Ramirez Apan TO, Hidemi Aguilar M, Bye R, Analgesic and antipyretic activities of an aqueous extract and of the flavone Linarin of Buddleia cordata. In: PM 62:137-140. 1996.

Reinhard KH, Uncaria tomentosa (WILLD.) DC. - Cat's claw, Una de gato oder Katzenkralle Protrait einer Arzneipflanze. In: ZPT 18(2)00132-121. 1997.

Sandberg F, Thorsen R (1962) Lloydia 25(3):201.

Schulz V, Hübner WD, Ploch M, Klinische Studien mit Psycho-Phytopharmaka. In: ZPT 18(3):141-154. 1997.

Winkler C and Wichtel M (1985) Pharm Acta Helv 60(9/10): 234.

Further information in:

Frohne D, Pfänder HJ, Giftpflanzen - Ein Handbuch für Apotheker, Toxikologen und Biologen, 4. Aufl., Wiss. Verlags-Ges Stuttgart 1997.

Hänsel R, Keller K, Rimpler H, Schneider G (Hrsg.), Hagers Handbuch der Pharmazeutischen Praxis, 5. Aufl., Bde 4-6 (Drogen), Springer Verlag Berlin, Heidelberg, New York, 1992-1994.

Lewin L, Gifte und Vergiftungen, 6. Aufl., Nachdruck, Haug Verlag, Heidelberg 1992.

Madaus G, Lehrbuch der Biologischen Arzneimittel, Bde 1-3, Nachdruck, Georg Olms Verlag Hildesheim 1979.

Roth L, Daunderer M, Kormann K, Giftpflanzen, Pflanzengifte, 4. Aufl., Ecomed Fachverlag Landsberg Lech 1993.

Schulz R, Hänsel R, Rationale Phytotherapie, Springer Verlag Heidelberg 1996.

Steinegger E, Hänsel R, Pharmakognosie, 5. Aufl., Springer Verlag Heidelberg 1992.

Teuscher E, Lindequist U, Biogene Gifte - Biologie, Chemie, Pharmakologie, 2. Aufl., Fischer Verlag Stuttgart 1994.

Teuscher E, Biogene Arzneimittel, 5. Aufl., Wiss. Verlagsges. Stuttgart 1997.

Wagner H, Wiesenauer M, Phytotherapie. Phytopharmaka und pflanzliche Homöopathika, Fischer-Verlag, Stuttgart, Jena, New York 1995.

Adrue

See Cyperus Articulatus

Aegle Marmelos

Bael

DESCRIPTION

Medicinal Parts: The medicinal parts are the unripe fruit, the root, the leaves, and the branches.

Flower and Fruit: The plant has greenish white flowers. The yellow fruit is globular or ovoid, with a hard shell. The fruit is divided internally like an orange. The flesh is reddish, with numerous seeds covered in a layer of latex.

Characteristics: The taste is mucilaginous and slightly sour.

Habitat: This plant is native to India but has spread over wide areas of south-east Asia.

Other Names: Bel, Bengal Quince

ACTIONS AND PHARMACOLOGY

COMPOUNDS

Tannins

Saccharides

Starch

Fatty oil

Furocoumarins

Furoquinolin alkaloids

EFFECTS

Bael has a digestive and an astringent effect.

INDICATIONS AND USAGE

Bael is used, especially in Indian medicine, for constipation and diarrhea.

PRECAUTIONS AND ADVERSE REACTIONS

No health hazards or side effects are known in conjunction with the proper administration of designated therapeutic dosages. Digestive complaints and constipation are conceivable with the intake of large quantities, due to the constituent tannins.

DOSAGE

Mode of Administration: Available as a liquid extract.

LITERATURE

Oliver-Bever B (Ed., 1986), Medicinal Plants of Tropical West Africa, Cambridge University Press UK.

Sharma BR and Sharma P, (1981) Planta Med 43:102.

Schimmer O, Furochinolinalkaloide als biologisch aktive Naturstoffe. In: ZPT 12(5):151. 1991.

Aegopodium Podagraria

Goutweed

DESCRIPTION

Flower and Fruit: The flowers range from 50 to 100 cm. They have large white or reddish double umbels that are usually androgynous. The flowers have no involucre and no calyx. The petals are white or pink, about 1.5 mm long, obcordate and cuneate at the base. The fruit is oblong and brownish with pale veins. The fruit is slightly pressed in at the sides, unwinged, unstriped, with a 3 mm-long mericarp.

Leaves, Stem and Root: The stem is erect, angular, grooved, hollow, glabrous and branched. The lower leaves are double trifoliate, and the upper leaves trifoliate. The leaflets are ovate and crenate-serrate.

Characteristics: Propagates via underground runners.

Habitat: Indigenous to Europe (not Spain), West Asia.

Production: Goutweed is the aerial part of Aegopodium podagraria.

Other Names: Goutwort, Ground Elder, Gout Herb, Herb Gerard(e), Jack-jump-about, Goatweed, Ashweed, Achweed,

English Masterwort, Pigweed, Eltroot, Bishop's Elder, Weyl Ash, White Ash, Bishopsweed, Bishopswort.

ACTION AND PHARMACOLOGY

COMPOUNDS

Volatile oil

Polyynes: (only in freshly-harvested leaves)

Flavonol glycosides: including hyperoside, isoquercitrin

Caffeic acid derivatives: including chlorogenic acid

Ascorbic acid

EFFECTS

No information available.

INDICATIONS AND USAGE

The herb is used internally as an infusion for gout and rheumatic diseases. It is used externally in macerations for poultices and baths for hemorrhoids, gout and rheumatic diseases, as well as for kidney and bladder disorders and intestinal disorders.

PRECAUTIONS AND ADVERSE REACTIONS

No health hazards or side effects are known in conjunction with the proper administration of designated therapeutic dosages.

DOSAGE

Mode of Administration: Internally as a tea; externally, the fresh herb is squeezed for poultices.

Daily Dosage: There is no exact dosage. A daily recommended dose consists of 1 to 2 dessertspoonfuls (30ml) of the juice of the fresh plant.

LITERATURE

Bohlmann F et al., Chem Ber 93, 981. 1968.

Hänsel R, Keller K, Rimpler H, Schneider G (Hrsg.), Hagers Handbuch der Pharmazeutischen Praxis, 5. Aufl., Bde 4-6 (Drogen), Springer Verlag Berlin, Heidelberg, New York, 1992-1994.

Harborne JB, Williams CA, PH 11(5):1741-1750. 1972.

Schneider V, Ernähr-Umschau 31(2):54-57. 1984.

Aesculus Hippocastanum

Horse Chestnut

DESCRIPTION

Medicinal Parts: The medicinal parts are the dried horse chestnut leaves, the oil extracted from the peeled nuts and the dried chestnut seeds.

Flower and Fruit: The white flowers are in stiffly upright, clavate panicles. Most of the flowers are male, but a few are female or adrogynous. The calyx is fused and bell-shaped with 5 irregular tips. The petals are 10 to 15 mm long with a yellow spot, which turns red. There are 3 upward petals and 2 downward. They are folded at the edge, cilate and cordate at the base. There are 7 S-shaped, bending stamens with red anthers that are longer than the petals. The ovary is 3-valved, superior and velvety. There is 1 style. The fruit capsules are green and globular with soft spines and fine hairs. There are 1 to 3 red-brown seeds (chestnuts), which are shiny brown with a yellowish gray-brown naval and a tough shell.

Leaves, Stem and Root: The deciduous tree is up to 35 m high and has a large regular crown. The roots are smooth and spread widely. The trunk is initially smooth and later has thinly scaled, peeling and fissured bark. The young twigs are yellowish to red-brown and initially covered with brown hairs. The buds are thick, clavate, and extremely sticky with dark red bud scales. The leaves are long, 5 to 7 palmate, with a 20 cm long grooved petiole. The leaflets are initially red-haired, 20 cm long, cuneate-obovate, acute, dentate, rich-green above and light green beneath.

Habitat: Indigenous to the mountains of Greece, Bulgaria, the Caucasus, northern Iran and the Himalayas. Cultivated elsewhere, especially in northern Europe including the British Isles, Denmark, Scandinavia, Russia (Narva and St. Petersburg).

Production: Horse Chestnut leaf consists of the fresh or dried leaf of Aesculus hippocastanum. A dry extract is manufactured from horse chestnut seeds adjusted to a content of 16-20% triterpene glycosides (calculated as anhydrous aescin).

Not To Be Confused With: The leaves of the sweet chestnut

Other Names: Spanish Chestnut, Buckeye.

ACTION AND PHARMACOLOGY

COMPOUNDS: HIPPOCASTANI FOLIUM

Triterpene saponins

Hydroxycoumarins: chief components aesculin, in addition fraxin and scopolin

Flavonoids: including rutin, quercitrin, isoquercitrin

Tannins

EFFECTS: HIPPOCASTANI FOLIUM

Main active principle: courmarin glucosides, aesculin, flavonol glycosides.

COMPOUNDS: HIPPOCASTANI SEMEN

Triterpene saponins: (3-8%, saponine mixture known as aescin): chief components beta-aescin (diesterglycoside mixture of the protoaescigenins), through migration of an acetyl group into the more water-soluble, but hemolytically only somewhat cryptoaescigenin, alpha-aescin is an equilibrium mixture made up of beta-aescin and cryptoaescin.

Flavonoids: in particular biosides and triosides of the quercetins

Oligosaccharides: including 1-kestose, 2-kestose, stachyose

Polysaccharides: starch (50%)

Oligomeric proanthocyanidins, condensed tannins: (only in the seed-coat)

Fatty oil: (2-3%)

EFFECTS: HIPPOCASTANI SEMEN

As found in different animal tests, the principal ingredient in Horse Chestnut seed extract, the triterpene glycoside mixture, aescin (escin), has an antiexudative and vascular tightening effect. There are indications that Horse Chestnut seed extract reduces the activity of lysosomal enzymes which is increased in chronic pathological conditions of the veins, so that the breakdown of glycoacalyx (mucopolysaccharides) in the region of the capillary walls is inhibited. The filtration of low-molecular proteins, electrolytes and water into the interstitium is inhibited through a reduction of vascular permeability.

INDICATIONS AND USAGE

HIPPOCASTANI FOLIUM

Eczema, superficial and deep varicose veins, leg pains, phlebitis and thrombophlebitis, hemorrhoids, spastic pains before and during menstruation. In folk medicine, the leaves are used as a cough remedy as well as arthritis and rheumatism.

HIPPOCASTANI SEMEN

■ Venous conditions

Treatment of complaints found in pathological conditions of the veins of the legs (chronic venous insufficiency), for example pains and a sensation of heaviness in the legs, nocturnal systremma (cramps in the calves) pruritis and swelling of the legs.

Horse chestnut seeds are used for symptoms of chronic venous insufficiency as well as post-traumatic and post-operative soft tissue swelling. Further indications are painful injuries, sprains, bruising, pain syndrome of the spine and edema.

PRECAUTIONS AND ADVERSE REACTIONS

HIPPOCASTANI FOLIUM

Health risks or side effects following the proper administration of designated therapeutic dosages are not recorded. One case of liver damage following I.M. administration of an extract of the drug (origin details of the drug uncertain) is known.

HIPPOCASTANI SEMEN

Health risks following the proper administration of designated therapeutic dosages are not recorded. Susceptible patients may nevertheless experience mucous membrane irritations of the gastrointestinal tract following intake of the drug; kidney function limitations could be increased; and itching of the skin has been observed. I.V administration of Aescin can lead to anaphylactic reactions.

The intake of larger quantities of horse chestnut seeds (in one case of a child with 5 seeds) can bring about vomiting, diarrhea, severe thirst, reddening of the face, enlargement of pupils, vision and consciousness disorders. Following stomach and intestinal emptying (gastric lavage, sodium sulphate) and the administration of activated charcoal, therapy for poisonings consists of diazepam for spasms, atropine for colic, electrolyte replenishment and sodium bicarbonate infusions for any acidosis that may arise. Intubation and oxygen respiration may also be necessary.

DOSAGE

HIPPOCASTANI FOLIUM

Mode of Administration: Extracts of the drug are contained in 'vein teas' or 'hemorrhoid teas' as well as in pharmaceutical preparations for the treatment of venous symptoms.

HIPPOCASTANI SEMEN

Mode of Administration: Liquid and dry preparations for oral application.

Daily Dosage: 30-150 mg aescin (escin)

LITERATURE

HIPPOCASTANI FOLIUM

Konoshima T, Lee KH (1986) J Nat Prod 49(4):650.

Preziosi P, Manca P (1965) Arzneim Forsch 15:404.

Proserpio G et al. (1980) Fitoterapia 2:113.

Rao GS et al. (1974) J Pharm Sci 63:471.

Further information in:

Chan, EH et al. (Eds), Advances in Chinese Medicinal Materials Research, World Scientific Pub. Co. Singapore 1985.

Hänsel R, Keller K, Rimpler H, Schneider G (Hrsg.), Hagers Handbuch der Pharmazeutischen Praxis, 5. Aufl., Bde 4-6 (Drogen), Springer Verlag Berlin, Heidelberg, New York, 1992-1994.

Madaus G, Lehrbuch der Biologischen Arzneimittel, Bde 1-3, Nachdruck, Georg Olms Verlag Hildesheim 1979.

Wichtl M (Hrsg.), Teedrogen, 4. Aufl., Wiss. Verlagsges. Stuttgart 1997.

HIPPOCASTANI SEMEN

Aizawa X, Fukui, Yamada K, Kogo H, Aescin, antiinflammatory action of Aescin (1, intravenous injection). In: Pharmacometrics (Tokyo) 8:211. 1974.

Alter H (1973), Zur medikamentösen Therapie der Varikosis. Z Allg Med 49(17):1301-1304.

Annoni F, Mauri A, Marincola Resele LF (1979), Venotonic activity of Escin on the human saphenous vein. Arzneim Forsch/Drug Res 29:672.

Arnold M, Przerwa M, Die therapeutische Beeinflußbarkeit experimentell erzeugter Ödeme. In: Arzneim Forsch 26:402-409. 1976.

Auster F, Wirkung eines Roßkastanienpräparates auf die Resistenz der Hautkapillaren. In: Pharmazie 11:726-730. 1956.

Bisler H, Pfeifer R, Klüken N, Pauschinger P (1986), Wirkung von Roßkastaniensamenextrakt auf die transkapilläre Filtration bei chronischer venöser Insuffizien. Z Dtsch Med Wschr 111: 1321-1328.

Büechi S, Antivirale Saponine, pharmakologische und klinische Untersuchungen. In: DAZ 136(2):89-98. 1996.

Daub B, Chronische Veneninsuffizienz: Roßkastanienextrakt oder Kompressionsstrumpf - gleiche Wirkung. In: DAZ 136(12):946. 1996.

Ehringer H, Objektivierbare Venentonisierung nach oraler Gabe eines Kombinationspräparates mit Roßkastanienextrakt. In: Arzneim Forsch 18:432. 1968.

Felix W, Schneider E, Schmidt A, Grimm G, Vasoaktive Wirkung von alpha-Aescin. In: Fischer H (Hrsg) Ergebnisse der Angiologie: Chronische Veneninsuffizienz. Pathogenese und medikamentöse Therapie, Schattauer, Stuttgart, 30:93-105. 1984.

Felix W, Spektrum Venenmittel. In: Arzneimitteltherapie heute. Bd. 45. Spektrum Venenmittel. Aesopus Verlag Zug S 29. 1986.

Felix W, Wirkungsmechanismen der internen Therapie mit "Venopharmaka". In: Dt med J 21:458-465. 1970.

Fink Serralde C, Dreyfus Cortes GO, Colo Hernandesz, Marquez Zacarias LA (1975), Valoracion de la escina pura en el tratamiento del sindrome des estasis venosa cronica. Münch Med Wschr (mex. Ausgabe) 117(1):41-46.

Fischer H, Pflanzliche Venentherapeutica. In: Therapiewoche 34:4101-4106. 1984.

Fricke U (1995) Venenmittel. In: Schwabe U, Paffrath D (Hrsg), Arzneiverordnungs-Report '95. Gustav Fischer Verlag Stuttgart, Jena, S 421-430.

Friederich HC, Vogelsberg H, Neiss A (1978), Ein Beitrag zur Bewertung von intern wirksamen Venenpharmaka. Z Hautkrankheiten 53(11):369-374.

Girerd I, DiPasquale, Steinetz G, Beach BG, Pearl VLW, The anti-edema properties of aescin. In: Arch internat Pharmacodyn Thér, Bruxelles 133:127-137. 1961.

Hampel H, Hofrichter G, Liehn HD, Schlemmer W, Zur Pharmakologie der Aescin-Isomere unter besonderer Berücksichtigung von alpha-Aescin. In: Arzneim Forsch 20:209-215. 1970.

Hitzenberger G (1989), Die therapeutische Wirksamkeit des Roßkastaniensamenextraktes. Wien Med Wschr 139(17):385-389.

Hübner G, Wray V, Nahrstedt A, Flavonolglycosides in Aesculus hippocastanum L.: Isolation, structure elucidation and quantification. In: PM 62, Abstracts of the 44th Ann Congress of GA, 139. 1996.

Jacker HJ, Zur Pharmakologie der Roßkastanie. In: PZH 116(9):959-968. 1977.

Konoshima T, Lee KH (1986) J Nat Prod 49(4):650.

Locks H, Baumgartner H, Konzett H (1974), Zur Beeinflussung des Benentonus durch Roßkastanienextrakte. Arzneim Forsch 24:1347.

Lohr E, Garanin G, Jesau P, Fischer H (1986), Ödemprotektive Therapie bei chronischer Veneninsuffizienz mit Ödemneigung. Münch Med Wschr 128:579-581.

Longiave D, Omini C, Nicosia S, Berti F (1978), The Mode of Action of Escin on Isolated Veins, Relationship with PGF2. Pharmacol Res 10:145.

Lorenz D, Marek ML (1960), Das therapeutisch wirksame Prinzip der Roßkastanie (Aesculus hippocastanum). Arzneim Forsch 10:263-272.

Marshall M, Dormandy JA (1987), Oedema of long distant flights. Phlebol 2:123-124.

Marshall M, Loew D (1994), Diagnostische Maßnahmen zum Nachweis der Wirksamkeit von Venentherapeutika. Phlebol 23:85-91.

Marshall M, Wüstenberg P, Klinik und Therapie der chronischen venösen Insuffizienz. In: Klinik und Therapie der chronischen venösen Insuffizienz, Braun Fachverlage, Karlsruhe 1994.

Neiss A, Böhm C (1976), Zum Wirksamkeitsnachweis von Roßkastaniensamenextrakt beim varikösen Symptomenkomplex. Münch Med Wschr 7:213-216.

Pauschinger P (1987), Klinisch experimentelle Untersuchungen zur Wirkung von Roßkastaniensamenextrakt auf die transkapilläre Filtration und das intravasale Volumen an Patienten mit chronisch venöser Insuffizien. Z Phlebol Proktol 16:57-61.

Preziosi P, Manca P, (1965) Arzneim Forsch 15:404.

Proserpio G et al., (1980) Fitoterapia 2:113.

Rao GS et al., (1974) J Pharm Sci 63:471.

Rothkopf M, Vogel G, Neue Befunde zur Wirksamkeit und zu Wirkungsmechanismen des Roßkastanien-Saponins Aescin. In: Arzneim Forsch 26:225-235. 1976.

Rudofsky G, Neiß A, Otto K, Seibel K (1986), Ödemprotektive Wirkung und klinische Wirksamkeit von Roßkastaniensamenextrakt im Doppelblindversuch. Phlebol Proktol 15:47-54.

Steiner M, Hillemanns HG (1986), Untersuchung zur ödemprotektiven Wirkung eines Venentherapeutikums. Münch Med Wschr 31:551-552.

Steiner M, Untersuchung zur ödemvermindernden und ödemprotektiven Wirkung von Roßkastanienextrakt. In: Phlebol Proktol 19:239-242. 1990.

Vayssairat M et al., Horse-chestnut seed extract for chronic venous insufficiency. In: Lancet 347(9009):182-183. 1996.

Vogel G, Aesculus hippocastanum L. - Die Roβkastanie. In: ZPT 10:102 - 106. 1989.

Vogel G, Marek ML, Stoeckert J, Weitere Untersuchungen zum Wirkungsmechanismus des Roβkastanien-Saponins Aescin. In: Arzneim Forsch 13:59. 1963.

Further information in:

Chan, EH et al. (Eds), Advances in Chinese Medicinal Materials Research, World Scientific Pub. Co. Singapore 1985.

Frohne D, Pfänder HJ, Giftpflanzen - Ein Handbuch für Apotheker, Toxikologen und Biologen, 4. Aufl., Wiss. Verlagsges. mbH Stuttgart 1997.

Hänsel R, Keller K, Rimpler H, Schneider G (Hrsg.), Hagers Handbuch der Pharmazeutischen Praxis, 5. Aufl., Bde 4-6 (Drogen), Springer Verlag Berlin, Heidelberg, New York, 1992-1994.

Madaus G, Lehrbuch der Biologischen Arzneimittel, Bde 1-3, Nachdruck, Georg Olms Verlag Hildesheim 1979.

Roth L, Daunderer M, Kormann K, Giftpflanzen, Pflanzengifte, 4. Aufl., Ecomed Fachverlag Landsberg Lech 1993.

Schulz R, Hänsel R, Rationale Phytotherapie, Springer Verlag Heidelberg 1996.

Steinegger E, Hänsel R, Pharmakognosie, 5. Aufl., Springer Verlag Heidelberg 1992.

Teuscher E, Lindequist U, Biogene Gifte - Biologie, Chemie, Pharmakologie, 2. Aufl., Fischer Verlag Stuttgart 1994.

Teuscher E, Biogene Arzneimittel, 5. Aufl., Wiss. Verlagsges. mbH Stuttgart 1997.

Wagner H, Wiesenauer M, Phytotherapie. Phytopharmaka und pflanzliche Homöopathika, Fischer-Verlag, Stuttgart, Jena, New York 1995.

Wichtl M (Hrsg.), Teedrogen, 4. Aufl., Wiss. Verlagsges. Stuttgart 1997.

Aethusa Cynapium

Fool's Parsley

DESCRIPTION

Medicinal Parts: The medicinal parts are whole of the fresh plant and the dried aerial parts (herb).

Flower and Fruit: White long-stemmed umbels with many florets, no involucre, calyx has 5 fused sepals; 5 white, sometimes reddish, obcordate, irregular petals; 5 stamens; 2-valved ovate ovary; fruit, 3 to 5 mm wide, globose schizocarp, straw yellow when ripe with red-brown stripes and opens easily. Each section has 5 triangular ribs with 1 or 2 oil grooves in the hollow and 2 in the joints.

Leaves, Stem and Root: The plant is a leafy, 60 cm high annual or biennial plant. The root is thin spindle-shaped and whitish. The stem is erect, round, grooved, hollow, glabrous and usually forked with a bluish bloom which rubs off. The leaves are glossy, dark green above, light green beneath. Leaflets are serrate with a triangular outline, double to treble pinnatifid; they give off an unpleasant garlic odor when rubbed.

Characteristics: Poisonous, 3 or 4 leafed pendulous bracteole; the plant can be mistaken for Parsley because of its similar appearance, but the plant is poisonous and this can have fatal consequences. This similarity has resulted in its being given the name Fool's Parsley. It also bears a resemblance to Hemlock, though it is not as poisonous.

Habitat: The plant is indigenous to northern and central Europe, introduced into North America; cultivated and used as an ornamental plant for meadows in southern Germany.

Not To Be Confused With: Young garden parsley is very similar. However, it differs in the glossiness of the underside surface of the leaf and pungent, burning, garlic-like smell of the leaves when rubbed.

Other Names: Dog Poison, Fool's-cicely, Small Hemlock, Dog Parsley, Lesser Hemlock

ACTIONS AND PHARMACOLOGY

COMPOUNDS

Polyynes: (only in freshly-harvested leaves), including aethusin, aethusanol A, aethusanol B

Flavone glycosides: including rutoside, narcissine, camphor oil-3-glucorhamnoside

Ascorbic acid

EFFECTS

No information is available.

INDICATIONS AND USAGE

Fool's-parsley has been used for gastroenteric complaints in children, infantile cholera, summer diarrhea, and convulsions.

PRECAUTIONS AND ADVERSE EFFECTS

Fool's parsley is considered a toxic plant. The older literature contains descriptions of poisonings, sometimes fatal ones, occurring as a result of confusing garden parsley with the freshly-harvested drug. Probably, however, these had to do with poisonings by spotted hemlock. Caution should nevertheless be exercised.

DOSAGE

Mode of Administration: The juice of the fresh drug is used in poultices; also available as alcoholic extracts.

LITERATURE

Bohlmann F et al., Chem Ber 93:981. 1968.

Bohlmann F et al., Chem Ber 88:1245. 1960.

Teuscher E et al., PA 45:537. 1990.

Further information in:

Frohne D, Pfänder HJ, Giftpflanzen - Ein Handbuch für Apotheker, Toxikologen und Biologen, 4. Aufl., Wiss. Verlags-Ges Stuttgart 1997.

Hänsel R, Keller K, Rimpler H, Schneider G (Hrsg.), Hagers Handbuch der Pharmazeutischen Praxis, 5. Aufl., Bde 4 - 6 (Drogen), Springer Verlag Berlin, Heidelberg, New York, 1992-1994.

Lewin L, Gifte und Vergiftungen, 6. Aufl., Nachdruck, Haug Verlag, Heidelberg 1992.

Madaus G, Lehrbuch der Biologischen Arzneimittel, Bde 1-3, Nachdruck, Georg Olms Verlag Hildesheim 1979.

Roth L, Daunderer M, Kormann K, Giftpflanzen, Pflanzengifte, 4. Aufl., Ecomed Fachverlag Landsberg Lech 1993.

Teuscher E, Lindequist U, Biogene Gifte - Biologie, Chemie, Pharmakologie, 2. Aufl., Fischer Verlag Stuttgart 1994.

Aframomum Melegueta

Grains of Paradise

DESCRIPTION

Medicinal Parts: The medicinal parts are the ripe seeds.

Flower and Fruit: The flowers are solitary, mauve and wax-like. The fruit is 10 cm long, pear-shaped and scarlet. The seeds are small, hard, shiny, reddish-brown and oyster-shaped. They have an aromatic and pungent taste and smell.

Leaves, Stem and Root: Aframomum melegueta is a reed-like plant, 1 to 2.5 m high. The leaves are long and narrow.

Habitat: The plant is indigenous to the tropical West Africa.

Not To Be Confused With: The seeds can be mistaken for peppercorns.

Other Names: Guinea Grains, Melegueta Pepper, Mallaguetta Pepper

ACTIONS AND PHARMACOLOGY

COMPOUNDS

Volatile oil

Pungent substances: including hydroxyphenylalkanones and hydroxyphenylalkanoles

Tannins

Starch

Fatty oil

EFFECTS

The seed is a stimulant.

INDICATIONS AND USAGE

Grains of Paradise was used as a stimulant. Now obsolete as a drug.

PRECAUTIONS AND ADVERSE REACTIONS

No health hazards or side effects are known in conjunction with the proper administration of designated therapeutic dosages. Due to the constituent pungent substances, the intake of larger dosages may well lead to irritations of the stomach and the urinary drainage passages.

LITERATURE

Connell WD, J Chem 23:369. 1970.

Further information in:

Hoppe HA (1975-1987) Drogenkunde, 8. Aufl., Bde 1-3, W. de Gruyter Verlag, Berlin, New York.

Kern W, List PH, Hörhammer L (Hrsg.), Hagers Handbuch der Pharmazeutischen Praxis, 4. Aufl., Bde. 1-8, Springer Verlag Berlin, Heidelberg, New York, 1969.

Aga

See Amanita Muscaria

Agar

See Gelidium Amansii

Agrimonia Eupatoria

Agrimony

DESCRIPTION

Medicinal Parts: The drug consists of the flowering plant which is cut a few fingers width above the ground and dried.

Flower and Fruit: Yellow, small, spike-like racemes, epicalyx, 5 sepals, 5 ovate petals, 5 to 20 stamens, 2 ovaries, roughly-haired calyx, deep furrows; fruit is obconical and thorny (burdocks).

Leaves, Stem and Root: Fifty to 100 cm high plant, erect stem, villous; leaves alternate; irregularly pinnate; deeply serrate leaflets, downy beneath.

Characteristics: Agrimony has a slight pleasant fragrance and a tangy, bitter taste.

Habitat: The plant is indigenous to middle and northern Europe, temperate Asia, and North America.

Production: Agrimony herb consists of the dried, above-ground parts of Agrimonia eupatoria and/or Agrimonia procera Wallroth, gathered just before or during flowering, as well as its preparations in effective dosage.

Other Names: Stickwort, Cocklebur, Liverwort, Common Agrimony, Philanthropos, Church Steeples, Sticklewort

ACTIONS AND PHARMACOLOGY

COMPOUNDS

Catechin tannins

EFFECTS

Agrimony is an astringent.

INDICATIONS AND USAGE

- Diarrhea
- Inflammation of the skin
- Inflammation of the mouth and pharynx

Agrimony is used internally for mild, nonspecific, acute diarrhea, and inflammation of oral and pharyngeal mucosa; externally for mild and superficial inflammation of the skin.

PRECAUTIONS AND ADVERSE REACTIONS

No health hazards or side effects are known in conjunction with the proper administration of designated therapeutic dosages. Because of the constituent tannins, the intake of larger quantities could well lead to digestive complaints and constipation.

DOSAGE

Daily Dosage: The average daily dose is 3 gm of herb or equivalent preparations.

LITERATURE

Bilai AR et al., A flavonol glycoside from Agrimonia eupatoria. In: PH 32:1078. 1993.

Chon SC et al., (1987) Med Pharmacol Exp 16(5):407-413.

Drozd GA et al., (1983) Khim Prir Soed 1:106.

Patrascu V et al., (1984) Ser. Dermato-Venerol 29(2):153-157.

Peter-Horvath M et al., (1964) Rev Med 10(2):190-193.

Further information in:

Kern W, List PH, Hörhammer L (Hrsg.), Hagers Handbuch der Pharmazeutischen Praxis, 4. Aufl., Bde. 1-8, Springer Verlag Berlin, Heidelberg, New York, 1969.

Madaus G, Lehrbuch der Biologischen Arzneimittel, Bde 1-3, Nachdruck, Georg Olms Verlag Hildesheim 1979.

Teuscher E, Biogene Arzneimittel, 5. Aufl., Wiss. Verlagsges. Stuttgart 1997.

Wichtl M (Hrsg.), Teedrogen, 4. Aufl., Wiss. Verlagsges. Stuttgart 1997.

Agrimony

See Agrimonia Eupatoria

Ailanthus Altissima

Tree of Heaven

DESCRIPTION

Medicinal Parts: The medicinal parts are the dried trunk and root bark.

Flower and Fruit: The small, greenish-yellow flower is in branched, axillary or terminal panicles. Some of the flowers are male, some female and some androgynous. The calyx is short and has 5 glandular, fused sepals. The sepals are much longer than the corolla and have 5 hollow, splayed petals. There are 10 stamens, often only 5 in the androgynous and rudimentary remains in the female flowers. There are 5 obovate, compressed ovaries with 5 splayed stigmas. There is a narrow, oblong-lanceolate schizocarp, 4 to 5 cm by 1 cm. It is winged above and below, first green then brown-red and finally brown. The seed is orbicular and found in the middle of the fruit section. It is thin-skinned, without any recognizable endosperm and has an ovate, flat cotyledon.

Leaves, Stem and Root: Ailanthus altissima is a beautiful, fast growing tree, up to 30 m high. The bark is smooth, pale and vertically striated. The branches are initially fine-haired, yellow or red brown. The leaves are up to 1 m long and odd-pinnate. The upper surface of the leaves is dark green and the under-surface is light gray-green. Both sides of the leaf are glandular-haired. The leaflets are ovate to oblong-lanceolate. The shallow, cordate base of the leaflets has 1 to 3 small lobes at either side, each with 1 gland. The wood surface is satin-like and white.

Characteristics: The flowers have a strong elder flower scent. The fresh bark and leaves give off an unpleasant, nauseating smell.

Habitat: The tree was originally indigenous to China. Today it grows in the wild and is cultivated in tropical and subtropical eastern Asia, northern Europe and North America.

Production: Tree of Heaven bark is the trunk and branch bark of Ailanthus altissima. The bark is gathered the whole year round. The outer bark is removed and dried in the sun. After drying, there is a process of sorting and removing foreign bodies, washing, macerating and a second drying.

Other Names: Ailanto, Chinese Sumach, Vernis de Japon

ACTIONS AND PHARMACOLOGY

COMPOUNDS

Quassinoids: including ailanthone, quassin

Indole alkaloids of the beta-carbolic type

Tannins

EFFECTS

An antimalarial action is being tested in an in-vitro vitro trial. The active agents also have astringent, antipyretic, and antispasmodic properties.

INDICATIONS AND USAGE

In Chinese medicine, the drug is used for pathological leukorrea, diarrhea, chronic diarrhea, chronic dysentery and dysmenorrhea. In Africa, it is also used for cramps, asthma, fast heart rate, gonorrhea, epilepsy and tapeworm infestation. It is increasingly used in the treatment of malaria.

Efficacy has not been proven.

PRECAUTIONS AND ADVERSE REACTIONS

Large doses of the drug are said to lead to queasiness, dizziness, headache, tingling in the limbs and diarrhea.

OVERDOSAGE

Fatal poisonings have been observed in animal experiments.

DOSAGE

Mode of Administration: Tree of Heaven is still being researched as a drug, up until now it has only been used in folk medicine.

Daily Dose: 6 to 9 g.

Storage: Keep in a dry, well-ventilated area away from moths.

LITERATURE

Bray DH et al., (1987) Phytother Res 1(1):22.

Casinovi CG et al., (1964) Tetrahedron Lett: 3991.

Casinovi CG et al., Tetrahedron Lett: 2273. 1965.

Furuno T et al., Bull Chem Soc Jpn 57:2484-2489. 1984.

Geissmann T, (1964) Ann Rev Pharmacol 4:305.

Ghosh P et al, (1977) Lloydia 40(4):636.

Ishibashi M et al., Bull Chem Soc Jpn 56:3683-3693. 1983.

Ishibashi M et al., Bull Chem Soc Jpn 57:2013-2014. 1984.

Ishibashi M et al., Bull Chem Soc Jpn 58:2723-2724. 1985.

Ishibashi M et al., Chem Pharm Bull 31:2179-2182. 1983.

Ishibashi M et al., Tetrahedron Lett:1205-1206. 1985.

Naora H et al., Bull Chem Soc Jpn 56:3694-3698. 1983.

Niimi Y et al., Chem Pharm Bull 35:4302-4306. 1987.

Ohmoto T et al., Chem Pharm Bull 29:390-395. 1981.

Ohmoto T et al., Chem Pharm Bull 32:170-173. 1984.

Polonski J, (1985) Prog Chem Org Nat Prod 47:221.

Polonsky J, (1973) Fortschr Chem Org Naturst 30:101.

Rücker G, Malariawirksame Verbindungen aus Pflanzen, insbesondere Peroxide. In: PUZ 24(4):189-195. 1995.

Varga E et al., (1980) Planta Med 40:337-339.

Varga E et al., Fitoterapia 52:183-186. 1981.

Further information in:

Hänsel R, Keller K, Rimpler H, Schneider G (Hrsg.), Hagers Handbuch der Pharmazeutischen Praxis, 5. Aufl., Bde 4 - 6 (Drogen), Springer Verlag Berlin, Heidelberg, New York, 1992-1994.

Lewin L, Gifte und Vergiftungen, 6. Aufl., Nachdruck, Haug Verlag, Heidelberg 1992.

Madaus G, Lehrbuch der Biologischen Arzneimittel, Bde 1-3, Nachdruck, Georg Olms Verlag Hildesheim 1979.

Roth L, Daunderer M, Kormann K, Giftpflanzen, Pflanzengifte, 4. Aufl., Ecomed Fachverlag Landsberg Lech 1993.

Ajuga Chamaepitys

Ground Pine

DESCRIPTION

Flower and Fruit: The plant has 2 to 4 flowers at each node. The petals are 4 to 6 mm. The tips of the petals are as long as or shorter than the tube. The corolla is yellow with red or purple markings, rarely entirely purple. The lower lip is entire and the stamens are exerted. The filaments are hairy. The mericarps are 2 to 5 mm long, obovate, reticulate-wrinkled and have a pitted surface.

Leaves, Stem and Root: Ground Pine is an annual or short-lived perennial. The stem is 5 to 30 cm long. It is usually heavily branched, glabrous to densely villous. The leaves are 3-partite with linear segments. They are 0.5 to 4 mm wide. The segments are sometimes 3-pinnatifid. The bracts are similar to the leaves.

Habitat: Sandy, stony areas of southern Britain and parts of Europe.

Other Names: Yellow Bugle

ACTIONS AND PHARMACOLOGY

COMPOUNDS

Volatile oil

Diterpene bitter principles

Caffeic acid derivatives: including rosemary acid

EFFECTS

Emmenagogue (stimulates menstrual flow), stimulant, diuretic.

INDICATIONS AND USAGE

Ground Pine is used for gout, rheumatism and gynecological disorders.

PRECAUTIONS AND ADVERSE REACTIONS

No health hazards or side effects are known in conjunction with the proper administration of designated therapeutic dosages.

DOSAGE

Mode of Administration: Mostly in combinations, as a liquid extract.

LITERATURE

Camps F et al., (1985) An Quim 81C(1):74-75.

Kooiman P, (1972) Acta Bot Nederl 21(4):417.

Ajuga Reptans

Bugle

DESCRIPTION

Medicinal Parts: The medicinal parts are the aerial parts collected during the flowering season and dried.

Flower and Fruit: The flowers are from 1 to 1.5 cm long. The flowers are in spikes. They are located in the axils of undivided bracts at the end of the stem. The 5-tipped, hairy calyx is short-stemmed, erect, labiate and campanulate. The tips are triangular and about as long as the tube. The corolla is bright violet-blue, pink or white. It is downy-haired on the outside with a long straight tube, which has a circle of hairs under the stamen. There are 4 stamens with yellow anthers. The 4 mericarps are 2 mm long and finely reticulate.

Leaves, Stem and Root: Ajuga Reptans is a shrub, up to 30 cm high with overground rooting runners sprouting from the rosette-like basal leaves. The flower stem is quadrangular, villous above and glabrous below. The rest of the plant is glabrous. The basal leaves are large, long-petioled, spatulate and dentate. The cauline leaves are crossed opposite, short-petioled, small and oval. The lowest or at least the third lowest stem is flower-bearing. There are some upper false whorls, which are compressed into a false spike.

Habitat: The plant is found in Europe, Britain, parts of Asia and northern Africa.

Production: The aerial parts of Ajuga reptans are picked when in bloom and dried. Gathered in uncultivated areas (the wild).

Other Names: Bugula, Middle Comfrey, Middle Confound, Sicklewort, Carpenter's Herb

ACTIONS AND PHARMACOLOGY

COMPOUNDS

Iridoid glycosides and ajugols

Phytoecdysone: ajugalactone

Diterpene bitter principles

Caffeic acid derivatives: including rosemary acid

EFFECTS

There is no information available.

INDICATIONS AND USAGE

Internally, Bugle is used as an astringent for inflammation of the mouth and larynx. It is also used for gallbladder and stomach disorders. Externally, the plant is used for the treatment of wounds.

Efficacy has not been proven.

PRECAUTIONS AND ADVERSE REACTIONS

No health hazards or side effects are known in conjunction with the proper administration of designated therapeutic dosages.

DOSAGE

Mode of Administration: Bugle is used topically, in alcoholic extracts, as a water infusion and in teas.

LITERATURE

Breschi M, Martinotti E, Catalano S, Flamini G, Morelli I, Pagni A, Vasoconstrictor activity of 8-O-Acetylharpagide from Ajuga reptans. In: JNP 55: 1145-1148. 1992.

Camps F et al., (1985) An Quim 81C(1):74-75.

Camps F et al., Rev Latinoamj Quim 12:81-88. 1981.

Camps F, Coll J, Insect allochemicals from Ajuga plants. In: PH 32:1361. 1993.

Komissarenko NF et al., Khim Prir Soedin 11:109-110. 1976.

Kooiman P, (1972) Acta Bot Nederl. 21(4):417.

Ruhdorfer J, Rimpler H, Z Naturforsch 36c:697-707. 1981.

Further information in:

Hänsel R, Keller K, Rimpler H, Schneider G (Hrsg.), Hagers Handbuch der Pharmazeutischen Praxis, 5. Aufl., Bde 4-6 (Drogen), Springer Verlag Berlin, Heidelberg, New York, 1992-1994.

Alcea Rosea

Hollyhock

DESCRIPTION

Medicinal Parts: The medicinal parts are the dried flowers of plants bearing dark purple flowers.

Flower and Fruit: Six to 10 cm flowers sit in the axils of the cauline leaves singly or in groups of 2 or 4, with the upper ones forming long spikes. Sepals of the epicalyx are broadly triangular and sharp-edged. The epicalyx is significantly shorter than the calyx and both are gray-green haired.

Leaves, Stem and Root: Alcea rosea is a biennial plant, which produces in the second year, a spire-like, hairy stem up to 3 m tall. Leaves are cordate-orbicular to rhomboid, weakly 3- to 5-lobed, and slightly scabrid-setulose. The sepals are epiclyx-subacute and triangular. The flowers are found in the leaf axils with short peduncles. The petals are 30 to 50 mm, contiguous, usually pink but sometimes white or violet. The mericarps are 7 mm long. The dorsal face has a deep, narrow furrow with rugose angles produced into parallel wings. The lateral faces are appressed-setose.

Habitat: Originally indigenous to southwest and central Asia. A few species were probably introduced into southeast central Europe as ornamental plants and then spread in the wild. Cultivated in Europe and temperate regions of Asia.

Other Names: Althea rose, Malva flowers, Rose mallow

ACTIONS AND PHARMACOLOGY

COMPOUNDS

Mucilages (acetylated galacturonorhamane)

Anthocyans (termed althaein): delphinidine- and malvidine-mono glycosides

EFFECTS

No information is available.

INDICATIONS AND USAGE

Hollyhock flower is used as mucilage for prophylaxis and therapy of diseases and discomforts of the respiratory tract and the gastrointestinal tract. The effectiveness for the claimed applications is not verified.

PRECAUTIONS AND ADVERSE REACTIONS

No health hazards or side effects are known in conjunction with the proper administration of designated therapeutic dosages.

LITERATURE

Hänsel R, Keller K, Rimpler H, Schneider G (Hrsg.), Hagers Handbuch der Pharmazeutischen Praxis, 5. Aufl., Bde 4-6 (Drogen), Springer Verlag Berlin, Heidelberg, New York, 1992-1994 (unter Alcea rosea).

Steinegger E, Hänsel R, Pharmakognosie, 5. Aufl., Springer Verlag Heidelberg 1992 (unter Alcea rosea).

Teuscher E, Biogene Arzneimittel, 5. Aufl., Wiss. Verlagsges. Stuttgart 1997.

Alchemilla Vulgaris

Lady's Mantle

DESCRIPTION

Medicinal Parts: The medicinal part is the herb collected in the flowering season and dried.

Flower and Fruit: The plant has inflorescences of small, insignificant, yellow-green many-flowered cymes. The perianth is 4-leaved. The flower has 4 stamens, 1 ovary and an inferior style. The fruit is enclosed in the calyx. The flowers are infertile.

Leaves, Stem and Root: Alchemilla vulgaris is a hardy, half-rosette shrub which grows from 30 to 50 cm. It has a branched stem which is villous to glabrous. The basal leaves are round, 7 to 9-lobed (dew cup); cauline leaves are short-petioled to sessile, 5 to 7 lobed, crenate or serrate and villous. Even the older leaves remain more or less folded.

Characteristics: Lady's Mantle is odorless and has an astringent taste.

Habitat: The plant grows in the whole of the northern hemisphere from North America, Greenland and Europe to the Mediterranean and Iceland; and Asia from the Caucasus and the Himalayas to Siberia.

Production: Lady's Mantle herb consists of the fresh or dried above-ground parts of Alchemilla vulgaris gathered at flowering time, as well as its preparations. It is produced mostly through cultivation.

Other Names: Bear's Foot, Leontopodium, Lion's Foot, Nine Hooks, Stellaria

ACTIONS AND PHARMACOLOGY

COMPOUNDS

Bitter principles

Flavonoids

Tannins

EFFECTS

Lady's Mantle herb has astringent properties, due to the presence of tannins. It has also been shown to inhibit tumor growth. In mice the total retardation of breast neoplasm-induced tumors was achieved using agrimoniin and the average life expectancy of the animals was increased. An extract of the drug hinders the enzymes elastase, trypsin, and a-chymotrysin.

INDICATIONS AND USAGE

■ Diarrhea

Lady's Mantle is used for mild and non-specific diarrhea and gastrointestinal disorders.

In folk medicine the drug is used internally for menopausal complaints, dysmenorrhea, gastrointestinal disorders, and as a gargle for mouth and throat inflammation. Externally, it is used for ulcers, eczema and other skin rashes and as an additive in baths for the treatment of lower-abdominal ailments.

PRECAUTIONS AND ADVERSE REACTIONS

No health hazards or side effects are known in conjunction with the proper administration of designated therapeutic dosages.

DOSAGE

Mode of Administration: Lady's Mantle herb is administered as a cut herb for infusions and decoctions, as well as other galenic preparations for internal use.

Daily Dosage: Lady's Mantle herb is administered in 2 to 4 gm single doses as an infusion; the average daily dose is 5 to 10 gm of herb. The tea is taken 3 times daily between meals.

LITERATURE

Dorne AJ et al., PH 25:65-68. 1986.

Filípek J, The effect of Alchemilla xanthochlora on lipid peroxidation and superoxide anion scavenging acticity. In: PA 47:717-718. 1992.

Geiger C, Rimpler H, PM 56:585-586. 1990.

Geiger C, Ellagitannine aus Alchemilla xanthochlora ROTHMALER und Potentilla erecta (L.) RAEUSCHEL. Beiträge zur Analytik und Strukturaufklärung. In: Dissertation Universität Freiburg. 1990.

Schimmer O, Felser C, Alchemilla xanthochlora ROTHM.- Der Frauenmantel. In: ZPT 13(6):207. 1993.

Schimmer O, Lindenbaum M, Tannins with antimutagenic properties in the herb of Alchemilla species and Potentilla anserina. In: PM 61(2):141-145. 1995.

Further information in:

Hänsel R, Keller K, Rimpler H, Schneider G (Hrsg.), Hagers Handbuch der Pharmazeutischen Praxis, 5. Aufl., Bde 4-6 (Drogen), Springer Verlag Berlin, Heidelberg, New York, 1992-1994.

Madaus G, Lehrbuch der Biologischen Arzneimittel, Bde 1-3, Nachdruck, Georg Olms Verlag Hildesheim 1979.

Wagner H, Wiesenauer M, Phytotherapie. Phytopharmaka und pflanzliche Homöopathika, Fischer-Verlag, Stuttgart, Jena, New York 1995.

Wichtl M (Hrsg.), Teedrogen, 4. Aufl., Wiss. Verlagsges. Stuttgart 1997.

Aletris Farinosa

True Unicorn Root

DESCRIPTION

Medicinal Parts: The medicinal part is the dried Aletris farinosa rhizome with roots. Fresh underground parts dug up after flowering are also used.

Flower and Fruit: The plant has numerous white, tubular-oblong, campanulate flowers. The flowers, with a few small bracts are in terminal, spike-like racemes on stalks that reach up to 1 m. The perianth is tubular, covered in scales and shrinks when ripe. Later, the perianth springs open in a beak shape. The fruit is an ovoid capsule containing many oblong ribbed seeds.

Leaves, Stem and Root: The leaves are erect-oblong, lanceolate and 2 to 20 cm long. The rhizome is brownish-gray, flattened and has a diameter of up to 1 cm, but is usually less. The upper part is covered in leaf bases and stem scars. The fracture is floury and white.

Characteristics: The plant has a sweet taste, becoming bitter and soapy. The odor is mild.

Habitat: The plant is found in the northeast U.S., south to Gulf of Mexico, southern Canada.

Production: True Unicorn root is the rhizome of Aletris farinosa. It is gathered in the wild, and air-dried in the shade.

Other Names: Star Grass, Colic-root, Starwort, Blazing Star, Ague-root, Aloe-root, Ague Grass, Black-root, Bitter Grass, Crow Corn, Bettie Grass, Devil's Bit, True Unicorn Star-Grass

ACTIONS AND PHARMACOLOGY

COMPOUNDS

Saponins

Volatile oil

Resins

Bitter principles

Starch

EFFECTS

The active agents increase motility, and act as a tonic. There may be an estrogenic principle but a possible estrogenic effect has not been sufficiently researched.

INDICATIONS AND USAGE

No clinical trial reports or documented observations are available.

In the U.S., the plant is used for gynecological disorders or ''female complaints'', in particular dysmenorrhea, amenorrhea and complaints associated with prolapses vaginae.

Preparations of False Unicorn Root are also used for loss of appetite, venous dyspepsia, flatulence and nervous digestive complaints. In Argentina, it is used to treat chronic bronchitis.

PRECAUTIONS AND ADVERSE REACTIONS

No health hazards or side effects are known in conjunction with the proper administration of designated therapeutic dosages.

DOSAGE

Mode of Administration: Available in the forms of powdered root, liquid extract and infusions for internal use.

Preparation: To prepare an infusion, 1.5 gm of the drug is added to 100 ml of water. A fluid extract (1:1) is produced with ethanol water (45%).

Daily Dosage: The recommended dose is 0.3 to 0.6 gm to be taken 3 times daily.

LITERATURE

Costello CH, Lynn EV, (1950) J Am Pharm Ass 39:117.

Marker RE et al., (1940) J Chem Soc 60:2620.

Further information in:

Hänsel R, Keller K, Rimpler H, Schneider G (Hrsg.), Hagers Handbuch der Pharmazeutischen Praxis, 5. Aufl., Bde 4 - 6 (Drogen), Springer Verlag Berlin, Heidelberg, New York, 1992-1994.

Madaus G, Lehrbuch der Biologischen Arzneimittel, Bde 1-3, Nachdruck, Georg Olms Verlag Hildesheim 1979.

Wagner H, Wiesenauer M, Phytotherapie. Phytopharmaka und pflanzliche Homeopathika, Fischer-Verlag, Stuttgart, Jena, New York 1995.

Alfalfa

See Medicago Sativa

Alisma Plantago-aquatica

Water Plantain

DESCRIPTION

Medicinal Parts: The medicinal part is the fresh rhizome.

Flower and Fruit: The peduncle is triangular. There are long-pedicled, white or reddish flowers in leafless, loose panicles. There are 3 sepals, 3 petals and 3 stamens in the flower. The fruit is small and obtuse and is formed by 15 to 30 ovaries.

Leaves, Stem and Root: The water leaves are ribbon-like. There are long stemmed, swimming leaves. The aerial leaves are basal, long-stemmed, cordate or oblong-ovate, and spoon-like.

Characteristics: Water Plantain has a bitter taste in rootstock. It is poisonous when fresh.

Habitat: The plant is distributed widely throughout Europe, northern Asia, and North America.

Other Names: Mad-Dog Weed

ACTIONS AND PHARMACOLOGY

COMPOUNDS

Triterpenes: including: alisol-A, alisol-B, alisol-C and their monoacetates

Sesquiterpenes

Flavone sulfate

Caffeic acid derivatives: chlorogenic acid sulfate

EFFECTS

No information is available.

INDICATIONS AND USAGE

The drug is used for diseases of the bladder and urinary tract.

PRECAUTIONS AND ADVERSE REACTIONS

No health hazards or side effects are known in conjunction with the proper administration of designated therapeutic dosages.

DOSAGE

Mode of Administration: The drug is available as an extract for oral use. The root is also used in homeopathy.

LITERATURE

Murata T et al., (1968) Tetrahedron Letteers 103:849.

Murata T et al., Chem Pharm Bull 18:1369. 1970.

Oshima Y et al., PH 22:183. 1983.

Further information in:

Kern W, List PH, Hörhammer L (Hrsg.), Hagers Handbuch der Pharmazeutischen Praxis, 4. Aufl., Bde 1-8, Springer Verlag Berlin, Heidelberg, New York, 1969.

Alkanna Tinctoria

Alkanna

DESCRIPTION

Medicinal Parts: The medicinal part is the root of the plant (the dried roots and rhizomes).

Flower and Fruit: The calyx is 4 to 5 mm in the flower, 5 to 6 mm in the fruit and eglandular. The corolla is blue and glabrous outside. The funnel is as long as or slightly longer than the calyx. The limb is 6 to 7 mm in diameter. There are 5 stamens and the anthers are fused with the corolla tube. The nutlets are 2 mm in diameter, irregularly reticulate and tuberculate.

Leaves, Stem and Root: Alkanna is a short-bristled, perennial half-rosette shrub. The stems are 10 to 20 cm, procumbent or ascending and glandular. The basal leaves are 6 to 15 cm by 0.7 to 1.5 cm, linear-lanceolate; the lower ones are cauline, oblong-linear and cordate at base. The bracts are slightly longer than calyx and oblong-lanceolate. The neck of the root is covered with the remains of leaves and the stems. The root is spindle-shaped, curved, up to 25 cm long and 1.5 cm thick, with purplish root bark.

Habitat: The plant is indigenous to southeastern Europe and some parts of Turkey and Hungary; cultivated in other parts of Europe, Britain, and northern Africa.

Production: Alkanna rhizomes are the dried roots and rhizomes of Alkanna tinctoria Tausch.

Other Names: Anchusa, Dyer's Bugloss, Spanish Bugloss, Alkanet root

ACTIONS AND PHARMACOLOGY

COMPOUNDS

Naphthazarine derivatives: including the ester of the (-)-alkannin (stained red)

Pyrrolizidine alkaloids

Tannins

EFFECTS

Antimicrobial action: In the agar diffusion test, Alkanna root extracts and Alkannin esters impaired the growth of *Staphylococcus aureus* and *Staphylococcus epidermidis*, however Alkannin worked only against *Candida albicans*.

Healing action for wounds: in a double-blind study, 72 patients, suffering from ulcers of the leg (Ulcus cruris) caused by varicose veins, were treated with Histoplastin Red® over a period of three years. After 5 to 6 weeks' daily administration, 80% of the patients' ulcers had healed or were considerably reduced in size.

The results are difficult to assess, as details concerning the patients, the treatment pattern and control groups are unavailable.

INDICATIONS AND USAGE

Used by the ancient Greeks to heal wounds; also for skin diseases and diarrhea.

Efficacy has not been adequately proven.

PRECAUTIONS AND ADVERSE REACTIONS

Hepatotoxicity and carcinogenity are expected, due to the pyrrolizidine alkaloids with 1,2-unsaturated necic parent substances in its makeup. Alkanna should not be taken internally for this reason.

DOSAGE

Mode of Administration: Seldom used as a drug. Taking internally is not to be recommended in any way, due to its toxic characteristics and its uncertain efficacy. Alkannin and extracts of the root are used externally in pharmacy.

Preparations: Extractum alcannae: almost black, green glistening mass (no extraction information).

Histoplastin Red® ointment: the ointment approved in Greece, contains 76.5g loosely defined ethereal oily alkanna root extract with lipophil ointment base (beeswax, mastic rubber and olive oil q.s. ad 100g).

LITERATURE

Majlathova L (1971) Nahrung 15:505.

Papageorgiou VP (1980) Planta Med 38(3):193-203.

Papageorgiou VP, PM 31:390-394. 1977.

Papageorgiou VP, Digenis GA, PM 39:81-84. 1980.

Röder E, Pyrrolizidinhaltige Arzneipflanzen. In: DAZ 132(45):2427-2435. 1992.

Röder E et al., PH 23:2125-2126. 1984.

Wiedenfield H et al., (1985) Arch Pharm 318(4):294.

Further information in:

Hänsel R, Keller K, Rimpler H, Schneider G (Hrsg.), Hagers Handbuch der Pharmazeutischen Praxis, 5. Aufl., Bde 4-6 (Drogen), Springer Verlag Berlin, Heidelberg, New York, 1992-1994.

Wichtl M (Hrsg.), Teedrogen, 4. Aufl., Wiss. Verlagsges. Stuttgart 1997.

Allium Cepa

Onion

DESCRIPTION

Medicinal Parts: The medicinal part is the bulb.

Flower and Fruit: The peduncles are up to 3 cm long. The flowers are greenish-white, in orbicular umbels, with 6 free flower bracts that are shorter than the 6 stamens. The pedicles are eight times as long as the flowers. The fruit is a thin-skinned capsule. The seeds are black and angular. The flowers are in globular umbels, before blooming in membranous sheaths.

Leaves, Stem and Root: The plant is perennial or biennial. There are many varieties and can be compressed-globose, ovate or oblong. Most varieties have secondary bulbs. Leaves are shorter than the peduncle, tubular or swollen and blue-green. There is a hollow scape, which is gray-blue, expanded and bloated below the middle.

Habitat: Central Asia is considered to be the region of origin; introduced to the Mediterranean; cultivated worldwide.

Production: Onion consists of the fresh or dried, thick and fleshy leaf sheaths and stipules of Allium cepa.

ACTIONS AND PHARMACOLOGY

COMPOUNDS

Alliins (alkylcysteine sulphoxides): in particular allylalliin (allyl-L-(+)-cysteine sulphoxide) and its gamma-glutamyl conjugates, that in the course of cutting up either the freshly-harvested bulbs or those that have been already dried and then re-moistened, are transformed into the so-called alliaceous oils.

Fructosans (polysaccharides)

Saccharose and other sugars

EFFECTS

The thiosulphinate exhibits an antimicrobial effect, and is effective against *Bacillus subtilis*, *Salmonella typhi*, *Pseudomonas aeroginosa* and *Escherichia coli*.

Lipid and blood pressure lowering effect: certain constituents function similarly to those in garlic, although this is not yet clinically proven.

Inhibits thrombocyte aggregation: dimethyl and diphenylthiosulphinateboth retard thrombocyte biosynthesis using thrombase stimulation.

Antiasthmatic and antiallergic effect: guinea pigs sensitized using ovalbumin were protected from asthma attack through the oral administration of onion juice. Administration of an ethanol onion extract significantly reduced allergy-induced bronchial constriction in asthma patients.

INDICATIONS AND USAGE

- Loss of appetite
- Arteriosclerosis
- Dyspeptic complaints
- Fevers and colds
- Cough/bronchitis
- Hypertension
- Tendency to infection
- Inflammation of the mouth and pharynx
- Common cold

In folk medicine the drug is administered internally for cough, whooping cough, bronchitis, asthma and angina; to stimulate gallbladder functions, for digestive disorders with bloating and colic pain, for dehydration, as an aid at the introduction of menstruation, for ascariasis, high blood pressure, arteriosclerosis and in the treatment of diabetes. Externally the drug is used for insect bites, wounds, light burns, furuncles, warts, and in the after-care of bruises.

The efficacy of Onion in folk medicine is unproved.

PRECAUTIONS AND ADVERSE REACTIONS

No health hazards or side effects are known in conjunction with the proper administration of designated therapeutic dosages. The intake of large quantities can lead to stomach complaints. Frequent contact with the drug leads on rare occasion to allergic reactions (hand eczema).

DOSAGE

Mode of Administration: Cut onions, pressed juice from fresh onions and other oral galenic preparations.

Preparation: Onion oil maceration: same as garlic maceration drug extract 1:1

Old recipe: Siripus Cepae: freshly grated onions 15 g; water 60 ml; ethanol 90%(V/V) 15 ml; saccharose 150 g; the ethanolic extract is boiled with the saccharose.

Popular: pressed juice and onion syrup: made of 500 g onions, 500 g water, 100 g honey and 350 g sugar.

Onion tincture: 100 g minced onions in 300 g ethanol 70% macerated for 10 days.

Daily Dosage: Raw drug is used therapeutically.

Externally the juice is spread or laid on as a poultice or in slices.

Internally: onion tincture 4 to 5 teaspoonfuls daily; onion syrup 4 to 5 tablespoons daily.

Average daily dose: 50 g of fresh onions or 20 g of dried drug.

LITERATURE

Agarwal RH, Controlled trial of the effect of cycloalliin on the fibrinolytic activity of venous blood. In: Atherosclerosis 27:347-351. 1977.

Augusti KT, Benaim ME, (1974) Clin Chim Acta 60:121.

Augusti KT, (1976) Curr Sci 45:863.

Dorsch W, et al., (1984) Eur J Pharmacol 107(1):17.

Jain RC, Vyas CR (1974) Brit Med J 2:730.

Kabelik J, (1970) Pharmazie 25:266.

Koch HP, Hormonwirkungen bei Allium-Arten. In: ZPT 13(6):177. 1992.

Kumari K, Augusti KT, Antidiabetic effects of S-methylcystein sulphoxide on alloxan diabetes. In: PM 61(1):72-74. 1995.

Liakopoulou-Kyriakides M et al., (1985) Phytochemistry 24: 600 and 1593.

Maugh TH, (1979) Science 204:293.

Spare CG, Virtanen AI, (1963) Acta Chem Scand 17:641.

Tverskoy L, Dmetriev A, Kozlovsky A, Grodzinsky D, Two phytoalexins from Allium-cepa bulbs. In: PH 30:799. 1991.

Vollhardt BR, Zwiebelölmazerat (z.B. Alligerol). In: Intern Praxis 32(1):201. 1992.

Wagner H, Bayer Th, Dorsch W, Das antiasthmatische Wirkprinzip der Zwiebel (Allium cepa L.). In: ZPT 9(6):165. 1988.

Whitaker JR (1976) Adv Food Res 22:73.

Zwiebeln gegen Durchfall. In: Medical Tribune 14:26. 1993.

Further information in:

Hänsel R, Keller K, Rimpler H, Schneider G (Hrsg.), Hagers Handbuch der Pharmazeutischen Praxis, 5. Aufl., Bde 4 - 6 (Drogen), Springer Verlag Berlin, Heidelberg, New York, 1992-1994.

Madaus G, Lehrbuch der Biologischen Arzneimittel, Bde 1-3, Nachdruck, Georg Olms Verlag Hildesheim 1979.

Wagner H, Wiesenauer M, Phytotherapie. Phytopharmaka und pflanzliche Homöopathika, Fischer-Verlag, Stuttgart, Jena, New York 1995.

Allium Sativum

Garlic

DESCRIPTION

Medicinal Parts: The medicinal parts are the whole fresh bulb, the dried bulb, and the oil of garlic.

Flower and Fruit: The long-pedicled flowers have a cyme with few florets. The numerous bulbils shed simultaneously. The flowers usually remain in bud form and often do not produce any seed. The petals are reddish or greenish white and longer than the stamens. The anthers of the middle stamens are spread at the base and have fan-shaped tips.

Leaves, Stem and Root: Allium sativum is a perennial. The plant is 25 to 70 cm high with an erect, rigid or crook-like stem, which is leafy to the middle. The leaves are flat, 4 to 25 mm, broad-linear, rough or smooth-edged, with a wedge-shaped tip. The sheath is beaked and longer than the inflorescence. The garlic bulb is usually a compound bulb; secondary bulbs are ovate. The bulb skin is silky white or green.

Habitat: Central Asia is considered to be the region of origin; introduced to the Mediterranean; cultivated worldwide.

Production: Bulbous garlic, consists of fresh or carefully dried bulbs which consist of the main bulb with several secondary bulbs (cloves). Garlic may be harvested in September and October when the leaves and bulbs are dry.

Other Names: Poor Man's Treacle, Clove Garlic

ACTIONS AND PHARMACOLOGY

COMPOUNDS

Alliins (alkylcysteine sulfoxides): in particular allylalliin (allyl-L-(+)-cysteine sulfoxide) and its gamma-glutamyl conjugates, that in the course of cutting up either the freshly-harvested bulbs or those that have been already dried and then re-moistened, are transformed into the so-called alliaceous oils: for example, into allicin (diallyl-disulphide-mono-S-oxide), cycloalliin, vinyl dithiins and diallyl-di- and trisulphides

Fructosans (polysaccharides)

Saponins

EFFECTS

The antibacterial, antimycotic, and lipid-lowering effects of garlic are proven. The drug also inhibits platelet aggregation, prolongs bleeding and clotting time, and enhances fibrinolytic activity.

INDICATIONS AND USAGE

- Arteriosclerosis
- Common cold
- Cough/bronchitis
- Fevers and colds
- Inflammation of the mouth and pharynx
- Tendency to infection

Garlic is used as a supportive to dietetic measures for elevated lipid levels in blood. The drug is also used as a preventative measure for age-related vascular changes.

In folk medicine, garlic is utilized internally for arteriosclerosis, high blood pressure, colds, coughs, whooping cough, and bronchitis. Garlic is also used for gastrointestinal ailments, particularly for digestive disorders with bloating and convulsive pain. Other uses include: menstrual pains, treatment of diabetes, and as a tonic for diverse illnesses and debilities; externally for corns, warts, calluses, otitis, muscle pain, neuralgia, arthritis, and sciatica.

PRECAUTIONS AND ADVERSE REACTIONS

No health hazards or side effects are known in conjunction with the proper administration of designated therapeutic dosages. The intake of large quantities can lead to stomach complaints. Frequent contact with the drug leads on rare occasion to allergic reactions (hand eczema).

DOSAGE

Mode of Administration: The minced bulb and preparations are for internal use and external treatment. Garlic oil in the form of a maceration or as a result of steam distillation is widely available.

Preparation: Garlic oil maceration - bulbs are homogenized and stirred in fatty oil (1:1) for 48 hours, and filtered.

Solid garlic extract - an extraction of the chopped bulbs with ethanol or methanol is allowed to evaporate.

Aqueous extract - fresh bulbs are macerated in cold water (1:1).

Fermented garlic - the minced drug is soaked over a long duration in a water-ethanol mixture, volatile agents escape and the garlic becomes odorless. Steam distillations and tinctures are also possible.

Daily Dosage: The average daily dose is 4 gm of fresh garlic or 8 mg of essential oil. One fresh garlic clove, 1 to 2 times daily.

Storage: Garlic should be hung in plaits in a dry place.

LITERATURE

Anonym, Knoblauch: Blockade der Cholesterinsynthese in der Leber. In: DAZ 134(45):4468. 1994.

Apitz-Castro R et al., (1983) Thromb Res 32:155.

Augusti KT, Benaim ME, (1974) Clin Chim Acta 60:121.

Augusti KT, Mathew PT, (1974) Experientia 30:468.

Block E et al., (1984) J Am Chem Soc 106:8295.

Brahmachar MD, Augusti KT, (1962) J Pharm Pharmacol 14: 254 and 617.

Chaudhuri BN et al., (1984) Biomed Biochim Acta 41:1045.

Ide N et al., Aged garlic extract and its constituents inhibit Cu++-induced oxidative modification of low density lipoproteins. In: PM 63(3):263-264. 1997.

Imai J et al., Antioxidant and radical scavenging effects of aged garlic extracts and its constituents. In: PM 60(5):417. 1994.

Jain AK, Can garlic reduce levels of serum lipids? In: JAMA 94:632-635. 1993.

Jain RC, Vyas CR, (1974) Brit Med J 2:730.

Jung F, Kiesewetter H, Mrowietz C, Pindur G, Heiden M, Miyashita C, Wenzel E, Akutwirkungen eines zusammengesetzten Knoblauchpräparates auf die Fließfähigkeit des Blutes. In: ZPT 10(3):87. 1989.

Kabelik J, (1970) Pharmazie 25:266.

Koch HP, Der lange Weg zum ''geruchlosen Knoblauch''. In: PUZ 25(4):186-191. 1996.

Koch HP, Epidemiologie der Knoblauchforschung. In: DAZ 132(40):2103. 1992.

Koch HP, Hormonwirkungen bei Allium-Arten. In: ZPT 13(6):177. 1992.

Koch HP, Metabolismus und Pharmakokinetik der Inhatsstoffe des Knoblauchs. Was wissen wir darüber? In: ZPT 13(3):83. 1992.

Koch HP, Saponine in Knoblauch und Küchenzwiebel. In: DAZ 133(41):3733. 1993.

Koch HP, Wie ''sicher'' ist Knoblauch? Toxische, allergische und andere unerwünschte Nebenwirkungen. In: DAZ 132(27):1419. 1992.

Koch B, In: Koch HP, Lawson LD: Garlic - The Science and Therapeutic Application of Allium sativum L. and Related Species, Williams & Wilkins, Baltimore. 1996.

Kubitschek J, Knoblauch blockiert Cholesterolsynthese in der Leber. In: ZPT 16(2):74, s. auch (3):146. 1995.

Lawson LD, Wang ZJ, Pre-hepatic fate of the organosulfur compounds derived from garlic (Allium sativum). In: PM 59(7):A688. 1993.

Mütsch-Eckner M, Erdelmeier CAJ, Sticher O, A novel amino acid glycoside and three amino acids from Allium sativum. In: JNP 56(6):864. 1993.

Nagae, S et al., Pharmacokinetics of the garlic compound S-allylcystein. In: PM 60(3):241. 1994.

Reuter HD, 6. Kongreβ der Gesellschaft für Phytotherapie:Satelliten-Symposium ''International Garlic Research''. In: ZPT 17(1):13-25. 1996.

Reuter HD, Chemie, Pharmakologie und medizinische Anwendung von Knoblauch. In: ZPT 10(4):124. 1989.

Reuter HD, II. Internationales Knoblauch-Symposium. In: ZPT 12(3):83. 1991.

Schiewe FP, Hein T, Knoblauch bei Hyperlipidämie. In: ZPT 16(6):343-348. 1995.

Schoetan A et al., (1984) Experientia 40(3):261.

Sendl A, Phytotherapie: Bärlauch und Knoblauch im Vergleich. In: DAZ 133(5):392. 1993.

Siegers CP, Neues zur arteriosklerotischen Wirkung des Knoblauchs. In: ZPT 14(1):21. 1993.

Walper A et al., Effizienz einer Diätempfehlung und einer zusätzlichen Phytotherapie mit Allium sativum bei leichter bis mäβiger Hypercholesterinämie. In: Medwelt 45(7/8):327. 1994.

Wenkert E et al., (1971) Experientia 28:377.

Whitaker JR, (1976) Adv Food Res 22:73.

Wichtl M, Pflanzliche Pille für die ewige Jugend. In: DAZ 131(17):837. 1991.

Further information in:

Chan H, But P, Pharmacology and Applications of Chinese Materia Medica Vol 1, World Scientific, Singapore 1986.

Frohne D, Pfänder HJ, Giftpflanzen - Ein Handbuch für Apotheker, Toxikologen und Biologen, 4. Aufl., Wiss. Verlags-Ges Stuttgart 1997.

Hänsel R, Keller K, Rimpler H, Schneider G (Hrsg.), Hagers Handbuch der Pharmazeutischen Praxis, 5. Aufl., Bde 4-6 (Drogen), Springer Verlag Berlin, Heidelberg, New York, 1992-1994.

Hausen BM, Allergiepflanzen - Pflanzenallergene, Ecomed Fachverlag Landsberg Lech 1988.

Madaus G, Lehrbuch der Biologischen Arzneimittel, Bde 1-3, Nachdruck, Georg Olms Verlag Hildesheim 1979.

Schulz R, Hänsel R, Rationale Phytotherapie, Springer Verlag Heidelberg 1996.

Steinegger E, Hänsel R, Pharmakognosie, 5. Aufl., Springer Verlag Heidelberg 1992.

Tang W, Eisenbrand G, Chinese Drugs of Plant Origin, Springer Verlag Heidelberg 1992.

Teuscher E, Biogene Arzneimittel, 5. Aufl., Wiss. Verlagsges. Stuttgart 1997.

Wagner H, Wiesenauer M, Phytotherapie. Phytopharmaka und pflanzliche Homöopathika, Fischer-Verlag, Stuttgart, Jena, New York 1995.

Allium Schoenoprasum

Chive

DESCRIPTION

Medicinal Parts: The medicinal parts are the fresh or dried aerial parts of the plant.

Flower and Fruit: The cyme has numerous florets. The sheath of the inflorescence has 2 or 3 flaps. The flap is broad-ovate and shorter than the inflorescence and is white or reddish. The florets are dense and globose with no bulbils. The petals of the perianth are lanceolate-ovate and acute or pointed. They are 7 to 11 mm long, bluish or white to yellowish and have a dark middle stripe. The stamens are shorter than the perianth. They are awl-shaped and fused with each other and the perianth petals at the base. The perianth surrounds the capsule like a balloon.

Leaves, Stem and Root: Allium schoenoprasum is a perennial, 15 to 30 cm high plant. The base is branched with numerous erect, closely packed leaves. Thin sheaths form incomplete, oblong bulbs. The bulb skin is thin, white and splitting when mature. The stem is round, usually smooth and leafy from the lower third. The leaves are completely hollow, round, somewhat elastic, gray or gray-green and compact.

Habitat: The plant grows wild in rocky pastures throughout temperate northern Europe and the U.S., otherwise it is cultivated.

Production: Chives are the complete aerial part of Allium schoenoprasum, which are harvested before flowering.

Other Names: Cives

ACTIONS AND PHARMACOLOGY

COMPOUNDS

Alliins (alkylcysteine sulfoxides): in particular methyl alliin (methyl-L-(+)-cysteine sulfoxide) and pentylalliin (pentyl-L-(+)-cysteine sulfoxide), as well as its gamma-glutamyl conjugates, that in the course of cutting up either the freshly-harvested bulbs or those that have been already dried and then re-moistened are transformed into the so-called alliaceous oils, dialkyl-disulphide-mono-S-oxides and diallyl-di- and trisulphides

EFFECTS

No information is available.

INDICATIONS AND USAGE

The drug is used as a vermifuge.

Efficacy has not been proven.

PRECAUTIONS AND ADVERSE REACTIONS

No health hazards or side effects are known in conjunction with the proper administration of designated therapeutic dosages. The intake of large quantities can lead to stomach complaints.

DOSAGE

Mode of Administration: Chive is used fresh or dried and as a powdered drug.

LITERATURE

Kameoka H, Hashimoto S, Two sulfur containing constituents from Allium schoenoprasum. In: PH 22:294-295. 1983.

Hashimoto S et al., Food Sci 48:1858. 1983.

Further information in:

Hänsel R, Keller K, Rimpler H, Schneider G (Hrsg.), Hagers Handbuch der Pharmazeutischen Praxis, 5. Aufl., Bde 4-6 (Drogen): Springer Verlag Berlin, Heidelberg, New York, 1992-1994.

Allium Ursinum

Bear's Garlic

DESCRIPTION

Medicinal Parts: The fresh herb and fresh bulb are the medicinal parts.

Flower and Fruit: The sheath of the terminal inflorescence is made up of 3 ovate-lanceolate, acute, early-falling leaves, which are almost as long as the peduncle. The inflorescence is a loose, flat, 2.5 to 6 cm wide cyme with 6 to 20 florets. The florets are erect, outward-inclined, pointed or blunt. They are pure white and have six, star-shaped, splayed petals. Six stamens are wedge-shaped, only fused at the base and only half as long as the involucre. One superior ovary is formed out of 3 carpels and 3 deep grooves. The 3-valved capsule contains black, angular seeds.

Leaves, Stem and Root: The plant has an upright, 10 to 50 cm high, double-edged, half-cylindrical, or triangular to round and compact stem. The leaf blade is flat, narrow-elliptical-lanceolate to narrow-ovate and acute. It is 6 to 20 cm long, thin, and the base is rounded to cordate, narrowing suddenly to a 5 to 20 cm long petiole. The dark-green underside is covered with irregular horizontal veins. They face upwards leaving the paler upper surface facing toward the ground. The bulb is almost cylindrical, 2 to 6 cm long, about 1 cm wide and surrounded by transparent or white skins.

Characteristics: Bear's garlic forms many onions and has a distinctive leek odor.

Habitat: Indigenous to almost all of Europe and Turkey. Bear's Garlic is also found in the Caucasus and Siberia as far as Kamtschatka; but not in the Hungarian plain and the evergreen Mediterranean region.

Not To Be Confused With: One case was reported of confusion with colchicum leaves.

Other Names: Ramsons, Broad-leaved Garlic

ACTIONS AND PHARMACOLOGY

COMPOUNDS

Alliins (alkylcysteine sulphoxides): in particular methyl alliin (methyl-L-(+)-cysteine sulphoxide) and allylalliin (allyl-L-(+)-cysteine sulphoxide) and presumably their gamma-glutamyl conjugates, that readily transform into the so-called alliaceous oils, for example into dimethyl-disulphide-mono-S-oxide, allicin (diallyl-disulphide- mono-S-oxide) and allyl-methyl-disulphide mono-S-oxide and the corresponding dialkyldi- or trisulphides

INDICATIONS AND USAGE

The drug is used for gastrointestinal complaints, fermentative dyspepsia, flatulence, high blood pressure, and arteriosclerosis; externally for chronic rashes.

Efficacy has not been proven.

PRECAUTIONS AND ADVERSE REACTIONS

No health hazards or side effects are known in conjunction with the proper administration of designated therapeutic dosages.

DOSAGE

Mode of Administration: The drug is used internally as well as externally.

Preparation: Extract of bear's garlic.

Daily Dosage: Due to low concentration of the active substance, the drug must be administered in higher doses than Allium sativum.

LITERATURE

Landshuter J et al., Comparative biochemical studies on a purified C-S-lyase preparation from wild garlic. In: PM 58(7):A666. 1992.

Sendl A, Bärlauch: Alternative zu Knoblauch. In: Naturw. Rdsch 7/94. 1994.

Sendl A, Phytotherapie: Bärlauch und Knoblauch im Vergleich. In: DAZ 133(5):392. 1993.

Veit M, Bärlauch (Allium ursinum) als Ersatz für Knoblauch (Allium sativum). In: ZPT 13(6):201. 1993.

Wagner H, Ebl G, Lotter H, Guinea M, Evaluation of natural products as inhibitors of angiotensin I-converting enzyme (ACE). In: Pharm Pharmacol Letters 1(1):15-18. 1991.

Wagner H, Sendl A, Bärlauch und Knoblauch. In: DAZ 130(33):1809. 1990.

Further information in:

Hänsel R, Keller K, Rimpler H, Schneider G (Hrsg.), Hagers Handbuch der Pharmazeutischen Praxis, 5. Aufl., Bde 4-6 (Drogen), Springer Verlag Berlin, Heidelberg, New York, 1992-1994.

Madaus G, Lehrbuch der Biologischen Arzneimittel, Bde 1-3, Nachdruck, Georg Olms Verlag Hildesheim 1979.

Teuscher E, Biogene Arzneimittel, 5. Aufl., Wiss. Verlagsges. Stuttgart 1997.

Wagner H, Wiesenauer M, Phytotherapie. Phytopharmaka und pflanzliche Homöopathika, Fischer-Verlag, Stuttgart, Jena, New York 1995.

Wichtl M (Hrsg.), Teedrogen, 4. Aufl., Wiss. Verlagsges. Stuttgart 1997.

Almond

See Prunus Amygdalus

Alnus Glutinosa

Black Alder

DESCRIPTION

Medicinal Parts: The medicinal part is the bark.

Flower and Fruit: Black Adler is monoecious. Male flowers are arranged in stemmed catkins and are produced in the previous year. Female flowers form ovoid fruit, which turns woody and remains on the tree the whole year.

Leaves, Stem and Root: Alnus glutinosa is a shrub or tree up to 25 m high with gray branches and orange-colored wood. The obovate leaves have double-serrate margins; the young leaves are very sticky.

Habitat: Black Adler grows in the Northern Hemisphere.

Production: Black Alder bark is the bark and branch rind of Alnus glutinosa. It is gathered in uncultivated areas.

Other Names: Common Alder, Owler, Tag Alder

ACTIONS AND PHARMACOLOGY

COMPOUNDS

Tannins

Flavonoids: in particular hypericin

Steroids: beta-sitosterol

Triterpenes

EFFECTS

The decoction is a tonic and has astringent and hemostatic properties.

INDICATIONS AND USAGE

Alnus glutinosa is used as a decoction for gargles in the treatment of streptococcal sore throat and pharyngitis, and for intestinal bleeding. Its efficacy has not been proven.

PRECAUTIONS AND ADVERSE REACTIONS

No health hazards or side effects are known in conjunction with the proper administration of designated therapeutic dosages.

DOSAGE

Mode of Administration: As an infusion for gargling.

Preparations: The bark is prepared as a decoction.

LITERATURE

Freudenberg K, Weinges K (1967) Tetrahedron Letters 17: 19.

Further information in:

Hänsel R, Keller K, Rimpler H, Schneider G (Hrsg.), Hagers Handbuch der Pharmazeutischen Praxis, 5. Aufl., Bde 4-6 (Drogen), Springer Verlag Berlin, Heidelberg, New York, 1992-1994.

Hoppe, HA (1975-1987) Drogenkunde, 8. Aufl., Bde 1-3, W. de Gruyter Verlag, Berlin, New York.

Aloe Barbadensis

Aloe

DESCRIPTION

Medicinal Parts: The dried and fresh juice of the leaves, the whole leaves, the gel from the water storing tissue and the roots.

Flower and Fruit: The inflorescence is forked once or twice and is 60 to 90 cm high. The raceme is dense, cylindrical and narrows towards the top. The terminal raceme is up to 40 cm high while the lower ones are somewhat shorter. Bracts are almost white; the flowers are yellow, orange or red, and 3 cm long.

Leaves, Stem and Root: The lily-like succulent-leafed rosette shrub has no stem or a 25 cm stem with about 25 leaves in an upright dense rosette. The leaf is thick and fleshy, 40 to 50 cm long, 6 to 7 cm wide at the base and lanceolate. The upper surface is concave; gray-green, often with a reddish tinge; these are sometimes patches in young plants. The leaf margin has a pale pink edge and 2 mm long pale teeth.

Habitat: Aloe is probably indigenous to Sudan and the Arabian peninsula. Today the species is found cultivated and wild in northern Africa, the Near East, Asia, and in the southern Mediterranean region. It has been introduced into America. Aloe ferox is indigenous to South Africa. Agave americana, known as American Aloe, is not a true Aloe.

Production: Curacao aloe consists of the dried latex of the leaves of Aloe barbadensis (syn. Aloe vera), as well as its preparations. Aloe is harvested from August until October. The juice is dried in various ways.

Cape aloe consists of the dried latex of the leaves of several species of the genus Aloe, especially Aloe ferox and its hybrids. The leaves are gathered by hand, and the collected liquid is thickened.

Not To Be Confused With: Aloe barbadensis and Aloe capensis have different properties.

ACTION AND PHARMACOLOGY

COMPOUNDS: ALOE BARBADENSIS

Anthracene derivatives: particularly anthrone-10-C-glykosyls, including aloin A, aloin B, 7-hydroxyaloins and 1,8-dihydroxyanthraquinones, including aloe-emodin

2-alkylchromones: including aloe resins B, C and D

Flavonoids

EFFECTS: ALOE BARBADENSIS

1,8-dihydroxy-anthracene derivatives have a laxative effect. This effect is primarily caused by the influence on the motility of the colon, an inhibition of stationary and stimulation of propulsive contractions; this results in an accelerated intestinal passage and, because of the shortened contraction time, a reduction in liquid absorption.

In addition, stimulation of active chloride secretion increases the water and electrolyte content, thereby strengthening the filling pressure of the bowels, and stimulating intestinal peristalsis. The drug functions antibacterially and is effective against Herpes Simplex viruses.

COMPOUNDS: ALOE CAPENSIS

Anthracene derivatives: particularly anthrone-10-C-glykosyls, including aloins A, and B, 5-hydroxyaloin A, 1,8-dihydroxyanthraquinones, including aloe-emodin, and mixed anthrone-C- and O-glycosides

Aloinosides A and B

2-alkylchromones: including aloe resins A, B, C and D

Flavonoids

EFFECTS: ALOE CAPENSIS

1,8-dihydroxy-anthracene derivatives have a laxative effect. This effect is primarily caused by the influence on the motility of the colon, an inhibition of stationary and stimulation of propulsive contractions. This results in accelerated intestinal passage and, because of the shortened contraction time, a reduction in liquid absorption. In addition, stimulation of active chloride secretion increases the water and electrolyte content, thereby strengthening the filling pressure of the bowels, and stimulating the intestinal peristalsis.

INDICATIONS AND USAGE

ALOE BARBADENSIS

■ Constipation

The drug is used for constipation, evacuation relief in the presence of anal fissures, hemorrhoids, and after recto-anal operations or for the preparation of diagnostic interventions in the gastrointestinal tract.

In folk medicine the drug is employed in Europe for its ability to influence digestion. In other cultures it is more widely deployed for worm infestation, stomach disorders, diabetes, arteriosclerosis, amenorrhea, menstrual complaints, infections, tumors, skin diseases, and colic. These uses are unsubstantiated.

ALOE CAPENSIS

■ Constipation

In central Europe, Aloe capensis is favored over Aloe barbadensis and is employed similarly. It is used for constipation, evacuation relief with anal fissures, hemorrhoids, treatment following recto-anal intervention, and for preparation of diagnostic operations in the gastrointestinal tract.

In folk medicine the drug is used as a constituent of the so-called ''Swedish herbs'', which, in Germany are widely used as a cure-all. In South Africa, the fresh juice finds use for eye inflammation and for syphilis. In Lesotho it is used by medicine men.

CONTRAINDICATIONS

Aloe is contraindicated in cases of intestinal obstruction, acutely inflamed intestinal diseases (e.g., Crohn's disease, ulcerative colitis), appendicitis and abdominal pain of unknown origin.

PRECAUTIONS AND ADVERSE REACTIONS

General: In single incidents, cramp-like discomforts of the gastrointestinal tract occur. These cases require a dosage reduction.

Long-term use leads to losses of electrolytes, in particular potassium, and as a result of this to hyperaldosteronism, inhibition of intestinal motility and enhancement of the effect of cardioactive steroids. In rare cases, heart arrhythmias, nephropathies, edemas and accelerated bone deterioration may occur. Long-term use can also lead to albuminuria and hematuria.

Pigmentation in the intestinal mucosa (pseudomelanosis coli) can also occur. This harmless side effect usually reverses upon discontinuation of the drug.

The possibility that long-term use of anthracene drugs increases the probability of colon carcinoma has not been fully clarified. Recent studies show no connections between the administration of anthracene drugs and the frequency of carcinomas in the colon.

Drug Interactions: Chronic use of aloe can lead to potassium loss, which can affect the actions of cardiac glycosides and antiarrhythmic drugs. There is an increase in the possibility of potassium deficiency when Aloe is used along with thiazide diuretics, licorice and corticosteroids.

Pregnancy: Aloe should not be used during pregnancy.

Pediatric Use: Aloe should not be prescribed to children under 12 years of age.

DOSAGE

ALOE BARBADENSIS

Mode of Administration: Due to the side effects of the drug, it is rarely used and is not recommended. Aloe powder, aqueous- and aqueous-alcoholic extracts in powdered or liquid form are available for oral use.

Daily Dosage: The recommended daily dosage is 20 to 30 mg hydroxyanthracene derivatives/day, calculated as anhydrous aloin. The individually correct dosage is the smallest dosage necessary to maintain a soft stool. Stimulating laxatives must not be used over an extended period of time (1 to 2 weeks) without medical advice.

Storage: Aloe should be protected from light and moisture.

ALOE CAPENSIS

Mode of Administration: Aloe capensis is available as aloe powder, aqueous and aqueous-alcoholic extracts in powdered or liquid form, for oral use.

Daily Dosage: The recommended daily dosage is 20 to 30 mg hydroxyanthracene derivatives/day, calculated as anhydrous aloin. The individually correct dosage is the smallest dosage necessary to maintain a soft stool. Stimulating laxatives must not be used over an extended period of time (1 to 2 weeks) without medical advice.

Storage: Aloe capensis must be protected from light; the extract should be stored over silica gel, away from light sources.

LITERATURE

ALOE BARBADENSIS

Anonym, Aloe und Aloine - Aktuelles über weltweit verwendete Arzneistoffe. In: DAZ 135(39):3644-3645. 1995.

BGA, Arzneimittelrisiken: Anthranoide. In: DAZ 132(21):1164. 1992.

Che QM, Akao T, Hattori M, Kobashi K, Namba T, Metabolism of barbaloin by intestinal bacteria. 2. Isolation of human intestinal bacterium capable of tranforming barbaloin to Aloe-emodin anthrone. In: PM 57:15. 1991.

Hutter JA et al., Antiinflammatory C-glucosyl chromone from Aloe barbadensis. In: JNP 59(5):541-543. 1996.

Klimpel BE et al., Anthranoidhaltige Laxantien - ein Risiko für die Entwicklung von Tumoren der ableitenden Harnwege. In: PUZ 26(1):33, Jahrestagung der DPhG, Berlin, 1996. 1997.

Koch A, Investigations on the laxative action of aloin in the human colon. In: PM 59(7):A689. 1993.

Koch A, Metabolisierung von Aloin. Korrelation zwischen In-vitro- und in-vivo-Versuchen. In: DAZ 135(13):1150-1152. 1995.

Park MK et al., Neoaloesin A: A new C-glucofuranosyl chromone from Aloe barbadensis. In: PM 62(4):363-365. 1996.

Shida T et al., (1985) Planta Med 51(3):273.

Tzeng SH, Ko WC, Ko FN, Teng CM, Inhibition of platelet aggregation by some flavonoids. In: Thromobosis Res 64:91. 1991.

Westendorf J, Phytotherapie: Anthranoide in Arzneipflanzen. In: DAZ 133(25):2345. 1993.

Yoig A, Egusa T, Arase M, Tanabe M, Tsujitt, Isolation and characterization of the glycoprotein fraction with proliferation-promotory activity on human and hamster cells in vitro. In: PM 63:18-21. 1997.

Further information in:

Hänsel R, Keller K, Rimpler H, Schneider G (Hrsg.), Hagers Handbuch der Pharmazeutischen Praxis, 5. Aufl., Bde 4-6 (Drogen), Springer Verlag Berlin, Heidelberg, New York, 1992-1994.

Hausen BM, Allergiepflanzen - Pflanzenallergene, Ecomed Fachverlag Landsberg Lech 1988.

Hoppe HA, (1975-1987) Drogenkunde, 8. Aufl., Bde 1-3, W. de Gruyter Verlag, Berlin, New York.

Lewin L, Gifte und Vergiftungen, 6. Aufl., Nachdruck, Haug Verlag, Heidelberg 1992.

Steinegger E, Hänsel R, Pharmakognosie, 5. Aufl., Springer Verlag Heidelberg 1992.

Teuscher E, Biogene Arzneimittel, 5. Aufl., Wiss. Verlagsges. Stuttgart 1997.

Wagner H, Wiesenauer M, Phytotherapie. Phytopharmaka und pflanzliche Homöopathika, Fischer-Verlag, Stuttgart, Jena, New York 1995.

Wichtl M (Hrsg.), Teedrogen, 4. Aufl., Wiss. Verlagsges. Stuttgart 1997.

ALOE CAPENSIS

Anonym, Aloe und Aloine - Aktuelles über weltweit verwendete Arzneistoffe. In: DAZ 135(39):3644-3645. 1995.

BGA, Arzneimittelrisiken: Anthranoide. In: DAZ 132(21):1164. 1992.

Che QM, Akao T, Hattori M, Kobashi K, Namba T, Metabolism of barbaloin by intestinal bacteria. 2. Isolation of human intestinal bacterium capable of tranforming barbaloin to Aloe-emodin anthrone. In: PM 57:15. 1991.

Klimpel BE et al., Anthranoidhaltige Laxantien - ein Risiko für die Entwicklung von Tumoren der ableitenden Harnwege. In: PUZ 26(1):33, Jahrestagung der DPhG, Berlin, 1996. 1997.

Koch A, Investigations on the laxative action of aloin in the human colon. In: PM 59(7):A689. 1993.

Koch A, Metabolisierung von Aloin. Korrelation zwischen In-vitro- und in-vivo-Versuchen. In: DAZ 135(13):1150-1152. 1995.

Shida, T et al., (1985) Planta Med 51(3):273.

Speranza G et al., Studies on Aloe, 12. Furoaloesone, a new 5-methylchromene from cape aloe. In: JNP 56(7):1089. 1993.

Speranza G, Manitto P, Monti D, Pezzuto D, Studies on Aloe, part 10: Feroxins A and B, two O-glycosylated 1-methyltetralins from cape Aloe. In: JNP 55:723-729. 1992.

Tzeng SH, Ko WC, Ko FN, Teng, CM, Inhibition of platelet aggregation by some flavonoids. In: Thromobosis Res 64:91. 1991.

Westendorf J, Phytotherapie: Anthranoide in Arzneipflanzen. In: DAZ 133(25):2345. 1993.

Yoig A, Egusa T, Arase M, Tanabe M, Tsujitt, Isolation and characterization of the glycoprotein fraction with proliferation-promotory activity on human and hamster cells in vitro. In: PM 63:18-21. 1997.

van Wyk BE et al., Geographical variation in the major compounds of Aloe ferox leaf exudate. In: PH 61(3):250-253. 1995.

Further information in:

Hänsel R, Keller K, Rimpler H, Schneider G (Hrsg.), Hagers Handbuch der Pharmazeutischen Praxis, 5. Aufl., Bde 4-6 (Drogen), Springer Verlag Berlin, Heidelberg, New York, 1992-1994.

Lewin L, Gifte und Vergiftungen, 6. Aufl., Nachdruck, Haug Verlag, Heidelberg 1992.

Madaus G, Lehrbuch der Biologischen Arzneimittel, Bde 1-3, Nachdruck, Georg Olms Verlag Hildesheim 1979.

Roth L, Daunderer M, Kormann K, Giftpflanzen, Pflanzengifte, 4. Aufl., Ecomed Fachverlag Landsberg Lech 1993.

Schulz R, Hänsel R, Rationale Phytotherapie, Springer Verlag Heidelberg 1996.

Steinegger E, Hänsel R, Pharmakognosie, 5. Aufl., Springer Verlag Heidelberg 1992.

Teuscher E, Biogene Arzneimittel, 5. Aufl., Wiss. Verlagsges. Stuttgart 1997.

Wagner H, Wiesenauer M, Phytotherapie. Phytopharmaka und pflanzliche Homöopathika, Fischer-Verlag, Stuttgart, Jena, New York 1995.

Wichtl M (Hrsg.), Teedrogen, 4. Aufl., Wiss. Verlagsges. Stuttgart 1997.

Aloysia Triphylla

Lemon Verbena

DESCRIPTION

Medicinal Parts: The medicinal part is the oil of vervain as a distillate of the fresh twigs and the dried leaves and stems.

Flower and Fruit: The plant has numerous small flowers in panicle-like spikes. The hairy calyx is about 3 mm long with 4 tips. The petals are white or bluish, and fused to a 4 to 5 mm long funnel at the base. There are 2 short and 2 long stamens in the funnel.

Leaves, Stem and Root: Aloysia triphylla is an up to 3 m tall shrub. The branches are striate and scabrous. They bear leaves in whorls of 3 or 4 on the stem. The leaves are entire-margined, short-petioled, lanceolate and about 7 to 10 cm long. They have lateral veins almost at right angles to the midrib, and are dotted on the underside with oil-bearing glands.

Characteristics: The leaves have a lemony fragrance.

Habitat: Originated in Argentina, Chile and Peru. The plant is cultivated in most other warmer countries. Main countries of cultivation are Algeria, Chile, Israel and Morocco.

Production: Lemon Verbena leaves are the leaves and stems, in whole and ground form, of Aloysia triphylla. The shrubs are propagated by runners or cuttings. They are cut from the second year of growth, in the month of July, before flowering. The young lateral branches appear in October. They are dried rapidly in thin layers or bundles. The dried leaves are then stripped off. The harvest consists of approximately 10,000 kg of the leaf drug per hectare.

Other Names: Herb Louisa, Lemon-scented Verbena

ACTION AND PHARMACOLOGY

COMPOUNDS

Volatile oil: main constituents are geraniol and neral

Flavonoids: including apigenin-, diosmetin- and luteolin-7-O-glucosides, beyond that, mono-, di- and trimethoxyflavones, including eupatorin

Iridoid glycosides

EFFECTS

The leaves are antispasmodic, sedative and are a febrifuge. There are no up-to-date studies available.

INDICATIONS AND USAGE

In France, Lemon Verbena is used in the symptomatic treatment of digestive disorders, agitation and insomnia. It has also been used in the treatment of febrile hemorrhoids, varicose veins and impure skin. In Morocco it is also used for chills and constipation. Efficacy has not been proven in any of these areas. The plant is used as an inactive ingredient to improve the flavor in medicinal teas.

PRECAUTIONS AND ADVERSE REACTIONS

No health hazards or side effects are known in conjunction with the proper administration of designated therapeutic dosages.

DOSAGE

Mode of Administration: In France, the infusion is available in various restaurants under the name ''Vervaine oderante''. Used in various medicinal preparations and tea mixtures.

Preparation: To prepare an infusion, use 5 to 29 g of the leaf per 1 liter of water.

Daily Dosage: Drink 2 to 5 cups of the infusion during the course of the day.

Storage: The drug must be stored in sealed containers, protected from light and dampness.

LITERATURE

Breitweiser K, (1943) Pharmaz Ind 10:76.

Killacky J et al., (1976) Planta Med 30:310.

Rimpler H, Sauerbier H, Biochem Syst Ecol 14:307-310. 1986.

Skalta H, Shammas G, PM 54:265. 1988.

Tomás-Barberán FA, Harborne JB, Self R, PH 26:2281-2284. 1987.

Torrent Marti MT, Rev R Acad Farm (Barcelona) 14:39-55. 1976.

Further information in:

Hänsel R, Keller K, Rimpler H, Schneider G (Hrsg.), Hagers Handbuch der Pharmazeutischen Praxis, 5. Aufl., Bde 4-6 (Drogen), Springer Verlag Berlin, Heidelberg, New York, 1992-1994.

Alpine Cranberry

See Vaccinium Vitis-Idaea

Alpinia Officinarum

Galangal

DESCRIPTION

Medicinal Parts: The medicinal part is the rhizome.

Flower and Fruit: Galangal is a perennial plant. It is similar in appearance to the sword lily, with a dark, reddish-brown, cylindrical rhizome about 1 to 2 cm in diameter and 3 to 6 cm long. The stem is marked at short intervals with raised rings, which are the scars of the leaf bases. Stems are up to 1.5 m with long narrow lanceolate leaves bearing racemes of orchid-shaped flowers, white and veined red; fracture of rhizome hard and tough, showing a pale inside with a darker central column.

Characteristics: Taste is pungent and spicy; odor is aromatic, rather like ginger.

Habitat: India, Thailand, southern China

Production: Galangal consists of the dried rhizome of Alpinia officinarum.

Not To Be Confused With: The rhizome of Kaempferia galanga and other Alpina species

Other Names: Galanga, East India Root, Chinese Ginger, China Root, India Root, East India Catarrh Root, Gargaut, Colic Root, Catarrh Root

ACTION AND PHARMACOLOGY

COMPOUNDS

Volatile oil: chief components-sesquiterpene hydrocarbons, sesquiterpene alcohols

Diarylheptanoids: (mixture termed galangol, some of them pungent substances)

Gingerole: (phenyl alkanones, pungent substances)

Starch

Tannin

Flavonoids: including galangin, galangin-3-methylether, kaempferide

EFFECTS

Antispasmodic, antiphlogistic, antibacterial.

INDICATIONS AND USAGE

- Loss of appetite
- Dyspeptic complaints
- Fevers and colds
- Cough/bronchitis
- Tendency for infections
- Liver and gallbladder complaints
- Inflammation of the mouth and pharynx
- Common cold

Galangal has also been used for loss of appetite, painful upper abdominal syndrome of the Roemheld complex type, and for sluggish digestion.

PRECAUTIONS AND ADVERSE REACTIONS

Health risks or side effects following the proper administration of designated therapeutic dosages are not reported.

DOSAGE

Mode of Administration: Comminuted drug and powder, as well as other galenic preparations for oral administration.

Preparation: Infusion - Pour boiling water over 0.5 to 1 g drug and strain after 10 minutes.

Daily Dosage: 2 to 4 grams. The infusion dosage is 1 cup 1/2 hour before meals.

LITERATURE

Collins KR, Pat EP 25649 (1981) Europe.

De Pooter HL et al., PH 24:93. 1985.

Haraguchi H et al., Antifungal activity from Alpinia galanga and the competition for incorporation of unsaturated fatty acids in cell growth. In: PM 62(4):308-313. 1996.

Haraguchi H et al., PM 62:308. 1996.

Itokawa H et al., (1987) Planta Med 53(1):32.

Mitsui S et al., (1976) Chem Pharm Bull 24:2377.

Further information in:

Fenaroli's Handbook of Flavor Ingredients, Vol. 1, 2nd Ed., CRC Press 1975.

Kern W, List PH, Hörhammer L (Hrsg.), Hagers Handbuch der Pharmazeutischen Praxis, 4. Aufl., Bde. 1-8, Springer Verlag Berlin, Heidelberg, New York, 1969.

Madaus G, Lehrbuch der Biologischen Arzneimittel, Bde 1-3, Nachdruck, Georg Olms Verlag Hildesheim 1979.

Steinegger E, Hänsel R, Pharmakognosie, 5. Aufl., Springer Verlag Heidelberg 1992.

Teuscher E, Biogene Arzneimittel, 5. Aufl., Wiss. Verlagsges. mbH Stuttgart 1997.

Wichtl M (Hrsg.), Teedrogen, 4. Aufl., Wiss. Verlagsges. Stuttgart 1997.

Alstonia Constricta

Fever Bark

DESCRIPTION

Medicinal Parts: The medicinal parts are the bark of the root and trunk.

Flower and Fruit: The flowers are creamy white and star-shaped.

Leaves, Stem and Root: Alstonia are evergreen trees, which grow to a height of 15 m. The leaves are glossy, oblong, and petiolate. The tree has a 2 to 7 cm rusty-brown, rugose periderm, which is deeply fissured. The inner surface is yellowish brown and coarsely striated longitudinally, fracture fibrous.

Characteristics: The tree is a protected species in some countries. The taste is very bitter, the odor, slightly aromatic.

Habitat: Alstonia constricta is indigenous to Australia; Alstonia scholaris is indigenous to India and the Philippines.

Production: Alstonia bark is the trunk and branch bark of Alstonia constricta.

Other Names: Australian Quinine, Australian Febrifuge, Alstonia Bark, Devil Tree, Dita Bark, Pale Mara, Devil's Bit, Australian Fever Bush, Pali-mara

ACTIONS AND PHARMACOLOGY

COMPOUNDS

Indole alkaloids: including reserpine, deserpidine, alstonine, tetrahydroalstonine, alstonidine, yohimbine

EFFECTS

The drug is said to be a febrifuge, antispasmodic, and antihypertensive. The antihypertensive effect is due to the reserpine and echitamin content.

INDICATIONS AND USAGE

The drug is used as a febrifuge and stimulant and for its reserpine content. In the past, it was used to treat rheumatism. In the Far East, it is used for diarrhea and malaria. It has also been used as a uterine stimulant.

PRECAUTIONS AND ADVERSE REACTIONS

No health hazards or side effects are known in conjunction with the proper administration of designated therapeutic dosages. Due to the presence of pharmacologically active indole alkaloids of the beta-carbolin-type, side effects that may resemble those of Rauwolfiae radix, and symptoms of poisoning following intakes of higher dosages are conceivable.

DOSAGE

Mode of Administration: The forms available are: powder, liquid extract, infusion and tincture. Up-to-date information on usage is not available.

Preparations: Fever Bark is available as an infusion, 1:20, a tincture, 1:8 or 1:10 and as a liquid extract, 1:1.

Daily Dosage: The average daily dose of infusion is 15 to 20 ml; tincture, 2 to 4 ml; liquid extract, 4 to 8 ml.

LITERATURE

Atta-ur-Rahman AM et al., (1985) Phytochemistry 24:2771.

Chopra RN et al., (Eds.) Chopra's Indigeneous Drugs of India, Vol 1, Dhur and Sons Calcutta 1938.

Goyal H et al., (1981) J Res Ayur Siddha. 2 (3):286.

Khan I, Qureshi Z (1967) J Pharm Pharmacol 19:815.

Kucera MV et al., (1973) Afric J Pharm Pharm Sci: 3228.

Oliver-Bever B (Ed.), Medicinal Plants of Tropical West Africa, Cambridge University Press Cambridge, London 1986.

Sharp TM, (1934) J Chem Soc 287.

Further information in:

Kern W, List PH, Hörhammer L (Hrsg.), Hagers Handbuch der Pharmazeutischen Praxis, 4. Aufl., Bde. 1-8, Springer Verlag Berlin, Heidelberg, New York, 1969.

Althaea Officinalis

Marshmallow

DESCRIPTION

Medicinal Parts: The medicinal parts are the mallow flowers, leaves, and roots.

Flower and Fruit: The reddish-white flowers are usually in axillary or terminal clusters. The 6 to 9 sepals of the epicalyx are fused at the base, pointed and 8 to 10 mm long. There are 5 sepals, 5 heart-shaped petals, and numerous stamens fused together with the anthers to a column. The ovaries are in a ring. There are numerous styles. The mericarps are smooth and downy. The 5 to 8 mm fruit is disc-like and breaks up into the mericarps, which are downy on the outside and often have fine, branched, and radiating ribs. The seeds are dark-brown, glabrous, kidney-shaped and somewhat compressed.

Leaves, Stem and Root: The 60 to 120 cm high hardy, velvety plant has an up to 50 cm long by a few cm thick erect root with secondary roots. The erect, succulent stem is usually woody at the base but unbranched. The leaves are short-petioled with an ovate, acute leaf-blade. The secondary leaves are narrow and dropping. The lower leaves are 5-lobed, and the upper cauline leaves are often triangular, more wide than long, and irregularly and roughly dentate.

Habitat: Originally indigenous to Asia and spread westward to southeast Europe and eastward to China. In temperate latitudes Althaea officinalis is established as a garden plant.

Production: Marshmallow root consists of the dried root, unpeeled or peeled, of Althaea officinalis. Marshmallow leaves consist of the dried leaves of Althaea officinalis. The root cultures are harvested from October to November, and after cleaning, are carefully dried at a maximum of 35°C.

Not To Be Confused With: May be confused with other Althea species.

Other Names: Althea, Mortification Root, Sweet Weed, Wymote, Mallards, Schloss Tea

ACTIONS AND PHARMACOLOGY

COMPOUNDS

Mucilages: mixture of collodially soluable polysaccharides, particularly galacturonic rhamnans, arabinogalactans, arabans, and glucans

Pectins

Starch

EFFECTS

The drug alleviates local irritation, inhibits mucociliary activity, stimulates phagocytosis, and functions as an anti-inflammatory and anticomplementary agent, immune stimulant, and hypoglycemic.

INDICATIONS AND USAGE

■ Cough/bronchitis

The drug is used for irritation of the oral and pharyngeal mucosa and associated dry cough; mild inflammation of the gastric mucosa; as cataplasm for light inflammations and skin burns.

In folk medicine, marshmallow is employed for catarrh of the mouth, throat, gastrointestinal tract and urinary tract, and for inflammation, ulcers, abscesses, burns, constipation, and diarrhea.

PRECAUTIONS AND ADVERSE REACTIONS

General: No health hazards or side effects are known in conjunction with the proper administration of designated therapeutic dosages.

Drug Interactions: The absorption of other drugs taken simultaneously may be delayed.

DOSAGE

Mode of Administration: Cut leaves for aqueous extracts as well as other galenic preparations for internal use. Cut or ground root for aqueous extracts as well as other galenic preparations for internal use. Marshmallow syrup is to be used only for treatment of dry coughs.

Note: Diabetics need to consider sugar concentration of the marshmallow syrup.

Preparation: To prepare a tea, use 10 to 15 gm with 150 ml of cold water and allow to stand for one and one-half hours, then warm to drink.

Daily Dosage: The average daily dose is 6 gm of the root and 5 gm of the leaf.

Marshmallow syrup: single dose is 10 gm.

Tea: freshly prepared tea taken several times daily.

Storage: The drug should be protected from light sources and insects.

LITERATURE

Blaschek W, Franz G, (1986) Planta Med 6:76P.

Capek P et al., Carbohydr Res 164:443. 1987.

Franz G, Madaus A, Stabilität von Polysacchariden. Untersuchungen am Beispiel des Eibischschleims. In: DAZ 130(40):2194. 1990.

Franz G, PM 14:90. 1966.

Franz G, PM 55:493. 1989.

Gudej J, (1981) Acta Pol Pharm 38:385.

Gudej J, Bieganowska HL, Chromatographia 30:333. 1990.

Gudej J, PM 57:284. 1991.

Hahn-Deinstrop E, Eibischwurzel Identifizierung von Eibischwurzel-Extrakt und Gehaltsbestimmung in einem Instant-Tee. In: DAZ 135(13):1147-1149. 1995.

Kardosova A et al., (1983) Coll Czech Commun 45:2082.

Kochich P et al., (1983) Sov J Bioorg Chem 9(2):121.

Nosál'ova G, Strapková A, Kardosova A, Capek P, Zatureck'y L, Bukovska E, Antitussive Wirkung des Extraktes und der Polysaccharide aus Eibisch (Althaea officinalis L. var. robusta). In: PA 47(3):224-226. 1992.

Nosolova G et al., PA 47:224. 1993.

Shimizu N, Tomoda T, Chem Pharm Bull 33:5539. 1985.

Tomoda M et al., (1980) Chem Pharm Bull 28:824.

Tomoda M et al., (1987) Planta Med 53(1):8.

Tomoda M et al., Chem Pharm Bull 25:1357. 1977.

Wunderer H, Zentral und peripher wirksame Antitussiva: eine kritische Übersicht. In: PZ 142(11):847-852. 1997.

Further information in:

Hänsel R, Keller K, Rimpler H, Schneider G (Hrsg.), Hagers Handbuch der Pharmazeutischen Praxis, 5. Aufl., Bde 4-6 (Drogen), Springer Verlag Berlin, Heidelberg, New York, 1992-1994.

Madaus G, Lehrbuch der Biologischen Arzneimittel, Bde 1-3, Nachdruck, Georg Olms Verlag Hildesheim 1979.

Schulz R, Hänsel R, Rationale Phytotherapie, Springer Verlag Heidelberg 1996.

Steinegger E, Hänsel R, Pharmakognosie, 5. Aufl., Springer Verlag Heidelberg 1992.

Teuscher E, Biogene Arzneimittel, 5. Aufl., Wiss. Verlagsges. Stuttgart 1997.

Wagner H, Wiesenauer M, Phytotherapie. Phytopharmaka und pflanzliche Homöopathika, Fischer-Verlag, Stuttgart, Jena, New York 1995.

Wichtl M (Hrsg.), Teedrogen, 4. Aufl., Wiss. Verlagsges. Stuttgart 1997.

Amanita Muscaria

Aga

DESCRIPTION

Medicinal Parts: Homeopathic dilutions are prepared from the fungus.

Flower and Fruit: Belongs to the group of lamella fungi, genus Amanita. The hymenium in the inside of the fruiting body is exposed by unfolding the cap on the underside.

Characteristics: Basidia is dirty white as are the cuffs and underside of the cap. The cap is orange at first then strong red with a few dirty white to yellow spots. The fungus is poisonous.

Habitat: Aga is found in the northern hemisphere in sandy, acid soils as far as the northern tundra.

Production: Aga is the above-ground part of Amanita muscaria.

Other Names: Fly Agaric

ACTIONS AND PHARMACOLOGY

COMPOUNDS

Ibotenic acid

Muscimol

Muscarine (traces)

Betalains (skin pigment)

EFFECTS

Hallucinogenic, toxic.

INDICATIONS AND USAGE

In homeopathy for the treatment of neuralgias, fever, anxiety, alcohol poisoning and joint pains.

PRECAUTIONS AND ADVERSE REACTIONS

The drug is highly toxic. Signs of poisoning include dizziness, vomiting, abdominal pain, movement disorders, muscle cramps and psychic stimulation, followed by deep sleep.

OVERDOSAGE

The intake of more than 10 gm of the fresh mushroom can lead to coordination disorders, confusion, illusions and manic attacks. Higher dosages (over 100 gm of fresh mushrooms) lead to unconsciousness, asphyxiation, coma and death.

The treatment of poisonings includes emptying the gastrointestinal tract and the use of sedatives. In case of shock, a plasma volume expander should be used. Artificial respiration should be carried out in case breathing ceases.

DOSAGE

Mode of Administration: In homeopathy dilutions of the mother tincture are used.

LITERATURE

Hastings MH et al., Brain Res 360:248. 1985.

Hatfield GM, Brady LR, JNP 38:36, 1975.

Marmo E, Med Res Rev 8:441, 1988.

Schwarz B, Ein Männlein steht im Walde. In: PZ 139(13):1040. 1994.

Further information in:

Bresinsky A, Bresl H, Giftpilze. Ein Handbuch für Apotheker, Ärzte und Biologen, Wiss. Verlagsges. mbH, Stuttgart 1885.

Lewin L, Gifte und Vergiftungen, 6. Aufl., Nachdruck, Haug Verlag, Heidelberg 1992.

Madaus G, Lehrbuch der Biologischen Arzneimittel, Bde 1-3, Nachdruck, Georg Olms Verlag Hildesheim 1979.

Roth L, Daunderer M, Kormann K, Giftpflanzen, Pflanzengifte, 4. Aufl., Ecomed Fachverlag Landsberg Lech 1993.

Teuscher E, Lindequist U, Biogene Gifte - Biologie, Chemie, Pharmakologie, 2. Aufl., Fischer Verlag Stuttgart 1994.

Amaranth

See Amaranthus Hypochondriacus

Amaranthus Hypochondriacus

Amaranth

DESCRIPTION

Medicinal Parts: Amaranth is the complete plant of Amaranthus hypochondriacus.

Flower and Fruit: The inflorescence is bifurcated, solitary and oblong-spicate in dense spike-like terminal clusters with very short internodes often composed of twigs. In some species they are all in the leaf axils. The plant is monoecious, dioecious or mixed. Bracteoles are (2-4-6) mm, ovate, with a very long mucro, about twice as long as the perianth. The perianth-segments are narrowly ovate, usually acute and about as long as the fruit. The segments are dry-skinned, whitish- or reddish-green to red. The ovary is ovate. The fruit is one-seeded, ovate, dry-skinned and forms a transversely-dehiscing capsule. Seeds are lentil-shaped, erect, circular, smooth and usually black.

Leaves, Stem and Root: The plant is a tall glabrous annual, occasionally perennial up to 2 m tall. It is erect, glabrous or sparsely pubescent above. The leaves are rhomboid-ovate and alternate with occasionally undulating or ruffled margins.

Habitat: Common in temperate and warm climates.

Other Names: Lady Bleeding, Lovely Bleeding, Love-Lies-Bleeding, Red Cockscomb, Velvet Flower, Pilewort, Prince's Feather

ACTIONS AND PHARMACOLOGY

COMPOUNDS

Saponins

EFFECTS

Astringent.

INDICATIONS AND USAGE

Amaranth has been used for diarrhea, ulcers and inflammation of the mouth and throat.

PRECAUTIONS AND ADVERSE REACTIONS

No health hazards or side effects are known in conjunction with the proper administration of designated therapeutic dosages.

DOSAGE

Mode of Administration: Orally as a liquid extract.

LITERATURE

Martindale. The Extra Pharmacopoeia, 27th Ed. Pub. The Pharmaceutical Press (1977) UK.

American Adder's Tongue

See Erythronium Americanum

American Bittersweet

See Celastrus Scandens

American Hellebore

See Veratrum Viride

American Ivy

See Parthenocissus Quinquefolia

American Pawpaw

See Asimina Triloba

American White Pond Lily

See Nymphaea Odorata

Ammi Visnaga

Bishop's Weed

DESCRIPTION

Medicinal Parts: The medicinal part is the dried ripe fruit.

Flower and Fruit: The rays are 150 cm, slender and patent in the flower, becoming erect, thickened and indurate in the fruit. The bracts are 1 to 2-pinnatisect, equaling or exceeding the rays, and the bracteoles are subulate. The pedicels are erect, stout and rigid in the fruit. The fruit is 2 to 2.5 mm.

Leaves, Stem and Root: Bishop's Weed is a robust annual or biennial up to 100 cm tall. The lower leaves are pinnate, the others are 2 to 3 pinnate. All of the leaves have narrow linear or filform lobes.

Habitat: Ammi Visnaga grows in the Mediterranean region, and is cultivated in the U.S., Mexico, Chile and Argentina.

Production: Bishop's Weed fruit consists of the dried, ripe fruits of Ammi Visnaga.

Other Names: Khella, Khella Fruits

ACTIONS AND PHARMACOLOGY

COMPOUNDS

Furochromones: particularly khellin, visnagin, khellol and khellol glucoside

Pyranocumarins: particularly visnadin and samidin

Flavonoids: including quercetin and isohamnetin and their 3-sulfates

Volatile oil

Fatty oil

EFFECTS

Intensification of the coronary and myocardial circulation, mild positive ionotrope; antispasmodic on smooth muscles

INDICATIONS AND USAGE

Bishop's Weed has been used for angina pectoris, cardiac insufficiency, paroxysmal tachycardia, extra systoles, hypertonia, asthma, whooping cough and cramp-like complaints of the abdomen.

PRECAUTIONS AND ADVERSE REACTIONS

Infrequently, a cholestatic jaundice (reversible) is observed following administration of the drug. The drug also possesses a phototoxic effect.

OVERDOSAGE

Long-term use or overdose of the drug can lead to queasiness, dizziness, loss of appetite, headache, sleep disorders, and with very high dosages (corresponding to over 100 mg khellin), elevated levels (reversible) of liver enzymes in blood plasma.

DOSAGE

No information is available.

LITERATURE

Duarte J et al., Effects of visnadine on rat vascular smooth muscle. In: PM 63(3):233-236. 1997.

Greinwald R, Stobernack HP, Ammi visnaga - Das Bischhofskraut. In: ZPT 11(2):65. 1990.

Le Quesne PW et al., JNP 48:496. 1985.

Martelli P et al., J Chromatogr 301:297. 1984.

Trunzler G, Phytotherapeutische Möglichkeiten bei Herz- und arteriellen Gefäßerkrankungen. In: ZPT 10(5):147. 1989.

Further information in:

Kern W, List PH, Hörhammer L (Hrsg.), Hagers Handbuch der Pharmazeutischen Praxis, 4. Aufl., Bde. 1-8, Springer Verlag Berlin, Heidelberg, New York, 1969.

Madaus G, Lehrbuch der Biologischen Arzneimittel, Bde 1-3, Nachdruck, Georg Olms Verlag Hildesheim 1979.

Schulz R, Hänsel R, Rationale Phytotherapie, Springer Verlag Heidelberg 1996.

Steinegger E, Hänsel R, Pharmakognosie, 5. Aufl., Springer Verlag Heidelberg 1992.

Teuscher E, Biogene Arzneimittel, 5. Aufl., Wiss. Verlagsges. Stuttgart 1997.

Wagner H, Wiesenauer M: Phytotherapie. Phytopharmaka und pflanzliche Homöopathika, Fischer-Verlag, Stuttgart, Jena, New York 1995.

Wichtl M (Hrsg.), Teedrogen, 4. Aufl., Wiss. Verlagsges. Stuttgart 1997.

Anacardium Occidentale

Cashew

DESCRIPTION

Medicinal Parts: The medicinal parts are the finely chopped bark, the cashew nut, the fresh leaves and the cashew shell oil.

Flower and Fruit: Flowers are in terminal, cyme-like, 10 to 20 cm long panicles and are polygamous. The pedicles are 2 to 3 mm long. The calyx is deeply divided into five sepals which are lanceolate, erect, imbricate, glabrous inside and covered on the outside with short, thick, gray hairs. The corolla is 5 petaled. The petals are lineal-lanceolate, 7 to 8 mm long by 1 mm wide, acute, soft and gray-haired on the outside. The petals are glabrous and yellow with a red stripe on the inside that curls outwards in the later stages. Seven to 10 stamens are fused at the base, but only one 8 to 9 mm long stamen is fertile; the sterile ones are shorter. Anthers are yellowish-white, oblong-ovate and burst open along a vertical slit. The gynoecium is obovate, 2 mm long, one-valved and elongates to a 4 mm long wedge-shaped style with a spot-like stigma. The flowers are followed by a fleshy, edible receptacle, which partly encloses the fruit. The fruit is reniform, with a smooth, pale grayish-brown drupe, about 2 to 3 cm long and 1 cm thick.

Leaves, Stem and Root: Anacardium occidentale is a broad evergreen tree from 6 to 10 m high with smooth glabrous branches, densely leafed towards the tops. It has short-petioled leaves that are alternate, coriaceous and entire-margined. The leaf blade is obovate, 12 to 14 cm by 6 to 8 cm with a prominent midrib and 10 to 14 almost parallel veins.

Habitat: The plant grows in the Caribbean and Central and South America; it is cultivated everywhere in the tropics especially in Africa and India.

Production: Fruit of the cashew tree is harvested with the stem removed.

Other Names: East Indian Almond

ACTIONS AND PHARMACOLOGY

COMPOUNDS

In the seed case:

Alkyl phenoles

Anacardic acid

Cardol

Methyl cardol

In the seeds:

Fatty oil

Chief fatty acids: oleic acid and linolenic acid

Proteins

Starch

EFFECTS

It has been demonstrated in vitro, that the dried extract prepared with ethanol is effective against the gram-positive bacteria *Bacillus subtilis* and *Staphylococcus aureus.* It is also mildly astringent.

INDICATIONS AND USAGE

Cashew is used as a skin stimulant and cauterizing agent for ulcers, warts and corns. It is also used for gastrointestinal ailments. Efficacy for these indications has not been documented.

PRECAUTIONS AND ADVERSE REACTIONS

The alkyl phenoles contained in the seed case of the nut are strong skin irritants. Contact between the seed case and skin can lead to erythemas with nodule and blister formation. Frequent contact can lead to rimose exanthemas. The roasted seeds eaten as cashew nuts are free of alkyl phenoles as is the plant stalk.

DOSAGE

Mode of Administration: Available preparations include acajou oil, cashew oil, oleum anacardiae and fatty oil extracted from the seeds.

Preparation: In combination preparations, particularly in homeopathy.

LITERATURE

Barroso MAT, Hort Sciences: 8:99. 1973.

Behl, Buch. In: Behl PN, Captain RM, Bedi BMS, Gupta S: Skin Irritant and Sensitizing plants found in India, PN Behl, India. 1967.

Kubo I et al., Tyrosinase inhibitors from Anacardium occidentale. In: JNP 57(4):545. 1994.

Laurens A, Paris RR (1976) Plant Med Phytother 11:16

Nagaraja KV, Plant Foods Hum Nutr 37:307-311. 1987.

Nagaraja KV, Qual Plat - Plant Foods Hum Nutr 37:69-75. 1987.

Neuwinger HD, Arzneipflanzen Schwarzafrikas. In: DAZ 134(6):453. 1994.

Ogunlana EO, Ramstad E (1975) Planta Med 27:354.

Paul VJ, Yeddanapalli LM, J Am Chem Soc 78:5675-5678. 1956.

Samant SK, Rege DV, Lebensm-Wiss Technol 22:164-168. 1989.

Sullivan JT et al. (1982) Planta Med 44:175.

Tyman JHP, Anal Chem 48:30-34. 1976.

Tyman JHP, Kiong LS, Lipids 13:525-532. 1978.

Further information in:

Hausen B, Allergiepflanzen, Pflanzenallergene, ecomed Verlagsgesellsch. mbH, Landsberg 1988.

Hänsel R, Keller K, Rimpler H, Schneider G (Hrsg.), Hagers Handbuch der Pharmazeutischen Praxis, 5. Aufl., Bde 4-6 (Drogen), Springer Verlag Berlin, Heidelberg, New York, 1992-1994.

Lewin L, Gifte und Vergiftungen, 6. Aufl., Nachdruck, Haug Verlag, Heidelberg 1992.

Madaus G, Lehrbuch der Biologischen Arzneimittel, Bde 1-3, Nachdruck, Georg Olms Verlag Hildesheim 1979.

Oliver-Bever B (Ed.), Medicinal Plants of Tropical West Africa, Cambridge University Press Cambridge, London 1986.

Roth L, Daunderer M, Kormann K, Giftpflanzen, Pflanzengifte, 4. Aufl., Ecomed Fachverlag Landsberg Lech 1993.

Anacyclus Pyrethrum

Pellitory

DESCRIPTION

Medicinal Parts: The medicinal part is the root.

Flower and Fruit: Each stem bears a 1 cm wide flower. The bracts are fused. The ray florets are white and tinged purple beneath. The disc florets are pointed. The fruit has transparent wings.

Leaves, Stem and Root: It is a perennial grass plant whose thickened, hollow stems grow a little along the ground before they turn up. They grow to about 45 cm high and have double-pinnate, tough leaves. The root is almost cylindrical, easily twisted and tapered and crowned with a tuft of gray hair. Brown and fissured on the outside with shiny black markings.

Habitat: The plant grows in North Africa and is cultivated in the Mediterranean.

Other Names: Pellitory of Spain, Pyrethre, Pyrethrum, Roman Pellitory, Spanish Camomile

ACTION AND PHARMACOLOGY

COMPOUNDS

Alkamides: including deca-2,4-dien acid-isobutylamide, anacycline, dehydroanacycline

Lignane: including sesamine

Inulin (fructosan)

Tannins

EFFECTS

Application to the skin stimulates the nerve ends, resulting in redness and irritation (hot, burning sensation).

INDICATIONS AND USAGE

Pellitory is used for rheumatic conditions, the external treatment of toothache, as a tonic to aid digestion and as an insecticide.

PRECAUTIONS AND ADVERSE REACTIONS

No health hazards or side effects are known in conjunction with the proper administration of designated therapeutic dosages. Signs of irritation are possible in connection with overdoses due to the mucous-membrane-stimulating character of the alkamides.

DOSAGE

Mode of Administration: No precise information is available.

LITERATURE

Kern W, List PH, Hörhammer L (Hrsg.), Hagers Handbuch der Pharmazeutischen Praxis, 4. Aufl., Bde 1-8, Springer Verlag Berlin, Heidelberg, New York, 1969.

Anagallis Arvensis

Scarlet Pimpernel

DESCRIPTION

Medicinal Parts: The medicinal part is the dried, flowering herb without the roots.

Flower and Fruit: The plant has 6 to 10 brick red flowers in the leaf axils, which are up to 2.5 times as long as the bracts. The symmetrically radiating flower has a double perianth. It has 5 sepals which are 4 to 5 mm long, entire-margined, narrow-lanceolate and acute. The wheel-shaped corolla is usually vermilion, but occasionally blue-flesh colored, lilac or white. The tip of the corolla is obovate to oval, about 7 mm long by 6 mm wide, overlapping at the base, entire-margined or slightly crenate with 50 to 70 glandular hairs. It has 5 stamens with a distinct awn that are fused to a funnel at the tube. The anthers are short, ellipsoid and cordate at the base. The superior ovary is globose and one-valved with an oblong style and head-like stigma. The fruit is a globose pyxidum, 4 to 5 mm in diameter, that contains 20 to 22 rough wart-like, brown seeds 1.3 mm long by 1 mm wide.

Leaves, Stem and Root: Anagallis arvensis is an annual herb with prostrate, creeping, square stems up to 30 cm long, and thinner, branched, ascending stems 6 to 30 cm long. The square shoots, like the leaves, are covered thickly when young with short hairs, which later become glabrous. The leaves are opposite, occasionally in whorls of 3, ovate to lanceolate, up to 20 mm long by 10 mm wide, sessile, entire-margined, acute and spotted black on the underside.

Characteristics: The flowers close at night and open at about 9 in the morning. They are poisonous.

Habitat: The plant is widely distributed throughout Europe, Asia, the U.S. and non-tropical South America.

Production: Scarlet Pimpernel herb is the dried herb in flower of Anagallis arvensis, without the root and occasionally the whole plant.

Not To Be Confused With: The blue flowering form of Anagallis arvensis is often confused with Anagallis foemina and occasionally with Stellaria media.

Other Names: Adder's Eyes, Poor Man's Weatherglass, Red Chickweed, Red Pimpernel, Shepherd's Barometer

ACTIONS AND PHARMACOLOGY

COMPOUNDS

Triterpene saponins: including anagalline, chief sapogenine 13,28-epoxy-16- oxooleanan

Cucurbitacins: including cucurbitacins E, B, D, I and L

Flavonoids

Caffeic acid derivatives

EFFECTS

The aqueous extract of the dried leaves is fungitoxic. Triterpenglycoside, anagalloside and aglycon anagalligenones, isolated from the drug, displayed inhibitory results against numerous micro-organisms. Aqueous extracts showed uterine contracting activity in rats, guinea pigs, rabbits, and on strips of human uterine material. The triterpene saponins isolated from the drug demonstrated action against human sperm. The methanol extract of the drug demonstrated estrogen activity in the Allen-Doisy-test. The saponins isolated from the powder drug with ethanol demonstrated hemolytic activity in human blood. The methanol extract of the dried powdered drug is antiviral against *Herpes simplex Type I, Adenovirus Type II* and *Polio Type II*, among others. The saponins are the active constituents. The acetyl-saponin isolated from the drug acts as a teniacide.

INDICATIONS AND USAGE

The drug is used to treat depression, disorders of the mucous membranes, hemorrhoids, herpes, painful kidney disorders, (in particular inflammation of the kidney and an increase in urination), liver disorders, poorly healing wounds and pruritus. The herb is used as a supporting treatment in various carcinomas. It is used both internally and externally to treat pains in the joints.

The efficacy of Scarlet Pimpernal in the treatment of these conditions has not been proven.

PRECAUTIONS AND ADVERSE REACTIONS

No health hazards or side effects are known in conjunction with the proper administration of designated therapeutic dosages. Large doses or long-term administration could lead to gastroenteritis and nephritis, due to the cucurbitacins content of the drug.

DOSAGE

Mode of Administration: Topically as a poultice, internally as an infusion.

Preparation: For the treatment of liver and kidney disorders as well as dropsy, add one-half teaspoonful of the drug to a glass of hot water and let it steep for 10 minutes. Drink throughout the day.

Daily Dosage: The usual dosage is 1.8 gm of the powder 4 times a day.

LITERATURE

Alimbaeva PK, Mukhamedziev MM, Rast Resur 5:380-385. 1969.

Aliotta G, De Napoli L, Giordano F, Piccialli G, Piccialli V, Santacroce C, An oleanen triterpene from Anagallis arvensis. In: PH 31(3):929-933. 1992.

Amoros M and Girre RL, (1977) Phytochemistry 26(3):787.

Amoros M et al., (1979) PlantMed Phytother 13:122.

Amoros M, Fauconnier B, Girre RL, In vitro antiviral activity of a saponin from Anagallis arvensis, Primulaceae, against herpes simplex virus and poliovirus. In: Antiviral Res 8:13-25. 1987.

Banerji R et al., (1981) Indian Drugs 19:121.

Büechi S, Antivirale Saponine, pharmakologische und klinische Untersuchungen. In: DAZ 136(2):89-98. 1996.

Yamada Y et al., (1978) Phytochemistry 17:1798.

Yamada Y et al., Chem Pharm Bull 26:3107-3112. 1978.

Further information in:

Hänsel R, Keller K, Rimpler H, Schneider G (Hrsg.), Hagers Handbuch der Pharmazeutischen Praxis, 5. Aufl., Bde 4-6 (Drogen), Springer Verlag Berlin, Heidelberg, New York, 1992-1994.

Hausen B, Allergiepflanzen, Pflanzenallergene, ecomed Verlagsgesellsch. mbH, Landsberg 1988.

Madaus G, Lehrbuch der Biologischen Arzneimittel, Bde 1-3, Nachdruck, Georg Olms Verlag Hildesheim 1979.

Roth L, Daunderer M, Kormann K, Giftpflanzen, Pflanzengifte, 4. Aufl., Ecomed Fachverlag Landsberg Lech 1993.

Anamirta Cocculus

Cocculus Indicus

DESCRIPTION

Medicinal Parts: The medicinal part is the ripe, dried fruit.

Flower and Fruit: Petiolate inflorescences are panicle-like, 16 to 40 cm long and usually inserted in the stem. Male flowers are occasionally axillary. The two outer petals are smaller and about 1 mm long. The inner ones are whitish or yellowish-green, broad-elliptoid, 2 to 3 mm long, in 2 alternating, triple whorls and are imbricate. The synandria are formed from a short-stemmed, globose cluster of about 30 to 35 anthers. The pollen is round and tricolporate. The female flowers also have 3+3 tepals as well as small staminoids. The 3 or 4 carpels are set sideways on a central, erect fruit axis that becomes conically oblong when the fruit ripens. The style is inserted in the side and the stigma is turned back. The drupes are globose to reniform, 9 to 11 mm long, glabrous and sit on the short, spreading branches of the fruit axis. The fruit is about 1 cm long, blackish and contains a horseshoe-shaped seed.

Leaves, Stem and Root: Anamirta cocculus are hardy, woody lianas with ash-gray to straw-yellow striped bark. The leaves are ovate to cordate. The leaf blade is 16 to 28 cm long and 10 to 24 cm wide and coriaceous. The main veins are arranged in palmate fashion at the base with parallel secondary veins. The 6 to 18 cm petiole is thickened at both ends.

Characteristics: The fruit shell is tasteless, the seed is bitter and oily.

Habitat: The plant grows in India, Sri Lanka and Malaysia.

Production: Cocculus Indicus seeds are the fruit of the false myrtle Anamirta cocculus.

Other Names: Fish Berries, Levant Nut

ACTIONS AND PHARMACOLOGY

COMPOUNDS

Sesquiterpens: picrotoxin, a mixture of picrotoxinine and its hydratisation by-product picrotin, picrotoxin acid methyl ester

Isoquinoline alkaloids: menispermine, paramenispermine

Fatty oil

EFFECTS

The central ends of the parasympathetic nerves are stimulated. The drug stimulates the medulla oblongata. Breathing frequency is primarily increased and secondarily decreased. The pulse slows down due to the stimulation of the vagus and an increase in blood pressure. Central nervous system-stimulated vomiting, increase in perspiration and saliva are probably due to the action of picrotoxin.

INDICATIONS AND USAGE

In the past, the drug was used as an insecticide in powder form for scabies. The picrotoxin, which was to paralyze fish in the fishing industry, was formerly used in cases of barbituric acid poisoning. In more recent times, it has been used in the treatment of peripheral and vestibular nystagmus and in both long and short-term therapy for peripherally based dizziness.

PRECAUTIONS AND ADVERSE REACTIONS

The drug is very poisonous. Mild poisonings cause headache, dizziness, nausea, coordination disturbances, general depression and spastic twitching.

OVERDOSAGE

High dosages lead to frequent vomiting, sleepiness and tonic-clonic spasms. Death follows, often not until days later, through asphyxiation and heart failure. Two to three Cocculus kernels can be fatal.

Treatment consists of inducing vomiting and/or gastric lavage, purging with sodium sulphate, instillation of activated charcoal and forced diuresis. The spasms should be suppressed with as much diazepam as is absolutely necessary. In case of fever, the patient should be wrapped in ice packs, administered high-caloric infusions and possibly oxygen respiration. Phenothiazines and analeptics should be avoided.

DOSAGE

Mode of Administration: In combination preparations.

Daily Dosage: One to 5 mg can be taken by healthy patients that do not experience side effects.

Storage: Store in tightly closed containers, protected from the light. The drug should be safely stored since it is poisonous.

LITERATURE

Frohne D, Pikrotoxin - Renaisssance eines ''obsoleten'' pflanzlichen Arzneistoffes. In: ZPT 10(3):101. 1989.

Further information in:

Hänsel R, Keller K, Rimpler H, Schneider G (Hrsg.), Hagers Handbuch der Pharmazeutischen Praxis, 5. Aufl., Bde 4-6 (Drogen), Springer Verlag Berlin, Heidelberg, New York, 1992-1994.

Hoppe HA, (1975-1987) Drogenkunde, 8. Aufl., Bde 1-3, W. de Gruyter Verlag, Berlin, New York.

Lewin L, Gifte und Vergiftungen, 6. Aufl., Nachdruck, Haug Verlag, Heidelberg 1992.

Madaus G, Lehrbuch der Biologischen Arzneimittel, Bde 1-3, Nachdruck, Georg Olms Verlag Hildesheim 1979.

Roth L, Daunderer M, Kormann K, Giftpflanzen, Pflanzengifte, 4. Aufl., Ecomed Fachverlag Landsberg Lech 1993.

Steinegger E, Hänsel R, Pharmakognosie, 5. Aufl., Springer Verlag Heidelberg 1992.

Teuscher E, Biogene Arzneimittel, 5. Aufl., Wiss. Verlagsges. mbH Stuttgart 1997.

Teuscher E, Lindequist U, Biogene Gifte - Biologie, Chemie, Pharmakologie, 2. Aufl., Fischer Verlag Stuttgart 1994.

Wagner H, Wiesenauer M, Phytotherapie. Phytopharmaka und pflanzliche Homöopathika, Fischer-Verlag, Stuttgart, Jena, New York 1995.

Andira Araroba

Goa Powder

DESCRIPTION

Medicinal Parts: The medicinal part is the dried and pulverized latex of the trunk and branches.

Flower and Fruit: Andira araroba is a large smooth tree whose yellowish wood has vertically running channels and spaces. The latex collects increasingly in these spaces as the tree ages. The bark forms in long flat pieces about 3 mm thick and is grayish-white and fissured externally. The inner surface is brownish and striated. The fracture is laminated with yellow fibers.

Characteristics: The taste is mucilaginous and bitter and the odor is slight but disagreeable.

Habitat: The tree grows in Brazil.

Production: Goa powder is exuded from the nuclear cavity of Andira araroba. The exuded substance is purified by recrystalization in benzol, thus producing raw chrysarobin.

Other Names: Araroba, Bahia Powder, Brazil Powder, Chrysatobine, Crude Chrysarobin, Ringworm Powder

ACTIONS AND PHARMACOLOGY

COMPOUNDS

Anthrone derivatives: in particular chrysophanolanthrone

EFFECTS

The powder is a strong reducing agent. It causes severe erythema upon contact with the skin. It inhibits glucose-6-phosphate-dehydrogenisation in psoriatic skin conditions. The drug easily absorbs through the skin.

INDICATIONS AND USAGE

Goa Powder is used for psoriasis in chrysarobin ointments and for various kinds of dermatomycosis. It has been widely replaced by synthetic anthranol.

PRECAUTIONS AND ADVERSE REACTIONS

The drug is severely irritating to skin and mucous membranes (redness, swelling, pustules and conjunctivitis, even without eye contact). Internal administration leads to vomiting, diarrhea and kidney inflammation (with as little as 0.01 gm). External administration on large skin areas could cause resorptive poisonings.

DOSAGE

Mode of Administration: Topically in emulsions, the synthetic anthranol cignolin is also used in the treatment of psoriasis.

LITERATURE

Anonym, Abwehr von Arzneimittelrisiken, Stufe II. In: DAZ 136(38):3253-2354. 1996.

BGA, Arzneimittelrisiken: Anthranoide. In: DAZ 132(21):1164. 1992.

Müller K, Wiegrebe W, Psoriasis und Antipsoriatika. In: DAZ 137(22):1893-1902. 1997.

Further information in:

Kern W, List PH, Hörhammer L (Hrsg.), Hagers Handbuch der Pharmazeutischen Praxis, 4. Aufl., Bde. 1-8, Springer Verlag Berlin, Heidelberg, New York, 1969.

Lewin L, Gifte und Vergiftungen, 6. Aufl., Nachdruck, Haug Verlag, Heidelberg 1992.

Thomson RH, Naturally Occurring Quinones, 2nd Ed., Academic Press New York 1971.

Anemone Hepatica

Liverwort

DESCRIPTION

Medicinal Parts: The drug is the herb, without roots, harvested at flowering season.

Flower and Fruit: The flowering stems are axillary, numerous, pubescent and erect. They are usually reddish and have 3, up to 1 cm long, entire-margined, ovate, unpetiolate, calyx-like bracts directly under the upright flower. The 6 to 8 bracts are sky blue, paler on the outside, occasionally pink or white, narrow-ovate, entire-margined and dropping. The are no nectaries. The stamens are almost white with red connective. The stigma is head-like. The fruit is oblong with a short beak fitted into the semi-globular receptacle.

Leaves, Stem and Root: The herb is a 7 to 15 cm high, hardy perennial with a short, fibrous, dark brown rhizome. The numerous leaves are basal, long-petioled, coriaceous, green above and usually more or less violet beneath. They are cordate and 3-lobed at the base, deeply indented, broadly ovate, with blunt to acute lobes. The young leaves, including the stems, are densely covered in silky white hairs. The leaves later become glabrous, and appear after flowering. Liverwort is a protected species in Germany, Austria, Switzerland, Italy, The Czech Republic, Slovakia, and Hungary.

Habitat: The plant is indigenous to almost all of Europe except the Atlantic regions, Denmark and northwest Germany. It is also indigenous to Korea, Japan and temperate North America.

Production: Liverwort consists of the fresh or dried aboveground parts of Hepatica nobilis. The herb is harvested when in bloom, and is air-dried in the shade. The roots must be left in the ground because they are a protected species.

Other Names: Herb Trinity, Kidneywort, Liverleaf, Liverweed, Round-leaved Hepatica, Trefoil

ACTIONS AND PHARMACOLOGY

COMPOUNDS

Precursors yielding protoanemonines: presumably ranunculin, (only in the freshly-harvested plant)

Flavonoids: including isoquercitrin, astragalin, quercimeritrin

Saponins

EFFECTS

The main active agents are lactone-forming glycosides, flavo-glycosides and anthocyane. The fresh plant contains protoanemonin, which causes skin irritation.

INDICATIONS AND USAGE

Preparations of Liverwort herb are used for liver ailments, liver diseases of all origins, jaundice, gallstones and gravel. The claimed efficacy has not been documented.

PRECAUTIONS AND ADVERSE REACTIONS

Health risks or side effects following the proper administration of designated therapeutic dosages are not recorded.

Extended skin contact with the freshly-harvested, bruised plant can lead to blister formation and cauterizations which are difficult to heal due to the resulting protoanemonine, which is severely irritating to the skin and mucous membranes. If taken internally, severe irritation to the gastrointestinal tract, combined with colic and diarrhea, as well as irritation of the urinary drainage passages, are possible.

Symptomatic treatment for external contact consists of mucilaginosa, following irrigation with diluted potassium permanganate solution. In case of internal contact, administration of activated charcoal should follow gastric lavage.

DOSAGE

Mode of Administration: The drug can be taken internally or used externally as a rinse.

Preparation: To make a rinse, a cataplasm can be made of the squeezed fresh plant; alcohol can be used if necessary. A liniment can be made with added fats, oils or alcohol.

Daily Dosage: When used internally, a single dose consists of 2 to 4 gm as an infusion, or 2 to 3 cups from a 3 to 6% infusion. The daily dosage is 4 teaspoonfuls, or 3.8 gm drug.

LITERATURE

Ruijgrok HWL, PM 11:338-347. 1963.

Further information in:

Hänsel R, Keller K, Rimpler H, Schneider G (Hrsg.), Hagers Handbuch der Pharmazeutischen Praxis, 5. Aufl., Bde 4-6 (Drogen), Springer Verlag Berlin, Heidelberg, New York, 1992-1994.

Madaus G, Lehrbuch der Biologischen Arzneimittel, Bde 1-3, Nachdruck, Georg Olms Verlag Hildesheim 1979.

Roth L, Daunderer M, Kormann K: Giftpflanzen, Pflanzengifte, 4. Aufl., Ecomed Fachverlag Landsberg Lech 1993.

Teuscher E, Lindequist U, Biogene Gifte - Biologie, Chemie, Pharmakologie, 2. Aufl., Fischer Verlag Stuttgart 1994.

Anemone Nemorosa

Wood Anemone

DESCRIPTION

Medicinal Parts: The medicinal parts are the aerial parts of the plant.

Flower and Fruit: The white flowers are solitary and located at the end of a long stem. The stem is erect when in flower, white to reddish-violet and have a diameter of 1.5 to 4 cm. The usually 6 (also 5 to 9) bracts are oblong-ovate, entire-margined, and glabrous. The flowers have numerous yellow stamens. The 10 to 20 carpels are oblong with a short curved beak. They are downy and 4 to 5 mm long. The fruit is a drooping compound with a roughly haired fruitlet.

Leaves, Stem and Root: Anemone nemorosa is a perennial plant, 6 to 30 cm high with a horizontally creeping yellow to dark brown, roundish rhizome. The stems are usually solitary, erect, glabrous or sparsely pubescent. There is usually a long-stemmed basal leaf. The leaf is tri-pinnate and pinnatifid-serrate. The first row of pinna are stemmed and have horizontal pinna sections, each with 1 pinna of the second level. There are cauline rosettes of 3 leaf-like bracts, which have a 2 cm long petiole. The bracts do not generally have axillary buds, are palmate and pinnatifid-serrate.

Habitat: The plant is spread almost all over Europe as far as the Volga region except in the Mediterranean and northern Lappland.

Production: Wood Anemone is the aerial part of Anemone nemorosa, collected shortly before the flowers open.

Other Names: Pasque Flower, Crowfoot, Wind Flower, Smell Fox

ACTIONS AND PHARMACOLOGY

COMPOUNDS

Protoanemonine-forming substance: in the freshly-harvested plant, presumably the glycosides ranunculin, that changes enzymatically when the plant is cut into small pieces, and probably also when it is dried, into the pungent, volatile protoanemonine that quickly dimerizes to anemonine; when dried, the plant is not capable of protoanemonine-formation

EFFECTS

No information is available.

INDICATIONS AND USAGE

In Russian folk medicine, the drug is used for stomach pains, delayed menstruation, gout, whooping cough, and asthma. In homeopathy, it is used for gynecological disorders.

No useful documentation on the efficacy of the drug is available.

PRECAUTIONS AND ADVERSE REACTIONS

No health hazards or side effects are known in conjunction with the proper administration of designated therapeutic dosages of the dehydrated drug.

Prolonged skin contact with the freshly-harvested, bruised plant can lead to blister formation and cauterizations, which are slow to heal due to the resulting protoanemonine, which is severely irritating to skin and mucous membranes. If taken internally, severe irritation to the gastrointestinal tract, combined with colic and diarrhea, as well as irritation of the urinary drainage passages, are possible.

Symptomatic treatment for external contact should consist of mucilage after irrigation with diluted potassium permanganate solution.

OVERDOSAGE

In case of internal contact, activated charcoal should follow gastric lavage. Death by asphyxiation following the intake of large quantities of protoanemonine-forming plants has been observed in animal experiments. Thirty freshly-harvested plants are believed to represent the fatal level for humans.

DOSAGE

Mode of Administration: The drug has application in highly dilute homeopathic preparations.

LITERATURE

Bonora A et al., PH 26:2277. 1987.

Ruijgrok HWL, PM 11:338-347. 1963.

Further information in:

Frohne D, Pfänder HJ, Giftpflanzen - Ein Handbuch für Apotheker, Toxikologen und Biologen, 4. Aufl., Wiss. Verlags-Ges Stuttgart 1997.

Hänsel R, Keller K, Rimpler H, Schneider G (Hrsg.), Hagers Handbuch der Pharmazeutischen Praxis, 5. Aufl., Bde 4-6 (Drogen): Springer Verlag Berlin, Heidelberg, New York, 1992-1994.

Lewin L, Gifte und Vergiftungen, 6. Aufl., Nachdruck, Haug Verlag, Heidelberg 1992.

Madaus G, Lehrbuch der Biologischen Arzneimittel, Bde 1-3, Nachdruck, Georg Olms Verlag Hildesheim 1979.

Roth L, Daunderer M, Kormann K, Giftpflanzen, Pflanzengifte, 4. Aufl., Ecomed Fachverlag Landsberg Lech 1993.

Teuscher E, Lindequist U, Biogene Gifte - Biologie, Chemie, Pharmakologie, 2. Aufl., Fischer Verlag Stuttgart 1994.

Anethum Graveolens

Dill

DESCRIPTION

Medicinal Parts: The medicinal part is the seed, the fresh or dried leaves and the upper stem.

Flower and Fruit: The yellow flowers are in large, 20 to 50 rayed umbels. There is no involucre or calyx. The petals have an inward-curving point, which is not indented. The fruit is flattened and oval with a rib on the back, which is sharp-edged. Ribs that appear on the edge have a winged edge.

Leaves, Stem and Root: The plant is 40 to 120 cm tall. The stem is erect, round, smooth, dark green and white striped. The stem is branched above, with a bluish bloom. The leaves are double and more pinnate, feathery, white-tipped leaflets with a deep groove on the upper surface. The leaf sheath is oblong with a thick-skinned edge.

Characteristics: Dill has an aromatic scent.

Habitat: Mediterranean region, southern Russia.

Production: Dill herb consists of the fresh or dried leaf and upper stem of Anethum graveolens. Dill seed consists of the dried fruit of Anethum graveolens.

Other Names: Dilly

ACTIONS AND PHARMACOLOGY

COMPOUNDS: ANETHI HERBA

Volatile oil

Furanocoumarins

EFFECTS: ANETHI HERBA

No information available.

COMPOUNDS: ANETHI FRUCTUS

Volatile oil

Furanocoumarins

EFFECTS: ANETHI FRUCTUS

Antispasmodic, bacteriostatic.

INDICATIONS AND USAGE

ANETHI HERBA

Dill herb is used for prevention and treatment of diseases and disorders of the gastrointestinal tract, kidney and urinary tract, for sleep disorders, as well as for spasms.

ANETHI FRUCTUS

- Loss of appetite
- Fevers and colds
- Cough
- Bronchitis
- Tendency to infection
- Liver and gallbladder complaints
- Inflammation of the mouth and pharynx
- Common cold

Dill is also used in Dyspepsia.

PRECAUTIONS AND ADVERSE REACTIONS

ANETHI HERBA

No health hazards or side effects are known in conjunction with the proper administration of designated therapeutic dosages.

ANETHI FRUCTUS

No health hazards or side effects are known in conjunction with the proper administration of designated therapeutic dosages. Photodermatosis is possible after contact with the juice of the freshly-harvested plant.

DOSAGE

ANETHI FRUCTUS

Mode of Administration: Whole seeds for teas and other galenic preparations for internal application.

Daily Dosage: The average daily dosage of the seeds is 3 gm; essential oil daily dose is 0.1 to 0.3 gm.

LITERATURE

ANETHI HERBA

Badoc A, Contribution à l'étude du genre Anethum. In: Mémoire Diplome supérieur Rech Biol et Physiol, Univ Sci Techn Lille Flandres Artois No. 122, Dec. 1986.

Debelmas AM, Rochat J, (1967) Plant Med Phytother 1:23.

Dranik LI, (1970) Khim Prir Soed 6:268.

Gijbels MJ et al., (1983) Sci Pharm 51:414.

Harborne JB, (1969) Phytochemistry 8:1729.

Kosawa M et al., (1976) Chem Pharm Bull 24:220.

Poggendorf A, Göckeritz D, Pohloudek-Fabini R, Der Gehalt an ätherischem Öl in Anethum graveolens. In: PA 32(10):607. 1977.

Varo PT, Heinz DE, (1970) J Agric Food Chem 18:234 et 239.

Further information in:

Kern W, List PH, Hörhammer L (Hrsg.), Hagers Handbuch der Pharmazeutischen Praxis, 4. Aufl., Bde. 1-8, Springer Verlag Berlin, Heidelberg, New York, 1969.

Madaus G, Lehrbuch der Biologischen Arzneimittel, Bde 1-3, Nachdruck, Georg Olms Verlag Hildesheim 1979.

ANETHI FRUCTUS

Badoc A, Contribution à l'étude du genre Anethum. In: Mémoire Diplome supérieur Rech Biol et Physiol, Univ Sci Techn Lille Flandres Artois No. 122, Dec. 1986.

Debelmas AM, Rochat J, (1967) Plant Med Phytother 1:23.

Dranik LI, (1970) Khim Prir Soed 6:268.

Gijbels MJ et al., (1983) Sci Pharm 51:414.

Harborne JB, (1969) Phytochemistry 8:1729.

Kosawa M et al., (1976) Chem Pharm Bull 24:220.

Poggendorf A, Göckeritz D, Pohloudek-Fabini R, Der Gehalt an ätherischem Öl in Anethum graveolens. In: PA 32(10):607. 1977.

Varo PT, Heinz DE, (1970) J Agric Food Chem 18:234 et 239.

Further information in:

Kern W, List PH, Hörhammer L (Hrsg.), Hagers Handbuch der Pharmazeutischen Praxis, 4. Aufl., Bde. 1-8, Springer Verlag Berlin, Heidelberg, New York, 1969.

Madaus G, Lehrbuch der Biologischen Arzneimittel, Bde 1-3, Nachdruck, Georg Olms Verlag Hildesheim 1979.

Angelica Archangelica

Angelica

DESCRIPTION

Medicinal Parts: The medicinal parts are the seed, whole herb and root.

Flower and Fruit: The flowers are greenish-white to yellowish and are arranged in 20 to 40 rayed compact umbels without an involucre. The tiny epicalyx has numerous sepals and the tips of the sepals are minute. The petals have an indented, indistinguishable tip. The elliptic fruit is 7 mm long by 4 mm wide and winged. The outer fruit membrane separates from the inner one.

Leaves, Stem and Root: The plant grows from 50 to 250 cm. The rhizome is short, strong, fleshy and has long fibrous roots. The stem is erect, often as thick as an arm at the base, round, finely grooved, hollow and tinged reddish below. The leaves are very large, 60 to 90 cm and tri-pinnate with a hollow petiole. Leaflets are ovate and unevenly serrate. The leaf sheaths are large and swollen.

Characteristics: The plant has a strong tangy odor. The taste is sweetish to burning tangy.

Habitat: Angelica is thought by some botanists to be indigenous to Syria. Today it is found growing in the wild on the coasts of the North and Baltic Seas as far north as Lapland. It is cultivated in other regions. Other species are found in America (A. atropurpurea), in Europe (A. sylvestris) and in China/Asia (A. sinensis).

Production: Angelica seed consists of the fruit of Angelica archangelica. Angelica herb consists of the above-ground parts of Angelica archangelica. Angelica root consists of the dried root and rhizome of Angelica archangelica.

Other Names: European Angelica, Garden Angelica

ACTIONS AND PHARMACOLOGY

COMPOUNDS: ANGELICAE FRUCTUS ET HERBA

Volatile oil

Furocoumarins

EFFECTS: ANGELICAE FRUCTUS ET HERBA

No information available.

COMPOUNDS: ANGELICAE RADIX

Volatile oil: chief components are alpha- and beta-phellandrenes, alpha-pinenes, macrocyclic lactones, including penta- and heptadecanolide

Furocoumarins: including. bergaptene, xanthotoxin, scopoletin, umbelliferone

Caffeic acid derivatives: including chlorogenic acid

Flavonoids

EFFECTS: ANGELICAE RADIX

Antispasmodic, cholagogue, stimulatory for secretion of gastric juices.

INDICATIONS AND USAGE

ANGELICAE FRUCTUS ET HERBA

Preparations of angelica seed and herb are used as a diuretic and diaphoretic.

The effectiveness for these applications is not documented.

ANGELICAE RADIX

- Loss of appetite
- Dyspeptic complaints

Loss of appetite, peptic discomfort such as mild spasms of the gastrointestinal tract, feeling of fullness, flatulence.

PRECAUTIONS AND ADVERSE REACTIONS

ANGELICAE FRUCTUS ET HERBA

No health hazards or side effects are known in conjunction with the proper administration of designated therapeutic dosages. Photodermatosis is possible following contact with the plant juice.

ANGELICAE RADIX

No health hazards or side effects are known in conjunction with the proper administration of designated therapeutic dosages. Photodermatosis is possible following intake of large quantities of the drug, in particular in the form of ethanolic extracts, due to the photosensitizing character of furanocoumarin.

DOSAGE

ANGELICAE RADIX

Mode of Administration: Comminuted herb and other oral galenic preparations for internal use.

Daily Dosage: 4.5 gm of drug, 0.5 to 3.0 gm of liquid extract (1:1); 1.5 gm of tincture (1:5); 10 to 20 drops of essential oil.

LITERATURE

ANGELICAE FRUCTUS ET HERBA

Amling R, Phytotherapeutika in der Neurologie. In: ZPT 12(1):9. 1991.

Ashraf M et al., (1980) Pak J Sci Ind Res 23 (1-2):73.

Chang, EH et al., (Eds), Advances in Chinese Medicinal Materials Research, World Scientific Pub. Co. Singapore 1985.

Escher S, Keller U et al., (1979) Helv Chim Acta 62 (7):2061.

Glowniak K et al., Localisation and seasonal chenges of psoralen in Angelica fruits. In: PM 62, Abstracts of the 44th Ann Congress of GA, 76. 1996.

Lemmich J et al., (1983) Phytochemistry 23 (2):553-555.

Leung AY, Encyclopedia of Common Natural Ingredients used in Food Drugs and Cosmetics, John Wiley & Sons Inc. New York, 1980.

Opdyke DLJ, (1975) Food Cosmet Toxicol: 13, Suppl 713.

Sethi OP, Shah AK, (1979) Ind J Pharm Sci 42 (6): C11.

Shimizu M, Matsuzawa T, Suzuki S, Yoshizaki M, Morita N, Evaluation of Angelicae radix (Touki) by inhibitory effect on platelet aggregation. In: Chem Pharm Bull 39:2046. 1991.

Taskinen J, (1975) Acta Chem Scan 29 (5):637 et (7) 757.

Tastrup O et al., (1983) Phytochemistry 22 (9):2035.

Zotikov YM et al., (1978) Rastit Resur 14 (4):579.

Further information in:

Kern W, List PH, Hörhammer L (Hrsg.), Hagers Handbuch der Pharmazeutischen Praxis, 4. Aufl., Bde. 1-8, Springer Verlag Berlin, Heidelberg, New York, 1969.

Madaus G, Lehrbuch der Biologischen Arzneimittel, Bde 1-3, Nachdruck, Georg Olms Verlag Hildesheim 1979.

ANGELICAE RADIX

Amling R, Phytotherapeutika in der Neurologie. In: ZPT 12(1):9. 1991.

Ashraf M et al., (1980) Pak J Sci Ind Res 23 (1-2):73.

Chang, EH et al., (Eds), Advances in Chinese Medicinal Materials Research, World Scientific Pub. Co. Singapore 1985.

Chalchat JC, Garry RPh, J Essent Oil Res 5:447. 1993.

Escher S, Keller U et al., (1979) Helv Chim Acta 62 (7):2061.

Glowniak K et al., Localisation and seasonal chenges of psoralen in Angelica fruits. In: PM 62, Abstracts of the 44th Ann Congress of GA, 76. 1996.

Harkar S, Razdan TK, Waight ES, Steroids, chromoines and coumarins from Angelica officinalis. In: PH 23:419-426. 1983.

Härmälä P, Kaltia S, Vuorela H, PM 58:287. 1992.

Lemmich J et al., (1983) Phytochemistry 23 (2):553-555.

Leung AY, Encyclopedia of Common Natural Ingredients used in Food Drugs and Cosmetics, John Wiley & Sons Inc. New York, 1980.

Nykanen I et al., Essent Oil Res 3:229. 1991.

Opdyke DLJ, (1975) Food Cosmet Toxicol: 13, Suppl 713.

Sethi OP, Shah AK, (1979) Ind J Pharm Sci 42 (6):C11.

Shimizu M, Matsuzawa T, Suzuki S, Yoshizaki M, Morita N, Evaluation of Angelicae radix (Touki) by inhibitory effect on platelet aggregation. In: Chem Pharm Bull 39:2046. 1991.

Sun H, Jakupovic J, PA 41:888. 1986.

Taskinen J, (1975) Acta Chem Scan 29 (5):637 et (7) 757.

Tastrup O et al., (1983) Phytochemistry 22 (9):2035.

Zotikov YM et al., (1978) Rastit Resur 14 (4):579.

Further information in:

Hausen B, Allergiepflanzen, Pflanzenallergene, ecomed Verlagsgesellsch. mbH, Landsberg 1988.

Kern W, List PH, Hörhammer L (Hrsg.), Hagers Handbuch der Pharmazeutischen Praxis, 4. Aufl., Bde. 1-8, Springer Verlag Berlin, Heidelberg, New York, 1969.

Madaus G, Lehrbuch der Biologischen Arzneimittel, Bde. 1-3, Nachdruck, Georg Olms Verlag Hildesheim 1979.

Roth L, Daunderer M, Kormann K, Giftpflanzen, Pflanzengifte, 4. Aufl., Ecomed Fachverlag Landsberg Lech 1993.

Schulz R, Hänsel R, Rationale Phytotherapie, Springer Verlag Heidelberg 1996.

Steinegger E, Hänsel R, Pharmakognosie, 5. Aufl., Springer Verlag Heidelberg 1992.

Teuscher E, Lindequist U, Biogene Gifte - Biologie, Chemie, Pharmakologie, 2. Aufl., Fischer Verlag Stuttgart 1994.

Teuscher E, Biogene Arzneimittel, 5. Aufl., Wiss. Verlagsges. Stuttgart 1997.

Wagner H, Wiesenauer M, Phytotherapie. Phytopharmaka und pflanzliche Homöopathika, Fischer-Verlag, Stuttgart, Jena, New York 1995.

Wichtl M (Hrsg.), Teedrogen, 4. Aufl., Wiss. Verlagsges. Stuttgart 1997.

Angostura

See Galipea Officinalis

Anise

See Pimpinella Anisum

Antennaria Dioica

Cat's Foot

DESCRIPTION

Medicinal Parts: The medicinal part is the flower.

Flower and Fruit: The plant has bright red and white, dioecious composite flowers. They are very small and are in terminal cymes. The female flowers are bright red with thread-like, cylindrical corolla. The male flowers are white with a tubular-funnel-shaped corolla. The bracts of the male are white, the female, pink. The fruit has a tuft of hair.

Leaves, Stem and Root: The plant is 7 to 20 cm tall, with leafy rooting runners. The stem is erect with basal leaves that are spatulate, green above, gray beneath, cauline, linear and erect.

Habitat: Europe, Asia, America as far as the Arctic.

Production: Cat's foot flower consists of the fresh or dried flowers of Antennaria dioica.

Not To Be Confused With: The flower heads of Helichrysum stoechas or Helichrysum angustifolium.

Other Names: Mountain Everlasting, Life Everlasting, Cudweed

ACTIONS AND PHARMACOLOGY

COMPOUNDS

Anthracene derivatives

Flavonoids: including luteolin and its glucosides

Bitter substances

Mucilages

Tannins

EFFECTS

In animal tests a mild spasmolytic and choleric effect was reported.

INDICATIONS AND USAGE

Preparations of Cat's Foot flower are used for intestinal diseases. In folk medicine, Cat's Foot is used as a diuretic.

Efficacy for the claimed applications are not documented.

PRECAUTIONS AND ADVERSE REACTIONS

No health hazards or side effects are known in conjunction with the proper administration of designated therapeutic dosages.

DOSAGE

Mode of Administration: Since the efficacy for the claimed uses is not documented, a therapeutic application cannot be recommended. There is no objection to its use as a brightening agent in teas.

Preparation: To prepare an infusion, pour boiling water over 1 gm finely cut drug, strain after 5 to 10 minutes.

LITERATURE

Delaveau P, et al., (1980) Planta Med 40:49.

Didry N et al., (1982) Ann Pharm Fr 40 (1):75.

Swiatek L et al., (1982) Planta Med 30:153, 12P.

Further information in:

Kern W, List PH, Hörhammer L (Hrsg.), Hagers Handbuch der Pharmazeutischen Praxis, 4. Aufl., Bde. 1-8, Springer Verlag Berlin, Heidelberg, New York, 1969.

Anthoxanthum Odoratum

Sweet Vernal Grass

DESCRIPTION

Medicinal Parts: The medicinal part is the whole plant.

Flower and Fruit: The plant size ranges from 15 to 50 cm. The green, solitary, flowered spikelet has 4 spelts, the lower half of which are as large as the upper and taller than the flowers. Both of the upper spelts are awned, with 2 stamens. The style is long, the stigma pinnate, and spikelets form an oblong false ear.

Leaves, Stem and Root: Grows as thick grass. The leaves are ciliate at the base of the lamina. The leaf sheath is deeply grooved and hairy.

Characteristics: Sweet Vernal Grass has a scent of dried woodruff and tangy taste.

Habitat: The plant is indigenous to Britain, Europe, and temperate Asia.

ACTIONS AND PHARMACOLOGY

COMPOUNDS

Hydroxy cinnamic acid glycosides: that form coumarin through dehydration of the plant

EFFECTS

No information is available.

INDICATIONS AND USAGE

The drug is used for headache, nausea, sleeplessness, and conditions of the urinary tract.

PRECAUTIONS AND ADVERSE REACTIONS

The freshly-harvested plant contains glycosidic precursors of coumarin, that release coumarin in the process of dehydration (contains up to 1.5% coumarin in the drug). No health hazards or side effects are known in conjunction with the proper administration of designated therapeutic dosages.

OVERDOSAGE

The administration of higher levels of the drug can lead to headache and dizziness. Liver injuries are possible among susceptible patients in long-term treatment. The abnormal liver values disappear when the drug is discontinued (recommend observation of liver enzyme values of the blood).

DOSAGE

Mode of Administration: The drug is used externally, as an extract.

LITERATURE

Brown SA, Cand J Biochem Physiol 38:143. 1960.

Fentem JH, Fry JR, Thomas NW, Species differences in the hepatotoxicity of coumarin-a comparision of rat and Mongolian gerbil. In: Toxicology 71(1-2):129. 1992.

Further information in:

Kern W, List PH, Hörhammer L (Hrsg.), Hagers Handbuch der Pharmazeutischen Praxis, 4. Aufl., Bde. 1-8, Springer Verlag Berlin, Heidelberg, New York, 1969.

Lewin L, Gifte und Vergiftungen, 6. Aufl., Nachdruck, Haug Verlag, Heidelberg 1992.

Poisonous Plants in Britain and their effects on Animals and Man, Ministry of Agriculture Fisheries and Food, Pub; HMSO (1984) UK.

Roth L, Daunderer M, Kormann K, Giftpflanzen, Pflanzengifte, 4. Aufl., Ecomed Fachverlag Landsberg Lech 1993.

Teuscher E, Lindequist U, Biogene Gifte - Biologie, Chemie, Pharmakologie, 2. Aufl., Fischer Verlag Stuttgart 1994.

Anthyllis Vulneraria

Woundwort

DESCRIPTION

Medicinal Parts: The medicinal parts are the flowers of the plant.

Flower and Fruit: The many-floreted capitula are in the upper bract axils. The papilonaceous flowers are almost sessile and have an upright corolla up to 20 mm long. The calyx is membranous and up to 17 mm long. It is tubular-bottle-shaped and shaggy to felt-haired. The color is yellow to white at the bottom, turning violet towards the top. The petals are whitish-yellow to yellow or occasionally crimson. They have a free standard, slightly shorter wings, and an acute, often red carina. Ten stamens are fused into a tube. The ovaries are stemmed with a thickened style and rounded stigma. The pod-fruit is enclosed in the dried calyx. It is ovate, reticulate, dark brown, single-seeded, and does not spring open. The seed is ovate, smooth, shiny, and checkered yellow-green.

Leaves, Stem and Root: Anthyllis vulneraria is a 15 to 30 cm high half-rosette shrub with a sturdy tap-root and a short, entire or often branched rhizome. The stem is upright, unbranched or branched, and tomentose. The leaves, depending where they are on the stem, are variously pinnate. All leaves are entire-margined, glabrous or slightly pubescent above, and thickly tomentose beneath. The stipules are small and generally connected to a clasping sheath.

Characteristics: Woundwort has a weak aromatic odor and dry taste.

Habitat: The plant is found all across Europe to the Caucasus and the Near East. It is found in the south from the Sahara to Ethiopia.

Other Names: Kidney Vetch, Ladies's Fingers, Lamb's Toes, Staunchwort

ACTIONS AND PHARMACOLOGY

COMPOUNDS

Tannins

Saponins

Flavonoids

Isoflavonoids

Lectins

EFFECTS
No information is available.

INDICATIONS AND USAGE
Woundwort tea is used in the treatment of ulcers and wounds both internally and externally. The drug is also used in a tea preparation with ribwort for coughs, as an ingredient of blood purifying teas, and for exposure and vomiting. It is used internally for diseases of the mouth and throat.

The efficacy of the above treatments has not been sufficiently proven.

PRECAUTIONS AND ADVERSE REACTIONS
No health hazards or side effects are known in conjunction with the proper administration of designated therapeutic dosages.

DOSAGE
Mode of Administration: Preparations are available for internal and external use.

Preparation: To prepare tea, use 1 dessertspoonful of the flowers per 250 ml of water.

LITERATURE
Sile A, Vanaga A, Nauka-Prakt Farm: 82-85. 1974.

Vetter J, Seregelyes-Csomos A, Magy Allatory Lapja 43(8):479-482. 1988.

Further information in:

Hänsel R, Keller K, Rimpler H, Schneider G (Hrsg.), Hagers Handbuch der Pharmazeutischen Praxis, 5. Aufl., Bde 4-6 (Drogen), Springer Verlag Berlin, Heidelberg, New York, 1992-1994.

Aphanes Arvensis

Parsley Piert

DESCRIPTION
Flower and Fruit: The flowers are in axillary clusters of 10 to 20. They are encircled by stipules. The sepals are erect, acuminate-ovate and pubescent on the outside and on the margins. They are glabrous on the inside and draw together when the fruit ripens. The fruit is 1 mm long, ovate, keeled, flat and jug-shaped. The calyx is vertically wrinkled and pubescent.

Leaves, Stem and Root: The plant is an annual or hardy annual 2 to 30 cm long and dull green in color. The root is thin, branched and fusiform. The stem is generally branched, and decumbent with short internodes. The leaves are 3 to 5 lobed fan- or diamond-shaped. The upper ones are short-petioled. The lower leaves are sessile and usually rough-haired, occasionally only ciliate. The stipules are semi-ovate, indentate-serrate, leafy and pubescent.

Habitat: Britain, Europe, northern Africa, U.S.

Production: Parsley Piert herb is the above-ground part of Aphanes arvensis.

Other Names: Parsley Breakstone, Field Lady's Mantle, Parsley Piercestone

ACTION AND PHARMACOLOGY
COMPOUNDS
Tannin

EFFECTS
The herb is claimed to be effective as a diuretic and refrigerant.

INDICATIONS AND USAGE
Parsley Piert is used in folk remedies in the treatment of urinary tract disorders, especially kidney and bladder stones, and as a diuretic.

PRECAUTIONS AND ADVERSE REACTIONS
No health hazards or side effects are known in conjunction with the proper administration of designated therapeutic dosages.

DOSAGE
Mode of Administration: The fresh or dried drug and the liquid extract are used.

LITERATURE
Kern W, List PH, Hörhammer L (Hrsg.), Hagers Handbuch der Pharmazeutischen Praxis, 4. Aufl., Bde 1-8, Springer Verlag Berlin, Heidelberg, New York, 1969.

Apium Graveolens

Celery

DESCRIPTION
Medicinal Parts: The medicinal parts are the above ground parts, the fruit, and the root of the plant.

Flower and Fruit: The umbels are greenish-white, small, 6 to 12 rayed, star-shaped and splayed. Some of them are top-heavy, short petioled or sessile, and some of them are terminal, more or less long-petioled with no involucre. Petals are usually 0.5 mm, white or greenish to yellowish, cordate at the base and have indented tips. The fruit is almost spherical and somewhat compressed at the side. The 5 mm mericarps are rounded in section. They are 5-cornered with 5 equal, weakly protruding, bow-shaped main ribs. The edge of the ribs form the edge of the mericarps. The fruit axis is bristly and slightly crenate at the tip.

Leaves, Stem and Root: The glabrous plant is a biennial and reaches a height of 30 to 100 cm. The root of the wild variety is fusiform, about 5 to 7 mm thick, branched and woody in the second year. The root of the cultivated variety is fleshy, roundly tuberous and reaches a diameter of over 15 cm. The stem is erect, with edged grooves, often hollow and branched. The leaves are glossy and rich green. The basal and lower cauline leaves are more or less long-petioled and pinnatifid. The upper cauline leaves are sometimes opposite. They are on short white-membrane edged sheaths and are almost sessile and tri-pinnate. The lower leaves are roundish, almost blunt at the base with broad, lozenge-shaped, indented-serrate, blunt, and short-thorned tips. The upper cauline leaves are wedge-shaped and acuminate, also 3-lobed or pinnate or lanceolate and entire-margined.

Characteristics: The plant has a strong odor.

Habitat: Celery is found in Europe from England and Lappland to southern Russia. It is also found in western Asia as far as eastern India as well as northern and southern Africa and South America. It is both cultivated and grows wild in North America, Mexico and Argentina.

Other Names: Smallage

ACTIONS AND PHARMACOLOGY

COMPOUNDS

Volatile oil, chief constituents (+)-limes: limonene, β-selinene, phthalides (among them 3-butylidenphthalide, 3-butylphthalide, 3-isobutylidendihydrophthalide)

Flavonoids: among them graveobioside A and B, apiin, isoquercitrin

Furocumarins: including bergapten

Also fatty oil: in the berries (also polyines in the root)

EFFECTS

No information is available.

INDICATIONS AND USAGE

Preparations of celery are used as a diuretic, for blood purification, for regulating elimination of the bowels, for glandular stimulation, rheumatic complaints, gout, gall and kidney stones. Celery is also used for weight loss due to malnutrition, for loss of appetite, exhaustion and as a prophylactic for nervous unrest.

The efficacy for the claimed applications is not documented.

CONTRAINDICATIONS

Because of the kidney-irritating effect of the volatile oil, the drug should not be administered in the presence of kidney infections.

PRECAUTIONS AND ADVERSE REACTIONS

No health hazards or side effects are known in conjunction with the proper administration of designated therapeutic dosages.

Because the furocumarin content of the freshly-harvested root can rise to 200 times the original level under storage conditions, due to latent yeast infections within the plant, relatively large amounts of furocumarins are frequently contained in stored celeriac bulbs or incorrectly dehydrated drug samples. The increase of furocumarin in this case can lead to phototoxicoses.

DOSAGE

Mode of Administration: The drug is available in a few combination preparations for internal use.

Storage: Should be kept sealed, away from light and moisture.

LITERATURE

Beier RS, Oertli EH, Psoralen and other phytoalexins in celery. In: PH 22(11):2595. 1983.

Bjeldanes LF, Kim I, (1977) J Org Chem 42:2333.

Fehr D, (1979) Pharmazie 29(5):349 et 34 (10):658.

Garg SK et al., (1979) Phytochemistry 18:1580 et 1764.

Garg SK et al., (1980) Planta Med 38:363.

Gijbels MJM et al., Phthalides in roots of Apium graveolens, A. graveolens var. rapeceum, Bifora testiculata and Petroselinum crispum var. tuberosum. In: Fitoterapia 56:17. 1985.

Harborne JB, in ''The Biology and Chemistry of the Umbelliferae'', Ed. V. N. Heywood. Pub. Academic Press, London 1971.

Lewis DA et al., (1985) Int J Crude Drug Res 28 (1):27.

Mac Leod G, Ames JM, Volatile components of celery and celeriac. In: PH 28(7):1817-1824. 1989.

Nigg HN, Strandberg JO, Beier RC, Petersen HD, Harrison JM, Furanocoumarins in Florida celery varieties increased by fungicide treatment. In: J Agricult Food Chem 45(4):1430-1436. 1997.

Tsi D et al., Effects of aqueous celery (Apium graveolens) extract on lipid parameters of rats fed a high fat diet. In: PM 61(1):18-21. 1995.

Uhlig, JW, Chang A, Jen JJ, Effect of phthalides on celery flavor. In: J Food Sci 52(3):658-660. 1987.

Yu RS, You SQ, (1984) Acta Pharm Sinica 19 (8):566.

Further information in:

Frohne D, Pfänder HJ, Giftpflanzen - Ein Handbuch für Apotheker, Toxikologen und Biologen, 4. Aufl., Wiss. Verlags-Ges Stuttgart 1997.

Hänsel R, Keller K, Rimpler H, Schneider G (Hrsg.), Hagers Handbuch der Pharmazeutischen Praxis, 5. Aufl., Bde 4-6 (Drogen), Springer Verlag Berlin, Heidelberg, New York, 1992-1994.

Hausen B, Allergiepflanzen, Pflanzenallergene, ecomed Verlagsgesellsch. mbH, Landsberg 1988.

Leung AY, Encyclopedia of Common Natural Ingredients Used in Food Drugs and Cosmetics, John Wiley & Sons Inc., New York 1980.

Madaus G, Lehrbuch der Biologischen Arzneimittel, Bde 1-3, Nachdruck, Georg Olms Verlag Hildesheim 1979.

Teuscher E, Lindequist U, Biogene Gifte - Biologie, Chemie, Pharmakologie, 2. Aufl., Fischer Verlag Stuttgart 1994.

Wagner H, Wiesenauer M, Phytotherapie. Phytopharmaka und pflanzliche Homöopathika, Fischer-Verlag, Stuttgart, Jena, New York 1995.

Wichtl M (Hrsg.), Teedrogen, 4. Aufl., Wiss. Verlagsges. Stuttgart 1997.

Apocynum Cannabinum

Canadian Hemp

DESCRIPTION

Medicinal Parts: The medicinal parts are the root and the juice obtained from the fresh plant.

Flower and Fruit: The small whitish-green, occasionally pink to violet flowers are on long pods. The calyx is deeply lobed and half as long as the corolla. The petals are oblong-lanceolate. The tufts of hair on the seeds are 2 to 3 cm long.

Leaves, Stem and Root: Apocynum cannabinum is a perennial up to 2 m tall. It has an erect stem, which branches at the top. The whole plant is glabrous or downy. The short-petioled leaves are 5 to 11 cm long, yellowish-green and oblong or oblong-ovoid. The tips of the leaves are initially rounded and then terminate abruptly in a thorny tip.

Characteristics: The plant has an acrid taste and is to a certain degree poisonous.

Habitat: Mostly in U.S. and Canada. It is cultivated in Russia.

Not To Be Confused With: Indian Hemp (Cannabis indica), though both species contain latex and their tough, fibrous bark can be used as a substitute for Hemp, hence the name.

Production: Canadian Hemp root is the root of Apocynum cannabinum. The plant is cultivated as a crop in Germany.

Other Names: Indian-Hemp, Dogbane, Milkweed, Fly-Trap, Bitterroot, Catchfly, Honeybloom, Milk Ipecac, Wallflower, Wild Cotton

ACTIONS AND PHARMACOLOGY

COMPOUNDS

Cardioactive steroid glycosides (cardenolids): in particular cymarin, k-strophantoside, apocannoside, cynocannoside

EFFECTS

The high content of cardenolide glycosides causes bradycardia and increased contraction of the heart. Blood pressure is lowered, and rebound vagotonia hypertension can occur. The drug increases diuresis and stimulation of the vasomotor centers. It causes more severe irritation of the intestinal mucous membrane than digitalis and strophantus preparations. It has a lower therapeutic effect on atrial fibrillation than digitalis.

Cardenollide glycoside cymine has a similar effect to glycoside strophantine but in general is weaker, with the exception of the stronger diuretic effect in edema. It is less cumulative.

INDICATIONS AND USAGE

The juice of the fresh plant is used in the treatment of condylomatosis and warts. American Indians use the roots for asthma, dropsy, coughs, syphilis, and rheumatism.

In folk medicine, the root is used to strengthen weak heart muscles following pneumonia, valvular insufficiency, senile heart. It is also used as a diuretic.

Efficacy in these areas has not been proven.

PRECAUTIONS AND ADVERSE REACTIONS

Topical irritation of the mucous membrane of the alimentary canal, accompanied by nausea and vomiting, is more common than in other drugs containing cardenolid glycosides. Vomiting and gastrointestinal irritations can occur, even with the administration of therapeutic doses of the drug (mucous membrane-irritating resin fraction).

OVERDOSAGE

For possible symptoms of overdose and treatment of poisonings see Digitalis folium. Despite the strong efficacy of the drug's cardioactive steroid glycosides in parenteral application, serious poisoning in the course of peroral administration is hardly to be expected, due to the low resorption rate.

DOSAGE

Daily Dosage: The average daily dose of the liquid extract is 10 to 30 drops to be taken 3 times daily; tincture (1:10), 0.3 to 0.6 ml.

Storage: Store in secure area as the drug is poisonous.

LITERATURE

Belkin M et al., (1952) J Nat Cancer Inst 13:742.

Desruelles J et al., Therapie 28:103-113. 1973.

Kupchan SM et al., J Med Chem 7:803-805. 1964.

Further information in:

Hänsel R, Keller K, Rimpler H, Schneider G (Hrsg.), Hagers Handbuch der Pharmazeutischen Praxis, 5. Aufl., Bde 4-6 (Drogen): Springer Verlag Berlin, Heidelberg, New York, 1992-1994.

Lewin L, Gifte und Vergiftungen, 6. Aufl., Nachdruck, Haug Verlag, Heidelberg 1992.

Madaus G, Lehrbuch der Biologischen Arzneimittel, Bde 1-3, Nachdruck, Georg Olms Verlag Hildesheim 1979.

Roth L, Daunderer M, Kormann K, Giftpflanzen, Pflanzengifte, 4. Aufl., Ecomed Fachverlag Landsberg Lech 1993.

Teuscher E, Lindequist U, Biogene Gifte - Biologie, Chemie, Pharmakologie, 2. Aufl., Fischer Verlag Stuttgart 1994.

Teuscher E, Biogene Arzneimittel, 5. Aufl., Wiss. Verlagsges. Stuttgart 1997.

Wagner H, Wiesenauer M, Phytotherapie. Phytopharmaka und pflanzliche Homöopathika, Fischer-Verlag, Stuttgart, Jena, New York 1995.

Apple Tree

See Malus Domestica

Aquilegia Vulgaris

Columbine

DESCRIPTION

Medicinal Parts: The medicinal parts are the complete aerial parts of the plant.

Flower and Fruit: The long-stemmed flowers are terminal, hanging, dark blue, dark violet, pink or white. The 5 sepals spread like petals. They are broadly ovate, and end in a blunt, green tip. The 5 petals are hood-shaped with long inwardly hooked spurs. There are numerous stamens and usually 5 ovaries. The follicle is oblong, erect, and glandular-downy. The seeds are glossy black, oval, 2.2 to 2.5 cm long by 1.5 cm wide. They are thick, blunt-tipped, and anatropous. The raphe on the side is a distinct line.

Leaves, Stem and Root: The 30 to 60 cm high plant has a many-headed, light brown and branched rhizome. The stems are erect and usually branched. They are glabrous or soft-haired. The basal leaves are long-petioled and trifoliate. The leaflets are wedge-shaped to ovoid, blunt, irregularly crenate to serrate, and bluntly lobed. The underside of the leaves are usually light green and pubescent. The cauline leaves are smaller than the basal leaves and simpler. The highest leaves are usually made up of a few elongate-ovate, entire-margined lobes.

Habitat: Originally indigenous to central and southern Europe. Today the plant is also found in Asia and in the eastern states of the U.S.

Production: Aquilegia vulgaris is a completely protected plant.

Other Names: Culverwort

ACTIONS AND PHARMACOLOGY

COMPOUNDS

Cyanogenic glycosides: trigloquinine

EFFECTS

Columbine acts as a cholagogue (no recent research work has been carried out).

INDICATIONS AND USAGE

Columbine is used for regulation of gallbladder contraction and general gastrointestinal disorders. The drug is also used internally for scurvy and jaundice and to treat states of agitation due to its supposedly tranquilizing effect.

Efficacy has not been proven.

PRECAUTIONS AND ADVERSE REACTIONS

No health hazards or side effects are known in conjunction with the proper administration of designated therapeutic dosages.

OVERDOSAGE

Poisonings from the leaves because of the cyanogenic glycoside content have not been observed. The quantities of hydrocyanic acid releasable from the leaves are apparently too small for toxicities.

DOSAGE

Mode of Administration: Columbine is available in various combination preparations for internal use.

LITERATURE

Bonora A et al., PH 26:2277. 1987.

Fat LTS, Proc Kon Nederl Akad Wetensch Ser C82:197. 1979.

Further information in:

Hänsel R, Keller K, Rimpler H, Schneider G (Hrsg.), Hagers Handbuch der Pharmazeutischen Praxis, 5. Aufl., Bde 4-6 (Drogen). Springer Verlag Berlin, Heidelberg, New York, 1992-1994.

Madaus G, Lehrbuch der Biologischen Arzneimittel, Bde 1-3, Nachdruck, Georg Olms Verlag Hildesheim 1979.

Roth L, Daunderer M, Kormann K, Giftpflanzen, Pflanzengifte, 4. Aufl., Ecomed Fachverlag Landsberg Lech 1993.

Arachis Hypogaea

Peanuts

DESCRIPTION

Medicinal Parts: The oil has medicinal applications.

Flower and Fruit: The flowers are 5 to 7 cm long, monosymmetrical and have a large golden-yellow standard. The flowers have lemon-yellow wings and a pure white carina. They are arranged singularly or in pairs in the leaf axils. They blossom at sunrise and wilt in the same morning during which time they stretch from 5 to 20 cm and act negatively phototropically downwards. After pollination, a meristem develops at the base of the ovary, from which the fruit axis grows. The fruit only starts to grow when the stem is 5 to 10 cm underground where it grows horizontally. The fruit is a 4 cm long by 1.5 cm thick closed pod with a fibrous, reticulate-wrinkled wall and 1 to 4 large seeds with no endosperm and a thin, red shell.

Leaves, Stem and Root: It is an annual herbaceous 30 to 70 cm high legume, with glabrous, double pinnate leaves and a decumbent to upright stem.

Habitat: Peanuts were originally indigenous to tropical and sub-tropical South America. Today, Arachis hypogaea is cultivated in all tropical and sub-tropical regions worldwide apart from the rain forests.

Production: Peanut oil is the fatty oil extracted from the seeds of Arachis hypogaea. It is extracted by means of a "cold press" method or by hexane extraction and refining.

Not To Be Confused With: Inexpensive Soya oil is sometimes added.

Other Names: Arachis, Groundnuts, Monkey Nuts

ACTIONS AND PHARMACOLOGY

COMPOUNDS

Fatty oil: chief fatty acids, oleic acid, linolic acid, palmitin acid, in small quantities also longer-chained fatty acids such as eicosanoic acid, tetracosanoic acid

EFFECTS

No information is available.

INDICATIONS AND USAGE

Peanut oil is added to ointments and medicinal oils, and applied rectally in rectal constipation. It is also used in dermatology for crusting and scaling of the scalp (with hair), baby care, and dry skin. Other applications include use as a bath additive for subacute and chronic eczema, for atrophic eczema and ichthyosis.

The pharmaceutical and medical industries use peanut oil as a vehicle for medication in external, enteral or parenteral preparations and the cosmetics industry uses it in skin, sun, and massage oil. Domestically, it is used as a salad or cooking oil that is said to lower blood cholesterol levels.

PRECAUTIONS AND ADVERSE REACTIONS

No health hazards or side effects are known in conjunction with the proper administration of designated therapeutic dosages.

DOSAGE

Mode of Administration: As an enema, oil, bath additive, medical and cosmetic vehicle.

Daily Dosage: As a rectal enema, 130 ml of oil is used at body temperature. For use in a bath, the recommended concentration is 4 ml per 10 liters of water. Adults should bathe for 15 to 20 minutes 2 to 3 times weekly. Children and babies should bathe for a few minutes 2 to 3 times weekly.

Storage: Protect from light in well-sealed, filled containers. Oils from different deliveries should not be stored together. Oils with a tocopherol content less than 50 mg/100mg do not store well.

LITERATURE

Adrian J, Jacquot R in, Valeur Alimentaire de l'Arachide et ses Derives, Maisonneuve et Larose, Paris 1968.

Boudreaux HB, Frampton VL (1960) Nature 185:469.

Codex Alimentarius Commission, Alinorm 79/17, Report 10th Session. Codex Committee on Fats and Oils, London 1987.

Further information in:

Hänsel R, Keller K, Rimpler H, Schneider G (Hrsg.), Hagers Handbuch der Pharmazeutischen Praxis, 5. Aufl., Bde 4-6 (Drogen): Springer Verlag Berlin, Heidelberg, New York, 1992-1994.

Roth L, Daunderer M, Kormann K, Giftpflanzen, Pflanzengifte, 4. Aufl., Ecomed Fachverlag Landsberg Lech 1993.

Steinegger E, Hänsel R, Pharmakognosie, 5. Aufl., Springer Verlag Heidelberg 1992.

Teuscher E, Biogene Arzneimittel, 5. Aufl., Wiss. Verlagsges. Stuttgart 1997.

Aralia Racemosa

Spikenard

DESCRIPTION

Medicinal Parts: The medicinal parts are the fresh and dried rhizome and roots.

Flower and Fruit: The inflorescence is a large panicle, each branch of which carries a simple, round, 10 to 15 flower umbel. The flowers are small and have greenish-white petals. The drupes are dark red to crimson, roundish and 5-ribbed.

The seeds are compressed and have a similarly formed endosperm.

Leaves, Stem and Root: Araliae racemosae is a herbaceous, bushy, stiffly branched perennial. The stem of which is woody at the base, up to 2 m high, glabrous and grooved. The leaflets are thin and oval. The leaflets can grow up to 20 cm long and 16 cm wide but are usually much smaller and cordate at the base. The rhizome is up to 15 cm long and has a diameter of roughly 2.5 cm with prominent concave scars. The roots are about 2 cm thick at the base, pale brown, and wrinkled. The root fracture is short and whitish.

Characteristics: The taste and odor are aromatic.

Habitat: The plant grows in North America from central Canada to Virginia.

Production: Araliae racemosae radix et rhizoma is the chopped up fresh or dried rhizome and root of Aralia racemosa, which is gathered in summer and autumn. The freshly chopped roots are either dried or processed immediately to form a thick paste.

Not To Be Confused With: It is possible to confuse Spikenard with the Aralia nudicaulis root. However, they can be distinguished by its lack of spotted hypodermis cells.

Other Names: Indian Root, Life of Man, Old Man's Root, Pettymorell, Spignet

ACTIONS AND PHARMACOLOGY

COMPOUNDS

Polyynes: including falcarinole, falcarindiole

Triterpene saponins

Volatile oil (very little)

EFFECTS

Due to its saponin content, the drug's effectiveness as a reflex expectorant for colds seems plausible. It is also diaphoretic and stimulates tissue renewal. Its efficacy has not been proven.

INDICATIONS AND USAGE

Preparations are used internally for colds, chronic coughs and asthma. It is used as an alternative to sarsaparilla in the treatment of skin diseases. The drug is also used for rheumatic conditions.

PRECAUTIONS AND ADVERSE REACTIONS

No health hazards or side effects are known in conjunction with the proper administration of designated therapeutic dosages. Because of the polyyne spectrum, sensitization connected with the plant is also possible through skin contact.

DOSAGE

Mode of Administration: The drug is administered internally as a fluid extract.

Preparation: It is prepared as a liquid extract (1:1); information on the ethanol content is unavailable.

Daily Dosage: When the drug is prepared as an infusion, the recommended daily dosage is approximately 15 gm per 500 ml, to be drunk, one cup at a time, during the course of the day. The recommended dosage of the liquid extract is 0.9 gm to 1.8 gm.

LITERATURE

Ahn Y-J, Kim M-J, Yamamoto T, Fujiwawa T, Mitsouka T (1990) Selective growth responses of human intestinal bacteria to Araliaceae extracts. Microbial Ecol Health Disease 3:223-229.

Hansen L and Boll PM (1986) Phytochemistry 25 (2):285.

Further information in:

Hänsel R, Keller K, Rimpler H, Schneider G (Hrsg.), Hagers Handbuch der Pharmazeutischen Praxis, 5. Aufl., Bde 4-6 (Drogen): Springer Verlag Berlin, Heidelberg, New York, 1992-1994.

Hoppe HA (1975-1987) Drogenkunde, 8. Aufl., Bde 1-3, W. de Gruyter Verlag, Berlin, New York.

Madaus G, Lehrbuch der Biologischen Arzneimittel, Bde 1-3, Nachdruck, Georg Olms Verlag Hildesheim 1979.

Roth L, Daunderer M, Kormann K, Giftpflanzen, Pflanzengifte, 4. Aufl., Ecomed Fachverlag Landsberg Lech 1993.

Teuscher E, Lindequist U, Biogene Gifte - Biologie, Chemie, Pharmakologie, 2. Aufl., Fischer Verlag Stuttgart 1994.

Wagner H, Wiesenauer M, Phytotherapie. Phytopharmaka und pflanzliche Homöopathika, Fischer-Verlag, Stuttgart, Jena, New York 1995.

Arctium Lappa

Burdock

DESCRIPTION

Medicinal Parts: The medicinal part is the fresh or dried root.

Flower and Fruit: The crimson flowers grow in long-peduncled, loose cymes. The heads are fairly large, globose and almost glabrous. All flowers are funnel-shaped and androgynous. The bracts are coriaceous, green and have a barb-shaped inward-curving tip. The fruit separate from their stems on ripening. The fruit is compressed and has a bristly tuft, which falls off easily.

Leaves, Stem and Root: The plant grows to a height of 80-150 cm. The stem is erect, rigid, grooved, branched and downy to wooly. The leaves are alternate, petiolate, broad to ovate-cordate. They are blunt and slightly wooly to hairy on the underside. The lowest leaves are very large and have a latex-filled stem.

Habitat: Burdock grows in Europe, north Asia and North America.

Production: Burdock root consists of the fresh or dried underground parts of Arctium lappa, Arctium minus, and/or Arctium tomentosum.

Other Names: Bardana, Beggar's Buttons, Burr Seed, Clot-Bur, Cockle Buttons, Cocklebur, Fox's Clote, Great Burr, Happy Major, Hardock, Hareburr, Lappa, Love Leaves, Personata, Philanthropium, Thorny Burr

ACTIONS AND PHARMACOLOGY

COMPOUNDS

Small amount of volatile oil of very complex make-up: including, among others, phenylacetaldehyde, benzaldehyde, 2-alkyl-3-methoxy-pyrazines

Sesquiterpene lactones

Polyynes: chief components trideca-1,11-dien-3,5,7,9-tetrain

Caffeic acid derivatives: including chlorogenic acid, isochlorogenic acid

Polysaccharides: inulin (fructosan), mucilages (xyloglucans, acidic xylans)

EFFECTS

No information is available.

INDICATIONS AND USAGE

Preparations of burdock root are used for ailments and complaints of the gastrointestinal tract, as a diaphoretic and diuretic, and for blood purifying. Externally, they are used for ichthyosis and psoriasis. The claimed efficacies have not been documented.

PRECAUTIONS AND ADVERSE REACTIONS

No health hazards or side effects are known in conjunction with the proper administration of designated therapeutic dosages. There is a small potential for sensitization via skin contact with the drug.

DOSAGE

Mode of Administration: The drug is used internally and externally.

LITERATURE

Bryson PD et al., (1978) J Am Med Ass 239 (20):2157.

Dombradi G, (1970) Chemotherapy 15:250.

Ichihara A et al., (1968) Tetrahedron 44:3961.

Ichihara A et al., (1978) Tetrahedron Letters 33:305.

Morita K et al., (1984) Mutat Res 129(1):25.

Naya K et al., (1972) Chem Letters 3:235.

Schulte K et al., (1967) Arzneim Forsch 17:829.

Takeda H, Kiriyami S, (1979) J Nutr 109(3):388.

Tsujita J et al., (1979) Nutr Rep Int 20(5):635.

Yamada Y et al., (1975) Phytochemistry 14:582.

Yamanouchi S et al., (1976) Yakugaku Zasshi 96(12):1492.

Further information in:

Hausen B, Allergiepflanzen, Pflanzenallergene, ecomed Verlagsgesellsch. mbH, Landsberg 1988.

Kern W, List PH, Hörhammer L (Hrsg.), Hagers Handbuch der Pharmazeutischen Praxis, 4. Aufl., Bde. 1-8, Springer Verlag Berlin, Heidelberg, New York, 1969.

Leung AY, Encyclopedia of Common Natural Ingredients Used in Food Drugs and Cosmetics, John Wiley & Sons Inc., New York, 1980.

Madaus G, Lehrbuch der Biologischen Arzneimittel, Bde 1-3, Nachdruck, Georg Olms Verlag Hildesheim 1979.

Wichtl M (Hrsg.), Teedrogen, 4. Aufl., Wiss. Verlagsges. Stuttgart 1997.

Arctostaphylos Uva-Ursi

Uva-Ursi

DESCRIPTION

Medicinal Parts: The medicinal part is the leaf.

Flower and Fruit: The flowers are in 3 to 12 short, terminal and hanging racemes. The pedicle has 2 small, ovate, ciliate bracteoles at the base. The calyx is 1 mm long, palmate and has 5 membranous tips. The corolla is ovoid to jug-shaped, white or reddish with a red border, 5 to 6 mm long with 5 short revolute tips. The 10 stamens are half as long as the corolla tube. The filaments are heavily thickened at the base. The anthers have porous openings, are crimson and have a long whip-like, curling appendage. The ovaries are 5 to 7 valved and the style is longer than the stamens. The fruit is a globose, pea-sized, scarlet, floury drupe. The fruit has 5 to 7 stone seeds, 4 mm in length, which are kidney-shaped and compressed at the sides.

Leaves, Stem and Root: The plant is a decumbent, up to 1.5 m long, creeping espalier with elastic, red-brown branches. The leaves are alternate, coriaceous, short petioled, spatulate-obovate or wedge-shaped, entire-margined and slightly revolute. They are 12 to 30 mm long by 4 to 15 mm wide, glabrous, glossy and evergreen. The underside is distinctly reticulate and the midrib and the margins are often downy.

Characteristics: The leaves have a more bitter, astringent than metallic sweetish taste. They are distinguished from the cranberry by the reticulate vein structure and the non-glandular spots beneath.

Habitat: The plant has spread from the Iberian peninsula across Central Europe northwards to Scandinavia and eastwards to Siberia. The plant is also found in the Altai mountains, the Himalayas and North America.

Production: Uva-Ursi (bearberry) leaves consist of the dried leaves of Arctostaphylos Uva-Ursi.

Other Names: Arberry, Bearsgrape, Kinnikinnick, Mealberry, Mountain Box, Mountain Cranberry, Redberry Leaves, Sagackhomi, Sandberry, Bearberry

ACTIONS AND PHARMACOLOGY

COMPOUNDS

Hydroquinone glycosides: arbutin (arbutoside, 5-12%), methyl arbutin (up to 2.5%), further 2- O-galloylarbutin, 6-O-galloylarbutin

Tannins (15-20%): gallo tannins, ellagic tannins, condensed tannins

Iridoide monoterpenes: monotropein

Flavonoids: including, among others, hyperoside (0.8-1.5%), quercitrin, isoquercitrin, myricitrin

Triterpenes: including, among others, ursolic acid (0.4-0.8%), uvaol

EFFECTS

Preparations made from Uva-Ursi act antibacterially in vitro. The antimicrobial effect is associated with the aglycon hydroquinone released from arbutin (transport form) or arbutin waste products in the alkaline urine. A methanol extract of the drug (50%) is said to have an inhibiting effect on tyrosinase activity. The forming of melanin from DOPA using tyrosinase as well as from DOPA-CHROM through auto-oxidation is also said to be inhibited by the drug. The maximum antibacterial effect is expected 3 to 4 hours after administration.

INDICATIONS AND USAGE

■ Infections of the urinary tract

Uva-Ursi is used for inflammatory disorders of the efferent urinary tract. The drug should not be taken over a long period of time without consulting a doctor.

CONTRAINDICATIONS

The drug is contraindicated in pregnant women, nursing mothers and children under 12 years of age.

PRECAUTIONS AND ADVERSE REACTIONS

General: No health hazards are known in conjunction with the proper administration of designated therapeutic dosages. Individuals with gastric sensitivity may experience queasiness and vomiting following intake of preparations made from the drug with high tannin content.

Use in Pregnancy: The drug is contraindicated during pregnancy.

Use in Nursing Mothers: The drug is contraindicated in nursing mothers.

Pediatric Use: Liver damage is conceivable in connection with administration of the drug over extended periods, particularly with children, due to the possible hepatotoxicity of the hydroquinones released. The drug is contraindicated in children under 12 years of age.

Drug Interactions: Uva-Ursi preparations should not be administered with any substance that causes acidic urine since this reduces the antibacterial effect. Because the urine-disinfecting effect of the hydroquinones released in the urinary tract only occurs in an alkali environment, the simultaneous administration of medication or food that increase uric acid levels in the bladder is to be avoided.

OVERDOSAGE

Overdosage can lead to inflammation and irritation of the bladder and urinary tract mucous membranes. Liver damage is conceivable in connection with administration of the drug over extended periods, particularly with children, due to the possible hepatotoxicity of the hydroquinones released.

DOSAGE

Mode of Administration: Uva-Ursi is available as comminuted drug, drug powder or dried extract for infusions or cold macerations and as extracts and solid forms for oral administration. It is a component of urologic combination preparations and is also available in mono-preparations.

Preparation: To make an infusion, pour boiling water over 2.5 gm finely cut or coarse powdered drug or place the drug in cold water which is rapidly brought to a boil, and strain after 15 minutes. (1 teaspoonful is equivalent to 2.5 gm drug.)

Daily Dosage: 3 gm drug to 150 ml water as an infusion or cold maceration up to 4 times a day or 400-840 mg hydroquinone derivatives calculated as water-free arbutin. The urine should be alkaline.

LITERATURE

Britton G, Haslam E, J Chem Soc (London): 7312. 1965.

Denford KE, (1973) Experientia 29:939.

Frohne D, (1970) Planta Med 18:1.

Frohne D, (1986) Arctostaphylos uva-ursi: Die Bärentraube. Z Phytother 7:45-47.

Frohne D, PM 18:1. 1970.

Hiller K, Pharmazeutische Bewertung ausgewählter Teedrogen. In: DAZ 135(16):1425-1440. 1995.

Ihring M, Blume H, Zur pharmazeutischen Qualität von Phytopharmaka 2. Mitt.: Vergleichende Bewertung von Arbutin enthaltenden Urologika. In: PZW 135(6)267. 1990.

Jahodar L et al., (1978) Pharmazie 33(8):536.

Jahodar L et al., (1981) Pharmazie 36(2):294.

Jahodar L et al., (1985) Cesk Farm. 34(5):174.

Kraus L, DAZ 111:1225. 1974.

Ng TB et al., Examination of coumarins, flavonoids and polysaccharopeptides for antibacterial activity. In: General Pharmacology 27(7):1237-1240. 1996.

Paper DH, Koehler J, Franz G, Bioavailalibilty of drug preparations containing a leaf extract of Arctostaphylos uva-ursi (Uvae Ursi Folium). In: PM 59(7):A589. 1993.

Thesen R, Phytotherapeutika-nicht immer harmlos. In: ZPT 9(49):105. 1988.

Thieme H, Winkler HJ, PA 26:235 et 419. 1971.

Further information in:

Hänsel R, Keller K, Rimpler H, Schneider G (Hrsg.), Hagers Handbuch der Pharmazeutischen Praxis, 5. Aufl., Bde 4-6 (Drogen): Springer Verlag Berlin, Heidelberg, New York, 1992-1994.

Madaus G, Lehrbuch der Biologischen Arzneimittel, Bde 1-3, Nachdruck, Georg Olms Verlag Hildesheim 1979.

Roth L, Daunderer M, Kormann K, Giftpflanzen, Pflanzengifte, 4. Aufl., Ecomed Fachverlag Landsberg Lech 1993.

Schulz R, Hänsel R, Rationale Phytotherapie, Springer Verlag Heidelberg 1996.

Steinegger E, Hänsel R, Pharmakognosie, 5. Aufl., Springer Verlag Heidelberg 1992.

Teuscher E, Biogene Arzneimittel, 5. Aufl., Wiss. Verlagsges. Stuttgart 1997.

Wagner H, Wiesenauer M, Phytotherapie. Phytopharmaka und pflanzliche Homöopathika, Fischer-Verlag, Stuttgart, Jena, New York 1995.

Wichtl M (Hrsg.), Teedrogen, 4. Aufl., Wiss. Verlagsges. Stuttgart 1997.

Areca Catechu

Areca Nut

DESCRIPTION

Medicinal Parts: The medicinal part is the nut.

Flower and Fruit: The plant is an erect palm up to 30 m high. The trunk has a girth of about 50 cm. The numerous feathery leaflets are 30 to 60 cm long, confluent and glabrous. The flowers are on branching spadix. The male flowers are numerous and above, the female are solitary and below. The ovoid drupe has a fibrous layer under the yellow shell and one-seeded stone. The seeds are conical or nearly spherical and about 2.5 cm in diameter. They are very hard, and contain a deep brown testa showing fawn marbling.

Characteristics: The taste is slightly acrid, astringent and the odor faint.

Habitat: The plant is found in the East Indies, cultivated in parts of Asia and eastern Africa.

Production: Areca or betel nuts are the fresh seeds of Areca catechu.

Not To Be Confused With: Piper betel which is also called Betel, the leaf of which is chewed.

Other Names: Betel Nut, Pinang

ACTIONS AND PHARMACOLOGY

COMPOUNDS

Pyridine alkaloids: arecoline, guvacoline (ester alkaloids), besides arecaidine, guvacine

Tannins: catechin type

EFFECTS

The drug acts on the parasympathetic nervous system with an effect that is more muscarinic than nicotinic. It stimulates secretion in the salivary, bronchial and intestinal glands and causes tremors and bradycardia. It also causes cramps in the muscles of intestinal parasites and stimulates the vagus nerve. Euphoria has been observed on chewing betel nuts. CNS stimulation has been observed in mice.

INDICATIONS AND USAGE

Seldom used as a miotic. The drug is rarely used in human medicine.

In veterinary medicine, the drug is used as a vermifuge for tape worms in cattle and dogs as well as for intestinal colic in horses.

The drug is widely taken as a recreational drug. Fresh slices of the seed are part of the ''betel titbit'' used in eastern Asia. (Arecoline is converted in the central nervous system to the stimulant arecaidine through chewing). It is taken by an estimated 450 million people.

PRECAUTIONS AND ADVERSE REACTIONS

Due to its arecoline content, the drug appears parasympathomimetic. It leads to increased salivation, in high doses to bradycardia, tremor, reflex excitability, spasms and eventual paralysis. Long-term use of the drug as a stimulant can result in malignant tumors of the oral cavity through formation of nitrosamines. When the nuts are chewed, the mouth and lips are stained red as are the feces.

OVERDOSAGE

The toxic dose for humans is 8 to 10 g of the drug. Atropine is given as the antidote. Chewing the ''nut'' leads to a saponification of the ester alkaloids. The resulting arecaidine has a euphoric effect.

DOSAGE

Mode of Administration: In the past, Areca Nut was used in chewing balm for gum disease and as a vermifuge. Today, it is only used as a vermifuge in veterinary medicine for house pets. Therapeutic use is insignificant.

Storage: Must be stored separately, protected from light and in well-sealed containers.

LITERATURE

Aue W, Pharm Zentralhalle 136:728. 1967.

Hirono I, J Environ Sci Health C3(2):145. 1985.

Huang JL, McLeish MJ, J Chromatogr 475:447. 1989.

Juptner H, (1968) Z Tropenmed Parasit 19:254.

Lewin L, Über Areca catechu, Chavica Betle und das Betelkauen. In: Monographie, Stuttgart, F. Enke, 1889.

Schneider E, PUZ 15:161. 1986.

Further information in:

Frohne D, Pfänder HJ, Giftpflanzen - Ein Handbuch für Apotheker, Toxikologen und Biologen, 4. Aufl., Wiss. Verlags-Ges Stuttgart 1997.

Kern W, List PH, Hörhammer L (Hrsg.), Hagers Handbuch der Pharmazeutischen Praxis, 4. Aufl., Bde. 1-8, Springer Verlag Berlin, Heidelberg, New York, 1969.

Lewin L, Gifte und Vergiftungen, 6. Aufl., Nachdruck, Haug Verlag, Heidelberg 1992.

Roth L, Daunderer M, Kormann K, Giftpflanzen, Pflanzengifte, 4. Aufl., Ecomed Fachverlag Landsberg Lech 1993.

Tang W, Eisenbrand G, Chinese Drugs of Plant Origin, Springer Verlag Heidelberg 1992.

Teuscher E, Lindequist U, Biogene Gifte - Biologie, Chemie, Pharmakologie, 2. Aufl., Fischer Verlag Stuttgart 1994.

Arenaria Rubra

See Spergularia Rubra

Aristolochia Clematitis

Birthwort

DESCRIPTION

Medicinal Parts: The medicinal parts are the aerial portion and the root.

Flower and Fruit: The plant has dirty yellow flowers, usually in axillary groups of 7. The perigone forms a straight tube, which is bulbous beneath and has a linguiform, oblong-ovate, obtuse border. There are 6 stamens, the style is upward growing and the stigma is 6-lobed. The flower is pollinated by insects and traps them briefly. The fruit is a globose, pear-shaped capsule.

Leaves, Stem and Root: The plant grows to a height of 30 to 100 cm. The stem is erect, simple, grooved and glabrous. The leaves are alternate, long-petioled, cordate-reniform, yellow-green with prominent ribs.

Characteristics: The plant has a fruit-like fragrance and is poisonous.

Habitat: Indigenous to Mediterranean regions, Asia Minor and the Caucasus, but is found in numerous other regions.

ACTIONS AND PHARMACOLOGY

COMPOUNDS

Aristolochic acids (10-nitro-phenanthrene-1-acids): in particular aristolochic acids I and II

Isoquinoline alkaloids: including magnoflorin, corytuberin

EFFECTS

Activation of phagocytes has been demonstrated in animal tests in rabbits and guinea pigs, along with an increase in serum bactericides and stimulation of β-lysine. In the ring test, stimulation and formation of granulation tissue was demonstrated in rats. In mice, there was a clear increase in the survival rate in cases of general infection. No significant results were recorded in cases where infections had no or only a low leucocytic immune reaction.

Pure aristolochic acid acts similarly to colchicine.

INDICATIONS AND USAGE

Birthwort is used to stimulate the immune system and in the treatment of allergically caused gastrointestinal and gallbladder colic. In homeopathy, the drug is used for gynecological disorders, climacteric symptoms, in addition to the treatment of wounds and ulcers. It is also used as a treatment after major surgery and in ear-nose-throat treatments. It is used in veterinary medicine for hormone-based sterility.

PRECAUTIONS AND ADVERSE REACTIONS

Birthwort drug is highly toxic. The intake of acutely toxic doses leads to vomiting, gastroenteritis, spasms, severe kidney damage and eventually to death by kidney failure. The chronic intake of low dosages in laboratory animals led to the development of tumors. Because of the genotoxic and cancerogenic effects of the aristolochic acids, the drug is not to be administered even in small dosages.

DOSAGE

Mode of Administration: Birthwort is used as a tincture in an ethanol solution. No further information is available.

LITERATURE

Che CT et al., (1984) J Nat Prod 47(2):331.

Fanselow G, Der Einfluβ von Pflanzenextrakten (Echinacea purpurea, Aristolochia clematitis) und homöopathischen Medikamenten auf die Phagocytoseleistung humaner Granulocyten in vitro. In: Dissertation Berlin. 1981.

Henrickson CU, (1970) Z Immunitäts Forsch 5:425.

Mengs U, Klein M, Genotoxic Effects of Aristolochic Acid in the Mouse Micronucleus Test. In: PM 52(6):502. 1988.

Mix DB et al., (1982) J Nat Prod 45(6):657.

Siess M, Seybold G, Untersuchungen über die Wirkung von Pulsatilla pratensis, Cimicifuga racemosa und Aristolochia clematis auf den Östrus infantiler und kastrierter weiβer Mäuse. In: Arzneim Forsch 10:514. 1960.

Strauch R, Hiller K, (1974) Pharmazie 29(10/11):656.

Tympner KD, (1981) Z Angew Phytother 5:181.

Further information in:

Chan H, But P (Eds.), Pharmacology and Applications of Chinese Materia Medica, Vol. 1, Ed. World Scientific Singapore 1986.

Frohne D, Pfänder HJ, Giftpflanzen - Ein Handbuch für Apotheker, Toxikologen und Biologen, 4. Aufl., Wiss. Verlags-Ges Stuttgart 1997.

Kern W, List PH, Hörhammer L (Hrsg.), Hagers Handbuch der Pharmazeutischen Praxis, 4. Aufl., Bde. 1-8, Springer Verlag Berlin, Heidelberg, New York, 1969.

Lewin L, Gifte und Vergiftungen, 6. Aufl., Nachdruck, Haug Verlag, Heidelberg 1992.

Madaus G, Lehrbuch der Biologischen Arzneimittel, Bde. 1-3, Nachdruck, Georg Olms Verlag Hildesheim 1979.

Roth L, Daunderer M, Kormann K, Giftpflanzen, Pflanzengifte, 4. Aufl., Ecomed Fachverlag Landsberg Lech 1993.

Steinegger E, Hänsel R, Pharmakognosie, 5. Aufl., Springer Verlag Heidelberg 1992.

Teuscher E, Lindequist U, Biogene Gifte - Biologie, Chemie, Pharmakologie, 2. Aufl., Fischer Verlag Stuttgart 1994.

Armoracia Rusticana

Horseradish

DESCRIPTION

Flower and Fruit: The inflorescence is made up of numerous, richly flowered racemes (cymes). The fragrant flowers are on 5 to 7 mm long, upright pedicles. The sepals are 2.5 to 3 mm long, broadly ovate, with a membranous white margin. The white petals are 5 to 7 mm long and broadly obovate. The inner stamens are 2.5 mm long; the outer ones 1.5 mm long. The stigma is broad, round and gently 2-lobed. The small pods are on 20 mm long, upright spreading stems. They are globose to obovate and 4 to 6 mm long. The seeds are smooth.

Leaves, Stem and Root: The plant is 40 to 120 cm high. It is a sturdy and glabrous perennial. The root is quite thick and woody. In cultivated varieties it is thick and fleshy, with numerous root heads, which are light yellowish white and have horizontal underground runners. The sometimes solitary stems are upright, branched above, grooved and hollow. The leaves are log-petioled, oblong-ovate, cordate at the base, 30 to 100 cm long and unevenly crenate. The lower cauline leaves have shorter petioles and are lobed or comb-shaped-pinnate with liner-oblong, entire-margined or serrate sections. The upper cauline leaves with narrowed bases are sessile, oblong or lanceolate, unevenly crenate to serrate and obtuse. The uppermost leaves are linear or almost entire-margined.

Characteristics: The rootstock has a strong and irritating odor and a sharp burning taste.

Habitat: The plant is indigenous to the Volga-Don region but has spread to almost all of Europe and outer parts of the world.

Production: Horseradish consists of the fresh or dried roots of Armoracia rusticana (syn. Cochlearia armoracia).

Other Names: Mountain Radish, Red Cole, Great Raifort

ACTIONS AND PHARMACOLOGY

COMPOUNDS

Glucosinolates sinigrin and gluconasturtin: In the freshly-harvested root, yields allyl mustard oil and a little 2-phenyl mustard oil when the root is cut up. The dehydrated root contains both of these mustard oils.

EFFECTS

Horseradish works antimicrobially against gram-positive and gram negative pathogens. It is an antispasmodic. In animal experiments, it is hyperaemic on skin and mucous membranes and carcinostatic.

INDICATIONS AND USAGE

- Infections of the urinary tract
- Cough/bronchitis

Internally, Horseradish is used to treat catarrh of the respiratory tract and as supportive therapy for infections of the urinary tract. Externally, the drug is used for catarrh of the respiratory tract and for hyperemic treatment for minor muscle aches. In folk medicine, horseradish is administered for influenza, respiratory ailments, digestion, gout, rheumatism, and liver and gallbladder disorders.

CONTRAINDICATIONS

Because of the mucous membrane-irritating effect of the mustard oils, the intake of the drug should not be carried out in the presence of stomach or intestinal ulcers or in patients with a history of kidney disease.

PRECAUTIONS AND ADVERSE REACTIONS

General: No health hazards or side effects are known in conjunction with the proper administration of designated therapeutic dosages.

Pediatric Use: Preparations of horseradish should not be administered to children under 4 years of age.

DOSAGE

Mode of Administration: Fresh or dried, cut or ground root, freshly pressed juice as well as other galenic preparations for internal or external applications.

Daily Dose: The average dose for internal use is 20 g fresh root; for external use, oinments with maximum 2% mustard oils may be used.

Storage: Fresh roots should be buried in soil or in sand.

LITERATURE

Stoll A, Seebeck E, Helv Chim Acta 31:1432-1434. 1948.

Further information in:

Hänsel R, Keller K, Rimpler H, Schneider G (Hrsg.), Hagers Handbuch der Pharmazeutischen Praxis, 5. Aufl., Bde 4-6 (Drogen), Springer Verlag Berlin, Heidelberg, New York, 1992-1994.

Lewin L, Gifte und Vergiftungen, 6. Aufl., Nachdruck, Haug Verlag, Heidelberg 1992.

Teuscher E, Lindequist U, Biogene Gifte - Biologie, Chemie, Pharmakologie, 2. Aufl., Fischer Verlag Stuttgart 1994.

Teuscher E, Biogene Arzneimittel, 5. Aufl., Wiss. Verlagsges. Stuttgart 1997.

Wagner H, Wiesenauer M, Phytotherapie. Phytopharmaka und pflanzliche Homöopathika, Fischer-Verlag, Stuttgart, Jena, New York, 1995.

Arnica Montana

Arnica

DESCRIPTION

Flower and Fruit: The terminal composite flower is found in the leaf axils of the upper pair of leaves. They have a diameter of 6 to 8 cm, are egg yolk yellow to orange-yellow and occasionally light yellow. The receptacle and epicalyx are hairy. The 10 to 20 female ray flowers are lingui-form. There are about 100 disc flowers, which are tubular. The 5-ribbed fruit is black-brown and has a bristly tuft of hair.

Leaves, Stem and Root: Arnica Montana is a 20 to 50 cm herbaceous plant with a 0.5 cm thick by 10 cm long usually unbranched, 3-sectioned, sympodial, brownish rhizome. The rhizome may also be 3-headed with many yellow-brown secondary roots. Leaves are in basal rosettes. They are in 2 to 3 crossed opposite pairs and are obovate and entire-margined with 5 protruding vertical ribs. The glandular-haired stem has 2 to 6 smaller leaves, which are ovate to lanceolate, entire-margined or somewhat dentate.

Characteristics: The flower heads are aromatic, the taste is scratchy.

Habitat: Found in Europe from Scandinavia to southern Europe. Also found in southern Russia and central Asia.

Production: Arnica flower consists of the fresh or dried inflorescence of Arnica montana or Arnica chamissonis. The flower should be dried quickly at 45°C.

Not To Be Confused With: Other yellow-flowering Asteracea.

Other Names: Mountain Tobacco, Leopard's Bane, Wolfsbane, Arnica Flowers, Arnica Root

ACTIONS AND PHARMACOLOGY

COMPOUNDS

Sesquiterpene lactones of the pseudo-guaianolid-type: particularly esters of the helenalin- and 11,13-dihydrohelenalins with short-chained fatty acids, for example acetic acid, isobutyric acid, 2- methyl-butyric acid, isovaleric acid

Volatile oil: with thymol, thymol esters, free fatty acids

Polyynes

Hydroxycumarine

Helenaline derivatives

EFFECTS

Especially when applied topically, arnica preparations have an antiphlogistic effect. In cases of inflammation, arnica preparations also show analgesic and antiseptic activity.

In animal experiments, Arnica influenced cardiovascular activity by increasing coronary flow and cardiac output and by reducing peripheral resistance.

INDICATIONS AND USAGE

- Fevers and colds
- Inflammation of the skin
- Cough/bronchitis
- Tendency to infection
- Inflammation of the mouth and pharynx
- Rheumatism

- Common cold
- Blunt injuries

For external use in injury and for consequences of accidents, such as hematoma, dislocations, contusions, edema due to fracture, rheumatic muscle and joint problems. Inflammation of the oral and throat region, furunculosis, inflammation caused by insect bites, phlebitis.

In Russian folk medicine the drug is used to treat uterus hemorrhage. Furthermore, the drug is utilized for myocarditis, arteriosclerosis, Angina pectoris, fatigue, cardiac insufficiency, sprains, contusions and for hair loss due to psychological causes. The various folk medicinal uses are unproven.

PRECAUTIONS AND ADVERSE REACTIONS

The risks connected with the external, appropriate administration of therapeutic dosages of the drug are minimal. Frequent administration, in particular of the undiluted tincture, as well as with contacts with the plant, can nevertheless lead to sensitization.

Repeated contact with, among other things, cosmetics containing Arnicae flos or other composite (for example tansy, chrysanthemums, sunflowers) leads to allergy-related skin rashes with itching, blister formation, ulcers and superficial necroses. External application of very high concentrations can also result in toxic-conditioned primary blister formation and necroses.

OVERDOSAGE

Overdoses taken internally can lead to poisonings, characterized by severe mucous membrane irritation (vomiting, diarrhea, mucous membrane hemorrhage) and cardiac muscle palsy following a brief stimulation of cardiac activity. For that reason, one is strongly advised against internal administration of the drug.

DOSAGE

Mode of Administration: Whole herb, cut herb, herb powder for infusions; liquid and semi-solid forms of medication for external application.

Preparation: Arnica tincture (3 to 10x dilution with water) is used to prepare a poultice. A tincture is prepared using 1 part Arnica flowers and 10 parts ethanol 70% v/v (according to DAB 10). Ointment with up to 15% Arnica oil or 20 to 25% tincture are common preparations. Arnica oil is an extract of 1 part herb and 5 parts fatty oil.

Daily Dose: Tincture for cataplasm: tincture in 3x to 10x dilution. For mouth rinses: tincture in 10x dilution.

Storage: The drug should be stored using all well known measures.

LITERATURE

Anonym, Arnikablüten nur äußerlich. In: DAZ 131(38):1949. 1991.

Beekman AC et al., Structure-cytotoxicity relationship of some helenanolide-type sesquiterpene lactones. In: JNP 60(3):252-257. 1997.

Brandt L, (1967) Scand J Haematol Suppl 2.

Brock FE, Arnica montana bei Venenleiden. In: ZPT 12(5):141. 1992.

Hall, IH et al., (1979) J Pharm Sci 68:537.

Halub M et al., (1975) Phytochemistry 14:1659.

Hörmann HP, Kortin HC (1995) Allergic acute contact dermatitis due to Arnica tincture self-medication. Phytomedicine 4:315-317.

Kaziro, GSN et al., (1984) Br. J Oral Maxillofacial Surg 22:42.

Merfort I, (1984) Planta Med 50 (1):107.

Merfort I, (1985) Planta Med 51 (2):136.

Schmidt Th J et al., Sesquiterpen lactones and inositol esters from Arnica angustifolia. In: PM 61(6):544-550. 1995.

Thesen R, Phytotherapeutika - nicht immer harmlos. In: ZPT 9(49):105. 1988.

Weil D, Reuter HD, Einfluß von Arnika-Extrakt und Helenalin auf die Funktion menschlicher Blutplättchen. In: ZPT 9(1):26. 1988.

Willuhn G et al., (1984) Planta Med 50 (1):35.

Willuhn G, Leven W, Luley C, Arnikablüten DAB 10. Untersuchung zur qualitativen und quantitativen Variabilität des Sesquiterepnelactongehaltes der offizinellen Arzneidroge. In: DAZ 134(42):4077. 1994.

Willuhn G, Leven W, Qualität von Arnikazubereitungen. In: DAZ 135(21):1939-1942. 1995.

Woerdenbag HJ et al., Cytotoxicity of flavonoids and sesquiterpene lactones from Arnica species. In: PM 59(7):A681. 1993.

Further information in:

Frohne D, Pfänder HJ, Giftpflanzen - Ein Handbuch für Apotheker, Toxikologen und Biologen, 4. Aufl., Wiss. Verlags-Ges Stuttgart 1997.

Hänsel R, Keller K, Rimpler H, Schneider G (Hrsg.), Hagers Handbuch der Pharmazeutischen Praxis, 5. Aufl., Bde 4-6 (Drogen): Springer Verlag Berlin, Heidelberg, New York, 1992-1994.

Hausen B, Allergiepflanzen, Pflanzenallergene, ecomed Verlagsgesellsch. mbH, Landsberg 1988.

Leung AY, Encyclopedia of Common Natural Ingredients Used in Food Drugs and Cosmetics, John Wiley & Sons Inc., New York 1980.

Lewin L, Gifte und Vergiftungen, 6. Aufl., Nachdruck, Haug Verlag, Heidelberg 1992.

Madaus G, Lehrbuch der Biologischen Arzneimittel, Bde 1-3, Nachdruck, Georg Olms Verlag Hildesheim 1979.

Roth L, Daunderer M, Kormann K, Giftpflanzen, Pflanzengifte, 4. Aufl., Ecomed Fachverlag Landsberg Lech 1993.

Schulz R, Hänsel R, Rationale Phytotherapie, Springer Verlag Heidelberg 1996.

Steinegger E, Hänsel R, Pharmakognosie, 5. Aufl., Springer Verlag Heidelberg 1992.

Teuscher E, Lindequist U, Biogene Gifte - Biologie, Chemie, Pharmakologie, 2. Aufl., Fischer Verlag Stuttgart 1994.

Teuscher E, Biogene Arzneimittel, 5. Aufl., Wiss. Verlagsges. Stuttgart 1997.

Wagner H, Wiesenauer M, Phytotherapie. Phytopharmaka und pflanzliche Homöopathika, Fischer-Verlag, Stuttgart, Jena, New York 1995.

Wichtl M (Hrsg.), Teedrogen, 4. Aufl., Wiss. Verlagsges. Stuttgart 1997.

Arrach

See Chenopodium Vulvaria

Arrowroot

See Maranta Arundinaceae

Artemisia Absinthium

Wormwood

DESCRIPTION

Medicinal Parts: The medicinal parts are the aerial parts of the plant.

Flower and Fruit: The plant grows from 60 to 120 cm in height. The numerous flower heads are short-stemmed and hang in a many-flowered panicle. The capitula are small, globular, inclined and 3 to 4 mm wide and almost as long. The bracts are gray, silky-pubescent with a rounded tip. The outer ones are linear-oblong and pubescent while the inner ones are ovate, obtuse, broad and have a transparent, membranous margin. The receptacle is rough-haired. The flowers are yellow and fertile. The disc florets are androgynous and the ray florets are female with an extending style stem. The fruit is about 1.5 mm long.

Leaves, Stem and Root: The plant is a semi-shrub with a woody, hardy rosette stem that is up to 1 m high. The stem is usually erect, branched and leafy. The alternate, long-petioled leaves are silky pubescent on both sides. The lower ones are abrupt pinnate and the upper ones simple. The leaf tips are lanceolate to linear-lanceolate, obtuse to acuminate and 2 to 3 mm wide.

Characteristics: The plant has an aromatic odor and a very bitter taste.

Habitat: Europe, northern Africa, parts of Asia, North and South America.

Production: Wormwood consists of the fresh or dried upper shoots and leaves, the fresh or dried basal leaves, or a mixture of the aerial plant parts from Artemisia absinthium, harvested during flowering season.

Not To Be Confused With: The drug will at times contain additions of Artemisiae herba.

Other Names: Green Ginger, Absinthe

ACTIONS AND PHARMACOLOGY

COMPOUNDS

Volatile oil with a high level of (+)-thujone

Sesquiterpene bitter principles: including absinthine, anabsinthine, artabsine and matricine

EFFECTS

In patients with liver disorders, a suspension of 20 mg extract in 10 ml water is administered with a stomach probe after which a significant increase of alpha-amylase, liapse, bilirubin and cholesterol was observed after 70 to 100 minutes.

In rabbits, fever induced through yeast injection could be reduced with the application of diverse fractions of the drug, using an esophageal probe.

A watery extract of the whole drug is supposed to retard the growth of *Plasmodium falciparum.* The essential oil of the drug may possess an antimicrobial effect. The drug also stimulates the bitter receptors in the taste buds of the tongue. When bitter agents are introduced into the mouth, they trigger a reflexive increase of stomach secretion with higher acid concentration.

INDICATIONS AND USAGE

- Loss of appetite
- Dyspeptic complaints
- Liver and gallbladder complaints

The drug is administered for loss of appetite, dyspeptic disorders, bloating, meteorism and for dyspepsia as a result of convulsive gallbladder disorders.

In folk medicine, wormwood preparations are used internally for gastric insufficiency, intestinal atonia, gastritis, stomachache, liver disorders, bloating, anemia, irregular menstruation, intermittent fever, loss of appetite, and worm infestation.

Externally, the drug is applied for poorly healing wounds, ulcers, skin blotches, and insect bites.

The above mentioned popular indications are insufficiently documented.

PRECAUTIONS AND ADVERSE REACTIONS

Due to the drug's thujone content, the internal administration of large doses can lead to vomiting, stomach and intestinal cramps, headache, dizziness and disturbances of the central nervous system. Continuous use is not advisable. The use of volatile oils and spirituous extracts from the drug for the manufacture of alcoholic drinks is forbidden in many countries because of possible injuries to health.

DOSAGE

Mode of Administration: Comminuted herb is used for infusions and decoctions. Powdered herb, extracts and tinctures in liquid or solid forms are used for oral administration. Combination with other bitters or aromatics is common.

Preparation: To prepare an infusion, pour 150 ml boiling water over 1/2 teaspoonful of the drug, strain after 10 minutes. A decoction is prepared by adding 1 handful of drug to 1 liter of boiling water for 5 minutes. To prepare a tea, use 1 g drug in 1 cup water.

Daily Dose: The total daily dose is 3 to 5 g of the herb as an aqueous extract. Internal dose of the infusion is 1 cup freshly prepared tea taken 30 minutes before each meal. The tincture dosage is 10 to 30 drops in sufficient water taken 3 times daily. The liquid extract dosage is 1 to 2 ml taken 3 times daily.

Externally, a decoction is used for healing of wounds and insect bites.

Storage: Wormwood must be kept in sealed containers and protected from light.

LITERATURE

Akhmedov IS et al., (1970) Khim Prir Soedin 6:691.

Akhmedov IS et al., (Artabin, a new lactone from Artemisia absinthium). In: Khim Prid Soed 5:622. 1970.

Baumann IC et al., (1975) Z Allg Med 51 (17):784.

Beauhaire J et al., (1981) Tetrahedron Letters 22 (24):2269.

Beauhaire J, Fourrey JL, (1982) J Chem Soc Perk Trans: 861.

Del Castillo J et al., (1975) Nature 253:365.

Dermanovic S et al., (1976) zit CA 87:98796h.

Greger H, Hofer O, New unsymmetrically substituted tetrahydrofuran lignans from Artemisia absinthium. In: Tetrahedron 36(24):3551. 1980.

Greger H, (1978) Phytochemistry 17:806.

Hoffman B, Herrmann K, (1982) Z Lebensm Unters Forsch 174 (3):211.

Kasimov Ah Z et al., (Anabsin-a new diguaianolide from Artemisia absinthium). In: Khim Prid Soed 4:495. 1979.

Kasymov SZ et al., (1979) Khim Prir Soed 5:658.

Kennedy AI et al., Volatile oils from normal and transformed roots of Artemisia absinthium. In: PH 32:1449. 1993.

Kinloch JD, (1971) Practitioner 206:44.

Lemberkovics E et al., Some phytochemical characteristics of essential oil ot Artemisia absinthium L. In: Herba hung 21(3):197-215. 1982.

Marles RJ, Kaminski J, Arnason JT, Pazos-Sanou L, Heptinstall S, Fischer NH, Crompton CW, Kindack DG, A bioassay for inhibition of serotonin release from bovine platelets. In: JNP 55:1044-1056. 1992.

Rucker G, Manns D, Wilbert S, Peroxides as constituents of plants. 10. Homoditerpene peroxides from Artemisia-absinthium. In: PH:31(1):340. 1992.

Schneider Von G, Mielke B, (1979) Deutsch Apoth Ztg 119 (25):977.

Stahl E, Gerard D, (1983) Z Lebensm Unters Forsch 176 (1):1.

Swiatek L, Dombrowicz E, (1984) Farm Pol 40 (2):729.

Vostrowski O et al., (1981) Z NaturForsch (C) 36 (5/6):369.

Vostrowski O et al., Über die Komponenten des ätherischen Öls aus Artemisia absinthium L.. In: Z Naturforsch 36(5/6):369. 1981.

Zafar MM, Hamdard ME, Hameed A, Screening of Artemisia absinthium for antimalarial effects on Plasmodium berghei in mice: Preliminary report. In: ETH 30(2):223. 1990.

Zakirov SK et al., (1976) Khim Prir Soedin 4:548.

Further information in:

Hänsel R, Keller K, Rimpler H, Schneider G (Hrsg.), Hagers Handbuch der Pharmazeutischen Praxis, 5. Aufl., Bde 4-6 (Drogen): Springer Verlag Berlin, Heidelberg, New York, 1992-1994.

Lewin L, Gifte und Vergiftungen, 6. Aufl., Nachdruck, Haug Verlag, Heidelberg 1992.

Madaus G, Lehrbuch der Biologischen Arzneimittel, Bde 1-3, Nachdruck, Georg Olms Verlag Hildesheim 1979.

Roth L, Daunderer M, Kormann K, Giftpflanzen, Pflanzengifte, 4. Aufl., Ecomed Fachverlag Landsberg Lech 1993.

Schulz R, Hänsel R, Rationale Phytotherapie, Springer Verlag Heidelberg 1996.

Steinegger E, Hänsel R, Pharmakognosie, 5. Aufl., Springer Verlag Heidelberg 1992.

Teuscher E, Lindequist U, Biogene Gifte - Biologie, Chemie, Pharmakologie, 2. Aufl., Fischer Verlag Stuttgart 1994.

Teuscher E, Biogene Arzneimittel, 5. Aufl., Wiss. Verlagsges. Stuttgart 1997.

Wagner H, Wiesenauer M, Phytotherapie. Phytopharmaka und pflanzliche Homöopathika, Fischer-Verlag, Stuttgart, Jena, New York 1995.

Wichtl M (Hrsg.), Teedrogen, 4. Aufl., Wiss. Verlagsges. Stuttgart 1997.

Artemisia Cina

Wormseed

DESCRIPTION

Medicinal Parts: The medicinal parts are the flowers.

Flower and Fruit: The numerous flower heads are about 2 mm long with a diameter of 1.5 mm. They are ovoid and greenish-yellow when fresh, later brownish-green. They contain three to five minute, tubular, androgynous florets with a slim, cylindrical, and glabrous receptacle. The epicalyces have numerous oblong-obtuse, imbricate scales.

Leaves, Stem and Root: Artemisia cina is an evergreen, perennial semi-shrub, 30 to 60 cm high with many slim sprouting stems. The knarled rhizome produces numerous leaf and flower branches. The stems are smooth and woody and the leaves pinnatifid on the non-flowering branches. The leaves on the flowering branches are small and entire-margined.

Characteristics: The odor is aromatic and characteristic, the taste bitter.

Habitat: The plant is indigenous to Iran, Turkestan, and the Kirghizin Steppes around Buchara.

Production: Wormwood flowers are the inflorescent buds of Artemisia cina. Occasionally, incorrectly named as wormseed.

Not To Be Confused With: Refined mustard flour.

Other Names: Levant, Santonica, Sea Wormwood

ACTIONS AND PHARMACOLOGY

COMPOUNDS

Sesquiterpene lactones: alpha-santonin, as well as artemisin, beta-santonin

EFFECTS

There are no pharmacological studies available because the active agent santonin was isolated as early as 1830. The drug has a vermifuge action, for ascarids in particular. Their muscles are paralyzed by santonin and they are forced into the large intestine where they are removed by means of a laxative.

In rats, the rectal temperature was lowered during fevers, which had been induced by brewer's yeast injections. This leads to the speculation that santonin effects body temperature in a similar manner to dopamine.

INDICATIONS AND USAGE

The drug is used for ascarid and oxyuris infestations.

PRECAUTIONS AND ADVERSE REACTIONS

No health hazards or side effects are known in conjunction with the proper administration of designated therapeutic dosages. However, any side effects may resemble those of the alpha-santonins: kidney irritation, gastroenteritis, stupor, visual disorders (xanthopsia), muscle twitchings, and epileptiform spasms.

OVERDOSAGE

Deadly poisonings following the intake of less than 10 gm of the drug are known. Administration in allopathic dosages is to be avoided.

DOSAGE

Preparation: Wormwood is completely obsolete as a drug, occasionally available as a powder for use when more modern antithelmintic agents fail. Symptoms of poisoning are possible in therapeutic dosages.

Daily Dosage: The drug is always used in combination with a laxative. The average single dose is 0.025 gm for adults, for children, take the child's age in years, double this amount in milligrams of the drug.

According to the Austrian pharmacopoeia, the single dose is 1 to 2 gm. The powder is administered in the morning and followed later by a castor oil or sodium sulfate. The remedy is repeated on the following day.

LITERATURE

Frohne D, Pfänder HJ: Giftpflanzen - Ein Handbuch für Apotheker, Toxikologen und Biologen, 4. Aufl., Wiss. Verlagsges. mbH Stuttgart 1997.

Hänsel R, Keller K, Rimpler H, Schneider G (Hrsg.), Hagers Handbuch der Pharmazeutischen Praxis, 5. Aufl., Bde 4-6 (Drogen): Springer Verlag Berlin, Heidelberg, New York, 1992-1994.

Lewin L, Gifte und Vergiftungen, 6. Aufl., Nachdruck, Haug Verlag, Heidelberg 1992.

Madaus G, Lehrbuch der Biologischen Arzneimittel, Bde 1-3, Nachdruck, Georg Olms Verlag Hildesheim 1979.

Roth L, Daunderer M, Kormann K: Giftpflanzen, Pflanzengifte, 4. Aufl., Ecomed Fachverlag Landsberg Lech 1993.

Teuscher E, Lindequist U, Biogene Gifte - Biologie, Chemie, Pharmakologie, 2. Aufl., Fischer Verlag Stuttgart 1994.

Teuscher E, Biogene Arzneimittel, 5. Aufl., Wiss. Verlagsges. mbH Stuttgart 1997.

Artemisia Dracunculus

Tarragon

DESCRIPTION

Medicinal Parts: The medicinal parts are the dried aerial parts of the plant.

Flower and Fruit: The flowers are drooping, almost globular and 2 to 3 mm across. The flowers are whitish, later reddish and clustered in loose panicles. The sepals of the epicalyx are oblong-elliptic, mostly green and the inner ones are ovate with a broad membranous edge. The ray florets are female. The disc florets are androgynous and infertile. The corolla is yellow and the receptacle glabrous.

Leaves, Stem and Root: The plant is a glabrous, 60 to 120 cm high herbaceous perennial. There are numerous stems, which are bushily branched with flowering branches at the top. The leaves are simple, lanceolate-linear, 2 to 10 cm by 2 to 10 mm, thorn-tipped, entire or slightly serrate, and somewhat glossy.

Characteristics: The odor is aromatic and intense.

Habitat: The plant is indigenous to Russia (Russian Tarragon) and Mongolia and is cultivated widely.

Production: Tarragon leaves or herbs are picked when in bloom and carefully dried.

Other Names: Little Dragon, Mugwort, Estragon

ACTIONS AND PHARMACOLOGY

COMPOUNDS

Volatile oil: of complex organization, according to breed, including alpha-pinenes, beta-pinenes, camphene, limonene, linalool, ocimene, myrcene, chavicol methyl ether

Flavonoids

Hydroxycoumarins

Polyynes

EFFECTS

No information is available.

INDICATIONS AND USAGE

Tarragon is considered to be an appetite stimulant.

PRECAUTIONS AND ADVERSE REACTIONS

No health hazards or side effects are known in conjunction with the proper administration of designated therapeutic dosages.

DOSAGE

Mode of Administration: Both the fresh and dried plant is used, mostly as a culinary herb.

LITERATURE

Balza F, Jamieson L, Towers GHN, Chemical constituents of teh aerial parts of Artemisia dracunculus. In: JNP 48:339. 1985.

Greger H, Bohlmann F, Zdero Ch, Neue Isocumarine aus Dracunculus. In: PH 16:795. 1977.

Lakupovic J, Tan RX, Bohlmann F, Jia ZJ, Huneck S, Acetylenes and other constituents from Artemisia dracunculus. In: PM 57:450. 1992.

Marco JA et al., Sesquiterpenes lactones from Artemisia species. In: PH 32:460. 1993.

Schormüller B, In: Schormüller J: Alkaloidhaltige Genußmittel, Gewürze, Kochsalz, Springer Verlag, Berlin, Heidelberg, New York. 1970.

Thieme H, Nguyen TT, PA 27:255-265. 1972.

Vostrowsky O et al., Über die Komponenten des ätherischen Öls aus Estragon (Artemisia dracunculus L.). In: Z Lebensm Untersuch Forsch 173:365-367. 1981.

Further information in:

Hänsel R, Keller K, Rimpler H, Schneider G (Hrsg.), Hagers Handbuch der Pharmazeutischen Praxis, 5. Aufl., Bde 4-6 (Drogen). Springer Verlag Berlin, Heidelberg, New York, 1992-1994.

Artemisia Vulgaris

Mugwort

DESCRIPTION

Medicinal Parts: The medicinal parts are the root and the above-ground parts of the plant.

Flower and Fruit: The flower heads are ovoid, 3 to 4 mm long by 2 mm wide. The numerous flowers are short stemmed, erect or slightly drooping. They are in dense, heavily branched panicles with numerous lanceolate bracts. The bracts are downy white with a green midrib. The inner ones are lanceolate and acuminate. The outside ones are oblong and obtuse with broad membranous margin. The flowers are yellowish or red-brown and almost glabrous. The inner ones are androgynous and the outside ones are female. The receptacle is glabrous. The fruit has an indistinct margin.

Leaves, Stem and Root: The plant is a long-stemmed, 70 to 150 cm high shrub with a branched, many-headed, and creeping rhizome without runners or rosette. The shoots are slightly pubescent, often red-tinged, and have a weak unpleasant smell. The stems are erect or ascending, edged, coriaceous, and die off each year. They are in branched panicles and downy. The leaves are 5 to 10 cm long, coriaceous, and the margins are often rolled back. The upper surface is usually dark green and glabrous, occasionally pubescent, and the lower surface is tomentose. The basal leaves are short-petioled and almost lobed like a lyre with a large 3 to 5 end section and 1 to 2 pairs of small side leaflets. The rest of the leaves are sessile or almost sessile with a slit base. The lower ones are double-pinnate, the middle and upper ones are pinnatifid and lanceolate, acuminate, entire-margined or slightly serrated.

Characteristics: Mugwort has a pleasant tangy taste. The root is sweet and pungent, the herb is aromatic and bitter.

Habitat: The plant is indigenous to Asia and North America. It is distributed all over Europe except in the south.

Not To Be Confused With: Asinthii herba.

Other Names: Wormwood, Felon Herb, St. John's Plant

ACTIONS AND PHARMACOLOGY

COMPOUNDS

Volatile oil: of very complex organization, chief constituents, according to breed, 1,8- cineol, camphor, linalool or thujone

Sesquiterpene lactones

Lipophilic flavonoids

Polyynes

Hydroxycoumarins: for example umbelliferone, aesculetin

EFFECTS

The aqueous extract and essential oil show antimicrobial activity in laboratory tests.

INDICATIONS AND USAGE

Mugwort is used in complaints and problems involving the gastrointestinal tract. The plant is also used for worm infestations, epilepsy, persistent vomiting, to promote circulation, and as a sedative. The root is used for asthenic states as a tonic, and in combination with other remedies also for psychoneuroses, neurasthenia, depression, hypochondria, autonomic neuroses, general irritability and restlessness, insomnia, and anxiety states.

The efficacy of Mugwort for the listed indications has not been substantiated.

PRECAUTIONS AND ADVERSE REACTIONS

No health hazards or side effects are known in conjunction with the proper administration of designated therapeutic dosages. Sensitization through skin contact has been observed, although very rarely.

DOSAGE

Mode of Administration: Since the efficacy for the claimed applications is not verified, a therapeutic administration is not recommended.

Preparation: "Moxibustion" (China, Japan) leaves are ground with water in a mortar and after the removal of the larger remnants, small cones are formed and dried to be later burnt onto the skin of the patient.

LITERATURE

Hoffmann B, Herrmann K, (1982) Z Lebensm Unters Forsch 174 (3):211.

Jork H, Juel S, (1979) Arch Pharm 312:540.

Juel S et al., (1976) Arch Pharm 309:458.

Kaul VK et al., (1976) Ind J Pharm 38 (1):21.

Marco JA et al., Sesquiterpenes lactones from Artemisia species. In: PH 32:460. 1993.

Marco JA, Sanz JF, Hierro P, Two eudesmane acids from Artemisia vulgaris. In: PH 30: 2403-2404. 1991.

Michaelis K et al., On the essential oil components from blossoms of Artemisia vulgaris L. In: Z Naturfosch 37(3/4):152. 1982.

Nano GM et al., (1976) Planta Med 30:211.

Nano GM et al., Composition of some oils from Artemisia vulgaris. In: PM 30(3):211. 1976.

Stefanovic M et al., (1982) Glas Khem Drush Beogr 47 (3):7.

Wallnöfer B, Hofer O, Greger H, Polyacetylenes from Artemsia "Vulgares" Group. In: PH 28(10):2687. 1989.

Further information in:

Hänsel R, Keller K, Rimpler H, Schneider G (Hrsg.), Hagers Handbuch der Pharmazeutischen Praxis, 5. Aufl., Bde 4-6 (Drogen): Springer Verlag Berlin, Heidelberg, New York, 1992-1994.

Hausen B, Allergiepflanzen, Pflanzenallergene, ecomed Verlagsgesellsch. mbH, Landsberg 1988.

Madaus G, Lehrbuch der Biologischen Arzneimittel, Bde 1-3, Nachdruck, Georg Olms Verlag Hildesheim 1979.

Wichtl M (Hrsg.), Teedrogen, 4. Aufl., Wiss. Verlagsges. Stuttgart 1997.

Artichoke

See Cynara Scolymus

Arum Maculatum

Arum

DESCRIPTION

Medicinal Parts: The medicinal part is the root of the plant.

Flower and Fruit: The flowers are pale yellowish-green. They are surrounded by a bulbous spath and therefore are not visible. A violet or brown-red spadix emerges from the bract with 2 circles of bristles underneath. Under the bristles are the male flowers, and under these again the female. The spath doubles the length of the spadix. The whole structure forms a typical insect trap. The fruit is a scarlet berry.

Leaves, Stem and Root: Arum maculatum is a 30 to 60 cm spit- to arrow-shaped plant. It is long-stemmed, glossy, often brown speckled, and basal. The petiole is spread to a sheath at the base. The root-stock is tuberous, ovoid, and floury-fleshy. The size varies between that of a hazelnut and a pigeon's egg.

Characteristics: Arum is a poisonous plant.

Habitat: The plant is indigenous to Europe, Britain, and the U.S.

Other Names: Lords and Ladies, Starchwort, Adder's Root, Bobbins, Friar's Cowl, Kings and Queens, Parson and Clerk, Ramp, Quaker, Wake Robin, Cocky Baby, Cuckoo Pint, Cypress Powder, Dragon Root, Gaglee, Ladysmock, Portland Arrowroot

ACTIONS AND PHARMACOLOGY

COMPOUNDS

Oxalates: partially in the form of calcium oxalate glands, partially in soluble form (cyanogenic glycosides (trigloquinine)

Mucilages: glucomannane

EFFECTS

The drug has diaphoretic and expectorant effects.

INDICATIONS AND USAGE

Arum is used for colds and inflammation of the throat.

PRECAUTIONS AND ADVERSE REACTIONS

The intake of plant parts leads to severe mucous membrane irritations (swelling of the tongue, bloody vomiting, bloody diarrhea), presumably due to lesions of the membrane from the very sharp-edged oxalate glands and the introduction of impurities into the wounds. Decoctions of the roots can be taken without risk in therapeutic dosages. The level of cyanogenic glycosides is too low to be able to bring about signs of poisoning; other soluble poisonous substances have not been shown to be present. Caution is nevertheless advised.

DOSAGE

No dosage information is available.

LITERATURE

Akhtardziev K et al., (1984) Farmatsiya 34(3):1.

Koch H, Steinegger E, Components of Arum maculatum L. (woven arrowroot). In: Pharm Acta Helv 54(2):33-36. 1979.

Mladenov IV, (1982) C R Acad Bulg Sci 35(8):116.

Moore THS, Vet Rec 89:569. 1971.

Nahrstedt A, Triglochinin in Arum maculatum. In: PH 14(12):1870-1871. 1975.

Poisonous Plants in Britain and their effects on Animals and Man, Ministry of Agriculture Fisheries and Food, Pub; HMSO (1984) UK.

Proliac A, Chaboud A, Raynaud J, Isolement et identification de trois C- glycosylflavonews dans les tiges feuilleés d'Arum dracunculus. In: PA:47:646-647. 1992.

Further information in:

Frohne D, Pfänder HJ, Giftpflanzen - Ein Handbuch für Apotheker, Toxikologen und Biologen, 4. Aufl., Wiss. Verlags-Ges Stuttgart 1997.

Lewin L, Gifte und Vergiftungen, 6. Aufl., Nachdruck, Haug Verlag, Heidelberg 1992.

Madaus G, Lehrbuch der Biologischen Arzneimittel, Bde. 1-3, Nachdruck, Georg Olms Verlag Hildesheim 1979.

Roth L, Daunderer M, Kormann K, Giftpflanzen, Pflanzengifte, 4. Aufl., Ecomed Fachverlag Landsberg Lech 1993.

Teuscher E, Lindequist U, Biogene Gifte - Biologie, Chemie, Pharmakologie, 2. Aufl., Fischer Verlag Stuttgart 1994.

Arundinaria Japonica

Bamboo

DESCRIPTION

Medicinal Parts: The medicinal parts are the young shoots of the plant.

Flower and Fruit: Greenish-yellow, round culms exceeding 3 m in height are surrounded at the culm nodes by dry leaf sheaths, which do not fall off. The upper surface of the leaves are shiny and dark green; the underside is matte and gray-green. The leaf margins are sharply serrated.

Habitat: The plant is indigenous to tropics, southern subtropics and Asia.

Production: Bamboo sprouts are the young shoots of Arundinaria japonica.

ACTIONS AND PHARMACOLOGY

COMPOUNDS

Soluble mono, oligo- and polysaccharides

Silicic acid: to some extent water-soluble

EFFECTS

No information is available.

INDICATIONS AND USAGE

In oriental medicine, the drug is used for asthma, coughs, and disorders of the gallbladder.

PRECAUTIONS AND ADVERSE REACTIONS

No health hazards or side effects are known in conjunction with the proper administration of designated therapeutic dosages.

DOSAGE

Preparation: The juice from the young shoots is hardened as bamboo sugar.

LITERATURE

No literature is available.

Asa Foetida

See Ferula Foetida

Asarum

See Asarum Europaeum

Asarum Europaeum

Asarum

DESCRIPTION

Medicinal Parts: The medicinal part is the root of the plant.

Flower and Fruit: The end of the stem forms a short-pedicled, slightly hanging flower. The perigone forms a campanulate tube with a 3 to 4 lobed margin. It is brownish on the outside, dark and purple on the inside. There are 2 x 6 stamens on the ovaries which are fused with the tube and are flattened above. The style is thick, short and not hollow, the stigma is 6-rayed. The fruit is a many-seeded, indehiscent capsule, and divided into many chambers by false membranes. In each capsule there are numerous, boat-shaped seeds with a spongy appendage.

Leaves, Stem and Root: Asarum europaeum is a perennial, 4 to 10 cm high, shaggy-haired plant. It has a thin, creeping rhizome which is branched, nodded and usually has 3 to 4 scale-like, brownish green stipules. It has an ascending short-scaled stem, with the terminal flower at the tip. There are 2 to 4 long-petioled, almost opposite, broad, reniform leaves, which are entire-margined, coriaceous, dark-green glossy above, pale and matte beneath, deeply reticulate, and evergreen.

Characteristics: The rhizome has a pepper-like smell, the leaves and flowers have an unpleasant camphor smell. Asarum europaeum is a protected species.

Habitat: The plant is indigenous to the northern parts of southern Europe, central and east-central Europe as far as the Crimea and eastwards into western Siberia as well as an enclave in the Atai; cultivated in the U.S.

Production: The root is gathered in August and air-dried in the shade.

Not To Be Confused With: Can be confused with other valerian types and with Arnica montana, Genum urbanum, Valeriana officinalis, and Viola ordorata. The mistaken powder can be identified by the presence of fibers, stone cells, oxalate filament agglomerations, and the absence of starch.

Other Names: Asarabacca, Hazelwort, Wild Nard, Snake-root, Public House Plant, Wild Ginger, Coltsfoot, False Coltsfoot

ACTIONS AND PHARMACOLOGY

COMPOUNDS

Volatile oil: composition depending very much upon breed, chief constituents asarone trans-isoasarone, trans-isoeugenol methyl ether, trans-isoelemicin or eudesmol, further sesquiterpene hydrocarbons, -alkohols, -furans,- carbonyl compounds

Caffeic acid derivatives: including chlorogenic acid, isochlorogenic acid

Flavonoids

EFFECTS

Asarum is an expectorant, bronchial spasmolytic, superficial relaxant, and local anesthetic. It has the following effects:

Emetic action: Useful studies of the nauseous effect only exist for Asari rhizoma cum herba in terms of the whole plant. However, self-experiment with 100 gm trans-isoasaron taken orally caused severe vomiting.

Reduction of surface tension: The surface-tension-reducing effect of trans-isoasaron and trans-isomethyleugenol were studied in vitro, using stalagmometry. Both substances showed a concentration-dependent surface activity, which surpassed the effect of the control substance tyloxapol in a normal treatment concentration.

Spasmolytic effect: The bronchial spasms, which are induced in a guinea pig by histamine, are inhibited in vivo, depending on the dose, by trans-isoasaron. The survival rate is determined subsequent to the addition of a histamine-containing aerosol 30 minutes after trans-isoasarin has been administered. The control substance here is clemizole hydrochloride, which has a similarly inhibiting effect.

Local anesthetic effect: The action of trans-isoasaron and of isomethyleugenol was tested on 10 volunteer subjects, in order to compare it with benzocaine (anesthetic index AI = 1). The results showed a dose-related action for both drugs, with the following anesthetic indexes of A=0.72 for trans-isoasarin and A=0.47 for trans-isomethyleugenol.

Antibacterial effect: The only studies available are those carried out on Asari rhizoma cum herba.

A double-blind clinical trial with a placebo as alternative was carried out on 30 patients with acute bronchitis; a further 30 with chronic bronchitis and an additional 30 with bronchial asthma. Eighty percent of the patients with acute bronchitis, 58% of the patients with chronic bronchitis, and 68% of the patients with bronchial asthma were cured or showed improvement in both their subjective and objective states.

The contrast with the placebo groups was significant. The treatment consisted of a daily dose of 3 x 2 tablets, purified dry (GB) or powdered (US) extract (30 mg phenylpropanol derivatives) taken over an average of 7 days. However, to obtain conclusive results, further trials are needed over a longer period and with more patients. The drug's efficacy was also tested in a multicentric field trial, a clinically controlled study, and an open bicentric study.

However, the results are only useful to a small extent, as there is an absence of details about placebo groups, trial parameters, and statistical analysis.

INDICATIONS AND USAGE

The purified dry extract of Asarum europaeum rootstock is used for inflammatory conditions of the lower respiratory system (acute and chronic bronchitis), for various causes of bronchial spasms and for bronchial asthma.

Asari rhizoma and Asari rhizoma cum herba are used for similar indications in folk medicine. In the past, the drugs were used as emetics. Some other uses are as antitussives (cough remedies), sneezing-powder for chronic rhinitis, for inflammation of the eye, for pneumonia, angina pectoris, migraines, liver disease and jaundice, for dehydration, as an emmenagogue (menstrual stimulant) and for artificial abortion.

Efficacy of the listed indications has not been adequately proven.

PRECAUTIONS AND ADVERSE REACTIONS

Older scientific literature contains reports of signs of poisoning (burning of the tongue, gastroenteritis, diarrhea, erysipeloid skin rashes, hemiparesis). An extremely susceptible mouse strain developed hepatoma after exposure to asarone. Administration of the drug is not advised.

DOSAGE

Mode of Administration: To be taken as a sneezing-powder, or orally as a purified dry extract in the form of coated tablets and pills. It is obsolete as a drug.

Preparation: The air-dried root-stock is extracted with an organic solvent, which can be mixed with water. The liquid extract is separated from the solvent by means of vacuum distillation. The watery remaining portion is diluted with an equal amount of distilled water, and further extraction takes place. The organic liquid extract is mixed with a suitable excipient according to the desired percentage of trans-isoasaron.

Trans-isoasaron can also be produced from asarylaldehyde by means of Perkin's cinnamic synthesis.

Daily Dosage: The average daily oral dose of the dry extract for adults and children aged 13 and over is 30 mg.

Phenylpropane derivatives (daily administration) should be spread over 2 to 3 doses per day. Children aged 2 and over can take an extract corresponding to 5 mg phenylpropanol derivatives 3 times daily. The average single dose of the drug is 0.1 gm.

As sneezing-powder, the average content of the drug is 20%.

Storage: Coated tablets and pills that contain the purified dry extract or the tincture from the rhizome, can be stored for a period of 28 days in conditions of high temperature, humidity, and light. Under normal conditions (i.e. brown glass, away from light), they can be stored for up to 2 years, after which period, stability should be checked.

LITERATURE

Doskotch RW, Vanevenhoven PW (1967) Lloydia 30:141.

Gracza L, (1987) Pharmazie 42 (2):141.

Gracza L, In vitro studies on the expectorant effect of the phenylpropane derivatives from hazlewort. 12. The active agents in Asarum europaeum. In: PM 42(2):155. 1981.

Gracza L, Phytobiological (phytophamacological) studies on phenylpropane derivatives from Asarum europaeum L. 10. Actice principles of Asarum europaeum L. In: Arzneim Forsch 30(5):767-771. 1980.

Gracza L, Über die Wirkstoffe von Asarum europaeum. 16. Mitt., Die lokalanästhetische Wirkung der Phenylprpanderivate. In: PM 48(3):153-157. 1983.

Mose JR, Lukas G, (1961) Arzneim Forsch 11:33.

Rosch A, (1984) Z Phytother 5(6):964.

Trennheuser L, Dissertation Saarbrücken. 1961.

Further information in:

Frohne D, Pfänder HJ, Giftpflanzen - Ein Handbuch für Apotheker, Toxikologen und Biologen, 4. Aufl., Wiss. Verlags-Ges Stuttgart 1997.

Hänsel R, Keller K, Rimpler H, Schneider G (Hrsg.), Hagers Handbuch der Pharmazeutischen Praxis, 5. Aufl., Bde. 4-6 (Drogen), Springer Verlag Berlin, Heidelberg, New York, 1992-1994.

Lewin L, Gifte und Vergiftungen, 6. Aufl., Nachdruck, Haug Verlag, Heidelberg 1992.

Madaus G, Lehrbuch der Biologischen Arzneimittel, Bde. 1-3, Nachdruck, Georg Olms Verlag Hildesheim 1979.

Roth L, Daunderer M, Kormann K, Giftpflanzen, Pflanzengifte, 4. Aufl., Ecomed Fachverlag Landsberg Lech 1993.

Teuscher E, Lindequist U, Biogene Gifte - Biologie, Chemie, Pharmakologie, 2. Aufl., Fischer Verlag Stuttgart 1994.

Asclepias Incarnata

Swamp Milkweed

DESCRIPTION

Medicinal Parts: The medicinal parts are the rhizome with roots.

Flower and Fruit: The flowers are reddish purple. They are located on terminal umbels in clusters of 2 to 6 on a 5 cm long peduncle. The umbels consist of 10 to 20 small florets. The fruit is a long pod.

Leaves, Stem and Root: The herbaceous plant is up to 80 cm high. The stem is erect and smooth. The upper part is branched and very leafy. The leaves are opposite, petiolate, oblong, lanceolate, hairy, acute, and cordate at the base. They are 10 to 18 cm long, 2.5 to 5 cm long, and sharp-edged. The rhizome is about 2 to 3 cm in diameter, yellowish-brown, irregularly globular or oblong, hard and knotty. The rhizome is covered with a thin, tough bark and is surrounded by light brown rootlets that are about 10 cm long.

Characteristics: The taste is sweetish, acrid and bitter. There is no odor.

Habitat: The plant is indigenous to America, Canada, and Asia.

Other Names: Swamp Silkweed, Rose-colored Silkweed

ACTIONS AND PHARMACOLOGY

COMPOUNDS

Cardioactive steroids (cardenolids)

EFFECTS

The cardiac glycosides are without therapeutic significance. The drug has an emetic effect.

INDICATIONS AND USAGE

Similar to other Asclepiadaceae, Swamp Milkweed is mainly used for digestive disorders.

PRECAUTIONS AND ADVERSE REACTIONS

No health hazards or side effects are known in conjunction with the proper administration of designated therapeutic dosages. The drug has an emetic effect in higher dosages, and digitalis-like poisonings are possible due to the cardioactive steroid content. For possible symptoms and treatments for poisonings see *Digitalis folium.*

LITERATURE

Kern W, List PH, Hörhammer L (Hrsg.), Hagers Handbuch der Pharmazeutischen Praxis, 4. Aufl., Bde. 1-8, Springer Verlag Berlin, Heidelberg, New York, 1969.

Asclepias Tuberosa

Pleurisy Root

DESCRIPTION

Medicinal Parts: The medicinal part is the pulverized root.

Flower and Fruit: The plant bears panicles of deep yellow and orange petalous flowers.

Leaves, Stem and Root: The plant is perennial, erect, 50 to 100 cm high with a fleshy root-stock bearing a few stout hairy stems. The leaves are alternate, oblong, glabrous, narrowly lanceolate, and dark green. The under surface is somewhat lighter. The root stock is mildly ring-shaped with a branched crown. The roots are grooved lengthwise, grayish brown on the outside and whitish on the inside. The tissue is made up of concentric rings, which divide easily. The root is tough, short and starchy. A. tuberosa is devoid of the latex typical of the genus (see A.incarnata).

Characteristics: The taste is nutty, bitter, with faint odor.

Habitat: Indigenous to America and Canada.

Production: Pleurisy root is the root of Asclepias tuberosa.

Other Names: Butterfly Weed, Canada Root, Flux Root, Orange Swallow-wort, Tuber Root, White Root, Wind Root, Swallow-wort, Orange Milkweed

ACTIONS AND PHARMACOLOGY

COMPOUNDS

Cardioactive steroids (cardenolids)

EFFECTS

Expectorant, tonic, diaphoretic, antispasmodic.

INDICATIONS AND USAGE

Pleurisy Root is used for coughs, pleurisy, disorders of the uterus, as an analgesic and to ease breathing.

PRECAUTIONS AND ADVERSE REACTIONS

No health hazards or side effects are known in conjunction with the proper administration of designated therapeutic dosages.

OVERDOSAGE

The drug has an emetic effect in higher dosages, and digitalis-like poisonings are possible due to the cardioactive steroid content. For possible symptoms and treatments for poisonings, see *Digitalis folium.*

DOSAGE

Mode of Administration: The drug is used internally as a liquid extract and is also available in combination preparations.

LITERATURE

Costello CH, Butler CL, (1950) J Am Pharm Ass Sci Ed 39:233.

Pagani F, (1975) Boll Chim Farm 114(8):450.

Petricic J, (1966) Arch Pharm Ber Dtsch. Pharm Ges 299(12):1007.

Further information in:

Kern W, List PH, Hörhammer L (Hrsg.), Hagers Handbuch der Pharmazeutischen Praxis, 4. Aufl., Bde. 1-8, Springer Verlag Berlin, Heidelberg, New York, 1969.

Madaus G, Lehrbuch der Biologischen Arzneimittel, Bde. 1-3, Nachdruck, Georg Olms Verlag Hildesheim 1979.

Roth L, Daunderer M, Kormann K, Giftpflanzen, Pflanzengifte, 4. Aufl., Ecomed Fachverlag Landsberg Lech 1993.

Ash

See Fraxinus Excelsior; Sorbus Torminalis

Asimina Triloba

American Pawpaw

DESCRIPTION

Medicinal Parts: The medicinal parts are the seeds, bark and leaves.

Flower and Fruit: The axillary flowers are dull purple and solitary. They are 3.5 cm wide. The petals are round, ovate, and marbled. The outer ones are almost circular and 3 to 4 times as long as the sepals. The fruit is yellowish, oblong-ovoid. The fleshy pods contain 3 flat, brown seeds. These are slightly polished with darker brown lines on the surface. They are oblong-oval, with a grayish hilum at one end. They taste and smell resinous.

Leaves, Stem and Root: Tree is up to 6 m in height. The young shoots and leaves are covered in rust-colored down and later become glabrous. The leaves are thin, smooth, entire, ovate, acuminate, 20-25 cm long and 7 cm wide. The leaves and flowers appear simultaneously.

Characteristics: The fruit has an unpleasant smell when unripe, but when ripe after frost, smell deliciously if faintly of custard, a characteristic which gives rise to one of its common names - Custard Apple.

Habitat: The plant is found in the west, south and central U.S., also India and parts of Asia and Africa.

Production: American Pawpaw seeds are the seeds of Asimina triloba.

Other Names: Custard Apple

ACTIONS AND PHARMACOLOGY

COMPOUNDS

Benzyl isoquinoline alkaloids

Polyketides

Fatty oil

EFFECTS

No information is available.

INDICATIONS AND USAGE

In homeopathy, American Pawpaw is used in the treatment of scarlet fever, fevers, vomiting, as well as mouth and throat inflammation.

PRECAUTIONS AND ADVERSE REACTIONS

The drug has a nauseant effect. Susceptible individuals may be susceptible to severe urticaria.

DOSAGE

Mode of Administration: The mother tincture is used in homeopathic dilutions.

LITERATURE

Kern W, List PH, Hörhammer L (Hrsg.), Hagers Handbuch der Pharmazeutischen Praxis, 4. Aufl., Bde. 1-8, Springer Verlag Berlin, Heidelberg, New York, 1969.

Lewin L, Gifte und Vergiftungen, 6. Aufl., Nachdruck, Haug Verlag, Heidelberg 1992.

Oliver-Bever B (Ed.) Medicinal Plants of Tropical West Africa, Cambridge University Press Cambridge, London 1986.

Asparagus Officinalis

Asparagus

DESCRIPTION

Medicinal Parts: The medicinal parts are the herb and the rhizome with roots.

Flower and Fruit: Thin pedicles measuring from 2 to 20 mm long grow 1 to 3 flowers from the nodes. The plants are usually dioecious. The perigone of the male flowers is about 5 mm long, funnel-shaped and whitish to green-yellowish. The perigone is longer than the cauline leaves and have oblanceolate sections which are twice as long as the perigone tube. The stamens are oblong and almost as long the filaments. The perigone of the female flowers is much smaller. The fruit is a pea-sized, brick-red, up to 8 mm thick, round berry. The seeds are black with wrinkly stripes and are 3 to 4 mm wide.

Leaves, Stem and Root: Asparagus officinalis is a perennial, 30 to 100 cm high plant (in cultivation up to 150 cm), with a short, woody root stock. The stem is erect, glabrous and smooth, later inclined with numerous erect to leaning branches. The scale sections at the base have short spurs. The phylloclades in clusters of 4 to 15 are round, needle-like, 5 to 25 cm long and about 0.5 cm thick. The root-stock is short and thick. It produces a few ascending shoots which are as thick as a finger, fleshy, white, and red or blue-reddish tinged. The female plants are often slimmer than the male, which are shorter and stockier.

Habitat: The plant grows in central and southern Europe, the Near East, western Siberia and northern Africa. It is cultivated in many places.

Production: Asparagus herb consists of the above-ground parts of Asparagus officinalis. Asparagus root consists of the rhizome with roots of Asparagus officinalis.

Other Names: Sparrow Grass

ACTIONS AND PHARMACOLOGY

COMPOUNDS: ASPARAGI HERBA

Flavonoids: including rutin, hyperoside, isoquercitrin

Steroid saponins

EFFECTS: ASPARAGI HERBA

Animal experiments indicate the herb has a mild diuretic action.

COMPOUNDS: ASPARAGI RHIZOMA CUM RADIX

Steroid saponins: including asparagosides A, B, D, F, G, H, I, the bitter steroid saponins, aspartic saponin I

Amino acids: among them, sulphur-containing aspartic acid, the esters 3-mercapto- butyric acid, 3-methylthio-isobutyric acid, diisobutyric acid disulphide

EFFECTS: ASPARAGI RHIZOMA CUM RADIX

Animal tests indicate a diuretic effect.

INDICATIONS AND USAGE

ASPARAGI HERBA

Preparations of Asparagus herb are used as a diuretic, although the effectiveness for the claimed application has not been sufficiently documented.

ASPARAGI RHIZOMA CUM RADIX

- Infections of the urinary tract
- Kidney and bladder stones

The root is used as a flushing-out therapy for inflammatory diseases of the urinary tract and for prevention of renal gravel.

CONTRAINDICATIONS

ASPARAGI RHIZOMA CUM RADIX

Because of the irritating effect of saponin, the drug should not be administered in the presence of kidney diseases. In the case of reduced cardiac and/or kidney function, irrigation therapy should not be attempted.

PRECAUTIONS AND ADVERSE REACTIONS

ASPARAGI HERBA

No health hazards or side effects are known in conjunction with the proper administration of designated therapeutic dosages. The plant has a low sensitization potential through skin contact. The berries are considered poisonous, although there is no proof of this.

ASPARAGI RHIZOMA CUM RADIX

No health hazards or side effects are known in conjunction with the proper administration of designated therapeutic dosages. There is a low sensitization potential, particularly among workers in canning factories who are prone to asparagus scabies.

DOSAGE

ASPARAGI RHIZOMA CUM RADIX

Mode of Administration: The cut rhizome is used for teas, as well as other galenic preparations for internal use. When used in flushing-out therapy, ensure ample fluid intake.

Daily Dosage: The daily dosage is 45 to 80 gm.

LITERATURE

ASPARAGI HERBA

Goryanu GM et al., (1976) Khim Prir Soed 3: 400 et 6: 762.

Kawano K et al., (1975) Agric Biol Chem 39: 1999.

Shiomi N et al., (1976) Agric Biol Chem 40: 567.

Tagasuki M et al., (1975) Chem Letters 1: 43.

Woeldecke M, Hermann K, (1974) Z Lebensm Forsch Unters 25: 459.

Further information in:

Frohne D, Pfänder HJ, Giftpflanzen - Ein Handbuch für Apotheker, Toxikologen und Biologen, 4. Aufl., Wiss. Verlags-Ges Stuttgart 1997.

Hänsel R, Keller K, Rimpler H, Schneider G (Hrsg.), Hagers Handbuch der Pharmazeutischen Praxis, 5. Aufl., Bde 4-6 (Drogen), Springer Verlag Berlin, Heidelberg, New York, 1992-1994.

Hausen B, Allergiepflanzen, Pflanzenallergene, ecomed Verlagsgesellsch. mbH, Landsberg 1988.

Lewin L, Gifte und Vergiftungen, 6. Aufl., Nachdruck, Haug Verlag, Heidelberg 1992.

Madaus G, Lehrbuch der Biologischen Arzneimittel, Bde 1-3, Nachdruck, Georg Olms Verlag Hildesheim 1979.

Roth L, Daunderer M, Kormann K, Giftpflanzen, Pflanzengifte, 4. Aufl., Ecomed Fachverlag Landsberg Lech 1993.

Teuscher E, Lindequist U, Biogene Gifte - Biologie, Chemie, Pharmakologie, 2. Aufl., Fischer Verlag Stuttgart 1994.

ASPARAGI RHIZOMA CUM RADIX

Goryanu GM et al., (1976) Khim Prir Soed 3: 400 et 6: 762.

Kawano K et al., Agric Biol Chem (Tokyo) 41:1. 1977.

Lazurevskii GV et al., Doklady Akademii Nauk SSSR 231:1479. 1976.

Pant G et al., PH 27:3324. 1988.

Shao Y et al., Steroidal saponins from Asparagus officinalis and their cytotoxic activity. In: PM 63(3):258-262. 1997.

Shiomi N et al., (1976) Agric Biol Chem 40: 567.

Tagasuki M et al., (1975) Chem Letters 1: 43.

Woeldecke M, Hermann K (1974) Z Lebensm Untersuch Forsch 25: 459

Further information in:

Frohne D, Pfänder HJ, Giftpflanzen - Ein Handbuch für Apotheker, Toxikologen und Biologen, 4. Aufl., Wiss. Verlags-Ges Stuttgart 1997.

Hänsel R, Keller K, Rimpler H, Schneider G (Hrsg.), Hagers Handbuch der Pharmazeutischen Praxis, 5. Aufl., Bde 4-6 (Drogen), Springer Verlag Berlin, Heidelberg, New York, 1992-1994.

Hausen B, Allergiepflanzen, Pflanzenallergene, ecomed Verlagsgesellsch. mbH, Landsberg 1988.

Leung AY, Encyclopedia of Common Natural Ingredients Used in Food Drugs and Cosmetics, John Wiley & Sons Inc., New York 1980.

Lewin L, Gifte und Vergiftungen, 6. Aufl., Nachdruck, Haug Verlag, Heidelberg 1992.

Madaus G, Lehrbuch der Biologischen Arzneimittel, Bde 1-3, Nachdruck, Georg Olms Verlag Hildesheim 1979.

Roth L, Daunderer M, Kormann K, Giftpflanzen, Pflanzengifte, 4. Aufl., Ecomed Fachverlag Landsberg Lech 1993.

Teuscher E, Lindequist U, Biogene Gifte - Biologie, Chemie, Pharmakologie, 2. Aufl., Fischer Verlag Stuttgart 1994.

Aspidosperma Quebracho-Blanco

Quebracho

DESCRIPTION

Medicinal Parts: The medicinal part is the bark.

Flower and Fruit: The inflorescences, which grow from the upper leaf axils, are opposite or in threes. They are shaped like a thyrsus and are warty to almost glabrous with numerous flowers. The flowers are 1 to 3 cm long. The bracts, which fall off, are very small and have a 2 to 3 mm stem. The sepals are ovate, obtuse, 1 to 2 mm long and uneven. The corolla is white, yellow or yellowish-green, smooth or uneven on the outside. The tube is 3 to 5 mm long and has long, narrow, lanceolate petals. The stamens are in the middle of the corolla tube. The anthers are 1 mm long. The follicles are cylindrical to ovoid, 4 to 10 cm long and 1 to 7 cm wide. They are very woody, slightly warty, with or without a midrib, uneven and stemless.

Leaves, Stem and Root: The tree grows to a height of 20 m and has slim branches. The young branches are warty. The older branches are smooth with thin orange-brown bark. The leaves are opposite or trifoliate, oblong-elliptoid, ovate-lanceolate to lanceolate, acuminate and gradually narrow at the base. They are 3 to 5 cm long by 0.5 to 1.5 cm wide, coriaceous often yellow-green and smooth. The leaves have 20 to 30 pairs of steeply ascending secondary ribs, which are very close to each other and sunk into a thick mesophyll. The bark is grayish and deeply fissured externally. The inner surface is yellowish-brown, often with a reddish tint and is grooved. The transverse fracture shows a coarsely granular outer layer and a fibrous or splintery, darker inner layer.

Characteristics: The bark has a bitter taste and is odorless.

Habitat: The plant grows in Chile, Argentina, southeast Bolivia, and southeast Brazil.

Production: Quebracho bark is the bark of Aspidosperma quebracho-blanco.

ACTIONS AND PHARMACOLOGY

COMPOUNDS

Indole alkaloids (0.5-1.5%): chief alkaloids aspidospermine (30%), yohimbine (quebrachine, 10%), further including, among others, (-)-quebrachamine, akuammidine

Tannins

EFFECTS

Quebracho bark works as an expectorant and stimulates the respiratory center.

INDICATIONS AND USAGE

Quebracho is used for bronchial asthma and conditions of the lower respiratory tract.

PRECAUTIONS AND ADVERSE REACTIONS

No health hazards are known in conjunction with the proper administration of designated therapeutic dosages. Side effects can include, among others, salivation, headache, outbreaks of sweating, vertigo, stupor, and sleepiness.

OVERDOSAGE

Intakes of larger dosages lead to queasiness and vomiting.

DOSAGE

Mode of Administration: The drug is rarely used as a drug in asthma remedies. It is available in extract or powder form and is often used in combination bronchial preparations.

LITERATURE

Biemann K et al., J Am Chem Soc 85:631. 1963.

Lyon RL et al., (1973) J Pharm Sci 62: 218.

Markey S et al., Tetrahedron Lett 157. 1967.

Willaman JJ, Hui-Li L, (1970) Lloydia 33 (3A): 1.

Wilson E et al., Rev farm (Buenos Aires) 125:9 (via CA 100: 109175. 1983.

Further information in:

Hänsel R, Keller K, Rimpler H, Schneider G (Hrsg.), Hagers Handbuch der Pharmazeutischen Praxis, 5. Aufl., Bde 4-6 (Drogen): Springer Verlag Berlin, Heidelberg, New York, 1992-1994.

Leung AY, Encyclopedia of Common Natural Ingredients Used in Food Drugs, Cosmetics, John Wiley & Sons Inc., New York 1980.

Lewin L, Gifte und Vergiftungen, 6. Aufl., Nachdruck, Haug Verlag, Heidelberg 1992.

Madaus G, Lehrbuch der Biologischen Arzneimittel, Bde 1-3, Nachdruck, Georg Olms Verlag Hildesheim 1979.

Roth L, Daunderer M, Kormann K: Giftpflanzen, Pflanzengifte, 4. Aufl., Ecomed Fachverlag Landsberg Lech 1993.

Steinegger E, Hänsel R, Pharmakognosie, 5. Aufl., Springer Verlag Heidelberg 1992.

Teuscher E, Biogene Arzneimittel, 5. Aufl., Wiss. Verlagsges. Stuttgart 1997.

Wichtl M (Hrsg.), Teedrogen, 4. Aufl., Wiss. Verlagsges. Stuttgart 1997.

Astragalus Gummifer

Tragacanth

DESCRIPTION

Medicinal Parts: The gum-like exudation from the stem, when dried, forms flakes which swell in water, forming a gelatinous mass.

Flower and Fruit: The axillary flowers are solitary or in groups of 2 or 3 and are sessile. The calyx is 6 to 7 mm long and densely pubescent. The corolla is yellowish to white and sometimes has bluish or reddish veins. The standard, wings and carina are each 9 to 10 mm long. The fruit is ovoid, 4 mm long with dense, silky hairs. The seed is oval, smooth and about 3 mm long.

Leaves, Stem and Root: Astralagus gummifer is a low, up to 30 cm high shrub with gray branches which become glabrous. The older branches have scale-like remains of the stipules from the previous year, which disappear later and a 1 to 4 cm long perennial, thorny leaf column. The 8 to 14 leaflets are folded, oblong-ovate, 2.5 to 6 mm long and 0.7 to 2.5 mm wide, blue-gray and glabrous or sparsely pubescent beneath.

Habitat: The plant grows in Turkey, Syria, Lebanon, northwest Iraq and the border area between Iran and Iraq.

Production: Tragacanth is the latex, which exudes from the bark of Astralagus gummifer and other varieties.

Other Names: Gum Dragon

ACTIONS AND PHARMACOLOGY

COMPOUNDS

Polysaccharides (water-soluble): approximately 40% tragacanthine, divisible into tragacanthic acid (galacturonane with side chains consisting of D-xylose, L-fucose, D-galactose) and an arabino-galactane-protein complex

Polysaccharides (non-water soluble): approximately 60% bassorin, similar make-up as with tragacanthine

EFFECTS

Tragacanth stimulates stretching of the intestinal wall, which results in increased peristalis.

INDICATIONS AND USAGE

Tragacanth is used as a laxative.

PRECAUTIONS AND ADVERSE REACTIONS

No health hazards or side effects are known in conjunction with the proper administration of designated therapeutic dosages. Allergic reactions have been observed in rare cases. Insufficient fluid supply following intake of large quantities of tragacanth can lead to obstruction ileus, as well as to esophageal closure.

DOSAGE

Mode of Administration: Tragacanth is used in various combinations and preparations.

LITERATURE

Anderson DMW, Bridgeman MME, PH 24:2301-2304. 1985.

Aspinall GO, Baillie J, J Chem Soc: 1702-1714. 1963.

Fang S et al., (1982): You Ji Hua Xue 2: 26.

Gralen N, Kärrholm M, J Colloid Sci 5:21-36. 1950.

Osswald H, (1968) Arzneim Forsch 18: 1495.

Srimal RC, Dhawan CN, (1973) J Pharm Pharmacol 25: 447.

Whistler RL et al., (1976) Adv Carbohydr Chem Biochem 32: 235.

Further information in:

Hänsel R, Keller K, Rimpler H, Schneider G (Hrsg.), Hagers Handbuch der Pharmazeutischen Praxis, 5. Aufl., Bde 4-6 (Drogen): Springer Verlag Berlin, Heidelberg, New York, 1992-1994.

Leung AY, Encyclopedia of Common Natural Ingredients Used in Food Drugs, Cosmetics, John Wiley & Sons Inc., New York 1980.

Steinegger E, Hänsel R, Pharmakognosie, 5. Aufl., Springer Verlag Heidelberg 1992.

Teuscher E, Biogene Arzneimittel, 5. Aufl., Wiss. Verlagsges. Stuttgart 1997.

Athyrium Filix-Femina

Lady Fern

DESCRIPTION

Medicinal Parts: The medicinal part is the rhizome with the roots.

Leaves, Stem and Root: Athyrium filix-femina or polypodium vulgare is a 10 to 40 cm high fern. The pencil-thick, creeping rhizome is densely covered with dark-brown hairs. Numerous tomentose, long, branched, dark-brown root fibbers sprout from the rhizome. The not-so-numerous leaves are in rigid, upright, double rows. They are coriaceous, glabrous, oblong-lanceolate or oblong, deeply pinnatifid and winter-green. The petioles are semi-round, smooth and whitish. On the underside of the leaf tips there are 2 parallel rows of large groups of filmless sporangia, which are initially yellowish and later turn dark brown.

Habitat: Lady fern is indigenous to Britain, parts of Europe, and the U.S.

Other Names: Common Polypody, Brake Root, Rock Brake, Rock of Polypody, Oak Fern

ACTIONS AND PHARMACOLOGY

COMPOUNDS

Steroid saponins: polypodosaponin I and II

Caffeic acid derivatives: including, among others, oslandin (glucocaffeic acid, sweet-tasting)

Free fatty acids

Methyl salicylate

Triterpenes

Ecdysterone: polypodine A (ecdysterone) and B (5-beta-hydroxyecdysterone)

Tannins and precursors: including, among others, catechin - 7-L-arabinofuranoside, catechin tannins

EFFECTS

The active agents are bitter substances, saponin and small amounts of essential oil. The drug is a mild expectorant; a choleric type effect is questionable.

INDICATIONS AND USAGE

The drug is used for respiratory and gastrointestinal tract illnesses.

PRECAUTIONS AND ADVERSE REACTIONS

No health hazards or side effects are known in conjunction with the proper administration of designated therapeutic dosages.

DOSAGE

Daily Dosage: As a digestive, in the treatment of functional gastrointestinal illnesses, 1 to 2 tablets or 10 to 20 drops to be taken 3 times daily.

LITERATURE

Abraham H, Zucker und Süβstoff. In: PTA 7(10):744. 1993.

Anonym, Niedere Pflanzen ganz groβ - 39. Jahrestagung der Gesellschaft für Arzneipflanzenforschung in Saarbrücken. In: DAZ 131(37):1899.

Constantinescu E et al., (1966) Pharmazie 21:121.

Jizba J et al., (1971) Tetrahedron Lett 18:1329.

Further information in

Hegnauer R, Chemotaxonomie der Pflanzen, Bde 1-11, Birkhäuser Verlag Basel, Boston, Berlin 1962-1997.

Kern W, List PH, Hörhammer L (Hrsg.), Hagers Handbuch der Pharmazeutischen Praxis, 4. Aufl., Bde 1-8, Springer Verlag Berlin, Heidelberg, New York, 1969.

Madaus G, Lehrbuch der Biologischen Arzneimittel, Bde 1-3, Nachdruck, Georg Olms Verlag Hildesheim 1979.

Atropa Belladonna

Belladonna

DESCRIPTION

Medicinal Parts: The medicinal parts are the leaves and roots.

Flower and Fruit: The flowers are solitary and hanging. The calyx is fused at the base, has 5 divisions and is spread like a star when the fruit ripens. The corolla is a campanulate tube, 2.5 to 3.5 cm long, violet, dirty yellow on the inside and has crimson veins. There are 5 stamens and 1 style with a 2-lobed stigma. The ovary is superior. The fruit is a cherry-sized globose berry. The fruit is initially green then black and glossy with numerous black, ovoid seeds.

Leaves, Stem and Root: Atropa belladonna is a perennial, herbacious plant 1 m to 2 m high with a many-headed cylindrical rhizome. The woody stem is erect, branched, bluntly angular and hairy. The leaves are ovately pointed, entire-margined, downy and up to 15 cm long. The lower ones are alternate. Near the inflorescence they are in pairs of 1 large and 1 small.

Characteristics: Belladonna has a strong narcotic smell, a sharp and bitter taste, and is poisonous.

Habitat: The plant is distributed throughout western, central and southern Europe, in the Balkans, southeast Asia, Iran, northern Africa, Denmark, Sweden and Ireland and is cultivated in other countries.

Production: Belladonna leaf consists of the dried leaves, or the dried leaves together with the flowering branch tips of Atropa belladonna. The leaves are collected in the wild from May to July. They are dried at maximum 60°C. Belladonna root consists of the dried roots and rhizomes of Atropa belladonna. The root of 2 to 4 year-old plants is dug up in mid-October to mid-November or shortly before the start of the flowering season. It is cleaned and dried at a maximum temperature of 50°C.

Not To Be Confused With: Belladonna leaf should not be confused with Ailanthus altissimus, Phytolacca americana or Scopolia carniolica. Belladonna root should not be confused with Atropa acuminata. It is sometimes adulterated with Phytolacca americana and Scopolia cariolica.

Other Names: Deadly Nightshade, Devil's Cherries, Devil's Herb, Divale, Dwale, Dwayberry, Great Morel, Naughty Man's Cherries, Poison Black Cherry

ACTIONS AND PHARMACOLOGY

COMPOUNDS: BELLADONNAE FOLIUM

Tropan alkaloids: chief alkaloid (-)-hyoscyamine, in drying transformed to some extent into atropine, furthermore apoatropine, scopolamine, tropine

Flavonoids

Hydroxycoumarins: including scopoline, scopoletine

Tannins

COMPOUNDS: BELLADONNAE RADIX

Tropan alkaloids: chief alkaloid (-)-hyoscyamine, in drying transformed to some extent into atropine, furthermore apoatropine, 3alpha-phenylacetoxytropane, tropine, cuskhygrine, scopolamine, pseudotropine

EFFECTS: BELLADONNAE FOLIUM AND RADIX

Atropa belladonna preparations act as a parasympatholytic or anticholinergic via a competitive antagonism of the neuromuscular transmitter acetylcholine. This antagonism concerns mainly the muscarine-like effect of acetylcholine and less the nicotine-like effects on the ganglions and the neuromuscular end plate. Atropa belladonna preparations release peripheral effects targeted on the vegetative nervous system and the smooth muscle system, as well as the central nervous system.

Because of the parasympatholytic properties, the drug can cause relaxation of organs with smooth muscles and relieve spastic conditions, especially in the gastrointestinal tract and bile ducts. Additionally, Belladonna use may result in muscular tremor or rigidity due to effects on the central nervous system. Atropa belladonna preparations have a positive dromotropic as well as a positive chronotropic effect on the heart.

INDICATIONS AND USAGE

BELLADONNAE FOLIUM

- Arrhythmia
- Cardiac insufficiency NYHA I and II
- Liver and gallbladder complaints
- Nervous heart complaints

Belladonna leaf is used for spasms and colic-like pain in the gastrointestinal tract and bile ducts. In folk medicine, the drug is contained in medicinal plasters and is applied for neuro-vegetative disorders, hyperkinesis, hyperhidrosis, and bronchial asthma.

BELLADONNAE RADIX

- Arrhythmia
- Cardiac insufficiency NYHA I and II
- Nervous heart complaints

The drug is used for colic-like pains in the gastrointestinal tract and bile ducts. In folk medicine, a drug from the leaves is preferred for pain in the gastrointestinal area, for asthma, bronchitis and muscular pain. (Also see Belladonnae folium.)

PRECAUTIONS AND ADVERSE REACTIONS

BELLADONNAE FOLIUM AND RADIX

No health hazards are known in conjunction with the proper administration of designated therapeutic dosages. The 4 early signs of poisoning include dryness of the mouth, mydriasis, and tachycardiac arrhythmias. The following symptoms could also occur as side effects, in particular with overdoses: hypocycloses, heat accumulation through reduction of perspiration, micturation difficulties, and obstipation.

Pediatric Use: The fatal dose in children is considerably less than that of adults.

Drug Interactions: Tricyclic antidepressants, amantadine and quinidine will increase the anticholinergic effect.

OVERDOSAGE

BELLADONNAE FOLIUM AND RADIX

High dosages lead to central excitation (restlessness, compulsion to talk, hallucinations, delirium, manic attacks, followed by exhaustion and sleep). The fatal dose depends on the atropine content; asphyxiation can occur with 100 mg atropine, which corresponds to 5 to 50 gm of belladonna. Treatment of poisonings consists of gastric lavage, application of wet cloths to reduce body temperature (avoid antipyretics), oxygen respiration for breathing distress, intubation, parenteral physostigmine salts as an antidote, diazepam for spasm and chlorpromazine for serious excitation.

DOSAGE

BELLADONNAE FOLIUM

Mode of Administration: The comminuted drug is used for decoctions and dried extracts and the powdered drug is used internally for galenic preparations. Due to the toxicity, the drug must be handled with care.

Daily Dosage: When using Belladonna powder (belladonnae pulvis normatus-total alkaloid content 0.28% to 0.32% German pharmacopoeia 10), the average single dose is 0.05 to 0.10 gm. The maximum single dose is 0.20 gm, which is equivalent to 0.60 mg total alkaloids, calculated as hyoscyamine. The maximum daily dosage is 0.60 gm, which is equivalent to 1.8 mg total alkaloids, calculated as hyoscyamine.

For Belladonna extract, the average single dose is 0.01 gm. The maximum single dose is 0.05 gm, which is equivalent to 0.73 mg total alkaloids, calculated as hyoscyamine. The maximum daily dosage is 0.150 gm, which is equivalent to 2.2 mg total alkaloids, calculated as hyoscyamine.

Storage: Should be carefully stored away form light sources.

BELLADONNAE RADIX

Mode of Administration: As a comminuted drug for infusions and dried extracts and as a powdered drug for other galenic preparations for internal use.

Daily Dosage: The average daily dosage is 0.3 gm, which is equivalent to 1.5 mg total alkaloids, calculated as hyoscyamine. Single doses range from 0.05 gm to a maximum of 0.1 gm.

For Belladonna extract, the total alkaloids range from 1.3% to 1.45% (German pharmacopoeia 10). Single doses of the extract range from 0.01 gm to 0.05 gm. The maximum daily dosage is 0.15 gm, which is equivalent to 2.2 mg total alkaloids, calculated as hyoscyamine.

Storage: The drug should be stored for a maximum of 3 years in well-sealed containers protected from light and insects.

LITERATURE

BELLADONNAE FOLIUM

Fintelmann V, Phytopharmaka in der Gastroenterologie. In: ZPT 15(3):137. 1994.

Hartmann Th et al., Reinvestigation of the alkaloid composition of Atropa belladonna plants, roots cultures, and cell suspension. In: PM 53:390-395. 1986.

Phillipson JD et al., (1975) Phytochemistry 14: 999-1003.

Further information in:

Frohne D, Pfänder HJ, Giftpflanzen - Ein Handbuch für Apotheker, Toxikologen und Biologen, 4. Aufl., Wiss. Verlags-Ges Stuttgart 1997.

Hänsel R, Keller K, Rimpler H, Schneider G (Hrsg.), Hagers Handbuch der Pharmazeutischen Praxis, 5. Aufl., Bde 4-6 (Drogen), Springer Verlag Berlin, Heidelberg, New York, 1992-1994.

Leung AY, Encyclopedia of Common Natural Ingredients Used in Food Drugs and Cosmetics, John Wiley & Sons Inc., New York 1980.

Lewin L, Gifte und Vergiftungen, 6. Aufl., Nachdruck, Haug Verlag, Heidelberg 1992.

Madaus G, Lehrbuch der Biologischen Arzneimittel, Bde 1-3, Nachdruck, Georg Olms Verlag Hildesheim 1979.

Roth L, Daunderer M, Kormann K, Giftpflanzen, Pflanzengifte, 4. Aufl., Ecomed Fachverlag Landsberg Lech 1993.

Steinegger E, Hänsel R, Pharmakognosie, 5. Aufl., Springer Verlag Heidelberg 1992.

Teuscher E, Biogene Arzneimittel, 5. Aufl., Wiss. Verlagsges. Stuttgart 1997.

Teuscher E, Lindequist U, Biogene Gifte - Biologie, Chemie, Pharmakologie, 2. Aufl., Fischer Verlag Stuttgart 1994.

Wagner H, Wiesenauer M, Phytotherapie. Phytopharmaka und pflanzliche Homöopathika, Fischer-Verlag, Stuttgart, Jena, New York 1995.

BELLADONNAE RADIX

Fintelmann V, Phytopharmaka in der Gastroenterologie. In: ZPT 15(3):137. 1994.

Hartmann Th et al., Reinvestigation of the alkaloid composition of Atropa belladonna plants, roots cultures, and cell suspension. In: PM 53:390-395. 1986.

Phillipson JD et al., (1975) Phytochemistry 14: 999.

Further information in:

Frohne D, Pfänder HJ, Giftpflanzen - Ein Handbuch für Apotheker, Toxikologen und Biologen, 4. Aufl., Wiss. Verlags-Ges Stuttgart 1997.

Hänsel R, Keller K, Rimpler H, Schneider G (Hrsg.), Hagers Handbuch der Pharmazeutischen Praxis, 5. Aufl., Bde 4-6

(Drogen), Springer Verlag Berlin, Heidelberg, New York, 1992-1994.

Leung AY, Encyclopedia of Common Natural Ingredients Used in Food Drugs and Cosmetics, John Wiley & Sons Inc., New York 1980.

Lewin L, Gifte und Vergiftungen, 6. Aufl., Nachdruck, Haug Verlag, Heidelberg 1992.

Madaus G, Lehrbuch der Biologischen Arzneimittel, Bde 1-3, Nachdruck, Georg Olms Verlag Hildesheim 1979.

Roth L, Daunderer M, Kormann K, Giftpflanzen, Pflanzengifte, 4. Aufl., Ecomed Fachverlag Landsberg Lech 1993.

Steinegger E, Hänsel R, Pharmakognosie, 5. Aufl., Springer Verlag Heidelberg 1992.

Teuscher E, Lindequist U, Biogene Gifte - Biologie, Chemie, Pharmakologie, 2. Aufl., Fischer Verlag Stuttgart 1994.

Teuscher E, Biogene Arzneimittel, 5. Aufl., Wiss. Verlagsges. Stuttgart 1997.

Wagner H, Wiesenauer M, Phytotherapie. Phytopharmaka und pflanzliche Homöopathika, Fischer-Verlag, Stuttgart, Jena, New York 1995.

Avena Sativa

Oats

DESCRIPTION

Medicinal Parts: The medicinal parts are the fresh or dried above-ground parts, the ripe, dried fruits, and the dried, threshed leaf and stem.

Flower and Fruit: The green flower is a loose panicle hanging on all sides and is 15 to 20 cm long. The spikelet has 2 to 3 flowers. The outer glume has no awn, is 18 to 30 mm long and has 7 to 11 ribs. The top glumes have 2 divisions and a dentate tip and are 12 to 24 mm long. They have 7 ribs and can either be awned or unawned. The awn is 15 to 40 mm long, upright and rough. The double ribbed husks are 10 to 20 mm long and are thickly ciliate on the short ridge. The 3 stamens are 2.5 to 4 mm long. The ovary has a pinnatifid stigma. The fruit is 7 to 12 mm long, narrowly elliptoid and pubescent.

Leaves, Stem and Root: Oat is an annual, light green grass with a bushy root. The stalks are 60 to 100 cm high, smooth and glabrous. The linear-lanceolate tapering, flat leaves are in double rows and the leaf sheath is clasping. The ligula is short, ovate with triangular pointed teeth. The leaf blade is linear-lanceolate and is 45 cm long by 5 to 15 mm wide.

Habitat: Oats are cultivated worldwide.

Production: Wild oat herb consists of the fresh or dried above-ground parts of Avena sativa, harvested during flowering season. The herb is air-dried. Oats consist of the ripe, dried fruits of Avena sativa. Oat bran is taken from the outer layer of the de-furred fruit. To make rolled oats, the de-furred fruit is treated with steam, then crushed. Oat straw consists of the dried, threshed leaf and stem of Avena sativa.

Other Names: Grain, Groats, Oatmeal, Straw

ACTIONS AND PHARMACOLOGY

COMPOUNDS: AVENAE HERBA

Soluble oligo- and polysaccharides: including saccharose, kestose, neokestose, beta- glucans, galactoarabinoxylans

Silicic acid: to some extent water-soluble

Steroid saponins: avenacoside A and B

Unusual amino acids: avenic acid A and B

Flavonoids

EFFECTS: AVENAE HERBA

In a doubtful experimental investigation, the drug was said to lower the uric acid level and to display an antihepatoxin effect in animal experiments.

COMPOUNDS: AVENAE FRUCTUS

Starch

Soluble polysaccharides: in particular beta-glucans and arabinoxylans

Proteins: including gliadin, avenin, avenalin

Peptides

Steroid saponins: avenacoside A and B

Sterols: including beta-sitosterol

Fatty oil

Vitamins of the B-group

EFFECTS: AVENAE FRUCTUS

De-furred oats are, according to various studies, able to lower serum cholesterol and to hinder prostaglandin biosynthesis.

COMPOUNDS: AVENAE STRAMENTUM

Soluble oligo- and polysaccharides: including saccharose, kestose, neokestose, beta-glucans, galactoarabinoxylans

Silicic acid: to some extent water-soluble

Steroid saponins: avenacoside A and B (unusual amino acids, avenic acid A and B)

Flavonoids

EFFECTS: AVENAE STRAMENTUM

There is no information available concerning the efficacy of oat straw.

INDICATIONS AND USAGE

AVENAE HERBA

Wild oat herb preparations are used for acute and chronic anxiety, atonia of the bladder and connective tissue, connective tissue deficiencies, excitation, gout, kidney ailments in Kneipp therapy, neurasthenic and pseudoneurasthenic syndromes, old age symptoms, opium and tobacco withdrawal treatment, rheumatism, skin diseases, sleeplessness, stress, weakness of the bladder, and as a tonic and roborant. The efficacy for the claimed applications is not documented.

AVENAE FRUCTUS

Oat preparations are used for diseases and complaints of the gastrointestinal tract, gallbladder and kidneys, for cardiovascular disorders, constipation, diabetes, diarrhea, physical fatigue, rheumatism, and as a gruel for chest and throat complaints. The claimed efficacy has not been substantiated.

AVENAE STRAMENTUM

- Inflammation of the skin
- Warts

The drug is employed externally for inflamed and seborrheic skin disorders, especially those accompanied by itch. Oat straw is used for abdominal fatigue, bladder and rheumatic disorders, eye ailments, frostbite, gout, impetigo and metabolic diseases. It is used in foot baths for chronically cold or tired feet. It is also used as a tea for flu and coughs.

PRECAUTIONS AND ADVERSE REACTIONS

AVENAE HERBA, FRUCTUS AND STRAMENTUM

No health hazards or side effects are known in conjunction with the proper administration of designated therapeutic dosages.

DOSAGE

AVENAE HERBA

Mode of Administration: The herb is used in homeopathy, in combination therapy and as a tea for internal use.

Preparation: To make a tea, 3 gm drug is boiled in 250 ml water, which is strained after cooling.

Daily Dosage: The tea is taken repeatedly throughout the day and shortly before going to bed.

Storage: The herb should be protected from light and moisture.

AVENAE FRUCTUS

Mode of Administration: The fruit is used in homeopathy and in combination preparations.

AVENAE STRAMENTUM

Mode of Administration: As a comminuted herb for decoctions and other galenic preparations as bath additives.

Preparations: To make oat straw bath, 100 gm chopped drug is boiled with 3 liters water for 20 minutes and the decoction is added to the bath.

Daily Dosage: 100 gm of herb is used for one full bath.

LITERATURE

AVENAE HERBA

Anand CL, (1971) Nature 233: 496.

Connr J et al., (1975) J Pharm Pharmacol 27: 92.

Effertz B et al., (1979) Z Pflanzenphysiol 92: 319.

Gabrinowicz JW, (1974) Med J Aust Ii: 306.

Kim et al., (1978) Biochim Biophys Acta 537: 22.

Schneider E, Lösliche Silikate im grünen Hafer. In: ZPT 11(4):129. 1990.

Willuhn G, Pflanzliche Dermatika. Eine kritische Übersicht.. In: DAZ 132(37):1873. 1992.

Further information in:

Hänsel R, Keller K, Rimpler H, Schneider G (Hrsg.), Hagers Handbuch der Pharmazeutischen Praxis, 5. Aufl., Bde 4-6 (Drogen), Springer Verlag Berlin, Heidelberg, New York, 1992-1994.

Madaus G, Lehrbuch der Biologischen Arzneimittel, Bde 1-3, Nachdruck, Georg Olms Verlag Hildesheim 1979.

Teuscher E, Lindequist U, Biogene Gifte - Biologie, Chemie, Pharmakologie, 2. Aufl., Fischer Verlag Stuttgart 1994.

Wichtl M (Hrsg.), Teedrogen, 4. Aufl., Wiss. Verlagsges. Stuttgart 1997.

AVENAE FRUCTUS

Connr J et al., (1975) J Pharm Pharmacol 27: 92.

Effertz B et al., (1979) Z Pflanzenphysiol 92: 319Anand CL (1971) Nature 233: 496.

Gabrinowicz JW, (1974) Med J Aust Ii: 306.

Kim et al., (1978) Biochim Biophys Acta 537: 22.

Schneider E, Lösliche Silikate im grünen Hafer. In: ZPT 11(4):129. 1990.

Willuhn G, Pflanzliche Dermatika. Eine kritische Übersicht.. In: DAZ 132(37):1873. 1992.

Further information in:

Hänsel R, Keller K, Rimpler H, Schneider G (Hrsg.), Hagers Handbuch der Pharmazeutischen Praxis, 5. Aufl., Bde 4-6 (Drogen), Springer Verlag Berlin, Heidelberg, New York, 1992-1994.

Madaus G, Lehrbuch der Biologischen Arzneimittel, Bde 1-3, Nachdruck, Georg Olms Verlag Hildesheim 1979.

Wagner H, Wiesenauer M, Phytotherapie. Phytopharmaka und pflanzliche Homöopathika, Fischer-Verlag, Stuttgart, Jena, New York 1995.

AVENAE STRAMENTUM

Kim et al., (1978) Biochim Biophys Acta 537: 22.

Anand CL, (1971) Nature 233: 496.

Connr J et al., (1975) J Pharm Pharmacol 27: 92.

Effertz B et al., (1979) Z Pflanzenphysiol 92: 319.

Gabrinowicz JW, (1974) Med J Aust Ii: 306.

Jaspersen-Schib R, Ballaststoffe als Lipidsenker. In: DAZ 132(39):1991. 1992.

Schneider E, Lösliche Silikate im grünen Hafer. In: ZPT 11(4):129. 1990.

Willuhn G, Pflanzliche Dermatika. Eine kritische Übersicht.. In: DAZ 132(37):1873. 1992.

Further information in:

Hänsel R, Keller K, Rimpler H, Schneider G (Hrsg.), Hagers Handbuch der Pharmazeutischen Praxis, 5. Aufl., Bde 4-6 (Drogen), Springer Verlag Berlin, Heidelberg, New York, 1992-1994.

Madaus G, Lehrbuch der Biologischen Arzneimittel, Bde 1-3, Nachdruck, Georg Olms Verlag Hildesheim 1979.

Teuscher E, Lindequist U, Biogene Gifte - Biologie, Chemie, Pharmakologie, 2. Aufl., Fischer Verlag Stuttgart 1994.

Wichtl M (Hrsg.), Teedrogen, 4. Aufl., Wiss. Verlagsges. Stuttgart 1997.

Avocado

See Persea Americana

Azadirachta Indica

Azedarach

DESCRIPTION

Medicinal Parts: The medicinal parts are the bark, the leaves, the branches, the seeds and the latex.

Flower and Fruit: The plant has small white flowers.

Leaves, Stem and Root: Deciduous tree up to 16 m high with compound, alternate, oblong, ovate-lanceolate, and pointed leaves. The bark is grayish-brown, externally fissured, with a buff inner surface and fibrous fracture.

Characteristics: The taste is bitter and odorless.

Habitat: Indigenous to the woods of India and Sri Lanka. Found today in other tropical regions such as Indonesia, Australia and west Africa.

Production: Azedrach bark, leaves and seeds are the trunk and branch bark, leaves and seeds of Azadirachta indica or of the closely related variety (in the literature often given as a synonym) of Melia azedarach.

Other Names: Neem, Nim, Margosa, Indian Lilac, Bead Tree, Pride of China, Holy Tree, Persian Lilac

ACTIONS AND PHARMACOLOGY

COMPOUNDS

Triterpenes and tetranortriterpenes (limonoids and protolimonoids of the gedunin-group) in seed oil: for example nimbolin A and B, nimbin, gedunin

Tannin and volatile oil in the bark and the leaves

EFFECTS

A. indica is an anti-inflammatory and febrifuge. Melia azedarach is also an anthelmintic.

INDICATIONS AND USAGE

Azedarach is used in inflammatory and febrile diseases (including malaria although unconfirmed). Melia azedarach is also used for worm infestation.

PRECAUTIONS AND ADVERSE REACTIONS

No health hazards or side effects are known in conjunction with the proper administration of designated therapeutic dosages.

DOSAGE

Mode of Administration: The drug is available as a tincture.

LITERATURE

Adnrei GM et al., (1986) Experientia 42 (7): 843.

Bray DH et al., (1985) Trans Royal Soc Trop Med Hyg 79: 426.

Ekong DEU, (1967) Chem Comm 808.

Ekong DEU, Ibiyemi SA, (1971) Chem Comm: 1177.

El Said et al., (1968), Study of certain Nigerian plants used in Fever. Communication at the Inter-Africa Symposium Dakar.

Garg GP, Nigam SK, Ogle CW, The gastric antiulcer effects of the leaves of Neem tree. In: PM 59(3): 215. 1993.

Godvindachari T et al., JNP 55:596-601. 1992.

Kraus W, Bokel M, (1981) Chemische Berichte 114: 267.

Lavie D, Levy EC, (1969) Tetrahedron Letters 3525.

Okpanyi SN, Ezenkwu GC, (1981) Planta Med 41: 34.

Pat. Appl 83/234, 294 Japan (1983).

Rojatkar SR et al., 1-Tigloyl-3-acteyl-11-hydroxy-4β-methylmeliacarpin from Azadirachta indica. In: PH 32:213. 1993.

Rücker G, Malariawirksame Verbindungen aus Pflanzen, insbesondere Peroxide. In: PUZ 24(4):189-195. 1995.

Siidiqui S et al., JNP 55:303-310. 1992.

Further information in:

Hänsel R, Keller K, Rimpler H, Schneider G (Hrsg.), Hagers Handbuch der Pharmazeutischen Praxis, 5. Aufl., Bde 4-6 (Drogen), Springer Verlag Berlin, Heidelberg, New York, 1992-1994.

Kern W, List PH, Hörhammer L (Hrsg.), Hagers Handbuch der Pharmazeutischen Praxis, 4. Aufl., Bde. 1-8, Springer Verlag Berlin, Heidelberg, New York, 1969.

Lewin L, Gifte und Vergiftungen, 6. Aufl., Nachdruck, Haug Verlag, Heidelberg 1992.

Madaus G, Lehrbuch der Biologischen Arzneimittel, Bde 1-3, Nachdruck, Georg Olms Verlag Hildesheim 1979.

Oliver-Bever B (Ed.), Medicinal Plants of Tropical West Africa, Cambridge University Press Cambridge, London 1986.

Azedarach

See Azadirachta Indica

Bael

See Aegle Marmelos

Ballota Nigra

Horehound

DESCRIPTION

Flower and Fruit: The clearly stemed flowers are 1 to 1.5 cm long. They are arranged in 4 to 10 fairly loose and often short-stemmed cymes in the axils of the cauline leaves. The bracteoles are arrow-shaped and soft. They are half as long as the funnel-shaped, downy to silky-shaggy haired calyx. The calyx has 5 awned tips. The corolla is reddish-lilac, occasionally white. It contains a straight tube which has a ring of hairs at the base and which grows out of the calyx tube. It has an elliptoid, slightly domed upper lip, which is slightly compressed from the outside. There is an equally long, downward hanging, white-marked lower lip, and an obovate, often edged or weakly dentate middle lip. The stamens are slightly hairy at the base, and have small, distinctly spreading pollen sacks. The plant produces a hard fruit. The nuts are ovoid, 12 mm long and quite smooth.

Leaves, Stem and Root: Horehound is a perennial 0.30 to 1 m high shrub with a short creeping rhizome and upright, sturdy, angular, branched stems. The whole plant is pubescent and fresh green. In the autumn, the plant often tinged brown-violet. The opposite leaves have a 0.5 to 1 cm long petiole. The lower ones are larger and have an ovate to almost round, 2 cm long to 1.5 to 3.5 cm wide leaf blade. They are weakly cordate, blunt or wedge-shaped at the base and finely crenate to roughly and unevenly serrate. Both sides are pubescent, the upper surface often becoming glabrous and somewhat glossy.

Characteristics: The whole plant has an unpleasant smell of essential oil.

Habitat: The plant is considered to be a weed in western, central and northern Europe; it was introduced to America.

Production: Black Horehound is the aerial part of Ballota nigra, gathered when in bloom. It is produced by sowing or planting out of cuttings at the end of winter. The harvest is in July and August. There are no special conditions for drying.

Not To Be Confused With: The drug can be confused with Folia melissae. Adulterations with hybrids of Marubium vulgare have been found on the market.

Other Names: Black Stinking Horehound

ACTIONS AND PHARMACOLOGY

COMPOUNDS

Diterpenes, marrubiin: 7-acetoxymarrubiin (to some extent bitter principles)

Volatile oil (traces, unpleasant smell)

Caffeic and ferulic acid derivatives: including chlorogenic acid

Tannin

EFFECTS

According to past literature, a drop in arterial blood pressure and bradycardia occurred in a dog when it was injected intravenously with an infusion (2.5g infusion per kg body weight). When a decoction of the fresh plant was administered intravenously the volume of gall secretions tripled within 30 minutes. Horehound also acts as a stimulant, antiemetic, and antispasmodic.

INDICATIONS AND USAGE

Internally, Horehound is used as a sedative in cases of hysteria and hypochondria, as a spasmolytic for stomach cramps and complaints, for whooping cough, and to increase bile flow. Horehound is also used to treat nervous, upset stomach, nausea and vomiting. In France, it is traditionally used in the symptomatic treatment of nervous disorders in adults and children, especially for mild sleep disorders and for the symptomatic treatment of coughs. Furthermore, Horehound enemas are used against ascaridae and suppositions, on the basis of the thickened fresh plant juice, which acts against oxyurene. Externally, Horehound is used for gout.

The drug's efficacy has not been adequately proven.

PRECAUTIONS AND ADVERSE REACTIONS

No health hazards or side effects are known in conjunction with the proper administration of designated therapeutic dosages.

DOSAGE

Mode of Administration: The drug is used internally and externally.

Preparation: Liquid extract: 1:1 in 25% ethanol. Tincture: 1:10 with 45% ethanol.

Daily Dose: Single dose of the drug is 2 to 4 g of the infusion; Liquid extract: 1 to 3 ml; Tincture: 1 to 2 ml.

LITERATURE

Balansard J, Compt Rend Soc Biol 115:1295-1297. 1933.

Kooiman P, (1972) Acta Bot Nederl 21 (4): 417.

Savona G et al., (1976) J Chem Soc (P) 1: 1607-1609.

Savona G et al., (1977) J Chem Soc (P) 1: 322-324 et 497-499.

Savona G et al., La chimica e líndustria 58:378. 1976.

Seidel V et al., Phenylpropanoid glycosides from Ballota nigra. In: PM 62(2):186-187. 1997.

Further information in:

Hänsel R, Keller K, Rimpler H, Schneider G (Hrsg.), Hagers Handbuch der Pharmazeutischen Praxis, 5. Aufl., Bde 4-6 (Drogen), Springer Verlag Berlin, Heidelberg, New York, 1992-1994.

Bamboo

See Arundinaria Japonica

Baneberry

See Actaea Spicata

Baptisia Tinctoria

Wild Indigo

DESCRIPTION

Medicinal Parts: The medicinal part is the root.

Flower and Fruit: The flowers are terminal and axillary in 7 to 10 cm long, lightly flowered racemes. The pedicles are 3 to 5 cm long. The calyx is 4 to 5 mm long and glabrous but has a slight fringe. The corolla is yellow. The standard is circular with convilute sides and is slightly shorter than the oblong wings. The 10 stamens are free-standing. The ovary is stemmed, elliptoid, drawn together at the style and stigma and is glabrous. The fruit is a blue-black, ovoid, slightly swollen pod, 7 to 15 mm long with a sharp tip. The seeds are yellowish brown, kidney-shaped and 2 mm long.

Leaves, Stem and Root: The plant is a many-branched, up to 1 m high shrub with a woody rootstock with knotty branches. The stem is 1 to 3 mm thick, round, slightly grooved and glabrous. The alternating leaves are trifoliate and have a 1 to 3 mm long petiole. The stipules are small and arrow-shaped and drop early. The 1 to 4 cm long, and 0.6 to 1 cm wide leaflets are ovate, almost sessile, entire-margined. They are wedge-shaped at the base and rounded at the tip. The distinct midrib on the lower surface is pubescent. The leaves are brittle. The roots vary in diameter from 0.2 to 1.5 cm. The outer surface is brownish, vertically wrinkled and grooved. It is also warty due to root fibers sticking to the surface. The tissue is solid and fibrous. The transverse fracture shows a thick bark and whitish wood with concentric rings.

Characteristics: The taste is bitter, acrid, and disagreeable; the odor is faint.

Habitat: Indigenous to southern Canada and the eastern and northeastern U.S.

Production: Wild indigo root is the subterranean part of Baptisia tinctoria, which is dug up in autumn. The plant is produced from uncultivated areas.

Not To Be Confused With: Wild Indigo can be confused or adulterated with the root of Baptisia australis (bluer, incorrect indigo) and Baptisia alba. They are also used as a substitute.

Other Names: Horse-fly Weed, Rattlebush

ACTIONS AND PHARMACOLOGY

COMPOUNDS

Water-soluble polysaccharide: in particular arabinogalactans

Glycoproteins

Quinolizidine alkaloids: including cytisine, N-methyl cytisine, anagyrine, sparteine isoflavonoids, formononetin

Hydroxycumarins: including scopoletine

EFFECTS

Stimulation of immune system. The ethanol extract has had a significantly positive effect on the phagocytosis of human erythrocytes. It has also been found to raise the leukocyte count and to improve the endogenous defense reaction. Wild Indigo has a mild estrogenic effect.

INDICATIONS AND USAGE

Wild Indigo root is used for septic and typhoid cases with prostration and fever, such as diphtheria, influenza, malaria, septic angina, and typhus. It is used internally for infections of the upper respiratory tract, the common head cold, tonsillitis, stomatitis, throat and mouth inflammation of the mucous membrane (catarrh), fever, lymphadenitis and furunculosis. It is used externally as an ointment for painless ulcers, inflamed nipples, and as a douche for leucorrhea. In North America, the root has long been taken as a tea against fever, scarlet fever, typhoid, and pharyngitis and externally as an ointment for sores. The water, in which the root is soaked, is used to clean open and inflamed wounds.

The efficacy of the drug has not been proven.

PRECAUTIONS AND ADVERSE REACTIONS

No health hazards or side effects are known in conjunction with the proper administration of designated therapeutic dosages.

OVERDOSAGE

Only very high dosages (for example 30 g of the drug) can lead to signs of poisoning (vomiting, diarrhea, gastrointestinal complaints, spasms), due to the quinolizidine alkaloid content.

DOSAGE

Mode of Administration: Wild Indigo is not common as a drug, but is found in combination preparations. Taken internally as a tea and tincture. Used externally as an ointment.

Preparation: To prepare an ointment, use 1 part liquid extract to 8 parts ointment base.

Daily Dose: Dosage for a single dose is 0.5 g to 1 g of the dried drug as decoction, to be taken 3 times daily.

LITERATURE

Beuscher H, Kopanski L, Modulation of the immune response by polymeric substances from Baptisia tinctoria and Echinacea angustifolia. In: Pharm Weekblad Sci Ed. 9:229. 1987.

Beuscher N, Beuscher HU, Bodinet C, Enhanced Release of Interleukin-1 from Mouse Macrophages by Glykoproteins and Polysaccharides from Baptisia tinctoria and Echinacea Species. In: PM, Abstracts of the 37th Annual Congress on Medicinal Plant Research Braunschwe.

Beuscher N, Bodinet C, Willigmann I, Harnischfeger G, Biologiocal activity of Baptisia tinctoria extracts. In: Inst. für Angew. Botanik der Univ. Hamburg, Angewandte Botanik, Berichte 6, 46-61. 1997.

Beuscher N, Kopanski L, Erwein C, Modulation der Immunantwort durch polymere Substanzen aus Baptisia tinctoria und Echinacea purpurea. In: Adv in the Biosc 68:329. 1987.

Beuscher N, Kopanski L, Stimulation der Immunantwort durch Inhaltsstoffe aus Baptisia tinctoria. In: PM 1985:381-384. 1985.

Beuscher N, Scheit KH, Bodinet C, Egert D, Modulation der körpereigenen Immunabwehr durch polymere Substanzen aus Baptisia tinctoria und Echinacea purpurea. In: Immunotherapeutic prospects of infectious diseases, Hrsg. Masihi KN, Lange W. Springer, Heidel.

Beuscher N, Scheit KH, Bodinet C, Kopanski L, Immunologisch aktive Glykoproteine aus Baptisia tinctoria. In: PM 55:358-363. 1989.

Bodinet C, Beuscher N, Kopanski L, Purification of Immunologicaly Active Glycoproteins from Baptisia tinctoria Roots by Affinity Chromatography and Isoelectric Focussing. In: PM, Abstracts of the 37th Annual Congress on Medicinal Plant Research Braunschwe.

Harnischfeger, Buch, Harnischfeger G, Stolze H, Bewährte Pflanzendrogen in Wissenschaft und Medizin, Notabene-Verlag, Bad Homburg. 1983.

Vömel T, Arzneim-Forsch 35:1437-1439. 1985.

Vömel T, Der Einfluβ eines pflanzlichen Immunstimulans auf die Phagozytose von Erythrozyten durch das retikulohistiozytäre System der isolierte perfundierten Rattenleber. In: Arzneim Forsch 35(II): 1437-1439. 1985.

Wagner H, Proksch A, Riess-Mauer I, Vollmar A, Odenthal S, Stuppner H, Jurcic K, LeTurdu M, Fang JN, Arzneim-Forsch 35: 1069-10750. 1985.

Further information in:

Hänsel R, Keller K, Rimpler H, Schneider G (Hrsg.), Hagers Handbuch der Pharmazeutischen Praxis, 5. Aufl., Bde 4-6 (Drogen), Springer Verlag Berlin, Heidelberg, New York, 1992-1994.

Madaus G, Lehrbuch der Biologischen Arzneimittel, Bde 1-3, Nachdruck, Georg Olms Verlag Hildesheim 1979.

Roth L, Daunderer M, Kormann K, Giftpflanzen, Pflanzengifte, 4. Aufl., Ecomed Fachverlag Landsberg Lech 1993

Steinegger E, Hänsel R, Pharmakognosie, 5. Aufl., Springer Verlag Heidelberg 1992.

Teuscher E, Biogene Arzneimittel, 5. Aufl., Wiss. Verlagsges. Stuttgart 1997.

Wagner H, Wiesenauer M, Phytotherapie. Phytopharmaka und pflanzliche Homöopathika, Fischer-Verlag, Stuttgart, Jena, New York 1995.

Barberry

See Berberis Vulgaris

Barley

See Hordeum Distychum

Barosma Species

Buchu

DESCRIPTION

Medicinal Parts: The leaves have a peppermint odor.

Flower and Fruit: The pentamerous flowers of B. betulina form a white or pink corolla 12 mm in diameter with lanceolate petals. The fruit is a 7 mm long capsule with 5 chambers and one seed per chamber. The upper surface is greenish-brown and rough. The fruit springs open at the 5 valves. The seeds are ovoid, oblong, about 5 mm long and 2 mm wide, glossy black, hard and have no endosperm. The flowers of B. crenulata are pink or white and are attached to short leafy side branches.

Leaves, Stem and Root: B. betulina is a small shrub with light green to yellowish leaves. The leaves are 12 to 20 mm in length, opposite, rigid and coriaceous. They are rhomboid or obovate, short-petioled with an oil gland in each indentation. The oil glands form small raised structures on the leaf surface. The stem is about 2 to 3 mm in diameter, red-brown, rough due to the oil glands and has 4 long grooves. The internodes are 8 to 20 mm long. B. crenulata is a slender glabrous bush 2 to 3 m high. It is branched and the branches are somewhat angular. The bark is violet-brown. The leaves of B. crenulata vary in form, are opposite and pubescent on both surfaces and are somewhat longer, i.e. up to 3 cm and have an obtuse, but not a revolute tip. The B. serratifolia bush is very similar although the leaves are longer, obtuse at the tip and narrowed on both edges. They are lanceolate, have a long serrated, saw-shaped margin and a blunt apex. They are yellowish green and up to 4 cm long. They all have an oil gland at the apex and indentations on the margin. There are smaller oil glands spread over the leaf blade.

Characteristics: The taste and odor are very characteristic.

Habitat: Indigenous to South Africa, Cape region.

Production: Buchu leaf consists of the dried leaves of Barosma betulina.

Not To Be Confused With: Other Barosma and Diosma species.

ACTIONS AND PHARMACOLOGY

COMPOUNDS

Volatile oil: chief components diosphenol and psi-diosphenol (mixture known as buccocamphor), limonene, (+)-menthone, (-)-isomenthone, pulegone, furthermore (-)- cis- and (+)-trans-8-mercapto-p-menth-3-one (odor-determining, so-called cassis aroma)

Flavonoids: including rutin and diosmetin

EFFECTS

At present no studies of the drug are available.

INDICATIONS AND USAGE

Buchu leaf is used for inflammation and infection of the kidneys and urinary tract, for bladder irritation, as a disinfectant of the urinary tract, and as a diuretic. In Europe the drug has been in use since the 16th century for the treatment of gout, various bladder disorders, rheumatism, and for the prostate gland. In South Africa it is still widely used.

The efficacy for the claimed applications is not documented.

PRECAUTIONS AND ADVERSE REACTIONS

No health hazards or side effects are known in conjunction with the proper administration of designated therapeutic dosages. The volatile oil lead to signs of irritation.

DOSAGE

Mode of Administration: Since the claimed efficacy has not been documented, the application of Buchu leaf cannot be recommended. Buchu is used in various preparations and combinations.

Preparation: Buchu is available as an extract, tincture, and infusion.

Daily Dose: The daily dose of the drug is 1 g to 2 g.

Storage: The drug must be kept cool and dry away from the light in sealed containers.

LITERATURE

Didry N, Pinkas M, (1982) Plant Med Phytother 16 (4): 249.

Kaiser R et al., (1975) J Agric Food Chem 23: 943-950.

Further information in:

Hänsel R, Keller K, Rimpler H, Schneider G (Hrsg.), Hagers Handbuch der Pharmazeutischen Praxis, 5. Aufl., Bde 4-6 (Drogen), Springer Verlag Berlin, Heidelberg, New York, 1992-1994.

Leung AY, Encyclopedia of Common Natural Ingredients Used in Food Drugs and Cosmetics, John Wiley & Sons Inc., New York 1980.

Madaus G, Lehrbuch der Biologischen Arzneimittel, Bde 1-3, Nachdruck, Georg Olms Verlag Hildesheim 1979.

Steinegger E, Hänsel R, Pharmakognosie, 5. Aufl., Springer Verlag Heidelberg 1992.

Wichtl M (Hrsg.), Teedrogen, 4. Aufl., Wiss. Verlagsges. Stuttgart 1997.

Basil

See Ocimum Basilicum

Bean

See Phaseolus Vulgaris

Bear's Garlic

See Allium Ursinum

Beet

See Beta Vulgaris

Belladonna

See Atropa Belladonna

Bellis Perennis

Wild Daisy

DESCRIPTION

Medicinal Parts: The medicinal part is the whole flowering plant.

Flower and Fruit: The flower heads are usually found singly at the end of the usually sharply angular stem. The flower is quite small to medium-sized and heterogamous. The epicalyx is semi-spherical to broadly-campanualte. The sepals of the epicalyx are more or less double-rowed. The receptacle is conical and glabrous when fruit bearing. The 1 to 2-rowed female ray flowers are linguiform, white, pink, purple or bluish and distinctly longer than the epicalyx. The disc flowers are androgynous, tubular, and have 5 tips. The achaenes are obovate, very flattened, ribless, and have side veins. There is no pappus or may only have short, brittle bristles.

Leaves, Stem and Root: The perennial leafy plant has basal leaves in rosettes or alternate leaves at the lower part of the stem. There are short cylindrical roots. The rosette leaves are circular to spatulate or circular-cordate, dentate or occasionally entire-margined with a single rib. They have vertical hairs on both sides. The plant is around 10 to 15 cm high.

Habitat: The plant is distributed from Portugal to the Moscow region and Asia Minor. It is also found from Great Britain to Ireland and southern Scandinavia, and as far as the Mediterranean. It is not found however on the Balearics, Sardinia, Sicily, Crete, and Cyprus.

Production: The capitula and short stems of the plant are picked and dried in either the sun or shade.

Other Names: Bruisewort

ACTIONS AND PHARMACOLOGY

COMPOUNDS

Triterpene saponins: polygalacturonic acid (acylated)

Polyynes: including trans-lachnophyllum ester

Flavonoids

EFFECTS

The drug is an astringent, reduces mucous production, and also has an anti-inflammatory effect.

INDICATIONS AND USAGE

Formerly, the drug was used to treat chest conditions and wounds. Today, it is used in folk medicine as an expectorant; also for wounds, skin diseases, coughs and bronchitis, disorders of the liver and kidneys, and inflammation. It eases diarrhea and gastrointestinal catarrh. It is also used in homeopathy.

PRECAUTIONS AND ADVERSE REACTIONS

No health hazards or side effects are known in conjunction with the proper administration of designated therapeutic dosages.

DOSAGE

Mode of Administration: The drug is used topically, as an extract, in teas and in poultices of pressed leaves in the treatment of skin diseases.

Preparation: An infusion is prepared by pouring 2 cups of water onto 2 teaspoonfuls of the drug, and allow to draw for 20 minutes. A decoction is prepared from the green leaves.

Daily Dosage: The daily dose of the infusion is 2 to 4 cups per day. Use a decoction for wound poultices.

LITERATURE

Avato P, Vitali C, Tava A, New acetylenic compounds from Bellis perennis L. and their antimicrobial activity. In: PM 61(Abstracts of 43rd Ann Congr):49. 1995.

Schöpke T, Wray V, Hiller K, Triterpenoid saponins of plants of the Asteraeae tribe (Asteraceae). In: PM 59(7):A591. 1992.

Schöpke Th et al., Saponin composition of the Bellis genus and related species. In: PM 61(Abstracts of 43rd Ann Congr):68. 1995.

Willigmann I et al., Antimycotic compounds from different Bellis perennis varieties. In: PM 58(Suppl.7):A636. 1993.

Further information in:

Hänsel R, Keller K, Rimpler H, Schneider G (Hrsg.), Hagers Handbuch der Pharmazeutischen Praxis, 5. Aufl., Bde 4-6 (Drogen): Springer Verlag Berlin, Heidelberg, New York, 1992-1994.

Madaus G, Lehrbuch der Biologischen Arzneimittel, Bde 1-3, Nachdruck, Georg Olms Verlag Hildesheim 1979.

Wagner H, Wiesenauer M, Phytotherapie. Phytopharmaka und pflanzliche Homöopathika, Fischer-Verlag, Stuttgart, Jena, New York 1995.

Bennet's Root

See Geum Urbanum

Berberis Vulgaris

Barberry

DESCRIPTION

Medicinal Parts: The medicinal part is the fruit and the root bark.

Flower and Fruit: The flowers are 5 to 7 cm long in yellow, dense, hanging clusters. The 6 sepals are yellow and the 6 petals have orange-colored honey glands at the base. The 6 stamens burst open at the side. The ovary is superior with a flat stigma. The edible fruit is a bright scarlet, oblong-cylindrical berry, 10 to 12 mm long and 6 mm thick. The exocarp is membranous-coriaceous. There are usually 2 seeds.

Leaves, Stem and Root: Barberry is a deciduous, heavily branched, thorny bush up to 2 m high. The thorny branches are angular, deeply grooved, initially brownish yellow, later more white-gray. The thorns are 1 to 2 cm long and stick out horizontally. The leaves are in bushels and are obovate to elliptoid, 2 to 4 cm long and narrowed into the 1 cm long petiole. They are dark green and reticulate, the margin is dentate.

Characteristics: The flowers have a repulsive smell; the stamens lie on the carpels at the slightest touch. The flesh of the fruit is juicy and sour.

Habitat: Europe, northern Africa, parts of America and central Asia.

Production: Barberries are the ripe fruit of Berberis vulgaris. Barberry root bark or berberis bark is the dried root bark of Berberis vulgaris.

Not To Be Confused With: There is a possiblity of confusion with the fruits of other berberidis types. The commercial drug often consists of admixtures; between 15% and 50% of branch and trunk bark.

Other Names: Berberry, Pipperidge, Jaundice Berry, Sow Berry, Mountain Grape, Oregon Grape

ACTIONS AND PHARMACOLOGY

COMPOUNDS: BERBERIDIS FRUCTUS

Isoquinoline alkaloids (at the most, traces)

Anthocyans

Chlorogenic acid

Malic acid, acetic acid

EFFECTS: BERBERIDIS FRUCTUS

Source of Vitamin C. In various metabolic processes, Vitamin C increases immune system activity, stimulates iron absorption, and prevents scurvy. There is a mild diuretic effect due to the acid content.

COMPOUNDS: BERBERIDIS RADICIS CORTEX

Isoquinoline alkaloids: in particular berberine, berbamine, oxyacanthin, further to include columbamine, palmatine, jatrorrhizine, magnoflorine.

EFFECTS: BERBERIDIS RADICIS CORTEX

Cardiovascular effect: Fractions from the root extracts, which contain 80% berberine and other alkaloids, have been shown to reduce the blood pressure of cats for several hours. With varying doses, both positive and negative inotropic effects on the cats' hearts were revealed.

Cholagogue effect: A homeopathic mother tincture separated from the ethanol and by using water, reduced to half its original volume, increased the bile flow in guinea pigs by an average of 20%. An extract with 80% berberine and additional alkaloids stimulated the bile excretion of rats by 72%.

Effect on the muscular system: A homeopathic mother tincture, separated from the ethanol and by using water, reduced to half its original volume, caused an increase in amplitudes at isolated sections in the small intestine of a rabbit. High concentrations resulted in a temporary tonus increase in guinea pig and rat intestines.

Antipyretic effect: Aqueous tinctures have a clear anti-febrile effect on a feverish rabbit.

Antibiotic effect

Stimulation of intestinal peristalsis

INDICATIONS AND USAGE

BERBERIDIS FRUCTUS

Decoction or alcoholic extract for lung, spleen and liver diseases. Jam or wine made from the fresh berries can relieve constipation and lack of appetite. Alcoholic extract for heartburn and stomach cramps. Also used for susceptibility to infection, feverish colds, and diseases of the urinary tract. Used in the pharmaceutical industry as a syrup for masking flavor.

BERBERIDIS RADICIS CORTEX

Medical use: For opium or morphine withdrawal. In folk medicine, the bark is used for liver malfunctions, gallbladder disease, jaundice, splenopathy, indigestion, diarrhea, especially linked to scrofulosis and tuberculosis, piles, renal disease, urinary tract disorders, gout, rheumatism, arthritis, lumbago, malaria, and leishmaniasis.

Efficacy has not been proven. Use for these indications is not advised.

PRECAUTIONS AND ADVERSE REACTIONS

BERBERIDIS FRUCTUS

No health hazards or side effects are known in conjunction with the proper administration of designated therapeutic dosages.

BERBERIDIS RADICIS CORTEX

No health hazards or side effects are known in conjunction with the proper administration of designated therapeutic dosages.

OVERDOSAGE

BERBERIDIS RADICIS CORTEX

Dosages over 4 mg will bring about light stupor, nose bleeds, vomiting, diarrhea and kidney irritation. The treatment for poisonings is to be carried out symptomatically.

DOSAGE

BERBERIDIS FRUCTUS

Mode of Administration: Internally: In tea mixtures and combination preparations.

Preparation: To prepare a tea infusion, pour approximately 150 ml of hot water into 1 to 2 teaspoons of whole or squashed Barberries and strain after 10 to 15 minutes.

BERBERIDIS RADICIS CORTEX

Mode of Administration: Mostly obsolete as a drug, occasionally in tea mixtures. Its use is often advised against.

Preparation: A tincture 1:10 is prepared according to the German Pharmacopeia 10th ed.

To extract the pure alkaloids from berberis roots, use 0.3% sulphuric acid mixed with 10% sodium chloride. The precipitated berberine hydrochloride is washed with mildly hydrochloric water and dried. It is then dissolved in water (pH 8) and filtered. The filtrate is heated to 70°C and set to pH 2.0 using hydrochloric acid. The precipitate of pure berberine hydrochloride is then washed and dried.

Daily Dose: The dosage of the infusion is 2 g in 250 ml water, to be sipped. The tincture dosage is 20 to 40 drops daily.

LITERATURE

BERBERIDIS FRUCTUS

Andronescu E et al., (1973) Clujul. Med 46: 627.

Chen MQ et al., (1965) Acta Pharm Sinica 12 (3): 185.

Cordell GA, Farnsworth NR, (1977) Lloydia 40: 1.

Ikram M, (1975) Planta Med 28: 253.

Lahiri SC et al., (1958) Ann Biochem Exp Med India 18: 95.

Liu CX et al., (1979) Chinese Traditional and Herbal Drugs Communications 9: 36.

Naidovich LP et al., (1976) Farmatsiya 24: 33.

Shapiro DK et al., Rastit Resur 19(1):84-89. 1983.

Subbaiah TV, Amin AH, (1967) Nature 215: 527.

Ubebaba K et al., (1984) Jpn J Pharmacol 36 (Suppl): 352.

Willaman JJ, Hui-Li L, (1970) Lloydia 33 (3A): 1.

Further information in:

Frohne D, Pfänder HJ, Giftpflanzen - Ein Handbuch für Apotheker, Toxikologen und Biologen, 4. Aufl., Wiss. Verlags-Ges Stuttgart 1997.

Hänsel R, Keller K, Rimpler H, Schneider G (Hrsg.), Hagers Handbuch der Pharmazeutischen Praxis, 5. Aufl., Bde 4-6 (Drogen), Springer Verlag Berlin, Heidelberg, New York, 1992-1994.

Leung AY: Encyclopedia of Common Natural Ingredients Used in Food Drugs and Cosmetics, John Wiley & Sons Inc., New York 1980.

Roth L, Daunderer M, Kormann K, Giftpflanzen, Pflanzengifte, 4. Aufl., Ecomed Fachverlag Landsberg Lech 1993.

BERBERIDIS RADICIS CORTEX

Andronescu E et al., (1973) Clujul. Med 46: 627.

Chen MQ et al., (1965) Acta Pharm Sinica 12 (3): 185.

Cordell GA, Farnsworth NR, (1977) Lloydia 40: 1.

Ikram M, (1975) Planta Med 28: 253.

Lahiri SC et al., (1958) Ann Biochem Exp Med India 18: 95.

Liu CX et al., (1979) Chinese Traditional and Herbal Drugs Communications 9: 36.

Naidovich LP et al., (1976) Farmatsiya 24: 33.

Subbaiah TV, Amin AH, (1967) Nature 215: 527.

Ubebaba K et al., (1984) Jpn J Pharmacol 36 (Suppl): 352.

Willaman JJ, Hui-Li L, (1970) Lloydia 33 (3A): 1.

Further information in:

Frohne D, Pfänder HJ, Giftpflanzen - Ein Handbuch für Apotheker, Toxikologen und Biologen, 4. Aufl., Wiss. Verlags-Ges Stuttgart 1997.

Hänsel R, Keller K, Rimpler H, Schneider G (Hrsg.), Hagers Handbuch der Pharmazeutischen Praxis, 5. Aufl., Bde 4-6 (Drogen), Springer Verlag Berlin, Heidelberg, New York, 1992-1994.

Madaus G, Lehrbuch der Biologischen Arzneimittel, Bde 1-3, Nachdruck, Georg Olms Verlag Hildesheim 1979.

Roth L, Daunderer M, Kormann K, Giftpflanzen, Pflanzengifte, 4. Aufl., Ecomed Fachverlag Landsberg Lech 1993.

Teuscher E, Lindequist U, Biogene Gifte - Biologie, Chemie, Pharmakologie, 2. Aufl., Fischer Verlag Stuttgart 1994.

Wagner H, Wiesenauer M, Phytotherapie. Phytopharmaka und pflanzliche Homöopathika, Fischer-Verlag, Stuttgart, Jena, New York 1995.

Beta Vulgaris

Beet

DESCRIPTION

Medicinal Parts: The root is the medicinal part.

Flower and Fruit: The flowers are in clusters of 2 to 4 in panicle-like leafy inflorescences.

Leaves, Stem and Root: The beet is a 0.5 to 1.5 m perennial with a swollen, edible, red or white tuber. The leaves are basal, in rosettes, long-petioled, upright and large. They are deep green and tinged with red.

Habitat: Beet is indigenous to the coastal regions of Europe, North Africa and Asia from Turkey to India. The red beets as well as the sugar beets and the white variety are all widely cultivated.

Other Names: Chard

ACTIONS AND PHARMACOLOGY

COMPOUNDS

Saccharose

Other oligosaccharides: refined sugar, ketose

Polysaccharides: including galactans, arabans, pectin

Fruit acids: including L(-)-malic acid, D(+)-tartaric acid, oxaluric acid, adipic acid, citric acid, glycolic acid, glutaric acid

Amino acids: including asparagine, glutamine

Betaine (trimethylglycine)

Triterpene saponins

EFFECTS

In animal tests, the drug is effective against depositing fat in the liver. Betaine is a methyl group donor in the transmethylation process in the liver.

INDICATIONS AND USAGE

Beet is used as a supportive therapy in diseases of the liver and fatty liver.

PRECAUTIONS AND ADVERSE REACTIONS

No health hazards or side effects are known in conjunction with the proper administration of designated therapeutic dosages.

OVERDOSAGE

An intake of very large quantities of the drug could lead to hypocalcemia and to kidney damage because of the oxaluric acid content.

DOSAGE

Mode of Administration: Beet is available as a granular powder in standardized form.

LITERATURE

Kern W, List PH, Hörhammer L (Hrsg.), Hagers Handbuch der Pharmazeutischen Praxis, 4. Aufl., Bde 1-8, Springer Verlag Berlin, Heidelberg, New York, 1969.

Betel Nut

See Piper Betle

Beth Root

See Trillium Erectum

Betonica Officinalis

Wood Betony

DESCRIPTION

Medicinal Parts: The medicinal part is the herb, including the basal leaves.

Flower and Fruit: The flowers are crimson and labiate in terminal, spike-like, irregular formation. The calyx, with 5 even, triangular tips, has long ciliate hairs and is shorter than the corolla tube. The corolla is curled downward and the white tube has no ring of hair. The upper lip is erect and the lower lip is 3-lobed with a broad middle lobe. There are 4 stamens.

Leaves, Stem and Root: The plant grows to a height of about 30 to 100 cm. The stem is erect, unbranched, quadrangular, bristly-haired and usually only has 2 distal pairs of leaves. The basal leaves are rosette-like. The leaves are elongate-ovate with a cordate base and crenate. The lower ones are larger and long-petioled and the upper ones are smaller and shorter.

Habitat: The plant grows in Europe.

Production: Wood Betony is the flowering plant of Betonica officinalis. The herb, including the basal leaves, is collected and dried in the shade at a maximum temperature of 40°C.

Not To Be Confused With: Stachys alpina

Other Names: Betony, Bishopswort

ACTIONS AND PHARMACOLOGY

COMPOUNDS

Betaine: including betonicine [(-)-oxystachydrine), (-)- stachydrine), (+)-oxystachydrine]

Caffeic acid derivatives: including chlorogenic acid, isochlorogenic acid, rosemary acid iridoid glycosides

Diterpene lactone

Flavonoids

EFFECTS

The drug is said to act as a tranquilizer, a disinfectant, and an astringent. It contains glycosides with hypotensive characteristics.

INDICATIONS AND USAGE

Wood Betony is an astringent. As an expectorant, it is used for coughs, bronchitis and asthma. It is contained in combination preparations as a sedative and for the treatment of neuralgia and anxiety. In folk medicine, it is used as an antidiarrheal agent, a carmative, and a sedative, and for catarrh, lung catarrh, heartburn, gout, nervousness, bladder and kidney stones, and inflammation of the bladder.

PRECAUTIONS AND ADVERSE REACTIONS

No health hazards or side effects are known in conjunction with the proper administration of designated therapeutic dosages.

DOSAGE

Mode of Administration: The herb is used topically, as an extract and an infusion. The fresh leaves are also used.

Daily Dosage: The infusion can be taken daily. The total daily dosage of the powder is 1 to 2 gm, to be taken in 3 separate doses. The fresh leaves may be boiled and used for wounds and swelling.

LITERATURE

Hoppe HA, (1975-1987) Drogenkunde, 8. Aufl., Bde 1-3, W. de Gruyter Verlag, Berlin, New York.

Kern W, List PH, Hörhammer L (Hrsg.), Hagers Handbuch der Pharmazeutischen Praxis, 4. Aufl., Bde. 1-8, Springer Verlag Berlin, Heidelberg, New York, 1969.

Madaus G, Lehrbuch der Biologischen Arzneimittel, Bde 1-3, Nachdruck, Georg Olms Verlag Hildesheim 1979.

Betula Species

Birch

DESCRIPTION

Medicinal Parts: Birch wine and Birch tea are made from the sap and leaves respectively.

Flower and Fruit: Betula pendula: The male flowers are sessile, oblong-cylindrical 6 to 10 cm long. The female catkins are petioled, cylindrical and 2 to 4 cm long by 8 to 10 mm thick when fully grown. They are densely flowered, first yellow-green, later light-green. The fruit scales are brownish and pubescent or glabrous. The middle lobes are small, short-triangular and shorter than the broad, always revolute side lobes. The fruit wings are half-oval and 2 to 3 times as broad as the fruit.

Betula pubescens: The male catkins are sessile, oblong-cylindrical, initially upright. Later hanging, 2.5 to 4 cm long and 6 to 10 mm thick, greenish to light brown. The middle lobes of the fruit scales protrude clearly, are usually linguiform-elogated and are generally longer than the usually sharp-cornered, clearly evolute side lobes. The fruit scales are about as broad as the fruit.

Leaves, Stem and Root: Betula pendula is an up to 30 cm high tree with a snow white bark, which usually peels off in horizontal strips or changes into a black, stony hard bark. Young branches are glabrous and thickly covered in warty, resin glands. The petioled leaves are dark green above, a lighter gray-green below and have serrate margins and particularly tightly packed veins. The lamina are about 3 to 7 cm long by 2 to 5 cm wide, rhomboid-triangular, acuminate, glabrous, densely covered in glands and have a doubly serrate margin.

Betula pubescens is a tree or a bush, which grows up to 30 m high. The bark usually remains white and only changes later into fissured, black, thinly flaking bark. The branches are upright or spread. The young branches are downy, have no glands and are later almost glabrous. The leaves usually have a cordate, rounded or broadly wedge-shaped base and are ovate or rhoimboid and short-tipped; they are 3 to 5 cm long by 0.5 to 3.5 cm wide, with rounded corners, a serrate margin and a tough consistency. They are dark green and glabrous above and a lighter green below; they are initially downy and later pubescent in the vein axils.

Habitat: B. pendula and B. pubescens are indigenous to Europe from the northern Mediterranean regions to Siberia and to temperate regions of Asia.

Production: Birch leaf consists of the fresh or dried leaf of Betula pendula (syn. Betula verrucosa), or Betula pubescens, or of both species. The leaves are collected in spring and dried at room temperature in the shade. Birch tar from B. pendula or B. pubescens.

ACTIONS AND PHARMACOLOGY

COMPOUNDS: BETULAE FOLIUM

Triterpene alcohol ester with saponin-like effect: betula-triterpene saponins

Flavonoids: including hyperoside, quercetin, myricetin digalactosides

Proanthocyanidins

Volatile oil

Monoterpene glucosides: including betula alboside A and B

Caffeic acid derivatives: including chlorogenic acid

EFFECTS: BETULAE FOLIUM

Birch leaves increase the amount of urine, have a mild saluretic effect and are antipyretic.

COMPOUNDS: PIX BETULINA

Phenols (6%): including among others guaiacol, cresole, catechol, pyrogallol, 5-propyl-pyrogallol dimethyl ether and 5-methyl- pyrogallol dimethyl ether

EFFECTS: PIX BETULINA

Birch tar is a skin irritant and antiparasitic.

INDICATIONS AND USAGE

BETULAE FOLIUM

- Infections of the urinary tract
- Kidney and bladder stones

The leaves are used in flushing-out therapy for bacterial and inflammatory diseases of the urinary tract and for kidney gravel. They are also used in adjunct therapy for rheumatic ailments, for increasing amount of urine. In folk medicine, the leaves are used as a blood purifier, and for gout and rheumatism. Externally, the leaves are used for hair loss and dandruff. The folk medicinal effect is not documented.

PIX BETULINA

The tar is used for skin diseases.

CONTRAINDICATIONS

BETULAE FOLIUM

The drug should not be used for edema when there is reduced cardiac or kidney function.

PRECAUTIONS AND ADVERSE REACTIONS

BETULAE FOLIUM

No health hazards or side effects are known in conjunction with the proper administration of designated therapeutic dosages.

PIX BETULINA

No health hazards are known in conjunction with the proper administration of designated therapeutic dosages. Birch tar can cause irritations on sensitive skin. Administration of the drug is not advisable, due to the possible presence of cancerogenic hydrocarbons.

DOSAGE

BETULAE FOLIUM

Mode of Administration: Comminuted herb or dry extracts for teas, as well as other galenic preparations and freshly-pressed plant juices for internal use.

Daily Dose: The average daily dose is 2 to 3 g drug several times a day, ensure ample intake of fluid (minimum 2 liters per day). The infusion is used between meals 3 to 4 times a day

Storage: In well sealed containers protected from light and moisture.

PIX BETULINA

Mode of Administration: In combination preparations as ointments and liniments. The preparations ''Buenoson ointment'' and ''Discmigon'' ointment contain birch tar. In addition, birch tar is a constituent of ''Unguentu'' for the treatment of scabies.

LITERATURE

BETULAE FOLIUM

Anonym, Phytotherapie: Pflanzliche Antirheumatika - was bringen sie. In: DAZ 136(45):4012-4015. 1996.

Hiller K, Pharmazeutische Bewertung ausgewählter Teedrogen. In: DAZ 135(16):1425-1440. 1995.

Hörhammer L, Wagner H, Luck R, Arch Pharm 290:338-341. 1957.

Karatodorof K, Kalarova R, (1977) Izn Durzh Inst Kontrol Lek Sredstva 10:103-9.

Pisha E et al., Discovery of betulinic acid as a selective inhibitor of human melanoma that functions by induction of apoptosis. In: Nature Medicine 1:1046-1051. 1995.

Rickling B, Glombitza KW, Saponins in the leaves of birch? Hemolytic dammarane triterpenoids esters of Betula pendula. In: PM 59(1):77. 1993.

Schilcher H, Boesel R, Effenberger ST Segebrecht S, Neuere Untersuchungsergebnisse mit aquaretisch, antibakteriell und prostatotrop wirksamen Arzneipflanzen. In: ZPT 10(3):77. 1989.

Sökeland J, Phytotherapie in der Urologie. In: ZPT 10(1):8. 1989.

Tschesche R, Ciper F, Breitmeier E, Chem Ber 110:3111-3117. 1977.

Further information in:

Hänsel R, Keller K, Rimpler H, Schneider G (Hrsg.), Hagers Handbuch der Pharmazeutischen Praxis, 5. Aufl., Bde 4-6

(Drogen), Springer Verlag Berlin, Heidelberg, New York, 1992-1994.

Madaus G, Lehrbuch der Biologischen Arzneimittel, Bde 1-3, Nachdruck, Georg Olms Verlag Hildesheim 1979.

Steinegger E, Hänsel R, Pharmakognosie, 5. Aufl., Springer Verlag Heidelberg 1992.

Teuscher E, Biogene Arzneimittel, 5. Aufl., Wiss. Verlagsges. Stuttgart 1997.

Wagner H, Wiesenauer M, Phytotherapie. Phytopharmaka und pflanzliche Homöopathika, Fischer-Verlag, Stuttgart, Jena, New York 1995.

Wichtl M (Hrsg.), Teedrogen, 4. Aufl., Wiss. Verlagsges. Stuttgart 1997.

PIX BETULINA

Kreitmair H, PA 8:534-536. 1953.

Nowak GA, Am Perf Cosmet 81:37-39. 1966.

Further information in:

Hänsel R, Keller K, Rimpler H, Schneider G (Hrsg.), Hagers Handbuch der Pharmazeutischen Praxis, 5. Aufl., Bde 4-6 (Drogen), Springer Verlag Berlin, Heidelberg, New York, 1992-1994.

Leung AY, Encyclopedia of Common Natural Ingredients Used in Food Drugs and Cosmetics, John Wiley & Sons Inc., New York 1980.

Bidens Tripartita

Burr Marigold

DESCRIPTION

Flower and Fruit: The flower heads are solitary, erect or inclined 15 to 25 mm long and wide and generally have no lingual blossoms. There are two rows of bracts. The inner row is ovate, brown-yellow; the outer ones are oblong and green. The petals are brown-yellow. The fruit is glabrous, distinctly compressed, brown-green, with thorny edges and 2 to 4 awns.

Leaves, Stem and Root: Bidens tripartita is an annual, erect, 15 to 100 cm high plant with a fibrous fusiform root. The stem is erect, heavily branched, glabrous or somewhat downy and often brown-red. The leaves are dark green, opposite and narrow to a short, winged petiole. The leaves are usually 3 to 5 lobed, ovate-rhomboid to lanceolate with pointed, roughly dentate tips and straight or narrowly curved teeth.

Habitat: The plant is found in damp regions throughout Europe.

Production: Burr Marigold is the aerial part of Bidens tripartita.

Other Names: Water Agrimony

ACTIONS AND PHARMACOLOGY

COMPOUNDS

Polyynes (tridecane derivatives): including trideca-1,12-dien-3,5,7,9-tetrain

Water-soluble polysaccharides

Bitter principles

Tannins

Volatile oil

EFFECTS

Astringent, diaphoretic, and diuretic.

INDICATIONS AND USAGE

Used for gout, hematuria, and colitis. According to unconfirmed reports, Burr Marigold is also in the treatment of alopecia.

PRECAUTIONS AND ADVERSE REACTIONS

No health hazards or side effects are known in conjunction with the proper administration of designated therapeutic dosages.

DOSAGE

No information is available.

LITERATURE

Bauer R, Neues von ''immunmodulierenden Drogen'' und ''Drogen mit antiallergischer und antiinflammatorischer Wirkung''. In: ZPT 14(1):23-24. 1993.

Ben'ko GN, (1983) Rastit Resur 19 (4),516.

Morozova SS et al., (1981) Rastit Resur 17 (1),101.

Further information in:

Kern W, List PH, Hörhammer L (Hrsg.), Hagers Handbuch der Pharmazeutischen Praxis, 4. Aufl., Bde. 1-8, Springer Verlag Berlin, Heidelberg, New York, 1969.

Bilberry

See Vaccinium Myrtillus

Birch

See Betula Species

Birthwort

See Aristolochia Clematitis

Bishop's Weed
See Ammi Visnaga

Bistort
See Polygonum Bistorta

Bitter Apple
See Citrullus Colocynthis

Bitter Milkwort
See Polygala Amara

Bitter Orange
See Citrus Aurantium

Bitter Wood
See Quassia Amara

Bittersweet Nightshade
See Solanum Dulcamara

Black Alder
See Alnus Glutinosa

Black Bryony
See Tamus Communis

Black Cherry
See Prunus Serotina

Black Cohosh
See Cimicifuga Racemosa

Black Elder
See Sambuscus Nigra

Black Haw
See Viburnum Prunifolium

Black Hellebore
See Helleborus Niger

Black Mulberry
See Morus Nigra

Black Mustard
See Brassica Nigra

Black Nightshade
See Solanum Nigrum

Black Pepper
See Piper Nigrum

Black Root
See Leptandra Virginica

Blackberry
See Rubus Fruticosus

Blackcurrant

See Ribes Nigrum

Blackthorn

See Prunus Spinosa

Bladderwort

See Utricularia Vulgaris

Bladderwrack

See Fucus Vesiculosus

Bloodroot

See Sanguinaria Canadensis

Blue Cohosh

See Caulophyllum Thalictroides

Bog Bilberry

See Vaccinium Uliginosum

Boldo

See Peumus Boldo

Boneset

See Eupatorium Perfoliatum

Borage

See Borago Officinalis

Borago Officinalis

Borage

DESCRIPTION

Flower and Fruit: The flowers are in separate, terminal, erect, leafy racemes. The calyx is divided almost to the base into 5 rough-haired tips. The 1.5 to 2.5 cm wide corolla is sky blue, occasionally white and has a short tube. The scales of the tube are white. The 5 stamens have a broadened filament and a violet, spur-like appendage. The anthers are black-violet. The style is thread-like with a head-like stigma. The ovary is divided into 4 valves. The small nut is elonagte-ovate, about 7 to 10 mm long, light brown, keeled, ribbed, warty and rough.

Leaves, Stem and Root: Borage is an annual, succulent, bristly haired, herb, 15 to 60 cm high. The erect, vertically grooved stems are covered in rough, whitish hairs. The leaves are alternate, clasping, solitary, entire-margined and hairy. They are also folded, curved in at the margins, green above and whitish beneath. They are 3 to 10 cm long and elliptoid to ovate.

Characteristics: Borage has a cucumber-like taste.

Habitat: Originally indigenous to the Mediterranean region, now found all over Europe and the U.S.

Production: Borage oil is the fatty oil of the seeds of Borago officinalis. Borage leaves are the dried leaves and inflorescence of Borago officinalis. The herb is harvested during the flowering period. Due to the plant's very high water content it should be artificially dried at 40°C.

Not To Be Confused With: The herb can be confused with Echium vulgare.

Other Names: Burrage, Bugloss, Burage

ACTIONS AND PHARMACOLOGY

COMPOUNDS: BORAGINIS OLEUM

Fatty oil: chief fatty acid is gamma-linolenic acid (17-25%), linoleic acid

EFFECTS: BORAGINIS OLEUM

The drug acts as an astringent and as a sequestering agent.

COMPOUNDS: BORAGINIS HERBA

Pyrrolizidine alkaloids: supinin, lycopsamin, 7-acetyl-lycopsamin, intermedin, 7-acetyl- intermedin

Silicic acid: to some extent water-soluble

Mucilages

Tannins

EFFECTS: BORAGINIS HERBA

Tannins have an astringent effect. Mucilage acts as sequestering agent.

INDICATIONS AND USAGE

BORAGINIS OLEUM

The oil is used for neurodermatitis and as a food supplement.

BORAGINIS HERBA

In folk medicine, Borage is used as a sequestering and mucilaginous agent for coughs and throat illnesses. It is also used as an anti-inflammatory agent for kidney and bladder disorders, as an astringent and as a substance for treating rheumatism. Preparations using Borage are also used for blood purification and dehydration, for the prevention of chest and peritoneal inflammation, rheumatism of the joints, as a pain-relieving, cardiotonic, sedative, sudorific and performance-enhancing agent, as well as for phlebitis and menopausal complaints. Borage is also used as a bronchial treatment.

Efficacy has not been proven.

PRECAUTIONS AND ADVERSE REACTIONS

BORAGINIS OLEUM

No health hazards or side effects are known in conjunction with the proper administration of designated therapeutic dosages.

BORAGINIS HERBA

Because of the hepatotoxic and hepatocarcinogenic pyrrolizidine alkaloid content, though small, the drug should not be administered.

DOSAGE

BORAGINIS OLEUM

Mode of Administration: In combination with vitamins as capsules.

BORAGINIS HERBA

Storage: The drug should be protected from light and moisture.

LITERATURE

BORAGINIS OLEUM

Fell KR, Peck JM, (1968) Planta Med 4: 411.

Ippen H, Gamma-Linolensäure besser aus Nachtkerzen- oder aus Borretschöl? In: ZPT 16(3):167-170. 1995.

Luthy J et al., (1984) Pharm Acta Helv 59 (9/10): 242.

Further information in:

Hänsel R, Keller K, Rimpler H, Schneider G (Hrsg.), Hagers Handbuch der Pharmazeutischen Praxis, 5. Aufl., Bde 4-6 (Drogen), Springer Verlag Berlin, Heidelberg, New York, 1992-1994.

BORAGINIS HERBA

Dodson CD, Stermitz FR, JNP 49(4):727-728. 1986.

Larson KM, Stermitz FR, JNP 47(4):747-748. 1984.

Röder E, Pyrrolizidinhaltige Arzneipflanzen. In: DAZ 132(45):2427-2435. 1992.

Further information in:

Frohne D, Pfänder HJ, Giftpflanzen - Ein Handbuch für Apotheker, Toxikologen und Biologen, 4. Aufl., Wiss. Verlags-Ges Stuttgart 1997.

Hänsel R, Keller K, Rimpler H, Schneider G (Hrsg.), Hagers Handbuch der Pharmazeutischen Praxis, 5. Aufl., Bde 4-6 (Drogen), Springer Verlag Berlin, Heidelberg, New York, 1992-1994.

Teuscher E, Lindequist U, Biogene Gifte - Biologie, Chemie, Pharmakologie, 2. Aufl., Fischer Verlag Stuttgart 1994.

Boswellia Carteri

Frankincense

DESCRIPTION

Medicinal Parts: The medicinal parts are the bark and trunk of the plant.

Flower and Fruit: The flowers are solitary and of a white or pale-white hue. The fruit is a capsule divided into 3 parts with a seed in each section.

Leaves, Stem and Root: Boswellia carteri is a richly foliated tree whose leaves alternate on the branches to the tips. It grows on few roots, which appear to be fused with the stony soil via an inert mass.

Habitat: Somalia, parts of Saudi Arabia.

Production: (Indian) Frankincense or Olibanum is the hardened gum resin of Boswellia carteri, which exudes when incisions are made in the trunk.

Other Names: Olibanum

ACTIONS AND PHARMACOLOGY

COMPOUNDS

Volatile oil (5-9%): chief components are pinene, dipentene, phellandrene

Resins (60%): components including, among others, alpha-boswellic acid, 3-acetyl-β-boswellic acid

Mucilages (12%)

EFFECTS

Externally, Frankincense can cause mild irritation of the skin. Internally, it is a mild carminative.

INDICATIONS AND USAGE

Obsolete as a drug.

In traditional Indian medicine, Indian Frankincense is used to treat chronic rheumatic inflammation. The black kohl powder with which Egyptian women paint their eyelids is traditionally made from charred Frankincense. It is also the ingredient of a perfumed hand paste.

PRECAUTIONS AND ADVERSE REACTIONS

No health hazards or side effects are known in conjunction with the proper administration of designated therapeutic dosages.

DOSAGE

Preparation: The Frankincense resin is obtained by tapping the bark, leaving the exudate for about three months during which time it hardens slightly, allowing the resin to be collected.

LITERATURE

Ammon HPT, Entzündliche Darmerkrankungen: Weihrauch bei Colitis ulcerosa, siehe auch folgenden Artikel. In: DAZ 137(3):125. 1997.

Ammon HPT, Hemmstoffe der Leukotrienbiosynthese. In: DAZ 137(3):139-40. 1997.

Ammon HPT, Weihrauch - ein neuer Weg in der Therapie der Entzündungen. In: DAZ 132(45).2442. 1991.

Ammon S, Ein pflanzliches Antirheumaticum. In: DAZ 131(19):972. 1991.

Ammon T, Lipoxygenasehemmer aus Weihrauch. In: DAZ 133(37):3295. 1993.

Anonym, Weihrauchtherapie. In: DAZ 134(4):324-325. 1995.

Hoernlein RF et al., Die Hemmung der 5-Lipoxygnesae durch Acetyl-11-keto-β-Boswelliasäure (AKBA): Struktur-Wirkungsbeziehungen. In: 8. Frühjahrstagung der DPhG, Salzau, Abstracts, in PUZ 25(3):140. 1996.

Kreymeier J, Rheumatherapie mit Phytopharmaka. In: DAZ 137(8):611-613. 1997.

Martinetz D, Der Indische Weihrauch - neue Aspekte eines alten Harzes. In: ZPT 13(4):121. 1992.

Müller-Bohn T, Chemie und Pharmakologie des Weihrauchs: Boswelliasäuren gegen chronische Polyarthritis und Colitis ulcerosa. In: DAZ 136(48):4324-4325. 1996.

Pfister-Hotz G, Phytotherapie in der Geriatrie. In: ZPT 18(3):165-162. 1997.

Rall B et al., Boswellic acids and protease activity (s.auch folgende Abstracts). In: PM 61(Abstracts of 43rd Ann Congr):105. 1995.

Wasielewski S, Maligne G, Weihrauchextrakt bei bösartigen Hirntumoren. In: DAZ 137(26):2250-2251. 1997.

Further information in:

Kern W, List PH, Hörhammer L (Hrsg.), Hagers Handbuch der Pharmazeutischen Praxis, 4. Aufl., Bde. 1-8, Springer Verlag Berlin, Heidelberg, New York, 1969.

Madaus G, Lehrbuch der Biologischen Arzneimittel, Bde 1-3, Nachdruck, Georg Olms Verlag Hildesheim 1979.

Wagner H, Wiesenauer M, Phytotherapie. Phytopharmaka und pflanzliche Homöopathika, Fischer-Verlag, Stuttgart, Jena, New York 1995.

Boxwood

See Buxus Sempervirens

Brassica Nigra

Black Mustard

DESCRIPTION

Flower and Fruit: The inflorescences are terminal or axillary and compressed into a semi-sphere. The flowers have 4 free sepals and 4 free petals, 6 stamens and 1 ovary. The sepals are 3.5 to 4.5 mm long and appear linear because of slits on the edge. They are yellow-green, usually glabrous, upright and slightly splayed. The yellow petals are twice as long as the calyx, obovate, rounded at the tip and narrowed to a stem at the base. The ovary is on the receptacle. The style is thin and has a semi-globose, cushion-like stigma. The fruit is an erect pod, which is linear and rounded or angular with a thin dividing wall. It is 10 to 25 mm long and pressed onto the stem. The seed is globose, brown, matte and punctate.

Leaves, Stem and Root: Black Mustard is an annual, tall-growing, slim-branched plant with thin fusiform roots. The stem grows up to 1 m. It is almost round and bristly-haired at the base, with a bluish bloom towards the top. It is glabrous with upright branches almost in bushels. The leaves are petiolate, up to 12 cm long and 5 cm wide. The lower ones are grass-green and are covered in 1 mm long bristles. They are pinnatifid with 2 to 4 obtuse lobes on each side and a large end section and are densely dentate. The upper stem and branch leaves are smaller, usually glabrous and blue-green, ovate or lanceolate and slightly dentate.

Habitat: Distributed worldwide in all temperate regions.

Production: Mustard seeds are the seeds of Brassica nigra.

ACTIONS AND PHARMACOLOGY

COMPOUNDS

Glucosinolates: chiefly sinigrin (allylglucosinolates, 1-5%), grinding the seeds into powder and then rubbing with warm water (not with hot water - enzymes would be destroyed), as well as chewing, releases the volatile mustard oil allylisothiocyanate

Fatty oil (30-35%)

Proteins (40%)

Phenyl propane derivatives: including, among others, sinapine (choline ester of sinapic acid, 1%)

EFFECTS

The enzymatic volatile oil allyisothcyanate is produced from sinigrin. This causes a stabbing pain and an intense reddening of the skin. Upon contact with the skin, Allylsen oil causes the severity of the inflammation to increase, to the extent were blisters and necrosis are possible.

INDICATIONS AND USAGE

Externally: in bronchial pneumonia and pleurisy (mustard poultice). As antirheumatic (mustard spirit 2%).

CONTRAINDICATIONS

Gastrointestinal ulcers and inflammatory kidney diseases.

PRECAUTIONS AND ADVERSE REACTIONS

General: No health hazards or side effects are known in conjunction with the proper administration of designated therapeutic dosages. Gastrointestinal complaints (and, rarely, kidney irritation) could occur following internal administration, due to the mucus-membrane-irritating effect of the mustard oil. The drug possesses minimal potential for sensitization; contact allergies have been observed. The draining effect associated with the drug's administration makes it inadvisable in the presence of varicosis and venous disorder. Sneezing, coughing and possible asthmatic attacks can result from breathing the allylisothiocyanate that arises with the preparation and application of mustard poultices. The vapors lead to signs of irritation in the eyes. Long-term external application or too-intensive reactions upon the skin can lead to injury (blister formation, suppurating ulcerations, necroses). Mustard poultices are to be removed after no more than 30 minutes.

Pediatric Use: No administration to children under 6 years of age.

OVERDOSAGE

Overdosage can lead to vomiting, stomach pain, diarrhea, in severe cases to somnolence, cardiac weakness and breathing difficulties, even to death through coma. Following installation of activated charcoal and shock prophylaxis (suitable body position, quiet, warmth), the therapy for poisonings consists of administering mucilaginosa for the protection of mucus membranes, generous amounts of fluids and treating possible cases of acidosis with sodium bicarbonate infusions. In case of shock, plasma volume expanders should be infused. Cardiac massage, intubation and oxygen respiration may also be necessary.

DOSAGE

Mode of Administration: Used externally as a mustard plaster. On rare occasions used as constituent in antirheumatic preparations and cardiac ointments.

Preparation: To prepare a mustard poultice, use approximately 100 g mustard flour and mix with lukewarm water, pack in linen.

Daily Dose: The poultice is placed on the chest for about 10 minutes (with a maximum of 3 to 5 minutes for children).

LITERATURE

Halva S et al., Agric Sci Finl 58:157. 1986.

Hill CB et al., J Am Soc Hort Sci 112(2):309. 1987.

Further information in:

Hänsel R, Keller K, Rimpler H, Schneider G (Hrsg.), Hagers Handbuch der Pharmazeutischen Praxis, 5. Aufl., Bde 4-6 (Drogen): Springer Verlag Berlin, Heidelberg, New York, 1992-1994.

Leung AY, Encyclopedia of Common Natural Ingredients Used in Food Drugs, Cosmetics, John Wiley & Sons Inc., New York 1980.

Madaus G, Lehrbuch der Biologischen Arzneimittel, Bde 1-3, Nachdruck, Georg Olms Verlag Hildesheim 1979.

Roth L, Daunderer M, Kormann K, Giftpflanzen, Pflanzengifte, 4. Aufl., Ecomed Fachverlag Landsberg Lech 1993.

Steinegger E, Hänsel R, Pharmakognosie, 5. Aufl., Springer Verlag Heidelberg 1992.

Teuscher E, Lindequist U, Biogene Gifte - Biologie, Chemie, Pharmakologie, 2. Aufl., Fischer Verlag Stuttgart 1994.

Teuscher E, Biogene Arzneimittel, 5. Aufl., Wiss. Verlagsges. Stuttgart 1997.

Wichtl M (Hrsg.), Teedrogen, 4. Aufl., Wiss. Verlagsges. Stuttgart 1997.

Brassica Oleracea Var. Capitata

Cabbage

DESCRIPTION

Flower and Fruit: The inflorescences have long-pedicled flowers. The flowers are large and have 4 erect, narrowly elliptoid sepals 6 to 12 mm long. The 4 petals are about twice as long as the calyx and are sulphur yellow. The margin broadens at the tip and narrows at the base to an equally long wedge-shaped funicle stem. The stamens are erect and close to the ovary. The central honey gland is almost erect. The fruit is oblong, pod-like, almost cylindrical and has a domed lid. The dividing wall of the fruit is thin as well as being pitted and folded between the seeds, which have a diameter of 1.5 to 4 mm and are dark brown.

Leaves, Stem and Root: The plant can be annual, biennial or perennial. It is about 2 m high and has thin roots. The stem is woody from the first year and is covered in leaf nodes. It has a bluish bloom and is branched towards the top. The leaves are fleshy, blue-green and glabrous. The lower ones are petiolate, lyre-shaped, pinnatifid or simple. The upper leaves are oblong to linear-oblong, usually entire-margined and narrowed to rounded at the base and sessile.

Habitat: Originally from the Mediterranean region. Today wild cabbage grows as far as southern England and Helgoland. Cultivated varieties are found in temperate and damp climates worldwide.

Production: White cabbage juice is the juice of Brassica oleracea var. capitata f. alba.

Other Names: Colewort

ACTIONS AND PHARMACOLOGY

COMPOUNDS

Mustard oils (breakdown products of the glucosinolates accompanying cell destruction): allyl mustard oil, methyl sulfinyl alkyl isothiocyanates, methyl sulfonyl alkyl isothiocyanates

3-hydroxy-methyl-indole

5-vinyl-oxazolidine-2-thion (goitrin)

Rhodanides

Alkyl nitriles

Amino acids: including S-methyl cysteine sulphoxide, S-methyl methionine sulphoxide when extracted from red cabbage, also anthocyans, including cyanidine-5-glucoside-3-sophoroside

EFFECTS

Cabbage protects the mucous membrane of the stomach from gastric hydrochloric acid.

INDICATIONS AND USAGE

Roemheld syndrome, gastritis, gastric and duodenal ulcers, gastralgia, subacidity. Contained in homeopathic preparations.

PRECAUTIONS AND ADVERSE REACTIONS

No health hazards or side effects are known in conjunction with the proper administration of designated therapeutic dosages.

DOSAGE

Mode of Administration: As a standard preparation or prepared from chopped and pressed Cabbage for internal use. Also available in homeopathic preparations.

Daily Dose: To augment a bland diet take 1 liter of juice daily as a dietary additive.

For gastralgia and subacidity, the dose is 1 teaspoonful to be taken before meals, 3 times daily.

LITERATURE

Josefsson E, PH 6:1617-1627. 1967.

Kaoulla N et al., PH 19:1053-1056. 1980.

Larson KM, Stermitz FR, JNP 47(4):747-748. 1984.

Petroski RJ, Tookey HL, PH21:1903-1905. 1982.

Slominski BA, Campbell LD, J Agric Food Chem 37:1297-1302. 1989.

Further information in:

Hänsel R, Keller K, Rimpler H, Schneider G (Hrsg.), Hagers Handbuch der Pharmazeutischen Praxis, 5. Aufl., Bde 4-6 (Drogen), Springer Verlag Berlin, Heidelberg, New York, 1992-1994.

Kern W, List PH, Hörhammer L (Hrsg.), Hagers Handbuch der Pharmazeutischen Praxis, 4. Aufl., Bde. 1-8, Springer Verlag Berlin, Heidelberg, New York, 1969.

Teuscher E, Lindequist U, Biogene Gifte - Biologie, Chemie, Pharmakologie, 2. Aufl., Fischer Verlag Stuttgart 1994.

Brewer's Yeast

See Saccharomyces Cerevisiae

Broad Bean

See Vicia Faba

Brooklime

See Veronica Beccabunga

Broom

See Cytisus Scoparius

Broom Corn

See Sorghum Vulgare

Brunfelsia Hopeana

Manaca

DESCRIPTION

Medicinal Parts: The medicinal parts are the roots and stem.

Flower and Fruit: The flowers are large, conical and very fragrant. They are blue or white. The calyx is divided into 5, with rounded lobes and 2 lips covering the bud. There are 4 fertile anthers, which fuse together above where they divide into 2 stigma-like lobes. The fruit is a fleshy or leathery capsule with numerous large seeds embedded in it.

Leaves, Stem and Root: Manaca is a shrub with obovate deciduous leaves. The roots are about 1.5 cm in diameter and are very woody and tough. They are yellow in the center and have a papery, pale brown epidermis. The stems have a small yellow medulla.

Habitat: South America, West Indies, Brazil.

Production: Manaca root is the root of Brunfelsia hopeana.

Other Names: Pohl, Vegetable Mercury

ACTIONS AND PHARMACOLOGY

COMPOUNDS

The active ingredients of the drug have not yet been adequately investigated. The spasmogenic brunfelsamidine (pyrrole-3-carboxamidine, identical with Nierembergia toxin) has been demonstrated in the related species Brunfelsia grandiflora.

EFFECTS

Diuretic and antirheumatic.

INDICATIONS AND USAGE

Manaca is used in the treatment of rheumatic conditions.

PRECAUTIONS AND ADVERSE REACTIONS

No health hazards or side effects are known in conjunction with the proper administration of designated therapeutic dosages. In animal experiments, anxiety states, restlessness, increase in cardiac and pulmonary frequency, elevated salivation, vomiting, muscle tremors, and tonic-clonic spasms were observed following intake of plant parts of Brunfelsia-species, as well as death.

DOSAGE

Mode of Administration: Liquid extract.

LITERATURE

Lloyd HA et al., Brunfeslamidine: A novel convulsant from the medicinal plant Brunfelsia grandiflora. In: Tetrahedron Letters 26(22):2623-2624. 1985.

Further information in:

Frohne D, Pfänder HJ, Giftpflanzen - Ein Handbuch für Apotheker, Toxikologen und Biologen, 4. Aufl., Wiss. Verlags-Ges Stuttgart 1997.

Kern W, List PH, Hörhammer L (Hrsg.), Hagers Handbuch der Pharmazeutischen Praxis, 4. Aufl., Bde. 1-8, Springer Verlag Berlin, Heidelberg, New York, 1969.

Roth L, Daunderer M, Kormann K, Giftpflanzen, Pflanzengifte, 4. Aufl., Ecomed Fachverlag Landsberg Lech 1993.

Bryonia Alba

White Bryony

DESCRIPTION

Medicinal Parts: The medicinal part is the root.

Flower and Fruit: The plant is monoecious, occasionally dioecious. The male flowers are in long-peduncled racemes, which are 10 to 12 mm wide and shed easily. The female flowers are in short-stemmed umbel-like clusters. The sepals are almost as long as the corolla. The 5 petaled corolla is yellowish white and has green veins. The 3 styles are almost completely free. The stigmas are glabrous. There are 2 fused, inferior, 3-valved ovaries. The fruit is a 1 to 2-seeded, thin-skinned, 7 to 8 mm thick, globose black berry.

Leaves, Stem and Root: White Bryony is a perennial, extremely fast-growing plant. It has a thick, up 2.5 kg, tuberous root. The root is fleshy, wrinkled horizontally, yellowish-gray on the outside and white and slimy on the inside. The grooved, angular stems are climbing, branched and have long internodes and simple screw-like climbers. They grow up to 4 m long. The leaves are short-petioled, broadly cordate, pentagonal to 5-lobed and covered with short bristles on both sides.

Characteristics: The root is bitter and spicy. The plant is categorized as extremely poisonous.

Habitat: Indigenous to eastern and southeastern Europe as far as Iran.

Production: Bryonia root consists of the dried taproot of Bryonia alba.

Other Names: Tetterberry, Wild Hops, Wild Vine, Wood Vine, English Mandrake, Devil's Turnip, Wild Nep, Tamus, Ladies's Seal

ACTIONS AND PHARMACOLOGY

COMPOUNDS

Cucurbitacins: including cucurbitacins B, D, E, I, J, K, L, 23,24-dihydro-cucurbitacins, 1,2,23,24-tetrahydrocucurbitacins, 22-deoxycucurbitacins

Cucurbitacin glycosides

Triterpenes with unusual structure

Sterols with unusual structure

Polyhydroxy fatty acids: including 9,12,13-Trihydroxy-octadeca-10(E)-15(Z)-dienic acid.

Lectins

EFFECTS
Various aqueous extracts of the drug display an antitumoral effect. The resin is a drastic purgative. The methanol extracts have a strong hypoglycemic affect.

INDICATIONS AND USAGE

Bryonia root is used as a laxative, emetic and diuretic in the treatment of various disorders of the gastrointestinal tract and respiratory tract and for rheumatic disorders. It is also prophylacticaly and therapeutically for metabolic disorders, liver disease, acute and chronic infectious disease.

PRECAUTIONS AND ADVERSE REACTIONS

The drug is highly toxic when freshly-harvested. The toxicity of the drug declines rapidly with dehydration and in storage, because of the instability of the cucurbitacins. Due to the cucurbitacin content, the drug has a severely irritating effect on skin and mucuous membranes. Contact between skin and the juice of the plant can lead to rash, infection, blister formation and necroses.

OVERDOSAGE

The intake of toxic dosages can lead to vomiting, bloody diarrhea, colic, kidney irritation, anuria, collapse, spasms, paralysis, and under certain conditions, to death.

Following gastric lavage, the treatment for poisonings should proceed symptomatically. 40 berries are presumed fatal for an adult, 15 for a child.

DOSAGE

Mode of Administration: Since the efficacy of Bryonia preparations for the claimed applications is not documented, and since the use of it as a drastic laxative and emetic is obsolete, a therapeutic administration cannot be justified because of the risks involved.

Bryonia is found occasionally in some pharmaceutical preparations.

Preparation: A decoction is prepared by adding 0.5 to 1 g drug to 1 cup water.

Daily Dose: Dosage of the powder is 0.3 to 0.5 g as an emetic and purgative.

LITERATURE

Hylands PJ, Mansour ESS, PH 21(11):2703-2707. 1982.

Konopa J et al., (1974) Arzneim Forsch 24(10), 1554.

Oobayashi K, Yoshikawa K, Arihara S, Structural revision of Bryonoside and structure elucidation of minor saponins from Bryonia dioica. In: PH 31:943-946. 1992.

Panossian AG et al., (1983) Planta Med 47(1), 17-25.

Pohlmann J, The cucurbitacins in Bryonia alba and Bryonia dioica. In: PH 14(7):1587-1589. 1980.

Suganda AG et al., (1983) J Nat Prod 46(5), 626.

Vartanian GS et al., (1984) Byull Eksp Biol Med 97(3), 295.

Further information in:

Frohne D, Pfänder HJ, Giftpflanzen - Ein Handbuch für Apotheker, Toxikologen und Biologen, 4. Aufl., Wiss. Verlags-Ges Stuttgart 1997.

Hänsel R, Keller K, Rimpler H, Schneider G (Hrsg.), Hagers Handbuch der Pharmazeutischen Praxis, 5. Aufl., Bde 4-6 (Drogen), Springer Verlag Berlin, Heidelberg, New York, 1992-1994.

Lewin L, Gifte und Vergiftungen, 6. Aufl., Nachdruck, Haug Verlag, Heidelberg 1992.

Madaus G, Lehrbuch der Biologischen Arzneimittel, Bde 1-3, Nachdruck, Georg Olms Verlag Hildesheim 1979.

Roth L, Daunderer M, Kormann K, Giftpflanzen, Pflanzengifte, 4. Aufl., Ecomed Fachverlag Landsberg Lech 1993.

Steinegger E, Hänsel R, Pharmakognosie, 5. Aufl., Springer Verlag Heidelberg 1992.

Teuscher E, Lindequist U, Biogene Gifte - Biologie, Chemie, Pharmakologie, 2. Aufl., Fischer Verlag Stuttgart 1994.

Teuscher E, Biogene Arzneimittel, 5. Aufl., Wiss. Verlagsges. Stuttgart 1997.

Wagner H, Wiesenauer M, Phytotherapie. Phytopharmaka und pflanzliche Homöopathika, Fischer-Verlag, Stuttgart, Jena, New York 1995.

Buchu

See Barosma Species

Buck Bean

See Menyanthes Trifoliata

Buckthorn

See Rhamnus Cathartica

Buckthorn Bark

See Rhamnus Frangula

Buckwheat

See Fagopyrum Esculentum

Bugle

See Ajuga Reptans

Bugleweed

See Lycopus Virginicus

Bulbous Buttercup

See Ranunculus Bulbosus

Burdock

See Arctium Lappa

Burnet Saxifrage

See Pimpinella Major

Burning Bush

See Dictamnus Albus

Burr Marigold

See Bidens Tripartita

Butcher's Broom

See Ruscus Aculeatus

Buttercup

See Ranunculus Acris

Butternut

See Juglans Cinerea

Buxus Sempervirens

Boxwood

DESCRIPTION

Medicinal Parts: The leaves are the medicinal part.

Flower and Fruit: Clusters of axillary yellow flowers open in early spring. The male flowers are evenly shaped and have 4 tepals, 4 stamens and a small rudimentary ovary. The female flowers have 4 to 8 tepals, 3 fused carpels with 3 free, short, thick styles. The fruit is a capsule with oblong, 5 to 6 mm long seeds.

Leaves, Stem and Root: Boxwood is an evergreen monoecious shrub or tree growing to a height of 6 m with variable form and leaf shape. The green branches are initially pubescent, later glabrous, olive green, angular and densely covered with ovate leaves which are usually opposite. The upper surface of the leaves is smooth, coriaceous, dark green and very glossy. The lower surface is lighter in shade and the lamina margin is smooth.

Characteristics: The leaves have a nauseous taste.

Habitat: The plant is found mainly in southern and central Europe with a clear division into an east and west regions, i.e., northwest Spain and southern France in the west and the Balkans to northern Greece and Asia minor in the east. It is otherwise extensively cultivated.

Production: Boxwood leaves are the leaves of Buxus sempervirens.

Other Names: Dudgeon, Bush Tree

ACTIONS AND PHARMACOLOGY

COMPOUNDS

Steroid alkaloids

EFFECTS

No information available.

INDICATIONS AND USAGE

Formerly used as a blood purifier and in the treatment of rheumatic conditions.

PRECAUTIONS AND ADVERSE REACTIONS

No health hazards or side effects are known in conjunction with the proper administration of designated therapeutic dosages. Contact dermatitis, in particular through contact with the freshly-harvested plant, are possible.

OVERDOSAGE

The intake of toxic dosages of the drug leads to vomiting, diarrhea, severe clonic spasms, eventually to signs of paralysis and ultimately to fatal asphyxiation. The fatal dosage in dogs is 0.1 g of the alkaloid mixture/kg body weight (approximately 5 to 10 g of the drug/kg body weight). The treatment for poisonings proceeds through suppression of the spasms with diazepam or barbiturates (no more than absolutely necessary) followed by gastric lavage, and possible oxygen respiration. Phenothiazines and analeptics are not to be administered.

DOSAGE

Mode of Administration: Boxwood is obsolete as a drug.

LITERATURE

Atta-ur-Rahman et al., Alkaloids from Buxus species. In: PH 31(8):2933-2935. 1992.

Atta-ur-Rahman et al., New alkaloids from Buxus sempervirens. In: JNP 52:1319-1322. 1989.

Atta-ur-Rahman et al., Steroidal alkaloids from leaves of Buxus sempervirens. In: PH 30(4):1295-1298. 1991.

Khodshaev BU et al., (1984) Khim Prir Soedin 6:802.

Willaman JJ, Hui-Li L, (1970) Lloydia 33(3A):1.

Further information in:

Frohne D, Pfänder HJ, Giftpflanzen - Ein Handbuch für Apotheker, Toxikologen und Biologen, 4. Aufl., Wiss. Verlags-Ges Stuttgart 1997.

Hänsel R, Keller K, Rimpler H, Schneider G (Hrsg.), Hagers Handbuch der Pharmazeutischen Praxis, 5. Aufl., Bde 4-6 (Drogen), Springer Verlag Berlin, Heidelberg, New York, 1992-1994.

Lewin L, Gifte und Vergiftungen, 6. Aufl., Nachdruck, Haug Verlag, Heidelberg 1992.

Roth L, Daunderer M, Kormann K, Giftpflanzen, Pflanzengifte, 4. Aufl., Ecomed Fachverlag Landsberg Lech 1993.

Teuscher E, Lindequist U, Biogene Gifte - Biologie, Chemie, Pharmakologie, 2. Aufl., Fischer Verlag Stuttgart 1994.

Cabbage

See Brassica Oleracea Var. Capitata

Caesalpinia Bonducella

Divi-Divi

DESCRIPTION

Flower and Fruit: The flowers are dorsiventrally zygomorphous in dense clusters. The sepals are free or fused at their base, or fused to the base of the petals or stamens to form the corolla. The petals are separate from each other but have an ascending bud covering. There are twice as many stamens as petals, usually 10. The ovary always has only 1 carpel. The fruit is indehiscent or a legume with yellow nuts.

Leaves, Stem and Root: Divi-Divi is a tree or shrub, which grows to a height of 9 m with alternate entire-margined or double-pinnate thorny leaves.

Habitat: Sri Lanka, Brasil, South America.

Production: Nikkar nuts are the seeds of Caesalpinia bonducella.

Other Names: Nikkar Nuts, Nichol Seeds

ACTIONS AND PHARMACOLOGY

COMPOUNDS

Fatty oil: chief fatty acids are linoleic acid, oleic acid, palmitic acid, stearic acid

Proteins

Starch

Diterpenes: including, among others, alpha-, beta-, gamma-, eta-caesalpine

Saponins

EFFECTS

Divi-Divi is a febrifuge and tonic.

INDICATIONS AND USAGE

Febrile illnesses. The roasted seeds are also used in the treatment of diabetes.

PRECAUTIONS AND ADVERSE REACTIONS

No health hazards or side effects are known in conjunction with the proper administration of designated therapeutic dosages.

DOSAGE

Mode of Administration: Seed ground and roasted for internal use.

LITERATURE

Balmain et al., Tetrahedron 1967:5027. 1967.

Further information in:

Hoppe HA, (1975-1987) Drogenkunde, 8. Aufl., Bde 1-3, W. de Gruyter Verlag, Berlin, New York.

Kern W, List PH, Hörhammer L (Hrsg.), Hagers Handbuch der Pharmazeutischen Praxis, 4. Aufl., Bde 1-8, Springer Verlag Berlin, Heidelberg, New York, 1969.

Cajuput

See Melaleuca Leucadendron

Calabar Bean

See Physostigma Venenosum

Calamint

See Calamintha Ascendens

Calamintha Ascendens

Calamint

DESCRIPTION

Flower and Fruit: The medium-sized to large flowers are 5 to 20 blossomed cymes. The pedicle is 0 to 22 mm long and the tubular calyx is 3 to 7 mm by 1 to 1.5 mm in size and slightly downy to very downy on the inside. The upper tips are 0.5 to 1.5 mm and the lower ones are 1 to 2 mm, downy, and occasionally have long ciliate hairs. The corolla is white to lilac and purple.

Leaves, Stem and Root: Calamint is a perennial, 30 to 80 cm high, slightly to densely downy shrub. The leaves are oval, obtuse, almost entire-margined or lightly to deeply crenate-serrate, with 9 teeth on each side.

Habitat: Britain, Europe, northern Africa.

Production: Calamint is the above-ground part of Calamintha ascendens.

Other Names: Basil Thyme, Mountain Mint, Mountain Balm, Mill Mountain

ACTIONS AND PHARMACOLOGY

COMPOUNDS

Volatile oil: including pulegone, menthone, menthol and its ester, β-bisobolen, cineol, thymol

Triterpenes: including calaminthadiol, ursolic acid

EFFECTS

Diaphoretic and expectorant.

INDICATIONS AND USAGE

Febrile colds and respiratory diseases.

PRECAUTIONS AND ADVERSE REACTIONS

No health hazards or side effects are known in conjunction with the proper administration of designated therapeutic dosages.

DOSAGE

No information is available.

LITERATURE

Kokkalo E, Stefanaou E, Flavour Fragrance J 5(1):23-26. 1990.

de Pooter HL, Goetghebeur P. Schamp P, PH 26(12):3355-3356. 1987.

Further information in:

Hänsel R, Keller K, Rimpler H, Schneider G (Hrsg.), Hagers Handbuch der Pharmazeutischen Praxis, 5. Aufl., Bde 4-6 (Drogen), Springer Verlag Berlin, Heidelberg, New York, 1992-1994.

Calamus

See Acorus Calamus

Calendula Officinalis

Marigold

DESCRIPTION

Flower and Fruit: On the tip of each stem there is a 5 to 7 cm composite flower head consisting of an epicalyx of numerous narrow-lanceolate sepals, which are densely covered on both sides with glandular hairs. The inner section of the flower head is made up of orange-yellow tubular florets. The disc florets are pseudohermaphrodites, the female sterile. The zygomorphic ray florets at the edge are female, their stamens are completely absent and their inferior ovaries are much more developed than those of the tubular florets. Fruit only form in the female ray flowers. The heterocarp achaens are sickle-shaped, curved and ringed.

Leaves, Stem and Root: The plant is usually an annual, seldom biennial. It grows to between 30 and 50 cm high and have a 20 cm long tap root and numerous thin, secondary roots. The stem is erect, angular, downy and branched from the base up or higher. The alternate leaves are almost spatulate at the base, oblong to lanceolate above and are all tomentose.

Characteristics: The plant has a strong, unpleasant smell.

Habitat: Central and southern, Europe, western Asia and the U.S.

Production: Marigold flowers are the ray florets of the completely unfolded, collected and dried capitula of Calendula officinalis. Harvest begins in July. Drying is carried out in the shade at a maximum of 45°C. Calendula herba consists of the fresh or dried above-ground parts of Calendula officinalis harvested during flowering season.

Not To Be Confused With: Other Asteraceae; arnica and saffron are often adulterated with marigold.

Other Names: Calendula, Holligold, Goldbloom, Golds, Mary Bud, Ruddes, Mary Gowles, Holigold, Marybud, Gold-bloom

ACTIONS AND PHARMACOLOGY

COMPOUNDS: CALENDULAE FLOS

Triterpene saponins: oleanolic acid mono- and diglycosides (triterpene mono-, di- and triole, mono- and diesters, mainly lauric, myristic and palmitic acids as acid components)

Flavonoids

Hydroxycoumarins: including umbelliferone, scopoletine

Carotinoids: chief components lutein, zeaxanthin

Sesquiterpene glycosides

Volatile oil

Water-soluble polysaccharides: rhamnoarabinogalactans, arabinogalactans

Polyynes

EFFECTS: CALENDULAE FLOS

The results of numerous studies are available. The flowers are antimicrobial, antifungal, antibacterial, antiviral, antiphlogistic and vulnerary. They stimulate the immune system, inhibit tumors, have an inhibitory effect on the CNS and are estrogenic, choleretic and hemolytic.

COMPOUNDS: CALENDULAE HERBA

Triterpene saponins

Flavonoids

Carotinoids

Volatile oil

EFFECTS: CALENDULAE HERBA

No information available.

INDICATIONS AND USAGE

CALENDULAE FLOS

- Inflammation of the mouth and pharynx
- Wounds and burns

Externally, Marigold is used for inflammation of the oral and pharyngeal mucosa, poorly healing wounds, Ulcus cruris, to clean wounds, enlarged and inflamed lymph glands, artheroma and acute and chronic skin inflammation. Marigold is very important in folk medicine where it is used externally for varicosis, phlebitis, thrombophlebitis, skin changes, wounds, furunculosis, anal eczema, proctitis, conjunctivitis, dry dermatosis, eczema, and acne. It is a constituent in treatments for dry skin, bee stings and frostbite.

Marigold is used internally in folk remedies for inflammatory conditions of internal organs, gastrointestinal ulcers, and dysmenorrhea. It is also used as a diuretic and diaphoretic in convulsions, fever and obstipation; as well as for liver disease, toothache, tired limbs, eye inflammation, as a cardiotonic, for worm infestation and formerly as a cancer therapy (no longer in use).

CALENDULAE HERBA

Preparations are used for circulation, ulcers, spasms, swelling of the glands, jaundice and for wounds and eczema. The herb is used in Russia for strep throat, on the Canaries for coughs and cramps and in China for irregular menstruation.

Efficacy in the claimed applications has not been demonstrated.

PRECAUTIONS AND ADVERSE REACTIONS

CALENDULAE FLOS ET HERBA

No health hazards or side effects are known in conjunction with the proper administration of designated therapeutic dosages. There is a low potential for sensitization through frequent skin contact with the drug.

DOSAGE

CALENDULAE FLOS

Mode of Administration: Comminuted drug for decoctions, and other preparations to be applied topically. It is available as tinctures, liquid extracts and infusions.

Preparation: An infusion for internal use is prepared using 1 to 2 g of drug to 1 cup water. For external use, a tincture (1:9) is prepared using a 20% alcohol/water mixture. An ointment is prepared by adding 2 to 5 g drug in 100 g ointment.

Daily Dose: Internally, the infusion is taken several times a day

Storage: Protected from light and moisture; maximum 3 years.

CALENDULAE HERBA

Mode of Administration: Since efficacy has not been proven the therapeutic value is uncertain.

Preparation: Contained in Kneipp's calendula ointment®.

LITERATURE

CALENDULAE FLOS

Ahmed AA et al., Sesquiterpene glycosides from Calendula officinalis. In: JNP 56(10):1821. 1993.

Antibiotika und Immunabwehr. In: Symbiose 4(2):20. 1992.

Della Loggia R et al., The Role of triterpenoids in the topical antiinflammatory activity of Calendula officinalis flowers. In: PM 60(6):516-520. 1994.

Della Logia R et al., The role of triterpenoids in the topological anti-inflammatory activity of Calendula officinalis flowers. In: PM 60(6):516-520. 1994.

Isaac O, Calendula officinalis L.- Die Ringelblume, Portrait einer Arzneipflanze. In: ZPT 15(6):357-370. 1994.

Isaac O, Die Ringelblume. Botanik, Chemie, Pharmakologie, Toxikologie, Pharmazie und therapeutsche Verwendung, Wissenschaftl. Verlagsges. mbH Stuttgart, 1992.

Kasprzyk Z, Pyrek J, (1968) Phytochemistry 7:1631.

Kasprzyk Z, Wilkomyrski B, (1973) Phytochemistry 13:2299.

Mennet-von Eiff M, Meier B, Phytotherapie in der Dermatologie. In: ZPT 16(4):201-210. 1995.

Pyrek J, (1977) Roczniki Chemii 51:1141:2331 et 2493.

Samochowiec E et al. (1979) Wiad Parazytol 25(1):77.

Vecherko LP et al., (1975) Khim Prir Soed 11(3):366.

Wilkomirski B, (1985) Phytochemistry 24(12):3067.

Willuhn G, Ringenblumenblüten (Calendulablüten). In: Tägl Praxis 33(3):685. 1992.

Further information in:

Hänsel R, Keller K, Rimpler H, Schneider G (Hrsg.), Hagers Handbuch der Pharmazeutischen Praxis, 5. Aufl., Bde 4-6 (Drogen), Springer Verlag Berlin, Heidelberg, New York, 1992-1994.

Hausen B, Allergiepflanzen, Pflanzenallergene, ecomed Verlagsgesellsch. mbH, Landsberg 1988.

Madaus G, Lehrbuch der Biologischen Arzneimittel, Bde 1-3, Nachdruck, Georg Olms Verlag Hildesheim 1979.

Steinegger E, Hänsel R, Pharmakognosie, 5. Aufl., Springer Verlag Heidelberg 1992.

Teuscher E, Biogene Arzneimittel, 5. Aufl., Wiss. Verlagsges. Stuttgart 1997.

Wagner H, Wiesenauer M, Phytotherapie. Phytopharmaka und pflanzliche Homöopathika, Fischer-Verlag, Stuttgart, Jena, New York 1995.

Wichtl M (Hrsg.), Teedrogen, 4. Aufl., Wiss. Verlagsges. Stuttgart 1997.

CALENDULAE HERBA

Isaac O, Die Ringelblume. Botanik, Chemie, Pharmakologie, Toxikologie, Pharmazie und therapeutsche Verwendung, Wissenschaftl. Verlagsges. mbH Stuttgart, 1992.

Kasprzyk Z, Pyrek J, (1968) Phytochemistry 7:1631.

Kasprzyk Z, Wilkomyrski B, (1973) Phytochemistry 13:2299.

Pyrek J, (1977) Roczniki Chemii 51:1141:2331 et 2493.

Samochowiec E et al., (1979) Wiad Parazytol 25(1):77.

Vecherko LP et al., (1975) Khim Prir Soed 11(3):366.

Wilkomirski B, (1985) Phytochemistry 24(12):3067.

Further information in:

Hänsel R, Keller K, Rimpler H, Schneider G (Hrsg.), Hagers Handbuch der Pharmazeutischen Praxis, 5. Aufl., Bde 4-6 (Drogen), Springer Verlag Berlin, Heidelberg, New York, 1992-1994.

Madaus G, Lehrbuch der Biologischen Arzneimittel, Bde 1-3, Nachdruck, Georg Olms Verlag Hildesheim 1979.

California Poppy

See Eschscholtzia Californica

Calluna Vulgaris

Heather

DESCRIPTION

Medicinal Parts: The medicinal parts are the complete herb with leaves, the flowers, and the growing shoots of the plant.

Flowers and Fruit: The inflorescence is turned to one side, dense, and hanging. The short-pedicled flowers are nodding, pale-violet-pink, occasionally white and have 4 small, oval, fringed bracts. The calyx has 4 violet-pink, glossy, and petaloid sepals, which have the consistency of straw. The 8 stamens form a brown-red club. The superior ovary has 4 sections and the style is larger than the calyx. The style has a thick, button-like 4-knobbed stigma. The fruit capsule is globose, 1.5 mm long and 4 sectioned. The fruit is covered in thick white bristles and is many-seeded. The dividing walls break off easily.

Leaves, Stem and Root: Calluna vulgaris is a dwarf shrub, 0.2 to 1 m high with decumbent, rooting shoots and ascending branches. The small stems are thin, gray-brown, heavily branched and have numerous upright branches. The leaves are linear-lanceolate, in groups of 4 rows. They are imbricate, 1 to 3.5 mm long, revolute, sessile and have 2 mm long points at the base. The margins are glandular with downward-pointing spurs.

Habitat: With the exception of a few Mediterranean islands the plant is distributed throughout most of Europe, Russia, and Asia minor as well as on the Atlantic coast of North America.

Production: The herb is harvested from July to October and dried.

Not To Be Confused With: Erica tetralix.

Other Names: Ling

ACTIONS AND PHARMACOLOGY

COMPOUNDS

Flavonoids: including kaempferol, quercetin, myricetin, taxifolin

(+)-catechin

Catechin tannins

Oligomere proanthocyanidins

Triterpenes: including ursolic acid

Steroids: beta-sitosterol

EFFECTS

Heather is said to be a diuretic, antimicrobial, cholagogic, antirheumatic, and vulnary.

These effects have not yet been documented.

INDICATIONS AND USAGE

Preparations of heather and/or heather flowers are used as a diuretic for diseases and ailments of the kidneys, the lower urinary tract and for enlargement of the prostate. They are also used for gastrointestinal disorders, colic, diarrhea, liver and gallbladder disease, gout, rheumatism, respiratory complaints, insomnia, agitation, and wounds.

The efficacy for the claimed uses is not documented.

PRECAUTIONS AND ADVERSE REACTIONS

No health hazards or side effects are known in conjunction with the proper administration of designated therapeutic dosages.

DOSAGE

Mode of Administration: Preparations are available for internal and external use.

Preparation: A decoction is prepared by adding 1.5 gm of the drug to 1/4 liter of water and then boiling for 3 minutes. For a bath additive, 500 gm of the drug is boiled in a few liters of water, strained, and added to the bath. A liquid extract 1:1 is also used.

Daily Dosage: The average daily dose of the decoction is 3 cups daily between meals; liquid extract, 1 to 2 teaspoonfuls daily.

Externally, the drug is used for full baths.

Storage: The drug should be stored in well dried, sealed containers.

LITERATURE

Jaläl MAF, Read DJ, Haslam E, Phenolic composition and its seasonal variation in Calluna vulgaris. In: PH 21(6):1397. 1982.

Mantilla JLG, Vieitez E, An Edafol Agrobiol 34:765-774. 1975.

Simon A et al., Further flavonoid glycosides from Calluna vulgaris. In: PH 32:1045. 1993.

Simon A et al., Two flavonol 3-[triacetylarabinosyl(1->6)glucosides] from Calluna vulgaris. In: PH 33:1237. 1993.

Further information in:

Hänsel R, Keller K, Rimpler H, Schneider G (Hrsg.), Hagers Handbuch der Pharmazeutischen Praxis, 5. Aufl., Bde 4-6 (Drogen): Springer Verlag Berlin, Heidelberg, New York, 1992-1994.

Madaus G, Lehrbuch der Biologischen Arzneimittel, Bde 1-3, Nachdruck, Georg Olms Verlag Hildesheim 1979.

Calotropis Procera

Calotropis

DESCRIPTION

Medicinal Parts: The bark with its outer cork layer removed is known as Mudar, and is the medicinal part.

Flower and Fruit: The fragrant flowers are 2.5 cm in diameter and form umbel-like flower clusters. The erect petals are whitish and have purple spots on the upper half. The bracts of the corolla are smooth or downy with a divided tip. The ovate folliclesare is 7.5 to 10 cm long by 5 to 7.5 cm wide. The seeds have a tuft of silky hair.

Leaves, Stem and Root: The upright herbacious perennial normally grows to a height of 1.8 to 2.4 m. The leaves are short-petioled, 6 to 15 cm long by 4.5 to 8 cm wide, oblong-elliptoid to broadly ovate. The bark occurs in irregular short pieces, slightly quilled or curved and about 0.3 - 0.5 cm thick. The external portion is grayish-yellow, soft and spongy. The internal portion is yellowish-white. The fracture is short.

Characteristics: The taste is acrid and bitter.

Habitat: Indigenous to parts of Asia, India, Africa, Pakistan and on the Sunda Islands.

Production: Calotropis bark are pieces of the dried root bark of Calotropis procera.

Other Names: Mudar Bark, Mudar Yercum

ACTIONS AND PHARMACOLOGY

COMPOUNDS

Cardioactive steroids (cardenolids)

EFFECTS

The cardenolid glycocides calotropine shows an antitumor effect in vitro on human epidermoid carcinoma cells of the rhinopharynx. It is also works as an expectorant and a diuretic.

INDICATIONS AND USAGE

The powdered root bark is used against dysentery. It has a similar effect to that of the ipecacuanha root. In Indian and African folk medicine, the bark is used to treat epilepsy, hysteria, cramps, cancer, warts, leprosy, elephantitis, worms, fever, gout, and snake bites. In particular, the milky juice is used against boils, ulcers, swellings, and rheumatism.

In Africa, it is used to treat toothache, syphilis, digestive disorders and diarrhea.

In India, the smoke (fumes) from the bark is used for coughs and asthma and as a sudorific.

The applications mentioned have yet to be proven.

PRECAUTIONS AND ADVERSE REACTIONS

No health hazards or side effects are known in conjunction with the proper administration of designated therapeutic dosages.

OVERDOSAGE

The drug is highly toxic. Higher dosages cause vomiting, diarrhea, bradycardia and convulsions. Very high dosages bring about death. Following gastric lavage, the treatment for poisonings proceed symptomatically (for further measures, see Digitalis folium).

DOSAGE

Mode of Administration: Calotropis is used in a ground form, as a powder, as smoke (fume) and also topically.

Daily Dosage: As an expectorant and diaphoretic 200 mg to 600 mg; as an emetic 2 g to 4 g.

LITERATURE

Seiber JN et al., (1982) Phytochemistry 21(9):2343.

Willaman JJ, Hui-Li L, (1970) Lloydia 33(3A):1.

Further information in:

Hänsel R, Keller K, Rimpler H, Schneider G (Hrsg.), Hagers Handbuch der Pharmazeutischen Praxis, 5. Aufl., Bde 4-6 (Drogen), Springer Verlag Berlin, Heidelberg, New York, 1992-1994.

Caltha Palustris

Marsh Marigold

DESCRIPTION

Medicinal Parts: The medicinal part is the dried aerial part of the flowering plant.

Flower and Fruit: The flowers are about 4 cm in diameter. The involucre is simple and has 5 or more yolk-yellow, 12 to 18 mm long ovate bracts, which are glossy greenish on the outside. There are numerous stamens and 5 to 8 ovaries. The fruit is a star-shaped follicle with a short beak. The seeds are dark brown to black, measuring about 2.5 cm long by 1.3 cm wide.

Leaves, Stem and Root: Caltha palustris is a 15 to 30 cm high perennial marsh plant with a sturdy, many headed rhizome. The glabrous, hollow stem is ascending or decumbent. The leaves are dark green and have an oily-glossy, cordate to reniform, crenate or serrate-margined leaf blade. The petioles are grooved. The cauline leaves have shorter petioles and are smaller, clasping, and often have a membranous leaf sheath.

Characteristics: The plant is classified as poisonous.

Habitat: Caltha palustris is distributed in all temperate regions of the Northern Hemisphere.

Other Names: Cowslip, Kingcups, Water Blobs, Horse Blobs, Bull's Eyes, Leopard's Foot, Meadow Routs, Verrucaria, Solsequia, Sponsa Solis, Palsy Root, Water Dragon

ACTIONS AND PHARMACOLOGY

COMPOUNDS

Protoanemonine-forming substances: in the freshly-harvested plant, presumably the glycoside ranunculin, that changes enzymatically when the plant is cut into small pieces, and probably also when it is dried, into the pungent, volatile protoanemonine that quickly dimerizes to anemonine; when dried, the plant is not capable of protoanemonine-formation

Triterpene saponins

Triterpene lactones: caltholid, palustrolid

Isoquinoline alkaloids (aporphine type, very small quantities): including corytuberin, magnoflorine, protopin

EFFECTS

The drug lowers cholesterol levels and raises blood sugar levels in rats subsequent to oral administration (according to unavailable Russian research). There are also reports of anti-inflammatory effects on formaldehyde-induced inflammation.

Insufficient information is available for an authoritative assessment of these effects.

INDICATIONS AND USAGE

In former times, marsh marigold application was used against jaundice, liver, and bilious complaints. Some native American tribes and those practicing Russian folk medicine used the plant for dressing and cleansing skin lesions and sores. When administered internally, it is meant to have a laxative and diuretic effect. The drug is still in use today to stop pain and cramps, for menstrual disorders, and bronchial catarrh.

PRECAUTIONS AND ADVERSE REACTIONS

No health hazards or side effects are known in conjunction with the proper administration of designated therapeutic dosages of the dehydrated drug.

Extended skin contact with the freshly-harvested, bruised plant can lead to blister formation and cauterizations that are difficult to heal due to the resulting protoanemonine, which is severely irritating to skin and mucous membranes.

OVERDOSAGE

If taken internally, large quantities can bring about severe irritation to the gastrointestinal tract, combined with colic and diarrhea, as well as with irritation of the urinary drainage passages.

Symptomatic treatment for external contact should consist of mucilage, after irrigation with diluted potassium permanganate solution; in case of internal contact, activated charcoal should follow gastric lavage. The dangers are less than with any of the other crowfoot family (Anemones nemorosae herba), due to the relatively low level of protoanemonine-forming substances in the plant.

LITERATURE

Bhandari P et al., Triterpenoid saponins from Caltha palsutris. In: PM 53(1):98-100. 1987.

Bhandari P et al., Two nortriterpene lactones from Caltha palustris. In: PH 23(8):1699- 1702. 1984.

Bonora A et al., PH 26:2277. 1987.

Bruni A et al., Protoanemonin detection in Caltha palustris. In: JNP 49(6):1172-1173. 1986.

Further information in:

Frohne D, Pfänder HJ, Giftpflanzen - Ein Handbuch für Apotheker, Toxikologen und Biologen, 4. Aufl., Wiss. Verlags-Ges Stuttgart 1997.

Hänsel R, Keller K, Rimpler H, Schneider G (Hrsg.), Hagers Handbuch der Pharmazeutischen Praxis, 5. Aufl., Bde 4-6 (Drogen): Springer Verlag Berlin, Heidelberg, New York, 1992-1994.

Lewin L, Gifte und Vergiftungen, 6. Aufl., Nachdruck, Haug Verlag, Heidelberg 1992.

Madaus G, Lehrbuch der Biologischen Arzneimittel, Bde 1-3, Nachdruck, Georg Olms Verlag Hildesheim 1979.

Roth L, Daunderer M, Kormann K, Giftpflanzen, Pflanzengifte, 4. Aufl., Ecomed Fachverlag Landsberg Lech 1993.

Teuscher E, Lindequist U, Biogene Gifte - Biologie, Chemie, Pharmakologie, 2. Aufl., Fischer Verlag Stuttgart 1994.

Calystegia Sepium

Greater Bindweed

DESCRIPTION

Medicinal Parts: The medicinal parts are the whole flowering plant and the root.

Flower and Fruit: The solitary white flowers are about 5 cm long, the pedicle is quadrangular. Under the calyx there are 2 cordate, pointed, red-bordered bracts, which extend to cover the calyx. There are 5 sepals. The corolla is fused and conical. There are 5 stamens and 1 superior ovary. The fruit is a capsule.

Leaves, Stem and Root: The plant is about 10 to 30 cm high and has a creeping rhizome. The stem is angular, glabrous, and twining. The leaves are alternate, petiolate, cordate or arrow-shaped. The base of the leaves are acuminate, and they often have dentate lobes. Most twining plants seem to follow the course of the sun and bind round a support from left to right, but the Convolvulus will always twine against the sun, confounding all attempts to train it, even dying in the process.

Characteristics: The flowers close in damp weather.

Habitat: The plant is indigenous to Europe and eastern U.S.

Production: The upper part of the herb is harvested during the flowering season and dried at temperatures of no more than 40°C in a well aired place.

Other Names: Devil's Vine, Hedge Lily, Lady's Nightcap, Rutland Beauty, Hedge Convolvulus, Old Man's Night Cap, Bearbind

ACTIONS AND PHARMACOLOGY

COMPOUNDS

Glycoretins: (polymeric, resinous glycosides of hydroxy fatty acids (C12-C16) with oligosaccharides, whose hydroxyl groups have been esterified with (among others) acetic, propionic, isobutyric, and valeric acid)

Tannins

EFFECTS

The drug has a powerful effect; activity in the smooth muscle area is stimulated, intestinal peristalsis is increased, and there is an increase in bile production.

INDICATIONS AND USAGE

Greater Bindweed is used for fevers, urinary tract diseases, as a purgative for constipation, and to increase the production of bile.

PRECAUTIONS AND ADVERSE REACTIONS

No health hazards or side effects are known in conjunction with the proper administration of designated therapeutic dosages. It is conceivable that an overdose of the drug would trigger intestinal colic.

DOSAGE

Mode of Administration: The pressed juice, powdered root and the infusion are used. Due to the strong action of the drug, it is not in much use today.

Preparation: An infusion is prepared by adding 1 to 2 spoonfuls of the cut drug per cup of water.

LITERATURE

Kern W, List PH, Hörhammer L (Hrsg.), Hagers Handbuch der Pharmazeutischen Praxis, 4. Aufl., Bde 1-8, Springer Verlag Berlin, Heidelberg, New York, 1969.

Roth L, Daunderer M, Kormann K, Giftpflanzen, Pflanzengifte, 4. Aufl., Ecomed Fachverlag Landsberg Lech 1993.

Camellia Sinensis

Green Tea

DESCRIPTION

Flower and Fruit: The flowers grow short-pedicled and singly or in cluster of a few flowers in the leaf axils. They are white or pale pink and have a diameter of 3 to 5 cm. The flowers have between 5 and 7 sepals and petals at a time. The petals are fused at the base with the numerous stamens. The ovary has 3 chambers. The fruit is a greenish-brown, woody capsule with a diameter of 1 to 1.5 cm and contains 1 to 3 smooth brown seeds.

Habitat: The plant does not originate from the wild. It was originally cultivated in China and is grown as a tea plant today in India, China, Sri Lanka, Japan, Indonesia, Kenya, Turkey, Pakistan, Malawi and Argentina.

Other Names: Black Tea, Tea, Chinese Tea

ACTIONS AND PHARMACOLOGY

COMPOUNDS

Purine alkaloids: caffeine (previously referred to as theine or teine; depending upon the development stage of the leaves, 2.9-4.2%, content declining with age), theobromine (0.15-0.2%), theophylline (0.02-0.04%)

Triterpene saponins: theafolia saponins, aglycones including, among others, barringtogenol C, R1-barringenol

Catechins: in unfermented (green) tea 10-25%, with fermentation partially changing over into oligomeric quinones with tannin character, including, among others, into theaflavine, theaflavin acid, thearubigene, or into non-water soluble polymeric- flavonoids: including, among others, quercetin, kaempferol, myrecetin

Caffeic acid derivatives: including, among others, chlorogenic acid, theogallin

Anorganic ions: high fluoride content- (130-160 mg/kg), potassium and aluminum ions

Volatile oil: chief components linalool, in fermented tea also including, among others, 2-methyl-hept-2-en-6-on, alpha-ionon and beta-ionon, more than 300 volatile compounds are involved in tea aroma

EFFECTS

Caffeine, as the active agent, results in stimulation of the CNS. Antidiarrheal (tannin containing substance).

INDICATIONS AND USAGE

Green Tea is used for stomach disorders, vomiting, and diarrhea when taken as a beverage.

PRECAUTIONS AND ADVERSE REACTIONS

General: No health hazards are known in conjunction with the proper administration of designated therapeutic dosages. Side effects of tea consumption are possible with persons who have sensitive stomachs, chiefly brought about by the chlorogenic acid and tannin content. Hyperacidity, gastric irritation, reduction of appetite, as well as obstipation or diarrhea could be the result of intense tea consumption. These side effects can be generally avoided through the addition of milk (reduction of the chlorogenic acid and other tannins).

Care should be taken with persons who have weakened cardiovascular systems, renal diseases, thyroid hyperfunction, elevated susceptibility to spasm and certain psychic disorders, for example panicky states of anxiety. With long-term intake of dosages above 1.5 g caffeine/day, non-specific symptoms occur, such as restlessness, irritability, sleeplessness, palpitation, vertigo, vomiting, diarrhea, loss of appetite and headache.

Pregnancy: Pregnant women should under no circumstances exceed a dosage of 300 mg/day (5 cups of tea spread out over the course of a day), and in fact should avoid caffeine altogether.

Nursing Mothers: Infants whose nursing mothers consume beverages containing caffeine could suffer from sleep disorders. The resorption of alkaline medications can be delayed because of chemical bonding with the tannins.

OVERDOSAGE

Overdosage (quantities corresponding to more than 300 mg caffeine, or 5 cups of tea as a beverage) can lead to restlessness, tremor and elevated reflex excitability. The first signs of poisoning are vomiting and abdominal spasm. Fatal poisonings are not possible with tea beverages.

DOSAGE

Mode of Administration: As an infusion, also occasionally in combinations. Proportionally contained in teas used to remove excess fat and for slimming purposes.

Preparation: The tannin containing substance (and with it the antidiarrheal action) increases when the tea is left to brew.

LITERATURE

Anonym, Grüner Tee schützt vor Krebs. In: DAZ 137(24):2045. 1997.

Büechi S, Antivirale Saponine, pharmakologische und klinische Untersuchungen. In: DAZ 136(2):89-98. 1996.

Graham B, In: Graham HN: Tea: The Plant and Its Manufacture, Chemistry, and Consumption of the Beverage. In: The Methylxanthine Beverages and Foods: Chemistry, Consumption, and Heath Effects, Alan R. Liss, New York, S.29-74. 1984.

Haslam E, Natural polyphenols (vegetable tannins) as drugs: possible modes of action. In: JNP 59(2):205-215. 1996.

Imai K, Nakachi K, Cross sectional study of effects of drinking green tea on cardiovascular and liver disease. In: Brit Med J 310:693-696. 1995.

Jain AK, Shimoi K, Nakamura Y, Kada T, Hana Y, Tomita J, Crude tea extracts decrease the mutagenic activity of N-methyl-N'-nitro-N-nitrosoguanidine in vitro an in gastric tract of rats. In: Mutat Res 210(1)1-8. 1989.

John TJ, Mukundan P, Antiviral property of tea. In: Curr Sci 47:159. 1978.

Ludewig R, (1995) Schwarzer und Grüner Tee als Genuβ- und Heilmittel. Dtsch Apoth Z 135:2203-2218.

Scholz E, Camellia sinensis (L.) O. KUNTZE. Der Teestrauch. In: ZPT 16(4):231-250. 1995.

Schröder B, In: Schröder R: Kaffee, Tee und Kardamom, Ulmer-Verlag, Stuttgart. 1991.

Sur P, Ganguly DK, Tea root extract (TRE) as an antineoplastic agent. In: PM 60(2):106. 1994.

Yoshizawa S et al., (1987) Phytother Res 1(1):44.

Further information in:

Hänsel R, Keller K, Rimpler H, Schneider G (Hrsg.), Hagers Handbuch der Pharmazeutischen Praxis, 5. Aufl., Bde 4-6 (Drogen): Springer Verlag Berlin, Heidelberg, New York, 1992-1994.

Leung AY, Encyclopedia of Common Natural Ingredients Used in Food Drugs, Cosmetics, John Wiley & Sons Inc., New York 1980.

Lewin L, Gifte und Vergiftungen, 6. Aufl., Nachdruck, Haug Verlag, Heidelberg 1992.

Oliver-Bever B (Ed.), Medicinal Plants of Tropical West Africa, Cambridge University Press, Cambridge 1986.

Roth L, Daunderer M, Kormann K, Giftpflanzen, Pflanzengifte, 4. Aufl., Ecomed Fachverlag Landsberg Lech 1993.

Steinegger E, Hänsel R, Pharmakognosie, 5. Aufl., Springer Verlag Heidelberg 1992.

Teuscher E, Lindequist U, Biogene Gifte - Biologie, Chemie, Pharmakologie, 2. Aufl., Fischer Verlag Stuttgart 1994.

Teuscher E, Biogene Arzneimittel, 5. Aufl., Wiss. Verlagsges. Stuttgart 1997.

Wagner H, Wiesenauer M, Phytotherapie. Phytopharmaka und pflanzliche Homöopathika, Fischer-Verlag, Stuttgart, Jena, New York 1995.

Wichtl M (Hrsg.), Teedrogen, 4. Aufl., Wiss. Verlagsges. Stuttgart 1997.

Camphor Tree

See Cinnamomum Camphora

Canadian Fleabane

See Erigeron Canadensis

Canadian Hemp

See Apocynum Cannabinum

Canella Alba

Canella

DESCRIPTION

Medicinal Parts: The medicinal part is the bark of the plant.

Flower and Fruit: The flowers are small and seldom open. They are violet and fused in clusters to the tips of the branches. The involucre is sometimes fused at the base. The stamens are fused to form a pollen tube. The fruit is an elongate berry with 4 reniform seeds. The fruit changes color from green to blue and then to a shiny black.

Leaves, Stem and Root: Canella alba is a tree which grows up to 15 m and is only branched at the top. The bark is whitish-yellowish on the outside and chalk-like on the inside. The leaves are alternate, oblong, thick, and are a dark, intense laurel-green shade.

Habitat: The plant is indigenous to the Caribbean and Florida.

Other Names: White Cinnamon, White Wood, Wild Cinnamon

ACTIONS AND PHARMACOLOGY

COMPOUNDS

Volatile oil: chief components eugenol, cineol, pinenes, caryophyllene

Resins

Bitter principles

EFFECTS

Canella has a stimulant and tonic effect. It also has an antimicrobial effect.

INDICATIONS AND USAGE

Canella currently only has use as a culinary spice.

PRECAUTIONS AND ADVERSE REACTIONS

No health hazards or side effects are known in conjunction with the proper administration of designated therapeutic dosages.

DOSAGE

No information is available.

LITERATURE

El Feraly M et al., (1980) J Nat Prod 43:407.

Morton JF, An Atlas of Medicinal Plants of Middle America, Charles C. Thomas USA 1981.

Further information in:

Kern W, List PH, Hörhammer L (Hrsg.), Hagers Handbuch der Pharmazeutischen Praxis, 4. Aufl., Bde 1-8, Springer Verlag Berlin, Heidelberg, New York, 1969.

Cannabis Sativa

Marijuana

DESCRIPTION

Flower and Fruit: Hemp is dioecious. The female flowers are reduced to the perigone with one bract. The complete inflorescences form a leafy, false spike. The male flowers form panicles rich in pollen. Pollination is by wind. The fruit is a gray-green, glossy achaene, 3.5 to 5 mm long and 2.5 to 4 mm wide. The seeds have little endosperm, are white, oily-fleshy and hooked.

Leaves, Stem and Root: The variety cannabis is an annual or biennial plant, which is usually branched and grows up to 5 m. The plant has erect, rough-haired and compressed bristles. The leaves are long-petioled and 3 to 7 pinnate. The leaflets are lanceolate and serrate.

Habitat: The plant probably originated in the Middle East. Today it is grown worldwide in temperate and tropical regions.

Production: Indian hemp is the dried flowering or fruiting branch tips of Cannabis sativa var. indica. Production depends on the origin. One method is by striping the leaves. Another method is stripping the resin exuded from the flowers and multiple fruit, which is shaped into balls or sheet forms. The final method involves cutting 5 cm to 10 cm long branch tips, which have just borne fruit, removing the leaves, pressing the shooting tips and gathering them into bundles.

Not To Be Confused With: Prior to being used as a narcotic, marijuana was often combined with Nicotiana tabacum, Lavandula officinalis, Nepeta catarina or Origanum vulgare. It is possible to confuse Marijuana with varieties of Urtica, Moraceae, Ulmaceae and Boraginaceae.

Other Names: Cannabis, Pot, Bhang, Grass, Indian Hemp, Weed, Ganja, Kif

ACTIONS AND PHARMACOLOGY

COMPOUNDS

Cannabinoids: chief active agent 9-tetrahydrocannabinol (9-THC = 1-THC), in addition to 60 additional cannabinoids

Volatile oil: of a very complex composition, with, among other things beta-caryophyllenes, humules, caryophyllene oxide, alpha-pinenes, beta-pinenes, limonene, myrcene, beta-ocimene

Flavonoids

EFFECTS

Psychotropic action: In most subjects the effect is registered following an oral dose of 20 mg d-9-tetrahydrocannabinol or after inhaling a cigarette with 2% d-9-tetrahydrocannabinol. The symptoms are mood swings, reduction in drive, inability to think clearly, confusion, lack of concentration, impairment of short term memory and perception of time. Sensory impressions become heightened or experienced differently.

Complex tasks become more difficult, the capacity to understand or empathize is impaired. Negative reactions such as anxiety, panic and psychosis can occur.

It is only possible to describe this effect in animal tests, on the basis of free behavioral and controlled behavioral tests. A stimulating effect has also been observed with lower doses. Not all cannaboids cause the same effect. CBC, CBD and CBG have no psychomimetic effect. Various interactions occur in combination with d-9-tetrahydrocannabinol.

Antiemetic action: has been reported in clinical studies involving cancer patients receiving chemotherapy.

Anticonvulsive action: d-9-tetrahydrocannabinol reduces the clinical and electrographic convulsion intensity in cats.

Analgesic characteristics: d-9-tetrahydrocannabinol displays analgesic characteristics, while at the same time partially increasing sensitivity to pain.

Body temperature: In animal tests, d-9-tetrahydrocannabinol and other cannaboids reduced body temperature. The maximum reduction was relatively small. A stronger hypothermic effect was observed in higher doses, which affected behavior.

Respiratory tract: The inhalation of marihuana smoke caused bronchial dilation in healthy subjects. Methacholine-induced asthma attacks can be terminated by inhaling marihuana, in this case only psychomimetic cannaboids are active.

Eyes: The ability of cannabis products to reduce intra-occular pressure was discovered accidentally during trials on the effect of inhaling high doses. During the tests, intra-occular pressure dropped by 45%. Eye drops applied locally had the same effect as standard medication but the effect lasted longer.

Immune system: In vitro and in animal testing, depending on the tissue, the immune system was significantly suppressed after cannaboid administration.

Antimicrobial action: CBC, CBDA, CBG and d-9-tetrahydrocannabinol displayed antibacterial effects. CBC and d-9-tetrahydrocannabinol are bacteriostatic and bactericidal against *streptococci* and *staphylococci.*

Tumor inhibiting effect: The in-vitro inhibiting effect of d-9-tetrahydrocannabinol, d-8-tetrahydrocannabinol and CBN on the growth of transplanted lung tumors has been documented.

Heart, circulation: Cannaboids increase heart frequency, peripheral vasodilatation causes an increase in systolic blood pressure in the prone position and a decrease in the supine position.

Other effects: d-9-tetrahydrocannabinol is said to be an appetite stimulant. Long term usage leads to a clear increase in tolerance for most of the pharmacological effects.

Mode of action: Most cannaboids act on the CNS. The multiplicity of effects does not point to just one receptor. Possible interaction with cell-wall lipids or effects on prostoglandin biosynthesis is under discussion at present.

When administered orally, the first psychotropic reactions take effect 30 to 60 minutes later. The effect is at its optimum between 2 to 3 hours later and lasts for a total of 8 hours. When inhaled the effect sets in within a few minutes, reaches its climax or maximum after 30 minutes and lasts for 3 hours.

INDICATIONS AND USAGE

Cannabis was first mentioned in the pharmacopoeia of the Chinese Emperor about 3,000 years ago. Cannabis resin was used for beriberi, constipation, female conditions, gout, malaria, rheumatism and absent-mindedness. In early Indian and Chinese medicine, it was used for nervous depressive states, insomnia, vomiting, tetanus and coughs.

In medieval herbals, it was mostly used externally. There are recipes for balms for healing contractures and for cooling poultices for the head and joints and for podagra.

In 1845, the herb tips were mentioned for internal administration for gonorrhea, angina pectoris and choking fits. It was not until the nineteenth century that Indian hemp was described as having a euphoric effect; it was used for insomnia, neuralgia, painful rheumatism, painful gastrointestinal disorders, cholera, tetanus, epilepsy, strychnine poisoning, acute bronchitis, whooping cough, asthma, impending abortion and weak contractions. The extract was used as a sedative and mild soporific.

Current literature on phytotherapeutic drugs cite as indications for Indian hemp: painful disorders of the alimentary canal such as ulcers or cancer; respiratory disorders such as asthma, emphysema or chronic bronchitis; neuralgia, migraine; urinary tract disorders; mental disorders such as anxiety, neurasthenia or hysteria.

Efficacy has not been proven.

PRECAUTIONS AND ADVERSE REACTIONS

No health hazards or side effects are known in conjunction with the proper administration of designated therapeutic dosages. The intake of toxic dosages, as is common with the smoking of cannabis, leads almost at once to euphoric states (pronounced gaiety, laughing fits) with exaggerated apprehension of sensual impressions. Alterations in the perception of time and space, as well as acoustical, visual and sensory hallucinations, lasting for 2 to 3 hours are common in higher dosages.

Driving ability can be disturbed for as long as 8 hours. Although only rarely reported, acute poisoning symptoms include nausea, vomiting, tear flow, hacking cough, disturbances of cardiac function and numbness of the limbs. Despite its widespread use as a deliriant, instances of death are very rare. The results of chronic abuse are laryngitis, bronchitis, apathy, psychic decline and disturbances of genital functions.

DOSAGE

Mode of Administration: As it is categorized as an illegal narcotic, neither a folk medicinal nor therapeutic usage is officially permitted. It is used illegally as a narcotic. The production of only certain varieties, those with lower levels of 9-tetrahydrocannabinol, is permitted for the extraction of the fibers.

Daily Dosage: The former average oral single dose of the drug was 0.1 g.

Narcotic: hash and tobacco are mixed. 1 cigarette contains 0.5 g to 1 g of the drug with at least 5 mg to 10 mg d-9-tetrahydrocannabinol for the psychotropic effect. More exact dosages are almost impossible to stipulate due to the varieties of action of the different cannaboids and because of varying breathing techniques.

Storage: Store with care, protected from light. Studies have shown that 9-tetrahydrocannabinol has a strong affinity with synthetics and rubber and is easily absorbed by them.

LITERATURE

Anonym, Cannabis: Hanf als Nutzpflanze. In: DAZ 135(27):2538-2541. 1995.

Anonym, Rezeptorforschung: Körpereigener Ligand des Cannabis-Rezeptors isoliert. In: DAZ 133(24):2214. 1993.

Clarke CC, Marijuana botany. In: And/Or Press, Berkeley, California. 1981.

Drogenmiβbrauch: Drogen im Straβenverkehr. In: DAZ 134(27):2575. 1994.

Evans AT et al., (1985) J Pharm Pharmacol.

Evans AT et al., (1987) FEBS 211: 119.

Evans AT et al., (1987) Biochem Pharmacol 36: 2035.

Evans FJ, Cannabinoids - The separation of central from peripheral effects on a structural basis. In: PM 57:60. 1991.

Fairbairn JW et al., J Pharm Pharmacol 28: 130.

Fairbairn JW, Pickens JT (1981) Br. J Pharmacol 72: 401.

Gil EW et al., (1970) Nature 228: 135.

Goedecke H, Karkos J, Die arzneiliche Verwendung von Cannabisprodukten. In: DAZ 136(34):2859-2862. 1996.

Jungmayr P, Rauschmittel: Macht Marihuana dumm? In: DAZ 136(34):2867-2868. 1996.

Kovar KA, Cannabis - was ist das? In: DAZ 132(43):2302. 1992.

Nahas, B, In: Marihuana in Science and Medicine. Nahas G (Ed.) Raven Press New York. 1984.

Paris RR et al., (1976) Plant Med Phytother 10:144.

Ross SA, ElSohly MA, The volatile oil composition of fresh and air-dried buds of Cannabis. In: JNP 59(1):49-51. 1996.

Segelman A et al., (1977) J Pharm Sci 66: 1358.

Täschner KL, Drogen und Straβenverkehr. In: DAZ 134(35):3299. 1994.

Turner CE et al., (1980) J Nat Prod 43: 169.

Yamaudi T, (1975) Phytochemistry 14: 2189.

Further information in:

Frohne D, Pfänder HJ, Giftpflanzen - Ein Handbuch für Apotheker, Toxikologen und Biologen, 4. Aufl., Wiss. Verlags-Ges. Stuttgart 1997.

Hänsel R, Keller K, Rimpler H, Schneider G (Hrsg.), Hagers Handbuch der Pharmazeutischen Praxis, 5. Aufl., Bde 4-6 (Drogen), Springer Verlag Berlin, Heidelberg, New York, 1992-1994.

Lewin L, Gifte und Vergiftungen, 6. Aufl., Nachdruck, Haug Verlag, Heidelberg 1992.

Madaus G, Lehrbuch der Biologischen Arzneimittel, Bde 1-3, Nachdruck, Georg Olms Verlag Hildesheim 1979.

Roth L, Daunderer M, Kormann K, Giftpflanzen, Pflanzengifte, 4. Aufl., Ecomed Fachverlag Landsberg Lech 1993.

Teuscher E, Lindequist U, Biogene Gifte - Biologie, Chemie, Pharmakologie, 2. Aufl., Fischer Verlag Stuttgart 1994.

Teuscher E, Biogene Arzneimittel, 5. Aufl., Wiss. Verlagsges. Stuttgart 1997.

Capsella Bursa Pastoris

Shepherd's Purse

DESCRIPTION

Medicinal Parts: The medicinal part is the aerial portion of the plant.

Flower and Fruit: The plant stays in bloom for almost the whole year. The flowers are white and about 4 to 6 mm long. The 4 sepals are 1 to 2 mm long and the 4 petals 2 to 3 mm long. There are 6 stamens. The inflorescence is extended after flowering. The many-seeded pod is 4 to 9 mm long and almost as wide. They are glabrous, flattened, long-stemmed, triangular and obcordate. The seeds are 0.8 to 1 mm long and red-brown with a short style.

Leaves, Stem and Root: Shepard's purse is a 2 to 40 cm high plant with a simple fusiform root and a simple upright stem. The stem is glabrous or has scattered hairs on the lower section. The basal leaves form a rosette and are petioled, entire-margined or pinnatifid. The few cauline leaves are alternate, smaller, sessile, entire, very wrinkled and involute.

Habitat: Worldwide, except tropical regions.

Production: Shepherd's purse herb consists of the fresh or dried, above-ground parts of Capsella bursa.

Other Names: Shepherd's Scrip, Shepherd's Sprout, Lady's Purse, Witches' Pouches, Rattle Pouches, Case-weed, Pick-Pocket, Blindweed, Pepper-and-Salt, Poor Man's Parmacettie, Sanguinary, Mother's Heart, Cocowort, St. James' weed, Shepherd's Heart, Toywort

ACTIONS AND PHARMACOLOGY

COMPOUNDS

Cardioactive steroids: presumably only in the seeds

Glucosinolates, sinigrin: 9-methyl sulfinyl nonyl glucosinolate, 9-methyl sulfinyl decyl glucosinolate

Flavonoids: including rutin, luteolin-7-rutinoside

Caffeic acid derivatives: including chlorogenic acid.

The plant very often acts as a host to endophytic fungi (Albugo candida, Peronospora parasitica), so the presence of mytotoxins is also to be reckoned with.

EFFECTS

A number of different studies have shown both a lowering and elevation of blood pressure, positive inotropic and chronotropic cardiac effects as well as increased uterine contraction. Despite numerous studies a clear therapeutic use could not be identified.

INDICATIONS AND USAGE

- Cardiac insufficiency NYHA I and II
- Arrhythmia
- Hypertension
- Hypotension
- Nosebleeds
- Nervous heart complaints
- Premenstrual syndrome (PMS)
- Wounds and burns

Internally, the plant is used for symptomatic treatment of mild menorrhagia and metrorrhagia. Externally, it is used for nosebleeds and superficially bleeding skin injuries. Shepherd's Purse is seldom used in folk medicine today. In America it is used for headaches.

PRECAUTIONS AND ADVERSE REACTIONS

No health hazards or side effects are known in conjunction with the proper administration of designated therapeutic dosages.

DOSAGE

Mode of Administration: Comminuted drug for tea and other galenic preparations for internal use and external administration.

Daily Dosage: Internally, the average daily dose is 10 to 15 g of drug. The liquid extract daily dose is 5 to 8 g drug. The infusion may be drunk throughout the day.

Storage: Protect from light and moisture.

LITERATURE

Farkas L, In ''Pharmacognosy and Phytochemistry 1st Int Cong. Munich 1971'', Springer-Verlag 1971.

Hill RK, in ''The Alkaloids Vol. 2'', Ed. SW Pelletier, John Wiley 1984.

Kuroda K, Tagaki K, (1968) Nature 220:707.

Kuroda K et al., (1976) Cancer Res 36:1900.

Kuroda K, Kaku T, (1969) Life Sci 8(1):151.

Kuroda K, Tagaki K, (1969) Arch Int Pharmacodyn 178(2): 382, 392.

Teuscher E, Lindequist U, Giftstoffe mikrobieller Endo- und Epiphyten. Gefahren für Mensch und Tier? In: DAZ 132(42):2231. 1992.

Vermathen M, Glasl H, Effect of the herb extract of Capsella bursa pastoris on blood coagulation. In: PM 59(7):A670. 1993.

Further information in:

Hänsel R, Keller K, Rimpler H, Schneider G (Hrsg.), Hagers Handbuch der Pharmazeutischen Praxis, 5. Aufl., Bde 4-6 (Drogen), Springer Verlag Berlin, Heidelberg, New York, 1992-1994.

Madaus G, Lehrbuch der Biologischen Arzneimittel, Bde 1-3, Nachdruck, Georg Olms Verlag Hildesheim 1979.

Teuscher E, Lindequist U, Biogene Gifte - Biologie, Chemie, Pharmakologie, 2. Aufl., Fischer Verlag Stuttgart 1994.

Wichtl M (Hrsg.), Teedrogen, 4. Aufl., Wiss. Verlagsges. Stuttgart 1997.

Capsicum Annuum

Cayenne

DESCRIPTION

Medicinal Parts: The milder varieties produce green or red Bell Peppers and Paprika, other varieties are much hotter and pungent.

Flower and Fruit: The flowers are usually solitary or occasionally in pairs or in threes. They are hanging and long-pedicled. The calyx is semi-globose to campanulate and has 5 to 7 tips. The corolla is wheel-shaped with a short tube, varying in color from white to yellow; occasionally from purple to violet with whitish-green or violet markings. There are 5 to 6 stamens with violet anthers and 5 small papillous staminoids in between. The ovary is superior. The dividing walls are partially underdeveloped. The seed carriers at the top are attached to the walls and fused to a column below. The berry is 1.5 to 5 cm long and up to 9 cm thick and varies in form. The calyx remains. The wall of the fruit is tough and leathery and may be red, yellow-green, or brownish. The seeds are numerous, light, yellowish-white, flat, disc, circular, or kidney-shaped and thickened at the margins. The surface is pitted.

Leaves, Stem and Root: Capsicum annum is an annual (in the tropics perennial) 20 to 100 cm high plant with an erect stem, which is somewhat woody and angular. It is sparsely branched higher up. The leaves are usually solitary, long-petioled, oval, lanceolate to ovate, obtusely accuminate, wedge-shaped at the base, entire-margined or slightly curved and glabrous.

Habitat: Indigenous to Mexico and Central America. Cultivated today in all warmer regions of the globe.

Production: Paprika consists of the dried ripe fruit of Capsicum anuum or Capsicum fructescens. The fruit is harvested when completely ripe and dried at a maximum temperature of 35°C.

Not To Be Confused With: Other varieties of Capsicum anuum.

Other Names: Capsicum, Grains of Paradise, African Pepper, Bird Pepper, Chilli Pepper, Sweet Pepper, Hungarian Pepper, Red Pepper, Goat's Pod, Zanzibar Pepper, Paprika

ACTIONS AND PHARMACOLOGY

COMPOUNDS

Capsaicinoids (amides of the vanillyl amine with C8 - C13-fatty acids): chief components capsaicin, dihydrocapsaicin

Carotinoids: in particular capsanthin (dark red)

Flavonoids

Steroid saponins (mixture = capsicidin)

EFFECTS

Many documented trials are based on observations of various extracts of the drug. The local effect is first pain, then warmth, then hypersensitivity; reversible or irreversible peripheral nerve damage is possible.

INDICATIONS AND USAGE

- Muscular tensions
- Rheumatism

Cayenne is used for painful muscle spasms in areas of shoulder, arm and spine, rheumatic conditions, arthritis, frostbite, chronic lumbago; as a gargle for hoarseness, sore throats, infected throats; in creams for circulation and as a female orgasm stimulant. Use should be limited to 2 days, longer usage can cause festering dermatitis, blistering and ulceration.

The drug is used internally for gastrointestinal disorders, loss of appetite, dyspepsia, diarrhea, alcoholism, seasickness; for malarial fever, yellow fever and other fevers, prophylatically for arteriosclerosis, stroke and heart disease as well as to increase potency.

PRECAUTIONS AND ADVERSE REACTIONS

General: There has not yet been a final determination of possible health hazards or side effects in conjunction with the proper administration of designated therapeutic dosages. Internal administration could show side effects through the elevation of the gastrointestinal peristalsis in the form of diarrhea, intestinal and gallstone colics. Besides the intended stimulating effect, external applications can lead to blister and ulcer formation. Investigations into mutagenicity, teratogenicity and carcinogenicity yielded contradictory results.

OVERDOSAGE

Toxic dosages lead to life-threatening hypothemias by affecting the thermoreceptors. High dosages of the drug (or the herb) administered over extended periods can bring about chronic gastritis, kidney damage, liver damage and neurotoxic effects. The treatment for poisonings proceeds symptomatically.

DOSAGE

Mode of Administration: Preparations of paprika are exclusively for external indications in antirheumatic ointments and plasters.

Preparation: A liquid extract is prepared by percolating 100g drug with 60g ethanol. Other formulations include: Capsicum-oleoresin with 90% ethanol and a tincture with 90% ethanol.

Daily Dosage: Externally: daily dose: 10 g drug; Tincture: (1:10); Semi-solid preparations: maximum 50 mg capsaicin in 100g neutral base.

Storage: Protected from light and well sealed.

LITERATURE

Anonym, Behandlung chronischer Schmerzen: Capsaicin - Lichtblick für Schmerzpatienten. In: DAZ 137(13):1027-1028. 1997.

Anonym, Phytotherapie:Pflanzliche Antirheumatika - was bringen sie? In: DAZ 136(45):4012-4015. 1996.

Bascom R, Kageysobotka A, Prous D, Effect of intranasal capsaicin on symptoms and mediator release. In: J Pharmacol Exp Ther 259(3):1323. 1991.

Camara B, Moneger R, (1978) Phytochemistry 17:91.

Gal IE, (1967) Pharmazie 22:120.

Kreymeier J, Rheumatherapie mit Phytopharmaka. In: DAZ 137(8):611-613. 1997.

Masada Y et al., (1971) J Food Sci 36:858.

Monsereenusorn Y et al., (1982) Crit Rev Toxicol 10:321.

Further information in:

Hänsel R, Keller K, Rimpler H, Schneider G (Hrsg.), Hagers Handbuch der Pharmazeutischen Praxis, 5. Aufl., Bde 4-6 (Drogen): Springer Verlag Berlin, Heidelberg, New York, 1992-1994.

Leung AY, Encyclopedia of Common Natural Ingredients Used in Food Drugs and Cosmetics, John Wiley & Sons Inc., New York 1980.

Lewin L, Gifte und Vergiftungen, 6. Aufl., Nachdruck, Haug Verlag, Heidelberg 1992.

Madaus G, Lehrbuch der Biologischen Arzneimittel, Bde 1-3, Nachdruck, Georg Olms Verlag Hildesheim 1979.

Roth L, Daunderer M, Kormann K, Giftpflanzen, Pflanzengifte, 4. Aufl., Ecomed Fachverlag Landsberg Lech 1993.

Steinegger E, Hänsel R, Pharmakognosie, 5. Aufl., Springer Verlag Heidelberg 1992.

Teuscher E, Lindequist U, Biogene Gifte - Biologie, Chemie, Pharmakologie, 2. Aufl., Fischer Verlag Stuttgart 1994.

Teuscher E, Biogene Arzneimittel, 5. Aufl., Wiss. Verlagsges. mbH Stuttgart 1997.

Wagner H, Wiesenauer M, Phytotherapie. Phytopharmaka und pflanzliche Homöopathika, Fischer-Verlag, Stuttgart, Jena, New York 1995.

Wichtl M (Hrsg.), Teedrogen, 4. Aufl., Wiss. Verlagsges. Stuttgart 1997.

Caraway

See Carum Carvi

Cardamom

See Elettaria Cardamomum

Carex Arenaria

German Sarsaparilla

DESCRIPTION

Medicinal Parts: The drug is the dried rhizome.

Flower and Fruit: The inflorescence is somewhat hanging and consists of 6 to 16 ovoid, 1 cm long, terminal, straight, greenish spikes. The lower ones are female and the middle ones are female at the base and male at the tip. The upper ones are only male. These are simple greenish unisexual flowers without a corolla. They have 1 husk with an ovary surrounded by a tubular-like involucre. The style has 2 stigmas, 3 stamens and a fruit oval. It is somewhat acute at both ends and the tube has a winged edge. The flowers form many blossomed spikelets, which in turn form a terminal, oblong ear. The middle spikelets contain male flowers at the tip and female flowers at the base. The upper spikelets are male.

Leaves, Stem and Root: Red Sedge is a 15 to 45 cm high plant with a 2 to 5 mm thick, horizontally creeping rhizome, which produces extremely long runners. The plant has black-brown basal leaves, which break up into long fibers. The stem is sturdy, upright and about 1 mm thick. It is sharply triangular, rough above, and surrounded by brown leaf sheaths at the base. The leaves are linear and usually grooved. The lamina are rigid and gradually tapering forward to the involute tip. The roots form such a thick mass that they prevent the water from getting in and thus prevent the washing away of dykes and dams.

Characteristics: The rootstock has an aromatic-turpentine odor.

Habitat: The plant grows in Europe mainly on the Atlantic, Baltic and southern Scandinavian coasts as far as central Germany. It was introduced to the American Atlantic coast.

Production: German sarsaparilla consists of the dried, underground parts of Carex arenaria. The root is dug up in March and April, dried and cut into pieces for sale.

Not To Be Confused With: Other Carex varieties.

Other Names: Red Sedge, Sand Sedge, Red Couchgrass, Sea Sedge

ACTIONS AND PHARMACOLOGY

COMPOUNDS

Saponins

Volatile oil: contents include methyl salicylate and cineol

Flavonoids

Tannins

EFFECTS

There are no studies available on efficacy.

INDICATIONS AND USAGE

There are no documented indications to date. In folk medicine, preparations of German sarsaparilla are used for the prevention of gout, rheumatism, inflammation of the joints, for skin ailments and as a diaphoretic and diuretic; further, for venereal disease, flatulence, colic, liver disorders, diabetes, edema, lung tuberculosis and amenorrhea.

PRECAUTIONS AND ADVERSE REACTIONS

No health hazards or side effects are known in conjunction with the proper administration of designated therapeutic dosages.

DOSAGE

Mode of Administration: Since the efficacy for the claimed uses are not documented, a therapeutic application cannot be recommended. The cold maceration and the decoction are used in folk medicine.

Preparation: A decoction is prepared by adding 3 g drug to 1 cup water. A cold maceration is made by adding 2 teaspoonfuls drug to 1/4 liter water.

Daily Dosage: The average daily dose is 3 g drug as a decoction. The cold maceration is dosed 1 cup, 2 to 3 times daily.

LITERATURE

Hänsel R, Keller K, Rimpler H, Schneider G (Hrsg.), Hagers Handbuch der Pharmazeutischen Praxis, 5. Aufl., Bde 4-6 (Drogen), Springer Verlag Berlin, Heidelberg, New York, 1992-1994.

Madaus G, Lehrbuch der Biologischen Arzneimittel, Bde 1-3, Nachdruck, Georg Olms Verlag Hildesheim 1979.

Carica Papaya

Papaya

DESCRIPTION

Medicinal Parts: The medicinal parts are the leaves and fruits.

Flower and Fruit: The plant has varying yellow to yellowish-white flowers of both sexes. The male flowers form many-branched, hanging panicles with small flowers. The female flowers are almost sessile in the leaf axils on the trunk. In addition there are androgynous, fertile flowers. The yellow to yellow-green berry fruit is up to 30 cm long, 15 cm thick and 2 to 5 kg. The fruit is clavate, lightly grooved and contains numerous peppercorn-sized seeds surrounded by orange-yellow, and melon-flavored flesh.

Leaves, Stem and Root: Carica papaya is a 4 to 8 m high bushy tree with an unbranched fleshy-woody trunk which is hollow in the middle. The leaves are long-petioled, very large and segmented into 5 to 7 palmate lobes which terminate in sharp tips.

Habitat: Indigenous to tropical America. Cultivated in all tropical regions today.

Production: Raw papain is the latex from Carica papaya which has been dried using various methods; where necessary it is decontaminated mechanically or by filtration. Papaya leaves consist of the fresh or dried leaves of Carica papaya harvested before the fruit appears.

Other Names: Melon Tree, Papaw, Mamaeire

ACTIONS AND PHARMACOLOGY

COMPOUNDS: PAPAINUM CRUDUM

Proteolytic enzymes (proteinases): papain, chymopapain A and B, proteinase A and B, papaya peptidase A

Other enzymes: lysozyme, chitotransferase, glycosidases, callase, pectinesterases, lipases, phosphatases, cycloligases

EFFECTS: PAPAINUM CRUDUM

The results of the analgesic and anti-inflammatory effects are contradictory. Experiments have shown that papain has an edema-reducing effect. The fibrinogenous effect has not been sufficiently proven.

COMPOUNDS: CARICAE PAPAYAE FOLIUM

Polyketide alkaloids: carpaine, pseudocarpaine

Glucosinolates

Cyanogenic glycosides (traces): including prunasin

Saponins

Proteolytic ferments (ficin)

EFFECTS: CARICAE PAPAYAE FOLIUM

No information is available.

INDICATIONS AND USAGE

PAPAINUM CRUDUM

Papaya is used for gastrointestinal digestion complaints, inflammations and ulcers in the gastro-duodenal area, and pancreas excretion insufficiency.

CARICAE PAPAYAE FOLIUM

Papaya leaf preparations are used singly or in combinations for prophylaxis and therapy of diseases and disorders of the gastro-intestinal tract, for infections with intestinal parasites. The effectiveness for the claimed applications has not been documented.

CONTRAINDICATIONS

Papaya is contraindicated in pregnancy.

PRECAUTIONS AND ADVERSE REACTIONS

PAPAINUM CRUDUM

General: No health hazards or side effects are known in conjunction with the proper administration of designated therapeutic dosages. An increase in hemorrhaging tendency is not to be ruled out where there are coagulation disorders. Allergic reactions are possible.

Drug Interactions: There has been some documented interactions with warfarin. Papaya extract has been shown to increase the international normalized ratio (INR) levels when used in conjunction with warfarin.

CARICAE PAPAYAE FOLIUM

No health hazards or side effects are known in conjunction with the proper administration of designated therapeutic dosages.

DOSAGE

Daily Dosage: No information is available.

LITERATURE

PAPAINUM CRUDUM

Buttle DJ et al., Affinity purification of the novel cysteine proteinase papaya proteinase IV, and papain from papaya latex. In: Biochem J 261(2):469-476. 1989.

Lohiya NK et al., Antifertility effects of aqueous extract of Carica papaya seeds in male rats. In: PM 60(5):400. 1994.

McKee RA, Smith H, Purification of proteinases from Carica papaya. In: PH 25:2283. 1986.

Zoch E, Über die Inhaltsstoffe des Handelspapains. In: Arzneim Forsch 19:1593. 1969.

Further information in:

Kern W, List PH, Hörhammer L (Hrsg.), Hagers Handbuch der Pharmazeutischen Praxis, 4. Aufl., Bde. 1-8, Springer Verlag Berlin, Heidelberg, New York, 1969.

Madaus G, Lehrbuch der Biologischen Arzneimittel, Bde 1-3, Nachdruck, Georg Olms Verlag Hildesheim 1979.

Shaw D, Leon C, Kolex S, Traditional remedies and food supplements: a 5-year toxicological study (1991-1995). Drug Saf 1997 Nov; 17(5):342-56.

Steinegger E, Hänsel R, Pharmakognosie, 5. Aufl., Springer Verlag Heidelberg 1992.

Teuscher E, Biogene Arzneimittel, 5. Aufl., Wiss. Verlagsges. Stuttgart 1997.

CARICAE PAPAYAE FOLIUM

Hegnauer R, Chemotaxonomie der Pflanzen, Bde 1-11, Birkhäuser Verlag Basel, Boston, Berlin 1962-1997.

Kern W, List PH, Hörhammer L (Hrsg.), Hagers Handbuch der Pharmazeutischen Praxis, 4. Aufl., Bde. 1-8, Springer Verlag Berlin, Heidelberg, New York, 1969.

Madaus G, Lehrbuch der Biologischen Arzneimittel, Bde 1-3, Nachdruck, Georg Olms Verlag Hildesheim 1979.

Oliver-Bever B (Ed.), Medicinal Plants of Tropical West Africa, Cambridge University Press Cambridge, London 1986.

Roth L, Daunderer M, Kormann K, Giftpflanzen, Pflanzengifte, 4. Aufl., Ecomed Fachverlag Landsberg Lech 1993.

Carlina Acaulis

Carline Thistle

DESCRIPTION

Medicinal Parts: The medicinal part is the root.

Flower and Fruit: The flowers are made up of individual heads that are 7 to 13 cm in diameter. The disc florets are androgynous, pink to violet, and have a 5-tipped radial corolla. The outer bracts are thorny. The middle bracts consist of glossy white, acuminate, 3 to 4 cm long leaves. The stamens have bristly tipped appendages. The styles are cylindrical with short stigma lobes. The fruit is 5 mm long, obclavate to cylindrical, and bluntly angular with bifurcated hairs at the tip.

Leaves, Stem and Root: Carlina acaulis is a 30 cm high thistle-like, leafy plant with milky latex. The stem is compressed and under 5 cm long. The whorled to alternate leaves are flat or slightly frilled and a little tough, 10 to 20 cm long, pinnatifid to pinnatisect with broad, thorny tips. The rhizome is finger thick and has 1 or more heads.

Habitat: The plant extends from Spain, Italy, and the Balkans across central Europe to central Russia.

Not To Be Confused With: Confusions occur through the addition of other Carlina species.

Other Names: Stemless Carlina Root, Dwarf Carline, Ground Thistle, Southernwood Root

ACTIONS AND PHARMACOLOGY

COMPOUNDS

Volatile oil

Inulin (fructosan)

Tannins

EFFECTS

The ethereal oil hinders the growth of *Staphylococcus aureus* up to a dilution of 1:2 X 105.

Carline Thistle has mild diuretic, spasmolytic, and diaphoretic effects.

INDICATIONS AND USAGE

The drug is used internally for cholecystopathy, digestive insufficiency, and also for spasms in the alimentary canal. In Spain, it is used to treat colds and illnesses accompanied by fever.

Externally, it is used as a wash for dermatosis, and to rinse wounds and ulcers; to alleviate cancer of the tongue.

Efficacy of the drug has not been sufficiently documented.

PRECAUTIONS AND ADVERSE REACTIONS

No health hazards or side effects are known in conjunction with the proper administration of designated therapeutic dosages.

DOSAGE

Mode of Administration: Carline Thistle is used both internally and externally.

Daily Dosage: Common preparations and doses are:

Decoction: boil 3 gm of drug in 150 ml of water for 5 minutes, drink 3 cups daily.

Infusion: 2 teaspoons of the drug to be boiled in 1 cup of water for 10 minutes, leave to draw for half an hour then take 3 to 4 cups daily between mealtimes.

Tincture: 20 gm of chopped drug, left to draw for 10 days in 80 gm of ethanol 60%, use 40 to 50 drops, 4 to 5 times daily.

Wine: add 50 gm of the drug to 1 L of white wine, leave to draw for a minimum of 12 days, then strain; drink one full small glass before mealtimes.

Externally it is used as a decoction; 30 gm of the drug added to 1 L of water.

Storage: To be stored in sealed containers.

LITERATURE

Schilcher H, Hagels H, Carlinae radix. Verfälschung, Verwechslung oder Ersatzdroge. In: DAZ 130(40):2186. 1990.

Further information in:

Hänsel R, Keller K, Rimpler H, Schneider G (Hrsg.), Hagers Handbuch der Pharmazeutischen Praxis, 5. Aufl., Bde 4-6 (Drogen), Springer Verlag Berlin, Heidelberg, New York, 1992-1994.

Wichtl M (Hrsg.), Teedrogen, 4. Aufl., Wiss. Verlagsges. Stuttgart 1997.

Carline Thistle

See Carlina Acaulis

Carob

See Ceratonia Siliqua

Carrageen

See Chondrus Crispus

Carrot

See Daucus Carota

Carthamus Tinctorius

Safflower

DESCRIPTION

Medicinal Parts: The medicinal parts are the flowers and the oil extracted from its embryos.

Flower and Fruit: Axillary flowers grow in the leaf axils. They are initially red-yellow, later bright orange. The heads are up to 4 by 3 cm and are encircled by upper leaves. The bracts are light green and have thorny tips with a thorny appendage. The fruit is 6 to 8 cm long, obovate or pear-shaped and bluntly wedge-shaped at the base with protruding long ribs; pappus consists of scales.

Leaves, Stem and Root: Carthamus tinctorius is an annual plant which grows up to 90 cm high; it has a thin fusiform root. The stem is erect, simple or branched at the top into stiff, glabrous, whitish-yellow, and glossy branches. The leaves are long, fairly soft, and glabrous with a thorny-serrate margin and tip.

Habitat: The plant is said to be indigenous to Iran, northwest India and possibly parts of Africa. It is also found in the Far East and North America. It is also cultivated.

Production: The flowers are gathered as they begin to wilt, the calyx and inferior ovary are removed, the remainder is put in the shade where it is mildly warm, and left to dry. Direct sunlight destroys the coloring pigment. Safflower or thistle oil is the oil extracted from the embryos of the fruits of Carthamus tinctorius.

Other Names: Dyer's Saffron, American Saffron, Fake Saffron, Bastard Saffron, Zaffer

ACTIONS AND PHARMACOLOGY

COMPOUNDS: CARTHAMI FLOS

Chalcones and their p-quinones

Flavonoids

EFFECTS: CARTHAMI FLOS

No information is available.

COMPOUNDS: CARTHAMI OLEUM

Fatty oil: chief fatty acids linoleic acid (55-88%), linolenic acid

Carotinoids

EFFECTS: CARTHAMI OLEUM

Safflower oil lowers the serum cholesterol levels.

INDICATIONS AND USAGE

CARTHAMI FLOS

In folk medicine, it is mainly used as a stimulant, purgative, antihydrotic, emmenagogue, abortifacient, expectorant, pneumonic, and for tumors. In China, it is given to women for hyperemia. It is also added to teas, which soothe coughs and bronchial conditions.

CARTHAMI OLEUM

Safflower oil is used for the prophylaxis of arteriosclerosis.

PRECAUTIONS AND ADVERSE REACTIONS

No health hazards or side effects are known in conjunction with the proper administration of designated therapeutic dosages.

DOSAGE

Daily Dosage: The average daily dose is 3 gm of decoction; single dose is 1 gm.

LITERATURE

CARTHAMI FLOS

Amling R, Phytotherapeutika in der Neurologie. In: ZPT 12(1):9. 1991.

Caldes G et al., (1981) J Gen Appl Microbiol 27, 157.

Thomson RH, Naturally Occurring Quinones, 2nd Ed., Academic Press New York 1971.

Further information in:

Chan, EH et al., (Eds.), Advances in Chinese Medicinal Materials Research, World Scientific Pub. Co. Singapore 1985.

Kern W, List PH, Hörhammer L (Hrsg.), Hagers Handbuch der Pharmazeutischen Praxis, 4. Aufl., Bde. 1-8, Springer Verlag Berlin, Heidelberg, New York, 1969.

CARTHAMI OLEUM

Caldes, G et al., (1981) J Gen Appl Microbiol 27, 157.

Xu SX, (1986) Chung Yao Tung Pao 11(2):42.

Further information in:

Chan, EH et al., (Eds.), Advances in Chinese Medicinal Materials Research, World Scientific Pub. Co. Singapore 1985.

Kern W, List PH, Hörhammer L (Hrsg.), Hagers Handbuch der Pharmazeutischen Praxis, 4. Aufl., Bde. 1-8, Springer Verlag Berlin, Heidelberg, New York, 1969.

Steinegger E, Hänsel R, Pharmakognosie, 5. Aufl., Springer Verlag Heidelberg 1992.

Teuscher E, Biogene Arzneimittel, 5. Aufl., Wiss. Verlagsges. mbH Stuttgart 1997.

Carum Carvi

Caraway

DESCRIPTION

Medicinal Parts: The medicinal part is the oil extracted from the seeds.

Flower and Fruit: The main trunk and the side branches each terminate in a compound flowering umbel of 8 to 16 umbel rays. The epicalyx and calyx are almost non-existent. The florets are white or reddish and very small. The fruit is a schizocarp, glabrous, oblong, and elliptoid. It consists of 2 mericarps which are 3 to 6 mm long, sickel-shaped, brownish with 5 lighter, angular main ribs (caraway seeds).

Leaves, Stem and Root: Carum carvi is usually a biennial, 30 to 100 cm high plant with a fleshy, fusiform tap root. The stem is erect, angular, grooved, filled with latex, glabrous, and branched from the ground up. The rosette leaves and the cauline leaves are glabrous and in part tri-pinnate. The lower pinna are typically crossed.

Characteristics: The plant has a caraway taste and an aromatic smell.

Habitat: Caraway is found in Europe, Siberia, the Caucasus, the Near East, the Himalayas, Mongolia, and Morocco. Found wild in North America after being introduced.

Production: Caraway is harvested when completely ripe and threshed 3 weeks later. The oil is recovered from the crushed seeds by a process of aqueous steam distillation.

Not To Be Confused With: Carvon is occasionally added in synthetic form.

ACTIONS AND PHARMACOLOGY

COMPOUNDS

In the berries: volatile oil, fatty oil, polysaccharides, proteins, furocoumarins (traces)

In volatile oil: in particular D-(+)-carvone and D-(+)-limonene

EFFECTS

In animal tests the drug had a spasmolytic effect. The antimicrobial effect has been demonstrated against *bacillus, pseudomonas*, and *candida*; *dermatomyces* are also inhibited. The choleretic effect has been described in a study which is not accessible.

INDICATIONS AND USAGE

- Common cold
- Cough/bronchitis
- Fevers and colds
- Inflammation of the mouth and pharynx
- Liver and gallbladder complaints
- Loss of appetite
- Tendency to infection

Caraway is used for dyspeptic complaints, meteorism, gastrointestinal cramps, flatulence, and feelings of fullness as well as nervous cardiac-gastric complaints.

In folk medicine, the drug is used in mouthwashes, to improve lactation in nursing mothers, as an emmenagogic, and also as a stomachic.

PRECAUTIONS AND ADVERSE REACTIONS

No health hazards or side effects are known in conjunction with the proper administration of designated therapeutic dosages.

OVERDOSAGE

An intake of larger dosages of the volatile oil (see for example in caraway liquor) for extended periods can lead to kidney and liver damage.

DOSAGE

Mode of Administration: Essential oil and its galenic preparations for internal use; comminuted fresh drug for infusions and other galenic preparations.

Preparation: An infusion is prepared by pressing 1 to 2 teaspoonfuls of seeds before using and pour 150 ml of hot water over it, drain after 10 to 15 minutes.

Daily Dosage: The average single dose of oil is 2 to 3 drops on sugar; caraway, 1 to 5 gm. The average daily dose of oil is 3 to 6 drops; caraway, 1.5 to 6 gm.

Storage: Protect from light and moisture in glass or metal containers.

LITERATURE

Debelmas AM, Rochat J, (1967) Plant Med Phytother 1:23.

Harries N et al., (1978) J Clin Pharm 2:171.

Hopf H, Kandler O, (1977) Phytochemistry 16:1715.

Koedam A, Scheffer JJC, Barheim Svendsen A, Z Lebensm Unters Forsch 168:106-111. 1979.

Salveson A et al., Sci Pharm 46(2):93-100. 1978.

Further information in:

Chan, EH et al. (Eds), Advances in Chinese Medicinal Materials Research, World Scientific Pub. Co. Singapore 1985.

Hänsel R, Keller K, Rimpler H, Schneider G (Hrsg.), Hagers Handbuch der Pharmazeutischen Praxis, 5. Aufl., Bde 4-6 (Drogen), Springer Verlag Berlin, Heidelberg, New York, 1992-1994.

Leung AY, Encyclopedia of Common Natural Ingredients Used in Food Drugs and Cosmetics, John Wiley & Sons Inc., New York 1980.

Madaus G, Lehrbuch der Biologischen Arzneimittel, Bde 1-3, Nachdruck, Georg Olms Verlag Hildesheim 1979.

Schulz R, Hänsel R, Rationale Phytotherapie, Springer Verlag Heidelberg 1996.

Simon JE, Chadwick AF, Craker LE (Eds.), Herbs. An Indexed Bibliography 1971-80. Archon Books, USA 1984.

Steinegger E, Hänsel R, Pharmakognosie, 5. Aufl., Springer Verlag Heidelberg 1992.

Teuscher E, Biogene Arzneimittel, 5. Aufl., Wiss. Verlagsges. mbH Stuttgart 1997.

Wichtl M (Hrsg.), Teedrogen, 4. Aufl., Wiss. Verlagsges. Stuttgart 1997.

Cascara Sagrada

See Rhamnus Purshianus

Cascarilla

See Croton Eleuteria

Cashew

See Anacardium Occidentale

Cassia Species

Senna

DESCRIPTION

Medicinal Parts: The medicinal parts are the leaves.

Flower and Fruit: The flowers are yellow, occasionally white or pink, and are axillary or terminal in ones, twos or threes in erect racemes. The calyx is deeply divided with a short tube and 5 regular, imbricate sepals. There are 5 layered petals. The 4 to 10 stamens are often irregular and partially sterile. The ovary is sessile or short-stemmed with a short or oblong style. The pod can be cylindrical or flat, angular or winged, opening or remaining closed and often has horizontal walls between the seeds. The seeds are numerous and horizontally or vertically compressed.

Leaves, Stem and Root: The genus Cassia comprises shrubs, subshrubs, and herbaceous perennials with paired-pinnate leaves. There are axes with stem glands either between the leaflets or on the petiole. The stipules have varying shapes.

Habitat: Cassia species is found in the tropical and subtropical regions of all continents except Europe. Most varieties are indigenous to North, Central, and South America.

Other Names: Tinnevelly Senna, India Senna, Alexandrian Senna

ACTIONS AND PHARMACOLOGY

COMPOUNDS

Anthracene derivatives: (in the leaves 2.5-3.5%, in the berries of Cassia senna 3.4%, of Cassia angustifolia 2.2-

6.0%) chief components sennosides A, A1 and B, further including among others sennosides C and D

Naphthacene derivatives: including among others 6-hydroxymusizin glucoside (in Cassia senna), tinnevellin-6-glucosides (in Cassia angustifolia)

EFFECTS

Senna has a laxative effect, due to the sennosides, and their active metabolite in the colon, rheinanthrone. The effect is primarily caused by the influence on the motility of the colon by inhibiting stationary and stimulating propulsive contractions. This results in an accelerated intestinal passage and, because of the shortened contact time, a reduction in liquid absorbed through the lumen. In addition, stimulation of active chloride secretion increases water and electrolyte content of the intestine.

INDICATIONS AND USAGE

■ Constipation

Senna is used for constipation, evacuation relief in cases of anal fissures, hemorrhoids, after recto-anal operations, and in preparation of diagnostic intervention in the gastrointestinal tract.

Stimulating laxatives must not be used over a period of more than 1 to 2 weeks without medical advice.

CONTRAINDICATIONS

The herb is not to be administered in the presence of intestinal obturation, acute inflammatory intestinal diseases, appendicitis, or to children under 12 years of age.

PRECAUTIONS AND ADVERSE REACTIONS

General: Spasmodic gastrointestinal complaints can occur as a side effect to the drug's purgative effect or through overdosage.

Long-term use leads to losses of electrolytes, in particular potassium ions, and as a result of this to hyperaldosteronism, albuminuria, hematuria, inhibition of intestinal motility, muscle weakness, enhancement of the effect of cardioactive steroids and an influence over the effects of antiarrhythmics. In rare cases this may lead to heart arrhythmias, nephropathies, edema and accelerated bone deterioration. The question of the increase in probability of the appearance of carcinomas in the colon following long-term administration of anthracene drugs has not yet been fully clarified; recent studies show no connections between the administration of anthracene drugs and the frequency of carcinomas in the colon.

Drug Interactions: In cases of chronic use or abuse, loss of potassium may potentiate cardiac glycosides and have an effect on antiarrhythmic medications.

Pregnancy: The drug should not be used during pregnancy or while nursing.

Pediatric Use: Not to be used by children under 12 years of age.

DOSAGE

Mode of Administration: Comminuted herb, powder or dried extracts for teas, decoctions, cold macerates, or elixirs. Liquid or solid forms of medication exclusively for oral use.

Preparation: To prepare an infusion, pour hot water (not boiling) over 0.5 to 2 gm of comminuted drug, steep for 10 minutes, then strain; or steep in cold water for 10 to 12 hours, then strain. The cold water method, according to various authors, should result in a solution containing less resin, which is responsible for abdominal pain. The drug takes effect after a latency period of 10 to 12 hours.

Daily Dosage: The average dose is 20 to 60 mg hydroxyanthracene derivatives.

LITERATURE

Anonym, Sennahaltige Laxanzien: Alte Arzneipflanze in neuem Licht? In: DAZ 133(28):2594. 1993.

BGA, Arzneimittelrisiken: Anthranoide. In: DAZ 132(21):1164. 1992.

Choi JS et al., In vitro antimutagenic effects of anthraquinone aglycones and naphthoquinones. In: PM 63(1):11-14. 1997.

Christ B et al., (1978) Arzneim Forsch 28:225.

Dufour P, Gendre P, (1988) Long-Termin mucosal alterations by sennosides, related compounds. Pharmacology 36(Suppl 1):194-202.

Fairbairn JW (1964) Lloydia 27:79.

Fairbairn JW (1976) Pharmacol 14(Suppl 1):48.

Fairbairn JW, Shrestha AB, (1967) Lloydia 30:67.

Jahn K et al., Toxicology of Cassia fikifiki Aubréville 6 Pellegrin in relation to other species of the genus Cassia (s.l.). In: PM 62, Abstracts of the 44th Ann Congress of GA, 57. 1996.

Klimpel BE et al., Anthranoidhaltige Laxantien - ein Risiko für die Entwicklung von Tumoren der ableitenden Harnwege. In: PUZ 26(1):33, Jahrestagung der DPhG, Berlin, 1996. 1997.

Lemli J, Cuveele J, (1975) Phytochemistry 14:1397.

Lemli, J et al., (1981) Planta Med 43:11.

Leng-Peschlow E, Mengs U, Sennalaxantien: Sicher und wirksam. In: PZ 140(8):668-676. 1995.

Schultze W, Jahn K, Richter R, Volatile constituents of the dried leaves of Cassia angustifolia and C. acutifolia (Sennae folium). In: PM 61(6):540-543. 1996.

Silber W, Sprühgetrockneter Senna-Extrakt. In: DAZ 131(9):349. 1991.

Sprecher E, Über die Qualität von Phytopharmaka. In: ZPT 12(4):105. 1991.

Sydiskis RJ, Owen DG, Lohr JL, Rosler KHA, Blosmster RN, Inactivation of enveloped viruses by anthraquinones extracted from plants. In: Antimicrob Agents Chemother 35:2463-2466. 1991.

Van Os FHL (1976) Pharmacol 14(Suppl 1):7.

Further information in:

Hänsel R, Keller K, Rimpler H, Schneider G (Hrsg.), Hagers Handbuch der Pharmazeutischen Praxis, 5. Aufl., Bde 4-6 (Drogen): Springer Verlag Berlin, Heidelberg, New York, 1992-1994.

Leung AY, Encyclopedia of Common Natural Ingredients Used in Food Drugs, Cosmetics, John Wiley & Sons Inc., New York 1980.

Lewin L, Gifte und Vergiftungen, 6. Aufl., Nachdruck, Haug Verlag, Heidelberg 1992.

Madaus G, Lehrbuch der Biologischen Arzneimittel, Bde 1-3, Nachdruck, Georg Olms Verlag Hildesheim 1979.

Roth L, Daunderer M, Kormann K, Giftpflanzen, Pflanzengifte, 4. Aufl., Ecomed Fachverlag Landsberg Lech 1993.

Schulz R, Hänsel R, Rationale Phytotherapie, Springer Verlag Heidelberg 1996.

Steinegger E, Hänsel R, Pharmakognosie, 5. Aufl., Springer Verlag Heidelberg 1992.

Teuscher E, Lindequist U, Biogene Gifte - Biologie, Chemie, Pharmakologie, 2. Aufl., Fischer Verlag Stuttgart 1994.

Teuscher E, Biogene Arzneimittel, 5. Aufl., Wiss. Verlagsges. Stuttgart 1997.

Wagner H, Wiesenauer M, Phytotherapie. Phytopharmaka und pflanzliche Homöopathika, Fischer-Verlag, Stuttgart, Jena, New York 1995.

Wichtl M (Hrsg.), Teedrogen, 4. Aufl., Wiss. Verlagsges. Stuttgart 1997.

Castanea Sativa

Chestnut

DESCRIPTION

Medicinal Parts: The medicinal parts are the leaves.

Flower and Fruit: The male, monoecious, yellowish-white flowers are in 12 to 20 cm long, erect catkins consisting of numerous, 7 flowered clusters. These are located in the leaf axils of the upper branches. There are 3 to 6 female flowers at the base of unopened male catkins. When the fruit ripens in October, the outer soft thorny husk bursts into 4 lobes, revealing a brown-skinned sweet chestnut which needs ''wine weather'' to ripen.

Leaves, Stem and Root: The tree grows from 15 to 30 m high. The bark is smooth at first, olive green, later dark brown, and vertically reticulate. The leaves are 8 to 25 cm long, coriaceous, oblong-lanceolate with long pointed, serrated teeth.

Habitat: Northern, temperate hemispheres; prefers maritime climate.

Production: The leaves are collected and air-dried.

Other Names: Sweet Chestnut, Husked Nut, Jupiter's Nut, Sardian Nut, Spanish-Chestnut

ACTIONS AND PHARMACOLOGY

COMPOUNDS

Tannins

Flavonoids: including rutin, quercitrin, myricetin

EFFECTS

No information is available

INDICATIONS AND USAGE

Chestnut leaves are used for complaints affecting the respiratory tract, such as bronchitis and whooping cough, leg pain, circulation, diarrhea, and as a gargle for sore throats.

Efficacy for the claimed indications has not been documented.

PRECAUTIONS AND ADVERSE REACTIONS

No health hazards or side effects are known in conjunction with the proper administration of designated therapeutic dosages.

DOSAGE

Preparation: An infusion is prepared by pouring boiling water over 5 gm of comminuted drug and then straining it.

Daily Dosage: The average single dose is 5 gm of drug or 5 gm of liquid extract.

LITERATURE

Haddock EA et al., PH 21:1049-1062. 1982.

Further information in:

Hänsel R, Keller K, Rimpler H, Schneider G (Hrsg.), Hagers Handbuch der Pharmazeutischen Praxis, 5. Aufl., Bde 4-6 (Drogen), Springer Verlag Berlin, Heidelberg, New York, 1992-1994.

Leung AY, Encyclopedia of Common Natural Ingredients Used in Food Drugs and Cosmetics, John Wiley & Sons Inc., New York 1980.

Madaus G, Lehrbuch der Biologischen Arzneimittel, Bde 1-3, Nachdruck, Georg Olms Verlag Hildesheim 1979.

Wichtl M (Hrsg.), Teedrogen, 4. Aufl., Wiss. Verlagsges. Stuttgart 1997.

Castor Oil Plant

See Ricinus Communis

Catechu

See Acacia Catechu

Catnip

See Nepeta Cataria

Cat's Foot

See Antennaria Dioica

Caulophyllum Thalictroides

Blue Cohosh

DESCRIPTION

Medicinal Parts: The root is the medicinal part.

Flower and Fruit: The inflorescence on the terminal leaf is panicled, 3 to 6 cm long and surrounded by a leaf like bract. The flowers are yellowish-green to purple and are 1 cm in diameter. The six sepals are arranged in 2 rows. The 6 petals are markedly reduced, inconspicuous, and gland-like. The 6 stamens are as long as the petals. The ovary opens before it is ripe and contains 2 dark blue 5 to 8 mm long, roundish seeds which are on solid stems and which resemble drupes because of the fleshy seed-shell.

Leaves, Stem and Root: The plant is a leafy, 30 to 70 cm high erect perennial with a brownish-gray, branched rhizome. The leaves are inserted in the middle of the shoot with a large, almost sessile leaf which is tri-pinnate and resembles 3 foliage leaves. The leaflets are stemmed, obovate, finely divided into 3 lobes, and wedge-shaped at the base.

Characteristics: Taste is sweetish, then bitter, almost odorless.

Habitat: The plant is found in the damp woods of the eastern part of North America.

Other Names: Papoose Root, Squawroot, Blueberry Root, Beechdrops, Blue Ginseng, Yellow Ginseng

ACTIONS AND PHARMACOLOGY

COMPOUNDS

Quinolizidine alkaloids: main alkaloids (-)-anagyrines, (-)-N-methyl-cytisines

Magnoflorine (isoquinoline alkaloid)

Triterpene saponins

Caulosapogenin

EFFECTS

An unspecified glycoside, which has been localized from the drug, and then injected into the ears of rabbits, causes a strong local irritation. Applying a solution into the rabbit's eyes leads to inflammation. Glycoside is supposed to have an oxytoxic effect.

The weak estrogenic, spasmolytic effect is probably caused by, as of yet, unknown constituents, the ensuing nicotine effect is possibly caused by N-methylcytisine.

INDICATIONS AND USAGE

In India, the drug is known as a treatment for gynecological disorders. In English and American medicine, the drug has been used since the beginning of the 20th century; for worm infestation, dehydration, menstrual ailments, cramps, and mainly to stimulate contractions and act as an antispasmodic during labor.

The above-mentioned applications have not been sufficiently proven medically.

PRECAUTIONS AND ADVERSE REACTIONS

General: No health hazards or side effects are known in conjunction with the proper administration of designated therapeutic dosages.

Pregnancy: The drug should not be taken during the first three months of pregnancy due to its estrogenic effect and possible teratogenic action of the anagyrines.

DOSAGE

Mode of Administration: The drug is used internally as a decoction or a liquid extract.

Preparation: Infusion (no specifications); Liquid Extract 1:1 in ethanol 70% (V/V)

Daily Dosage: The average single dose is 0.3 to 1 gm of drug; 0.5 to 1 ml of liquid extract.

LITERATURE

Benoit PS et al., (1976) Lloydia 39:160.

Di Carlo FI et al., (1964) J Reticuloendothelial Soc 1:224.

Flom MS et al., (1967) J Pharm Sci 56:1515-1517.

Strigina LI et al., (1975) Phytochemistry 15:1583.

Strigina LI et al., (1976) Khim Prir Soedin 5:619.

Further information in:

Hänsel R, Keller K, Rimpler H, Schneider G (Hrsg.), Hagers Handbuch der Pharmazeutischen Praxis, 5. Aufl., Bde 4-6 (Drogen), Springer Verlag Berlin, Heidelberg, New York, 1992-1994.

Hegnauer R, Chemotaxonomie der Pflanzen, Bde 1-11, Birkhäuser Verlag Basel, Boston, Berlin 1962-1997.

Madaus G, Lehrbuch der Biologischen Arzneimittel, Bde 1-3, Nachdruck, Georg Olms Verlag Hildesheim 1979.

Roth L, Daunderer M, Kormann K, Giftpflanzen, Pflanzengifte, 4. Aufl., Ecomed Fachverlag Landsberg Lech 1993.

Cayenne

See Capsicum Annuum

Ceanothus Americanus

New Jersey Tea

DESCRIPTION

Medicinal Parts: The medicinal parts are the dried leaves, the dried root bark as well as the fresh leaves.

Flower and Fruit: The inflorescences grow in the axils of the upper leaves and have long peduncles. They are 5 to 15 cm long, panicled, and have numerous cyme-like partial inflorescences. The flowers are white, the petals are 2 to 3 mm long and twice as long as the sepals. The fruit is a globose capsule with a diameter of about 7 mm.

Leaves, Stem and Root: Ceanothus americanus is a low deciduous shrub 40 to 100 cm high with greenish purple branches. The petioled leaves are alternate, 3 to 10 cm long by 1.5 to 5 cm wide, ovate or oblong-ovate, rounded at the base, lightly pointed at the tip, and with pinnatifid nerves. The upper surface is glabrous or has finely compressed silky hairs. The lower surface is densely gray and pubescent. The leaf blade is finely and irregularly serrated. The root is tough, woody, dark brown, and striated or finely wrinkled longitudinally. The bark is thin, brittle, and dark brown.

Characteristics: The taste is astringent; odorless.

Habitat: Indigenous to the eastern and central North America. It is also used for breeding garden hybrids.

Other Names: Red Root, Wild Snowball, Jersey Tea, Mountain-sweet, Walpole Tea, Redroot

ACTIONS AND PHARMACOLOGY

COMPOUNDS

Cyclic peptide alkaloids: cyclic peptines

Triterpenes: including ceanothusic acid, ceanothenic acid

EFFECTS

In blood taken from young rats, an aqueous-ethanol extract of the drug reduced blood-clotting time by 25%. However, the results are difficult to assess.

The drug is still useful as an astringent, expectorant, and antispasmodic.

INDICATIONS AND USAGE

Formerly, it was used as an astringent, in the clotting of the blood, for fever, gonorrhea, syphilis, and for colds and chills, especially of the respiratory organs.

The efficacy of the drug has not been proven.

DOSAGE

Mode of Administration: Orally as a liquid extract.

PRECAUTIONS AND ADVERSE REACTIONS

No health hazards or side effects are known in conjunction with the proper administration of designated therapeutic dosages.

LITERATURE

Lagarias JC et al., (1979) J Nat Prod 42:220 et 663

Mayo de P, Starratt AN, Canad J Chem 40:1632-1641. 1962.

Servis RE et al., J Am Chem Soc 91:5619-5624. 1969.

Further information in:

Hänsel R, Keller K, Rimpler H, Schneider G (Hrsg.), Hagers Handbuch der Pharmazeutischen Praxis, 5. Aufl., Bde 4-6 (Drogen), Springer Verlag Berlin, Heidelberg, New York, 1992-1994.

Cedar

See Cedrus Libani

Cedrus Libani

Cedar

DESCRIPTION

Medicinal Parts: The medicinal parts are the leaves, the wood and the oil.

Flower and Fruit: The male cones are 3 to 5 cm, the female 7 to 12 cm and almost cylindrical truncate or umbilicate at the apex.

Leaves, Stem and Root: The cedar is a majestic tree up to 40 m in height with a rigid leading shoot and a flat crown. The young branches are glabrous. The needle-like leaves are dark green and 20 to 30 mm long.

Habitat: The Lebanon cedar is indigenous to the Lebanese mountains and the southwest of Turkey. The tree is cultivated in Asia and Africa.

Production: Cedar oil is the essential oil extracted from the leaves and wood Cedrus libani.

ACTIONS AND PHARMACOLOGY

COMPOUNDS

When extracted from Cedrus libani (true cedarwood oil): borneol

When extracted from Cedrus atlantica (atlas cedarwood oil): cadinenes

When extracted from Cedrus deodora (Himalaya cedarwood oil): alpha- and gamma- atlantone, p-methyl-3-tetrahydroacetophenone

EFFECTS

Expectorant.

INDICATIONS AND USAGE

Cedar wood oil is used for catarrhal conditions of the respiratory tract.

PRECAUTIONS AND ADVERSE REACTIONS

No health hazards or side effects are known in conjunction with the proper administration of designated therapeutic dosages.

DOSAGE

Mode of Administration: As a rub (Bormelin balm), also as an inhalation.

LITERATURE

Kern W, List PH, Hörhammer L (Hrsg.), Hagers Handbuch der Pharmazeutischen Praxis, 4. Aufl., Bde. 1-8, Springer Verlag Berlin, Heidelberg, New York, 1969.

Celandine

See Chelidonium Majus

Celastrus Scandens

American Bittersweet

DESCRIPTION

Medicinal Parts: The medicinal parts are the root and the bark of the plant.

Flower and Fruit: The twining shrub is up to 8 m tall. The leaves are 5 to 12.5 cm long, ovate to ovate-lanceolate and serrate. There are numerous very small greenish flowers on terminal racemes 10 cm long. The orange-yellow seed capsules are 1 cm in diameter.

Habitat: The plant is indigenous to North America.

Other Names: Waxwork, False Bittersweet

ACTIONS AND PHARMACOLOGY

COMPOUNDS

Tannins

Celastrol (yellow quinoide nortriterpene)

EFFECTS

American Bittersweet has diuretic and diaphoretic effects.

INDICATIONS AND USAGE

The drug has been used for rheumatism, menstrual disorders, and liver disorders, but is rarely used today.

PRECAUTIONS AND ADVERSE REACTIONS

No health hazards or side effects are known in conjunction with the proper administration of designated therapeutic dosages.

DOSAGE

No information is available.

LITERATURE

Hegnauer R, Chemotaxonomie der Pflanzen, Bde 1-11, Birkhäuser Verlag Basel, Boston, Berlin 1962-1997.

Kern W, List PH, Hörhammer L (Hrsg.), Hagers Handbuch der Pharmazeutischen Praxis, 4. Aufl., Bde. 1-8, Springer Verlag Berlin, Heidelberg, New York, 1969.

Celery

See Apium Graveolens

Centaurea Cyanus

Cornflower

DESCRIPTION

Medicinal Parts: The medicinal parts are the fast-growing ray flowers and the dried ray florets which have been separated from the receptacle and epicalyx and to a lesser extent the tubular florets which have usually been separated from the ovaries.

Flower and Fruit: The 3 cm wide flowers are solitary and terminal. The tubular flowers are blue, the cultivated ones are usually all purple-violet, pale pink, or white. The lateral florets are larger, in rays and funnel-shaped. The oblong gray fruit is an achaene with the remains of a tuft of hair.

Leaves, Stem and Root: Twenty to 70 cm high annual or biennial plant with fusiform, pale tap roots. It has a rosette of basal leaves and an erect, branched, spider-web-pubescent, angular stem, covered in alternate, faintly linear-lanceolate leaves. The basal leaves are lyre-shaped, pinnatafid, and long-petioled. The upper leaves are non-compound.

Habitat: The plant is probably indigenous to the Middle East, but is cultivated worldwide because of grain production.

Production: The plant is harvested during the flowering season from June to August.

Other Names: Centaurea, Batchelor's Buttons, Bluebonnet, Bluebottle, Blue Centaury, Cyani, Bluebow, Hurtsickle, Blue Cap, Cyani-flowers

ACTIONS AND PHARMACOLOGY

COMPOUNDS

Anthocyans: chief components succinylcyanin (centaurocyanin, cyanidine-3-O-(6-O-succinyl-beta-D-glucosyl)-5-O-beta-D-glucoside)

Flavonoids

Bitter principles (structure unknown)

EFFECTS

In vitro, it is an antibacterial.

INDICATIONS AND USAGE

Cornflowers and their preparations are used for fever, menstrual disorders, vaginal candida, as a laxative, tonic, bitter, also as a diuretic and an expectorant, as well as a stimulant for liver and gall bladder function, also used in the preparation of eye washes for eye inflammation and conjunctivitis, eczema of the scalp, and coughs.

Efficacy in the claimed applications is not documented.

PRECAUTIONS AND ADVERSE REACTIONS

Health risks or side effects following the proper administration of designated therapeutic dosages are not recorded. The drug possesses a weak sensitization potential.

DOSAGE

Preparation: Infusion is prepared by adding 1 gm of drug per cup.

Storage: Store carefully and protect from light.

LITERATURE

Bandyukova V, Khalmatov K, (1967) Khim Prir Soedin 3:57.

Kakegawa K et al., PH 26:2261-2263. 1987.

Suljok G, László-Bencsik A, PH 24013021-1122. 1985.

Takeda K et al., PH 27:1228-1229. 1988.

Further information in:

Hänsel R, Keller K, Rimpler H, Schneider G (Hrsg.), Hagers Handbuch der Pharmazeutischen Praxis, 5. Aufl., Bde 4-6 (Drogen), Springer Verlag Berlin, Heidelberg, New York, 1992-1994.

Centaurium Umbellatum

Centaury

DESCRIPTION

Medicinal Parts: The medicinal parts are the dried, aerial parts of the flowering plant.

Flower and Fruit: The different-sized flowers form a dense or loose cyme. They are purple to pink-red, seldom white. The calyx tube pentangular with awl-shaped tips. There are 5 petals fused into a tube, 5 stamens mostly fused to the corolla and 1 superior, narrowly linear ovary. The stigma is 2-lobed. The fruit is a large, yellow, many-seeded capsule.

Leaves, Stem and Root: The plant is an annual which grows to between 5 and 30 cm high. The stem is erect, quadrangular, and unbranched. The cauline leaves are crossed opposite, fleshy, oblong-ovate to lanceolate, and sessile. The basal leaves are rosette-like, obovate, and narrowed to a petiole.

Characteristics: Centaury has a very bitter taste.

Habitat: Found in the Mediterranean region and as far as Britain and Scandinavia. Cultivated in the U.S.

Production: The plant is harvested during the flowering season, dried quickly to retain the flower color.

Not To Be Confused With: Other Centaurium varieties.

Other Names: Feverwort, Centaury Gentian, Filwort, Centory, Christ's Ladder, Bitter Herb, Bitterbloom, Bitter Clover, Eyebright, Rose Pink, Wild Succory, Canchalagua

ACTIONS AND PHARMACOLOGY

COMPOUNDS

Iridoide bitter principles (monoterpenes): in particular swertiamarin, including among others gentiopicrin, sweroside

Iridoide alkaloids

Xanthones

EFFECTS

Centaury increases gastric secretion and salivation because of the typical bitter reaction, also antiphlogistic and antipyretic effects have been studied in various animal experiments.

INDICATIONS AND USAGE

■ Loss of appetite

The drug is used for loss of appetite, dyspepsia, and poor gastric secretion.

In folk medicine, it is used for fever, worm infestation, diabetes in Mallorca, as a hypotensive in Egypt, and also for kidney stones; efficacy in these areas has not been proven.

CONTRAINDICATIONS

Because of its secretion-activating effect, the drug should not be administered in the presence of stomach or intestinal ulcers.

PRECAUTIONS AND ADVERSE REACTIONS

No health hazards or side effects are known in conjunction with the proper administration of designated therapeutic dosages.

DOSAGE

Mode of Administration: Comminuted herb for infusions and other bitter-tasting preparations for internal use.

Daily Dosage: The average daily dose is 6 gm of drug or 1 to 2 gm of extract; single dose is 1 gm.

The powdered drug is taken 3 times daily on a wafer with honey; the infusion is taken 1/2 hour before meals.

The daily dose of extractum Centaurii fluidum is 2 to 5 ml.

Storage: Protect from light and moisture in sealed containers.

LITERATURE

Bishay DW et al., (1978) Planta Med 33:422.

D'Agostino M et al., (1985) Boll Soc Ital Biol Sper 61 (2):165.

Do T et al., PM 53:580. 1987.

Lacroix R et al., (1973) Tunisie Med 51:327.

Neshta NM et al., (1983) Khim Prir Soed 1:106.

Schimmer O, Mauthner H, Centaurium erythraea RAFN. Tausendgüldenkraut. In: ZPT 15(5):299-304. 1994.

Schimmer O, Mauthner H, Polymethoxylated xanthones from the herb of Centaurium erythraea with strong antimutagenic properties in Salmonella typhimurium. In: PM 62(6):561-564. 1996.

Sluis van der WG, Plant Syst Evol 149:253-286. 1985.

Sluis WG van der et al., (1980) Planta Med 39:268.

Sluis van der WG, PM 41:221-231. 1981.

Further information in:

Hänsel R, Keller K, Rimpler H, Schneider G (Hrsg.), Hagers Handbuch der Pharmazeutischen Praxis, 5. Aufl., Bde 4-6 (Drogen), Springer Verlag Berlin, Heidelberg, New York, 1992-1994.

Leung AY, Encyclopedia of Common Natural Ingredients Used in Food Drugs and Cosmetics, John Wiley & Sons Inc., New York 1980.

Madaus G, Lehrbuch der Biologischen Arzneimittel, Bde 1-3, Nachdruck, Georg Olms Verlag Hildesheim 1979.

Schulz R, Hänsel R, Rationale Phytotherapie, Springer Verlag Heidelberg 1996.

Steinegger E, Hänsel R, Pharmakognosie, 5. Aufl., Springer Verlag Heidelberg 1992.

Teuscher E, Biogene Arzneimittel, 5. Aufl., Wiss. Verlagsges. mbH Stuttgart 1997.

Wagner H, Wiesenauer M, Phytotherapie. Phytopharmaka und pflanzliche Homöopathika, Fischer-Verlag, Stuttgart, Jena, New York 1995.

Wichtl M (Hrsg.), Teedrogen, 4. Aufl., Wiss. Verlagsges. Stuttgart 1997.

Centaury

See Centaurium Umbellatum

Centella Asiatica

Gotu Kola

DESCRIPTION

Medicinal Parts: The medicinal parts are the dried aerial parts, the fresh and dried leaves and stem.

Flower and Fruit: The pedicles are 1.2 to 4 cm long. The sepals of the epicalyx are oval to circular, with a membranous border and are about 2.5 to 3 mm long and 1.5 to 2.5 mm wide. The umbels have 2 or 3 sessile or short pedicled florets. The petals are white, to purple or pink. The calyx is not generally dentate. The fruit is oval to globose and has a diameter of 2 to 5 mm. The mericarps are clearly flattened at the sides and usually have 7 to 9 ribs and are raised rugose.

Leaves, Stem and Root: Centella asiatica is tender umbelliferous plant with numerous creeping stems which have roots at the nodes and are glabrous. The circular-reniform leaves are 2 to 6 cm long and 1.5 to 5 wide, with a crenate margin and 5 to 9 ribs. The petioles are 3 to 30 cm long.

Characteristics: Gotu Kola is almost tasteless and odorless.

Habitat: The plant is indigenous to southeast Asia, India, Sri Lanka, parts of China, western South Sea Islands, Madagascar, South Africa, southeast U.S., Mexico, Venezuela, Columbia, and eastern South America.

Production: The plant is gathered throughout the year and dried in the sun.

Other Names: Indian Pennywort, Marsh Penny, White Rot, Thick-leaved Pennywort, Hydrocotyle

ACTIONS AND PHARMACOLOGY

COMPOUNDS

Triterpene acids, including madasiatic acid

Triterpene acid ester from oligosaccharides (pseudosaponins): including asiaticoside, asiaticoside A, asiaticoside B

Volatile oil

EFFECTS

The psychotropic and europharmacological effects of an extract of the drug were investigated, using mice and rats in tests. In forced swimming behavioral tests, an extract of Centella caused a significant reduction in the duration of the immobilization phase. These tests show the sedative and antidepressive effects of Gotu Kola.

Ulcer-protective effect: Asiaticoid (suspended in propylene glycol) administered orally to rats, significantly reduced the formation of ulcers.

Antimicrobial effect: Using the puncture test procedure, asiaticoid showed the development of effectual zones with Pseudomonas pyocyaneus and Trichoderma mentagrophytes.

Healing effect: Asiaticoid mixture accelerated the healing process of wounds in rats in repeated skin injury tests.

Effect on vein tone: In a randomized, multi-center, double-blind versus placebo study of 94 patients with chronic insufficiency of the veins, the application of an asiaticoid mixture led to significant improvement in subjective (heaviness in the legs, pain in standing up, edema) and objective (plethysmographic measurements of vein tone) parameters.

The influence of asiaticoid on the formation of collagen is under discussion.

INDICATIONS AND USAGE

Clinical studies point to the effectiveness of triterpene fractions of the drug on vein insufficiency. Further experiments are still necessary to provide final affirmation of the therapeutic usefulness of the drug.

In India, the drug is used for skin diseases, syphilis, rheumatism, in the treatment of leprosy, for mental illness, epilepsy, hysteria, and for dehydration.

In southeast Asia, the drug is used to prompt bladder activity (urination), for physical and mental exhaustion, diarrhea, eye diseases, inflammations, asthma, and high blood pressure.

It is recommended to take the drug for rheumatism and skin diseases, and topically for poorly healing wounds, leprosy sores, and post-operative scarring.

Countless studies and reports are available on the Madecassol® therapy. However, these publications are difficult to interpret.

The efficacy of the drug has not been sufficiently proven.

PRECAUTIONS AND ADVERSE REACTIONS

No health hazards or side effects are known in conjunction with the proper administration of designated therapeutic dosages. The drug possesses a low potential for sensitization through skin contact.

DOSAGE

Daily Dosage: Drug; 0.6 gm of dried leaves or infusion to be taken 3 times daily, normal single dose is 0.33 to 0.68 gm.

Centasium®: 10 mg p.o. (tablets) 3 to 6 times daily; 10 mg i.m. daily (ampules); powder (2%) or ointment (1%), 1 to 2 times daily; 1 drop applied to the area under the eyelids, 6 times daily.

Centelase®: 3 to 6 tablets (10 mg) daily; 20 drops (10 mg/ml) 3 to 6 times daily; 1 ampule (10 mg/ml) i.m. daily; powder (2%) or ointment (1%), 1 to 2 times daily.

Emdecassol®: ointment twice daily.

Madecassol®: 3 to 6 tablets (10 mg) daily.

LITERATURE

Asakawa Y et al., (1982) Phytochemistry 21(10):2590.

Allegra G et al., (1981) Clin Terap. 99:507.

Bonte F et al., Influence of asiatic acid, madecassic acid, and asiaticosid on human collagen I synthesis. In: PM 60(2):133. 1994.

Bossé JP et al., (1979) Ann Plastic Surg 3(1):13.

Brevoort P, Der Heilpflanzenmarkt der USA - Ein Überblick. In: ZPT 18(3):155-162. 1997.

Castellani C et al., Boll Chim Farm 120:570-605. 1981.

Di Carlo FI et al., (1964) J Reticuloendothelial Soc 1:224.

Dutta T, Basu UP, (1968) Ind J Exp Biol 6(3):181.

Dutta T, Basu UP, (1967) Ind J Chem 5:586.

Dutta T, Basu UP, Bull Nat Inst Sci India 37:178-184. 1968.

Rao PS, Seshardri TR, (1969) Curr. Sci 38:77.

Vecchaio AD et al., (1984) Farm Ed Prat 39(10):355.

Further information in:

Hänsel R, Keller K, Rimpler H, Schneider G (Hrsg.), Hagers Handbuch der Pharmazeutischen Praxis, 5. Aufl., Bde 4-6 (Drogen), Springer Verlag Berlin, Heidelberg, New York, 1992-1994.

Hausen B, Allergiepflanzen, Pflanzenallergene, ecomed Verlagsgesellsch. mbH, Landsberg 1988.

Madaus G, Lehrbuch der Biologischen Arzneimittel, Bde 1-3, Nachdruck, Georg Olms Verlag Hildesheim 1979.

Roth L, Daunderer M, Kormann K, Giftpflanzen, Pflanzengifte, 4. Aufl., Ecomed Fachverlag Landsberg Lech 1993.

Steinegger E, Hänsel R, Pharmakognosie, 5. Aufl., Springer Verlag Heidelberg 1992.

Tang W, Eisenbrand G, Chinese Drugs of Plant Origin, Springer Verlag Heidelberg 1992.

Wagner H, Wiesenauer M, Phytotherapie. Phytopharmaka und pflanzliche Homöopathika, Fischer-Verlag, Stuttgart, Jena, New York 1995.

Centranthus Ruber

Red-Spur Valerian

DESCRIPTION

Medicinal Parts: The medicinal part is the root of the plant.

Flower and Fruit: The numerous flowers are in dense cymes, red, pink or seldom white. The corolla is tubular and spurred at the base. Each flower contains 1 stamen. The fruit is small and dry. The margin of the surrounding calyx forms a pinnatifid rosette or a papus.

Leaves, Stem and Root: The plant grows from about 30 to 80 cm high. The rhizome is perennial and very branched. The stems are tough, bushy at the base, hollow, and smooth. The leaves are 5 to 10 cm long in opposite pairs, somewhat fleshy, and entire-margined.

Habitat: The plant is indigenous to the countries bordering the Mediterranean. It is naturalized in southern England.

Other Names: Pretty Betsy, Bouncing Bess, Delicate Bess, Drunken Sailor, Bovisand Soldier

ACTIONS AND PHARMACOLOGY

COMPOUNDS

Valepotriate (iridoide epoxy compounds)

EFFECTS

The drug has sedative and equilibrate effects.

INDICATIONS AND USAGE

The drug is not in current use. In the past it was occasionally used as a sedative.

PRECAUTIONS AND ADVERSE REACTIONS

No health hazards or side effects are known in conjunction with the proper administration of designated therapeutic dosages.

DOSAGE

No information is available.

LITERATURE

Handjieva N et al., PM 34:203. 1978.

Marekow NL, PM 23A:48. 1977.

Schneider G, Valepotriat-Artefakte aus Centrantus ruber. In: Arch Pharmaz 318(6):515- 519. 1985.

Further information in:

Hegnauer R: Chemotaxonomie der Pflanzen, Bde 1-11, Birkhäuser Verlag Basel, Boston, Berlin 1962-1997.

Kern W, List PH, Hörhammer L (Hrsg.), Hagers Handbuch der Pharmazeutischen Praxis, 4. Aufl., Bde 1-8, Springer Verlag Berlin, Heidelberg, New York, 1969.

Cephaelis Ipecacuanha

Ipecac

DESCRIPTION

Medicinal Parts: The medicinal parts are the pulverized ipecacuanha root of the 3 to 4-year-old plant which have been dug up and dried quickly in the sun.

Flower and Fruit: The flowers are in terminal, capitulum-shaped inflorescences surrounded by 4 to 6 bracts. The individual florets have a 5-tipped calyx which is ciliated at the tips with a white campanulate-conical, 5-tipped corolla. A bitter dark purple, fleshy drupe develops from the 2 carpeled ovary.

Leaves, Stem and Root: Cephaelis ipecacuanha is a perennial, evergreen, leafy plant about 40 cm high with a 2 to 4 mm thick rhizome from which sprout numerous 20 cm long fibrous roots some of which develop into tubers. The creeping or ascending, simple or branched somewhat quadrangular green stem occasionally bears adventitious roots. The opposite leaves are entire-margined and the leaf blade narrows into the short petiole. There are stipules at the base of the leaf, which are slit like awls and are fused together with the petiole-like leaf sheath.

Habitat: Indigenous to the sparser woods of Brazil and is cultivated in India and on the Malaysian Archipelago.

Production: The subterranean parts of the 3 to 4-year-old plants are quickly dried in the sun and then cut into pieces of 5 to 10 cm in length.

Other Names: Ipecacuanha, Ipecacuanha Rio, Matto Grosso

ACTIONS AND PHARMACOLOGY

COMPOUNDS

Isoquinoline alkaloids of the emetine type (2-4%): chief alkaloids emetine and cephaelin

Starch

EFFECTS

The drug effects the sen.ory stomach nerves; it is secretory in small doses and emetic in larger doses. It is also spasmolytic and expectorant. It is partially effective in amoebic dysentery due to the action of the alkaloid emetin on the magna-form of the pathogen.

INDICATIONS AND USAGE

Ipecac is contained in expectorants and secretory preparations, it is used as a bronchial treatment and as an emetic in cases of poisoning. It is also used to soothe and assist in the coughing up of thick phlegm and in the treatment of croupous bronchitis in children.

PRECAUTIONS AND ADVERSE REACTIONS

No health hazards or side effects are known in conjunction with the proper administration of designated therapeutic dosages as an expectorant. Administration over extended periods can lead to myopathias. Frequent contact with the drug can trigger allergic reactions of the skin and the mucous membranes (''druggist's asthma'', the allergen is a glycoprotein).

OVERDOSAGE

Higher dosages of the drug (1 to 2 gm) have a nauseant effect (therapeutically used as an emetic). Toxic dosages can lead to mucous membrane erosion in the gastrointestinal tract, tachycardia, drop in blood pressure, cardiac rhythm disorders as well as to disorders in respiratory function and possibly to convulsions, states of shock, and coma.

Following intestinal emptying (sodium sulfate), the treatment for poisonings consists of the administration of generous amounts of liquids (warm tea), instillation of activated charcoal and shock prophylaxis (quiet, warmth), the treatment of spasms with diazepam (i.v.), electrolyte substitution and the countering of any acidosis imbalance that may appear through sodium bicarbonate infusions. In the event of shock, plasma volume expanders should be infused. Monitoring of kidney function is necessary. Intubation and oxygen respiration may also be required.

DOSAGE

Mode of Administration: Ipecac is used orally as a tincture, extract and fluid extract and in medicinal preparations with a standardized alkaloid content.

LITERATURE

Berrens L, Young E, (1963) Int. Arch All. Appl. Immunol. 22:51.

Garrettson LK, Ipecac home use- we need hope replaced with data- editoral comment. In: J Toxicol Clin Toxicol 29(4):515. 1991.

Kleinschartz W, Litovitz T, Overda GM, Bailey KM, Kuba A, The effect of milk on Ipecac-induced emesis. In: J Toxicol Clini Toxicol 29(4):505. 1991.

Kunkel N, Vergiftungen: Aktivkohle, Ipecacuanhasirup oder Magenspülung? In: DAZ 132(30):1587. 1992.

Nagakura N et al., Four tetrahydroisoquinoline-monoterpene glucosides from Cephaelis ipecacuanha. In: PH 32:761. 1993.

Wiegrebe W, Kramer WJ, Shamma M, The emetine alkaloids. In: JNP 47(3):397. 1984.

Further information in:

Hänsel R, Keller K, Rimpler H, Schneider G (Hrsg.), Hagers Handbuch der Pharmazeutischen Praxis, 5. Aufl., Bde 4-6 (Drogen), Springer Verlag Berlin, Heidelberg, New York, 1992-1994.

Leung AY, Encyclopedia of Common Natural Ingredients Used in Food Drugs and Cosmetics, John Wiley & Sons Inc., New York 1980.

Lewin L, Gifte und Vergiftungen, 6. Aufl., Nachdruck, Haug Verlag, Heidelberg 1992.

Madaus G, Lehrbuch der Biologischen Arzneimittel, Bde 1-3, Nachdruck, Georg Olms Verlag Hildesheim 1979.

Roth L, Daunderer M, Kormann K, Giftpflanzen, Pflanzengifte, 4. Aufl., Ecomed Fachverlag Landsberg Lech 1993.

Steinegger E, Hänsel R, Pharmakognosie, 5. Aufl., Springer Verlag Heidelberg 1992.

Teuscher E, Lindequist U, Biogene Gifte - Biologie, Chemie, Pharmakologie, 2. Aufl., Fischer Verlag Stuttgart 1994.

Teuscher E, Biogene Arzneimittel, 5. Aufl., Wiss. Verlagsges. Stuttgart 1997.

Wagner H, Wiesenauer M, Phytotherapie. Phytopharmaka und pflanzliche Homöopathika, Fischer-Verlag, Stuttgart, Jena, New York 1995.

Wichtl M (Hrsg.), Teedrogen, 4. Aufl., Wiss. Verlagsges. Stuttgart 1997.

Ceratonia Siliqua

Carob

DESCRIPTION

Medicinal Parts: The medicinal parts are the fruit and the bark.

Flower and Fruit: The inflorescences are erect and lateral in old wood, often bushy, clustered or catkin-like, unisexual with erect lignifying receptacles. There is no corolla. The male flowers have 5 long filaments with long slits and opening pollen tubes. The female flowers have short-stemmed ovaries. The pods are 10 to 20 cm by 2 cm, tough leathery, brown-violet, flat often rounded to a horn shape; numerous, lumpy, and glossy brown seeds.

Leaves, Stem and Root: Usually under 6 m high, broad crowned, walnut-like tree, sparsely branched and with cracked gray-brown bark; coriaceous, evergreen, 2 to 4 paired pinnate leaves; leaflets, obovate, 4 to 5 cm long, curved, glabrous, glossy dark green above, and red-brown beneath.

Habitat: Indigenous to southeastern Europe and West Asia, otherwise cultivated.

Production: Carob seed flour is the ground endosperm of the seeds of Ceratonia siliqua.

Not To Be Confused With: Carob Tree, Jacaranda procera or Jacaranda caroba.

Other Names: St. John's Bread, Locust Bean, Locust Pods, Sugar Pods

ACTIONS AND PHARMACOLOGY

COMPOUNDS

Mucilages: chiefly made up of galactomannanes

Proteins

EFFECTS

Carob is a dietary mucilaginous and binding agent; also an antidiarrheal.

INDICATIONS AND USAGE

Carob is used in dietary agents for acute nutritional disorders, diarrheal disorders, dyspepsia, entero-colitis, coeliac disease, and sprue. It is also used for habitual vomiting in babies, acetonaemic vomiting, rumination, retching cough, and vomiting.

Carob seed flour is used in the production of glutin-free starch bread where there is vomiting during pregnancy, coelica disease, and obesity.

PRECAUTIONS AND ADVERSE REACTIONS

No health hazards or side effects are known in conjunction with the proper administration of designated therapeutic dosages.

DOSAGE

Daily Dosage: For a 3 to 10% arabon preparation, add 20 to 30 mg of drug to water, tea, or milk, to be drunk during the course of the day. As a baking agent in glutin-free bread for babies, add 1/4 to 1/2 gm of drug (max. 2 gm) to 100 ml liquid; adults 1% to 3% additive to low calorie starters and desserts.

LITERATURE

McLeary BV, Biomass A Cellulose and Hemicellulose 160:523. 1988.

Further information in:

Kern W, List PH, Hörhammer L (Hrsg.), Hagers Handbuch der Pharmazeutischen Praxis, 4. Aufl., Bde 1-8, Springer Verlag Berlin, Heidelberg, New York, 1969.

Leung AY, Encyclopedia of Common Natural Ingredients Used in Food Drugs and Cosmetics, John Wiley & Sons Inc., New York 1980.

Steinegger E, Hänsel R, Pharmakognosie, 5. Aufl., Springer Verlag Heidelberg 1992.

Tang W, Eisenbrand G, Chinese Drugs of Plant Origin, Springer Verlag Heidelberg 1992.

Teuscher E, Biogene Arzneimittel, 5. Aufl., Wiss. Verlagsges. mbH Stuttgart 1997.

Cetraria Islandica

Iceland Moss

DESCRIPTION

Medicinal Parts: The medicinal part is the dried thallus commonly known as Iceland Moss.

Flower and Fruit: Cetraria Islandica is a lichen which grows on the ground and has a stiff curling thallus from 2 to 6 cm high, erect dichotomously branched, with a 1 to 10 cm wide section. The upper surface is olive-brown-green or brown, the underside whitish to light brownish, the margins are covered in 0.5 mm long papilla which contain the reproductive parts.

Characteristics: Iceland Moss tastes bitter and when wet, has a smell reminiscent of seaweed.

Habitat: Grows in the boreal, alpine, and arctic regions of the northern hemisphere and in some regions of the southern hemisphere.

Other Names: Iceland Lichen, Cetraria, Eryngo-leaved Liverwort

ACTIONS AND PHARMACOLOGY

COMPOUNDS

Mucilages, glucans (50%): lichenan (lichenan), isolichenan (isolichenan)

Aromatic lichen acids (2-3%)

Aliphatic lichen acids (1.0-1.5%)

EFFECTS

The bitter organic acids have an antibiotic effect. It is also a demulcent and a mild antimicrobial.

INDICATIONS AND USAGE

- Common cold
- Cough/bronchitis
- Dyspeptic complaints

- Fevers and colds
- Inflammation of the mouth and pharynx
- Loss of appetite
- Tendency to infection

Iceland Moss is also used for irritation of the oral and pharyngeal mucous membranes; loss of appetite and gastroenteritis (the bitter organic acids).

In folk medicine, the drug has been used for lung disease, kidney and bladder complaints, as well as externally for poorly healing wounds.

PRECAUTIONS AND ADVERSE REACTIONS

No health hazards or side effects are known in conjunction with the proper administration of designated therapeutic dosages. In rare cases, external administration of the drug led to sensitization.

DOSAGE

Mode of Administration: Comminuted herb for infusions and other galenic formulations for internal use; comminuted herb preferably for cold maceration and other bitter-tasting preparations for internal use.

Preparation: To prepare an infusion, pour boiling water over 1.5 to 2.5 gm of comminuted drug and strain after 10 minutes (1 teaspoonful = 1.3 gm of drug); infusion may be sweetened.

Daily Dosage: The average daily dose is 4 to 6 gm of herb.

LITERATURE

Anonym, Niedere Pflanzen ganz groβ - 39. Jahrestagung der Gesellschaft für Arzneipflanzenforschung in Saarbrücken. In: DAZ 131(37):1899.

Pengsuparp Th et al., Mechanistic evaluation of new plant-derived compounds that inhibit HIV-1 reverse transcriptase. In: JNP 58(7):1024-1031. 1995.

Wunderer H, Zentral und peripher wirksame Antitussiva: eine kritische Übersicht. In: PZ 142(11):847-852. 1997.

Further information in:

Fenaroli's Handbook of Flavor Ingredients, Vol. 1. 2nd Ed. Pub. CRC Press Boca Raton 1975.

Hänsel R, Keller K, Rimpler H, Schneider G (Hrsg.), Hagers Handbuch der Pharmazeutischen Praxis, 5. Aufl., Bde 4-6 (Drogen): Springer Verlag Berlin, Heidelberg, New York, 1992-1994 (unter Cetraria).

Steinegger E, Hänsel R, Pharmakognosie, 5. Aufl., Springer Verlag Heidelberg 1992.

Teuscher E, Biogene Arzneimittel, 5. Aufl., Wiss. Verlagsges. Stuttgart 1997.

Wichtl M (Hrsg.), Teedrogen, 4. Aufl., Wiss. Verlagsges. Stuttgart 1997.

Chamaemelum Nobile

Roman Chamomile

DESCRIPTION

Medicinal Parts: The medicinal parts are the Roman Chamomile oil extracted from the fresh or dried filled or unfilled flower heads and the dried aerial plant parts, the dried flower heads of the cultivated, filled varieties and the fresh aerial parts of the flowering plant.

Flower and Fruit: The stems end in 12 to 18 fruit-bearing, white florets, which are about 2 to 2.5 cm wide. The epicalyx is semi-globose. The bracts are in a number of rows and are lanceolate to spatulate with a broad membranous border. The receptacle is clavate, is filled with latex and is covered at the edge with slit bracts. The linguiform florets are female and silver-white. The tubular florets are androgynous and yellow. The corolla of every floret has a short appendage at the base, which surrounds the tip of the fruit. The achaenes are 2 mm long, light brown, almost triangular with vertical ribs. The achaenes are smooth and have no pappus.

Leaves, Stem and Root: The 15 to 30 cm high plant has a deeply buried rhizome. The rhizome sprouts numerous, ascending, occasionally upright, simple or branched, rounded, vertically grooved, pubescent stems. The stems are covered in alternating, heavily segmented, gray-green to rich-green, 2 to 4 cm long leaves.

Habitat: The plant is indigenous to southern and western Europe and northern Africa and is cultivated all over Europe. The main exporters are Belgium, France, Great Britain and Italy as well as Poland, the Czech and Slovakian Republics, North America and Argentina.

Production: Roman Chamomile consists of the dried flowers of the cultivated double flowered variety of Chamaemelum nobile. The plant is harvested in June and July, then dried at temperatures of 35°C.

Other Names: Ground Apple, Whig Plant

ACTIONS AND PHARMACOLOGY

COMPOUNDS

Volatile oil: chief components include ester of angelic- or tiglic acid with isobutanol, isoamyl alcohol or 3-methyl-pentan-1-ol, to some extent present as hydroperoxides

Sesquiterpene lactones: in particular nobilin, besides 3-epinobilin, 1,10-epoxynobilin, 3-dehydronobilin, present to some extent as hydroperoxides, including 1-beta-hydroperoxy-isonobilin, 4-alpha-hydroperoxy-manolide

Flavonoids

Caffeic and ferulic acid ester

Polyynes: Including cis- and trans-dehydromatricaria ester

EFFECTS

In contrast to true chamomile, there are few studies available. The essential oil is active against gram-positive bacteria and dermatomyces. The drug is also cytostatic and acts on the CNS causing a reduction of aggressive behavior in animal tests.

INDICATIONS AND USAGE

In folk medicine, it is used mainly in France for feelings of fullness, bloating and mild spasmodic gastrointestinal disturbances and sluggishness of the bowels. It is also used for menstrual complaints, nervousness, hysteria, and general debility. It is used topically for inflammation of the mouth and throat, rhinitis, toothache, earache, headache and influenza. The oil is used in mouthwashes.

PRECAUTIONS AND ADVERSE REACTIONS

No health hazards or side effects are known in conjunction with the proper administration of designated therapeutic dosages. The drug possesses a small potential for sensitization.

DOSAGE

Mode of Administration: Since the efficacy for the claimed uses is not documented and there is a certain risk involved, a therapeutic application cannot be recommended. Roman Chamomile is used in folk medicine as a fluid extract, tincture, elixir, wine, syrup and powder.

Preparation: To prepare a decoction, add 3 gm drug to 100 ml water. An infusion is prepared using 7 to 8 capitula per cup.

Daily Dosage: The average single dose of the drug is 1.5 gm at the main meals. The average daily dose of an infusion is 50 ml to 200 ml. When used as a bath additive, add 50 gm to 10 liters of water.

Storage: In well-sealed glass or metal containers protected from moisture.

LITERATURE

Damiani P et al., (1983) Fitoterapia 54:213.

Holub M, Samek Z, (1977) Collect Czech Chem Commun 42: 1053.

Herisset A et al., (1971) Plant Med Phytother 5(3):234.

Herisset A et al., (1974) Plant Med Phytother 8(4):306 and 287.

Isaac O, Chamaemelum nobile (L.) Allioni - Römische Kamille. In: ZPT 14(4):212. 1993.

Further information in:

Hänsel R, Keller K, Rimpler H, Schneider G (Hrsg.), Hagers Handbuch der Pharmazeutischen Praxis, 5. Aufl., Bde 4-6 (Drogen), Springer Verlag Berlin, Heidelberg, New York, 1992-1994.

Hausen B, Allergiepflanzen, Pflanzenallergene, ecomed Verlagsgesellsch. mbH, Landsberg 1988.

Leung AY, Encyclopedia of Common Natural Ingredients Used in Food Drugs and Cosmetics, John Wiley & Sons Inc., New York 1980.

Steinegger E, Hänsel R, Pharmakognosie, 5. Aufl., Springer Verlag Heidelberg 1992.

Teuscher E, Biogene Arzneimittel, 5. Aufl., Wiss. Verlagsges. mbH Stuttgart 1997.

Wichtl M (Hrsg.), Teedrogen, 4. Aufl., Wiss. Verlagsges. Stuttgart 1997.

Chamomile

See Matricaria Chamomilla

Chaste Tree

See Vitex Agnus-Castus

Chaulmoogra

See Hydnocarpus Species

Cheiranthus Cheiri

Wallflower

DESCRIPTION

Medicinal Parts: The medicinal parts are the dried flowers, the dried ripe seeds, and the fresh aerial parts of the erect plant before flowering.

Flower and Fruit: The flowers are golden yellow to orange-yellow in dense racemes on 10 to 14 cm long, pubescent, erect stems. The sepals are 9 to 11 mm long, linear-lanceolate, with a membranous border. The stigma is curled back. The fruit is a pod, which has no beak but has distinct ribs. The seeds are arranged in 1 row, are 3 mm long, oblong, narrowly winged, and light brown.

Leaves, Stem and Root: The plant grows from about 30 to 70 cm. The stems are woody below and semi-shrub-like with gray appressed hairs and thick foliage above. The leaves are lanceolate with revolute tip, short-petioled, entire-margined, and hairy.

Characteristics: The plant has a pleasant fragrance.

Habitat: The plant is probably only indigenous to the eastern Mediterranean region, but is cultivated today in Europe, northern Africa, western Asia, Japan, and New Zealand.

Production: Today, Wallflower can be obtained from commercial growers (cultivated regions).

Other Names: Gillyflower, Wallstock-gillofer, Giroflier, Handflower, Keiri, Beeflower

ACTIONS AND PHARMACOLOGY

COMPOUNDS

Cardioactive steroid glycosides (cardenolids): in particularly high concentration in the seeds, including cheirotoxin, glucoerysimoside, cheiroside A

Glucosinolates

Fatty oil (in the seeds)

EFFECTS

The drug has cardiac effects (similar to digitaloid drugs).

INDICATIONS AND USAGE

The seeds were formerly used for cardiac insufficiency, as a laxative, and to encourage menstruation. The plant was used to treat gallbladder and liver diseases because of its bitter content.

Efficacy has not been proven.

PRECAUTIONS AND ADVERSE REACTIONS

No health hazards or side effects are known in conjunction with the proper administration of designated therapeutic dosages.

OVERDOSAGE

For possible symptoms of overdose and treatment of poisonings see Digitalis folium. Despite the strong efficacy of the drug's cardioactive steroid glycosides in parenteral application, serious poisoning is hardly to be expected, due to the presumably low resorption rate following peroral administration.

DOSAGE

Mode of Administration: Wallflower is mostly obsolete as a drug. It is contained as an extract in some combination preparations.

LITERATURE

Belokon VF, Makarevich IF, Khim Prir Soedin 424. 1980.

Makarevich IF, Belokon VF, Khim Prir Soedin 662. 1975.

Moore IA, Tamm C, Reichstein T, Helv Chim Acta 37:755. 1954.

Schwarz H, Katz A, Reichstein T, Pharm Acta Helv 21:250. 1946.

Wagner P, Ber Dtsch Chem Ges 41:4467. 1908.

Further information in:

Hänsel R, Keller K, Rimpler H, Schneider G (Hrsg.), Hagers Handbuch der Pharmazeutischen Praxis, 5. Aufl., Bde 4-6 (Drogen): Springer Verlag Berlin, Heidelberg, New York, 1992-1994.

Madaus G: Lehrbuch der Biologischen Arzneimittel, Bde 1-3, Nachdruck, Georg Olms Verlag Hildesheim 1979.

Roth L, Daunderer M, Kormann K: Giftpflanzen, Pflanzengifte, 4. Aufl., Ecomed Fachverlag Landsberg Lech 1993.

Teuscher E, Lindequist U: Biogene Gifte - Biologie, Chemie, Pharmakologie, 2. Aufl., Fischer Verlag Stuttgart 1994.

Cheken

See Eugenia Chequen

Chelidonium Majus

Celandine

DESCRIPTION

Medicinal Parts: The medicinal parts are the aerial parts which have been collected during the flowering season and dried; the root which has been collected in late autumn and dried and the fresh rhizome.

Flower and Fruit: Yellow flowers in umbels, 2 sepals, 4 petals, numerous yellow stamens, and 1 ovary. The fruit is pod-like and many-seeded. The seeds are black-brown and glossy.

Leaves, Stem and Root: Thirty to 120 cm high plant with an erect stem, irregularly bifurcated, thickened nodes. The leaves are alternate, indent-pinnatifid, the upper ones pinnatisect, dull green above, sea-green beneath. The plant contains dark yellow latex.

Characteristics: Celandine is hot and has a bitter taste. The latex has a narcotic fragrance.

Habitat: The whole of Europe and the temperate and subarctic regions of Asia.

Production: The plant is collected in the wild during the flowering season and dried at higher temperatures. The herb is gathered in uncultivated regions and harvested commercially.

Other Names: Tetterwort

ACTIONS AND PHARMACOLOGY

COMPOUNDS: CHELIDONII HERBA

Isoquinoline alkaloids of the protoberberine type: including coptisine (main alkaloid), berberine

Isoquinoline alkaloids of the benzophenanthridine type: including chelidonine, sanguinarine

Isoquinoline alkaloids of the protopine type: including protopin, cryptopine

Caffeic acid derivatives: including 2-(-)-coffeoyl-D-glyceric acid, coffeoyl-L-malic acid

EFFECTS: CHELIDONII HERBA

Celandine has mild analgesic, cholagogic, antimicrobial, oncostatic, and central-sedative effects; also acts as a spasmolytic on smooth muscles. In animal tests, it is a cytostatic; nonspecific immune stimulation.

Note: the blood pressure-lowering effects and the therapeutic efficacy for mild forms of hypertonia (borderline hypertonia) need further investigation.

COMPOUNDS: CHELIDONII RADIX

Isoquinoline alkaloids of the protoberberine type: including coptisine (main alkaloid), berberine

Isoquinoline alkaloids of the benzophenanthridine type: including chelidonine, sanguinarine, Chelerythrin

Isoquinoline alkaloids of the protopine-type: including protopin, cryptopine

Caffeic acid derivatives: including 2-(-)-coffeoyl-D-glyceric acid, coffeoyl-L-malic acid

EFFECTS: CHELIDONII RADIX

Only clinical studies and experiments on the fresh plants are available. However, previous studies have shown that the extract, with an alkaloid content of 80%, should have similar effects to those of the fresh leaves: immobilization in mice, where it was applied subcutaneously and per orally; on rabbit intestines it caused limpness, and in higher doses, tone reduction; the rabbit uterus contracted. Positive inotropal effects were observed in isolated cat and frog hearts; in a canine heart-lung preparation it stimulated the heart, raised blood pressure and widened the arteries.

Experimental data are unavailable, therefore the results must be considered unofficial.

An oncostatic effect was observed through the cyto-toxic results of Eagle's 9 KB carcinoma of the naso-pharynx in cell cultures.

INDICATIONS AND USAGE

CHELIDONII HERBA

- Liver and gallbladder complaints
- Loss of appetite

Celandine is used for spasmodic pain of the bile ducts and the gastrointestinal tract.

In folk medicine, it was used for skin conditions such as blister rashes, scabies, and warts; it is said to be effective in the treatment of cholecystitis, chloelithiasis, catarrhal jaundice, gastroenteritis, and diffuse latent liver complaints; also for intestinal polyps, and breast lumps; recommended for angina pectoris, cramps, asthma, arteriosclerosis, high blood pressure, stomach cancer, gout, edema, and hepatitis.

CHELIDONII RADIX

In folk medicine, the fresh roots are chewed to alleviate toothache, and a powder derived from the roots is applied to ease tooth extraction.

In China, the drug is used in cases of irregular menstruation.

The efficacy of the drug has not been proven.

PRECAUTIONS AND ADVERSE REACTIONS

CHELIDONII HERBA

No health hazards or side effects are known in conjunction with the proper administration of designated therapeutic dosages. Older scientific literature credits the plant with toxicity (burning in the mouth, nausea, vomiting, bloody diarrheas, hematuria, stupor), but recent studies offer no clear proofs of this; animal experiments yielded no results.

No symptoms of inflammation were observed in the eyes of rabbits following introduction of the chyle, nevertheless contact between it and the eyes is to be avoided.

CHELIDONII RADIX

No health hazards or side effects are known in conjunction with the proper administration of designated therapeutic dosages. Older scientific literature credits the plant with toxicity (burning in the mouth, nausea, vomiting, bloody diarrheas, haematuria, stupor), but recent studies offer no clear proofs of this; animal experiments yielded no results.

DOSAGE

CHELIDONII HERBA

Mode of Administration: Comminuted and powdered drug for infusions and decoctions; dried extracts for liquid and solid medicinal forms for internal use.

Daily Dosage: The average daily dose is 2 to 4 gm of drug in liquid or solid extracts, equivalent to 12 to 30 mg total alkaloids calculated as chelidonine; fluid extract, 1 to 2 ml three times daily; decoction, 3 cups daily; infusion, 3 cups between meals.

Storage: Should be protected carefully from light.

CHELIDONII RADIX

Daily Dosage: The standard dose is 0.5 gm of drug.

Storage: It must be stored carefully.

LITERATURE

CHELIDONII HERBA

Äberlein H et al., Chelidonium majus L, Components with in vitro affinity for GABA A receptor: Positive cooperation of alkaloids. In: PM 62(3):227-231. 1996.

Anonym, Brennpunkt ZNS. In: DAZ 137(25):2166-2167. 1997.

Arnason JT, Gurein B, Kraml MM, Mehta B, Rehmond JC, Scaiano JC, Phototoxic and photochemical properties of sanguinarin. In: Photochemistry and Photobiology 55(1):35. 1992.

Baumann J (1975), Über die Wirkung von Chelidonium, Curcuma, Absinth und Carduus marianus auf die Galle- und Pankreassekretion bei Hepatopathien. Med Mschr 29:173.

Boegge SC et al., Reduction of ACh-induced contraction of rat isolated ileum by Coptisin, (+)-Caffeoylmalic acid, Chelidonium majus, and Corydalis lutea extracts. In: PM 62(2):173-174. 1997.

Diener H, Schöllkraut. In: PTA 8(2):145. 1994.

Dostál J et al., Structure of chelerythrine base. In: JNP 58(5):723-729. 1995.

Fulde G, Wichtl M, Analytik von Schöllkraut, Hauptalkaloid Coptisin. In: DAZ 134(12):1031. 1994.

Hahn R, Nahrstedt A, Hydroxycinnamic acid derivatives, caffeoylmalic and new caffeoylaldonic acid esters, from Chelidonium majus. In: PM 59(1):71. 1993.

Hamacher H, Haben Phytopharmaka eine Zukunft? In: DAZ 131(42):2155. 1991.

Kim DJ, Ahn B, Han BS, Tsuda H, Potential preventive effects of Chelidonium majus L (Papaveraceae) herb extract on glandular stomach tumor development in rats treated with N-methyl-N'-nitro-N nitrosoguanidine (MNNG) and hypertonic sodium chloride. In: Can.

Mitra S et al., Effect of Chelidonium majus L. on experimetal hepatic tissue injury. In: Phytother Res 10(4):354-356. 1996.

Reuter HD, Pflanzliche Gallentherapeutika (Teil I) und (Teil II). In: ZPT 16(1):13-20 u. 77-89. 1995.

Schilcher H, Pharmazeutische Aspekte pflanzlicher Gallentherapeutika. In: ZPT 16(4):211-222. 1995.

Schmidt M, Phytotherapie: Pflanzliche Gallenwegstherapeutika. In: DAZ 135(8):680-682. 1995.

Táborská E et al., The alkaloids of Chelidonium majus L. and their variability. In: PM 62, Abstracts of the 44th Ann Congress of GA, 145. 1996.

Vahlensiek U et al., The effect of Chelidonium majus herb extract on the choleresis in the isolated perfused rat liver. In: PH 61(3):267-270. 1995.

Vavreckova C, Gawlik I, Müller K, Benzophenanthridine alkaloids of Chelidonium majus: I. Inhibition of 5- and 12-lipoxygenase by a non-redox mechanism. In: PM 62(5):397-401. 1996.

Willaman JJ and Hui-Li L (1970) Lloydia 33 (3A):1.

Further information in:

Chan, EH et al., (Eds), Advances in Chinese Medicinal Materials Research, World Scientific Pub. Co. Singapore 1985.

Frohne D, Pfänder HJ, Giftpflanzen - Ein Handbuch für Apotheker, Toxikologen und Biologen, 4. Aufl., Wiss. Verlagsges. mbH Stuttgart 1997.

Hänsel R, Keller K, Rimpler H, Schneider G (Hrsg.), Hagers Handbuch der Pharmazeutischen Praxis, 5. Aufl., Bde 4-6 (Drogen): Springer Verlag Berlin, Heidelberg, New York, 1992-1994.

Lewin L, Gifte und Vergiftungen, 6. Aufl., Nachdruck, Haug Verlag, Heidelberg 1992.

Madaus G, Lehrbuch der Biologischen Arzneimittel, Bde 1-3, Nachdruck, Georg Olms Verlag Hildesheim 1979.

Roth L, Daunderer M, Kormann K, Giftpflanzen, Pflanzengifte, 4. Aufl., Ecomed Fachverlag Landsberg Lech 1993.

Schulz R, Hänsel R, Rationale Phytotherapie, Springer Verlag Heidelberg 1996.

Steinegger E, Hänsel R, Pharmakognosie, 5. Aufl., Springer Verlag Heidelberg 1992.

Teuscher E, Lindequist U, Biogene Gifte - Biologie, Chemie, Pharmakologie, 2. Aufl., Fischer Verlag Stuttgart 1994.

Teuscher E, Biogene Arzneimittel, 5. Aufl., Wiss. Verlagsges. mbH Stuttgart 1997.

Wagner H, Wiesenauer M, Phytotherapie. Phytopharmaka und pflanzliche Homöopathika, Fischer-Verlag, Stuttgart, Jena, New York 1995.

Wichtl M (Hrsg.), Teedrogen, 4. Aufl., Wiss. Verlagsges. Stuttgart 1997.

CHELIDONII RADIX

Hänsel R, Keller K, Rimpler H, Schneider G (Hrsg.), Hagers Handbuch der Pharmazeutischen Praxis, 5. Aufl., Bde 4-6 (Drogen): Springer Verlag Berlin, Heidelberg, New York, 1992-1994.

Literatur zu den Wirkungen der Inhaltsstoffe vgl. Chelidonii herba.

Chelone Glabra

Turtle Head

DESCRIPTION

Medicinal Parts: The fresh herb picked during the flowering season

Flower and Fruit: The inflorescence is a short terminal spike of bilabiate white, purple, cream or pink flowers. The lower lip is awned in the tube and the cordate anthers are downy. The seeds are round and bitter.

Leaves, Stem and Root: The plant is small, erect, and may reach up to 60 cm in height. It is a perennial herb with angular, smooth stems and a horizontally spreading root system. The leaves are opposite, oblong-lanceolate, on short petioles.

Characteristics: The leaves have a tea-like smell and an extremely bitter taste.

Habitat: Northeastern U.S. and Canada.

Production: Turtle Head is the above-ground part of Chelone glabra.

Other Names: Turtlebloom, Balmony, Chelone, Shellflower, Salt-rheum Weed, Bitter Herb, Hummingbird Tree, Snakehead

ACTION AND PHARMACOLOGY

COMPOUNDS

Iridoide monoterpenes: catalpol

Resin: (bitter-tasting)

EFFECTS

No information available.

INDICATIONS

In homoeopathy in the treatment of liver disorders, digestive disorders, worm infestation.

PRECAUTIONS AND ADVERSE REACTIONS

No health hazards or side effects are known in conjunction with the proper administration of designated therapeutic dosages.

DOSAGE

Mode of Administration: The herb is available in homoeopathic dilutions.

LITERATURE

Belofsky G et al., PH 28:1601. 1989.

Further information in:

Kern W, List PH, Hörhammer L (Hrsg.), Hagers Handbuch der Pharmazeutischen Praxis, 4. Aufl., Bde. 1-8, Springer Verlag Berlin, Heidelberg, New York, 1969.

Chenopodium Ambrosioides

Wormseed Oil

DESCRIPTION

Medicinal Parts: Seeds and the herb, including the flowers.

Flower and Fruit: The numerous small flowers are yellowish green and form small racemes or roundish spikes in the axils of the apical leaves. The calyx is divided into 5, the lobes are ovate and pointed. There are 5 stamens. The ovary has small, oblong, stemmed glands at the tip. The angular fruit is enclosed in the calyx. The seeds are achaenes and are smooth, small and black.

Leaves, Stem and Root: The plant is an annual plant which grows to about 1 m in height with a branched, reddish stem covered in alternate linear to lanceolate leaves. The whole plant gives off a pleasant fragrance.

Habitat: Mexico and South America but has spread to the eastern U.S.

Production: Wormseed oil is the seed oil of Chenopodium ambrosioides.

Other Names: Mexican Tea, American Wormseed, Jesuit's Tea

ACTION AND PHARMACOLOGY

COMPOUNDS

ascaridiole: chief constituent (80%), additionally including, according to variety and breed, p-cymene, L-pinocarvone, alpha-pinenes and/or alpha-terpenes (beware, the wormseed oil is explosive)

EFFECTS

Anthelmintic: it causes flight and defensive reactions in worms.

INDICATIONS AND USAGE

Used against roundworms and hookworms, if other more modern anthelmintic drugs fail.

PRECAUTIONS AND ADVERSE REACTIONS

Even the administration of therapeutic dosages can lead to disorders of the central nervous system (spasms, signs of paralysis, Pachymeningitis haemorrhagica). Damage to the Nervus cochlearis is frequent, leading to buzzing in the ears, and hearing impairment (sometimes lasting for years).

OVERDOSAGE

Cases of death have been observed following intake of 10 mg of the oil (much less for children). For that reason, an administration in allopathic dosages is to be strictly ruled out.

DOSAGE

Mode of Administration: It is obsolete as a drug. In clinically described cases, which are exceptional, it can be used in combination with a fast-acting and powerful purgative.

Daily Dosage: Two single doses of drops per day, with one drop per year of the child's age and a gap of 1 hour between doses. To be taken in the morning on an empty stomach. 2 hours later, a purgative is given. Adults should receive 20 drops.

LITERATURE

Bombardelli E et al., (1976) Fitoterapia 47:3.

Gupta GS, Behari M, (1972) J Ind Chem Soc 49:317.

Further information in:

Chan, EH et al., (Eds), Advances in Chinese Medicinal Materials Research, World Scientific Pub. Co. Singapore 1985.

Leung AY, Encyclopedia of Common Natural Ingredients Used in Food Drugs and Cosmetics, John Wiley & Sons Inc., New York 1980.

Lewin L, Gifte und Vergiftungen, 6. Aufl., Nachdruck, Haug Verlag, Heidelberg 1992.

Madaus G, Lehrbuch der Biologischen Arzneimittel, Bde 1-3, Nachdruck, Georg Olms Verlag Hildesheim 1979.

Roth L, Daunderer M, Kormann K, Giftpflanzen, Pflanzengifte, 4. Aufl., Ecomed Fachverlag Landsberg Lech 1993.

Chenopodium Vulvaria

Arrach

DESCRIPTION

Medicinal Parts: The whole fresh flowering plant.

Flower and Fruit: The flowers are small yellow-green and inconspicuous. They are in clusters in leafless compact spikes at the tip of the stem. The fruit is enclosed by the involucre. The seeds are black and glossy.

Leaves, Stem and Root: The plant is 15 to 40 cm high. The stems are branched from low down. The leaves are broad, rhomboid, entire-margined and petiolate. The whole plant is floury-dusty.

Characteristics: Distinctive smell of musty herring brine.

Habitat: Europe.

Production: Arrach is the complete flowering plant of Chenopodium vulvaria.

Other Names: Stinking Arrach, Stinking Goosefoot, Dog's Arrach, Goat's Arrach, Goosefoot, Stinking Motherwort, Netchweed, Oraches

ACTION AND PHARMACOLOGY

COMPOUNDS

Mono, di- and trimethylamine

Betaine

Tannins

EFFECTS

No information available.

INDICATIONS AND USAGE

Internally and externally to relieve cramps and as an emmenagogue.

PRECAUTIONS AND ADVERSE REACTIONS

No health hazards or side effects are known in conjunction with the proper administration of designated therapeutic dosages.

DOSAGE

Mode of Administration: Externally and as an extract.

LITERATURE

Roth L, Daunderer M, Kormann K, Giftpflanzen, Pflanzengifte, 4. Aufl., Ecomed Fachverlag Landsberg Lech 1993.

Cherry Laurel

See Prunus Laurocerasus

Chestnut

See Castanea Sativa

Chickweed

See Stellaria Media

Chicory

See Cichorium Intybus

Chimaphila Umbellata

Pipsissewa

DESCRIPTION

Medicinal Parts: The medicinal parts are the dried leaves, the fresh aerial parts of the flowering plant and the dried complete plant.

Flower and Fruit: The plant has 10 cm long terminal inflorescences with umbels of 2 to 7 flowers. The flowers which are initially bright pink and then white are nodding and mildly campanulate. The 5 sepals are obovate, dentate and about a third as long as the 5 petals. The petals are broadly ovate, domed, pink, and 5 to 6 mm long. The 10 stamens are thickened at the base, the edges are winged and ciliate. The anthers are short thick and red. The style is very short and the stigma broad and shorter than the anthers. The fruit is a 5-grooved capsule with erect stems.

Leaves, Stem and Root: The plant is a perennial, up to 25 cm high semi-shrub with an upright, angular stem and a creeping white rhizome. The evergreen, alternate leaves are short-petioled, coriaceous, ovate-spatulate to linear and wedge-shaped. The leaf margin is sharply serrate.

Habitat: Europe, Asia, Siberia, North and South America.

Production: Pipsissewa is the aerial part of Chimaphila umbellata.

Other Names: Prince's Pine, Ground Holly, Umbellate Wintergreen, Butter Winter, King's Cureall, Love in Winter, Rheumatism Weed, King's Cure

ACTION AND PHARMACOLOGY

COMPOUNDS

Hydroquinone derivatives: chief components isohomoarbutin, additionally homoarbutin (arbutin)

Naphthacene derivatives (naphthoquinone): chimaphilin (2,7-dimethyl-1,4-naphthoquinone)

Flavonoids: including among others hyperoside, avicularin

Tannins: (4-5%)

EFFECTS

Urinary antiseptic (see Uvae ursi folium).

INDICATIONS AND USAGE

See Uvae ursi herba.

PRECAUTIONS AND ADVERSE REACTIONS

No health hazards or side effects are known in conjunction with the proper administration of designated therapeutic dosages. The drug possesses a weak sensitizing effect, due to its chimaphilin content. The drug is not suitable for long-term use because of its hydroquinone glycoside content (see Uvae ursi folium).

DOSAGE

Mode of Administration: Constituent of homeopathic preparations in dilutions or as a mother tincture.

LITERATURE

Walewska E, Thieme H, (1969) Pharmazie 24:423.

Bolkart KH et al., (1968) Naturwissenschaften 55:445.

Further information in:

Hänsel R, Keller K, Rimpler H, Schneider G (Hrsg.), Hagers Handbuch der Pharmazeutischen Praxis, 5. Aufl., Bde 4-6 (Drogen), Springer Verlag Berlin, Heidelberg, New York, 1992-1994.

Madaus G, Lehrbuch der Biologischen Arzneimittel, Bde 1-3, Nachdruck, Georg Olms Verlag Hildesheim 1979.

Thomson RH, Naturally Occuring Quinones, 2nd Ed., Academic Press New York 1971.

Chinese Cinnamon

See Cinnamomum Aromaticum

Chionanthus Virginicus

Fringetree

DESCRIPTION

Medicinal Parts: The medicinal part is the dried root or tree bark.

Flower and Fruit: The tree bears long peduncles of white, snowdrop-like flowers with fringed petals the same size as magnolia flowers. The fruit is dark blue and oval.

Leaves, Stem and Root: Fringetree is a deciduous shrub or tree up to 10 m tall. The leaves are smooth or downy, oblong or oval, 7.5 to 20 cm long and opposite. The root bark is about 3 mm thick and consists of irregular, quilled pieces up to about 8 cm long. The bark is externally dull brown with concave scars. The inner surface is smooth and buff colored. The fracture is short and dense with projecting bundles of stone cells.

Characteristics: Fringetree is almost odorless and very bitter.

Habitat: Central and southern U.S. also in eastern Asia.

Production: Fringetree rootbark is the rootbark of Chionanthus virginicus.

Other Names: Gray Beard Tree, Old Man's Beard, Poison Ash, Snowflower, White Fringe, Chionanthus, Snowdrop Tree

ACTION AND PHARMACOLOGY

COMPOUNDS

Lignane glycosides

Saponins

EFFECTS

Hepatic, cholagogue, diuretic, tonic.

INDICATIONS AND USAGE

Fringetree is used in treatment of the liver and gallbladder conditions (including gallstones).

PRECAUTIONS AND ADVERSE REACTIONS

No health hazards or side effects are known in conjunction with the proper administration of designated therapeutic dosages.

DOSAGE

Mode of Administration: Liquid extract and preparations.

LITERATURE

Steinegger E, Jacober H, Pharm Acta Helv 34:585. 1959.

Further information in:

Kern W, List PH, Hörhammer L (Hrsg.), Hagers Handbuch der Pharmazeutischen Praxis, 4. Aufl., Bde. 1-8, Springer Verlag Berlin, Heidelberg, New York, 1969.

Madaus G, Lehrbuch der Biologischen Arzneimittel, Bde 1-3, Nachdruck, Georg Olms Verlag Hildesheim 1979.

Chiretta

See Swertia Chirata

Chive

See Allium Schoenoprasum

Chondrodendron Tomentosum

Pareira

DESCRIPTION

Medicinal Parts: The medicinal parts are the curare, i.e. the extract from the fresh or dried trunk with the bark and the dried roots.

Flower and Fruit: The flowers are in 10 to 15 cm long axillary clusters on stems that are often unbranched. There are 9 outer pubescent sepals about 1 mm long. The inner 6 sepals are about 3.5 mm long and glabrous. The petals are 0.4 mm long. The fruit is a drupe about 12 mm long and 9 mm wide on a 4 mm long stem.

Leaves, Stem and Root: The plant is a climber which climbs to about 30 m. The stems are velvety. The petioles are short-haired at the base, have long erect hairs near the leaf blade and are about 8 to 12 cm long. The leaves are somewhat coriaceous, entire-margined, sparse above, tomentose beneath. They are mildly cordate, triangular-ovate or roundish and obtuse, 10 to 15 cm long and the same width. The root is about 2 to 5 cm in diameter, tortuous, black, longitudinally furrowed with transverse ridges and some constrictions. Internally the root is grayish-brown, and the transverse section shows three or four concentric rings, traversed by wide medullary rays. The stem pieces are similar but the external surface is grayish and marked with numerous round, warty lenticels.

Characteristics: The taste is bitter, then slightly sweet and odorless.

Habitat: The plant is found in western Bolivia, Peru, Ecuador, central Columbia and Panama.

Production: Pareira root is the root of Chondrodendron tomentosum.

Other Names: Pereira Brava, Velvet Leaf, Ice Vine

ACTION AND PHARMACOLOGY

COMPOUNDS

Bibenzyl isoquinoline alkaloids: including, among others, D-tubocurarine, chondrocurarine, (-)-curine, (+)-chondrofoline, chondrocurine, isochondrodendrine

EFFECTS

Uncertain emmenagogic and diuretic actions.

INDICATIONS AND USAGE

Only the tubocurarine extracted from the bark and twigs is in use. It is a peripheral muscle relaxant, which inhibits the stimulation of transference in the neuromuscular, hence causing a paralysis of the skeletal muscles.

Tubocurare is used in modern anaesthetics.

PRECAUTIONS AND ADVERSE REACTIONS

No health hazards or side effects are known in conjunction with the oral administration of designated therapeutic dosages of the drug. The alkaloids with curare-like effect, such as tubocurarine, are not resorbed with oral administration of the drug.

DOSAGE

Mode of Administration: Drug not in use.

LITERATURE

Guha et al., (1979) J Nat Prod 42:1.

Further information in:

Hänsel R, Keller K, Rimpler H, Schneider G (Hrsg.), Hagers Handbuch der Pharmazeutischen Praxis, 5. Aufl., Bde 4-6 (Drogen), Springer Verlag Berlin, Heidelberg, New York, 1992-1994.

Madaus G, Lehrbuch der Biologischen Arzneimittel, Bde 1-3, Nachdruck, Georg Olms Verlag Hildesheim 1979.

Teuscher E, Lindequist U, Biogene Gifte - Biologie, Chemie, Pharmakologie, 2. Aufl., Fischer Verlag Stuttgart 1994.

Chondrus Crispus

Carrageen

DESCRIPTION

Medicinal Parts: The medicinal part is carrageen, the Irish seaweed which is the thallus that has been freed from the adhesive disc then dried and bleached in the sun.

Flower and Fruit: Gamatangia: The spematangia are colorless and are at the end of the younger thallus lobes. The spermatia are 7.5 to 10 m long and 4 to 5 m wide; the carposporangia are 20 to 20 m long and 14 to 25 m wide and has no outer threads. The tetrasporangia along with the cruciform arranged tatra spores are in the medulla of the short side branches.

Thallus: Chondrus crispus is a perennial red algae which grows in waters up to 25 m deep. The thallus is usually yellow-green to purplish-brown when fresh, white to yellow and translucent after drying; thallus (fronds) 10 to 30 cm long on an adhesive disc, arising from subcylindrical stem, becoming flattened, curled and sometimes bifid. The segments are linear and usually 3 to 8 mm wide. The margin is linguiform, later repeatedly dividing into bifid thallus lobes. The thallus is cartilaginous and double layered. The internal tissue is made up of reticulately-linked cells. The bark layer is at right angles to the thallus and the bifurcated cell strings are like strings of pearls, which are spread radially.

Habitat: From the coast of Iceland to the Baltic and northern Russia to the south of Spain, Morocco and the Cape Verde Islands as well parts of North America and some Japanese coastal regions.

Production: Carrageen is the dried and bleached thalli of Chondrus crispus as well as other varieties of Gigartina species.

Other Names: Irish Moss, Chondrus, Carrahan, Carragennan

ACTION AND PHARMACOLOGY

COMPOUNDS

Carrageenans: (carrageenine): in particular kappa-, iota- and lambda-carrageenan (muciform galactane sulphate)

Proteins

Mineral salts: including iodides and bromides

EFFECTS

As an expectorant (coughs) and secretory agent (diarrhea).

The drug is mucous-like, and hinders the effect of peptides in digestive enzymes. Carrageen is regarded as a mucilaginosum.

INDICATIONS AND USAGE

Bronchitis, diarrhea.

PRECAUTIONS AND ADVERSE REACTIONS

No health hazards or side effects are known in conjunction with the proper administration of designated therapeutic dosages. Intracutaneous injections of solutions can trigger local inflammations (inflammation model in medicinal research).

DOSAGE

Mode of Administration: Seldom used, as granules in combinations.

LITERATURE

Chapman, B, In: Chapman VJ, Chapman DJ, seaweeds and their uses. Chapmann and Hall, London, New York 1980.

Stancioff DJ, Renn DW, (1975) A C S Symp Ser. 15:282.

Thomson AW, Horne CHW, (1976) Brit J Exp Pathol 57:455.

Further information in:

Hänsel R, Keller K, Rimpler H, Schneider G (Hrsg.), Hagers Handbuch der Pharmazeutischen Praxis, 5. Aufl., Bde 4-6 (Drogen), Springer Verlag Berlin, Heidelberg, New York, 1992-1994.

Steinegger E, Hänsel R, Pharmakognosie, 5. Aufl., Springer Verlag Heidelberg 1992.

Teuscher E, Biogene Arzneimittel, 5. Aufl., Wiss. Verlagsges. mbH Stuttgart 1997.

Chrysanthemum Cinerariifolium

Pyrethrum

DESCRIPTION

Flower and Fruit: Solitary flower heads are at the end of long slender peduncles, consisting of white lingual florets and yellow tubular florets.

Leaves, Stem and Root: Pyrethrum is a perennial, 20 to 60 cm high plant with an erect stem covered in alternating, pinnate, roughly serrated leaves. The underside of leaves is downy.

Characteristics: The whole plant gives off a heavy perfume.

Habitat: Indigenous to the Balkan region, widely cultivated.

Production: Pyrethrum flowers are the dried compound flowers of Chrysanthemum cinerariifolium.

Other Names: Dalmatian Pellitory, Dalmation Insect Flowers

ACTION AND PHARMACOLOGY

COMPOUNDS

Pyrethrine: (ester of monoterpene acid with alkylcyclopentenolone, 1%): chief components pyrethrines I and II, additionally cinerines I and II, jasmoline I and II

EFFECTS

Neurotoxic effect on the sodium canal of insects.

INDICATIONS AND USAGE

Pyrethrum is used as an insecticide and antiscabies remedy. For head lice, crablice and their nits.

PRECAUTIONS AND ADVERSE REACTIONS

No health hazards or side effects are known in conjunction with the proper administration of designated therapeutic dosages. The pyrethrines possess only limited toxicity in humans (dosages up to 2 g of the drug are non-toxic).

OVERDOSAGE

Headache, ringing in the ears, nausea, paraesthesias, respiratory disturbances and other neurotoxic symptoms have been observed as signs of poisoning.

Following gastric lavage with burgundy-colored potassium permanganate solution and installation of activated charcoal, the therapy for poisonings consists in treating possible cases of acidosis with sodium bicarbonate infusions. In case of shock, plasma volume expanders should be infused. Monitoring of kidney function is essential. Intubation and oxygen respiration may also be necessary.

DOSAGE

Mode of Administration: Externally as a liquid extract (rinse after use!).

LITERATURE

Anonym, Bio-Insektensprays: Wirken Pyrethroide als Nervengifte? In: DAZ 132(31):1632. 1992.

Kern W, List PH, Hörhammer L (Hrsg.), Hagers Handbuch der Pharmazeutischen Praxis, 4. Aufl., Bde. 1-8, Springer Verlag Berlin, Heidelberg, New York, 1969.

Lewin L, Gifte und Vergiftungen, 6. Aufl., Nachdruck, Haug Verlag, Heidelberg 1992.

Pachaly P, Pflanzenschutzmittel in der Apotheke - Pyrethrum. In: DAZ 132(19):1032. 1992.

Roth L, Daunderer M, Kormann K, Giftpflanzen, Pflanzengifte, 4. Aufl., Ecomed Fachverlag Landsberg Lech 1993 (unter Chrysanthemum cinerariifolium).

Stüttgen G, Skabies und Läuse heute. In: DAZ 132(34):1745. 1992.

Teuscher E, Lindequist U, Biogene Gifte - Biologie, Chemie, Pharmakologie, 2. Aufl., Fischer Verlag Stuttgart 1994.

Teuscher E, Biogene Arzneimittel, 5. Aufl., Wiss. Verlagsges. Stuttgart 1997.

Chrysanthemum Leucanthemum

Ox-eye Daisy

DESCRIPTION

Flower and Fruit: Long pedicled flowers with a semi-globular calyx. Imbricate, green, wide sepals; golden-yellow orbicular corolla. Young flowers white, 1 to 2 cm long, top-shaped, 2.5 to 3 mm long fruit.

Leaves, Stem and Root: Perennial, 10 to 100 cm high somewhat hairy or glabrous plant with cylindrical knotted root. The stem is erect, glabrous, simple or divided into numerous oblong 1-headed branches. The leaves are tough, compound, glabrous or slightly pubescent. The cauline leaves are petiolate, linear to ovate-oblong, roughly dentate to almost pinnatisect.

Habitat: Britain and Europe, parts of Russia and Asia.

Production: Ox-eye Daisy is the above-ground part of Chrysanthemum leucanthemum.

Other Names: White Weed, Golden Daisy, Herb Margaret, Maudlinwort, White Daisy, Great Ox-eye, Goldenseal, Marguerite, Moon Daisy, Horse Gowan, Maudlin Daisy, Dun Daisy, Butter Daisy, Horse Daisy, Moon Flower, Moon Penny, Poverty Weed

ACTION AND PHARMACOLOGY

COMPOUNDS

Cyclitols: including meso-inositol, L(-)-quercitol

Polyynes: among them the strongly sensibilizing trideca-3,5,7,9,11-pentain-1-ol and its acetate

Flavonoids: including a C-glycosyl flavone, containing a cyclitol instead of a sugar

EFFECTS

Antispasmodic, diuretic, tonic.

As a tonic, it has a similar action to that of chamomile.

INDICATIONS AND USAGE

See Chamomile.

PRECAUTIONS AND ADVERSE REACTIONS

No health hazards or side effects are known in conjunction with the proper administration of designated therapeutic dosages. There is however a strong potential for sensitization via skin contact with the drug.

DOSAGE

Mode of Administration: See Chamomile.

LITERATURE

Hausen B, Allergiepflanzen, Pflanzenallergene, ecomed Verlagsgesellsch. mbH, Landsberg 1988.

Hegnauer R, Chemotaxonomie der Pflanzen, Bde 1-11, Birkhäuser Verlag Basel, Boston, Berlin 1962-1997.

Kern W, List PH, Hörhammer L (Hrsg.), Hagers Handbuch der Pharmazeutischen Praxis, 4. Aufl., Bde 1-8, Springer Verlag Berlin, Heidelberg, New York, 1969.

Teuscher E, Lindequist U, Biogene Gifte - Biologie, Chemie, Pharmakologie, 2. Aufl., Fischer Verlag Stuttgart 1994.

Cichorium Intybus

Chicory

DESCRIPTION

Medicinal Parts: The medicinal parts are the dried leaves and roots, which are collected in autumn, and the whole plant collected and dried in the flowering season as well as the fresh plant and root.

Flower and Fruit: Size: 30-100 cm. The numerous flower heads are 3 to 4 cm in diameter and are terminal or axillary, solitary or in groups, sessile or short-pedicled. The epicalyx bracts are bristly ciliate, often glandular-haired. The inner ones are oblong-lanceolate and erect, the outer ones ovate, splayed and half as long as the inner ones. The androgynous lingual florets are light blue, seldom white or pink. The fruit is an achaene 2 to 3 mm in length. It has no hair tuft and is straw yellow to blackish and ovate.

Leaves, Stem and Root: The plant can grow to a height of 2 m and has a hardy, 10 to 30 cm long, thick root. The stem is rigidly erect and is sparsely branched above and often bristly. The leaves are 10 to 30 cm long and 1 to 5 cm wide, obovate, oblong, shaped like a cross-cut saw or slit, with numerous stiff hairs beneath. The lowest leaves in a basal rosette are petiolate. The upper ones as well as those near the inflorescences are alternate, oblong to lanceolate, crenate-dentate and sessile.

Characteristics: Bitter taste.

Habitat: The plant is found in Europe, the Near East as far as Iran, north and South Africa, all of America, Australia and New Zealand.

Production: The dried, aerial parts and underground parts, collected in autumn, of Cichorium intybus.

Other Names: Succory, Hendibeh

ACTION AND PHARMACOLOGY

COMPOUNDS

Sesquiterpene lactones, guaianolid glycosides

Caffeic acid derivatives: chiroree acid, chlorogenic acid, isochlorogenic acid, dicoffeoly tartaric acid

Hydroxycoumarins: including umbelliferone

Flavonoids: including hyperoside

Polyynes

EFFECTS

In animal studies a distinct reduction of pulse rate and contractility; mildly cholagogic; lowered the cholesterin level in rats livers and plasma; antiexudative.

INDICATIONS AND USAGE

- Loss of appetite
- Dyspeptic complaints
- Liver and gallbladder complaints

In folk medicine: Recommended laxative for children.

PRECAUTIONS AND ADVERSE REACTIONS

No health hazards or side effects are known in conjunction with the proper administration of designated therapeutic dosages. There is a weak potential for sensitization via skin contact with the drug.

DOSAGE

Mode of Administration: Comminuted drug for infusions as well as other bitter-tasting preparations for internal use.

Preparation: Infusion: scald 2 to 4 g drug with boiling water and strain after 10 minutes.

Daily Dose: 3 to 5 g comminuted drug; single dose: 2 to 4 g whole herb for an infusion.

LITERATURE

Anonym, Abwehr von Arzneimittelrisiken, Stufe II. In: DAZ 136(38):3253-2354. 1996.

BGA, Arzneimittelrisiken: Anthranoide. In: DAZ 132(21):1164. 1992.

Balbaa S et al., (1973) Planta Med 24:133.

Benoit PS et al., (1976) Lloydia 39:160.

Kawabata S, Deki M, (1977) Kanzei Chuo Bunsek 17:63.

Müller K, Wiegrebe W, Psoriasis und Antipsoriatika. In: DAZ 137(22):1893-1902. 1997.

Noldenn U, Dissertation Universität Bonn. 1989.

Proliac A, Blanc M, (1976) Helv Chem Acta 58:2503.

Wagner, H, In "The Biology and Chemistry of the Compositae", Eds V. N. Heywood et al. Academic Press, London 1977.

Further information in:

Hänsel R, Keller K, Rimpler H, Schneider G (Hrsg.), Hagers Handbuch der Pharmazeutischen Praxis, 5. Aufl., Bde 4-6 (Drogen), Springer Verlag Berlin, Heidelberg, New York, 1992-1994.

Hausen B, Allergiepflanzen, Pflanzenallergene, ecomed Verlagsgesellsch. mbH, Landsberg 1988.

Madaus G, Lehrbuch der Biologischen Arzneimittel, Bde 1-3, Nachdruck, Georg Olms Verlag Hildesheim 1979.

Cicuta Virosa

European Water Hemlock

DESCRIPTION

Medicinal Parts: The medicinal part is the rhizome with roots.

Flower and Fruit: The flower is a white umbelliferous blossom with distinct calyx tips. The petals have indented tips. The style cushion is flat. The fruit is brown-yellow, 2.5 mm by 3 mm, and has dark-brown stripes.

Leaves, Stem and Root: The plant grows to a height of 30 to 120 cm. The leaves are 2 to 3-pinnate. The leaflets are lanceolate and sharply serrate. The whole plant is glabrous. The rhizome is tuberous, fleshy, and hollow. The stem is erect, round, hollow, glabrous, branched above, and forms adventitious roots at the nodes.

Characteristics: The rhizome has a disgusting smell and is extremely poisonous.

Habitat: The plant is indigenous to Europe and Asia.

Other Names: Cowbane

ACTIONS AND PHARMACOLOGY

COMPOUNDS

Polyynes: including cicutoxin, isocicutoxin

Furanocoumarins

Alkyl phthalides

EFFECTS

No information is available.

INDICATIONS AND USAGE

The drug is used in homeopathic dilutions for migraine, painful menstruation, worm infestation, and inflammation of the skin.

Efficacy has not been proven.

PRECAUTIONS AND ADVERSE REACTIONS

The freshly-harvested root stock is extremely poisonous, due to its cicutoxin content. The plant itself is weakly poisonous.

OVERDOSAGE

Two to 3 gm of the root stock is said to be fatal for an adult. The toxicity of the drug declines through dehydration and storage. Symptoms of poisoning, following the initial stupor and nausea, include severe tonic-clonic spasms, unconsciousness, canosis, and extremely widened pupils. Death occurs through asphyxiation at the peak of a convulsive attack or through heart failure.

Forced diuresis, hemodialysis and hemoperfusion are initiated as treatment for poisonings. Gastric lavage should only be carried out under anesthetic because of the danger of convulsion. Benzodiazepine or barbiturates are used to lessen the effects of the spasms.

DOSAGE

Mode of Administration: Topically and internally as a dilution of the mother tincture.

LITERATURE

Bilia AR, Ctalano S, Fontana C, Morelli I, Palme E, A new saponin from Potentilla tormentilla. In: PM 58(7):A723. 1992.

Wittstock U, Hadacek F, Wurz G, Teuscher E, Greger H, Polyacetylenes from water hemlock, Cicura virosa. In: PM 61(5):439-445. 1995.

Wittstock U, Lichtnow KH, Teuscher E, Effects of cicutoxin and related polyacetylenes from cicuta virosa on neuronal action potentials: a comparative study on the mechanism of the convulsive action. In: PM 63(2):120-124. 1997.

Wittstock U, Lichtnow KH, Teuscher E, Effects of polyacetylenes from Cicuta virosa on the electrical activity of molluscan giant neurones. In: PM 61(Abstracts of 43rd Ann Congr):84. 1995.

Wittstock U, Wurz G, Hadacek F, Greger H, Teuscher E, Biocative polyacetylens from Cicuta virosa. In: PM 58(7):A722. 1992.

Further information in:

Frohne D, Pfänder HJ: Giftpflanzen - Ein Handbuch für Apotheker, Toxikologen und Biologen, 4. Aufl., Wiss. Verlagsges. mbH Stuttgart 1997.

Kern W, List PH, Hörhammer L (Hrsg.), Hagers Handbuch der Pharmazeutischen Praxis, 4. Aufl., Bde 1-8, Springer Verlag Berlin, Heidelberg, New York, 1969.

Lewin L, Gifte und Vergiftungen, 6. Aufl., Nachdruck, Haug Verlag, Heidelberg 1992.

Madaus G: Lehrbuch der Biologischen Arzneimittel, Bde 1-3, Nachdruck, Georg Olms Verlag Hildesheim 1979.

Roth L, Daunderer M, Kormann K: Giftpflanzen, Pflanzengifte, 4.Aufl., Ecomed Fachverlag Landsberg Lech 1993.

Teuscher E, Lindequist U: Biogene Gifte - Biologie, Chemie, Pharmakologie, 2. Aufl., Fischer Verlag Stuttgart 1994.

Teuscher E: Biogene Arzneimittel, 5. Aufl., Wiss. Verlagsges. mbH Stuttgart 1997.

Cimicifuga Racemosa

Black Cohosh

DESCRIPTION

Medicinal Parts: The medicinal part is the fresh and dried root.

Flower and Fruit: The inflorescence is a long peduncled, drooping raceme, 30 to 90 cm long with white flowers. There are 3 to 8 petals without nectaries and the sepals enclose the flower bud.

Leaves, Stem and Root: The plant is 1 to 1.5 m high. It is leafy, with a sturdy, blackish rhizome which is cylindrical, tough and knotty. The straight, strong, dark brownish roots sprout from the underground rhizome and are roughly quadrangular and grooved. The transverse root section shows wedge-shaped bundles of white wood while the section of rhizome shows a large black medulla surrounded by a ring of paler, woodier wedges. The leaves are double-pinnate, smooth and crenate-serrate.

Habitat: Canada and U.S., cultivated in Europe.

Production: The medicinally used part of the plant consists of the dried rhizome with attached roots of Cimicifuga racemosa.

Other Names: Black Snake Root, Rattleroot, Rattleweed, Squaw Root, Bugbane, Bugwort, Cimicifuga, Richweed

ACTION AND PHARMACOLOGY

COMPOUNDS

Triterpene glycoside: including actein, 27-deoxyactein

Phenylpropane derivatives: including isoferulic acid

EFFECTS

The estrogen-like effect cannot be upheld any longer due to more recent results of research. In vitro and in vivo investigations demonstrate that compounds of the rootstock of Cimifuga racemosa couple to the estrogen-receptor, however, these results must be interpreted as a blockade of the receptor.

INDICATIONS AND USAGE

■ Climacteric complaints

Climacteric (menopausal) ailments, premenstrual and dysmenorrheic neurovegetative disorders.

PRECAUTIONS AND ADVERSE REACTIONS

No health hazards or side effects are known in conjunction with the proper administration of designated therapeutic dosages. An intake of very high dosages of the drug (5 g) or an extract (12 g) leads to vomiting, headache, dizziness, limb pains and lowered blood pressure.

Common adverse effects include gastric discomfort.

DOSAGE

Mode of Administration: Galenic preparations for internal use.

Daily Dosage: Alcoholic-aqueous extracts (ethanolic-aqueous 40-60% (V/V) or isopropanolic-aqueous 40% (V/V)) corresponding to 40 mg drug.

LITERATURE

Benoit, P S et al., (1976) Lloydia 39:160.

Berger S, Junior P, Kopanski L, 27-Desoxyactein: a New Polycyclic Triterpenoid Glycoside from Actaea racemosa. In: PM 54:579-780. 1988.

Beuscher N, Cimicifuga racemosa L. - Die Traubensilberkerze. In: ZPT 16(5):301-310. 1995.

Corsano S, Panizzi L, Sull' Acteina, principio attivo della Actaea racemosa. In: Atti Acca Nazl Lincei, Rend, Classe Sci, Fis. Mat. Nat 38:600-604. 1965.

Daiber W, Klimakterische Beschwerden: ohne Hormone zum Erfolg! In: Ärztl Praxis 35:1946-1947. 1983.

Düker EM, Kopanski L, Jarry H, Wuttke W, (1991) Effects of extracts from cimicifuga racemosa on gonadotropin release in menopausal women and ovariectomized rats. Planta Med 57:420-424.

Einer-Jensen N, Zhao J, Andersen KP, Kristoffersen K, Cimicifuga and Melbrosia lack oestrogenic effects in mice and rats. In: Maturitas 25(1995):149-153. 1996.

Földes J, Die Wirkungen eines Extraktes aus Cimicifuga racemosa. In: Ärztl Forsch 13:623-624. 1959.

Genazzani, E et al., (1962) Nature 194:544.

Gerhard I, Liske E, Wüstenberg P, Behandlung von psychovegetativen Beschwerden im Klimakterium mit Remifemin(R)plus (Poster). In: ZPT 16(5, Supplement):21, 6. Phytotherapiekongreβ in Berlin. 1995.

Görlich N, Behandlung ovarieller Störungen in der Allgemeinpraxis. In: Ärztl Praxis 14:1742-1743. 1962.

Harnischfeger G, Cillien N, Influence of Cimicifuga racemosa extract fractions on the proliferation of human carcinoma cells in vitro with regard to their estrogen receptor sensitivity. In: PM 62, Abstracts of the 44th Ann Congress of GA, 40. 1996.

Harnischfeger G, Stolze H, Bewährte Wirksubstanzen aus Naturstoffen. Traubensilberkerze. In: Notabene medici 10:446-450. 1980.

Jarry H, Gorkow Ch, Wuttke W, (1995) Treatment of Menopausal Symptoms with Extracts of Cimicifuga Racemosa, In vivo and in vitro Evidence for Estrogenic Activity. In, Loew D, Netbrock N (Hrsg) Phytopharmaka in Forschung und klinischer Anwendung. Steinkopff Verlag, Darmstadt, S 99-112.

Jarry H, Harnischfeger G, (1985) Studies on the endocrine effects of the contents of Cimicifuga racemosa, 1. Influence on the serum concentration of pituitary hormones in ovariectomized rats. Planta Med 51:46-49.

Jarry H, Harnischfeger G, Düker E, (1985) Studies on the endocrine effects of the contents of Cimicifuga racemosa, 2. In vitro binding of compounds to extrogen receptors. Planta Med 51:316-319.

Jarry H, Isolierung pharmakogologisch aktiver Substanzen aus Cimicifuga racemosa. In: Dissertation, math.-naturwiss. 1984.

Jarry H, Ludwig L, Stephan A, Wuttke W, Erste Beweise für eine direkte Wirkung von Inhaltsstoffen von Cimicifuga racemosa auf die in-vitro- Steroidsekretion von porcinen Granulosa- und Lutealzellen (Poster). In: ZPT 16(5, Supplement):7-8, 6. Phytotherapiek.

Kesselkauf O, Über die Behandlung klimakterischer Beschwerden mit Remifemin. In: Med Monatsschr 11:87-88. 1957.

Krämer H, Geisenhofer H, Erfahrungen mit dem Cimicifuga-Präparat Remifemin. In: Therapie der Gegenwart 97:238-239. 1958.

Lauritzen C, Nichthormonale Therapie klimakterischer Beschwerden. In: Gynäkol Praxis 14:43-56. 1990.

Neβelhut T, Schellhase C, Dietrich R, Kuhn W, Untersuchungen zur proliferativen Potenz von Phytopharmaka mit östrogenähnlicher Wirkung bei Mammakarzinomzellen. In: Arch Gynecol Obstetrics 254:817-818. 1993.

Pethö A, Umstellung einer Hormonbehandlung auf ein pflanzliches Gynäkologikum möglich? In: Ärztl Praxis 47:1551-1553. 1987.

Radics, L et al., (1975) Tetrahedron Letters 48:4287.

Shibata, M et al., (1980) Yakugaku Zasshi 100:1143.

Shibata, M, (1977) J Chem Soc Jpn 97:911.

Stoll W, (1987) Phytotherapeutikum beeinfluβ atrophisches Vaginalepithel, Doppelblindversuch Cimicifuga vs. Östrogenpräparat. Therapeutikon 1:23-32.

Stolze H, Der andere Weg klimakterische Beschwerden zu behandeln. In: Gyne 1:14-16. 1982.

Suntry L, (1984) Pat. JP 84/20298 Japan.

Vorberg G, Therapie klimakterischer Beschwerden. Erfolgreiche hormonfreie Therapie mit Remifemin R. In: ZFA 60:626-629. 1984.

Warnecke G, (1985) Beeinflussung klimakterischer Beschwerden durch ein Phytotherapeutikum. Erfolgreiche Therapie mit Cimicifuga- Monoextrakt. Med Welt 36:871-874.

Winterhoff H, (1993) Arzneipflanzen mit endokriner Wirksamkeit. Z Phytother 14:83-94.

Further information in:

Chan, EH et al., (Eds), Advances in Chinese Medicinal Materials Research, World Scientific Pub. Co. Singapore 1985.

Kern W, List PH, Hörhammer L (Hrsg.), Hagers Handbuch der Pharmazeutischen Praxis, 4. Aufl., Bde. 1-8, Springer Verlag Berlin, Heidelberg, New York, 1969.

Leung AY, Encyclopedia of Common Natural Ingredients Used in Food Drugs and Cosmetics, John Wiley & Sons Inc., New York 1980.

Lewin L, Gifte und Vergiftungen, 6. Aufl., Nachdruck, Haug Verlag, Heidelberg 1992.

Madaus G, Lehrbuch der Biologischen Arzneimittel, Bde 1-3, Nachdruck, Georg Olms Verlag Hildesheim 1979.

Roth L, Daunderer M, Kormann K, Giftpflanzen, Pflanzengifte, 4. Aufl., Ecomed Fachverlag Landsberg Lech 1993.

Schulz R, Hänsel R, Rationale Phytotherapie, Springer Verlag Heidelberg 1996.

Steinegger E, Hänsel R, Pharmakognosie, 5. Aufl., Springer Verlag Heidelberg 1992.

Teuscher E, Biogene Arzneimittel, 5. Aufl., Wiss. Verlagsges. mbH Stuttgart 1997.

Wagner H, Wiesenauer M, Phytotherapie. Phytopharmaka und pflanzliche Homöopathika, Fischer-Verlag, Stuttgart, Jena, New York 1995.

Cinchona Pubescens

Cinchona

DESCRIPTION

Medicinal Parts: The medicinal part is the dried bark of 6 to 8 year-old trees.

Flower and Fruit: The 35 cm long inflorescence is panicled, opposite, often leafy and densely blossomed. The flowers are almost sessile and the tube is thickly covered in silky hairs. The calyx has appressed hairs and the tips are short and widely acuminate. The corolla is red or pink and 10 to 12 mm long. The fruit is an oblong, glabrous and longitudinally grooved capsule.

Leaves, Stem and Root: The plant is an evergreen tree, sometimes a bush, which grows from 5 to 15 m high, with a dense crown. The branches are at right angles to the trunk. The young branches are usually pubescent. The stipules are large, ovate, obtuse or acuminate, silky-haired or glabrous. The leaves have an up to 8 cm long petiole. The leaf blade is 15 to 40 cm long and 7 to 25 cm wide, oblong-elliptoid to roundish with curved side ribs. The bark occurs in quills or flat pieces up to 30 cm long and 3 to 6 mm thick. The external surface is brownish-gray, usually fissured with an exfoliating cork. Lichens and mosses may be seen as grayish-white or greenish patches. The inner surface is yellowish to reddish-brown. The fracture is fibrous.

Characteristics: The bark has an astringent, bitter taste and the odor is slight.

Habitat: Indigenous to mountainous regions of the tropical U.S., cultivated elsewhere.

Production: Cinchona bark consists of the dried bark of Cinchona pubescens or other varieties. Trees are felled at between 6 and 12 years. They are dried slowly in the sun initially and then artificially dried at maximum temperatures of 70°C.

Not To Be Confused With: Yellow factory bark.

Other Names: Peruvian Bark, Jesuit's Bark

ACTIONS AND PHARMACOLOGY

COMPOUNDS

Quinoline alkaloids: main alkaloids are quinine, quinidine, cinchonine, cinchonidine bittere triterpene acid monoglycosides, in particular chinovic acid-3-chinovoside, chinovic acid-3-glucoside

Catechin tannins

EFFECTS

Stimulation of the secretion of saliva and gastric juices.

INDICATIONS AND USAGE

- Loss of appetite
- Dyspeptic complaints

Cinchona bark is used to correct loss of appetite, dyspepsia and flatulence with a sense fullness. In folk medicine, the bark is used for malaria, flu, enlarged spleen, muscle cramps, cancer, and gastric disorders. Externally it is used for scrapes and leg ulcers.

PRECAUTIONS AND ADVERSE REACTIONS

General: Sensitization to quinine and quinidine have been observed (eczema, itching). Even with therapeutic dosages, an enhanced pseudohemophilia can occur by the drug triggering thrombocytopenia.

Drug Interactions: Because of the possibility of thrombocytopenia, care must be taken when Cinchona preparations are administered along with other drugs that are known to precipitate thrombocytopenia.

OVERDOSAGE

In cases of overdosage (over 3 g quinine) or of long-term administration of the drug or its alkaloids, nausea, summer cholera, headache, fall of body temperature, intravascular hemolysis, cardiac arrhythmias, buzzing in the ears, hearing and visual disorders (all the way to complete deafness and blindness) may occur. Death comes with dosages of 10 to 15 g of quinine through heart failure and asphyxiation. Following gastric lavage, the symptomatic therapy for acute poisonings includes atropine for bradycardia and phenytoin in the presence of tachycardic heart rhythm disorders. Forced diuresis and hemodialysis are not suitable as therapeutic measures.

DOSAGE

Mode of Administration: Comminuted drug and other bitter-tasting galenic preparations to be taken internally.

Preparation: An infusion is prepared by pouring boiling water over 1/2 teaspoonful of the drug and allowing to draw for 10 minutes. A decoction is prepared by adding 0.5 g to 1 teacup of water. A tincture in the proportion of 1:5 in 75% ethanol is also used.

Other preparations involve various complicated extraction processes.

Daily Dosage: Total daily dose is 1 to 3 g of drug. The liquid extract daily dose is 0.6 to 3 g of cinchona liquid extract, which contains 4 to 5% total alkaloids. A daily dose of 0.15 to 0.6 g cinchona extract with 15 to 20% total alkaloids may also be used.

The standard single dose of the extract is 0.2 g. The liquid extract single dose is 0.5 to 1 g.

Storage: Keep protected from light and moisture.

LITERATURE

Chinidin: Photoallergische Reaktion. In: DAZ 133(30):2765. 1993.

Hämorrhoidenbehandlung: Ambulant oder stationär. In: DAZ 133(40):3616. 1993.

Risdale CE, Hasskarls cinchona barks. 1. Historical review. In: Reinwardtia 10, Teil 2: 245-264. 1985.

Schönfeld, Fleischer K, Eichenlaub D, Die Malariavorbeugung. Mückenschutz und Arzneimittel zur Kurzzeitprophylaxe und Notfallbehandlung. In: DAZ 133(21):1981. 1993.

Further information in:

Chan, EH et al., (Eds), Advances in Chinese Medicinal Materials Research, World Scientific Pub. Co. Singapore 1985.

Hänsel R, Keller K, Rimpler H, Schneider G (Hrsg.), Hagers Handbuch der Pharmazeutischen Praxis, 5. Aufl., Bde 4-6 (Drogen): Springer Verlag Berlin, Heidelberg, New York, 1992-1994.

Leung AY, Encyclopedia of Common Natural Ingredients Used in Food Drugs and Cosmetics, John Wiley & Sons Inc., New York 1980.

Lewin L, Gifte und Vergiftungen, 6. Aufl., Nachdruck, Haug Verlag, Heidelberg 1992.

Madaus G, Lehrbuch der Biologischen Arzneimittel, Bde 1-3, Nachdruck, Georg Olms Verlag Hildesheim 1979.

Manske RHF, Holmes HL, fortgeführt von Rodrigo RGA, Brossi A): The Alkaloids - Chemistry and Physiology, III:1, XIV:181, XXXIV:331, Academic Press New York 1950-1997.

Roth L, Daunderer M, Kormann K, Giftpflanzen, Pflanzengifte, 4. Aufl., Ecomed Fachverlag Landsberg Lech 1993.

Steinegger E, Hänsel R, Pharmakognosie, 5. Aufl., Springer Verlag Heidelberg 1992.

Teuscher E, Lindequist U, Biogene Gifte - Biologie, Chemie, Pharmakologie, 2. Aufl., Fischer Verlag Stuttgart 1994.

Teuscher E, Biogene Arzneimittel, 5. Aufl., Wiss. Verlagsges. mbH Stuttgart 1997.

Wagner H, Wiesenauer M, Phytotherapie. Phytopharmaka und pflanzliche Homöopathika, Fischer-Verlag, Stuttgart, Jena, New York 1995.

Wichtl M (Hrsg.), Teedrogen, 4. Aufl., Wiss. Verlagsges. Stuttgart 1997.

Cinnamomum Aromaticum

Chinese Cinnamon

DESCRIPTION

Medicinal Parts: The medicinal parts are the flowers collected and dried after they have finished blossoming, the young twigs and whole or partly peeled, dried bark of thin branches as well the oil extracted from them and the young dried branches.

Flower and Fruit: The flowers are small and are on short, slender, silky pedicles. They are arranged in threes in cymous panicles in the leaf axils and in larger panicles at the end of the branches. The perianth is slightly silky, about 3 mm long, with oblong-lanceolate petals. The fruit is a juicy, pea-sized, elliptoid, smooth drupe.

Leaves, Stem and Root: Evergreen tree up to 7 m tall with aromatic bark and angular branches. The bark is brown, in quilled pieces, sometimes with the remains of the outer layer present. The 7.5 to 10 cm long leaves are oblanceolate and are on 6 to 8 cm long petioles and are pubescent and more or less tapered towards the base. They are coriaceous, alternate and are brown underneath.

Habitat: Indigenous and cultivated in southern China, Vietnam and Burma.

Production: Chinese cinnamon consists of the completely or partly peeled, dried stem bark from the above ground axis of Cinnamomum aromaticum. The drug comes from 2 to 3 cm thick branches; it is peeled with horn knives and freed from cork and outer rind and dried in the sun within 24 hours.

Not To Be Confused With: Waste products from the production process or other barks and materials.

Other Names: Cassia, False Cinnamon, Bastard Cinnamon, Cassia Lignea, Cassia Bark, Cassia aromaticum, Canton Cassia

ACTION AND PHARMACOLOGY

COMPOUNDS

Volatile oil: chief components cinnamaldehyde, weiterhin cinnamylacetate, cinnamyl alcohol, o-methoxycinnamaldehyde, cinnamic acid, coumarin

Diterpenes

Tannins

Oligomere proanthocyanidins

Mucilages

EFFECTS

Antibacterial, fungistatic, improves immunity in animal tests, promotes motility, inhibits ulcers.

INDICATIONS AND USAGE

- Loss of appetite
- Dyspeptic complaints
- Fevers and colds
- Cough/bronchitis
- Tendency to infection
- Inflammation of the mouth and pharynx
- Common cold

Loss of appetite, dyspeptic complaints such as mild, colicky upsets of the gastrointestinal tract, bloating, flatulence; used in the symptomatic treatment of gastrointestinal disorders, temporary states of exhaustion and to increase weight.

Used in Chinese medicine for impotence, diarrhea, enuresis, rheumatic conditions, testicle hernia, menopause syndrome, amenorrhoea, abortion and to stabilize immunity.

PRECAUTIONS AND ADVERSE REACTIONS

General: No health hazards or side effects are known in conjunction with the proper administration of designated therapeutic dosages. The drug possesses a medium potential for sensitization. Sensitizations to cinnamaldehyde occur frequently.

Pregnancy: The drug is not to be administered in time of pregnancy.

DOSAGE

Mode of Administration: Comminuted bark for infusions; essential oil, as well as other galenic preparations for internal use.

Preparation: Tincture of cinnamon: moisten 200 parts cinnamon bark evenly with ethanol and percolate to produce 1000 parts tincture.

Daily Dosage: 2 to 4 g drug; 0.05 to 0.2 g essential oil; Average single dose: 1 g.

Storage: Cool, dry conditions in well-sealed containers.

LITERATURE

Hikino H, Economic and Medicinal Plant Research, Vol I., Academic Press UK 1985.

Lockwood GB, Die Hauptbestandteile des ätherischen Öls von Cinnamomum cassia BLUME. In: PM 36(4):380-381. 1979.

Nagai H et al., (1982) Jpn J Pharmacol 32(5):813.

Nohara T et al., (1982) Phytochemistry 21(8):2130.

Nohara T et al., (1985) Phytochemistry 24(8):1849.

Nohara T et al., Cinncassiol E, a diterpene from the bark of Cinnamomum cassia. In: PH 24:1849. 1985.

Nohara T et al., PH 21:2130-2132. 1982.

Otsuka H et al., (1982) Yakugaku Zasshi 102:162.

Sagara K et al., J Chromatogr 409:365-370. 1987.

Senayake UM et al., (1978) J Agric Food Chem 20:822.

Structure of potent antiulcerogenic compounds from Cinnamomum cassia, Tetrahedron 44:4703. 1988.

Further information in:

Chan, EH et al., (Eds), Advances in Chinese Medicinal Materials Research, World Scientific Pub. Co. Singapore 1985.

Hänsel R, Keller K, Rimpler H, Schneider G (Hrsg.), Hagers Handbuch der Pharmazeutischen Praxis, 5. Aufl., Bde 4-6 (Drogen), Springer Verlag Berlin, Heidelberg, New York, 1992-1994.

Tang W, Eisenbrand G, Chinese Drugs of Plant Origin, Springer Verlag Heidelberg 1992.

Cinnamomum Camphora

Camphor Tree

DESCRIPTION

Medicinal Parts: The medicinal part is camphor oil extracted from the tree.

Flower and Fruit: The flowers are small and white and are on 1 to 1.5 mm long pedicles. The petals are pubescent on the inside. The flowers are in long-peduncled axillary panicles. The stamens form 3 circles, are 1.5 mm long, pubescent with broad, sessile-cordate glands. The fruit is a purple-black, 1-seeded, 10 to 12 mm oval drupe.

Leaves, Stem and Root: The plant is an evergreen tree growing up to 50 m tall and 5 m in diameter. The trunk is erect at the lower part and is knottily branched above. The leaves are 5 to 11 cm long by 5 cm across, oval-lanceolate, alternate, acuminate, grooved, glossy and light yellowish green above, paler beneath.

Habitat: Found from Vietnam to southern China as far as southern Japan.

Production: Purified camphor is obtained from the wood of the camphor tree Cinnamomum camphora using steam distillation followed by sublimation.

Other Names: Gum Camphor, Laurel Camphor, Cemphire.

ACTION AND PHARMACOLOGY

COMPOUNDS

Camphora is a single substance: D(+)-camphor ((1R,4R)-1,7,7-Trimethyl-bicyclo[2.2.1]heptan-2-on), extracted from the volatile oil of the trunk of the camphor tree, Cinnamomum camphora. L(-)-camphor also occurs in nature. Synthetic camphor is DL-camphor.

EFFECTS

External: bronchial secretolytic, hyperemic.

Internal: circulatory tonic, respiratory analeptic, bronchial antispasmodic.

INDICATIONS

- Cardiac insufficiency NYHA I and II
- Arrhythmia
- Cough/bronchitis
- Hypertension
- Hypotension
- Nervous heart complaints
- Rheumatism

External: muscular rheumatism, catarrhal diseases of the respiratory tract, cardiac symptoms.

Internal: hypotonic circulatory regulation disorders, catarrhal diseases of the respiratory tract.

PRECAUTIONS AND ADVERSE REACTIONS

General: Local administration can lead to skin irritation, as well as to resorbent and/or airborne poisonings. Contact eczema occasionally appears following the application of oily salves containing camphor.

Pediatric Use: Camphor salves should not be administered to infants.

OVERDOSAGE

Symptoms of poisonings that have been seen particularly in children, include intoxicated states, delirium, spasms and respiratory control disturbances. Treatment proceeds symptomatically. The lethal dosage for children is approximately 1 g, for adults approximately 20 g (toxic dosage of camphor is 2 g).

DOSAGE

Mode of Administration: Locally or for inhalation; in liquid or semisolid form. Internally, in liquid or solid preparations.

Daily Dosage: Internal average daily dosage: 30 to 300 mg. For external use, depending on prescribed application, generally in concentrations of not higher than 25%, for small children not higher than 5%.

LITERATURE

Bean NE, Camphora -curriculum vitae of a perverse terpene. In: Chem in Brain 8(9):386. 1972.

Burrow A, Eccles R, Jones AS, (1983) The effects of camphor, eucalyptus and menthol vapur on nasal resistance to airflow and nasal sensation. Acta Otolaryng (Stockholm) 96:157-161.

Stone JE, Blundell MJ, (1951) Anal Chem 23:771.

Takaoka D et al., (1975) Nippon Kagaku Kaishi 12:2192.

Further information in:

Bruchhausen F von, Ebel S, Frahm AW, Hackenthal E (Hrsg.), Hagers Handbuch der Pharmazeutischen Praxis, 5. Aufl., Bde 7-9 (Stoffe), Springer Verlag Berlin, Heidelberg, New York, 1993.

Lewin L, Gifte und Vergiftungen, 6. Aufl., Nachdruck, Haug Verlag, Heidelberg 1992.

Madaus G, Lehrbuch der Biologischen Arzneimittel, Bde 1-3, Nachdruck, Georg Olms Verlag Hildesheim 1979.

Roth L, Daunderer M, Kormann K, Giftpflanzen, Pflanzengifte, 4. Aufl., Ecomed Fachverlag Landsberg Lech 1993.

Steinegger E, Hänsel R, Pharmakognosie, 5. Aufl., Springer Verlag Heidelberg 1992.

Teuscher E, Lindequist U, Biogene Gifte - Biologie, Chemie, Pharmakologie, 2. Aufl., Fischer Verlag Stuttgart 1994.

Teuscher E, Biogene Arzneimittel, 5. Aufl., Wiss. Verlagsges. Stuttgart 1997.

Wagner H, Wiesenauer M, Phytotherapie. Phytopharmaka und pflanzliche Homöopathika, Fischer-Verlag, Stuttgart, Jena, New York 1995.

Cinnamomum Verum

Cinnamon

DESCRIPTION

Medicinal Parts: The medicinal parts are the cinnamon oil extracted from the bark, the cinnamon bark of younger branches and the cinnamon leaf oil.

Flower and Fruit: The flowers are whitish green, inconspicuous and have an unpleasant smell. They are arranged in loose, axillary or terminal panicles; they are about 0.5 cm long and are covered in silky hairs. The fruit is berry-like, ovoid-oblong, short-thorned and half-enclosed by the epicalyx.

Leaves, Stem and Root: The plant is a heavily foliated evergreen tree 6.5 to 12 m tall with a pale brown bark in thin quills, several rolled inside one another. The branches are cylindrical with a gray-brown bark. The leaves are opposite, splayed horizontally to leaning, initially red, later green, tough. They are about 12 cm by 5 cm, roundish-ovate or ovate-lanceolate to oblong, more or less acuminate and entire-margined. The leaves smell like cloves.

Habitat: Indigenous to Sri Lanka and southwest India.

Production: The thin bark without the cork or outer rind is dried in the shade.

Not To Be Confused With: Other powdered cinnamon varieties

Other Names: Ceylon Cinnamon

ACTION AND PHARMACOLOGY

COMPOUNDS

Volatile oil: chief components - cinnamaldehyde, weiterhin eugenol, cinnamylacetate, cinnamyl alcohol, o-methoxycinnamaldehyde, cinnamic acid

Diterpenes

Oligomeric proanthocyanidins

Mucilages

EFFECTS

Antibacterial, fungistatic, promotes motility; mildly positive estrogen reactions on the genital system of animals in tests; increases gastric secretions and is an insecticide.

INDICATIONS AND USAGE

- Loss of appetite
- Dyspeptic complaints
- Fevers and colds
- Cough/bronchitis
- Tendency to infection
- Inflammation of the mouth and pharynx
- Common cold

Loss of appetite, dyspepsia.

Folk medicine: infantile diarrhea, chills, influenza and worm infestation; externally for cleaning wounds.

PRECAUTIONS AND ADVERSE REACTIONS

General: No health hazards or side effects are known in conjunction with the proper administration of designated therapeutic dosages. The drug possesses a medium potential for sensitization. Sensitizations to cinnamaldehyde occur frequently.

Pregnancy: The drug is not to be administered in time of pregnancy.

DOSAGE

Mode of Administration: Comminuted drug for infusions; essential oil, as well as other galenic preparations for internal use.

Daily Dosage: 2 to 4 g drug, 0.05 to 0.2 g essential oil;

Infusion: 1 cup 2 to 3 times daily at mealtimes

Liquid extract: 0.5 to 1 ml 3 times daily

Tincture: up to 4 ml 3 times daily

Storage: Protect from light and moisture in non-synthetic containers.

LITERATURE

Buchalter L (1971) J Pharm Sci 60: 144.

Isogai A et al. (1977) Agric Biol Chem 41: 1779.

Kato Y (1975) Koryo 113: 17, et 24.

Kaul R, Pflanzliche Procyanidine. Vorkommen, Klassifikation und pharmakologische Wirkungen. In: PUZ 25(4):175-185. 1996.

Schneider E, Cinnamomum verum - Der Zimt. In: ZPT 9(6):193. 1988.

Schröder, Buch. In: Schröder R: Kaffee, Tee und Kardamom, Ulmer-Verlag, Stuttgart. 1991.

Further information in:

Hänsel R, Keller K, Rimpler H, Schneider G (Hrsg.): Hagers Handbuch der Pharmazeutischen Praxis, 5. Aufl., Bde 4-6 (Drogen), Springer Verlag Berlin, Heidelberg, New York, 1992-1994.

Leung AY: Encyclopedia of Common Natural Ingredients Used in Food Drugs and Cosmetics, John Wiley & Sons Inc., New York 1980.

Madaus G: Lehrbuch der Biologischen Arzneimittel, Bde 1-3, Nachdruck, Georg Olms Verlag Hildesheim 1979.

Roth L, Daunderer M, Kormann K: Giftpflanzen, Pflanzengifte, 4. Aufl., Ecomed Fachverlag Landsberg Lech 1993.

Steinegger E, Hänsel R: Pharmakognosie, 5. Aufl., Springer Verlag Heidelberg 1992.

Teuscher E: Biogene Arzneimittel, 5. Aufl., Wiss. Verlagsges. mbH Stuttgart 1997.

Wichtl M (Hrsg.): Teedrogen, 4. Aufl., Wiss. Verlagsges. Stuttgart 1997.

Cinnamon

See Cinnamomum Verum

Citronella

See Cymbopogon Species

Citrullus Colocynthis

Bitter Apple

DESCRIPTION

Medicinal Parts: The medicinal part is the dried pulp.

Flower and Fruit: The flowers are yellow and appear singly in the leaf axils. The fruit is as large as an apple. It is yellow, smooth, dry, and very bitter. When it is ripe it contains white spongy flesh within the coriaceous peel with numerous ovate, white or brownish seeds which are 0.75 cm long and 0.5 cm wide, ovate, compressed, with an edge and oily.

Leaves, Stem and Root: The annual plant is similar to a normal watermelon. The stems are leafy and rough-haired. The leaves are alternate on long petioles. They are triangular, divided, variously indented, obtuse and pubescent. The upper surface is delicate green, the lower one rough and pale.

Habitat: Indigenous to Turkey found also in Sri Lanka, Egypt, Syria, and the Arabian Gulf.

Production: Bitter Apples are the ripe fruits of Citrullus colocynthis which have been removed from the harder outer layer.

Other Names: Colocynth Pulp, Bitter Cucumber

ACTION AND PHARMACOLOGY

COMPOUNDS

Cucurbitacins: including cucurbitacin E-, J-, L-glucosides

Caffeic acid derivatives: chlorogenic acid

EFFECTS

Increases liquid in the intestine. Irritates the intestinal mucous membrane.

INDICATIONS AND USAGE

Preparations of Bitter Apples are used exclusively in fixed combinations in the treatment of acute and chronic constipation with various causes as well as in pregnancy, also in the treatment of liver and gallbladder disorders. Bitter Apple preparations act as drastic laxatives. Efficacy in other claimed areas of use has not been proven.

PRECAUTIONS AND ADVERSE REACTIONS

The drug is severely poisonous. It has a strongly irritating effect on mucus membranes due to its cucurbitacin glycoside content, out of which cucurbitacins are released in watery environments.

OVERDOSAGE

Vomiting, bloody diarrhea, colic, kidney irritation follow the intake of toxic dosages (0.6 - 1 g), and then increased diuresis, leading on to anuria. Lethal dosages (starting at 2 g) lead to convulsions, paralyses, and, if untreated, to death through circulatory collapse.

The treatment for poisonings should proceed symptomatically following gastric lavage. Administration in allopathic dosages is no longer defensible.

LITERATURE

Habs M et al., (1984) J Cancer Res Clin Oncol 108(1):154.

Konopa J et al., In: Advances in Antimicrobial and Antineoplastic Chemotherapy, Vol. 2, Ed. M. Semonsky, Avicenna Press Prague 1972.

Lavie D et al., (1964) Phytochemistry 3:52.

Rawson MD, (1966) Lancet 1:1121.

Further information in:

Hegnauer R, Chemotaxonomie der Pflanzen, Bde 1-11, Birkhäuser Verlag Basel, Boston, Berlin 1962-1997.

Kern W, List PH, Hörhammer L (Hrsg.), Hagers Handbuch der Pharmazeutischen Praxis, 4. Aufl., Bde. 1-8, Springer Verlag Berlin, Heidelberg, New York, 1969.

Lewin L, Gifte und Vergiftungen, 6. Aufl., Nachdruck, Haug Verlag, Heidelberg 1992.

Madaus G, Lehrbuch der Biologischen Arzneimittel, Bde 1-3, Nachdruck, Georg Olms Verlag Hildesheim 1979.

Roth L, Daunderer M, Kormann K, Giftpflanzen, Pflanzengifte, 4. Aufl., Ecomed Fachverlag Landsberg Lech 1993.

Wagner H, Wiesenauer M, Phytotherapie. Phytopharmaka und pflanzliche Homöopathika, Fischer-Verlag, Stuttgart, Jena, New York 1995.

Citrus Aurantifolia

Lime

DESCRIPTION

Medicinal Parts: The medicinal part is the bergamot oil extracted from the plant.

Flower and Fruit: The fragrant flowers are small and pure white. The fruit is about half the size of a lemon but has a smoother, thinner peel, a greenish yellow color and is sweet.

Leaves, Stem and Root: The evergreen tree is small, bent and thorny and normally only grows to a height of 2.5 m. The leaves are ovate-lanceolate and acuminate.

Habitat: Indigenous to Southern Asia, cultivated in the West Indies, Florida, Central America.

Production: Lemons and limes are the fruit of Citrus aurantifolia.

Other Names: Limette, Italian Limetta, Adam's Apple

ACTION AND PHARMACOLOGY

COMPOUNDS

Volatile oil: including containing citral, (+)-limonene, pinenes, alkanes, alkanols, alkanals, also furocoumarins in pressed oils

Citric acid

Flavonoids

EFFECTS

Refrigerant, antiscorbutic.

INDICATIONS AND USAGE

Scurvy, Vitamin C source in cases of general low resistance.

PRECAUTIONS AND ADVERSE REACTIONS

No health hazards or side effects are known in conjunction with the proper administration of designated therapeutic dosages. There is a low potential for sensitization through skin contact with the juice of the fruit or with the volatile oil.

DOSAGE

Mode of Administration: Lime is used internally as a liquid extract or the fresh fruit.

LITERATURE

Kovats et al., Helv Chim Acta 46:2705. 1963.

Lund ED, Bryan WL, (1977) J Food Sci 42:385.

Natarajan S et al., (1976) Econ Bot 30:38.

Shaw PE, Coleman RL, (1971) J Agric Food Chem 19:1276.

Stanley et al., PH 6:585. 1967.

Strickler et al., Helv Chim Acta 49:2055. 1966.

Tatum JH, Berry RE, (1977) Phytochemistry 16:1091.

Wilson W, Shaw PE, (1977) J Agric Food Chem 25:211.

Further information in:

Kern W, List PH, Hörhammer L (Hrsg.), Hagers Handbuch der Pharmazeutischen Praxis, 4. Aufl., Bde. 1-8, Springer Verlag Berlin, Heidelberg, New York, 1969.

Leung AY, Encyclopedia of Common Natural Ingredients Used in Food Drugs and Cosmetics, John Wiley & Sons Inc., New York 1980.

Roth L, Daunderer M, Kormann K, Giftpflanzen, Pflanzengifte, 4. Aufl., Ecomed Fachverlag Landsberg Lech 1993.

Citrus Aurantium

Bitter Orange

DESCRIPTION

Medicinal Parts: The medicinal parts are the fresh and dried fruit peel, the flowers, the seeds and the essential oil.

Flower and Fruit: The flowers are arranged singly or in clusters in the axils, and are very fragrant. The calyx is cup-shaped and the 5 thick fleshy petals are of an intensive white shade and revolute. The fruit is about 7.5 cm in diameter, subglobose, slightly flattened at both ends, 10- to 12-locular. The peel is thick, rough, orange when ripe. The fruit pulp is acid. The core is hollow when ripe.

Leaves, Stem and Root: Evergreen tree with a rounded crown and smooth grayish-brown bark. The branches are angular when young, becoming terete and glabrous soon after, with slender axillary spines. The alternate leaves are 7.5 to 10 cm, broadly elliptoid, subacute at the apex, cuneate or rounded below. Petioles are broadly winged, tapering to a wingless base.

Habitat: The plant is indigenous to tropical Asia but is widely cultivated in other regions today such as the Mediterranean.

Production: Bitter Orange flower consists of the dried flowers of Citrus aurantium. The oil is obtained by steam distillation of the fresh, fully opened flowers. Bitter orange peel consists of the dried outer peel of ripe fruits of Citrus aurantium separated from the white pulp layer.

Other Names: Orange, Neroli, Bigarade Orange

ACTION AND PHARMACOLOGY

COMPOUNDS: AURANTII FLOS ET FLORIS AETHEROLEUM

Volatile oil: chief constituents linalool, linalyl acetate, alpha-pinenes, limonene, nerol, geraniol

Methyl anthranilate

Limonoids: (triterpenoide bitter principles)

Flavonoids

EFFECTS: AURANTII FLOS ET FLORIS AETHEROLEUM

No information available.

COMPOUNDS: AURANTII PERICARPIUM

Volatile oil: chief constituents limonene, nerol, geraniol, linalool, linalyl-, neryl-, geranyl- and citronellyl acetate, typical constituent methyl anthranilate

Flavonoids: among them the bitter compounds neohesperidin dyhydrochalcone and naringin as well as the lipophilic compounds sinensetin, nobiletin, tangeretin

Furocoumarins

EFFECTS: AURANTII PERICARPIUM

Mild spasmolytic

INDICATIONS AND USAGE

AURANTII FLOS ET FLORIS AETHEROLEUM

Preparations of orange flower and orange flower oil are used as a preventive measure for gastric and nervous complaints, gout, sore throat, as a sedative, for nervous tension and sleeplessness.

AURANTII PERICARPIUM

- Loss of appetite
- Dyspeptic complaints

PRECAUTIONS AND ADVERSE REACTIONS

AURANTII FLOS ET FLORIS AETHEROLEUM

No health hazards or side effects are known in conjunction with the proper administration of designated therapeutic dosages.

AURANTII PERICARPIUM

No health hazards or side effects are known in conjunction with the proper administration of designated therapeutic dosages. An elevation of the UV-sensitivity is possible with light-skinned individuals (phototoxic effect of the furocoumarins). Frequent contact with the drug or with the volatile oil can lead to a sensitization (liquor industry, erythemas, swellings, blisters, pustules, dermatoses leading to scab formation, pigment spots).

DOSAGE

AURANTII PERICARPIUM

Mode of Administration: Comminuted drug for teas, other bitter-tasting galenic preparations for oral application.

Daily Dosage: Drug: 4 to 6 g;

Tincture (according to DAB 7): 2 to 3 g.

Extract (according to Erg. B. 6): 1 to 2 g.

LITERATURE

AURANTII FLOS ET FLORIS AETHEROLEUM

Slater CA, (1961) J Sci Agric Food 12:732.

Stanley WL, Jurd L, (1971) J Agric Food Chem 19:1106.

Tatum JH, Berry RE, (1977) Phytochemistry 16:109.

Further information in:

Kern W, List PH, Hörhammer L (Hrsg.), Hagers Handbuch der Pharmazeutischen Praxis, 4. Aufl., Bde. 1-8, Springer Verlag Berlin, Heidelberg, New York, 1969.

Leung AY, Encyclopedia of Common Natural Ingredients Used in Food Drugs and Cosmetics, John Wiley & Sons Inc., New York 1980.

Madaus G, Lehrbuch der Biologischen Arzneimittel, Bde 1-3, Nachdruck, Georg Olms Verlag Hildesheim 1979.

Roth L, Daunderer M, Kormann K, Giftpflanzen, Pflanzengifte, 4. Aufl., Ecomed Fachverlag Landsberg Lech 1993.

Tang W, Eisenbrand G, Chinese Drugs of Plant Origin, Springer Verlag Heidelberg 1992.

Wichtl M (Hrsg.), Teedrogen, 4. Aufl., Wiss. Verlagsges. Stuttgart 1997.

AURANTII PERICARPIUM

Clavarano I, Essenze Deriv. Agrum 36:5. 1966.

Horowitz RM, Gentili B, Tetrahedron 19:773. 1963.

Slater CA, (1961) J Sci Agric Food 12:732.

Stanley WL, Jurd L, (1971) J Agric Food Chem 19:1106.

Tatum JH, Berry RE, (1977) Phytochemistry 16, 109.

Further information in:

Kern W, List PH, Hörhammer L (Hrsg.), Hagers Handbuch der Pharmazeutischen Praxis, 4. Aufl., Bde. 1-8, Springer Verlag Berlin, Heidelberg, New York, 1969.

Leung AY, Encyclopedia of Common Natural Ingredients Used in Food Drugs and Cosmetics, John Wiley & Sons Inc., New York 1980.

Lewin L, Gifte und Vergiftungen, 6. Aufl., Nachdruck, Haug Verlag, Heidelberg 1992.

Madaus G, Lehrbuch der Biologischen Arzneimittel, Bde 1-3, Nachdruck, Georg Olms Verlag Hildesheim 1979.

Roth L, Daunderer M, Kormann K, Giftpflanzen, Pflanzengifte, 4. Aufl., Ecomed Fachverlag Landsberg Lech 1993.

Steinegger E, Hänsel R, Pharmakognosie, 5. Aufl., Springer Verlag Heidelberg 1992.

Tang W, Eisenbrand G, Chinese Drugs of Plant Origin, Springer Verlag Heidelberg 1992.

Teuscher E, Biogene Arzneimittel, 5. Aufl., Wiss. Verlagsges. Stuttgart 1997.

Wichtl M (Hrsg.), Teedrogen, 4. Aufl., Wiss. Verlagsges. Stuttgart 1997.

Citrus Limon

Lemon

DESCRIPTION

Medicinal Parts: The fruit is the medicinal part.

Flower and Fruit: Flowers are arranged singly or in short, sparsely-flowered racemes, hermaphrodite or functionally male. The petals are purplish-suffused on the outer surface. There are 25 to 40 stamens in coherent groups. The fruit is 6.5 to 12.5 cm, 8- to 10-locular, yellow when ripe, oblong or ovoid, with a broad, low, mamilliform projection at the apex. The rind is somewhat rough to almost smooth.

Leaves, Stem and Root: It is a small tree 3 to 6 m tall whose twigs are angular when young and soon become rounded, glabrous, with stout axillary spines. The leaves are pale-green, broadly elliptical, acute, serrate or crenate. The petiole has a narrow wing or is merely margined and is distinctly articulated with the lamina.

Habitat: The tree is indigenous to northern India, cultivated in Mediterranean regions and worldwide in subtropical regions.

Production: Lemons are the fruit, lemon peel is the skin of the fruit and lemon oil the essential oil extracted from the skins of Citrus limon.

Other Names: Limon

ACTIONS AND PHARMACOLOGY

COMPOUNDS

Volatile oil: chief components (+)-limonene, furthermore citral as an odor-bearer, n-nonanal, n-decanal, n-dodecanal, linalyl acetate, geranyl acetat, citronellyl acetat, methyl anthranilate, also lipophilic flavonoids in pressed oils, including sinensetin and furocoumarins

Flavonoids: in particular the bitter neohesperidosides naringin and neohesperidin dyhydro chalcones, furthermore hesperidin, rutin

EFFECTS

Citroflavonoids affect vascular permeability, are anti-inflammatory, diuretic and are a source of Vitamin C.

INDICATIONS AND USAGE

Lemon is used as a source of Vitamin C in cases of general low resistance, scurvy, colds etc., also used as a food-flavoring agent.

PRECAUTIONS AND ADVERSE REACTIONS

No health hazards or side effects are known in conjunction with the proper administration of designated therapeutic dosages. There is a low potential for sensitization through skin contact with volatile oil.

DOSAGE

Mode of Administration: Lemon is used internally in the form of oil, tincture, or fresh fruit.

LITERATURE

Calomme M et al., Inhibition of bacterial mutagenisis by Citrus flavonoids. In: PM 62(3):222-226. 1996.

Calomme M et al., PM 62:222. 1996.

Clavarano I, Essenze Deriv. Agrum 36:5. 1966.

Horowitz RM, Gentili B, Tetrahedron 19:773. 1963.

Paris R (1977) Plant Med Phytother 11(Suppl):129.

Paris R, Delaveau P, (1977) Plant Med Phytother 11(Suppl):198.

Further information in:

Kern W, List PH, Hörhammer L (Hrsg.), Hagers Handbuch der Pharmazeutischen Praxis, 4. Aufl., Bde. 1-8, Springer Verlag Berlin, Heidelberg, New York, 1969.

Leung AY, Encyclopedia of Common Natural Ingredients Used in Food Drugs and Cosmetics, John Wiley & Sons Inc., New York 1980.

Madaus G, Lehrbuch der Biologischen Arzneimittel, Bde 1-3, Nachdruck, Georg Olms Verlag Hildesheim 1979.

Oliver-Bever B (Ed.), Medicinal Plants of Tropical West Africa, Cambridge University Press Cambridge, London 1986.

Roth L, Daunderer M, Kormann K, Giftpflanzen, Pflanzengifte, 4. Aufl., Ecomed Fachverlag Landsberg Lech 1993.

Steinegger E, Hänsel R, Pharmakognosie, 5. Aufl., Springer Verlag Heidelberg 1992.

Tang W, Eisenbrand G, Chinese Drugs of Plant Origin, Springer Verlag Heidelberg 1992.

Teuscher E, Biogene Arzneimittel, 5. Aufl., Wiss. Verlagsges. mbH Stuttgart 1997.

Wichtl M (Hrsg.), Teedrogen, 4. Aufl., Wiss. Verlagsges. Stuttgart 1997.

Citrus Sinensis

Sweet Orange

DESCRIPTION

Medicinal Parts: The medicinal parts are the fresh and dried peel as well as the oil extracted from the peel.

Flower and Fruit: The flowers are arranged singly or in short limp racemes, and are fragrant. The fruit is depressed-globose to shortly ovoid, 10- to 13-locular. The peel is thin to rather thick, nearly smooth, orange to orange-yellow when ripe. The pulp is sweet. The core remains solid when ripe.

Leaves, Stem and Root: Citrus sinensis is an evergreen tree with rounded crown. The branches are angular when young, soon after terete, with a few slender, rather flexible axillary spines. The leaves are acute, rounded below; petioles narrowly winged.

Habitat: Like other Citrus varieties the plant is indigenous to Asia and is cultivated in the Mediterranean and other subtropical regions.

Production: Orange peel consists of the fresh or dried outer peel of ripe fruits of Citrus sinensis, separated from the white pith layer, as well as its preparations in effective dosage.

Other Names: Orange, China Orange, Citrus dulcis

ACTIONS AND PHARMACOLOGY

COMPOUNDS

Volatile oil: chief components (+)-limonene, furthermore citral as an odor-bearer, citronellal, nootkatone, sinesal, n-nonanal, n-necanal, n-dodecanal, linalyl acetate, geranyl acetat, citronellyl acetat, methyl anthranilate, also lipophilic flavonoids and furocoumarins in pressed oils

Flavonoids

EFFECTS

Sweet orange has a digestive effect.

INDICATIONS AND USAGE

- Dyspeptic complaints
- Loss of appetite

PRECAUTIONS AND ADVERSE REACTIONS

No health hazards or side effects are known in conjunction with the proper administration of designated therapeutic dosages. There is a low potential for sensitization through skin contact with volatile oil.

DOSAGE

Mode of Administration: Comminuted herb for teas and other bitter-tasting galenic preparations for oral application.

Daily Dosage: 10 to 15 gm of drug.

LITERATURE

Ihrig M, Qualitätskontrolle von süßem Orangenschalenöl. In: PZ 140(26):2350-2353. 1995.

Further information in:

Hausen B, Allergiepflanzen, Pflanzenallergene, ecomed Verlagsgesellsch. mbH, Landsberg 1988.

Kern W, List PH, Hörhammer L (Hrsg.), Hagers Handbuch der Pharmazeutischen Praxis, 4. Aufl., Bde. 1-8, Springer Verlag Berlin, Heidelberg, New York, 1969.

Cladonia Pyxidata

Cupmoss

DESCRIPTION

Medicinal Parts: The medicinal part is the whole plant.

Flower and Fruit: The plant is a lichen, not a moss as the name suggests. The scyphi are grayish-white, about 2.5 cm long, wineglass shaped, with hollow stems and a terminal cup.

Characteristics: The taste is mucilaginous and slightly sweet. There is no odor.

Habitat: The plant is indigenous to northwest America and is also common in Britain.

Production: The wineglass-shaped scyphi of Cladonia pyxidata are used.

Other Names: Chin Cups

ACTIONS AND PHARMACOLOGY

COMPOUNDS

Lichen acids: including fumaroprotocetraric acid, barbatic acid, psoromic acid

Mucilages

EFFECTS

Expectorant and antitussive.

INDICATIONS AND USAGE

Cupmoss is used in coughs, bronchitis, and also in the treatment of whooping cough.

PRECAUTIONS AND ADVERSE REACTIONS

Health risks or side effects following the proper administration of designated therapeutic dosages are not recorded.

DOSAGE

Mode of Administration: Cupmoss is used internally as an infusion with honey.

LITERATURE

Hoppe HA (1975-1987): Drogenkunde, 8. Aufl., Bde 1-3, W. de Gruyter Verlag, Berlin, New York.

Kern W, List PH, Hörhammer L (Hrsg.), Hagers Handbuch der Pharmazeutischen Praxis, 4. Aufl., Bde 1-8, Springer Verlag Berlin, Heidelberg, New York, 1969.

Claviceps Purpurea

Ergot

DESCRIPTION

Medicinal Parts: The medicinal part is the ergot in the form of the sclerotium which has formed on the rye and been dried.

Flower and Fruit: Permanent form of a fungus which is a parasite on ripening rye, wheat and other grasses. It is black, hard, and much larger than the grains of rye. The cycle of the fungus begins with the infection of the ovary by an ascospore. The spore, usually deposited by a visiting insect, germinates on the stigma, the hyphae grows down into the ovary where it appropriates food destined for the grain. When the ovary has been completely destroyed the mycelium grows. Horizontal walls are formed and fat vacuoles become visible. The hyphae of the skin layer store purple pigment and 3 weeks after the infection a long, curved, black sclerotium grows out reaching a length of about 8 cm bearing minute condia made up of the remains of the ovary and the style embedded into the lose mycelium. The sclerotium usually falls to the ground before harvest and overwinters. In spring 1 to 3 cm long red-stemmed, capitula-like, pink fruiting bodies grow out of it which in turn produce 50 to 70 μm long thread-like ascospores.

Habitat: Claviceps purpurea grows as a parasite on rye and other grasses, and is widespread.

Production: Ergot consists of the sclerotium of Claviceps purpurea, grown on rye, as well as preparations thereof.

Other Names: Cockspur Rye, Hornseed, Mother of Rye, Smut Rye, Spurred Rye

ACTIONS AND PHARMACOLOGY

COMPOUNDS

Indole alkaloids (ergot alkaloids, 0-1.0%)

Chief alkaloid of the lysergic acid amide type: ergometrine (ergobasine)

Chief alkaloid of the lysergic acid ergopeptine type: ergotamine, ergovaline, ergosine, ergocristine, ergocornine, alpha- and beta-ergocryptine, further alkaloids of the clavine type: including among others agroclavine, elymoclavine

Xanthone derivatives (ergochromes): including, among others, secalonic acid A

Anthracene derivatives: including, among others, clavorubine, endocrocine

Amines: including, among others, trimethylamine, methylamine

Fatty oil

EFFECTS

No information is available.

INDICATIONS AND USAGE

Ergot and ergot preparations are used in gynecology and obstetrics, e.g., hemorrhages, climacteric hemorrhages, menorrhagia and metrorrhagia, before and after miscarriage, for removal of the placenta and shortening of the afterbirth period and for atonia of the uterus.

CONTRAINDICATIONS

Ergot is contraindicated in peripheral blood flow disorders such as Raynaud's disease, Thrombangitis obliterans, severe arteriosclerotic vascular changes, liver function disorders, severe coronary insufficiency, kidney damage, pregnancy, nursing, infectious diseases, sepsis, hypertonia, and severe hypotonia.

PRECAUTIONS AND ADVERSE REACTIONS

No health hazards are known in conjunction with the proper administration of designated therapeutic dosages. Among the side effects that may occur: queasiness, vomiting, feeling of weakness in the legs, muscle pain, numbness in the fingers, angina complaints, tachycardia or bradycardia, localized edema and itching.

OVERDOSAGE

Overdosage or long-term administration can lead to: thrombosis, damage to the vessels of the retina, combined with optic atrophy, gangrene of the extremities, hemiplagia, and convulsions.

Symptoms of acute poisonings include: queasiness, vomiting, diarrhea, thirst, skin coolness, itching of the skin, rapid, weak pulse, paresthesia, numbness of the extremities, confusion or also unconsciousness.

Chronic poisonings appear as:

- Ergotismus gangrenosus: characterized with painful arterial blood flow disorders of the extremities with dry gangrene, angina complaints, field of vision losses, aphasias.

- Ergotismus convulsivus: characterized by muscle twitching, later clonic spasm and ultimately tonic spasms, hemiplagia, loss of consciousness and death.

Drug overdose is managed by gastrointestinal emptying (inducement of vomiting, gastric lavage with burgundy-colored potassium permanganate solution, sodium sulphate), followed by installation of activated charcoal and shock prophylaxis (quiet, warmth), the therapy for poisonings consists of treating angiospasms with Nitrolingual-spray and vascular massage, sedatives for spasm (diazepam or chloral hydrate) administration of blocking agents, electrolyte substitution and treating possible cases of acidosis with sodium bicarbonate infusions. Intubation and oxygen respiration may also be necessary.

LITERATURE

Anonym, Hepetitis C - Hohes Riskiko für Medizinberufe. In: PUZ 25(6):344. 1996.

Anonym, Parkinson-Krankheit: Mehe Lebensqualität bei Kombination von L-DOPA mit Dopaminagonisten. In: PUZ 24(2):101. 1995.

Crespi-Perellino N et al., JNP 50:1065-1074. 1987.

Ergotamin. In: DAZ 134(20):1887. 1994.

Flieger M et al., JNP 47:970-976. 1984.

Frohne D, Pfänder HJ: Giftpflanzen - Ein Handbuch für Apotheker, Toxikologen und Biologen, 4. Aufl., Wiss. Verlags-Ges. Stuttgart 1997.

Hänsel R, Keller K, Rimpler H, Schneider G (Hrsg.), Hagers Handbuch der Pharmazeutischen Praxis, 5. Aufl., Bde 4-6 (Drogen): Springer Verlag Berlin, Heidelberg, New York, 1992-1994.

Kobel H, Sanglier JJ, Biotechnology 4:569-609. 1986.

Lewin L, Gifte und Vergiftungen, 6. Aufl., Nachdruck, Haug Verlag, Heidelberg 1992.

Madaus G, Lehrbuch der Biologischen Arzneimittel, Bde 1-3, Nachdruck, Georg Olms Verlag Hildesheim 1979.

Marshall M, Wüstenberg P, Klinik und Therapie der chronischen venösen Insuffizienz. In: Klinik und Therapie der chronischen venösen Insuffizienz, Braun Fachverlage, Karlsruhe 1994. 1994.

Milhahn HC et al., Contributions to the dissociation between antineoplastic and mutagenic activities of the ergot minor alkaloid festucalavine by substitution at C-2. In: PM 59(7):A&83. 1993.

Militz M, Antoniusfeuer, Mutterkron und Isenheimer Altar. In: PZ 141(9):720-721. 1996.

Neurotransmitter: Serotoninagonisten und -antagonisten in der Pharmakotherapie. In: DAZ 133(51/52):4895. 1993.

Perellino NC, et al., Identification of ergobine, a new natural peptide ergot alkaloid. In: JNP 56(4):489-493. 1993.

Pertz H, Naturally occuring clavines: Antagonism/partial agonism at 5-HT2alpha receptors and antogonism at alpha1-adrenoceptors in blood vessel. In: PM 62(5)387-392. 1996.

Roth L, Daunderer M, Kormann K: Giftpflanzen, Pflanzengifte, 4. Aufl., Ecomed Fachverlag Landsberg Lech 1993.

Schlenger R, 50 Jahre LSD. In: DAZ 133(32):2903. 1993.

Schmidt M, LSD, Psilocybe, Ololiuqui. In: PTA 8(3):186. 1994.

Seeger R, Neumann HG, D-(+)-Lysergsäurediethylamid (LSD). In: DAZ 132(42):2244. 1992.

Seiffer B, Therapie der Akromegalie. In: Med Mo Pharm 15(5):159. 1992.

Stadler PA, PM 46:131-144. 1982.

Steinegger E, Hänsel R, Pharmakognosie, 5. Aufl., Springer Verlag Heidelberg 1992.

Teuscher E, Lindequist U, Biogene Gifte - Biologie, Chemie, Pharmakologie, 2. Aufl., Fischer Verlag Stuttgart 1994.

Teuscher E, Biogene Arzneimittel, 5. Aufl., Wiss. Verlagsges. Stuttgart 1997.

Vom Ergolin-Pharmakophor zu selektiven Arzneistoffen. In: DAZ 132(23):1235. 1992.

Wagner H, Wiesenauer M, Phytotherapie. Phytopharmaka und pflanzliche Homöopathika, Fischer-Verlag, Stuttgart, Jena, New York 1995.

Wang BH, Polya GM, The fungal teratogen secalonic acid D is an inhibitor of protein kinase C and of cyclic AMP-dependent protein kinase. In: PM 62(2)01711-114. 1997.

Wenzlaff H, Dihydroergotamin. In: DAZ 136(26):2179-2181. 1996.

Clematis Recta

Clematis

DESCRIPTION

Medicinal Parts: The medicinal part is the fresh, flowering plant.

Flower and Fruit: The flowers are in many blossomed terminal cymes. The individual blossoms are white and similar to Clematis vitalba, except that the bracts are only downy on the edges. The nutlet is glabrous, with a thickened edge and a long tail.

Leaves, Stem and Root: The plant grows to about 50 to 125 cm high. The stem is non-climbing, erect, leafy and glabrous. The leaves are pinnatifid. The leaflets are smaller than those of Clematis vitalba.

Characteristics: The plant is poisonous.

Habitat: The plant grows in Europe.

Production: Clematis herb is the whole fresh flowering plant of Clematis recta. The herb is gathered when the plant is in full flower. It is turned regularly while being dried in the shade.

Other Names: Upright Virgin's Bower

ACTIONS AND PHARMACOLOGY

COMPOUNDS

Protoanemonine-forming agents in the freshly-harvested plant: presumably the glycoside ranunculin, that changes enzymatically when the plant is cut into small pieces, and probably also when it is dried, into the pungent, volatile protoanemonine that quickly dimerises to anemonine. Once dried, the plant may not be capable of protoanemonine formation.

Saponins

EFFECTS
The fresh plant induces blistering on the skin and mucous membranes and is a fungicide. Sun plants are more effective than shade plants.

INDICATIONS AND USAGE
Clematis was formerly used as a remedy for venereal diseases (syphilis), chronic skin conditions, gout, rheumatism and bone disorders, as well as a diuretic. In the pharmaceutical industry, it is used for rheumatic pains, headaches and varicose veins. In folk medicine, it is used for blisters and as a poultice for festering wounds and ulcers.

PRECAUTIONS AND ADVERSE REACTIONS
No health hazards or side effects are known in conjunction with the proper administration of designated therapeutic dosages of the dehydrated drug. Extended skin contact with the freshly-harvested, bruised plant can lead to blister formation and cauterizations which heal poorly, due to the released protoanemonine, which is severely irritating to the skin and mucous membranes. If taken internally, severe irritation to the gastrointestinal tract, combined with colic and diarrhea, as well as irritation of the urinary drainage passages, are possible.

Symptomatic treatment for external contact consists of mucilaginosa, after irrigation with diluted potassium permanganate solution. In case of internal contact, administration of activated charcoal should follow gastric lavage.

OVERDOSAGE
Death by asphyxiation following the intake of large quantities of protoanemonine-forming plants has been observed in animal experiments. The risk associated with use of this plant is less than that of many other Ranunculaceae (Anemones nemorosae herba), due to the relatively low levels of protoanemonine-forming agents.

DOSAGE
Mode of Administration: The drug is seldom used today. It is available in the form of extracts, drops and infusions. Infusions are used for poultices.

LITERATURE
Bonora A et al., PH 26:2277. 1987.

Ruijgrok HWL, PM 11:338-347. 1963.

Southwell IA et al., Protoanemonin in australian Clematis. In: PH 33:1099. 1993.

Further information in:

Kern W, List PH, Hörhammer L (Hrsg.), Hagers Handbuch der Pharmazeutischen Praxis, 4. Aufl., Bde. 1-8, Springer Verlag Berlin, Heidelberg, New York, 1969.

Lewin L, Gifte und Vergiftungen, 6. Aufl., Nachdruck, Haug Verlag, Heidelberg 1992.

Madaus G, Lehrbuch der Biologischen Arzneimittel, Bde 1-3, Nachdruck, Georg Olms Verlag Hildesheim 1979.

Roth L, Daunderer M, Kormann K, Giftpflanzen, Pflanzengifte, 4. Aufl., Ecomed Fachverlag Landsberg Lech 1993.

Teuscher E, Lindequist U, Biogene Gifte - Biologie, Chemie, Pharmakologie, 2. Aufl., Fischer Verlag Stuttgart 1994.

Wagner H, Wiesenauer M, Phytotherapie. Phytopharmaka und pflanzliche Homöopathika, Fischer-Verlag, Stuttgart, Jena, New York 1995.

Clematis Vitalba

Traveller's Joy

DESCRIPTION
Medicinal Parts: The medicinal parts of the plant are the fresh leaves.

Flower and Fruit: The flowers are arranged in leafy cymes. The blossoms are small and white with 4 downy, revolute or splayed bracts. The stamens and ovaries are numerous. The fruit is a red-brown, long-tailed nut.

Leaves, Stem and Root: The plant grows to about 1.5 to 5 m high. The leaves are petiolate, 5-pinnate. The leaflets are ovate or slightly cordate, acute, and lobed. The petioles are clinging and the stems climbing, grooved, at first leafy then woody.

Characteristics: The flowers have a slight white thorn scent. The plant is poisonous.

Habitat: The plant is indigenous to Europe.

ACTIONS AND PHARMACOLOGY
COMPOUNDS
Protoanemonine-forming agents: in the freshly-harvested plant, presumably the glycosides ranunculin, that changes enzymatically when the plant is cut into small pieces, and probably also when it is dried, into the pungent, volatile protoanemonine that quickly dimerises to anemonine; when dried, the plant is not capable of protoanemonine formation.

Saponins

EFFECTS
No information is available.

INDICATIONS AND USAGE
The drug causes blistering and was formerly used to treat diseases of the male genitals, as well as for poorly healing

wounds. Today, it is used in small doses, both internally and externally, for migraine.

PRECAUTIONS AND ADVERSE REACTIONS

No health hazards or side effects are known in conjunction with the proper administration of designated therapeutic dosages of the dehydrated drug.

Extended skin contact with the freshly-harvested, bruised plant can lead to blister formation and cauterizations, which are difficult to heal due to the protoanemonine released, that is severely irritating to skin and mucous membranes. If taken internally, severe irritation to the gastrointestinal tract, combined with colic and diarrhea, as well as with irritation of the urinary drainage passages are possible. Symptomatic treatment for external contact should consist of mucilage, after irrigation with diluted potassium permanganate solution.

OVERDOSAGE

Ingestion of the drug should be treated with activated charcoal should follow gastric lavage. Death by asphyxiation following the intake of large quantities of protoanemonine-forming plants has been observed in animal experiments. The toxicity of this plant is less than that of many other Ranunculaceae (Anemones nemorosae herba), due to the relatively low levels of protoanemonine-forming agents.

DOSAGE

Mode of Administration: The drug is used topically and is also available in alcoholic extracts.

LITERATURE

Bonora A et al., PH 26:2277. 1987.

Ruijgrok HWL, PM 11:338-347. 1963.

Southwell IA et al., Protoanemonin in australian Clematis. In: PH 33:1099. 1993.

Further information in:

Frohne D, Pfänder HJ: Giftpflanzen - Ein Handbuch für Apotheker, Toxikologen und Biologen, 4. Aufl., Wiss. Verlagsges. mbH Stuttgart 1997.

Kern W, List PH, Hörhammer L (Hrsg.), Hagers Handbuch der Pharmazeutischen Praxis, 4. Aufl., Bde 1-8, Springer Verlag Berlin, Heidelberg, New York, 1969.

Lewin L, Gifte und Vergiftungen, 6. Aufl., Nachdruck, Haug Verlag, Heidelberg 1992.

Madaus G, Lehrbuch der Biologischen Arzneimittel, Bde 1-3, Nachdruck, Georg Olms Verlag Hildesheim 1979.

Roth L, Daunderer M, Kormann K: Giftpflanzen, Pflanzengifte, 4. Aufl., Ecomed Fachverlag Landsberg Lech 1993.

Teuscher E, Lindequist U, Biogene Gifte - Biologie, Chemie, Pharmakologie, 2. Aufl., Fischer Verlag Stuttgart 1994.

Clivers

See Galium Aparine

Clove

See Syzygium Aromaticum

Club Moss

See Lycopodium Clavatum

Cnicus Benedictus

St. Benedict Thistle

DESCRIPTION

Medicinal Parts: The flowering plant is the medicinal part.

Flower and Fruit: The blossom is a pale yellow, solitary, composite flower. The florets are tubular. The few lateral florets are sterile and have 3-part border and are smaller than the numerous androgynous florets. The epicalyx is ovate. The inner bracts end in long, rigid, and pinnatifid thorn, the outer ones in a simple thorn. They are broad, leafy and connected with the cordate-oblong leaflets of the epicalyx by numerous, web-like hairs. The fruit has a tuft of hair.

Leaves, Stem and Root: The thistle can grow to about 30 to 50 cm high. The stems are heavily branched, thistle-like, villous and sticky. The leaves are oblong, crenate, thorny-dentate, and roughly reticulate.

Characteristics: The plant has a strong and bitter taste.

Habitat: The thistle comes from southern Europe but is cultivated in other regions of the continent.

Production: St. Benedict Thistle herb consists of the dried leaves and upper stems, including inflorescence, of Cnicus benedictus.

Not To Be Confused With: Confusion with other plants rarely occurs.

Other Names: Blessed Thistle, Cardin, Holy Thistle, Spotted Thistle

ACTIONS AND PHARMACOLOGY

COMPOUNDS

Sesquiterpene lactone-bitter principles: chief components cnicin, additionally, salonitenolide

Lignans (bitter as well): trachelogenin, arctigenin, nortracheloside

Volatile oil: components including dodeca-1,11-dien-3,5,7,9-tetrain, p-cymene, fenchon, citral, cinnamaldehyde

EFFECTS

Stimulation of the secretion of saliva and gastric juices.

INDICATIONS AND USAGE

- Dyspeptic complaints
- Loss of appetite

St. Benedict Thistle is used to treat loss of appetite, dyspepsia, and is also used as a cholagogue.

PRECAUTIONS AND ADVERSE REACTIONS

Health risks or side effects following the proper administration of designated therapeutic dosages are not recorded. The drug exhibits a strong potential for sensitization (cross-reactions with mugwort and cornflower, among others); allergic reactions have however been seen only rarely.

DOSAGE

Mode of Administration: Comminuted drug and dried extracts for infusions or other bitter-tasting galenic preparations for internal use.

Preparation: Infusions are prepared by pouring boiling water over 1.5 to 2 gm of drug and drawn for 5 to 10 minutes.

Daily Dosage: Four to 6 gm of drug. The dosage for the aromatic bitter is 1 cup 1/2 hour before meals.

LITERATURE

Banhaelen M, Vanhaelen-Fastre R, (1975) Phytochemistry 14: 2709.

Farnsworth NR et al. (1975) J Pharm Sci 64(4):535.

Harnischfeger G, Stolze H, notabene medici 11:652. 1981.

Urzúa A, Acuna P, (1983) Fitoterapia 4:175

Vanhaelen-Fastre R, PM 24:165. 1973.

Vanhaelen-Fastre R, Vanhaelen M, (1976) Planta Med 29:179.

Further information in:

Fenaroli's Handbook of Flavor Ingredients, Vol. 1, 2nd Ed., CRC Press 1975.

Hausen B, Allergiepflanzen, Pflanzenallergene, ecomed Verlagsgesellsch. mbH, Landsberg 1988.

Kern W, List PH, Hörhammer L (Hrsg.), Hagers Handbuch der Pharmazeutischen Praxis, 4. Aufl., Bde. 1-8, Springer Verlag Berlin, Heidelberg, New York, 1969.

Madaus G, Lehrbuch der Biologischen Arzneimittel, Bde 1-3, Nachdruck, Georg Olms Verlag Hildesheim 1979.

Roth L, Daunderer M, Kormann K, Giftpflanzen, Pflanzengifte, 4. Aufl., Ecomed Fachverlag Landsberg Lech 1993.

Steinegger E, Hänsel R, Pharmakognosie, 5. Aufl., Springer Verlag Heidelberg 1992.

Teuscher E, Biogene Arzneimittel, 5. Aufl., Wiss. Verlagsges. mbH Stuttgart 1997.

Wagner H, Wiesenauer M, Phytotherapie. Phytopharmaka und pflanzliche Homöopathika, Fischer-Verlag, Stuttgart, Jena, New York 1995.

Wichtl M (Hrsg.), Teedrogen, 4. Aufl., Wiss. Verlagsges. Stuttgart 1997.

Coca

See Erythroxylum Coca

Cocculus Indicus

See Anamirta Cocculus

Cochlearia Officinalis

Scurvy Grass

DESCRIPTION

Medicinal Parts: The medicinal parts of the plant are the harvested and dried basal leaves of the first or second year; the flowers harvested shortly before or during flowering; the dried aerial parts of the plant and the fresh aerial parts of the plant collected during flowering.

Flower and Fruit: The flowers are arranged in initially tight, somewhat hanging, later longer racemes. The flower is large, white, and fragrant. The sepals are about 1.5 to 2 mm long, narrowly elliptoid, with a white membranous edge. The petals are about 4 to 5 mm long, oblong-obovate. The stamens are yellow. The fruit is a 4 to 7 mm long, globular or ovate pod and is crowned by the short style. There are 2 to 4 seeds in each loculus which are roundish-elliptoid, a little compressed and 1 to 3 mm long. The seed shell is usually red-brown and finely warty.

Leaves, Stem and Root: The glabrous plant is 15 to 35 cm high, a biennial or perennial and evergreen. It has a fusiform, fibrous rhizome from which grows one or more stemmed shoots which are sterile and fertile. The stems are ascending or almost erect, simple or branched, angular and grooved, leafy. The long-petioled basal leaves are in loose whorls, the cauline leaves are juicy, fleshy, petiolate, ovate, angular-dentate and the upper ones are clasping.

Characteristics: Flowers have a strong fragrance and taste when rubbed.

Habitat: The plant is found in central and northern Europe, Asia, and North America.

Production: True Scurvy-Grass is the fresh flowering herb of Cochlearia officinalis annuals.

Other Names: Scrubby Grass, Spoonwort

ACTIONS AND PHARMACOLOGY

COMPOUNDS

Glucosinolates: in the freshly-harvested, unbruised plant, chief components glucocochlearin, yielding with the destruction of the cells secretions of butyl mustard oil, besides among others glucotropaeolin (yielding butyl mustard oil) and sinigrin (yielding allyl mustard oil).

Flavonoids

Tropane alkaloids: tropine, m-hydroxybenzoyl-tropine (cochlearin)

Vitamin C

EFFECTS

Externally irritates the skin, due to the presence of mustard oils in the drug, in ethereal oil and in an ethanol solution.

INDICATIONS AND USAGE

Scurvy grass is used internally for Vitamin C deficiency, ''blood-cleansing or purification'' cures, gout, diuretic, rheumatism, stomach ache, and externally, as a poultice. A spirit made from scurvy-grass is used for skin irritations and as a mouthwash for gum diseases.

Efficacy has not been proven.

PRECAUTIONS AND ADVERSE REACTIONS

Health risks or side effects following the proper administration of designated therapeutic dosages are not recorded. The administration of higher dosages can lead to mucous membrane irritations of the gastrointestinal tract.

DOSAGE

Mode of Administration: Alcoholic extracts of Scurvy grass are used topically. Freshly pressed juice is for internal use.

LITERATURE

Cole RA, PH 15:759-762. 1976.

Further information in:

Hänsel R, Keller K, Rimpler H, Schneider G (Hrsg.), Hagers Handbuch der Pharmazeutischen Praxis, 5. Aufl., Bde 4-6 (Drogen): Springer Verlag Berlin, Heidelberg, New York, 1992-1994.

Madaus G, Lehrbuch der Biologischen Arzneimittel, Bde 1-3, Nachdruck, Georg Olms Verlag Hildesheim 1979.

Cocoa

See Theobroma Cacao

Coffea Arabica

Coffee

DESCRIPTION

Medicinal Parts: The medicinal parts of the plant are the seeds in various forms and stages.

Flower and Fruit: The inflorescences are axillary dense clusters with 10 to 20 flowers. The sessile or very short pedicled partial inflorescences bear dense, overlapping apical leaves. The calyx is 2.5 to 3 mm long with a blunt 5-tipped border. The corolla is white and fragrant. The stamens come from the mouth of the tube and are exserted. The ripe fruit is elliptoid and shows flattened in cross-section, 12 to 18 mm long by 12 to 15 mm wide and has a 3 to 6 mm long stem. It is initially green, later yellow and dark red when ripe. The exocarp is tough, the mesocarp is fleshy and slightly sweet. The endocarp is hard. The seeds are convex with a groove on one side. They are 8 to 12 mm long, 5 to 8 mm wide and 3 to 5 mm thick. They are gray-green when fresh and brown after roasting.

Leaves, Stem and Root: Coffea arabica is an evergreen shrub or small tree up to 8 m high with many basal branches. The young branches are glabrous and flattened and nodes produce many shoots. The bark of the fruiting branches is ashy white. The leaves live for 2 to 3 years; are 6 to 20 cm long and 2.5 to 6 cm wide. They are glabrous, slightly coriaceous, dark green, glossy, elliptoid-lanceolate with a distinct leaf tip.

Habitat: Supposedly indigenous to Ethiopia, cultivated in many tropical regions.

Production: The coffee charcoal is produced by roasting outer seed parts of green, dried fruit, until almost black, and then grinding. The coffee beans are ripe for harvest nine months after flowering. Thereafter, they are processed using one of two methods. In the dry method, the fruit is dried for 3 to 4 weeks in the sun, or mechanically with air-stream dryers. In the wet method, the beans are placed in a water-filled tank, where the ripe ones sink to the bottom, and all remaining ones float on top. The ripe fruit is then mechanically crushed and subsequently fermented. Fermentation lasts for approximately 48 hours (for arabica varieties). Afterwards the coffee is dried in the sun, or mechanically, but this is unusual.

Not To Be Confused With: Coffeae Semen is not easily confused with other drugs. However, ground and roasted coffee may be mixed with coffee substitutes, such as: chicory, dandelion root, figs, sugar beet root, lupin seeds, rye kernels, and barleycorn.

Other Names: Arabica Coffee, Arabian Coffee, Caffea

ACTIONS AND PHARMACOLOGY

COMPOUNDS: COFFEAE CARBO

Purine alkaloids: main alkaloid caffeine

Trigonelline

Carbonisation products of hemicelluloses

EFFECTS: COFFEAE CARBO

Absorbent and astringent.

COMPOUNDS: COFFEAE SEMEN

Purine alkaloids: main alkaloid caffeine (0.6 - 2.2 %), with it theobromine, theophylline

Caffeic and ferulic acid ester of quinic acid: in particular chlorogenic acid

Trigonelline

Norditerpene glycoside ester

In roasted coffee beans: numerous aromatic substances yielded from carbohydrates, proteins, fats and aromatic acids through pyrolysis

EFFECTS: COFFEAE SEMEN

Coffee has the stimulatory effect on the central nervous system (CNS) and gastric secretions. It also increase the psychomotor stamina.

INDICATIONS AND USAGE

COFFEAE CARBO

- Diarrhea
- Inflammation of the mouth and pharynx

Coffee is used for nonspecific, acute diarrhea, and local therapy of mild inflammation of the oral and pharyngeal mucosa. In folk medicine coffee is also used for festering wounds.

COFFEAE SEMEN

Most of the indicated effects of coffee are due to the presence of caffeine. The primary effects of caffeine can be summarized as follows:

Caffeine has a positive inotropic effect. In higher concentrations, it has a positive chronotropic effect on the heart and CNS. It causes a relaxation of the smooth muscles of blood vessels (except for cerebral blood vessels) and the bronchial tubes. Moreover, caffeine works as a short-lived diuretic and produces an increase of gastric secretions and the release of catecholamines.

Caffeine works competitively to block adenosinal receptors which lie on cell surfaces in the brain, fat tissue, liver, kidneys, heart, and erythrocytes.

Heart, circulation, vessels: People who normally do not drink coffee, react 1 hour after an intake of 250 gm, with an increase of 10 mm Hg in their systolic blood pressure. Habitual coffee drinkers are tolerant in this regard.

Blood: After 9 weeks of an average daily intake of 5.6 cups of coffee (steeped for 10 min.), the overall and LDL cholesterol increases significantly. The use of coffee filters can reduce this by up to 80%.

Digestive tract: Oral intake of 200 mg of chlorogene acid doubles gastric secretion, as does caffeine alone.

Miscellaneous: A diet consisting of 20% green coffee, impedes the growth of DMBA induced tumors in hamsters by 90%.

Outcome of the stimulating effects of caffeine commence a few minutes subsequent to taking the drug. The maximum plasma concentration of caffeine is reached between 15 and 45 minutes later. The plasma half-life amounts to 4 to 6 hours.

The coffee extracts made from roasted and unroasted seeds are used analogously with other drugs containing caffeine for physical and mental fatigue. The drink can also be used therapeutically in cases of hypotonia, as an analeptic agent, in the treatment of influenza (flu) and migraine, as an additive to analgesia.

In folk medicine coffee is also used to increase performance capability.

PRECAUTIONS AND ADVERSE REACTIONS

COFFEAE CARBO

General: Health risks or side effects following the proper administration of designated therapeutic dosages are not recorded.

Drug Interactions: The drug can hinder the resorption of other medicines.

COFFEAE SEMEN

General: Health risks following the proper administration of designated therapeutic dosages are not recorded. Quantities corresponding to up to 500 mg caffeine daily (5 cups of coffee) spread out over the day are toxicologically harmless for healthy adults accustomed to drinking coffee. Caution is advised for persons with sensitive cardiovascular systems, kidney diseases, hyperfunction of the thyroid gland, higher disposition to convulsions and certain psychic disorders, for example panic anxiety states. Side effects of coffee intake, mainly caused by its chlorogenic acid content, can include hyperacidity, stomach irritation, diarrhea, reduced appetite. The first signs of poisonings are vomiting and abdominal spasms. Non-specific symptoms such as restlessness, irritability, sleeplessness, palpitations, dizziness, vomiting, diarrhea, loss of appetite, and headache appear with the long-term intake of dosages exceeding 1.5 gm caffeine/day. Caffeine can lead to psychic as well as physical dependency (caffeinism). Symptoms of withdrawal can include headache and sleeping disorders.

Pregnancy: Pregnant women should avoid caffeine, under no circumstances exceeding a dosage of 300 mg/day (3 cups of coffee spread out over the day).

Nursing Mothers: Infants whose nursing mothers take drinks containing caffeine may suffer from sleeping disorders.

OVERDOSAGE

Higher dosages lead to stiffness, arrhythmic spasms of different muscle groups, opisthotonus and arrhythmic tachycardia. Fatal poisonings with the drug are not conceivable. The lethal dosage (LD50) for an adult is approximately 150 to 200 mg caffeine/kg body weight (for which 50 kg body weight = 7.5 gm = 75 cups of coffee), although there are cases of survival also with 106 gm caffeine. The death of a child following the intake of 5.3 gm of caffeine has been reported. The therapy for caffeine poisoning should begin with the inducement of vomiting or gastric lavage. Afterwards activated charcoal and sorbitol to retard resorption should be given. Spasms are to be treated with diazepam.

DOSAGE

COFFEAE CARBO

Mode of Administration: Powdered coffee charcoal and its preparations intended for internal consumption or local application.

Daily Dosage: The average daily dose for internal use is 9 gm of ground drug. The average single dose is 3 gm of powder.

Storage: It should be stored in well-sealed containers.

COFFEAE SEMEN

Mode of Administration: The ground beans are used in different types of infusion, i.e. cooked coffee (filter, espresso etc.). Caffeine is used in various combinations and preparations for various therapeutic uses.

Preparation: The dried seeds are roasted until they procure a deep brown color and a characteristic aroma. This process is usually carried out in the country of consumption. During roasting, the beans float for 1.5 to 3 minutes in hot gas at 220°C to 270°C.

Storage: The beans should be stored in sealed containers away from light.

LITERATURE

COFFEAE CARBO

Kuhn A, Schäfer G, (Kaffeekohle). In: Dtsch Med Wochenschr 23:922-923. 1939.

Further information in:

Hänsel R, Keller K, Rimpler H, Schneider G (Hrsg.), Hagers Handbuch der Pharmazeutischen Praxis, 5. Aufl., Bde 4-6 (Drogen): Springer Verlag Berlin, Heidelberg, New York, 1992-1994.

COFFEAE SEMEN

Anonym, Wieviel Coffein ist in welchem Produkt? In: PTA 5(1):40. 1991.

Bättig K, Kaffee in wissenschaftlicher Sicht. In: ZPT 9(3):95. 1988.

Bornkessel B, Sind Kaffeetrinker stärker gefährdet? In: DAZ 131(5):189. 1991.

Butz S, Nurses'-Health-Studie: Kaffe - kein Risikofaktor für koronare Herzkrankheit? In: DAZ 136(19):1680-1582. 1996.

Coffein: Entzugssyndrom bei Kaffeetrinkern. In: DAZ 133(6):441. 1993.

Ferré, Buch. In: Ferré F. Kaffee-Eine Kulturgeschichte. 1992.

Garattini, Buch. In: Caffeine, Coffee, and Health. Garattini S. Monographs of the Mario Negri Institute for Pharmacological Research, Milan. Raven Press, New York. 1993.

"Kaffee erhöht den Cholesterinspiegel". In: Aga 19:10682. 1991.

Martin E, Cholesterolspiegel erhöhender Faktor in Kaffeelipiden. In: DAZ 130(42):2376. 1990.

Schröder, Buch. In: Schröder R: Kaffee, Tee und Kardamom, Ulmer-Verlag, Stuttgart. 1991.

Schröder-Rosenstock K, Kaffeegenuβ - ein medizinisches Problem. In: DAZ 130(35):1919. 1990.

Silnermann K et al., (Entzugssymptome nach regelmäβigem Kaffeegenuβ). In: New Engl J Med 327017409. 1992.

Further information in:

Hänsel R, Keller K, Rimpler H, Schneider G (Hrsg.), Hagers Handbuch der Pharmazeutischen Praxis, 5. Aufl., Bde 4-6 (Drogen): Springer Verlag Berlin, Heidelberg, New York, 1992-1994.

Leung AY, Encyclopedia of Common Natural Ingredients Used in Food Drugs and Cosmetics, John Wiley & Sons Inc., New York 1980.

Lewin L: Gifte und Vergiftungen, 6. Aufl., Nachdruck, Haug Verlag, Heidelberg 1992.

Madaus G: Lehrbuch der Biologischen Arzneimittel, Bde 1-3, Nachdruck, Georg Olms Verlag Hildesheim 1979.

Roth L, Daunderer M, Kormann K: Giftpflanzen, Pflanzengifte, 4. Aufl., Ecomed Fachverlag Landsberg Lech 1993.

Teuscher E, Lindequist U: Biogene Gifte - Biologie, Chemie, Pharmakologie, 2. Aufl., Fischer Verlag Stuttgart 1994.

Teuscher E: Biogene Arzneimittel, 5. Aufl., Wiss. Verlagsges. mbH Stuttgart 1997.

Coffee

See Coffea Arabica

Cola Acuminata

Cola

DESCRIPTION

Medicinal Parts: The seeds are the medicinal parts of the plant.

Flower and Fruit: The male flowers with a diameter of 1.5 cm or the androgynous flowers with a diameter of 2.5 cm are axillary or on branches in cymes of few flowers. The 5 part calyx is white to yellow and marked red on the inside. The star-shaped fruit have 5 coriaceous, dark brown, up to 20 cm long and 5 cm wide and thick, unkeeled follicles arranged at right-angled to the stem. There are up to 14 ovate or square seeds of about 2.5 diameter in 2 rows with a white fleshy seed shell and usually reddish or red occasionally white seed kernal.

Leaves, Stem and Root: The plant is an evergreen tree 15 to 20 m tall. The trunk is branched down as far as the base. The old bark breaks off in pieces. The bark is dark green and rough. There are leaves only at the ends of the branches. They are 15 to 18 cm long and 10 cm wide, elliptoid to ovate, ending in a curled and spiralled tip, tough coriaceous, both sides are dark green and glossy.

Habitat: The plant is indigenous to Togo, Sierra Leone and Angola; found today in all tropical regions and cultivated widely.

Production: Ripe fruit is harvested, the seeds removed and dried in large piles. Cola nut consists of the endosperm freed from the testa of various Cola species, particularly Cola nitida.

Not To Be Confused With: Other varieties of Cola, such as Male kola which contains no caffeine.

Other Names: Kola Tree, Guru Nut, Cola Nut, Cola Seeds, Bissy Nut

ACTIONS AND PHARMACOLOGY

COMPOUNDS

Purine alkaloids: main alkaloid caffeine (0.6 - 3.7%), additionally theobromine, theophylline

(+)-catechin, (-)-epicatechin

Catechin tannins

Oligomeric proanthocyanidins

Starch

EFFECTS

A strong CNS stimulant; in animal tests: analeptic, stimulates production of gastric acid, lipolytic, increases motility; in humans: respiratory analeptic, stimulates gastric acid, lipolytic, increases motility, mildly positively chronotropic, and mildly diuretic.

INDICATIONS AND USAGE

■ Lack of stamina

Cola is used in mental and physical fatigue. In folk medicine it is used for tiredness, chewed to suppress hunger, thirst, morning sickness, and migraine; ground in poultices for wounds and inflammations; it is an indigenous cult drug.

PRECAUTIONS AND ADVERSE REACTIONS

Health risks following the proper administration of designated therapeutic dosages are not recorded. Side effects that may occur include difficulty falling asleep, hyperexcitability, nervous states of restlessness and stomach complaints. Signs of poisoning following the intake of cola drinks (20 to 60 mg caffeine per glass) or medications or stimulants containing cola extracts are hardly conceivable (Coffeae semen). Small children should avoid the intake of larger quantities of cola drinks. No administration should be carried out in the presence of stomach or duodenal ulcers, due to the drug's stimulation of gastric juice secretion.

DOSAGE

Mode of Administration: Powdered drug and other galenic preparations are for internal use.

Preparation: Dry extract: from the percolation 1:1 with 45% ethanol; Fluid extract: percolation with 70% ethanol (V/V); Cola tincture: 1:5 with 70% ethanol; Cola wine: 50 parts fluid cola extract with 850 parts Xeres wine and 100 parts sugar syrup.

Daily Dosage: Two to 6 gm of cola nut; 0.25 to 0.75 gm of cola extract; 2.5 to 7.5 gm of cola liquid extract; 10.0 to 30.0 gm of cola tincture; 60.0 to 180.0 gm of cola wine.

Storage: Cola should be protected from light in sealed containers.

LITERATURE

Hänsel R, Keller K, Rimpler H, Schneider G (Hrsg.), Hagers Handbuch der Pharmazeutischen Praxis, 5. Aufl., Bde 4-6 (Drogen): Springer Verlag Berlin, Heidelberg, New York, 1992-1994.

Leung AY, Encyclopedia of Common Natural Ingredients Used in Food Drugs and Cosmetics, John Wiley & Sons Inc., New York 1980.

Lewin L, Gifte und Vergiftungen, 6. Aufl., Nachdruck, Haug Verlag, Heidelberg 1992.

Madaus G, Lehrbuch der Biologischen Arzneimittel, Bde 1-3, Nachdruck, Georg Olms Verlag Hildesheim 1979.

Morton, JF, An Atlas of Medicinal Plants of Middle America, Charles C. Thomas USA 1981.

Oliver-Bever B (Ed.), Medicinal Plants of Tropical West Africa, Cambridge University Press Cambridge, London 1986.

Roth L, Daunderer M, Kormann K, Giftpflanzen, Pflanzengifte, 4. Aufl., Ecomed Fachverlag Landsberg Lech 1993.

Steinegger E, Hänsel R: Pharmakognosie, 5. Aufl., Springer Verlag Heidelberg 1992.

Teuscher E, Lindequist U: Biogene Gifte - Biologie, Chemie, Pharmakologie, 2. Aufl., Fischer Verlag Stuttgart 1994.

Teuscher E, Biogene Arzneimittel, 5. Aufl., Wiss. Verlagsges. mbH Stuttgart 1997.

Colchicum Autumnale

Colchicum

DESCRIPTION

Medicinal Parts: The fresh flowers and the dried ripe seeds, collected in early summer and the sliced, dried tubers and the fresh tubers are the medicinal parts of the plant.

Flower and Fruit: The flowers usually bloom in autumn, are bright lilac-pink, large, solitary or in pairs from the corm. The 6 bracts of the involucre are fused into a long, narrow tube. There are 6 stamens and 3 thread-like styles. The ovaries are on the side of the corm. The 3-valved capsule is initially green, later brown and wrinkled, containing black seeds with sticky appendages.

Leaves, Stem and Root: The 3 to 4 broadly lanceolate, tulip-like leaves appear together with the fruit in spring. They overlap at the base to from a tube.

Characteristics: All parts of the plant are very poisonous, taste disgusting, bitter, and are scratchy.

Habitat: Colchicum autumnale is a central European plant found in northern Ireland, England, northern Germany, southern Poland, the Ukraine, Bulgaria, European Turkey, northern Spain, central Asia, and Albania.

Production: The drug consists of the dried seeds harvested in June or July, or the cut and dried tubers harvested in July or August, or the fresh flowers harvested in late summer and autumn.

Other Names: Meadow Saffron, Meadow Saffran, Autumn Crocus, Naked Ladies, Upstart

ACTIONS AND PHARMACOLOGY

COMPOUNDS: COLCHICUM AUTUMNALE BULB

Tropolone alkaloids: colchicine, colchicoside and N-deacetyl-N-formyl-colchicine

COMPOUNDS: COLCHICUM AUTUMNALE SEMEN

Starch

Trupolone alkaloids: colchicine and colchicoside

Fatty oil

COMPOUNDS: COLCHICUM AUTUMNALE FLORA

Tropolone alkaloids: colchicine and N-deacetyl-N-formyl-colchicine, additional alkaloids including demecolcine

EFFECTS

Colchicum is antichemotactic, antiphlogistic, and an inhibitor of mitosis.

INDICATIONS AND USAGE

- Gout
- Mediterranean fever

PRECAUTIONS AND ADVERSE REACTIONS

General: The drugs are severely poisonous. Signs of poisoning, including stomach aches, diarrhea, nausea, vomiting, less frequently stomach and intestinal hemorrhages, can occur even with the administration of therapeutic dosages.

Kidney and liver damage, hair loss, peripheral nerve inflammation, myopathias and bone marrow damage with their resulting symptoms (leukopenia, thrombocytopenia, megaloblastic anemia, more rarely aplastic anemia) have been observed following long-term administration.

Pregnancy: Teratogenic damage, including following the intake of the drug by the father, are possible.

OVERDOSAGE

Three to 6 hours following intake of acutely toxic dosages burning of the mouth, difficulty swallowing, and thirst appear. After 12 to 14 hours the following appear: nausea, severe stomach pains, vomiting, diarrhea, bladder spasms, haematuria, fall in blood pressure and spasms, later progressive paralysis. Death follows through exhaustion, asphyxiation or circulatory collapse. The fatal dosage for an adult is 5 gm of the seeds, 1 to 1.5 gm for a child. The fatal dosage of an intake of colchicine lies between 7 mg and 200 mg.

The treatment for poisonings, following gastric lavage and the administration of a saline purgative (such as sodium sulphate), proceeds symptomatically (diazepam for convulsion, atropine for intestinal spasm), and includes possible intubation and oxygen respiration.

DOSAGE

Mode of Administration: Comminuted drug, freshly-pressed juice and other galenic preparations taken orally.

Daily Dosage: For an acute attack of gout, an initial oral dose corresponding to 1 mg colchicine, followed by 0.5 to 1.5 mg every 1 to 2 hours until pain subsides.

Total daily dosage must not exceed 8 mg of colchicine.

For familial Mediterranean Fever, prophylactic and therapeutic purposes, dosage corresponding to 0.5 to 1.5 mg of colchicine.

LITERATURE

Fell KR, Ramsden D, (1967) Lloydia 30:123.

Gasisc O, Potesilova H, Santavy F, PM 30:75-81. 1976.

Gröbner W, Wlater-Sack I, Gicht und ihre medikamentöse Therapie. In: DAZ 131(35):1789. 1991.

Heide L, Traditionelle Arzneipflanzen in der Gesundsheitsversorgung der Dritten Welt. Möglichkeiten und Grenzen. In: DAZ 133(23):2067. 1993.

Potesilova H, Coll Czech Chem Comm 32:141-157. 1967.

Santavy F, Reichstein T, Helv Chim Acta 33:1606-1627. 1950.

Santavy F, Talas M, Coll Czech Chem Comm 19:141-152. 1954.

Santavy F et al., PM 43:153-160. 1981.

Santavy F et al., Coll Czech Chem Comm 48:2989-2993. 1983.

Santavy F (1957) Pharm Zentralhalle 96:307.

Ulrichová J et al., Biochemical evaluation of colchicine and related analogs. In: PM 59(29):144. 1993.

Further information in:

Frohne D, Pfänder HJ, Giftpflanzen - Ein Handbuch für Apotheker, Toxikologen und Biologen, 4. Aufl., Wiss. Verlagsges. mbH Stuttgart 1997.

Hänsel R, Keller K, Rimpler H, Schneider G (Hrsg.), Hagers Handbuch der Pharmazeutischen Praxis, 5. Aufl., Bde 4-6 (Drogen), Springer Verlag Berlin, Heidelberg, New York, 1992-1994.

Lewin L, Gifte und Vergiftungen, 6. Aufl., Nachdruck, Haug Verlag, Heidelberg 1992.

Madaus G, Lehrbuch der Biologischen Arzneimittel, Bde 1-3, Nachdruck, Georg Olms Verlag Hildesheim 1979.

Roth L, Daunderer M, Kormann K, Giftpflanzen, Pflanzengifte, 4. Aufl., Ecomed Fachverlag Landsberg Lech 1993.

Steinegger E, Hänsel R, Pharmakognosie, 5. Aufl., Springer Verlag Heidelberg 1992.

Teuscher E, Lindequist U, Biogene Gifte - Biologie, Chemie, Pharmakologie, 2. Aufl., Fischer Verlag Stuttgart 1994.

Teuscher E, Biogene Arzneimittel, 5. Aufl., Wiss. Verlagsges. mbH Stuttgart 1997.

Collinsonia Canadensis

Stone Root

DESCRIPTION

Medicinal Parts: The medicinal parts are the dried root and rhizome as well as preparations from fresh or dried below ground growing parts of the plant.

Flower and Fruit: The flowers are dirty yellow labiate flowers with red venation on the inside in richly blossomed panicles. The upper lip has an obtuse tip. The side tips of the lower lip are small and rounded, the middle tips are larger and fringed. The calyx is acuminate and has 2 stamens. The fruit is a small nutlet.

Leaves, Stem and Root: The plant is a perennial and 90 to 120 cm high. The rhizome is grayish-brown, very hard, fibrous and up to 8 cm long. The shoots are glabrous, often tinged red and with few side shoots. The bark is very thin. The leaves are light green above, pale green below, glabrous, broad, cordate or ovate below, becoming narrower and shorter above.

Characteristic: The smell is strongly aromatic, unpleasant, and numbing in large amounts. The taste is bitter and unpleasant.

Habitat: The plant is indigenous to North America, from Canada to the Carolinas.

Production: Stone Root, the rhizome of Collinsonia, is gathered and dried in autumn.

Other Names: Hardhack, Horseweed, Heal-all, Knob Grass, Knob Root, Richweed, Richleaf, Knobweed, Hardback

ACTIONS AND PHARMACOLOGY

COMPOUNDS

Volatile oil: chief components caryophyllene, germacrene D, limonene, alpha- and beta-pinenes

Caffeic acid derivatives: including rosmaric acid

EFFECTS

Stone Root has stomachic, tonic, and diuretic effects.

INDICATIONS AND USAGE

Stone Root is used for calculi, kidney stones, urea (bladder semolina), bladder inflammation, dropsy, and gastro-intestinal disorders.

Efficacy has not been proven.

PRECAUTIONS AND ADVERSE REACTIONS

Health risks or side effects following the proper administration of designated therapeutic dosages are not recorded.

OVERDOSAGE

Overdoses can lead to mucous membrane irritations of the intestinal tract (colic-like pain, nausea), furthermore to strangury and feelings of dizziness.

DOSAGE

Mode of Administration: The drug is used internally as an extract, infusion, or tincture.

Preparation: Liquid extract (1:1) 1 ml to 4 ml; Tincture (1:5) 2 ml to 8 ml

Daily Dosage: The drug is generally used as a single dose, 1 to 4 gm, internally as an infusion.

LITERATURE

Joshi BS, Moore KM, Pelletier SW, Saponins from Collinsonia canadensis. In: JNP 55(10):1468-1476. 1992.

Lawrence BM et al., PH 11:2636-2638. 1972.

Wolters B, Zierpflanzen aus Nordamerika. In: DAZ 137(26):2253-2261. 1997.

Further information in:

Hänsel R, Keller K, Rimpler H, Schneider G (Hrsg.), Hagers Handbuch der Pharmazeutischen Praxis, 5. Aufl., Bde 4-6 (Drogen), Springer Verlag Berlin, Heidelberg, New York, 1992-1994.

Madaus G, Lehrbuch der Biologischen Arzneimittel, Bde 1-3, Nachdruck, Georg Olms Verlag Hildesheim 1979.

Colombo

See Jateorhiza Palmata

Colt's Foot

See Tussilago Farfara

Columbine

See Aquilegia Vulgaris

Combretum Micranthum

Opium Antidote

DESCRIPTION

Medicinal Parts: The dry leaves and stems are the medicinal parts.

Leaves, Stem and Root: The leaves are 10 to 13 cm long and about 6 cm wide, with 8 to 10 lateral spreading veins, transparent in the axils. The surface of the young leaves has small scales.

Characteristics: The taste is astringent and strong.

Habitat: The plant is indigenous to China, Malaysia, and Indonesia.

Other Names: Combretum, Jungle Weed

ACTIONS AND PHARMACOLOGY

COMPOUNDS

Pyrrolidine alkaloid betaines: stachydrines, 4-hydroxystachydrines, combretin-A (betaines drawn from the proline)

Catechin tannins

Flavonoids: including vitexin, saponaretin, orietin

EFFECTS

The drug has mild choleric and astringent effects.

INDICATIONS AND USAGE

The drug has been used for cholecystopathy, dyspepsia, and liver disease. It is obsolete as a drug and only found in combination preparations.

PRECAUTIONS AND ADVERSE REACTIONS

Health risks or side effects following the proper administration of designated therapeutic dosages are not recorded.

LITERATURE

Bassène E, Plantes Med Phytotherapie 21:173. 1987.

Bassène E et al., Ann Pharm Franc 44:491. 1986.

Further information in:

Hegnauer R, Chemotaxonomie der Pflanzen, Bde 1-11, Birkhäuser Verlag Basel, Boston, Berlin 1962-1997.

Kern W, List PH, Hörhammer L (Hrsg.), Hagers Handbuch der Pharmazeutischen Praxis, 4. Aufl., Bde 1-8, Springer Verlag Berlin, Heidelberg, New York, 1969.

Comfrey

See Symphytum Officinale

Commiphora Molmol

Myrrh

DESCRIPTION

Medicinal Parts: The resin which has exuded from the bark and dried in the air is the medicinal part.

Myrrh is a granular secretion which is discharged into cavities in the bark when it is wounded. The pale yellow exudate hardens to a red-brown mass about the size of a walnut.

Flower and Fruit: The yellow red inflorescences are panicled. The fruit is brown, about 7 mm long, ovate, and acuminate.

Leaves, Stem and Root: Commiphora molmol is a stunted shrub or small tree up 3 m high with a thick trunk and numerous irregular knotted branches and smaller clustered branchlets. It has a few trifoliate leaves at the end of short branches, with very small lateral leaflets. The terminal leaflet is 1 cm long, obovate, and glabrous. The oleo-gum resin exudes from fissures or incisions in the bark and is collected as irregular masses or tears, varying in color from yellowish or reddish-brown, often with white patches.

Characteristics: The surface may be oily or covered with fine dust. The taste is bitter and acrid. The odor is aromatic.

Habitat: The plant is indigenous to eastern Mediterranean countries, Somalia.

Production: Myrrh consists of oleo-gum resin exuded from the stems of Commiphora molmol, then air-dried. Myrrh can also originate from other Commiphora species if the chemical composition is comparable to the official drug.

Not To Be Confused With: ''False myrrh'' or Commiphora mukul.

Other Names: Guggal Gum, Guggal Resin, Didin, Didthin

ACTIONS AND PHARMACOLOGY

COMPOUNDS

Volatile oil (2-10%): chief components sesquiterpenes, including among others delta-elemene, beta-eudesmol, alpha-copaene, furosesquiterpenes: including among others 5-acetoxy-2-methoxy-4,5-dienone (aroma-bearer), furadesma-1,3-dien, isofuranogermacren (curzeren), curzenenone, 2-methoxy-furanoguaia-9-ene

Triterpenes (30-50%): including among others 3-epi-alpha-amyrin, alpha-amyrenone

Mucilages (30-60%, chiefly methyl-glucurono-galactans)

EFFECTS

Myrrh has astringent, disinfectant, and granulate-forming effects.

INDICATIONS AND USAGE

■ Inflammation of the mouth and pharynx

Myrrh is used for the topical treatment of mild inflammations of the oral and pharyngeal mucosa. In folk medicine, Myrrh is occasionally used internally as a carminative and also as an expectorant.

PRECAUTIONS AND ADVERSE REACTIONS

No health hazards or side effects are known in conjunction with the proper administration of designated therapeutic dosages.

DOSAGE

Mode of Administration: Powdered resin, myrrh tincture, and other galenic preparations for topical use.

Daily Dosage: Myrrh tincture: 2 to 3 times daily with undiluted tincture (1:5)

As a rinse or gargle: 5 to 10 drops in a glass of water.

In dental powders: 10% of powdered resin.

Storage: The herb and its preparations should be protected from light and moisture, in sealed containers, with a drying agent, as the carbohydrate component of the drug easily absorbs water; should not be stored in powdered form.

LITERATURE

Arora RB et al., (1972) Ind J Med Res 60(6):929.

Bajaj AC, Dev S, (1982) Tetrahedron 38(19):2949.

Brieskorn CH (1980) Tetrahedron Lett 21(6):1511.

Brieskorn CH et al., (1983) Phytochemistry 22:187 et 1207.

Delaveau P et al., (1980) Planta Med 40:49.

Kodama M et al., (1975) Tetrahedron Lett 35:3065.

Malhotra SC, Ahuja MMS, (1971) Ind J Med Res 59(10):1621.

Mester L et al., (1979) Planta Med 37(4):367.

Mincione E, Iavarone C, (1972) Chim Ind 54:424 and 525.

Pernet R, (1972) Lloydia 35:280.

Ruecker G, (1972) Arch Pharm 305(7):486.

Srivastava M et al., (1984) J Biosci 6(3):277.

Tripathi SN et al., (1975) Ind. J Exp Biol 13(1):15.

Wiendl RM, Franz G, Myrrhe. Neue Chemie einer alten Droge. In: DAZ 134(1):25. 1994.

Wylegalla R, Biblische Botanik: Pflanzen und Früchte aus dem gelobten Land. In: DAZ 137(11):867-869. 1997.

Further information in:

Hänsel R, Keller K, Rimpler H, Schneider G (Hrsg.), Hagers Handbuch der Pharmazeutischen Praxis, 5. Aufl., Bde 4-6

(Drogen), Springer Verlag Berlin, Heidelberg, New York, 1992-1994.

Leung AY, Encyclopedia of Common Natural Ingredients Used in Food Drugs and Cosmetics, John Wiley & Sons Inc., New York 1980.

Madaus G, Lehrbuch der Biologischen Arzneimittel, Bde 1-3, Nachdruck, Georg Olms Verlag Hildesheim 1979.

Steinegger E, Hänsel R, Pharmakognosie, 5. Aufl., Springer Verlag Heidelberg 1992.

Teuscher E, Biogene Arzneimittel, 5. Aufl., Wiss. Verlagsges. Stuttgart 1997.

Wichtl M (Hrsg.), Teedrogen, 4. Aufl., Wiss. Verlagsges. Stuttgart 1997.

Common Stonecrop

See Sedum Acre

Condurango

See Marsdenia Cundurango

Conium Maculatum

Hemlock

DESCRIPTION

Medicinal Parts: The medicinal parts of the plant are the dried leaves and the flowering branches of the 2-year-old and the fresh flowering plant.

Flower and Fruit: The plant has white flowers in 10 to 20 rayed umbels. There are 3 to 5 triangular to lanceolate, acuminate bracts; 3 to 6 small bracts on the outside of the small umbels; five 1.5 mm petals. The fruit is ovate with undulating veins and shows deep indentations on the mericarp on the seam side. There are no oil marks in the indentations.

Leaves, Stem and Root: The plant can be annual or perennial and up to 2 m high. The stem is erect, tubular, hollow, round, finely grooved, branched above, glabrous with brown-red marks below. The leaves are dark green glossy, 3-pinnate. The root is whitish and fusiform or branched.

Characteristics: The wilting herb smells of mice; red marked stem; very poisonous.

Habitat: The plant is indigenous to Europe, temperate Asia, northern Africa, and North and South America.

Production: Hemlock is harvested in uncultivated areas (the wild) or in small areas of cultivation. The aerial parts are air-dried in the open, in the shade.

Not To Be Confused With: Hemlock may be confused with canine parsley, water hemlock, wild chervil, tuberous chervil, and with anaesthetizing Kälberkopf.

Other Names: Cicuta, Poison Parsley, Poison Root, Poison Snakeweed, Spotted Crowbane, Spotted Hemlock, Spotted Parsley, Water Parsley, Winter Fern, Herb Bennet, Spotted Corobane, Musquash Root, Beaver Poison, Kex, Kecksies

ACTIONS AND PHARMACOLOGY

COMPOUNDS

Piperidin alkaloids: main alkaloid coniine, including, among others, N-methyl coniine, gamma-coniceine

The piperidin alkaloids are volatile and are likely to be present in toxicologically harmful quantities only in the freshly harvested plant, particularly in its berries, and in the freshly dried plant.

Polyynes

EFFECTS

The effects of the drug are caused by coniine in particular.

Toxic doses given to mice, rats, guinea pigs, and cats provoked the autonomous ganglion, clonic and tonal contractions of individual limbs, cramps, and eventually, paralysis.

Small doses given to mice led to blood pressure reduction in the short term. Higher doses resulted in a rise in blood pressure. Smaller doses stimulated respiration in cats, while higher doses impeded or slowed down the initial stimulus. In isolated guinea pig ileum, Coniine brought on contractions. In isolated perfundierten rabbit hearts, Coniine effected a negative inotrope, with a stabile heartbeat. With anaesthetized cats, a suppression of the muscle contraction reflex took place. Feeding or injecting lethal doses of Coniine into cows, horses, pigs, sheep, and hamsters was initially stimulating, producing twitching of the eyes and ears, which was followed by muscular debility, collapse, limpness, and death through paralysis.

Coniine absorbed through the skin and mucous membranes, is stimulating at first, then causes gradual paralysis of the spinal marrow or cord and the medulla oblongata and nicotine-like muscular paralysis.

INDICATIONS AND USAGE

No clinically proven forms of application exist.

Formerly, in folk medicine, the drug was used internally for neuralgia, rheumatism of the muscles and joints, stiffness of the neck, tetanic and epileptic cramps, bronchial spasms and pylori spasms. Externally, the drug was used as an ointment for coughs, asthma, sciatica, backache, and neuralgia.

Use is inadvisable due to the uncontrollable amounts of Coniine.

Efficacy has not been proven.

PRECAUTIONS AND ADVERSE REACTIONS

General: The drug is severely poisonous.

Pregnancy: The drug has a teratogenic effect with chronic intake.

OVERDOSAGE

Symptoms of poisoning following intake of toxic quantities (corresponding to 150 mg Coniine, approximately 10 gm of the freshly dried berries, approximately 30 gm of the freshly dried leaves) include burning of the mouth, scratchy gullet, salivation, rolling of the eyes, visual disorders, and weakness in the legs. Lethal dosages (corresponding to approximately 500 mg Coniine) cause glossoplegia, mydriasis, pressure in the head, dizziness, nausea, vomiting, diarrheas, loss of orientation, rising central paralysis, dyspepsia, cyanosis, and ultimately death through central asphyxiation, in the cases of very high dosages also through curare-like paralysis of the breathing musculature.

Following stomach and intestinal emptying (gastric lavage, sodium sulphate) and the administration of activated charcoal, plasma volume expanders and sodium bicarbonate infusions should be given in case of shock or to restore acidosis balance. If necessary, intubation and respiration should be carried out.

DOSAGE

Daily Dosage: The maximum dose for internal use; 0.3 gm, not to exeed 1.5 gm per day. The standard dose is 0.1 gm.

Storage: Hemlock should be stored above caustic lime, well dried, in closed containers and kept for no more than one year.

LITERATURE

Cromwell BT, Biochem J 64:259-266. 1956.

Kreitmair H, PA 3:565-566. 1948.

Madaus S, Schindler H, Arch Pharm 276:280-290. 1938.

Roberts MF, (1975) Phytochemistry 14:2395.

Roberts MF, (1980) Planta Med 39:216.

Seeger R, Neumann HG, DAZ-Giftlexikon Coniin. In: DAZ 131(13):720. 1991.

Further information in:

Frohne D, Pfänder HJ, Giftpflanzen - Ein Handbuch für Apotheker, Toxikologen und Biologen, 4. Aufl., Wiss. Verlagsges. mbH Stuttgart 1997.

Hänsel R, Keller K, Rimpler H, Schneider G (Hrsg.), Hagers Handbuch der Pharmazeutischen Praxis, 5. Aufl., Bde 4-6 (Drogen), Springer Verlag Berlin, Heidelberg, New York, 1992-1994.

Lewin L, Gifte und Vergiftungen, 6. Aufl., Nachdruck, Haug Verlag, Heidelberg 1992.

Madaus G, Lehrbuch der Biologischen Arzneimittel, Bde 1-3, Nachdruck, Georg Olms Verlag Hildesheim 1979.

Roth L, Daunderer M, Kormann K, Giftpflanzen, Pflanzengifte, 4. Aufl., Ecomed Fachverlag Landsberg Lech 1993.

Teuscher E, Lindequist U, Biogene Gifte - Biologie, Chemie, Pharmakologie, 2. Aufl., Fischer Verlag Stuttgart 1994.

Teuscher E, Biogene Arzneimittel, 5. Aufl., Wiss. Verlagsges. mbH Stuttgart 1997.

Contrayerva

See Dorstenia Contrayerva

Convallaria Majalis

Lily-of-the-Valley

DESCRIPTION

Medicinal Parts: The medicinal parts are the dried flower tips and the dried inflorescence, the Lily-of-the-Valley herb, the dried root rhizome with the roots, the flowering aerial parts and the whole, fresh, flowering plant.

Flower and Fruit: The flowers are in racemes nodding to one side, usually with a triangular penduncle. The tips are campanulate, 6 petalled with ovoid revolute tips. The perigone is white or pink. The stamens are attached to the base of the perigone. The fruit is a bright red, globular berry with 2 blue seeds. The plant is autosterile.

Leaves, Stem and Root: The 15 to 20 cm high plant has 2 to 3 leaves at the tip of the runner-like, branched rhizome. The leaves are elliptoid and acute. They taper to a long, sharp petiole at the base, which is clasped by a membranous sheath.

Characteristics: Fragrant but poisonous (all parts).

Habitat: The plant is indigenous to Europe, introduced into the U.S. and northern Asia.

Production: The harvested parts of the plant must be dried quickly at a maximum temperature of 60°C.

Not To Be Confused With: Polygonatum odoratum.

Other Names: May Lily, May Bells, Convallaria, Our Lady's Tears, Convall-lily, Lily Constancy, Jacob's Ladder, Ladder-to-Heaven, Muguet

ACTIONS AND PHARMACOLOGY

COMPOUNDS

Cardioactive steroid glycosides (cardenolides): varying according to geographical source chief glycoside convallatoxin (western and northwestern Europe), convalloside (northern and eastern Europe) or convallatoxin + convallatoxol (central Europe)

EFFECTS

Only older studies are available. These studies show Lily-of-the-Valley to have the following effects:

Cardiac: Positive inotropic effect on the myocardium economizes heart performance, lowers the elevated left-ventricular diastolic pressure, as well as pathologically raised venous pressure.

Renal: In animal tests, natriuretic and diuretic.

Venous: A dose dependent veno-constrictive effect was demonstrated in animal experiments.

INDICATIONS AND USAGE

- Arrhythmia
- Cardiac insufficiency NYHA I and II
- Infections of the urinary tract
- Kidney and bladder stones
- Nervous heart complaints
- Venous conditions

The drug is used for mild cardiac insufficiency (stage I-II NYHA), heart insufficiency due to old age, chronic cor pulmonale.

In folk medicine, Lily-of-the-Valley is also used for weak contractions in labor, epilepsy, dropsy, strokes and ensuing paralysis, conjunctivitis, leprosy; no longer used because of toxic effect.

PRECAUTIONS AND ADVERSE REACTIONS

General: Health risks following the proper administration of designated therapeutic dosages are not recorded. Nausea, vomiting, headache, stupor, disorders of color perception and cardiac arrhythmias can occur as side effects, particularly with overdosages.

Drug Interactions: The simultaneous administration of quinidine, calcium salts, saluretics, laxatives and glucocorticoids enhance effects and side effects.

OVERDOSAGE

For symptoms of an acute poisoning and therapy see Digitalis folium. The dangers of poisoning are relatively low with oral application, due to the poor absorbability of the glycosides.

DOSAGE

All information is based on Lilly-of-the-Valley powder as specified in the German pharmacopoeia.

Mode of Administration: Comminuted herb, as well as galenic preparations for internal use; no longer considered safe because of the levels of toxins.

Preparation: Tincture 1:10, liquid extract: 1:1, dry extract: 4:1

Daily Dosage: The average daily dose of the drug: 0.6 gm of tincture; 0.6 gm of liquid extract; 0.15 gm of dried extract. The average single dose: 2 gm of tincture; 0.2 gm of liquid extract.

In intravenous application, the full effective dose of convaltoxin is 0.4 to 0.6 mg, the prepared dose 0.2 to 0.3 mg.

Storage: The preparations should be stored in well-sealed containers protected from light.

LITERATURE

Bleier W et al., (1965) Pharm Acta Helv 40:554.

Hölzl J, Franz C, PM 24:378. 1973.

Kopp B, Kubelka W, (1982) Planta Med 45:87.

Krenn L, Schlifelner L, Stimpfl T, Kopp B, HPLC separation and quantitative determination of cardenolides in Herba Convallariae. In: PM 58(7)A82. 1992.

Laufke R (1958) Planta Med 6:237.

Loew D, Phytotherapie bei Herzinsuffizienz. In: ZPT 18(2):92-96. 1997.

Loew DA, Loew AD, Pharmakokinetik von herzglykosidhaltigen Pflanzenextrakten. In: ZPT 15(4):197-202. 1994.

Tschesche R et al., (1959) Naturwissensch. 46:109.

Tschesche R, in Pharmacognosy and Phytochemistry, Ed. H. Wagner and L. Hörhammer, Springer-Verlag Heidelberg, Berlin 1971.

Further information in:

Frohne D, Pfänder HJ, Giftpflanzen - Ein Handbuch für Apotheker, Toxikologen und Biologen, 4. Aufl., Wiss. Verlagsges. mbH Stuttgart 1997.

Hänsel R, Keller K, Rimpler H, Schneider G (Hrsg.), Hagers Handbuch der Pharmazeutischen Praxis, 5. Aufl., Bde 4-6 (Drogen), Springer Verlag Berlin, Heidelberg, New York, 1992-1994.

Lewin L, Gifte und Vergiftungen, 6. Aufl., Nachdruck, Haug Verlag, Heidelberg 1992.

Madaus G, Lehrbuch der Biologischen Arzneimittel, Bde 1-3, Nachdruck, Georg Olms Verlag Hildesheim 1979.

Roth L, Daunderer M, Kormann K, Giftpflanzen, Pflanzengifte, 4. Aufl., Ecomed Fachverlag Landsberg Lech 1993.

Schulz R, Hänsel R, Rationale Phytotherapie, Springer Verlag Heidelberg 1996.

Steinegger E, Hänsel R, Pharmakognosie, 5. Aufl., Springer Verlag Heidelberg 1992.

Teuscher E, Lindequist U, Biogene Gifte - Biologie, Chemie, Pharmakologie, 2. Aufl., Fischer Verlag Stuttgart 1994.

Teuscher E, Biogene Arzneimittel, 5. Aufl., Wiss. Verlagsges. mbH Stuttgart 1997.

Wagner H, Wiesenauer M, Phytotherapie. Phytopharmaka und pflanzliche Homöopathika, Fischer-Verlag, Stuttgart, Jena, New York 1995.

Coolwort

See Tiarella Cordifolia

Copaiba Balsam

See Copaifera Langsdorffi

Copaifera Langsdorffi

Copaiba Balsam

DESCRIPTION

Medicinal Parts: The medicinal parts are the resin oil tapped from an incision in the trunk.

Flower and Fruit: The flowers are small and yellow.

Leaves, Stem and Root: Copaifera langsdorffi is an evergreen tree up to 18 m high with compound leaves.

Characteristics: The resin oil consists of resin and essential oil. The oleoresin ranges in viscosity from very liquid and pale yellow to a resin-like substance of a red or fluorescent tint. The taste is unpleasant and there is a characteristic smell. A single tree can yield some 40 liters.

Habitat: Indigenous to tropical regions of South America and South Africa.

Production: Copaiba balsam is extracted from Copaifera reticulata and other varieties.

Other Names: Copaiva

ACTIONS AND PHARMACOLOGY

COMPOUNDS

Volatile oil: chief constituent alpha- and beta-caryophyllene, L-cadinenes, copaene

Resins: in particular diterpenoid oleoresins

EFFECTS

Possible bacteriostatic effect on the urinary tract.

INDICATIONS AND USAGE

The drug has various uses as a stimulant, laxative, and diuretic. Also used in infections of the urinary tract.

Copaiba Balsam is obsolete as a drug, however, it is still used in some homeopathic preparations.

PRECAUTIONS AND ADVERSE REACTIONS

The drug is irritating to the mucous membranes. Toxic in large amounts. Stomach pains appear after the intake of 5 gm of the drug, repeated doses bring about summer cholera, shivers, tremor, pains in the groin, and insomnia. Skin contact can lead to contact dermatitis (erythema, papular or vesicular rash, urticaria, petechias, occasionally the rashes heal leaving brown spots).

LITERATURE

Delle Monache G et al., (1971) Tetrahedron Letters 8:659.

Ferrari M et al., (1971) Phytochemistry 10:905.

Further information in:

Fenaroli's Handbook of Flavor Ingredients, Vol. 1. 2nd Ed. CRC Press 1975.

Kern W, List PH, Hörhammer L (Hrsg.), Hagers Handbuch der Pharmazeutischen Praxis, 4. Aufl., Bde. 1-8, Springer Verlag Berlin, Heidelberg, New York, 1969.

Leung AY, Encyclopedia of Common Natural Ingredients Used in Food Drugs and Cosmetics, John Wiley & Sons Inc., New York 1980.

Lewin L, Gifte und Vergiftungen, 6. Aufl., Nachdruck, Haug Verlag, Heidelberg 1992.

Madaus G, Lehrbuch der Biologischen Arzneimittel, Bde 1-3, Nachdruck, Georg Olms Verlag Hildesheim 1979.

Roth L, Daunderer M, Kormann K, Giftpflanzen, Pflanzengifte, 4. Aufl., Ecomed Fachverlag Landsberg Lech 1993.

Steinegger E, Hänsel R, Pharmakognosie, 5. Aufl., Springer Verlag Heidelberg 1992.

Coptis Trifolia

Goldthread

DESCRIPTION

Medicinal Parts: The medicinal parts are the rhizome and sometimes the stems and leaves.

Flower and Fruit: The solitary flowers are small and white and are arranged on leafless scapes.

Leaves, Stem and Root: Goldthread is a perennial plant in bushes of up to 15 cm with yellowish, scaly leaves at the base and long-petioled, obovate, evergreen leaves. The rhizome is thread-like, golden yellow with a matte surface and very small roots.

Characteristics: Goldthread has a very bitter taste and slight odor.

Habitat: Coptis trifolia is indigenous to India and Coptis groenlandica, which is also used, is indigenous to Greenland and Iceland.

Production: Goldthread rhizome is the rhizome of Coptis trifolia.

Other Names: Mouth Root, Cankerroot, Yellowroot, Coptis, Coptide

ACTIONS AND PHARMACOLOGY

COMPOUNDS

Isoquinoline alkaloids: including coptin, berberine

EFFECTS

The herb is a bitter tonic.

INDICATIONS AND USAGE

Goldthread is used in digestive disorders.

PRECAUTIONS AND ADVERSE REACTIONS

Health risks or side effects following the proper administration of designated therapeutic dosages are not recorded.

DOSAGE

Mode of Administration: Internally as a powdered drug or a liquid extract.

LITERATURE

Hegnauer R, Chemotaxonomie der Pflanzen, Bde 1-11, Birkhäuser Verlag Basel, Boston, Berlin 1962-1997.

Kern W, List PH, Hörhammer L (Hrsg.), Hagers Handbuch der Pharmazeutischen Praxis, 4. Aufl., Bde 1-8, Springer Verlag Berlin, Heidelberg, New York, 1969.

Coral Root

See Corallorhiza Odontorhiza

Corallorhiza Odontorhiza

Coral Root

DESCRIPTION

Medicinal Parts: The medicinal parts are the roots of the parasite.

Flower and Fruit: The plant has 10 to 20 flowers in terminal panicles. The flower heads are hood-like, reddish or purplish on the outside, paler and flecked with purple lines on the inside. One petal forms a lip with purple spots and a purple rim. The fruit is a large, bent-back, ribbed, long capsule.

Leaves, Stem and Root: Coral Root is a perennial which is found growing around the roots of trees in woodlands. The rhizome is small, brown, coral-like, about 2 to 3 cm long and 2 mm in thickness, with minute warts and transverse scars. The fracture is short and horny.

Characteristics: The taste is sweetish then bitter, the odor strong and peculiar when fresh.

Habitat: The parasite is indigenous to the U.S.

Production: Coral Root is the rhizome of Corallorhiza odontorhiza.

Other Names: Crawley Root, Scaly Dragon's Claw, Chicken Toe, Crawley, Fever Root, Turkey Claw

ACTIONS AND PHARMACOLOGY

COMPOUNDS

Unknown

EFFECTS

Coral Root has diaphoretic, febrifuge, and sedative effects.

INDICATIONS AND USAGE

Coral Root is used for colds. It is very efficient at inducing perspiration. Its scarcity prevents its wider use.

PRECAUTIONS AND ADVERSE REACTIONS

Health risks or side effects following the proper administration of designated therapeutic dosages are not recorded.

DOSAGE

Mode of Administration: Internally as a liquid extract.

LITERATURE

No literature is available.

Coriander

See Coriandrum Sativum

Coriandrum Sativum

Coriander

DESCRIPTION

Medicinal Parts: The medicinal parts are the coriander oil and dried ripe fruit.

Flower and Fruit: White, compact 3 to 5 blossomed umbels with no involucre. The floret has a 3-bract epicalyx. The border of the calyx has 5 tips. The corolla of the androgynous lateral florets are splayed. The fruit is globular and has a diameter of 3 cm, is straw yellow to brownish, and drops without dividing.

Leaves, Stem and Root: Coriandrum sativum is a 20 to 70 cm high plant with a bug-like smell. The root is thinly fusiform. The stem is erect, round, glabrous, and branched above. The leaves are light green, they are entire below and double-pinnate above.

Characteristics: The fresh herb and unripe fruit has a bug-like smell, ripe fruit has a pleasant tangy smell and taste.

Habitat: The herb is found in the Mediterranean region, central and eastern Europe, eastern Asia, and North and South America.

Production: Coriander consists of the ripe, dried, spherical fruit of Coriandrum sativum and its varieties vulgare A. and microcarpum. The fruit is threshed when it is rust red and is dried in lofts.

Not To Be Confused With: Grains and legumes.

ACTIONS AND PHARMACOLOGY

COMPOUNDS

Volatile oil: chief components D-(+)-linalool (coriandrol), including among others borneol, p-cymene, camphor, geraniol, limonene, alpha-pinenes, the unusual smell is caused by the trans-tridec-2-enale content

Fatty oil: chief fatty acids petroselic acid, oleic acid, linolenic acid

Hydroxycoumarins: including umbelliferone, scopoletine

EFFECTS

The essential oil of coriander stimulates the secretion of gastric juices and is a carminative and spasmolytic; in vitro it has antibacterial and antifungal effects.

INDICATIONS AND USAGE

- Dyspeptic complaints
- Loss of appetite

Coriander is used for dyspeptic complaints, loss of appetite, and complaints of the upper abdomen.

In folk medicine, coriander is also used for digestive and gastric complaints; in other cultures for coughs, chest pains, bladder complaints, leprosy rash, fever, dysentery, externally for headaches, oral and pharyngeal disorders, halitosis, post-partal complications; the folk indications have not been proven.

PRECAUTIONS AND ADVERSE REACTIONS

Health risks or side effects following the proper administration of designated therapeutic dosages are not recorded. The drug possesses a weak potential for sensitization.

DOSAGE

Mode of Administration: Crushed and powdered drug, as well as other galenic preparations for internal indications as well as household usages.

Preparations: The coriander extract 1:2 is prepared by percolating 1 weight part of the drug with 45% ethanol so that 2 weights tincture are produced. The infusion is prepared by pouring 150 ml of boiling water over 2 tsp. of crushed drug and straining after 15 minutes.

Daily Dosage: The average daily dose is 3.0 gm of drug; single dose: 1 gm; infusion: 1 fresh cup between meals; tincture: 10 to 20 drops after meals.

Storage: The non-comminuted drug is stored at a maximum temperature of 25°C protected from light in well-sealed containers.

LITERATURE

Calcandi V, Ciropol-Calcandi I, Georgescu E, PA 16(6):331-334. 1961.

Diedreichsen A et al., Chemotypes of Coriandrum sativum L. in the Gatersleben Genebank. In: PM 62, Abstracts of the 44th Ann Congress of GA, 82. 1996.

Formacék, Buch. In: Formacék, V, Kubeczka KH: Essential Oils Analysis by Capillary Gas Chromatography and Carbon-13-NMR Spectroscopy, John Wiley & Sons, Chicester, New York, Brisbane, Toronto, Singapore 1982.

Gijbels MJM et al., (1982) Fitoterapia 53(1/2):17.

Mascolo, N et al., (1987) Phytother Res 1(1):28.

Ram AS, Devi HM, (1983) Indian J Bot 6(1):21.

Schratz E, Quadry SMJS, PM 14(3):310-325. 1966.

Further information in:

Fenaroli's Handbook of Flavor Ingredients, Vol. 1, 2nd Ed., CRC Press 1975.

Hänsel R, Keller K, Rimpler H, Schneider G (Hrsg.), Hagers Handbuch der Pharmazeutischen Praxis, 5. Aufl., Bde 4-6 (Drogen), Springer Verlag Berlin, Heidelberg, New York, 1992-1994.

Leung AY, Encyclopedia of Common Natural Ingredients Used in Food Drugs and Cosmetics, John Wiley & Sons Inc., New York 1980.

Simon JE, Chadwick AF, Craker LE (Eds.), Herbs. An Indexed Bibliography 1971-80. Archon Books, USA 1984.

Steinegger E, Hänsel R, Pharmakognosie, 5. Aufl., Springer Verlag Heidelberg 1992.

Teuscher E, Biogene Arzneimittel, 5. Aufl., Wiss. Verlagsges. mbH Stuttgart 1997.

Wichtl M (Hrsg.), Teedrogen, 4. Aufl., Wiss. Verlagsges. Stuttgart 1997.

Corn Poppy

See Papaver Rhoeas

Cornflower

See Centaurea Cyanus

Cornus Florida

Dogwood

DESCRIPTION

Medicinal Parts: The medicinal part is the dried and occasionally the fresh bark.

Flower and Fruit: The flowers are sessile, small, greenish, and in clusters of 12 to 20 at the splayed end of a tough, 3 cm long stem. The bracts are white or pale reddish, ovate to long and are longer than the inflorescence. The petals are about 4 mm long. The fruit is a scarlet berry.

Leaves, Stem and Root: The plant is a deciduous shrub or a 4 to 9 m high tree which is heavily branched and has a dark gray, thick, and rough bark. The branches are smooth and covered in leaf scars. The leaves are 7 to 10 cm long, opposite, petiolate, entire, ovate acuminate at both ends, and somewhat rough. The upper surface is dark green. In autumn the upper surface is bright red to violet. The underside is always whitish-green. They are slightly pubescent when young.

Habitat: Cornus florida is indigenous to eastern and southern North America, other varieties are found in Europe.

Production: American Boxwood bark and root-bark are the bark and root-bark of Cornus florida.

Other Names: Dog-Tree, Box Tree, Boxwood, Budwood, False Box, Cornelian Tree, Cornel, Bitter Redberry, Green Ozier, Swamp Dogwood, Silky Cornel, Osier, Rose Willow

ACTIONS AND PHARMACOLOGY

COMPOUNDS

Steroid saponins: including sarsapogenin-O-beta-D-galactoside, sarsapogenin-O-beta-D-xylosyl-(1(2)-beta-D-galactoside

Iridoide monoterpenes: cornin (verbenalin)

Tannins

EFFECTS

Effect on molluscs: The drug destroys the biomphalaria glabratus snails (carrier of bilharziose).

Cardiac effect: Heart activity, at different levels up to the cessation of heartbeat, is examined depending on the concentration of the methanol extract.

Antiplasmodic effect: Induced malaria on chicks and Peking ducks was treated for 5 days with a water-insoluble fraction. As a result, antiplasmodic activity towards *P. cathemerium* could be observed, similar to that deployed by quinine and sulfadiazine. To date, the results can not be sufficiently assessed.

The bark works as a tonic, an astringent, and as a stimulant.

INDICATIONS AND USAGE

In North America, the dried bark was used in folk medicine for strength, to stimulate appetite, for fever and for chronic diarrhea. It is used externally as an astringent for wounds and boils. Formerly, it was in use as a replacement for quinine. It is still used for headaches and fatigue.

PRECAUTIONS AND ADVERSE REACTIONS

Health risks or side effects following the proper administration of designated therapeutic dosages are not recorded.

DOSAGE

Mode of Administration: Formerly the drug was used internally as a tincture as an alternative to quinine and externally as a liquid extract.

Preparation: Decoction or infusion (no specifications).

LITERATURE

Jacobs, B, In: Jacobs ML, Burlage HM: Index of Plants of North Carolina with Reputed Medicinal Uses, USA. 1958.

Jensen SR, Kjaer A, Nielsen BJ, Biochem Syst Ecol 3:75-78. 1975.

Hostettmann K, Hostettmann-Kaldas M, Nakanishi K, Helv Chim Acta 61:1990. 1978.

Further information in:

Hänsel R, Keller K, Rimpler H, Schneider G (Hrsg.), Hagers Handbuch der Pharmazeutischen Praxis, 5. Aufl., Bde 4-6 (Drogen), Springer Verlag Berlin, Heidelberg, New York, 1992-1994.

Corydalis Cava

Corydalis

DESCRIPTION

Medicinal Parts: The medicinal parts are the tubers collected and dried when the plant is dormant. The fresh tuber collected just before flowering is also used.

Flower and Fruit: Flowers first appear in the fourth or fifth year. There are 4 to 5 racemes of 6 to 12 blooms which are symmetrically 2-sided. There are 2 entire-margined bracts under the racemes. The flowers are dull red or yellowish white, seldom lilac, brown-red, or dark blue. The sepals are very small. The upper petal drawn out into a downward curved spur, the front end is curved upward like a lip. The inner petals form a hood-like protective cover for the 6 stamens fused into 2 bundles. There is one ovary. The fruit is a pale green pod 20 to 25 cm long. The seeds are 3 mm wide, black, round, smooth, and glossy.

Leaves, Stem and Root: The plant is perennial and grows to about 15 to 30 cm. A number of erect stems grow from the tuberous rhizome which quickly becomes hollow. The stems bear the racemes and the 2 leaves. The 2 leaves under the racemes are long-petioled, double trifoliate, sea-green above, and whitish green beneath.

Characteristics: The flowers have a slight fragrance of resin.

Habitat: The plant is indigenous to southern and central Europe.

Production: The tubers are dug up in autumn or in spring, once the ground has thawed. They are thoroughly cleaned, the roots and greenery are removed and the remainder is sliced. The material is dried in a well aired place, turned regularly and kept in temperatures not exceeding 40°C.

Other Names: Early Fumitory, Turkey Corn, Squirrel Corn.

ACTIONS AND PHARMACOLOGY

COMPOUNDS

Isoquinoline alkaloids: very complex, breed-specific mixture of approximately 40 alkaloids, including (+)-bulbocapnine and (+)-corytuberin (aporphine-type) as well as (-)-corydaline (berberine-type)

EFFECTS

The full extract has a mildly sedative, sleep inducing, spasmolytic, tranquilizing, and hallucinogenic effect. It suppresses the CNS, reduces blood pressure, and impedes movement of the small intestine.

INDICATIONS AND USAGE

Formerly, it was used in hyper-kinetic conditions. Today, it is occasionally used to treat melancholia, pathological neuroses, and mild forms of depression, as well as for severe nerve damage, trembling limbs, and emotional disturbances.

PRECAUTIONS AND ADVERSE REACTIONS

Health risks or side effects following the proper administration of designated therapeutic dosages are not recorded. Poisonings among humans have not yet been observed.

OVERDOSAGE

Clonic spasms with musculature tremor are to be expected with considerable overdosages.

DOSAGE

Mode of Administration: The drug is available as a full extract in ready made preparations.

LITERATURE

Santavy F, in Manske RHF (Ed.) The Alkaloids, Vol XII, Academic Press New York, p. 333-354. 1970.

Slavík J, Slavíkova L, Collect Czech Chem Commun 44:2261-2273. 1979.

Further information in:

Frohne D, Pfänder HJ, Giftpflanzen - Ein Handbuch für Apotheker, Toxikologen und Biologen, 4. Aufl., Wiss. Verlagsges. mbH Stuttgart 1997.

Hänsel R, Keller K, Rimpler H, Schneider G (Hrsg.), Hagers Handbuch der Pharmazeutischen Praxis, 5. Aufl., Bde 4-6 (Drogen), Springer Verlag Berlin, Heidelberg, New York, 1992-1994.

Lewin L, Gifte und Vergiftungen, 6. Aufl., Nachdruck, Haug Verlag, Heidelberg 1992.

Madaus G, Lehrbuch der Biologischen Arzneimittel, Bde 1-3, Nachdruck, Georg Olms Verlag Hildesheim 1979.

Roth L, Daunderer M, Kormann K, Giftpflanzen, Pflanzengifte, 4. Aufl., Ecomed Fachverlag Landsberg Lech 1993.

Steinegger E, Hänsel R, Pharmakognosie, 5. Aufl., Springer Verlag Heidelberg 1992.

Teuscher E, Lindequist U, Biogene Gifte - Biologie, Chemie, Pharmakologie, 2. Aufl., Fischer Verlag Stuttgart 1994.

Cotton

See Gossypium Herbaceum

Couch Grass

See Elymus Repens

Cowhage

See Mucuna Pruriens

Crataegus Species

Hawthorn

DESCRIPTION

Medicinal Parts: The medicinal parts are generally white thorn flowers, leaves, fruit, and various mixtures of different plant parts.

Flowers and Fruit: The white flowers are in richly-blossomed cymes. The sepals are usually short, more or less triangular, entire-margined or, particularly the American variety, fairly long with glandular tips. The petals are usually separate, orbicular, crenate, white or occasionally red. There are 10 to 20 stamens and 1 to 5 carpels, which are more or less fused to the receptacle. There are 2 ovules, the upper one is sterile and covers the lower fertile one like a cap. There is 1 seed in each chamber. The false fruit is ovoid or globose and crowned by the remains of the sepals. It is red, black, or yellow and mealy.

Leaves, Stem and Root: Hawthorn is a bulky shrub or small tree, 1.5 to 4 m high with hard wood and usually thorny branches. The leaves have many forms, shallowly 3 to 5 lobed, lobes pointed forwards, unevenly serrate, obovate, yellowish-green, and glossy.

Characteristics: The flowers have an unpleasant smell and a slightly bitter taste; the fruit has a sour taste.

Habitat: The plant is indigenous to northern temperate zones of Europe, Asia, and North America.

Production: The medicinal parts of the Hawthorn plant are collected in the wild and dried at room temperature.

Not To Be Confused With: Flowers, leaves, and fruit of Robinia pseudoacacia, Sorbus aucuparia or Prunus spinosa.

Other Names: Haw, May, Whitethorn

ACTIONS AND PHARMACOLOGY

COMPOUNDS

Flavonoide

O-glycosides: including rutin, hyperoside

6-C- and 8-C-glycosyl compounds: including vitexin, vicenin-1, orientin

6-C- and 8-C-glycosyl compounds: additionally linked O-glycosidically with further monosaccharides, including vitexin-2''-O-alpha-L-rhamnoside, vitexin-2''-O-alpha-L-rhamnoside-4'''- acetate

Oligomeric proanthocyanidins

Biogenic amines: including tyramine

EFFECTS

The material available is only of limited value. The active principles are procyanidins and flavonoids. They cause an increase in coronary blood flow due to dilatory effects resulting in an improvement of myocardial blood flow. The drug is positively inotropic and positively chronotropic. The cardiotropic effect of Crataegus is said to be caused by the increased membrane permeability for calcium as well as the inhibition of phosphodiesterase with an increase of intracellular cylco-AMP concentrations. Furthermore, increased coronary and myocardial circulatory perfusion, reduction in peripheral vascular resistance were observed.

INDICATIONS AND USAGE

■ Decrease in cardiac output (Stage II NYHA)

Hawthorn is used in mild cardiac insufficiency (Stage I-II NYHA), senile heart, chronic cor pulmonale, and mild forms of bradycardial arrythmias. In folk medicine, Hawthorn is also used as a cardio and arterio treatment as well as a cardiotonic and to regulate blood pressure and as a sedative; efficacy in these areas has not been proven.

PRECAUTIONS AND ADVERSE REACTIONS

Health risks or side effects following the proper administration of designated therapeutic dosages are not recorded.

DOSAGE

Mode of Administration: The dried and comminuted drug for decoctions as well as liquid or dry extracts for oral intake.

Daily Dosage: The average daily dose is 5 gm of drug or 160 to 900 mg extract, (ethanol 45% V/V or methanol 70% V/V) standardized on procyanidin or flavonoids; single dose: 1 gm of drug several times daily. The duration of treatment is minimum 6 weeks.

Storage: Hawthorn should be protected form light in well-sealed containers.

LITERATURE

Ammon HPT, Händel M, (1981) Crataegus, Toxikologie und Pharmakologie. Teil 1, Toxizität. Planta Med 43:105-120.

Ammon HPT, Handel M, (1981) Planta Med 43:105, 209 et 313.

Anonym, 5. Kongreβ für Phytotherapie: Phytoforschung intensiviert. In: DAZ 133(48):4593. 1993.

Anonym, Behandlung der leichten Herzinsuffiziens: Weiβdornextrakt und ACE-Hemmer im Vergleich. In: DAZ 134(39):3749. 1994.

Anonym, Phytopharmaka für ältere Menschen: Ginkgo, Kava, Hypericum und Crataegus. In: DAZ 135(5):400-402. 1995.

Anonym, Weiβdorn bei Herzinsuffiziens und Angina pectoris. In: Symbiose 4(3):16. 1992.

Bahorun T, Gressier B, Trotin F, Brunet C, Dine Th, Luyckx M, Vasseur J, Cazin M, Cazin JC, Pinkas M, Oxygen species scavenging activity of phenolic activities, fresh plant organs and pharmaceutical preparations. In: Arzneim Forsch 46(11):1086-1089. 1996.

Bahorun T, Trotin F, Pommery J, Vasseur J, Pinkas M, Antioxydant activities of Crataegus monogyna extracts. In: PM 60(4):323-328. 1994.

Beretz A et al., (1980) Planta Med 39(3):241.

Ciplea AG, Richter KD, (1988) The protective effect of Allium sativum and Crataegus on isoprenaline-induced tissue necroses in rats. Arzneim Forsch/Drug Res 38:1588-1592.

Czygan FC, Crataegus-Arten- Weiβdorn, Portrait einer Arzneipflanze. In: ZPT 15(2)01937. 1994.

Dingermann T, Phytopharmaka im Alter: Crataegus, Ginkgo, Hypericum und Kava-Kava. In: PZ 140(23):2017-2024. 1995.

Eichstädt H, Bäder M, Danne O, Kaiser W, Stein U, Felix R, (1989) Crataegus-Extrakt hilft dem Patienten mit NYHA II-Herzinsuffizien Therapiewoche 39: 3288-3296.

Ficarra P et al., (1984) Farm Ed Prat 39(10)342.

Ficarra P et al., (1984) Farm Ed Prat 39(5)148.

Fischer K, Jung F, Koscielny J, Kiesewetter H, (1994) Crataegus-Extrakt vs. Methyldigoxin. Einfluβ auf Rheologie und Mikrozirkulation bei 12 gesunden Probanden. Münch Med Wschr 136 (Suppl 1), 35-38.

Förster A, Förster K, Bühring M, Wolfstädter HD, (1994) Crataegus bei mäβig reduzierter linksventrikulärer Auswurffraktion. Ergospirometrische Verlaufsuntersuchung bei 72. Patienten in doppelblindem Vergleich mit Plazebo. Münch Med Wschr 136 (Suppl 1), 21-26

Iwamoto M et al., (1981) Planta Med 42(1):1

Joseph G, Zhao Y, Klaus W (1995) Pharmakologisches Wirkprofil von Crataegus-Extrakt im Vergleich zu Epinephrin, Amrinon, Milrinon und Digoxin am isoliert perfundierten Meerschweinchenherzen. Arzneim Forsch/Drug Res 45: 1261-1265

Kaul R, Pflanzliche Procyanidine. Vorkommen, Klassifikation und pharmakologische Wirkungen. In: PUZ 25(4):175-185. 1996.

Klensch O, Nagell A, Die Darreichungsform Tee am Beispiel Weiβdornblätter mit Blüten. In: DAZ 134(32):3005. 1994.

Krzeminski T, Chatterjee SS, (1993) Ischemia and early reperfusion induced arrhythmias, beneficial effects of an extract of Crataegus oxyacantha L. Pharm Pharmacol Lett 3:45-48.

Kurcok A, (1992) Ischemia- and reperfusion-induced cardiac injury; effects of two flavonoids containing plant extracts possessing radical scavenging properties. Naunyn-Schmiedebergs's Arch Pharmacol 345 (Suppl RB 81) Abstr 322.

Kurzmann M, Schimmer O, Weiβdorn - Flavonoidmuster und DC-Identitätsprüfung. In: DAZ 136(33):2759-2764. 1996.

Loew D, (1994) Crataegus-Spezialextrakte bei Herzinsuffizien. Kassenarzt 15:43-52.

Loew D, Phytotherapie bei Herzinsuffizienz. In: ZPT 18(2):92-96. 1997.

Meier B, Neue Erkenntnisse zur Analytik und Wirksamkeit von Weiβdorn. In: DAZ 136(44):3877-3879. 1996.

Pöpping S, Rose H, Ionescu I, Fischer Y, Kammermeier H, (1995) Effect of a Hawthorn Extract on Contraction and Energy Turnover of Isolated Rat Cordiomyocytes. Arzneim Forsch/Drug Res 45:1157-1161.

Rehwald A et al., HPLC analysis of the flavonoids of Crataegi folium cum flore. In: PM 59(7)28. 1993.

Reuter HD, Crataegus als pflanzliches Kardiakum. In: ZPT 15(2):73. 1994.

Rewerski W et al., (1971) Arzneim Forsch 21:886.

Schlegelmilch R, Heywood R, (1994) Toxicity of Crataegus (Hawthorn) Extract (WS 1442). J Am Coll Toxicol 13:103-111.

Schmidt U, Kuhn U, Ploch M, Hübner WD, (1994) Wirksamkeit des Extraktes LI 132 (600 mg/Tag) bei 8wöchiger Therapie. Plazebokontrollierte Doppelblindstudie mit Weiβdorn an 78 herzinsuffizienten Patienten im Stadium II nach NYHA. Münch Med Wschr 136(Suppl 1):13-20.

Schüssler M et al., Effect of flavonoids from Crataegus species in Langendorf perfused isolated guinea pig heart. In: PM 58(7)46. 1992.

Schuessler M et al., Cardiac effects of flavonoids from Crataegus species. In: PM 59(7)88. 1993.

Siegel G, Casper U, (1995) Crataegi folium cum flore. In, Loew D, Rietbrock N (Hrsg) Phytopharmaka in Forschung und klinischer Anwendung. Steinkopff Verlag, Darmstadt, S. 1-14.

Siegel G, Casper U, Walter H, Hetzer R, (1994) Weiβdorn-Extrakt LI 132. Dosis- Wirkungs-Studie zum Membranpotential und Tonus menschlicher Koronararterien und des Hundepapillarmuskels. Münch med Wschr 136(Suppl 1):45-56.

Sprecher E, Pflanzliche Geriatrika. In: ZPT 9(2):40. 1988.

Sticher O, Rehwald A, Meier B, (1994) Kriterien der pharmazeutischen Qualität von Crataegus-Extrakten. Münch Med Wschr 136(Suppl 1):69-73.

Tauchert M, Loew D, (1995) Crataegi folium cum flore bei HerzinsuffizienZ In, Loew D, Rietbrock N (Hrsg) Phytopharmaka in Forschung und klinischer Anwendung. Steinkopff Verlag, Darmstadt, S. 137-144.

Tauchert M, Ploch M, Hübner WD, (1994) Wirksamkeit des Weiβdorn-Extraktes LI 132 im Vergleich mit Captopril. Multizentrische Doppelblindstudie bei 132 Patienten mit Herzinsuffizienz im Stadium II nach NYHA. Münch Med Wschr 136(Suppl 1):27-34.

Tauchert M, Siegel G, Schulz V, (1994) Weiβdorn-Extrakt als pflanzliches Cardiacum (Vorwort). Neubewertung der therapeutischen Wirksamkeit. Münch Med Wschr 136(Suppl 1):3-5.

Trunzler G, Phytotherapeutische Möglichkeiten bei Herz- und arteriellen Gefäβerkrankungen. In: ZPT 10(5):147. 1989.

Wagner H, Grevel J, (1982) Planta Med 45:98.

Wichtl M, Pflanzliche Geriatrika. In: DAZ 132(30):1576. 1992.

Further information in:

Hänsel R, Keller K, Rimpler H, Schneider G (Hrsg.), Hagers Handbuch der Pharmazeutischen Praxis, 5. Aufl., Bde 4-6 (Drogen), Springer Verlag Berlin, Heidelberg, New York, 1992-1994.

Madaus G, Lehrbuch der Biologischen Arzneimittel, Bde 1-3, Nachdruck, Georg Olms Verlag Hildesheim 1979.

Schulz R, Hänsel R, Rationale Phytotherapie, Springer Verlag Heidelberg 1996.

Steinegger E, Hänsel R, Pharmakognosie, 5. Aufl., Springer Verlag Heidelberg 1992.

Teuscher E, Biogene Arzneimittel, 5. Aufl., Wiss. Verlagsges. mbH Stuttgart 1997.

Wagner H, Wiesenauer M, Phytotherapie. Phytopharmaka und pflanzliche Homöopathika, Fischer-Verlag, Stuttgart, Jena, New York 1995.

Wichtl M (Hrsg.), Teedrogen, 4. Aufl., Wiss. Verlagsges. Stuttgart 1997.

Crithum Maritimum

Samphire

DESCRIPTION

Medicinal Parts: The aerial parts of the plant are the medicinal parts.

Flower and Fruit: The 10 to 20 radiating umbels are medium-sized, sturdy, and domed. The barely 1 mm long petals are yellow or greenish white. The style is very short and barely visible. The fruit is ovate-oblong. The fruit wall is thick and filled with a spongy, air-retaining tissue.

Leaves, Stem and Root: The plant is a perennial, glabrous shrub with woody base. The root is long, cylindrical, thick, hard, knotty, ringed, gray, branching upwards and polycephalous. The stem is erect, 20 to 50 cm high, round, tender, grooved, hollowed, woody, and with less branches higher up. The leaves are seagreen, fleshy, and glossy.

Habitat: The plant grows on the Atlantic, Mediterranean, and Baltic coasts.

Production: Samphire herb is the above-ground part of Crithmum maritimum.

Other Names: Sea Fennel, Sampier, Crest Marine, Pierce-Stone, Peter's Cress.

ACTIONS AND PHARMACOLOGY

COMPOUNDS

Volatile oil

Ascorbic acid

EFFECTS

Samphire is a diuretic and also a source of Vitamin C.

INDICATIONS AND USAGE

The herb is used in scurvy and states of general resistance.

PRECAUTIONS AND ADVERSE REACTIONS

Health risks or side effects following the proper administration of designated therapeutic dosages are not recorded.

DOSAGE

Mode of Administration: Samphire is used internally and is available as an extract and also as a food additive.

LITERATURE

Francke W, (1982) Econ Bot 36 (2):163.

Further information in:

Hegnauer R, Chemotaxonomie der Pflanzen, Bde 1-11, Birkhäuser Verlag Basel, Boston, Berlin 1962-1997.

Crocus Sativus

Saffron

DESCRIPTION

Medicinal Parts: The medicinal parts are stigma and style.

Flower and Fruit: The lilly-like flowers have two 2 bracts at the base. There is a pale violet-veined calyx, yellow anthers, and a white filament. The thread-like style is 10 mm long. The stigma is bright orange. The plant is non-fruit-bearing.

Leaves, Stem and Root: The grass-like plant is a perennial and 8 to 30 cm high. There is a large squat tuber, surrounded by reticulate, and fibrous sheaths. The leaves are erect or splayed, narrow, and have a ciliate margin and keel.

Habitat: The plant is indigenous to India, the Balkans and the eastern Mediterranean region and is cultivated in India, Spain, France, Italy, and in the Middle East.

Production: Saffron is produced by drying the brown-red stigma over fire.

Not To Be Confused With: The powdered drug is more or less always adulterated; Calsendula officinalis, Carthamus tinctorius are usually used.

ACTIONS AND PHARMACOLOGY

COMPOUNDS

Apocarotinoid glycosides: in particular crocin (crocetin-beta-digentiobioside), colored intensive yellow orange

Picrocrocin (glycosidic bitter principle): the apocarotinoids and picrocrocin are presumably breakdown products of a carotinoid-digentiobioside-diglucoside (protocrocin)

Volatile oil: components 4,5-dehydro-beta-cyclocitral (safranal), 4-hydroxy-beta-cyclocitral (breakdown products of the picrocrocin)

Carotinoids: lycopene, alpha-, beta-, gamma-carotene

EFFECTS

Small doses of Saffron stimulate the secretion of the gastric juices. Large doses in situ to stimulate the smooth muscle of the uterus.

INDICATIONS AND USAGE

Saffron is no longer of interest medicinally. It is used sometimes in folk medicine to stimulate digestion.

PRECAUTIONS AND ADVERSE REACTIONS

Health risks or side effects following the proper administration of designated therapeutic dosages are not recorded.

OVERDOSAGE

Lethal poisonings can occur with overdosages or through the abuse of larger doses as an abortient (abortive dosage approximately 10 gm, lethal dosage approximately 12 to 20 gm).

Symptoms of poisoning include vomiting, uterine bleeding, intestinal colic, bloody diarrheas, hematuria, severe schwere purpuras, hemorrhaging of skin of the nose, lips and eyelids, attacks of dizziness, stupor, yellowing of the skin and the mucous membranes (through inclusion of the apocarotinodermas), and central paralysis.

The treatment consists of stomach and intestinal emptying (gastric lavage, sodium sulfate) and the administration of activated charcoal; convulsions to be treated with diazepam, colics with atropine, and any eventual acidosis with sodium bicarbonate infusions. Intubation and oxygen respiration may also be necessary.

DOSAGE

Storage: It is stored in air-tight, non-synthetic containers, and protected from light.

LITERATURE

Dhingra VK et al. (1975) Ind J Chem 13:339.

Duquenois P, (1972) Bull Soc Pharm Strasbourg 15:149.

Morimoto S et al., Post-harvest degradation of carotenoid glucose esters in saffron. In: PM 60(5):438. 1994.

Thesen R, Phytotherapeutika - nicht immer harmlos. In: ZPT 9(49):105. 1988.

Wagner K, Dissertation Universität Saarbrücken. 1969.

Further information in:

Fenaroli's Handbook of Flavor Ingredients, Vol. 1, 2nd Ed., CRC Press 1975.

Frohne D, Pfänder HJ: Giftpflanzen - Ein Handbuch für Apotheker, Toxikologen und Biologen, 4. Aufl., Wiss. Verlagsges. mbH Stuttgart 1997.

Kern W, List PH, Hörhammer L (Hrsg.), Hagers Handbuch der Pharmazeutischen Praxis, 4. Aufl., Bde 1-8, Springer Verlag Berlin, Heidelberg, New York, 1969.

Leung AY, Encyclopedia of Common Natural Ingredients Used in Food Drugs and Cosmetics, John Wiley & Sons Inc., New York 1980.

Lewin L, Gifte und Vergiftungen, 6. Aufl., Nachdruck, Haug Verlag, Heidelberg 1992.

Madaus G, Lehrbuch der Biologischen Arzneimittel, Bde 1-3, Nachdruck, Georg Olms Verlag Hildesheim 1979.

Roth L, Daunderer M, Kormann K, Giftpflanzen, Pflanzengifte, 4. Aufl., Ecomed Fachverlag Landsberg Lech 1993.

Steinegger E, Hänsel R, Pharmakognosie, 5. Aufl., Springer Verlag Heidelberg 1992.

Tang W, Eisenbrand G, Chinese Drugs of Plant Origin, Springer Verlag Heidelberg 1992.

Teuscher E, Lindequist U, Biogene Gifte - Biologie, Chemie, Pharmakologie, 2. Aufl., Fischer Verlag Stuttgart 1994.

Teuscher E, Biogene Arzneimittel, 5. Aufl., Wiss. Verlagsges. mbH Stuttgart 1997.

Wichtl M (Hrsg.), Teedrogen, 4. Aufl., Wiss. Verlagsges. Stuttgart 1997.

Croton Eleuteria

Cascarilla

DESCRIPTION

Medicinal Parts: The medicinal part is the bark.

Flower and Fruit: The flowers are small, have white petals and a pleasant fragrance.

Leaves, Stem and Root: The plant is a small tree which rarely grows to more than 6 m. It has small, opposite, ovate-lanceolate leaves about 5 cm long. They are densely covered by scales beneath, giving them a silver-bronze appearance. Above, the scales are scattered and white. The bark occurs in short quilled pieces, usually with a chalky, more or less cracked, white surface, with black dots due to the fruit of lichens; transverse fracture reddish-brown.

Characteristics: The taste is aromatic and bitter.

Habitat: Indigenous to the West Indies, also grown in tropical areas of America.

Other Names: Sweet Wood Bark, Sweet Bark, Bahama Cascarilla

ACTIONS AND PHARMACOLOGY

COMPOUNDS

Volatile oil: chief components are p-cymene, limonene, alpha-thujone, pinenes, linalool, myrcene, terpeninol-4

Diterpene bitter principles: including Cascarillin

EFFECTS

Cascarilla is a stimulant and a tonic.

INDICATIONS AND USAGE

Cascarilla is used for digestive disorders, diarrhea and also for vomiting.

PRECAUTIONS AND ADVERSE REACTIONS

Health risks or side effects following the proper administration of designated therapeutic dosages are not recorded.

DOSAGE

Mode of Administration: Available as a powder, liquid extract, or tincture.

LITERATURE

Mc Echean CE et al., J Chem Soc 166B:633. 1966.

Further information in:

Fenaroli's Handbook of Flavor Ingredients, Vol. 1, 2nd Ed., CRC Press 1975.

Hegnauer R, Chemotaxonomie der Pflanzen, Bde 1-11, Birkhäuser Verlag Basel, Boston, Berlin 1962-1997.

Kern W, List PH, Hörhammer L (Hrsg.), Hagers Handbuch der Pharmazeutischen Praxis, 4. Aufl., Bde 1-8, Springer Verlag Berlin, Heidelberg, New York, 1969.

Leung AY, Encyclopedia of Common Natural Ingredients Used in Food Drugs and Cosmetics, John Wiley & Sons Inc., New York 1980.

Steinegger E, Hänsel R, Pharmakognosie, 5. Aufl., Springer Verlag Heidelberg 1992.

Croton Tiglium

Croton Seeds

DESCRIPTION

Medicinal Parts: The seeds are the medicinal parts. The oil is extracted from the seeds and is toxic; 1 ml can be fatal.

Flower and Fruit: Croton Tiglium is a shrub or tree up to 6 m. The leaves are alternate, smooth, ovate or acuminate. They are dark green above, paler beneath with an unpleasant smell. There are inconspicuous flowers in terminal racemes. The seeds have a brown, mottled appearance. The outer layer of the seed is easily removed, leaving a hard and black coat.

Characteristics: Croton seeds oil is yellowish or reddish-brown and rather viscid, with an unpleasant odor. It is toxic and should be handled with extreme care.

Habitat: The tree is found throughout in Asia and China.

Other Names: Tiglium, Tiglium Seeds

ACTIONS AND PHARMACOLOGY

COMPOUNDS

Diterpenes: phorbol ester, including 12-O-tridecane olyphorbol-13-acetate (TPA, myristoylphoarbolacetate, MPA)

Fatty oil

EFFECTS

Croton Seed oil is a drastic irritant. TPA is a carcinogen, affecting prostaglandin metabolism.

INDICATIONS AND USAGE

At present, it is used only in Chinese medicine and in very small doses as a remedy for gallbladder colic, obstruction of the bowels and malaria.

PRECAUTIONS AND ADVERSE REACTIONS

The phorbol esters of the oils are severe cocarcinogenics. Therapeutic uses as well as skin or mucous membrane contacts with the drug are to be strictly avoided. The drug possesses acute toxicity. When applied to the skin, it brings about itching, burning, and after a time blisters. If taken internally, it leads to burning in the mouth, vomiting, dizziness, stupor, painful bowel movements, and ultimately to collapse.

OVERDOSAGE

One to 2 drops are already acutely toxic; the lethal dosage is put at 20 drops. After stomach and intestinal emptying, treatment of poisonings can only proceed symptomatically.

DOSAGE

Mode of Administration: Croton Seed oil is obsolete as drug.

LITERATURE

Berenblum I, Shubik P (1947) Brit J Cancer 1:379.

Evans FJ (Ed.), Naturally Occurring Phorbol Esters, CRC Press 1986.

Evans FJ, Taylor SE, (1983) Prog Chem Org Nat Prod 44:1.

Hecker E, (1968) Cancer Res 28:2338.

Mc Echean CE et al., J Chem Soc 166B:633. 1966.

Nishizuka Y, (1984) Nature 308:693.

Further information in:

Chan, EH et al., (Eds): Advances in Chinese Medicinal Materials Research, World Scientific Pub. Co. Singapore 1985.

Kern W, List PH, Hörhammer L (Hrsg.), Hagers Handbuch der Pharmazeutischen Praxis, 4. Aufl., Bde 1-8, Springer Verlag Berlin, Heidelberg, New York, 1969.

Lewin L, Gifte und Vergiftungen, 6. Aufl., Nachdruck, Haug Verlag, Heidelberg 1992.

Madaus G, Lehrbuch der Biologischen Arzneimittel, Bde 1-3, Nachdruck, Georg Olms Verlag Hildesheim 1979.

Roth L, Daunderer M, Kormann K, Giftpflanzen, Pflanzengifte, 4. Aufl., Ecomed Fachverlag Landsberg Lech 1993.

Steinegger E, Hänsel R, Pharmakognosie, 5. Aufl., Springer Verlag Heidelberg 1992.

Teuscher E, Lindequist U, Biogene Gifte - Biologie, Chemie, Pharmakologie, 2. Aufl., Fischer Verlag Stuttgart 1994.

Wagner H, Wiesenauer M, Phytotherapie. Phytopharmaka und pflanzliche Homöopathika, Fischer-Verlag, Stuttgart, Jena, New York 1995.

Cubeb

See Piper Cubeba

Cucurbita Pepo

Pumpkin

DESCRIPTION

Medicinal Parts: The medicinal parts are the fresh and dried seeds.

Flower and Fruit: The flower is yellow, monoecious, very large, and solitary in the leaf axils. The male flower has a longer pedicle. The calyx is fused to the corolla except for the 5 awl-shaped tips. The corolla is 5-tipped and funnel-shaped. The interior is pubescent. There are 3 stamens fused to the anther. The ovary is inferior and 3-locular. The fruit is very large with many seeds. The flesh is fibrous, yellow-orange to white, and has a viscous placenta. The seeds are 7 to 15 mm long, narrow, broad or narrow-ovate with a shallow groove and flat ridge around the margin.

Leaves, Stem and Root: Annual plant 3 to 8 m long with decumbent or climbing, sharply-angular with longitudinal grooves and with hairy spines. The leaves are alternate, very large and bristly, petiolate 5 to 7 lobes from a cordate base.

Habitat: Pumpkin is indigenous to America and is widely cultivated especially in temperate climates.

Other Names: Field Pumpkin

ACTIONS AND PHARMACOLOGY

COMPOUNDS

Steroids: Delta5-, Delta7- and Delta8-phytosterols (24- alkyl sterols), including clerosterol, isofucosterol, sitosterol, stigmasterol, cholesterol, isoavenasterol, spinasterol

Fatty oil

Unusual amino acids: including cucurbitin (vermifuge)

Gamma-tocopherol

EFFECTS

There are no pharmacological studies that substantiate the empirically documented clinical efficacy; the empirical evidence indicates efficacy for prostate hyperplasia; also antiphlogistic and antioxidative.

INDICATIONS AND USAGE

- Irritable bladder
- Prostate complaints

Pumpkin is used for irritable bladder, micturition problems accompanying prostate adenoma stages I to II; this medication relieves only the difficulties associated with an enlarged prostate without reducing the enlargement; medical supervision is essential.

In folk medicine, it is also used for kidney inflammation, intestinal parasites, particularly tape worm, and vulnary.

PRECAUTIONS AND ADVERSE REACTIONS

Health risks or side effects following the proper administration of designated therapeutic dosages are not recorded.

DOSAGE

Mode of Administration: Whole and coarsely ground seed and other galenic preparations are for internal use.

Daily Dosage: The average daily dose is 10 gm of ground seeds, mornings and evenings, 1 to 2 heaping dessert spoons with liquid.

Storage: It should be protected from light and moisture.

LITERATURE

Anonym, Welche Bedeutung haben pflanzliche Prostatamittel. In: DAZ 133(9):720. 1993.

Koch E (1995) Pharmakologie und Wirkmechanismen von Extrakten aus Sabalfrüchten (Sabal fructus), Brennesselwurzeln (Urticae radix) und Kürbissamen (Cucurbitae peponis semen) bei der Behandlung der benignen Prostatahyperplasie. In: Loew D, Rietbrock N (Hrsg.) Phytopharmaka in Forschung und klinischer Anwendung. Steinkopff Verlag, Darmstadt, S 57-79.

Miersch WDE, Benigne Prostatahyperplasie. In: DAZ 133(29):2653. 1993.

Nahrstedt A (1993) Pflanzliche Urologica - eine kritische Übersicht. Pharm Z 138:1439-1450.

Schabort JC (1978) Phytochemistry 17:1062.

Schiebel-Schlosser, G., Kürbiskerne stärken die Blasenfunktion. In: PTA 4(11):552. 1990.

Schilcher H (1987a) Pflanzliche Diuretika. Urologe [B] 27:215-222; (1987b)n Möglichkeiten und Grenzen der Phytotherapie am Beispiel pflanzlicher Urologika. Urologe [B] 27:316-319.

Schilcher H, Boesel R, Effenberger ST Segebrecht S, Neuere Untersuchungsergebnisse mit aquaretisch, antibakteriell und prostatotrop wirksamen Arzneipflanzen. In: ZPT 10(3):77. 1989.

Schilcher H, Dunzendorfer U, Ascali F, Dekta-7-Sterole, das prostatatrope Wirkprinzip des Kürbis? In: Urologe (B) 27:316-319. 1987.

Tewary JP, Srivasta MC, (1968) J Pharm Sci 57:328.

Further information in:

Hänsel R, Keller K, Rimpler H, Schneider G (Hrsg.), Hagers Handbuch der Pharmazeutischen Praxis, 5. Aufl., Bde 4-6 (Drogen), Springer Verlag Berlin, Heidelberg, New York, 1992-1994.

Madaus G, Lehrbuch der Biologischen Arzneimittel, Bde 1-3, Nachdruck, Georg Olms Verlag Hildesheim 1979.

Oliver-Bever B (Ed.), Medicinal Plants of Tropical West Africa, Cambridge University Press, Cambridge, London 1986.

Steinegger E, Hänsel R, Pharmakognosie, 5. Aufl., Springer Verlag Heidelberg 1992.

Teuscher E, Biogene Arzneimittel, 5. Aufl., Wiss. Verlagsges. mbH Stuttgart 1997.

Wagner H, Wiesenauer M, Phytotherapie. Phytopharmaka und pflanzliche Homöopathika, Fischer-Verlag, Stuttgart, Jena, New York 1995.

Wichtl M (Hrsg.), Teedrogen, 4. Aufl., Wiss. Verlagsges. Stuttgart 1997.

Cudweed

See Gnaphalium Uliginosum

Cumimum Cyminum

Cumin

DESCRIPTION

Medicinal Parts: The medicinal parts are the cumin oil extracted from the ripe fruit and the ripe, dried fruit.

Flower and Fruit: The flowers are in umbels radiating in groups of 3 to 5. The petals are white or red, oblong, and deeply bordered with a long indented tip. The involucral bracts are long and simple. The style is short and turned outwards at the end. The ovary is inferior and 3-locular. The fruit is a schizocarp, about 6 mm long and 1.5 mm wide and is crowned with awl-shaped calyx tips. The mericarp is almost round in transverse section, with 5 thread-like, bristly main ribs and bristly secondary ribs.

Leaves, Stem and Root: The plant is a delicate, glabrous, annual 10 to 50 cm high. The stem is bifurcated at the base and glabrous. The leaves are glabrous and finely pinnatifid with oblong-linear tips of which the lower are mostly doubly trifoliate.

Habitat: The plant is indigenous to Turkestan (Hager) or northern Egypt (Grieve) but is cultivated today in the whole of the Mediterranean region as well as in Iran, Pakistan, India, China, the U.S. and South America.

Not To Be Confused With: Certain Indian products, such as Carum carvi and the fruit of the earth chestnut, Bunium bulbocastanium can be mistaken for or confused with cumin. Synthetic coloring is frequently added to Turkish products.

ACTIONS AND PHARMACOLOGY

COMPOUNDS

Volatile oil: chief components cuminaldehyde, gamma-terpenes, beta-pinenes, p-cymene, 1,3-p-menthandial

Fatty oil: chief fatty acids petroselic acid, palmitic acid

EFFECTS

Antimicrobial: A powder suspension of the drug has diverse inhibitory effects; it stunts mycelium growth, toxin production or afla-toxin production in *Aspergillus ochraceus*, *C. versicolor*, and *C. flavus*.

Influence on blood-clotting: A dried cumin ether extract inhibits (in vitro) arachidon acid induced plate aggregation in platelet-rich human plasma.

Mutagenic effect: In comparison to *Salmonella thyphimurum* TA 100, a mutagenic effect of the polar fractions of chloroform extract and methanol extract of cumin did appear.

Influence of pharmacological metabolism: An injection of a dried ether extract prolonged the phenobarbituate hypnosis of female albino mice, up to 120%; a higher dose shortened it to 83%.

Estrogenic effect: An acetone extract of cumin, administered to female albino rats (ovariectomised, ovaries have been removed) led, depending on the dosage, to an increase in the weight of the uterus, an increase in the amount of protein in the endometrium, and to an increase of alkali phosphates.

Other effects (for which there are no experimental results) include the following: obstructive influence on fertility, galactogen, antispasmodic, diuretic, and aphrodisiac.

Cumin also has carminative, stimulant, and analgesic effects.

INDICATIONS AND USAGE

In folk medicine, cumin is used as a carminative for stomach disorders, diarrhea, and colic, particularly in veterinary medicine.

In America, Africa, and India the drug is used as an abortive and as an emmenagogue.

In Indonesia, cumin is used in cases of bloody diarrhea, headache (paste is applied to the forehead), and is taken orally for rheumatic ailments.

PRECAUTIONS AND ADVERSE REACTIONS

Health risks or side effects following the proper administration of designated therapeutic dosages are not recorded.

DOSAGE

Mode of Administration: Cumin is used both internally and externally in ground form and as a pressed oil.

Daily Dosage: The average single dose is 300 to 600 gm (5 to 10 fruits) of drug.

LITERATURE

Harborne JB, Williams CE (1972) Phytochemistry 11:1741.

Tassan CG, Russel GF, J Food Sci 40020185-1188. 1975.

Varo PT, Heinz DE, (1970) J Agric Food Chem 18:234 et 239.

Further information in:

Hänsel R, Keller K, Rimpler H, Schneider G (Hrsg.), Hagers Handbuch der Pharmazeutischen Praxis, 5. Aufl., Bde 4-6 (Drogen): Springer Verlag Berlin, Heidelberg, New York, 1992-1994.

Leung AY, Encyclopedia of Common Natural Ingredients Used in Food Drugs and Cosmetics, John Wiley & Sons Inc., New York 1980.

Cumin

See Cumimum Cyminum

Cup Plant

See Silphium Perfoliatum

Cupmoss

See Cladonia Pyxidata

Cupressus Sempervirens

Cypress

DESCRIPTION

Medicinal Parts: The medicinal parts are the cones, branches, and the oil.

Leaves, Stem and Root: Cupressus sempervirens is a tree which grows up to 30 m tall. The leaves are 0.5 to 1 mm, dark green, and obtuse. The male cones are 4 to 8 mm, the female, 25 to 40 mm. They are elliptical-oblong (rarely, globose), green when young and shining yellowish-gray when ripe, with 8 to 14 short and obtusely spiked scales. There are 8 to 20 seeds on each scale.

Habitat: The plant is indigenous to Turkey and is cultivated throughout the Mediterranean region.

ACTIONS AND PHARMACOLOGY

COMPOUNDS

Chief components: alpha-pinenes, D-camphene, D-silvestren, p-cymene, L-cadinenes, cedrol, terpinenol-4, terpineol, acetyl- and isovalerianyl monoterpene ester

EFFECTS

Cypress acts as an expectorant.

INDICATIONS AND USAGE

The drug is used externally for head colds, coughs, and bronchitis.

PRECAUTIONS AND ADVERSE REACTIONS

Health risks or side effects following the proper administration of designated therapeutic dosages are not recorded. Kidney irritation is likely with intake of larger dosages.

DOSAGE

Mode of Administration: Occasionally, Cypress is used externally as an ointment.

LITERATURE

Kern W, List PH, Hörhammer L (Hrsg.), Hagers Handbuch der Pharmazeutischen Praxis, 4. Aufl., Bde 1-8, Springer Verlag Berlin, Heidelberg, New York, 1969.

Curcuma Domestica

Turmeric

DESCRIPTION

Medicinal Parts: The medicinal parts are the stewed and dried rhizome.

Flower and Fruit: The inflorescence is cone-like, 10 to 15 cm long, and is attached to a stem enclosed in a sheathing petiole. The flower has 2 pale green bracts, which are 5 to 6 cm long. The covering bracts are whitish, often red-tinged. The individual flowers are yellowish white or yellow. The flowers have a tubular, 3-lobed calyx and funnel-shaped, 3-tipped corolla. The fruit is a gobular capsule.

Leaves, Stem and Root: Curcuma domestica is a perennial, erect, and leafy plant with very large, lily-like leaves up to 1.2 m long. The leaf blade is ovate-lanceolate, thin, entire-margined, and narrows to a long sheath-like petiole. The main rhizome is thickened to a tuber and has numerous roots. The roots in turn terminate in partially elliptical tubers. The secondary rhizomes are digit-shaped with no roots. All rhizomes are yellowish-brown with stipules and appear transversely ringed when they die.

Habitat: Probably indigenous to India. Cultivated today in India and other tropical regions of southern Asia.

Production: Turmeric root consists of the finger-like, often tuber-like, scalded and dried rhizomes of Curcuma longa. The plant is harvested at the end of the growing season and sun dried.

Not To Be Confused With: Curcuma xanthorrhiza

ACTIONS AND PHARMACOLOGY

COMPOUNDS

Volatile oil: chief components alpha- and beta-tumerone, artumerone, alpha- and gamma- atlantone, curlone, zingiberene, curcumol

Curcuminoids: including curcumin, demethoxycurcumin, bidemethoxycurcumin

1,5-diaryl-penta-1,4-dien-3-on- derivatives

Starch

EFFECTS

Turmeric has choleretic, cholikinetic, antihepatotoxic, antihyperlipidemic and anti-inflammatory. It is also antioxidative, antitumoral and antimicrobial. It has insect repellent and antifertile effects. It also effects prostaglandin.

INDICATIONS AND USAGE

- Liver and gallbladder complaints
- Loss of appetite

Turmeric is used for dyspeptic disorders, particularly feelings of fullness after meals and regular meteorism. In folk medicine, the drug is used for diarrhea, intermittent fever, dropsy, bronchitis, colds, worms, leprosy, kidney inflammation and cystitis. Other uses include, headaches, flatulence, upper abdominal pains, chest infections, fever, diarrhea, colic, amenorrhea, and blood rushes. It is used externally for bruising, leech bites, festering eye infections, inflammation of the oral mucosa, inflammatory skin conditions, and infected wounds.

Efficacy of the folk indications are not proven.

PRECAUTIONS AND ADVERSE REACTIONS

Health risks or side effects following the proper administration of designated therapeutic dosages are not recorded. Stomach complaints can occur following extended use or in the case of overdose.

DOSAGE

Mode of Administration: Comminuted drug, as well as other galenic preparations for internal use.

Preparation: To prepare an infusion, scald 0.5 to 1 gm with boiling water, cover and draw for 5 minutes and then strain. The tincture strength is 1:10.

Daily Dosage: The average daily dose of the drug is 1.5 to 3 gm of powder, 2 to 3 times daily between meals. The infusion dose is 2 to 3 cups between mealtimes. The tincture dose is 10 to 15 drops 2 to 3 times daily.

Storage: Turmeric should be protected from light.

LITERATURE

Ammon HPT, Anazodo MI, Safayhi H, Dhawan BN, Srimal RC, PM 58:226. 1992.

Ammon HPT, Wahl MA, Pharmacology of Curcuma longa. In: PM 57:1-7. 1991.

Basu AB, (1971) Ind J Pharm 33:131.

Dhar ML et al., (1968) Ind J Exp Biol 6:232.

Garg SK, (1974) Planta Med 26:225.

Kiso Y et al., (1983) Planta Med 49:185.

Krishnamurthy N et al., (1976) Trop Sci 18:37.

Masuda T et al., Anti-oxidative and anti-inflammatory curcumin-related phenolics from rhizomes of Curcuma domestica. In: Phytochemistry 32:1557. 1993.

Nagarajan K, Arya VP, (1982) J Sci Ind Res 41:232.

Nakayama R et al., Two curcuminoid pigments from Curcuma domestica. In: PH 33:501. 1993.

Ravindranath V, Satyanarayana MN, (1980) Phytochemistry 19:2031.

Srimal RC, Dhawan CN, (1973) J Pharm Pharmacol 25:447.

Veit M, Beeinflussung der Leukotrien-Biosynthese durch Curcumin. In: ZPT 14(1):46. 1993.

Wagner H et al., (1986) 6th Int Conf. Prostaglandins and Related Compounds. Florence, Italy. June 3rd-6th. Pub. Fondzione Giovanni Lorenzini.

Further information in:

Hänsel R, Keller K, Rimpler H, Schneider G (Hrsg.), Hagers Handbuch der Pharmazeutischen Praxis, 5. Aufl., Bde 4-6 (Drogen): Springer Verlag Berlin, Heidelberg, New York, 1992-1994.

Leung AY, Encyclopedia of Common Natural Ingredients Used in Food Drugs and Cosmetics, John Wiley & Sons Inc., New York 1980.

Steinegger E, Hänsel R, Pharmakognosie, 5. Aufl., Springer Verlag Heidelberg 1992.

Tang W, Eisenbrand G, Chinese Drugs of Plant Origin, Springer Verlag Heidelberg 1992.

Teuscher E, Biogene Arzneimittel, 5. Aufl., Wiss. Verlagsges. mbH Stuttgart 1997.

Wichtl M (Hrsg.), Teedrogen, 4. Aufl., Wiss. Verlagsges. Stuttgart 1997.

Curcuma Xanthorrhizia

Curcuma

DESCRIPTION

Medicinal Parts: The medicinal parts are the dried, tuberous rhizomes cut into slices.

Flower and Fruit: The inflorescence is large, purple or crimson. The corolla has a red margin. Otherwise it is very similar to Curcuma domestica.

Leaves, Stem and Root: The plant is a perennial, 1.75 m high and leafy. The leaves are in long thin sheaths on the rhizome. The leaf blades are broadly lanceolate or oblong and have a narrow, purple mark on the midrib. The main rhizome is thickened like a tuber, ovate, the size of a fist with numerous roots and thin lateral rhizomes. The roots terminate partially in ovate tubers.

Habitat: Indigenous to the forests of Indonesia and the Malaysian peninsula. Cultivated mainly on Java, in Malaysia, Thailand and the Philippines.

Production: Curcuma is cultivated and harvested in the second year of growth. After the rhizome has been washed, the main thick root is isolated, cut and dried at a temperature of 50°C.

Not To Be Confused With: The rhizome of Curcuma domestica

Other Names: Tewon Lawa, Temu Lawak

ACTIONS AND PHARMACOLOGY

COMPOUNDS

Volatile oil: chief components ar-curcumene (alpha-curcumene), xanthorrhizol, beta-curcumene, germacrene, furanodien, furanodienone

Curcuminoids: including curcumin, demethoxycurcumin

Non-phenolic diarylheptanoids

Starch

EFFECTS

Curcuma acts in a similar manner to turmeric root but is mainly choleretic and antitumoral (animal testing).

INDICATIONS AND USAGE

- Liver and gallbladder complaints
- Loss of appetite

Curcuma is used for dyspepsia, particularly feelings of fullness after meals and meteorism.

In Indian folk medicine, it has long been used for liver and gallbladder complaints.

PRECAUTIONS AND ADVERSE REACTIONS

Health risks or side effects following the proper administration of designated therapeutic dosages are not recorded. Stomach complaints can occur following extended use or in the case of overdose. Because of the stimulating effect of the drug upon the biliary tract, it should not be administered if there is a bile duct blockage. Colic can occur when the patient suffers from gallstones.

DOSAGE

Mode of Administration: Comminuted drug for infusions and other galenic forms for internal use.

Preparation: The infusion is prepared by pouring 1 cup of boiling water over 1/2 tsp of drug and straining after 10 minutes.

Daily Dosage: The average daily dose is 2 gm of drug; Infusion: 2 to 3 times daily between meals.

Storage: It should be protected from light.

LITERATURE

Anonym, Brennpunkt ZNS. In: DAZ 137(25):2166-2167. 1997.

Baumann J (1975) Über die Wirkung von Chelidonium, Curcuma, Absinth und Carduus marianus auf die Galle- und Pankreassekretion bei Hepatopathien. MedMschr 29:173.

Claeson P et al., Non-phenolic linear diarylheptanoids from Curcuma xanthorrhiza: a novel type of topical anti-inflammatory agents: Structure-activity relationship. In: PM 62(3):236-240. 1996.

Guttenberg A (1926) Das Cholagogum Curcumen. Klein Wschr 5:1998-1999.

Maiwald L, Schwantes PA (1991) Curcuma xanthorrhiza Roxb., eine Heilpflanze tritt aus dem Schattendasein. Z Phytother 12:35-445.

Reuter HD, Pflanzliche Gallentherapeutika (Teil I) und (Teil II). In: ZPT 16(1):13-20 u. 77-89. 1995.

Sabieraj J, Wirkung von Curcuma xanthorrhiza. In: DAZ 131(13):609. 1991.

Schilcher H, Pharmazeutische Aspekte pflanzlicher Gallentherapeutika. In: ZPT 16(4):211-222. 1995.

Schmidt M, Phytotherapie: Pflanzliche Gallenwegstherapeutika. In: DAZ 135(8):680-682. 1995.

Veit M, Beeinflussung der Leukotrien-Biosynthese durch Curcumin. In: ZPT 14(1):46. 1993.

Further information in:

Hänsel R, Keller K, Rimpler H, Schneider G (Hrsg.), Hagers Handbuch der Pharmazeutischen Praxis, 5. Aufl., Bde 4-6

(Drogen), Springer Verlag Berlin, Heidelberg, New York, 1992-1994.

Madaus G, Lehrbuch der Biologischen Arzneimittel, Bde 1-3, Nachdruck, Georg Olms Verlag Hildesheim 1979.

Steinegger E, Hänsel R, Pharmakognosie, 5. Aufl., Springer Verlag Heidelberg 1992.

Tang W, Eisenbrand G, Chinese Drugs of Plant Origin, Springer Verlag Heidelberg 1992.

Teuscher E, Biogene Arzneimittel, 5. Aufl., Wiss. Verlagsges. mbH Stuttgart 1997.

Wichtl M (Hrsg.), Teedrogen, 4. Aufl., Wiss. Verlagsges. Stuttgart 1997.

Curcuma Zedoaria

Zedoary

DESCRIPTION

Medicinal Parts: The medicinal part is the dried tuberous part of the rhizome, cut in transverse slices or in longitudinal quarters.

Flower and Fruit: The inflorescences are on 5 to 15 cm long, obtuse, and silky involucre bracts. The spike-like inflorescences are 7.5 to 12.5 cm long and 5 to 7.5 cm wide. The bracts bearing the flowers are ovate with revolute tips, pale green with a reddish border, densely punctuated with glands, more or less stiff hairs on the surface in particular at the tip. The bracts at the tip of the inflorescence are 5 cm long, initially white, then pink to crimson. The flowers are pale yellow. The calyx is 8 mm long, obtuse, and 3-tipped. The tips of the corolly are broadly triangular and pale pink at the extreme tips. The labellum is light yellow, fluorescent yellow in the center with very slightly reddish tinged borders at the lower part. The ovary is 4 to 5 mm long and very weakly pubescent. The fruit is an ovate, thin, smooth, and irregularly opening capsule. The elliptical seeds have a white aril.

Leaves, Stem and Root: Curcuma zedoaria is a perennial, erect, and leafy plant. The rhizome has a grayish outer surface and is ovate to pear-shaped, thick and palmately branched downwards, whitish yellow, has a strong smell of camphor with numerous thin roots. The roots are partially thickened to ovate, white tubers. The leaves in groups of 4 and 6 on the rhizome are up to 1 m long. The 20 to 60 cm long and 8 to 10 cm wide leaf blade is oblong-ovate, glabrous, and has a purple mark in the middle of the leaf.

Characteristic: The taste is bitter, the smell is like camphor and is reminiscent of cardamom and ginger.

Habitat: The plant is indigenous to northeast India and is found in the Moluccas, the Philippines and New Guinea.

Other Names: Turmeric

ACTIONS AND PHARMACOLOGY

COMPOUNDS

Volatile oil (1.0-1.5%): chief components zingiberene, 1,8-cineole, D-camphor, D-camphene, D-borneol, alpha-pinene, further including among others curcumol, zederone, curcumeneol, curculone, furanodienone, isofuranodienone

Curcuminoids: curcumin, desmethoxycurcumin, bisdesmethoxycurcumin

Starch (50%)

EFFECTS

No information is available.

INDICATIONS AND USAGE

Zedoary is used as a stomachic for digestive debility, colic, and spasms (stomachic, carminative). In folk medicine, it is also used as a remedy for nervous diseases.

PRECAUTIONS AND ADVERSE REACTIONS

No health hazards or side effects are known in conjunction with the proper administration of designated therapeutic dosages.

DOSAGE

Preparation: Extracts of the drug are contained in numerous combination preparations for gastrointestinal indications and as cholagogues. Infusion: pour boiling water over 1 to 1.5 gm of comminuted or powdered drug, or put in cold water and strain after 3 to 5 minutes (1 teaspoonful = 3 gm of drug).

Daily Dosage: Drink 1 cup as an aromatic bitter at meals.

LITERATURE

Gupta SK et al., Lloydia 39:218-222. 1976.

Hikino H et al., (1970) Chem Pharm Bull 18:752.

Kuronayagi M, Natori S, Yakugaku Zasshi 90:1467-1470 (via CA 74:61612. 1970.

Latif MA et al., Br J Nutr 41:57. 1979.

Matthes HWD et al., (1980) Phytochemistry 19:2643.

Shiobara Y et al., (1985) Phytochemistry 24(11):2629.

Further information in:

Hänsel R, Keller K, Rimpler H, Schneider G (Hrsg.), Hagers Handbuch der Pharmazeutischen Praxis, 5. Aufl., Bde 4-6 (Drogen): Springer Verlag Berlin, Heidelberg, New York, 1992-1994.

Cuscuta Epithymum

Dodder

DESCRIPTION

Medicinal Parts: The medicinal parts are the aerial parts of the plant.

Flower and Fruit: The flowers are reddish, wax or flesh-colored. They are arranged in small clusters. The calyx is divided into 5 and the corolla is fused to a 4 to 5 tipped tube with fringed scales inside. There are 5 stamens and 1 ovary.

Leaves, Stem and Root: The plant is a leafless parasite up to 150 cm high. The stem is yellow or reddish, thread-like, branched, with sucking roots, and climbing.

Habitat: The plant grows in Europe, Asia, and South Africa.

Other Names: Lesser Dodder, Dodder of Thyme, Devil's Guts, Beggarweed, Hellweed, Strangle Tare, Scaldweed

ACTIONS AND PHARMACOLOGY

COMPOUNDS

Saponins

Tannins

A purgative principle (see Calystegiae sepii herba et radix)

The drug has been subjected to very little investigation.

EFFECTS

Dodder has hepatic and laxative effects.

INDICATIONS AND USAGE

Dodder is used for disorders of the urinary tract, spleen, and liver.

PRECAUTIONS AND ADVERSE REACTIONS

Health risks or side effects following the proper administration of designated therapeutic dosages are not recorded. It is conceivable that the drug triggers intestinal colic in cases of overdosage.

LITERATURE

Pagnani F, Ciarallo G, (1974) Boll Chim Farm 113(1):30.

Further information in:

Kern W, List PH, Hörhammer L (Hrsg.), Hagers Handbuch der Pharmazeutischen Praxis, 4. Aufl., Bde. 1-8, Springer Verlag Berlin, Heidelberg, New York, 1969.

Cyclamen Europaeum

Cyclamen

DESCRIPTION

Medicinal Parts: The medicinal part is the rhizome with the roots.

Flower and Fruit: The flowers are pinkish-red, solitary and nodding on erect stems. The 5 sepals are ovate, pointed, and dentate. The corolla is a short campanulate tube with 5 revolute tips and it is darker at the base. There are 5 stamens and 1 ovary. The fruit is a capsule, which opens on 5 sides.

Leaves, Stem and Root: The plant grows from about 5 to 10 cm. The rhizome is a disc-like tuber. The leaves are long-petioled, orbicular or cordate, crenate, glabrous, with a white edge above, and red beneath. The petioles and pedicles are roughly glandular.

Characteristics: The flowers are fragrant and poisonous.

Habitat: The plant is found in the Alps, and alpine regions of southern Europe.

Other Names: Groundbread, Sowbread, Swinebread, Ivy-leafed Cyclamen

ACTIONS AND PHARMACOLOGY

COMPOUNDS

Triterpene saponins: including cyclamin, deglucocyclamin I, deglucocyclamin II

EFFECTS

No information is available.

INDICATIONS AND USAGE

The drug is used to treat menstrual complaints, emotional disorders/nervous states, and digestive problems. In homeopathy, cyclamen is used for migraine and its autonomic accompanying symptoms, and in the treatment of PMS (premenstrual syndrome).

PRECAUTIONS AND ADVERSE REACTIONS

The intake of even small dosages (0.3 gm) can lead to nausea, vomiting, diarrhea, and stomach pain.

OVERDOSAGE

High dosages can cause spasm and asphyxiation. Following gastric lavage and the administration of activated charcoal, the treatment for poisonings proceeds symptomatically. (Treatment of convulsions with diazepam, of colic with atropine).

DOSAGE

Mode of Administration: Cyclamen is used in homeopathic treatments. It is also used topically and in alcoholic extracts.

LITERATURE

Tschesche R, Mercker HJ, Wulff G, Liebig Ann Chem 721:194. 1969.

Tschesche R, Striegler H, Fehlhaber HW, Liebig Ann Chem 691:165. 1966.

Further information in:

Frohne D, Pfänder HJ: Giftpflanzen - Ein Handbuch für Apotheker, Toxikologen und Biologen, 4. Aufl., Wiss. Verlagsges. mbH Stuttgart 1997.

Kern W, List PH, Hörhammer L (Hrsg.), Hagers Handbuch der Pharmazeutischen Praxis, 4. Aufl., Bde 1-8, Springer Verlag Berlin, Heidelberg, New York, 1969.

Lewin L, Gifte und Vergiftungen, 6. Aufl., Nachdruck, Haug Verlag, Heidelberg 1992.

Madaus G, Lehrbuch der Biologischen Arzneimittel, Bde 1-3, Nachdruck, Georg Olms Verlag Hildesheim 1979.

Roth L, Daunderer M, Kormann K, Giftpflanzen, Pflanzengifte, 4. Aufl., Ecomed Fachverlag Landsberg Lech 1993.

Steinegger E, Hänsel R, Pharmakognosie, 5. Aufl., Springer Verlag Heidelberg 1992.

Teuscher E, Lindequist U, Biogene Gifte - Biologie, Chemie, Pharmakologie, 2. Aufl., Fischer Verlag Stuttgart 1994.

Wagner H, Wiesenauer M, Phytotherapie. Phytopharmaka und pflanzliche Homöopathika, Fischer-Verlag, Stuttgart, Jena, New York 1995.

Cydonia Oblongata

Quince

DESCRIPTION

Medicinal Parts: The medicinal parts are the fruit and seeds.

Flower and Fruit: Relatively large, solitary, perfumed, pink flowers. The fruit is yellow, downy, and apple or pear-shaped.

Leaves, Stem and Root: Three to 6 m high tree or shrub with tomentose branches covered in alternate, ovate leaves. The undersurface of leaves is grass-green and tomentose.

Habitat: Indigenous to south-west and central Asia but has also spread to Europe, in particular the Mediterranean.

Production: The ripe quinces are picked, stored for a period, then cut and finally dried at temperatures not exceeding 50°C. The seeds are gathered up and used in whole or ground form.

ACTIONS AND PHARMACOLOGY

COMPOUNDS

Cyanogenic glycosides: amygdalin (corresponding to 0.4 - 1.5%, 27 to 75 mg HCN/100 g)

Mucilages

Fatty oil

EFFECTS

No information is available.

INDICATIONS AND USAGE

Quince is used as a demulcent in digestive disorders and diarrhea. As a lotion, it is used to soothe the eyes. The seeds are also used to treat coughs and gastrointestinal catarrh. Additionally used as compresses or poultices for injuries, inflammation of the joints, injuries of the nipples, and gashed or deeply cut fingers.

PRECAUTIONS AND ADVERSE REACTIONS

Health risks or side effects following the proper administration of designated therapeutic dosages are not recorded. Because quince mucilage is prepared from the whole seeds, and/or the whole seeds are taken internally, the cyanogenic glycosides are credited with a slight toxicological relevance.

DOSAGE

Preparation: The drug is used as a powder, a lotion, a decoction and an extract. Extract/decoction: 1 tsp. of whole seeds per cup of water. A viscous poultice is prepared from the ground seeds.

LITERATURE

De Tommasi N et al., New tetracyclic sesterterpenes from Cydonia vulgaris. In: JNP 59(3):267-270. 1996.

Huber P, Landw Versuchst 75:462. 1911.

Sommer W, Dissertation Universität Kiel. 1984.

Further information in:

Kern W, List PH, Hörhammer L (Hrsg.), Hagers Handbuch der Pharmazeutischen Praxis, 4. Aufl., Bde. 1-8, Springer Verlag Berlin, Heidelberg, New York, 1969.

Steinegger E, Hänsel R, Pharmakognosie, 5. Aufl., Springer Verlag Heidelberg 1992

Teuscher E, Lindequist U, Biogene Gifte - Biologie, Chemie, Pharmakologie, 2. Aufl., Fischer Verlag Stuttgart 1994.

Cymbopogon Species

Citronella

DESCRIPTION

Medicinal Parts: The medicinal parts are the dried leaves and the lemon grass oil of Cymbopogon citratus and the cintronella oil from Cymbopogon nardus.

CYMBOPOGON CITRATUS

Flower and Fruit: The flowers are 30 cm long false spikes with reddish brown sheaths 15 to 25 mm long. The racemes are 15 to 17 mm long. The sessile spikelet is 6 mm long and the upper spelts are 0.7 mm wide, lanceolate, narrowly winged, flattened at the back, slightly concave and ribless in the lower part. The stemmed spikelet is 4.5 mm long and the lower spelt is 0.7 mm wide. Inflorescences are rarely formed on this variety.

Leaves, Stem and Root: Cymbopogon citratus is a perennial plant with an up to 2 m, smooth glabrous stalk. The leaf blade is linear, acuminate, up to 90 cm long and 5 mm wide and smooth on both sides. The leaf sheaths are round, glabrous and smooth. The ligule is paper-like and less than 1 mm long.

CYMBOPOGON NARDUS

Flower and Fruit: The inflorescence is very large and consists of a 1 m long spike with numerous racemes up to 20 mm long and arranged in zigzag order. The sessile spike is 5 mm long. The lower spelt is oblong-lanceolate, usually flat, narrowly winged with 3 ribs. The awn, if there is one, is smooth and glabrous. The leaf blade is up to 1 m long and 1.5 cm wide and usually light green. The upper surface is smooth, the lower surface and the margin are rough. The leaf sheaths are glabrous and yellowish green. The basal leaf sheaths are also glabrous but green to reddish. The ligule is paper-like and about 1 mm long.

Characteristics: Cymbopogon species have essential oils in tube-like cells with corked walls.

Habitat: Citronella grass was originally indigenous to the tropics and the subtropics of the old world. Today it is cultivated in Central and South America and Queensland, Australia.

Production: Ceylon citronella grass consists of the above-ground parts of Cymbopogon nardus. West Indian lemon-grass consists of the above-ground parts of Cymbopogon citratus. West Indian lemongrass oil consists of the essential oil from Cymbopogon citratus. Java citronella oil consists of the essential oil from Cymbopogon winterianus.

Other Names: Lemongrass

ACTIONS AND PHARMACOLOGY

COMPOUNDS

The volatile oils have, as chief components, depending on origin:

Cymbopogon citratus (Cymbopogonis citrati aetheroleum): citral, myrcene

Cymbopogon winteranus (Citronellae aetheroluem): citro-nellal, geraniol, citronellol, geranyl acetate, citronellyl acetate

Cymbopogon nardus: geraniol, citronellal

EFFECTS

No information is available.

INDICATIONS AND USAGE

Citronella grass is used as a mild astringent and a tonic for the stomach. The effectiveness for other claimed applications is not documented.

PRECAUTIONS AND ADVERSE REACTIONS

The application of salves with the volatile oil upon the skin has led in rare cases to signs of allergy. A toxic alveolitis was observed in 2 cases following inhalation of the volatile oil.

DOSAGE

No information is available.

LITERATURE

De Silva MG, Mfg Chemist 30:415-416. 1959.

Sarer E, Scheffer JJC, Svendsen AB, Composition of the essential oil of Cymbopogon citratus (DC.) STAPF cultivated in turkey. In: Sci Pharm 51:58. 1983.

Further information in:

Hänsel R, Keller K, Rimpler H, Schneider G (Hrsg.), Hagers Handbuch der Pharmazeutischen Praxis, 5. Aufl., Bde 4-6 (Drogen), Springer Verlag Berlin, Heidelberg, New York, 1992-1994.

Leung AY, Encyclopedia of Common Natural Ingredients Used in Food, Drugs and Cosmetics, John Wiley & Sons Inc., New York 1980.

Steinegger E, Hänsel R, Pharmakognosie, 5. Aufl., Springer Verlag Heidelberg 1992.

Teuscher E, Biogene Arzneimittel, 5. Aufl., Wiss. Verlagsges. mbH Stuttgart 1997.

Cynanchum Vincetoxicum

German Ipecac

DESCRIPTION

Medicinal Parts: The medicinal parts of the plant are the leaves or rhizome with the attached roots.

Flower and Fruit: The plant has small white flowers in peduncled cymes, 5 sepals, and a wheel-shaped corolla. There is a 5-lobed secondary corolla. There are 5 stamens whose anthers are fused to a 5 sectioned wreath. The 2 superior ovaries have a common stigma. The fruit is a 5 cm long, glabrous, striped, clavate follicle. The seeds have silky tufts of hair.

Leaves, Stem and Root: The plant grows from 30 to 100 cm. The underground creeping rhizome has heavily branched runners. The stem is unbranched, thin and erect. The leaves are opposite, short petioled, ovate to oblong and entire-margined.

Characteristics: The fresh rhizome has an intensive odor. The taste is sweet, then bitter-hot. It is poisonous.

Habitat: The plant is indigenous to Europe.

Production: German Ipecac herb and rhizome are the leaves and rhizome (including attached roots), of Cynanchum vincetoxicum. The subterranean rhizome, including parts of the roots, are dug up in autumn, cleaned and quickly dried at temperatures of up to 50°C.

ACTIONS AND PHARMACOLOGY

COMPOUNDS

Saponin-like 15-oxasteroide glycosides (mixture termed vincetoxin): aglycones including hirundigenin, anhydrohirundigenin, vincetogenin

Isoquinoline alkaloids: including tylophorin

EFFECTS

The drug has a diuretic, diaphoretic, digestive and emmenagogic effects.

INDICATIONS AND USAGE

The drug was formerly used for dropsy. In folk medicine it was used as a diuretic, diaphoretic and emetic, for kidney complaints, dropsy, the plague, snake bite and dysmennorrhea. Today, it is used in the treatment of digestive and kidney disorders and for dysmenorrhea. The poultices heal swellings and bruising.

PRECAUTIONS AND ADVERSE REACTIONS

According to older scientific literature, ''Vincetoxin'' in high dosages brought about vomiting, apnea and cardiac paralysis in animal experiments. Seed extracts led to advancing paralysis of the central nervous system. Poisonings of humans have not been found in recent reports.

DOSAGE

Mode of Administration: As an infusion, powdered drug, and alcoholic extract.

Preparation: The drug is prepared as an infusion.

Daily Dosage: The infusion should be administered under medical supervision.

LITERATURE

Kennard O et al., Tetrahedron Letters 3799-3804. 1968.

Further information in:

Frohne D, Pfänder HJ, Giftpflanzen - Ein Handbuch für Apotheker, Toxikologen und Biologen, 4. Aufl., Wiss. Verlagsges. mbH Stuttgart 1997.

Hänsel R, Keller K, Rimpler H, Schneider G (Hrsg.), Hagers Handbuch der Pharmazeutischen Praxis, 5. Aufl., Bde 4-6 (Drogen), Springer Verlag Berlin, Heidelberg, New York, 1992-1994.

Lewin L, Gifte und Vergiftungen, 6. Aufl., Nachdruck, Haug Verlag, Heidelberg 1992.

Madaus G, Lehrbuch der Biologischen Arzneimittel, Bde 1-3, Nachdruck, Georg Olms Verlag Hildesheim 1979.

Roth L, Daunderer M, Kormann K, Giftpflanzen, Pflanzengifte, 4. Aufl., Ecomed Fachverlag Landsberg Lech 1993.

Steinegger E, Hänsel R, Pharmakognosie, 5. Aufl., Springer Verlag Heidelberg 1992.

Teuscher E, Lindequist U, Biogene Gifte - Biologie, Chemie, Pharmakologie, 2. Aufl., Fischer Verlag Stuttgart 1994.

Cynara Scolymus

Artichoke

DESCRIPTION

Medicinal Parts: The medicinal parts are the dried whole or cut basal leaves and the dried or fresh herb from the artichoke.

Flower and Fruit: Globose, thorny capitual of lingual florets grow at the end of the stem. The epicalyx is ovate to globose. The bracts are fleshy and taper into a flattened greenish or purple tip. The petals are blue, lilac, or white. The fruit is a pubescent achaene 4 to 5 mm in diameter and 7 to 8 mm long. They are flecked brown and are glossy.

Leaves, Stem and Root: Cynara scolymus is a perennial plant with a short rhizome and a strong, erect, glabrous stalk. The stalk is up to 2 m high, thickly covered in lanceolate, prickly pinnate to double pinnate leaves. The upper surface is bare and light green; the lower surface is grey and tomentose.

Habitat: The plant is found in the Mediterranean region, the Canary Islands and South America. It is cultivated elsewhere.

Production: Artichoke is cultivated and dried with extreme care. Artichoke root is the dried root of Cynara scolymus. Artichoke leaf consists of the fresh or dried basal leaves of Cynara scolymus

Other Names: Garden Artichoke, Globe Artichoke

ACTIONS AND PHARMACOLOGY

COMPOUNDS: CYNARAE FOLIUM

Caffeic acid derivatives: chlorogenic acid, neochlorogenic acid, cryptochlorogenic acid, cynarin

Flavonoids: in particular rutin

Sesquiterpene lactones: cynaropicrin, dehydrocynaropicrin, grossheimin, cynaratriol

COMPOUNDS: CYNARAE RADIX

Caffeic acid derivatives, including chlorogenic acid sesquiterpene lactones are not contained in the rhizome.

EFFECTS: CYNARAE FOLIUM AND RADIX

A choleretic effect has been observed in rats; the cholesterol levels were reduced in the rats, a hepatostimulating and bitter effect has also been documented.

INDICATIONS AND USAGE

- Liver and gallbladder complaints
- Loss of appetite

Artichoke is used for dyspeptic problems and also for prophylactic treatment against the return of gall stones.

In folk medicine, Artichoke is also used for digestion complaints and as a tonic in convalescence.

CONTRAINDICATIONS

Because of the stimulating effect of the drug upon the biliary tract, it should not be administered if there is a bile duct blockage. Colic can occur where the patient suffers from gallstones.

PRECAUTIONS AND ADVERSE REACTIONS

Health risks or side effects following the proper administration of designated therapeutic dosages are not recorded. The plant possesses a medium potential for sensitization through skin contact. Allergic reactions occur in particular when there is frequent on-the-job contact with artichokes. There are cross-reactions with other composite (including chrysanthemes, arnica pyrethrum).

DOSAGE

Mode of Administration: Dried, comminuted drug, pressed juice of fresh plant, and other galenical preparations for internal use.

Daily Dosage: The average daily dose is 6 gm of drug; single dose: 500 mg of dry extract.

Storage: Artichoke should be protected from light and insects in well-sealed containers.

LITERATURE

Adzet T, Puigmacia M, J Chromatogr 348:447-453. 1985.

Brand N, Cynara scolymus L. - Die Artischocke. In: ZPT 11(5):169. 1990.

Fintelmann V, Antidyspetische und lipidsenkende Wirkung von Artischockenblätterextrakt. In: ZPT 17(5) Beilage ZFA. Zeitschrift für Allgem Med. 1996.

Fintelmann V, Menβen HG, Artischockenblätterextrakt Aktuelle Erkenntnis zur Wirkung als Lipidsenker und Antidyspeptikum. In: DAZ 136(17):1405-1414. 1996.

Kirchhoff R, Beckers CH, Kirchhoff GM, Trinczek-Gärtner H, Petrowicz O, Reimann HJ (1994) Increase in choleresis by means of artichoke extract. Phytomedicine 1:107-115.

Reuter HD, Pflanzliche Gallentherapeutika (Teil I) und (Teil II). In: ZPT 16(1):13-20, 77-89. 1995.

Schilcher H, Pharmazeutische Aspekte pflanzlicher Gallentherapeutika. In: ZPT 16(4):211-222. 1995.

Schmidt M, Phytotherapie: Pflanzliche Gallenwegstherapeutika. In: DAZ 135(8):680-682. 1995.

Wasielewski S, Artischockenblätterextrakt: Prävention der Arteriosklerose?. In: DAZ 137(24):2065-2067. 1997.

Further information in:

Hänsel R, Keller K, Rimpler H, Schneider G (Hrsg.), Hagers Handbuch der Pharmazeutischen Praxis, 5. Aufl., Bde 4-6 (Drogen), Springer Verlag Berlin, Heidelberg, New York, 1992-1994.

Hausen B, Allergiepflanzen, Pflanzenallergene, ecomed Verlagsgesellsch. mbH, Landsberg 1988.

Schulz R, Hänsel R, Rationale Phytotherapie, Springer Verlag Heidelberg 1996.

Steinegger E, Hänsel R, Pharmakognosie, 5. Aufl., Springer Verlag Heidelberg 1992.

Teuscher E, Lindequist U, Biogene Gifte - Biologie, Chemie, Pharmakologie, 2. Aufl., Fischer Verlag Stuttgart 1994.

Teuscher E, Biogene Arzneimittel, 5. Aufl., Wiss. Verlagsges. mbH Stuttgart 1997.

Wagner H, Wiesenauer M, Phytotherapie. Phytopharmaka und pflanzliche Homöopathika, Fischer-Verlag, Stuttgart, Jena, New York 1995.

Cynoglossum Officinale

Hound's Tongue

DESCRIPTION

Medicinal Parts: The medicinal parts are the aerial parts (Cynoglossi herba) and root (Cynoglossi radix) of the herb.

Flower and Fruit: The flowers are on short, bent pedicles, which after flowering, grow to 1 cm. The corolla is cup-shaped and larger than the calyx. The corolla is initially dark violet, then dull brown. It is occasionally white with thickened, velvety purple or light red, tubular scales. The nutlets are flat, ovoid and light-brown. They are 5 to 7 mm wide, thickened at the edge, and covered with barbs.

Leaves, Stem and Root: The plant is a biennial. The tap root is 10 to 30 cm long and up to 1.5 cm thick. It is reddish colored with a few fibers. The shoots are gray-green and smell of mice. The stems are usually rigidly erect, angular, hairy and heavily foliated. They are 30 to 80 cm high and up to 1 cm thick. The lower leaves are in rosettes, which form a tough, coriaceous sheath at the base. The upper leaves are sessile and clasping.

Habitat: Especially common in Germany and Switzerland, now also found in the U.S. in areas where Germans and Swiss settled.

Production: Hound's Tongue herb consists of the above-ground parts of Cynoglossum officinale. The root is gathered in the second spring and then dried.

Other Names: Dog's Tongue, Dog-bur, Gypsy Flower, Sheep-lice, Woolmat

ACTIONS AND PHARMACOLOGY

COMPOUNDS: CYNOGLOSSI HERBA

Pyrrolizidine alkaloids: main alkaloids heliosupine, echinatine, also 7-angeloylheliotridine, acetylheliosupine

EFFECTS: CYNOGLOSSI HERBA

No information is available.

COMPOUNDS: CYNOGLOSSI RADIX

Pyrrolizidine alkaloids: main alkaloids presumably, as in the plant, heliosupine and echinatine

Tannins

EFFECTS: CYNOGLOSSI RADIX

According to previous reports, cynoglossin has a paralyzing effect on the peripheral nerve ends of frogs. The substances consolicin and consolidin have a paralyzing effect on the CNS, which is 3 times stronger than the effect of cynoglossin. The toxicity should disappear with storage.

The drug has been used externally to heal wounds and internally for diarrhea.

INDICATIONS AND USAGE

CYNOGLOSSI HERBA

Preparations of Hound's Tongue have been used as an antidiarrheal and an expectorant. The effectiveness of the herb for the claimed applications is not documented.

CYNOGLOSSI RADIX

In the past, it was used as an analgesic both internally and externally, as a cough sedative and for diarrhea.

The root is used externally in the treatment of wounds.

PRECAUTIONS AND ADVERSE REACTIONS

WARNING: The traditional folk medicinal preparations should not be used!

Because of its high pyrrolizidine alkaloid content with 1,2-unsaturated necine parent substances, the drug is both hepatotoxic and hepatocarcinogenic in effect. The drug should under no circumstances be taken internally.

DOSAGE

See Warning above regarding internal use.

Storage: The herb should be protected from light and kept dry above annealed calcium chloride in air-tight, sealed glass or chalk containers, with the possible addition of a few drops of chloroform or carbon tetrachloride as an insecticide. It should be renewed annually.

LITERATURE

CYNOGLOSSI HERBA

Knight AP, Kimberling CV, Stermitz FR, Roby MR, Cynoglossum officinale (hounds-tongue) - a cause of pyrrolizidine-alkaloid poisoning in horse. In: J Am Vet Med Assoc 185(6):647-650. 1984.

Mattocks AR, Pigott CD, Pyrrolizidine lakloids from Cynoglossum germanicum. In: PH 29(9):2871. 1990.

Further information in:

Frohne D, Pfänder HJ: Giftpflanzen - Ein Handbuch für Apotheker, Toxikologen und Biologen, 4. Aufl., Wiss. Verlagsges. mbH Stuttgart 1997.

Kern W, List PH, Hörhammer L (Hrsg.), Hagers Handbuch der Pharmazeutischen Praxis, 4. Aufl., Bde 1-8, Springer Verlag Berlin, Heidelberg, New York, 1969.

Lewin L, Gifte und Vergiftungen, 6. Aufl., Nachdruck, Haug Verlag, Heidelberg 1992.

Steinegger E, Hänsel R, Pharmakognosie, 5. Aufl., Springer Verlag Heidelberg 1992.

Teuscher E, Lindequist U, Biogene Gifte - Biologie, Chemie, Pharmakologie, 2. Aufl., Fischer Verlag Stuttgart 1994.

CYNOGLOSSI RADIX

Knight AP, Kimberling CV, Stermitz FR, Roby MR, Cynoglossum officinale (hounds-tongue) - a cause of pyrrolizidine-alkaloid poisoning in horse. In: J Am Vet Med Assoc 185(6):647-650. 1984.

Mattocks AR, Pigott CD, Pyrrolizidine lakloids from Cynoglossum germanicum. In: PH 29(9):2871. 1990.

Further information in:

Kern W, List PH, Hörhammer L (Hrsg.), Hagers Handbuch der Pharmazeutischen Praxis, 4. Aufl., Bde 1-8, Springer Verlag Berlin, Heidelberg, New York, 1969.

Cyperus Articulatus

Adrue

DESCRIPTION

Medicinal Parts: Adrue root is used in the West Indies for its anti-emetic properties.

Flower and Fruit: The tubers are blackish and top-shaped, with bristly remains of former leaves. The plant is sometimes connected in twos or threes by narrow underground stems. The transverse section is pale, showing a central column with darker vascular bundles.

Characteristics: Adrue has an aromatic odor and a bitter taste, reminiscent of Lavender.

Habitat: Turkey, region of the river Nile, Jamaica.

Production: Adrue root is the root of Cyperus articulatus.

Other Names: Guinea Rush

ACTIONS AND PHARMACOLOGY

COMPOUNDS

Volatile oil: containing above all sesquiterpene hydrocarbons and sesqiterpene alcohols, including cyperenone

EFFECTS

Adrue has anti-emetic, carminative and sedative properties.

INDICATIONS AND USAGE

Preparations of the root are used for digestive disorders, nausea, and flatulence.

PRECAUTIONS AND ADVERSE REACTIONS

Health risks or side effects following the proper administration of designated therapeutic dosages are not recorded.

DOSAGE

Mode of Administration: Available as a liquid extract for internal use.

LITERATURE

Pinder AR, (1976) Tetrahedron 23:2172.

Further information in:

Kern W, List PH, Hörhammer L (Hrsg.), Hagers Handbuch der Pharmazeutischen Praxis, 4. Aufl., Bde 1-8, Springer Verlag Berlin, Heidelberg, New York, 1969.

Cypress

See Cupressus Sempervirens

Cypress Spurge

See Euphorbia Cyparissias

Cypripedium Calceolus

Nerve Root

DESCRIPTION

Medicinal Parts: The medicinal parts are the dried rhizome with the roots, the fresh underground parts harvested in autumn and the fresh roots. The roots of several varieties are used as a sedative and antispasmodic.

Flower and Fruit: The plant develops terminal inflorescences with 1 to 2 flowers that have leaf-like bracts. The flowers are 4 to 9 cm long by 0.5 to 1 cm wide. They are linear-lanceolate and twisted. The petals are green, green-brown or yellow. The petals, including the protruding lip or shoe, are splayed. The shoe is 3 to 4 cm long in the shape of an inflated sack. It is lemon yellow to gold with purple spots and veins. The pollen is powdery. The pollen seeds are in 4 groups. The ovary is single-valved and pubescent.

Leaves, Stem and Root: Nerve Root is a perennial, 15 to 70 cm high. The plant has a horizontal rootstock with scales and thick root fibers. The stem is round with short hairs, and is covered at the base with scaly brown leaves. There are 3 to 4 leaves above these, which are broad, elliptical, sheath-like, folded and acute. The upper surface is bright green, the underside, paler.

Habitat: Indigenous to U.S. and Canada, cultivated in Europe.

Production: Lady's Slipper rhizome is the rhizome of Cypripedium calceolus.

Not To Be Confused With: Other Cypripedium varieties

Other Names: Lady's Slipper, American Valerian, Bleeding Heart, Moccasin Flower, Monkey Flower, Noah's Ark, Slipper Root, Venus Shoe, Yellows

ACTIONS AND PHARMACOLOGY

COMPOUNDS

Volatile oil

Phenanthrene quinones: including cypripedi

Tannins

EFFECTS

Nerve Root is astringent and styptic. No additional information is available.

INDICATIONS AND USAGE

In folk medicine, the drug is used for insomnia, emotional tension, states of agitation, nervousness and hysteria. It is also used internally in the treatment of menorrhagia and diarrhea, as well as externally in the treatment of pruritus vulvae. Efficacy has not been proven.

PRECAUTIONS AND ADVERSE REACTIONS

Health risks or side effects following the proper administration of designated therapeutic dosages are not recorded. The plant possesses a medium potential for sensitization through skin contact.

DOSAGE

Mode of Administration: The drug is administered in its dry form or as liquid extract. The supply of higher (concentrated)

doses should be avoided. This is a highly protected plant. The sale and cultivation of the drug is forbidden.

Preparation: Liquid extract: 1:1 in 45% alcohol.

Daily Dose: To be taken internally, 2 teaspoonfuls (2 to 4 g) of the dried drug as an infusion.

LITERATURE

Schmalle HW, Hausen BM, Naturwissenschaften: 66:527. 1979.

Further information in:

Hänsel R, Keller K, Rimpler H, Schneider G (Hrsg.), Hagers Handbuch der Pharmazeutischen Praxis, 5. Aufl., Bde 4-6 (Drogen), Springer Verlag Berlin, Heidelberg, New York, 1992-1994.

Hausen B, Allergiepflanzen, Pflanzenallergene, ecomed Verlagsgesellsch. mbH, Landsberg 1988.

Madaus G, Lehrbuch der Biologischen Arzneimittel, Bde 1-3, Nachdruck, Georg Olms Verlag Hildesheim 1979.

Cytisus Laburnum

Laburnum

DESCRIPTION

Medicinal Parts: The seeds are the medicinal parts.

Flower and Fruit: The flowers bow down in clusters of 10 to 30. There are 10 to 25 cm long racemes. The calyx is short, campanulate, pubescent and marked brown at the base. The anthers are orange. The pod is 5 to 8 cm by 8 to 9 cm, flat, lumpy, and silky-haired with wings. The seeds are flat and dark brown.

Leaves, Stem and Root: Cytisus laburnum is a small shrub or tree occasionally up to 7 m high with light gray branches and smooth, dark green, initially erect branchlets. The alternate leaves are almost in rosettes on short shoots with 2 to 7 cm long petioles. The leaflets are elliptical to ovate, rounded or thorn tipped, which are glabrous above and light gray pubescent beneath.

Habitat: The plant is indigenous to mountainous regions of Europe. It is also cultivated worldwide.

Other Names: Golden Chain, Pea Tree, Bean Trifoil

ACTIONS AND PHARMACOLOGY

COMPOUNDS

Quinolizidine alkaloids: main alkaloids (-)-cytisins, beyond that (-)-N-methylcytisins and epibaptifolin

Lectins

EFFECTS

No information is available.

INDICATIONS AND USAGE

Experiments in the use of cytisin as a pesticide (lice) have shown that in the necessary concentration the danger of poisoning is too high.

PRECAUTIONS AND ADVERSE REACTIONS

There are no indications for this drug. The drug is severely toxic. See Overdosage section.

OVERDOSAGE

Symptoms of poisoning include nausea, dizziness, salivation, pains in the mouth, in the throat and in the stomach area, outbreaks of sweat, headache as well as extended, severe, and sometimes bloody vomiting. If no vomiting occurs, excitatory states can come about from the centrally-stimulating effect of the drug, with tonic-clonic spasms, that later change over into paralyses. Anuria and uremia have also been observed. Death comes through asphyxiation.

Fifteen to 20 seeds or 3 to 4 unripe berries are considered fatal for an adult. While poisonings occur relatively frequently, cases of death have not been recorded in recent times. If no vomiting has occurred, poisonings are treated with gastric lavage, then through the administration of activated charcoal; spasms are to be treated with chlorpromazine or diazepam. In cases of asphyxiation, intubation and oxygen respiration are to be carried out.

LITERATURE

Greinwald R, Untersuchungen zur chemotaxonomischen Bedeutung von Leguminosenalkaloiden und zum Alkaloidstoffwechsel in transformierten Geweben und Zellkulturen. In: Dissertation Universität Würzburg. 1988.

Gresser G, Der Besenginster - Cytisus scoparius (L.) LINK. In: ZPT 17(5):320-330. 1996.

Seeger R, Neumann HG, Cytisin. In: DAZ 132(7):303. 1992.

Tschirch C, Kraus L, Goldregen-Alkaloid Cytisin. In: DAZ 132(47):2560. 1992.

Further information in:

Frohne D, Pfänder HJ, Giftpflanzen - Ein Handbuch für Apotheker, Toxikologen und Biologen, 4. Aufl., Wiss. Verlagsges. mbH Stuttgart 1997.

Hänsel R, Keller K, Rimpler H, Schneider G (Hrsg.), Hagers Handbuch der Pharmazeutischen Praxis, 5. Aufl., Bde 4-6 (Drogen), Springer Verlag Berlin, Heidelberg, New York, 1992-1994.

Lewin L, Gifte und Vergiftungen, 6. Aufl., Nachdruck, Haug Verlag, Heidelberg 1992.

Madaus G, Lehrbuch der Biologischen Arzneimittel, Bde 1-3, Nachdruck, Georg Olms Verlag Hildesheim 1979.

Roth L, Daunderer M, Kormann K, Giftpflanzen, Pflanzengifte, 4. Aufl., Ecomed Fachverlag Landsberg Lech 1993.

Teuscher E, Lindequist U, Biogene Gifte - Biologie, Chemie, Pharmakologie, 2. Aufl., Fischer Verlag Stuttgart 1994.

Teuscher E, Biogene Arzneimittel, 5. Aufl., Wiss. Verlagsges. mbH Stuttgart 1997.

Wagner H, Wiesenauer M, Phytotherapie. Phytopharmaka und pflanzliche Homöopathika, Fischer-Verlag, Stuttgart, Jena, New York 1995.

Cytisus Scoparius

Broom

DESCRIPTION

Medicinal Parts: The medicinal parts are the dried and stripped broom flowers, the dried aerial parts (broom herb) and freshly picked flowers.

Flower and Fruit: The bilabiate flowers are bright yellow, 20 to 25 mm long, large, solitary or in pairs. The flowers are on 2 or 3 obovate bracts on short stems, or singly in the leaf axils. They seem to form long racemes. The corolla is bright yellow, sometimes white. The standard is revolute, the wings obtuse. The ovary is short-stemmed and villous with a glabrous, strongly hooked style. The pod is oblong, compressed, glabrous on the surfaces, villous on the seams and is a matte black. There are numerous brown-black seeds.

Leaves, Stem and Root: Broom is a shrub, which grows from 0.5 to 2 m high. The tap root is very sturdy, woody and the bark of the root is brown. The branches are thick, usually crooked and the bark is also brown. Young shoots are glabrous, later pubescent. The branchlets are cane-like, erect and pentagular. The leaves are small, short-petioled, with 3 obovate to lanceolate, 1 to 2 cm long and 1.5 to 9 mm wide pointed leaflets. The leaflets, particularly on the undersurface, are silkly pubescent. After flowering, sessile and entire leaves form on the upper shoot.

Habitat: The herb is found in Europe, northern Africa, Canary Islands, North America, Chile, South Africa and Japan.

Production: Broom herb consists of the aerial parts of Cytisus scoparius. Broom flowers consist of the flowers of Cytisus scoparius.

Not To Be Confused With: The herb should not be confused with other Cystisus or Genista varieties. The flowers should not be confused with Spanish Broom.

Other Names: Broom, Broomtops, Besom, Scoparium, Irish Tops, Basam, Bizzom, Browme, Brum, Breeam

ACTION AND PHARMACOLOGY

COMPOUNDS: CYTISI SCOPARII HERBA

Quinolizidine alkaloids: main alkaloid (-)-sparteine, including, among others, 11, 12-dehydrosparteine, 17-oxosparteine, lupanine, alpha-isosparteine

Biogenic amines: including tyramine, epinine, dopamine

Flavonoids

Isoflavonoids: including genistein, sarothamnoside

EFFECTS: CYTISI SCOPARII HERBA

No specific studies are available. Tyramine acts indirectly on the sympathetic nervous system as a vasoconstrictor and hypertensive.

COMPOUNDS: CYTISI SCOPARII FLOS

Quinolizidine alkaloids (very small quantities): main alkaloid (-)-sparteine

Biogenic amines: including tyramine

Flavonoids: including scoparin (C-glycosylflavone)

EFFECTS: CYTISI SCOPARII FLOS

The drug can contain over 2% tyramine. It contains small amounts of alkaloids. The main alkaloid is sparteine. Tyramine acts as an indirect sympathicomimetic, vasoconstrictoral and hypotensive. Sparteine acts negatively inotropic and negatively chronotropic; because of the very minimal amounts of sparteine no intense effect can be expected.

INDICATIONS

CYTISI SCOPARII HERBA

- Hypertension

The herb is used for functional heart and circulatory disorders, as an adjunct in the stabilization of circulation and to raise blood pressure. Folk medicine uses include pathological edema, cardiac arrythmia, nervous cardiac complaints, low blood pressure, heavy menstruation, hemorrhaging after birth, as a contraction stimulant, for bleeding gums, hemophilia, gout, rheumatism, sciatica, gall and kidney stones, enlarged spleen, jaundice, bronchial conditions and snake bites. The efficacy of these indications has not been proven.

CYTISI SCOPARII FLOS

The use of the pure drug cannot be recommended except as an inactive ingredient in teas. In folk medicine, the flowers are used for edema, rheumatism, gout, kidney stones, jaundice, liver disorders, enlarged spleen and as a blood purifier.

CONTRAINDICATIONS

CYTISI SCOPARII HERBA ET FLOS

The drug is contraindicated in high blood pressure, A-V block, MAO inhibitors, and pregnancy.

PRECAUTIONS AND ADVERSE REACTIONS

CYTISI SCOPARII HERBA

General: Health risks or side effects following the proper administration of designated therapeutic dosages are not recorded. Common (Scotch) Broom preparations should not however be used in cases of high blood pressure or with atrioventricular blocks.

Drug Interactions: Use of Broom herb with monoamine oxidase inhibitors (amine content) may cause a hypertensive crisis.

Pregnancy: The herb should not be used during pregnancy (abortive efficacy).

CYTISI SCOPARII FLOS
Health risks or side effects following the proper administration of designated therapeutic dosages are not recorded. The drug should not be used in cases of high blood pressure or when the patient is being treated with monoamine oxidase inhibitors (amine content).

OVERDOSAGE

CYTISI SCOPARII HERBA
Doses corresponding to more than 300 mg sparteine (approximately 30 g of the drug), lead to dizziness, headache, palpitations, prickling in the extremities, feeling of weakness in the legs, outbreaks of sweat, sleepiness, pupil dilation and ocular palsy. If no vomiting has occurred, poisonings are treated with gastric lavage, and administration of activated charcoal. Spasms are to be treated with chlorpromazine or diazepam. In cases of asphyxiation, intubation and oxygen respiration are to be carried out. No deaths through poisonings with this drug have been proven beyond a doubt (though they certainly have been with sparteine).

DOSAGE

CYTISI SCOPARII HERBA
Mode of Administration: The herb is available in aqueous essential oil extracts for internal administration.

Daily Dosage: The daily dose of the infusion is 1 cup fresh infusion 3 times daily. The liquid extract dosage is 1 to 2 ml daily. The tincture internal use dosage is 0.5 to 2 ml. Aqueous-ethanol extracts corresponding to 1:1.5 drug are also used.

Storage: Carefully protect from light and moisture.

CYTISI SCOPARII FLOS
Mode of Administration: Since the efficacy for the claimed uses has not been documented, and considering the risks, a therapeutic application cannot be justified.

Daily Dosage: Infusion dosage is 1 cup daily. For pathological edema, 1l infusion per day are administered in 4 portions during meals for 1 month.

LITERATURE

CYTISI SCOPARII HERBA
Brum-Bousquet M, Delaveau P, (1981) Plant Med Phytother 15(4):201.

Brum-Bousquet M et al., (1981) Planta Med 43(4):367.

Kurihara T, Kikuchi M, (1980) Yakugaku Zasshi 100(10):1054.

Murakoshi I et al., (1986) Phytochemistry 25(2):521.

Seeger R, Neumann HG, Spartein. In: DAZ 132(30):1577. 1992.

Vixcardi P et al., (1984) Pharmazie 39(11):781.

Wink M, Heinen HJ, Vogt H, Schiebel HM, Plant Cell Rep 3:230-233. 1984.

Wink M et al., (1981) Planta Med 43(4):342.

Young N et al., (1984) Biochem J 222(1):41.

Further information in:

Chan EH, et al., (Eds.), Advances in Chinese Medicinal Materials Research, World Scientific Pub. Co. Singapore 1985.

Hänsel R, Keller K, Rimpler H, Schneider G (Hrsg.), Hagers Handbuch der Pharmazeutischen Praxis, 5. Aufl., Bde 4-6 (Drogen): Springer Verlag Berlin, Heidelberg, New York, 1992-1994.

Leung AY, Encyclopedia of Common Natural Ingredients Used in Food, Drugs and Cosmetics, John Wiley & Sons Inc., New York 1980.

Lewin L, Gifte und Vergiftungen, 6. Aufl., Nachdruck, Haug Verlag, Heidelberg 1992.

Madaus G, Lehrbuch der Biologischen Arzneimittel, Bde 1-3, Nachdruck, Georg Olms Verlag Hildesheim 1979.

Roth L, Daunderer M, Kormann K, Giftpflanzen, Pflanzengifte, 4. Aufl., Ecomed Fachverlag Landsberg Lech 1993.

Steinegger E, Hänsel R, Pharmakognosie, 5. Aufl., Springer Verlag Heidelberg 1992.

Teuscher E, Lindequist U, Biogene Gifte - Biologie, Chemie, Pharmakologie, 2. Aufl., Fischer Verlag Stuttgart 1994.

Teuscher E, Biogene Arzneimittel, 5. Aufl., Wiss. Verlagsges. mbH Stuttgart 1997.

Wagner H, Wiesenauer M, Phytotherapie. Phytopharmaka und pflanzliche Homöopathika, Fischer-Verlag, Stuttgart, Jena, New York 1995.

CYTISI SCOPARII FLOS
Brum-Bousquet M, Delaveau P, (1981) Plant Med Phytother 15(4):201.

Brum-Bousquet M et al., (1981) Planta Med 43(4):367.

Kurihara T, Kikuchi M, (1980) Yakugaku Zasshi 100(10):1054.

Murakoshi I et al., (1986) Phytochemistry 25(2):521-524.

Seeger R, Neumann HG, Spartein. In: DAZ 132(30):1577. 1992.

Vixcardi P et al., (1984) Pharmazie 39(11):781.

Wink M, Heinen HJ, Vogt H, Schiebel HM, Plant Cell Rep 3:230-233. 1984.

Wink M et al., (1981) Planta Med 43(4):342-352.

Young N et al., (1984) Biochem J 222(1):41.

Further information in:

Chan EH et al., (Eds.), Advances in Chinese Medicinal Materials Research, World Scientific Pub. Co. Singapore 1985.

Hänsel R, Keller K, Rimpler H, Schneider G (Hrsg.), Hagers Handbuch der Pharmazeutischen Praxis, 5. Aufl., Bde 4-6 (Drogen): Springer Verlag Berlin, Heidelberg, New York, 1992-1994.

Leung AY, Encyclopedia of Common Natural Ingredients Used in Food Drugs and Cosmetics, John Wiley & Sons Inc., New York 1980.

Lewin L, Gifte und Vergiftungen, 6. Aufl., Nachdruck, Haug Verlag, Heidelberg 1992.

Madaus G, Lehrbuch der Biologischen Arzneimittel, Bde 1-3, Nachdruck, Georg Olms Verlag Hildesheim 1979.

Roth L, Daunderer M, Kormann K, Giftpflanzen, Pflanzengifte, 4. Aufl., Ecomed Fachverlag Landsberg Lech 1993.

Steinegger E, Hänsel R, Pharmakognosie, 5. Aufl., Springer Verlag Heidelberg 1992.

Teuscher E, Lindequist U, Biogene Gifte - Biologie, Chemie, Pharmakologie, 2. Aufl., Fischer Verlag Stuttgart 1994.

Teuscher E, Biogene Arzneimittel, 5. Aufl., Wiss. Verlagsges. mbH Stuttgart 1997.

Wagner H, Wiesenauer M, Phytotherapie. Phytopharmaka und pflanzliche Homöopathika, Fischer-Verlag, Stuttgart, Jena, New York 1995.

Daemonorops Draco

Dragon's Blood

DESCRIPTION

Medicinal Parts: The medicinal part is the red resin from the fruit, which is extracted from both Daemonorops draco and Daemonorops propinquis.

Flower and Fruit: The flowers are arranged along the branch. The fruit is a cherry-sized berry ending in a point. When the fruit are ripe, they are covered in a reddish, resinous substance, which is separated in various ways.

Leaves, Stem and Root: Dragon's Blood is a tree with long, thin, flexible stems, which are inclined to climb when they are older. The leaves have thorny petioles, which grow into long appendages. The bark is covered in hundreds of flattened thorns.

Habitat: Malaysia, Indonesia.

Production: Dragon's Blood resin is the resin of Daemonorops draco.

Other Names: Dracorubin, Sanguis Draconis, Draconis Resina

ACTIONS AND PHARMACOLOGY

COMPOUNDS

Ester resins (dracoresin): benzoyl ester of dracoresinotannol

Dracoresen

Flavane quinones: including dracorubin (dracocarmin), dracorhodin, both colored an intense red

EFFECTS

Dragon's Blood has an astringent effect.

INDICATIONS AND USAGE

The resin is used for diarrhea, digestive disorders and as a coloring agent.

PRECAUTIONS AND ADVERSE REACTIONS

Health risks or side effects following the proper administration of designated therapeutic dosages are not recorded.

DOSAGE

Mode of Administration: The resin is used in a powder form.

LITERATURE

Merlini L, Gasini G, J Chem Soc Perkin I 1976:1570. 1976.

Rao SR et al., JNP 45:646. 1982.

Further information in:

Hegnauer R, Chemotaxonomie der Pflanzen, Bde 1-11, Birkhäuser Verlag Basel, Boston, Berlin 1962-1997.

Kern W, List PH, Hörhammer L (Hrsg.), Hagers Handbuch der Pharmazeutischen Praxis, 4. Aufl., Bde 1-8, Springer Verlag Berlin, Heidelberg, New York, 1969.

Daffodil

See Narcissus Pseudonarcissus

Damiana

See Turnera Diffusa

Dandelion

See Taraxacum Officinale

Daphne Mezereum

Mezereon

DESCRIPTION

Medicinal Parts: The medicinal part is the bark, which is collected before the flowering season.

Flower and Fruit: The flowers are dark pink. They appear before the leaves in irregular, sessile clusters usually in threes. There is a 4 tipped calyx with an external silky-haired tube. There are 8 stamens in 2 rows. There is 1 free ovary. The fruit consists of a bright red, pea-sized, juicy, ovoid, 1-seeded berry.

Leaves, Stem and Root: The plant is a 50 to 150 cm high perennial. It is a deciduous, sparsely branched shrub with reed-like, grayish or yellow-brown very tough branches. The leaves are short-petioled, lanceolate, narrowing towards the petiole and entire-margined.

Characteristics: Mezereon has a strong pleasant fragrance. The plant is poisonous and can be fatal if ingested. It is a protected species.

Habitat: Indigenous to Europe as far as Siberia, cultivated in the U.S., Canada and elsewhere.

Production: Mezereon root, root bark and bark are from Daphne mezereum. The bark of the trunk and the root are gathered before flowering, dried and rolled up but with the phloem facing outwards. Care should be taken not to destroy the plant during the harvest.

Other Names: Spurge Olive, Spurge Laurel, Daphne, Spurge Flax, Wild Pepper, Dwarf Bay, Camolea

ACTIONS AND PHARMACOLOGY

COMPOUNDS

Diterpenes: daphnane derivatives, including mezerein, daphnetoxin

EFFECTS

The drug acts as a powerful skin stimulant, hallucinogenic and a rubifacient.

INDICATIONS AND USAGE

In the past, Mezeron root was used to relieve headaches and toothache. It was also infrequently used for joint pains and to increase circulation in rheumatic complaints. In homeopathy, it is used for skin conditions such as cradle cap, shingles, weeping eczemas and encrusted (scab-like), weeping blisters.

PRECAUTIONS AND ADVERSE REACTIONS

External contact with the severely irritating toxic diterpenes of Daphne mezereon causes erysipeloid reddening of the skin, swelling, blister formation and shedding of the epidermis. Extended exposure leads to the formation of necroses. Contact with the eyes brings about severe conjunctivitis. If taken internally, reddening and swelling of the oral mucous membranes, feeling of thirst, salivation, stomach pains, vomiting and severe diarrhea occur.

Results of resorption include headache, dizziness, stupor, tachycardia, spasms and possibly death through circulatory collapse. Cool wrappings and anaesthetic salves are recommended for treatment of the skin injuries.

OVERDOSAGE

With poisonings resulting from intake of the drug, gastric lavage should precede calcium gluconate, I.V., and perhaps also administration of corticoids.

DOSAGE

Mode of Administration: The drug is seldom used today. Used in homeopathic dilutions, topically and internally.

Preparation: Ointment: 20% drug content.

Storage: The effect fades, if it is stored for too long. Therefore, do not store for a period of more than 2 years.

LITERATURE

Evans B, In: Evans FJ:Naturally Occuring Phorbolesters, CRC Press Inc., Boca Raton, Florida. 1986.

Kupchan SM, Baxter RL, (1974) Science 187:652.

Nyborg J, La Cour, T, (1975) Nature 257:824.

Ronlan A, Wickberg B, Tetrahedron Lett 4261. 1970.

Schildknecht H et al., (1970) Chem Ztg 94:347.

Schindler H, PM 10:232. 1962.

Stout GH et al., (1970) J Am Chem Soc 92:1070.

Further information in:

Frohne D, Pfänder HJ, Giftpflanzen - Ein Handbuch für Apotheker, Toxikologen und Biologen, 4. Aufl., Wiss. Verlagsges. mbH Stuttgart 1997.

Kern W, List PH, Hörhammer L (Hrsg.), Hagers Handbuch der Pharmazeutischen Praxis, 4. Aufl., Bde 1-8, Springer Verlag Berlin, Heidelberg, New York, 1969.

Lewin L, Gifte und Vergiftungen, 6. Aufl., Nachdruck, Haug Verlag, Heidelberg 1992.

Madaus G, Lehrbuch der Biologischen Arzneimittel, Bde 1-3, Nachdruck, Georg Olms Verlag Hildesheim 1979.

Roth L, Daunderer M, Kormann K: Giftpflanzen, Pflanzengifte, 4. Aufl., Ecomed Fachverlag Landsberg Lech 1993.

Teuscher E, Lindequist U, Biogene Gifte - Biologie, Chemie, Pharmakologie, 2. Aufl., Fischer Verlag Stuttgart 1994.

Wagner H, Wiesenauer M, Phytotherapie. Phytopharmaka und pflanzliche Homöopathika, Fischer-Verlag, Stuttgart, Jena, New York 1995.

Date Palm

See Phoenix Dactylifera

Datura Stramonium

Jimson Weed

DESCRIPTION

Medicinal Parts: The medicinal parts are the dried leaves or the dried leaves with the tips of the flowering branches. Occasionally the fruit, the ripe seeds and the fresh, aerial parts of the plant are used. Parts of the plant are regarded as poisonous.

Flower and Fruit: The flowers are large, white, solitary, terminal or in the branch bifurcations. The calyx has a long 5-edged and short 5-tipped tube. The corolla is funnel-shaped and folded with a short 5-sectioned border. There are 5 free stamens and 1 superior ovary. The fruit is a 5 cm long 4-valved capsule, which is densely thorny and walnut-sized. The numerous seeds are 3.5 mm long, flat, reniform and black.

Leaves, Stem and Root: The plant is an annual and grows to 1.2 m high. It has a simple or bifurcated, round, erect glabrous stem. The leaves are 20 cm long, long-petioled, ovate, dentate, glabrous and dark green.

Characteristics: The foliage has an unpleasant smell, the flowers are fragrant and poisonous.

Habitat: Most temperate and subtropical parts of the world, probably originated in Central America.

Production: Jimson Weed leaf consists of the dried leaf, or the dried leaves and flowering tops of Datura stramonium. Jimson weed seed consists of the ripe seed of Datura stramonium.

Other Names: Devil's Apple, Devil's Trumpet, Jamestown Weed, Mad-apple, Nightshade, Peru-apple, Stinkweed, Stinkwort, Stramonium, Thorn-apple, Datura

ACTIONS AND PHARMACOLOGY

COMPOUNDS: DATURA STRAMONIUM FOLLIUM

Tropane alkaloids (0.1-0.65%): chief alkaloids (-)-hyoscyamine, under drying conditions changing over to some extent into atropine, and scopolamine (ratio 4:1), furthermore including, among others, apoatropine, belladonnine, tigloylmeteloidin

Flavonoids

Hydroxycoumarins: including, among others, umbelliferone, scopolin, scopoletin

Withanolide: including, among others, withastramonolide

COMPOUNDS: DATURA STRAMONIUM SEMEN

Tropane alkaloids (0.4-0.6%): chief alkaloids (-)-hyoscyamine, under drying conditions changing over to some extent into atropine, and scopolamine (ratio 4:1).

Indole alkaloids (β-carboline type): including, among others, fluorodaturin (very fluorescent).

Lectins

Fatty oil (15-45%)

Proteins (12-25%)

EFFECTS

No information is available.

INDICATIONS AND USAGE

Jimson Weed preparations are used for asthma, spastic or convulsive cough, pertussis during bronchitis and influenza. Also, Jimson Weed is used as basic therapy for diseases of the autonomic nervous system.

CONTRAINDICATIONS

Glaucoma, suspicion of glaucoma, paralytic ileus, pyloric stenosis, enlarged prostate, tachycardic arrhythmias, acute pulmonary edema.

PRECAUTIONS AND ADVERSE REACTIONS

No health hazards are known in conjunction with the proper administration of designated therapeutic dosages. Restrictions on administration: for patients with urine retention, coronoary sclerosis. The intake of very high dosages leads to central excitation (restlessness, compulsive speech, hallucinations, delirium, manic episodes), followed by exhaustion and sleep.

OVERDOSAGE

The 4 early warning symptoms of a poisoning are: skin reddening, dryness of the mouth, tachycardic arrhythmias and mydriasis. Accomodation disorders, heat build-up through decline in sweat secretion, miction disorders and severe constipation can occur as side effects, particularly with overdosages.

Lethal dosages (for adults starting at 100 mg atropine, depending upon atropine content, 15 to 100 g of the leaf drug, 15 to 25 g of the seed drug, considerably less for children) carry with them the danger of asphyxiation. Treatment for poisonings include stomach emptying, temperature-lowering measures with wet cloths (no antipyretics), oxygen respiration for respiratory distress, intubation, parenteral physostigmine salts as antidote, diazepam for spasms and chlorpromazine for severe excitation.

DOSAGE

No information is available.

LITERATURE

Evans WC, PH 23:1717. 1984.

Friedmann M, Levin CE, J Agric Food Chem 37:998. 1989.

Itoh T et al., PH 17:971. 1978.

Kraft K, Europäische Rauschdrogen. In: ZPT 17(6):343-355. 1996.

Mechler E, Hann N, PM 42:102. 1981.

Mirazamatov RT et al., Khim Prir Soedin (3):381. 1986.

Sharova EG et al., Khim Prir Soedin (1):126. 1977.

Tursunova RL et al., Khim Prir Soedin (1):91. 1978.

Further information in:

Frohne D, Pfänder HJ, Giftpflanzen - Ein Handbuch für Apotheker, Toxikologen und Biologen, 4. Aufl., Wiss. Verlags-Ges. Stuttgart 1997.

Hänsel R, Keller K, Rimpler H, Schneider G (Hrsg.), Hagers Handbuch der Pharmazeutischen Praxis, 5. Aufl., Bde 4-6 (Drogen): Springer Verlag Berlin, Heidelberg, New York, 1992-1994.

Lewin L, Gifte und Vergiftungen, 6. Aufl., Nachdruck, Haug Verlag, Heidelberg 1992.

Madaus G, Lehrbuch der Biologischen Arzneimittel, Bde 1-3, Nachdruck, Georg Olms Verlag Hildesheim 1979.

Roth L, Daunderer M, Kormann K, Giftpflanzen, Pflanzengifte, 4. Aufl., Ecomed Fachverlag Landsberg Lech 1993.

Steinegger E, Hänsel R, Pharmakognosie, 5. Aufl., Springer Verlag Heidelberg 1992.

Teuscher E, Lindequist U, Biogene Gifte - Biologie, Chemie, Pharmakologie, 2. Aufl., Fischer Verlag Stuttgart 1994.

Teuscher E, Biogene Arzneimittel, 5. Aufl., Wiss. Verlagsges. Stuttgart 1997.

Wagner H, Wiesenauer M, Phytotherapie. Phytopharmaka und pflanzliche Homöopathika, Fischer-Verlag, Stuttgart, Jena, New York 1995.

Daucus Carota

Carrot

DESCRIPTION

Medicinal Parts: The medicinal part is the root.

Flower and Fruit: The flowers are in compact, terminal umbels or flattened, compound capitula. The peduncle divides in ray-like fashion from one particular point. Each ray divides and forms further umbels with white flowers. The outer flowers are irregular and larger than the others. The florets are small. When in bloom, the flower head is flattened or slightly convex. When they are ripe, the flowers draw together to form a cup-like structure. The double achaenes are formed in the fruit umbel. They are slightly flattened and have numerous bristles arranged in 5 rows.

Leaves, Stem and Root: The Carrot is a biennial, 30 cm to 1 m high cultivated plant with a fusiform, usually red root and numerous pinnate, segmented, hairy leaves. In the second year the plant produces a branched, angular stem with alternate jointed leaves, which terminates in the flowering umbels.

Habitat: Now found in its cultivated form all over the world.

Production: Carrots are the roots of Daucus carota. The ripe roots are harvested.

Other Names: Bird's Neat, Birds' Nest, Bees' Nest, Queen Annc's Lace, Philtron

ACTIONS AND PHARMACOLOGY

COMPOUNDS

Carotinoids: including alpha-, beta-, gamma-, zeta-carotene, lycopene

Volatile oil (very little): including, among others, p-cymene, limonene, dipenten, geraniol, alpha- and beta- caryophyllene

Polyynes: including falcarinol (carotatoxin)

Glucose: saccharose

EFFECTS

Carrot is a mild vermifuge. The essential oil has an initially stimulating, followed by a paralyzing effect on worms. In controlled animal tests, a temporary reduction of arterial blood pressure was observed. The pectin content is probably responsible for the severe constipating effect of the carrot. The essential oil has a mild bactericidal effect, especially on gram-positive bacteria. The drug has a positive effect on visual acuity and scotopic (twilight) vision, as well as being a mild diuretic.

INDICATIONS AND USAGE

The Carrot is an unreliable adjuvant in the treatment of oxyurias. It is a useful drug in pediatrics for tonsillitis, nutritional disorders and as a dietary agent for digestive disorders. It is also used in medicinal preparations for dermatological conditions such as photodermatosis and pigment anomalies. It is used in teas for intestinal parasites.

PRECAUTIONS AND ADVERSE REACTIONS

Health risks or side effects following the proper administration of designated therapeutic dosages are not recorded. The drug has a low potential for sensitization through skin contact.

DOSAGE

Mode of Administration: The drug is taken in a ground form or consumed as a juice or vegetable. It is found in ready made medicinal preparations.

Preparation: The carrot is finely grated and made into a juice or syrup.

LITERATURE

Gupta KR, Niranjan GS, (1982) Planta Med 46:240.

Harborne JB In: The Biology and Chemistry of the Umbelliferae, Ed. VN Heywood, Academic Press, London, 1971.

Ram AS, Devi HM, (1983) Indian J Bot 6(1):21.

Further information in:

Hausen B, Allergiepflanzen, Pflanzenallergene, ecomed Verlagsgesellsch. mbH, Landsberg 1988.

Kern W, List PH, Hörhammer L (Hrsg.), Hagers Handbuch der Pharmazeutischen Praxis, 4. Aufl., Bde 1-8, Springer Verlag Berlin, Heidelberg, New York, 1969.

Leung AY, Encyclopedia of Common Natural Ingredients Used in Food Drugs and Cosmetics, John Wiley & Sons Inc., New York 1980.

Delphinium Consolida

Larkspur

DESCRIPTION

Flower and Fruit: The flowers are in short racemes and are blue, pink or purple. The petals are fused to a helmet-like form with a honey spur at the back, which reaches into the back of the 5 sepals. There is usually only 1 glabrous ovary, but numerous stamens. The fruit is a follicle with black, flattened seeds, which have sharp edges and a scarred surface.

Leaves, Stem and Root: The plant grows from 15 to 40 cm. Larkspur is an annual and has a thin stem which is sparsely branched from the middle. The leaves are alternate and divided into narrow linear sections. The lowers ones are petioled and the upper ones sessile.

Habitat: Europe, U.S., especially the western U.S.

Production: Delphinium flower consists of the flowers of Delphinium consolida.

Not To Be Confused With: The flowers of Delphinium oriental.

Other Names: Knight's Spur, Lark Heel, Lark's Claw, Lark's Toe, Staggerweed

ACTIONS AND PHARMACOLOGY

COMPOUNDS

Diterpene alkaloids: including delphinine

EFFECTS

The presence of alkaloids has sometimes been described in the literature but they cannot always be found.

INDICATIONS AND USAGE

Preparations of delphinium flower are used as a diuretic and vermifuge, as a sedative and an appetite stimulant. In folk medicine, Larkspur is used occasionally as a diuretic. It was formerly as an anthelmintic.

The efficacy for the claimed applications is not documented.

PRECAUTIONS AND ADVERSE REACTIONS

Health risks or side effects following the proper administration of designated therapeutic dosages are not recorded.

OVERDOSAGE

Although the delphine has a paralyzing effect upon peripheral and motor nerve endings and the central nervous system, poisonings among humans by Delphinium consolida have never been observed.

Toxic dosages in animal experiments have led to death through asphyxiation (LD50 rabbits 1.5-3.0 mg/kg body weight, I.V.). Poisonings of animals with fatal results through Delphinium species are particularly frequent in the U.S.

DOSAGE

Mode of Administration: Since the efficacy of Delphinium and its preparations is not documented, a therapeutic administration cannot be recommended.

Preparation: Larkspur is found only in teas; often as an inactive ingredient.

Daily Dose: 1.5g.

LITERATURE

Gheorgiu A et al., Ann Pharm Frnac 22:49. 1964.

Further information in:

Kern W, List PH, Hörhammer L (Hrsg.), Hagers Handbuch der Pharmazeutischen Praxis, 4. Aufl., Bde 1-8, Springer Verlag Berlin, Heidelberg, New York, 1969.

Teuscher E, Lindequist U, Biogene Gifte - Biologie, Chemie, Pharmakologie, 2. Aufl., Fischer Verlag Stuttgart 1994.

Delphinium Staphisagria

Stavesacre

DESCRIPTION

Medicinal Parts: The medicinal parts are the ripe, dried seeds.

Flower and Fruit: The flowers are deep blue. The sections of the involucres are 13 to 20 mm long. The limb of the lateral honey-leaves gradually narrows to a claw. The follicles are 8 to 11 mm wide and swollen. The seeds are grayish-black, wrinkled and pitted. They are triangular or square and convex at the back. The seeds are about 2 cm long.

Leaves, Stem and Root: The plant is annual and has a 30 to 100 cm high stout, simple, patent-pilose stem. The leaves are

5 to 7 palmate or lobed, pubescent on both surfaces with a mixture of very short and longer hairs. The segments are entire-margined or 3-lobed, with ovate-lanceolate, or oblong, sharp-edged lobes.

Characteristics: The seeds are poisonous. They taste bitter and tingling and are odorless.

Habitat: The plant is found in Asia Minor and Europe and is cultivated in Italy and France.

Production: Stavesacre seeds are the seeds of Delphinium staphisagria.

Other Names: Lousewort

ACTIONS AND PHARMACOLOGY

COMPOUNDS

Diterpene alkaloids: main alkaloid delphinine, including, among others, the bi-diterpene alkaloids staphisine, staphisagroine

EFFECTS

Stavesacre has a similar effect to aconitine.

INDICATIONS AND USAGE

The plant was formerly used for neuralgia. Today, it is used almost exclusively in homeopathy for the treatment of various ailments. Washes and ointments are used for lice.

PRECAUTIONS AND ADVERSE REACTIONS

External administration of extracts of the drug leads to reddening, inflammation, and eczema. Internal administration could lead to inflammation of the throat, salivation, nausea, skin itching and urinary and stool urgency.

OVERDOSAGE

The intake of 2 teaspoonfuls of seeds leads to weakened pulse, stomach pain, labored breathing and collapse.

Treatment of poisoning consists of stomach and intestinal emptying (gastric lavage, sodium sulphate), and the administration of activated charcoal. Further treatment should proceed symptomatically (i.e. diazepam for spasms, sodium bicarbonate for acidoses, intubation and oxygen respiration may also be required).

DOSAGE

Mode of Administration: An extract from the seeds is used in homeopathic dilutions.

Storage: The drug should be stored cautiously, as it is poisonous.

LITERATURE

Micovic IV, J Serb Chem Soc 51:355. 1986.

Further information in:

Kern W, List PH, Hörhammer L (Hrsg.), Hagers Handbuch der Pharmazeutischen Praxis, 4. Aufl., Bde. 1-8, Springer Verlag Berlin, Heidelberg, New York, 1969.

Lewin L, Gifte und Vergiftungen, 6. Aufl., Nachdruck, Haug Verlag, Heidelberg 1992.

Madaus G, Lehrbuch der Biologischen Arzneimittel, Bde 1-3, Nachdruck, Georg Olms Verlag Hildesheim 1979.

Roth L, Daunderer M, Kormann K, Giftpflanzen, Pflanzengifte, 4. Aufl., Ecomed Fachverlag Landsberg Lech 1993.

Teuscher E, Lindequist U, Biogene Gifte - Biologie, Chemie, Pharmakologie, 2. Aufl., Fischer Verlag Stuttgart 1994.

Wagner H, Wiesenauer M, Phytotherapie. Phytopharmaka und pflanzliche Homöopathika, Fischer-Verlag, Stuttgart, Jena, New York 1995.

Devil's Claw

See Harpagophytum Procumbens

Dicentra Cucullaria

Turkey Corn

DESCRIPTION

Medicinal Parts: The medicinal part is the dried tuber.

Flower and Fruit: The inflorescence is racemous. The 4 to 10 flowers are odorless, white and often tinged pink. The flowers are hanging, with yellow to yellow-orange tips and widely splayed spurs. The fruit is oval and 9 to 13 mm long. The seeds are reniform, 2 mm long, black and glossy.

Leaves, Stem and Root: Turkey Corn is a delicate, glabrous, 15 to 40 cm high plant on a tawny yellow, tuberous rhizome. The rhizome has subglobular, pink, smaller tubers about 0.5 cm in diameter, with a scar on both depressed sides. All the leaves are basal and almost triangular in outline. They are 3-pinnate and bluish-green on the underside.

Characteristics: The taste of the tuber is bitter.

Habitat: Canada and U.S.

Production: Turkey Corn root is the root of Dicentra cucullaria.

Other Names: Squirrel Corn, Staggerweed, Bleeding Heart, Corydalis, Dutchman's Breeches

ACTIONS AND PHARMACOLOGY

COMPOUNDS

Isoquinoline alkaloids: including bicuculline, corlumine, protopine, cryptopine, cularine

EFFECTS

Diuretic and tonic.

INDICATIONS AND USAGE

Turkey corn is used for digestive disorders, urinary tract diseases, menstrual disorders, and skin rashes.

PRECAUTIONS AND ADVERSE REACTIONS

Health risks or side effects following the proper administration of designated therapeutic dosages are not recorded. Bicuculline is a centrally-acting, spasmogenic antagonist of gamma-aminobutyric acid (GABA). Poisonings are therefore conceivable with intakes of higher dosages, but nevertheless have not been observed.

DOSAGE

Mode of Administration: The drug is available as a liquid extract.

LITERATURE

Kanamori H, Sakamoto I, Mizuta M, Chem Pharm Bull 34:1826. 1986.

Manske RHF, Canad J Res 7:265-269. 1932.

Manske RHF, Canad J Res Sect B 16:81-90. 1938.

Tusboi NS, J Labelled compd Radiopharm 13:353. 1977.

Further information in:

Hänsel R, Keller K, Rimpler H, Schneider G (Hrsg.), Hagers Handbuch der Pharmazeutischen Praxis, 5. Aufl., Bde 4-6 (Drogen): Springer Verlag Berlin, Heidelberg, New York, 1992-1994.

Madaus G, Lehrbuch der Biologischen Arzneimittel, Bde 1-3, Nachdruck, Georg Olms Verlag Hildesheim 1979.

Roth L, Daunderer M, Kormann K, Giftpflanzen, Pflanzengifte, 4. Aufl., Ecomed Fachverlag Landsberg Lech 1993.

Steinegger E, Hänsel R, Pharmakognosie, 5. Aufl., Springer Verlag Heidelberg 1992.

Teuscher E, Lindequist U, Biogene Gifte - Biologie, Chemie, Pharmakologie, 2. Aufl., Fischer Verlag Stuttgart 1994.

Dictamnus Albus

Burning Bush

DESCRIPTION

Medicinal Parts: The medicinal parts are the dried and occasionally the fresh leaves, the fresh or dried root, and the fresh or dried root rind.

Flower and Fruit: The flowers are terminal racemes and pink with dark veins. They are large and irregular, with 5 sepals and 5 petals. There are 2 bracteoles and are slightly zygomorphous. The 10 stamens are long, threadlike, and bent forward. The ovaries have 5 carpels fused at the base, on a short gynophore. The fruit is capsule which bursts open into mericarps ejecting the seeds.

Leaves, Stem and Root: The plant is a 0.5 to 1.5 m high perennial. Numerous erect, unbranched, and sticky-glandular-haired shoots grow from the root. The leaves are alternate, odd, 7 to 11 pinnate, and transparently punctuated with oil glands.

Characteristics: The plant has a strong lemon or cinnamon fragrance. The oil is easily inflammable.

Habitat: The plant is indigenous to Central Europe, parts of Asia, and cultivated in the northern U.S.

Not To Be Confused With: The name of the herb can be confused with that of Herba Dictamni cretici. Confusion with Carophyllaceen roots has been mentioned by previous sources.

Other Names: Fraxinella, Dittany, Gas Plant, Diptam

ACTIONS AND PHARMACOLOGY

COMPOUNDS: DICTAMNI ALBI RADIX

Volatile oil: chief components are the fraxinellone derivatives, thymol methylether, beta-pinenes, pregeijerene, geijerene

Furoquinoline alkaloids: including skimmianine, gamma-fagarine, dictamnine

Limonoids: including limonin, obacunone, dictamdiol, limonin diosphenol

EFFECTS: DICTAMNI ALBI RADIX

The drug is a contraceptive. It has also been used to promote hair growth. In folk medicine, the drug is used as a diuretic and spasmolytic.

COMPOUNDS: DICTAMNI ALBI HERBA

Volatile oil: chief components (according to breed) anethole + estragole, anethole + myrcene, limonene, 1,8-cineol, p-cymene + estragole

Furoquinoline alkaloids: including skimmianine, gamma-fagarine, dictamnine

Furocoumarins: including psoralen, xanthotoxin, auraptene, bergapten

Limonoids: including limonin, obacunone, obacunone acid

Flavonoids: including rutin, diosmin

EFFECTS: DICTAMNI ALBI HERBA

When doses of the restricted extract were given to infected cats, this caused a 40% reduction in the laying of (its) eggs by Clonorchis sinensis.

INDICATIONS AND USAGE

DICTAMNI ALBI RADIX

The drug is used for digestive disorders and diseases of the urinary tract. In the middle ages, the drug was used for worm infestations, hysteria, epilepsy, desiccation, and to promote menstruation. Today, the drug is still employed in the treatment of uro-genital disorders and Fluor albus.

In China and Korea, the root is applied in cases of hepatitis, inflammation of the skin, rheumatic ailments, fever, hemorrhage of the womb, thread fungus, as a sedative, tonic, and for upset children crying (in a nervous state). Also found in decoctions for the external treatment of eczema, impetigo, and scabies. In India, diluted extracts are used for amenorrhea and birth control.

Efficacy of the listed applications has not been clinically proven.

DICTAMNI ALBI HERBA

In the middle ages, the drug was used as a cure or remedy for wounds, to promote menstruation, and to aid the expulsion of the afterbirth. It served as a urinary aid and was used in the treatment of epilepsy, in combination with mistletoe and peony.

At the end of the 19th century, the drug was applied as an ointment for rheumatism. The infusion is used to treat stomach disorders, cramps and as a remedy for worm infestation, and to promote menstruation. In Greece, it is used as a tonic and as a stimulant.

Efficacy has not been proven.

PRECAUTIONS AND ADVERSE REACTIONS

DICTAMNI ALBI RADIX AND HERBA

Health risks or side effects following the proper administration of designated therapeutic dosages are not recorded. The plant can trigger phototoxicoses through skin contact.

DOSAGE

DICTAMNI ALBI HERBA

Mode of Administration: The herb is used internally as an infusion, and is occasionally found in medicinal preparations.

Infusion is prepared by adding 20 gm of the dried herb to 1 liter of water, or 1 gm fresh or 2 gm dried drug to 1 cup of water.

Daily Dosage: Drink one cup of the infusion, 3 times daily; drink one cup after main meals, twice daily.

DICTAMNI ALBI RADIX

Mode of Administration: Mostly obsolete as a drug. Occasionally it is used in tea mixtures and as an ingredient found in Swedish herbal mixtures.

Preparation: To prepare a tea infusion, add 1 teaspoon of the drug to 2 glasses of hot water.

Daily Dosage: Drink the tea preparation during the course of the day.

LITERATURE

DICTAMNI ALBI RADIX

Kanamori H, Sakamoto I, Mizuta M, Chem Pharm Bull 34:1826. 1986.

Reisch J, PM 15:320. 1967.

Renner W, PA 12:763-776. 1962.

Renner W, PA 17:763. 1962.

Szenedrei K, Novak I, Varga E, Buzas G, PA 23:76-77. 1968.

Further information in:

Hänsel R, Keller K, Rimpler H, Schneider G (Hrsg.), Hagers Handbuch der Pharmazeutischen Praxis, 5. Aufl., Bde 4-6 (Drogen), Springer Verlag Berlin, Heidelberg, New York, 1992-1994.

Hausen B, Allergiepflanzen, Pflanzenallergene, ecomed Verlagsgesellsch. mbH, Landsberg 1988.

Madaus G, Lehrbuch der Biologischen Arzneimittel, Bde 1-3, Nachdruck, Georg Olms Verlag Hildesheim 1979.

Roth L, Daunderer M, Kormann K, Giftpflanzen, Pflanzengifte, 4. Aufl., Ecomed Fachverlag Landsberg Lech 1993.

Teuscher E, Lindequist U, Biogene Gifte - Biologie, Chemie, Pharmakologie, 2. Aufl. Fischer Verlag Stuttgart 1994.

DICTAMNI ALBI HERBA

Kanamori H, Sakamoto I, Mizuta M, Chem Pharm Bull 34:1826. 1986.

Reisch J, PM 15:320. 1967.

Renner W, PA 12:763-776. 1962.

Renner W, PA 17:763. 1962.

Szenedrei K, Novak I, Varga E, Buzas G, PA 23:76-77. 1968.

Further information in:

Hänsel R, Keller K, Rimpler H, Schneider G (Hrsg.), Hagers Handbuch der Pharmazeutischen Praxis, 5. Aufl., Bde 4-6 (Drogen), Springer Verlag Berlin, Heidelberg, New York, 1992-1994.

Hausen B, Allergiepflanzen, Pflanzenallergene, ecomed Verlagsgesellsch. mbH, Landsberg 1988.

Madaus G, Lehrbuch der Biologischen Arzneimittel, Bde 1-3, Nachdruck, Georg Olms Verlag Hildesheim 1979.

Roth L, Daunderer M, Kormann K, Giftpflanzen, Pflanzengifte, 4. Aufl., Ecomed Fachverlag Landsberg Lech 1993.

Teuscher E, Lindequist U, Biogene Gifte - Biologie, Chemie, Pharmakologie, 2. Aufl., Fischer Verlag Stuttgart 1994.

Digitalis Purpurea

Foxglove

DESCRIPTION

Medicinal Parts: The medicinal parts are the dried leaves (a powder of these), the ripe dried seeds, the fresh leaves of the 1-year-old plant or the leaves of the 2-year-old plant collected at the beginning of flowering. In the past, the drug of Digitalis purpurae was the raw material employed in isolating the cardiac glycosides. Today, Digitalis Iantana is used.

Flower and Fruit: The flowers are carmine red with white-edged spots on the inside. The flowers appear in long hanging racemes. They have 5 free, short-tipped sepals. The corolla is about 4 cm long, campanulate, bilabiate with an obtuse upper lip and an ovate tip on the lower lip. The flower is glabrous on the outside and has a white awn on the inside. There are 2 long and 2 short stamens and 1 superior ovary. The fruit is a 2-valved, ovate, glandular villous capsule.

Leaves, Stem and Root: The plant is a biennial with a branched tap root. In the first year it develops a leaf rosette. In the second it produces a 2 m high, erect, unbranched, gray, tomentose stem. The leaves are alternate, ovate, tapering upwards and petiolate. Almost all leaves are crenate; only the highest ones are entire-margined.

Characteristics: The plant is very poisonous; tastes hot-bitter with a slightly unpleasant odor.

Habitat: Foxglove is indigenous to Europe. Introduced to the east and the American continent.

Production: Foxglove leaves are the leaves of Digitalis purpurea or of Digitalis lanata. Digitalis lanata corresponds to Digitalis purpurea but has a milder effect. The rose leaves are harvested during the first period of vegetation in early autumn. The drying period is decisive for the content of cardenolide glycosides. The temperature for drying is 30°C to 50°C.

Not To Be Confused With: Confusion seldom occurs due to cultivation under controlled conditions.

Other Names: Digitalis, Dead Men's Bells, Dog's Finger, Fairy Fingers, Fairy Gloves, Finger Flower, Folks' Glove, Lion's Mouth, Ladies' Glove, Witches' Gloves, Gloves of Our Lady, Fairy Caps, Fairy Thimbles, Virgin's Glove

ACTIONS AND PHARMACOLOGY

COMPOUNDS

Cardioactive steroid glycosides (cardenolides): including from the A-sequence (aglycone digitoxigenin) purpurea glycoside A (primary glycoside), digitoxin (secondary glycoside)

B-sequence (aglycone gitoxigenin): purpurea glycoside B (primary glycoside), gitoxin (secondary glycoside), Digitalinum verum

E-sequence (aglycone gitaloxigenin): glucoverodoxin, glucogitaloxin, gitaloxin

Pregnane glycosides: including digipurpurin, diginin, digitalonin

Steroid saponin: including desgalactotigonin, digitonine, purpureagitoside

Anthraquinones

EFFECTS

Foxglove stimulates contraction of the heart muscles, reduces the frequency of heartbeat and lowers the oxygen requirement of the heart (in relation to performance).

INDICATIONS AND USAGE

In folk medicine, the drug's use originated in Ireland, then came to Scotland and England and finally to central Europe. It was used to treat ulcers in the lower abdomen, boils, headaches, abscesses, and paralysis. Externally, the drug was used for the granulation of poorly healing wounds and to cure ulcers. Furthermore, the drug was used for cardiac insufficiency, especially high blood pressure.

Efficacy of the listed applications has not been proven.

PRECAUTIONS AND ADVERSE REACTIONS

General: Because of the narrow therapeutic range of digitalis glycosides, a certain percentage of patients may experience side effects immediately upon administration of therapeutic dosages: hypertonia in gastrointestinal area, loss of appetite, vomiting, diarrhea and headache.

Drug Interactions: The simultaneous administration of arrhythmogenic substances (sympathomimetics, methylxanthines, phosphodiesterase inhibitors, quinidine) increases the risks of the appearance of cardiac arrhythmias.

OVERDOSAGE

With overdosage, in addition to the already-mentioned symptoms, the following can also occur:

Heart: cardiac rhythm disorders, all the way up to life-threatening ventricular tachycardia, atrial tachycardia with atrioventricular block

Central nervous system: stupor, visual disorders, depression, confused states, hallucinations, psychoses

Lethal dosages lead to heart failure or asphyxiation. Administration over extended periods leads in rare cases to gynecomastia. Because of the difficulties in standardizing the drug, the administration of pure glycosides is to be preferred (digitoxin).

The first measures to be taken in case of poisoning are gastric lavage and activated charcoal instillation. All other measures proceed according to the symptoms. For loss of potassium, careful replenishment is necessary. For ectopic irritation build-up in the ventricle, administration of phenytoin as an antiarrhythmatic is recommended. Lidocaine should be used in cases of ventricular extrasystole, and for partial atrioventricular block, atropine is recommended. The prophylactic installation of a pacemaker is often necessary. For elimination of the glycosides hemoperfusion is possible, the administration of cholestyramine for interrrupting the enterohepatic circulation and/or the application of digitoxin antibodies (antigen-binding fragments, digitalis antidote (Boehringer Mannheim), is very likely only fully effective with digitoxin poisoning).

The drugs and pure glycosides should be administered in the following situations (among others) atrioventricular block of the 2nd and 3rd degree, hypercalcaemia, hypocalcaemia, hypertrophic cardiomyopathy, carotid sinus syndrome, ventricular tachycardia, thoracic aortic aneurysm, WPW-syndrome.

DOSAGE

Mode of Administration: Today, the drug is obsolete. Due to the lack of reproductivity of content, the use of appropriate pure glycosides is advisable. Digitoxin is contained in mono preparations (extract) and used as an isolated pure substance.

Preparation: Tincture: shaken for 1 day in 25% ethanol at a ratio of 1:10.

The manufacture of the digoxin and digitoxin is a complicated process that involves fermentation, extraction, and evaporation.

Storage: Store carefully away from sources of light.

LITERATURE

Brisse B, Anwendung pflanzlicher Wirkstoffe bei kardialen Erkrankungen. In: ZPT 10(4):107. 1989.

Buschauer A, Entwicklung neuer positiv inotroper Arzneistoffe: Suche nach einm ''Digitalisersatz''. In: PZW 134(1)3. 1989.

Cohn JN, (1974) J Am Med Ass 229: 1911.

Höltje HD, Molecular Modelling von Digitaloiden. In: PZ 137(37):2812. 1992.

Ikeda Y et al., Quantitative HPLC analysis of cardiac glycosides in Digitalis purpurea. In: JNP 58(6):897-901. 1995.

Lichius JJ, Weber R, Kirschke M, Liedtke S, Brieger D, Neues vom Fingerhut und seinen Kaffeesäureestern. In: DAZ 135(40):3794-3800. 1995.

Lustenberger, B, In: Lustenberger J (Basler Dissertationen zur Geschichte der Pharmazie und Naturwissenschaften, Bd. 4), Der Weg zur Etablierung der Reinglykoside in der Digitalistherapie. Juris Druck - Verlag Dietikon. 1993.

Rall B, Herzinsuffizienz: Was bringt die Digitalis-Therapie? In: DAZ 137(3):126-27. 1997.

Thomas R et al., (1974) J Pharm Sci 63:1649.

Tschesche R, Brügmann G, Tetrahedron 20:1469-1475. 1964.

Voigt G, Hiller K, Sci Pharm 55:201-207. 1987.

Wichtl M, Bühl W, Huesmann G, DAZ 127:2391-2400. 1987.

Further information in:

Frohne D, Pfänder HJ, Giftpflanzen - Ein Handbuch für Apotheker, Toxikologen und Biologen, 4. Aufl., Wiss. Verlagsges. mbH Stuttgart 1997.

Hänsel R, Keller K, Rimpler H, Schneider G (Hrsg.), Hagers Handbuch der Pharmazeutischen Praxis, 5. Aufl., Bde 4-6 (Drogen), Springer Verlag Berlin, Heidelberg, New York, 1992-1994.

Lewin L, Gifte und Vergiftungen, 6. Aufl., Nachdruck, Haug Verlag, Heidelberg 1992.

Madaus G, Lehrbuch der Biologischen Arzneimittel, Bde 1-3, Nachdruck, Georg Olms Verlag Hildesheim 1979.

Roth L, Daunderer M, Kormann K, Giftpflanzen, Pflanzengifte, 4. Aufl., Ecomed Fachverlag Landsberg Lech 1993.

Steinegger E, Hänsel R, Pharmakognosie, 5. Aufl., Springer Verlag Heidelberg 1992.

Teuscher E, Lindequist U, Biogene Gifte - Biologie, Chemie, Pharmakologie, 2. Aufl., Fischer Verlag Stuttgart 1994.

Teuscher E, Biogene Arzneimittel, 5. Aufl., Wiss. Verlagsges. mbH Stuttgart 1997.

Wagner H, Wiesenauer M, Phytotherapie. Phytopharmaka und pflanzliche Homöopathika, Fischer-Verlag, Stuttgart, Jena, New York 1995.

Dill

See Anethum Graveolens

Dioscorea Villosa

Wild Yam

DESCRIPTION

Medicinal Parts: The medicinal part is the dried rhizome with the roots.

Flower and Fruit: The plant has small greenish-yellow flowers. The male flowers are in drooping panicles; the female ones in drooping spicate racemes.

Leaves, Stem and Root: Dioscorea villosa is a perennial vine. It has a pale brown, cylindrical, twisted, tuberous rhizome and a thin, woolly, reddish-brown stem that measures up to 12 m long. The leaves are broadly ovate, usually alternating, cordate and 6 to 14 cm long. The upper surface is glabrous and they are pubescent beneath. The fracture is short and hard.

Characteristics: The taste is insipid at first, then acrid. The leaves are odorless.

Habitat: The plant is indigenous to the Southern U.S. and Canada. It is now widely cultivated in many parts of the world in tropical, subtropical and temperate regions.

Other Names: China Root, Colic Root, Devil's Bones, Rheumatism Root, Yuma

ACTIONS AND PHARMACOLOGY

COMPOUNDS

Saponins: including dioscin (aglycone diosgenin)

Isoquinuclidine alkaloids: including dioscorin

EFFECTS

Anti-inflammatory, cholagogue, antispasmodic, and a mild diaphoretic.

INDICATIONS AND USAGE

Wild Yam is used for rheumatic conditions, gallbladder colic, dysmenorrhea and cramps.

Industrially used as an active agent in the half-synthesis of steroid hormones and for the manufacture of homeopathic preparations.

PRECAUTIONS AND ADVERSE REACTIONS

Health risks or side effects following the proper administration of designated therapeutic dosages are not recorded.

OVERDOSAGE

Poisoning is conceivable with overdosages because of the picrotoxin-like effect of dioscorin (see Cocculi fructus).

DOSAGE

Mode of Administration: Liquid extract.

LITERATURE

Hegnauer R, Chemotaxonomie der Pflanzen, Bde 1-11, Birkhäuser Verlag Basel, Boston, Berlin 1962-1997.

Kern W, List PH, Hörhammer L (Hrsg.), Hagers Handbuch der Pharmazeutischen Praxis, 4. Aufl., Bde 1-8, Springer Verlag Berlin, Heidelberg, New York, 1969.

Madaus G, Lehrbuch der Biologischen Arzneimittel, Bde 1-3, Nachdruck, Georg Olms Verlag Hildesheim 1979.

Dipsacus Silvestris

Teazle

DESCRIPTION

Medicinal Parts: The medicinal part is the whole flowering plant with root.

Flower and Fruit: The flowers are lilac with 8 cm long, cylindrical capitula. The bracts are lanceolate-awl-shaped, curved upwards, thorny and longer than the capitulum. The long outer bract with its straight tip is longer than the flowers. The calyx is basin-shaped and the corolla is fused with 4 tips. There are 4 stamens and 1 inferior ovary. The fruit is a nutlet.

Leaves, Stem and Root: The plant is a biennial that grows 80 to 150 cm high. The stem is erect, angular, and thorny. The basal leaves are rosette-like, crenate-serrate. The cauline leaves are oblong with a thorny midrib underneath.

Habitat: The plant grows in southern England.

Production: Common Teazle root is the underground part of Dipsacus silvestris.

Other Names: Barber's Brush, Brushes and Combs, Card Thistle, Church Broom, Venus' Basin

ACTIONS AND PHARMACOLOGY

COMPOUNDS

Iridoide monoterpenes: including cantleyoside, loganin, sweroside, sylvestroside III and IV

Caffeic acid derivatives: including chlorogenic acid

EFFECTS

No information is available.

INDICATIONS AND USAGE

Theazle is used externally for small wounds, fistulae, psoriasis and as a rub in the treatment of rheumatism.

PRECAUTIONS AND ADVERSE REACTIONS

Health risks or side effects following the proper administration of designated therapeutic dosages are not recorded.

DOSAGE

Mode of Administration: Teazle is used externally in alcoholic extracts.

LITERATURE

Hegnauer R, Chemotaxonomie der Pflanzen, Bde 1-11, Birkhäuser Verlag Basel, Boston, Berlin 1962-1997.

Kern W, List PH, Hörhammer L (Hrsg.), Hagers Handbuch der Pharmazeutischen Praxis, 4. Aufl., Bde. 1-8, Springer Verlag Berlin, Heidelberg, New York, 1969.

Madaus G, Lehrbuch der Biologischen Arzneimittel, Bde 1-3, Nachdruck, Georg Olms Verlag Hildesheim 1979.

Dipteryx Odorata

Tonka Beans

DESCRIPTION

Medicinal Parts: The medicinal part is the bean.

Flower and Fruit: The beans are usually 2 to 5 cm long and 1 cm in diameter. They have a grayish or black color.

Characteristics: The bean has a characteristic odor, like new mown hay of coumarin.

Habitat: South America.

Other Names: Tonquin Bean

ACTIONS AND PHARMACOLOGY

COMPOUNDS

Coumarin (1-3% to 10%)

Fatty oil

EFFECTS

Tonic and aromatic.

INDICATIONS AND USAGE

Whooping cough (no longer used).

PRECAUTIONS AND ADVERSE REACTIONS

Health risks or side effects following the proper administration of designated therapeutic dosages are not recorded. The therapeutic administration of drugs containing coumarin can lead to slight liver damage (elevated liver enzyme values in the blood) in a very small number of patients, that is, however, reversible following discontinuance of the drug.

OVERDOSAGE

The intake of very high dosages (4 g coumarin, equivalent to 150 g of the drug) could bring about stupor, headache, nausea and vomiting.

DOSAGE

Mode of Administration: Tonka Beans are obsolete as a drug.

LITERATURE

Sullivan G, (1968) J Agric Food Chem 30(3):609.

Further information in:

Lewin L, Gifte und Vergiftungen, 6. Aufl., Nachdruck, Haug Verlag, Heidelberg 1992.

Roth L, Daunderer M, Kormann K, Giftpflanzen, Pflanzengifte, 4. Aufl., Ecomed Fachverlag Landsberg Lech 1993.

Steinegger E, Hänsel R, Pharmakognosie, 5. Aufl., Springer Verlag Heidelberg 1992.

Teuscher E, Lindequist U, Biogene Gifte - Biologie, Chemie, Pharmakologie, 2. Aufl., Fischer Verlag Stuttgart 1994.

Divi-Divi

See Caesalpinia Bonducella

Dodder

See Cuscuta Epithymum

Dogwood

See Cornus Florida

Dorstenia Contrayerva

Contrayerva

DESCRIPTION

Medicinal Parts: The medicinal parts are the roots of a number of species.

Flower and Fruit: The plant has long-pedicled, greenish flowers.

Leaves, Stem and Root: The plant is a perennial, growing to a height of up to 30 cm. It is stemless with palmate leaves. The rhizome is about 2 to 4 cm long and 1 cm thick. It is reddish-brown on the outside, paler on the inside and rough with leaf scars. The rhizome is nearly cylindrical and tapers suddenly at the end into a tail-like root with numerous curled, wiry rootlets.

Characteristics: The taste is slightly aromatic, then acrid.

Habitat: Contrayerva is found in Mexico, Peru and the West Indies.

Production: Contrayerva root is the rhizome of Dorstenia contrayerva and related varieties.

ACTIONS AND PHARMACOLOGY

COMPOUNDS

Cardioactive steroids (cardenolides): syriogenin

Furocoumarins

EFFECTS

Diaphoretic and stimulant.

INDICATIONS AND USAGE

Preparations of the root are used as a stimulant to treat low stamina. Also has been used as an antidote for snakebite (uncertain mechanism).

PRECAUTIONS AND ADVERSE REACTIONS

Health risks or side effects following the proper administration of designated therapeutic dosages are not recorded. The plant can trigger phototoxicoses through skin contact.

DOSAGE

Mode of Administration: Ground root as an infusion.

LITERATURE

Casagrande C et al., Tetrahedron 30:3587. 1974.

Further information in:

Hegnauer R, Chemotaxonomie der Pflanzen, Bde 1-11, Birkhäuser Verlag Basel, Boston, Berlin 1962-1997.

Kanamori H, Sakamoto I, Mizuta M, Chem Pharm Bull 34:1826. 1986.

Renner W, PA 17:763. 1962.

Reisch J, PM 15:320. 1967.

Szenedrei K, Novak I, Varga E, Buzas G, PA 23:76-77. 1968.

Renner W, PA 12:763-776. 1962.

Lewin L, Gifte und Vergiftungen, 6. Aufl., Nachdruck, Haug Verlag, Heidelberg 1992.

Dragon's Blood

See Daemonorops Draco

Drimia Maritima

Squill

DESCRIPTION

Medicinal Parts: The medicinal parts come from the bulbs of the white latex variety collected after flowering and the fresh, fleshy bulb scales of the white variety and of the red variety.

Flower and Fruit: The flowering stem is erect and 50 to 150 cm high. It is often a washed purple color and glabrous. The flowers, which often number 100, are arranged in richly flowered, dense racemes up to 60 cm long. The bracts are membranous and pointed. They are shorter than the pedicles and drop early. The pedicles are up to 3 cm long, thin and smooth. The flowers are white, radial and star-shaped. The ovary is ovate to oblong triangular. The capsule is ovate to oblong, 3-valved, obtuse or almost pointed. Each chamber has 1 to 4 seeds, which are elongate, flattened, smooth, glossy and winged.

Leaves, Stem and Root: The plant is a perennial bulb plant. The bulbs are pear-shaped, about 15 to 30 cm in diameter. They are rarely sold whole commercially, as they tend to start growing. The fracture is short, tough and flexible.

Characteristics: The taste is bitter and acrid.

Habitat: Indigenous to the Mediterranean and is cultivated there too.

Production: Squill consists of the sliced, dried, fleshy middle scales of the onion of the white variety of Urginea maritima, harvested during the flowering season.

Other Names: Scilla

ACTIONS AND PHARMACOLOGY

COMPOUNDS

Cardioactive steroid glycosides (bufadienolides, 1-3%): chief components glucoscillarene A, proscillaridin A, scillarene A; including, among others, scillicyanoside, scilliglaucoside

Mucilage

EFFECTS

The drug is inotropic on myocardial work capacity and negatively chronotropic. The overall effect is economy of heart action. There is a lowering of increased, left ventricular diastolic pressure and pathologically elevated venous pressure.

INDICATIONS AND USAGE

- Cardiac insufficiency NYHA I and II
- Arrhythmia
- Nervous heart complaints
- Venous conditions

Squill is used for milder cases of cardiac insufficiency, also for reduced kidney capacity.

CONTRAINDICATIONS

The drug and pure glycosides, among others, should not be administered in the presence of second or third degree atrioventricular blocks, hypercalcaemia, hypokaliemia, hypertrophic cardiomyopathy, carotid sinus syndrome, ventricular tachycardia, thoracic aortic aneurysm, WPW-syndrome.

PRECAUTIONS AND ADVERSE REACTIONS

General: No health hazards are known in conjunction with the proper administration of designated therapeutic dosages. Because of the narrow therapeutic range of cardioactive steroid glycosides, side effects could appear among a variety of patients immediately upon receiving even therapeutic dosages: tonus elevation in the gastrointestinal area, loss of appetite, vomiting, diarrhea, headache and irregular pulse.

Contact with the juice of the fresh bulb can lead to skin inflammations (squill dermatitis). The administration of pure glycosides is preferable due to the difficulties of standardizing the drug (proscillaridin A).

Drug Interactions: Increase of effectiveness and thus also of side effects is possible with concomitant administration of quinidine, calcium, saluretics, laxatives and extended therapy with glucocorticoids.

The simultaneous administraton of arrhythmogenic substances (sympathomimetics, methylxanthines, phosphodiesterase inhibitors, quinidine) increases the risk of the appearance of cardiac arrhythmias.

OVERDOSAGE

Besides the already-mentioned symptoms, overdosage can lead to cardiac rhythm disorders, life-threatening ventricular tachycardias, atrial tachycardias with atrioventricular block, stupor, vision disorders, depression, confused states, hallucinations and psychosis. Fatal dosages lead to cardiac arrest or asphyxiation.

Treatment of poisoning includes gastric lavage and instillation of activated charcoal. All other measures are to be carried out according to the symptoms. In case of potassium loss, careful replenishment; for ectopic impulse formation in the ventricle, administration of phenytoin as antiarrhythmic drug; lidocaine for ventricular extrasystole; for pronounced bradycardia, atropine or orciprenaline. The prophylactic use of a pacemaker is recommended. Hemoperfusion for eliminating the glycosides or the administration of cholestyramine for interrupting the enterohepatic circulation are possible.

DOSAGE

Mode of Administration: Comminuted drug and other galenic preparations for internal use.

Daily Dose: Average daily dosage: 0.1 to 0.5 g of standardized sea onion powder.

LITERATURE

Brisse B, Anwendung pflanzlicher Wirkstoffe bei kardialen Erkrankungen. In: ZPT 10(4):107. 1989.

Eichstädt H, Hansen G, Danne O, Koch HP, Minge C, Richter W, Schröder R, Die positiv inotrope Wirkung eines Scilla-Extraktes nach Einmal-Applikation. In: ZPT 12(2):46. 1991.

Garcia-Casado P et al., (1977) Pharm Acta Helv 52:218.

Hakim FS, Evans FJ, (1976) Pharm Acta Helv 52:117.

Kamano Y, Satoh N, Nakayoshi H, Pettit GR, Smith CR, Rhinovirus inhibition by bufadienolides. In: Chem Pharm Bull 36:326-332. 1988.

Karawya MS et al., (1973) Planta Med 23:213.

Kopp B, Krenn L, Jurenitsch J, Bufadienolide in Meerzwiebeln. In: DAZ 130(40):2175. 1990.

Krenn L, Ferth R, Robien W, Kopp B, Bufadienolide aus Urginea-maritima-sensu-strictu. In: PM 57:560. 1991.

Krenn L, Kopp B, 9-Hydroxyscilliphaeosid, a new bufadienolide from Urginea maritima. In: JNP 59(6):612-613. 1996.

Loew D, Phytotherapie bei Herzinsuffizienz. In: ZPT 18(2):92-96. 1997.

Loew DA, Loew AD, Pharmakokinetik von herzglykosidhaltigen Pflanzenextrakten. In: ZPT 15(4):197-202. 1994.

Majinda RRT et al., Bufadienolides and other constituents of Urginea sanguinea. In: PM 63(2):188-190. 1997.

Mathic C, Ourrison G, (1964) Phytochemistry 3:115, 133, 377 et 379.

Sato, Muro T, Antiviral activity of scillarenin, a plant bufadienolide. In: Jap J Microbiol 18:441-448. 1974.

Vega FA, (1976) An Rev Acad Farm. 42(1):81.

Further information in:

Frohne D, Pfänder HJ, Giftpflanzen - Ein Handbuch für Apotheker, Toxikologen und Biologen, 4. Aufl., Wiss. Verlags-Ges. Stuttgart 1997.

Hänsel R, Keller K, Rimpler H, Schneider G (Hrsg.), Hagers Handbuch der Pharmazeutischen Praxis, 5. Aufl., Bde 4-6 (Drogen): Springer Verlag Berlin, Heidelberg, New York, 1992-1994.

Leung AY, Encyclopedia of Common Natural Ingredients Used in Food Drugs, Cosmetics, John Wiley & Sons Inc., New York 1980.

Lewin L, Gifte und Vergiftungen, 6. Aufl., Nachdruck, Haug Verlag, Heidelberg 1992.

Madaus G, Lehrbuch der Biologischen Arzneimittel, Bde 1-3, Nachdruck, Georg Olms Verlag Hildesheim 1979.

Roth L, Daunderer M, Kormann K, Giftpflanzen, Pflanzengifte, 4. Aufl., Ecomed Fachverlag Landsberg Lech 1993.

Schulz R, Hänsel R, Rationale Phytotherapie, Springer Verlag Heidelberg 1996.

Steinegger E, Hänsel R, Pharmakognosie, 5. Aufl., Springer Verlag Heidelberg 1992.

Teuscher E, Lindequist U, Biogene Gifte - Biologie, Chemie, Pharmakologie, 2. Aufl., Fischer Verlag Stuttgart 1994.

Teuscher E, Biogene Arzneimittel, 5. Aufl., Wiss. Verlagsges. Stuttgart 1997.

Wagner H, Wiesenauer M, Phytotherapie. Phytopharmaka und pflanzliche Homöopathika, Fischer-Verlag, Stuttgart, Jena, New York 1995.

Drimys Winteri

Winter's Bark

DESCRIPTION

Medicinal Parts: The medicinal part is the dried bark of the trunk and larger branches.

Flower and Fruit: The flowers are solitary or in umbels and often in clusters at the tips of the branches. They are fragrant and white. The sepals are membranous, broadly ovate to reniform. The 4 to 14 petals are also membranous, oblong to narrow-ovate. The 15 to 40 stamens are in 2 to 4 rows. The 2 to 10 carpels are free, ovate or elliptical. There are 9 to 18 ovules on a short seed stalk. The fruit is berry-like, black to violet, fleshy and usually contains 2 or 3 seeds in bushels.

Leaves, Stem and Root: The plant is an evergreen tree or shrub, with brownish or gray wrinkled branches. The bark is a romatic and smooth. The leaf blade is coriaceous, oblong-ovate to elliptical, with a somewhat revolute margin. The undersurface is usually punctate.

Characteristics: Astringent taste and mild smell.

Habitat: The plant is found from central Chile to Cape Horn and in neighboring Argentina.

Production: Genuine Winter's Bark is the bark of Drimys winteri, from the dried trunk or produced from the stronger branches.

Not To Be Confused With: The drug is often confused with Cortex Canellae albae and with the bark of Cinnamodendron corticosum.

Other Names: Pepper Bark, Winter's Cinnamon, Wintera Aromatica, Wintera

ACTIONS AND PHARMACOLOGY

COMPOUNDS

Volatile oil: chief components eugenol, caryophyllene, 1,8-cineol, pinenes

Sesquiterpenes: including drimenol, drimenin, confertifoline, polygodial, isodrimenine, winterin, valdiviolide, fuegin, futranolide, cryptomeridiol, 1beta-p-cumaroyloxypolygodial, a trimeric sesquiterpene lactone

EFFECTS

The drug has carminative, stomachic, and tonic effects.

INDICATIONS AND USAGE

In South America, the drug is used for toothache, as a stomachic and for dermatitis. Other uses include digestive disorders, flatulence and colic.

Efficacy has not been proven.

PRECAUTIONS AND ADVERSE REACTIONS

Health risks or side effects following the proper administration of designated therapeutic dosages are not recorded.

DOSAGE

Mode of Administration: As an infusion and domestic herb.

LITERATURE

Hänsel R, Keller K, Rimpler H, Schneider G (Hrsg.), Hagers Handbuch der Pharmazeutischen Praxis, 5. Aufl., Bde 4-6 (Drogen): Springer Verlag Berlin, Heidelberg, New York, 1992-1994.

Hegnauer R, Chemotaxonomie der Pflanzen, Bde 1-11, Birkhäuser Verlag Basel, Boston, Berlin 1962-1997.

Morton JF, An Atlas of Medicinal Plants of Middle America, Charles C. Thomas USA 1981.

Drosera Rotundifolia

Sundew

DESCRIPTION

Medicinal Parts: The medicinal part is the whole herb.

Flower and Fruit: Size: The plant is from 7 to 20 cm tall. The flowers are white and arranged in racemes turned to one side. There are 5 sepals, 5 petals and 1 ovary with 3 to 5 styles. The fruit is capsular.

Leaves, Stem and Root: The leaves are basal rosette, long-petioled and thickly covered in red glandular hairs. The thickened ends have a drop of viscid juice to trap insects.

Characteristics: The herb has a sour, bitter, hot taste.

Habitat: Europe, India, China, North and South America, on wet and peat ground.

Production: Sundew consists of the dried, above- and below-ground parts of Drosera ramentacea.

Not To Be Confused With: Asian varieties.

Other Names: Dew Plant, Lustwort, Youthwort, Red Rot

ACTIONS AND PHARMACOLOGY

COMPOUNDS

Naphthaquinone derivatives:

if the source is Drosera rotundifolia: plumbagin, ramentaceone

if the source is Drosera ramentacea: ramentone, ramentaceone, biramentaceone, plumbagin

if the source is Drosera madagascariensis: 7-methyl juglone, plumbagin

if the source is Drosera peltata: plumbagin, droserone, 8-hydroxydroserone

EFFECTS

The drug has ecretolytic, broncho-spasmolytic, and antitussive effects.

INDICATIONS AND USAGE

■ Cough/bronchitis

Used for respiratory problems, particularly for coughing fits and dry coughs. In folk medicine, Sundew is used for asthma and warts.

PRECAUTIONS AND ADVERSE REACTIONS

Health risks or side effects following the proper administration of designated therapeutic dosages are not recorded.

DOSAGE

Mode of Administration: Liquid and solid preparations for external and internal application. The plant is a highly protected species and is in danger of extinction.

Preparation: To prepare an infusion, pour boiling water over 1 to 2 g drug and strain after 10 minutes.

Daily Dose: The average daily dose is 3 g drug. The dosage of the infusion when used as a broncholytic is 1 cup, 3 to 4 times daily.

LITERATURE

Ayuga C et al., (1985) An R Acad Farm 51(2):321.

Budzianowski J et al., Ellagic acid derivatives and further naphthoquinones from Dionea muscipula and four species of the genus Drosera in vitro cultures. In: PM 59(7):A654. 1993.

Croft S et al., (1985) Ann Trop Med Parasitol 79(6):651.

Franz G, Workshop über Sonnentaukraut. In: DAZ 135(47):4431-4433. 1995.

Krenn L, Länger R, Kopp B, DAZ 135:867. 1995.

Langer R, Kopp B, Qualitätsprüfung von Sonnentaukraut. In: DAZ 135(8):657-664. 1995.

Schilcher H, Elzer M, Drosera - der Sonnentau, ein bewährtes Antitussivum. In: ZPT 14(1):50. 1993.

Vichnanova SA et al., (1973) Planta Med (Suppl):185.

Wunderer H, Zentral und peripher wirksame Antitussiva: eine kritische Übersicht. In: PZ 142(11):847-852. 1997.

Zenk MH, Fürbringer M, Steglich W, PH 8:2199. 1969.

Further information in:

Kern W, List PH, Hörhammer L (Hrsg.), Hagers Handbuch der Pharmazeutischen Praxis, 4. Aufl., Bde 1-8, Springer Verlag Berlin, Heidelberg, New York, 1969.

Madaus G, Lehrbuch der Biologischen Arzneimittel, Bde 1-3, Nachdruck, Georg Olms Verlag Hildesheim 1979.

Teuscher E, Biogene Arzneimittel, 5. Aufl., Wiss. Verlagsges. mbH Stuttgart 1997.

Thomson RH, Naturally Occurring Quinones, 2nd Ed., Academic Press New York 1971.

Wichtl M (Hrsg.), Teedrogen, 4. Aufl., Wiss. Verlagsges. Stuttgart 1997.

Dryopteris Filix-mas

Male Fern

DESCRIPTION

Medicinal Parts: The medicinal parts are the dried fronds, the dried rhizome collected in autumn with the leaf bases, the fresh rhizome and the fresh aerial parts.

Flower and Fruit: On the underside of the leaflets there are 2 rows of sori, covered by kidney-shaped, red-brown film. The spores are dark brown.

Leaves, Stem and Root: The root is a crooked half-underground fleshy rhizome, covered in the remains of dark brown petioles, which produces long branched root fibers. The remains of the petioles are linear-lanceolate and tomentose with red-brown scales. The foliage grows in a crown, with fronds arranged in spirals, 60 cm to 1.5 m high, 2-pinnate, oblong-lanceolate, alternate, sessile leaflets, subdivided with round segments. The young fronds are rolled in spirals and thickly covered in hairs and gradually open out as the fronds grow.

Habitat: The plant is found in the temperate zones of Europe, northern Asia and in North and South America.

Production: Male Fern leaf consists of the fresh or dried leaf of Dryopteris filix-mas. Male Fern herb consists of the fresh or dried above-ground parts of Dryopteris filix-mas. Male Fern rhizome consists of the fresh or dried rhizomes with leaf scars, separated from attached roots, harvested in autumn, of Dryopteris filix-mas. The root-stock is collected in autumn and gently dried.

Not To Be Confused With: The rhizomes of most European Dyopteris species.

Other Names: Aspidium, Bear's Paw Root, Fern, Knotty Brake, Male Shield Fern, Marginal Fern, Sweet Brake

ACTION AND PHARMACOLOGY

COMPOUNDS: DRYOPTERIS FILIX-MAS RHIZOME

Acylphloroglucinoles (2%, mixtures termed raw filicin or filicin): in particular, flavaspidic acids, filicinic acids, paraspidin, desaspidin

Tannins

COMPOUNDS: DRYOPTERIS FILIX-MAS LEAVES

Acylphloroglucinoles (0.2%, mixtures termed raw filicin or filicin): in particular, flavaspidic acids, filicinic acids, paraspidin, desaspidin

Flavonoids

EFFECTS

Male Fern rhizome has an anthelmintic effect and is strongly cytotoxic against band worms and liver flukes, although roundworm and oxyuris are resistant. It is also cell toxic, virostatic and antiviral.

INDICATIONS AND USAGE

Preparations of Male Fern herb are used externally for rheumatism, sciatica, muscle pain, neuralgia, earache and toothache, for teething in infants and sleep disorders, as well as internally for tapeworms and flukes. The efficacy for the claimed applications is not documented.

CONTRAINDICATIONS

The drug should not be administered in the presence of anemia, cardiac, liver or kidney diseases or diabetes. A forgoing of the drug in favor of a different vermifuge is strongly recommended.

PRECAUTIONS AND ADVERSE REACTIONS

General: The following can occur even with therapeutic dosages: queasiness, nausea, severe headache, vomiting, diarrhea.

Pregnancy: The drug should not be used during pregnancy.

Pediatric Use: The drug should not be administered to children under 4 years.

Use in the Elderly: The drug should not be administered to elderly persons.

OVERDOSAGE

Overdosages in susceptible patients can lead to liver, cardiac and kidney damage as well as central nervous system disorders such as spasms, more rarely also to psychoses and to permanent injuries such as paralysis and visual disorders, even blindness.

Cases of death, particularly among children, have been observed following administration of Filmaron oil (10% solution of volatile extracts of the rhizomic drug in cooking oil).

DOSAGE

Mode of Administration: **Warning: Dosages may be toxic!** Due to the risks, an internal application is not recommended; if possible other remedies should be used. Because the efficacy of the claimed applications is not documented, therapeutic usage is not recommended.

Daily Dosage: The single and daily dose of Extractum Filicus is 6 to 8 gm for adults and 4 to 6 gm for children. In case of an unsuccessful cure, the treatment may only be repeated after an interim of a few weeks. The single and daily maximum dose of Extractum Filicus siccum is 3 gm. The maximum daily dosage of Aspidinolfilicium oleo solutum is 20 gm.

Storage: The drug is stored over charcoaled calcium for a maximum duration of 1 year, with a relative humidity below 0.05 in sealed containers away from light sources.

LITERATURE

Bottari F et al., (1972) Phytochemistry 11:2519.

Calderwood JM et al., J Pharm Pharmacol 21:55 S.

Karl C, Pedersen PA, Müller G, Z Naturforsch 36C:607-610. 1981.

Widén CJ, Sarvela J, Britton OM, On the location and distribution of phloroglucinols (Filicins) in Ferns. In: Ann Bot Fennici 20:407. 1983.

Widén CJ, Vida G, Euw JV, Reichenstein T, Helv Chim Acta 54:2824-2850. 1971.

Further information in:

Frohne D, Pfänder HJ, Giftpflanzen - Ein Handbuch für Apotheker, Toxikologen und Biologen, 4. Aufl., Wiss. Verlagsges. mbH Stuttgart 1997.

Hänsel R, Keller K, Rimpler H, Schneider G (Hrsg.), Hagers Handbuch der Pharmazeutischen Praxis, 5. Aufl., Bde 4-6 (Drogen), Springer Verlag Berlin, Heidelberg, New York, 1992-1994.

Leung AY, Encyclopedia of Common Natural Ingredients Used in Food Drugs and Cosmetics, John Wiley & Sons Inc., New York 1980.

Roth L, Daunderer M, Kormann K, Giftpflanzen, Pflanzengifte, 4. Aufl., Ecomed Fachverlag Landsberg Lech 1993.

Teuscher E, Lindequist U, Biogene Gifte - Biologie, Chemie, Pharmakologie, 2. Aufl., Fischer Verlag Stuttgart 1994.

Duckweed

See Lemna Minor

Dusty Miller

See Senecio Cineraria

Dwarf Elder

See Sambucus Ebulus

Dyer's Broom

See Genista Tinctoria

Echinacea

Purple Coneflower

DESCRIPTION

Medicinal Parts: The medicinal parts are, depending on varieties, the roots, leaves or the whole plant in various stages of development.

Flower and Fruit: The flower-heads are large and solitary on terminal peduncles with spreading ray florets. The bracts are in a number of rows. The bracts are leafy, rigid, thorny tipped, and longer than the conical erect disc florets. The reddish or occasionally white florets are conspicuous. The ligual florets are usually sterile and 3 cm long. The pappus is small or absent.

Leaves, Stem and Root: Echinacea is usually a perennial herb up to 45 cm. in height. The leaves are sparse, solitary, lanceolate to linear, opposite or alternate. They are 7.5 to 20 cm long and have a rough surface. The leaves are entire-margined and are on slender petioles. The dried rhizome is grayish-brown, often twisted and longitudinally furrowed. The diameter of the rhizome is about 1 cm. The transverse section shows a thin bark and a yellowish, porous wood, which is flecked with black.

Characteristics: The taste is slightly sweet then bitter leaving a tingling sensation on the tongue. The odor is faintly aromatic.

Habitat: Echinacea purpurea grows in the middle or eastern U.S. and is cultivated in Europe. Echinaceae pallida grows in the middle or eastern U.S. Echinacea angustifolia grows in the western U.S. and in Europe.

Production: Echinacea purpurea herba consists of the fresh, above-ground parts, harvested at flowering time and freshly processed aerial parts harvested during the flowering season. Echinacea pallida consists of the fresh or dried above-ground parts, collected at the time of flowering. Echinacea angustifolia herba et radix consists of the fresh or dried roots, or the fresh or dried above-ground parts collected at the time of flowering. Echinacea purpurea radix consists of the underground parts of Echinacea purpurea, which is harvested mechanically. Echinacea pallida radix consists of fresh or dried root. For Echinaceae pallidae radix, the roots are cultivated using a plow and subsequently air-dried.

Not To Be Confused With: The herbs and roots of Echinacea purpurea, Echinacea angustifolia and Echinacea pallida have different medicinal properties. Some Echinacea species may be confused with or adulterated with Parthenium integrifoium.

Other Names: Black Sampson, Niggerhead, Rudbeckia, Sampson Root

ACTIONS AND PHARMACOLOGY

COMPOUNDS: ECHINACEAE PURPUREAE HERBA

Water-soluble immunostimulating polysaccharides (4-O-methylglucuronylarabinoxylans, acidic arabinorhamnogalactans)

Volatile oil (under 0.08-0.32%): components including germacrene alcohol, borneol, bornylacetate, pentadeca-8-en-2-on, germacrene D, caryophyllene, caryophyllene epoxide

Flavonoids: in particular rutin

Caffeic and ferulic acid derivatives: including cichoriic acid, cichoriic acid methyl ester, 2-O- caffeoyl-3-O-feruloyl-tartaric acid, 2,3-O-diferuloyl tartaric acid 2-O-caffeoyl tartaric acid

Alkamides, including undeca-2E,4Z-dien-8,10-diin acid- and dodeca-2E,4E-8Z,10E/Z- tetraen acid isobutylamide

EFFECTS: ECHINACEA PURPUREA HERBA

The drug is reported to accelerate the healing of wounds. Echinacea purpurea herba has produced immune effects when given internally or parenterally. Some of the effects include an increase of the number of white blood cells and spleen cells, activation of the capacity for phagocytosis by human granulocytes, elevations in body temperature, reproduction of T-helper cells and the production of cytokines such as interleukin-1, interleukin-6 and TNF-alpha.

COMPOUNDS: ECHINACEA PURPUREA RADIX

Water-soluble immunostimulating polysaccharides

Immunostimulating glyco proteins

Volatile oil (0.2%): components including caryophyllene, humules, caryophyllene epoxide, dodeca-2,4-dien-1-yl-isovalerate

Caffeic and ferulic acid derivatives: including cichoriic acid, cichoriic acid methyl ester, 2-O- caffeoyl tartaric acid

Alkamides: including undeca-2E,4Z-dien-8,10-diinacetyl- and dodeca-2E,4E-8Z,10E/Z-tetracetyliso- butylamide

Polyynes: including trideca-1-en-3,5,7,9,11-pentain, pontica epoxide

Non alkylatingly effective pyrrolizidine alkaloids: tussilagine, isotussilagine

EFFECTS: ECHINACEA PURPUREA RADIX

Echinacea purpura radix has been shown to be antibacterial, virostatic, immune-modulating, insecticidal and to affect arachidonic acid metabolism. In vitro, alcoholic root extracts show a 23% increase in phagocytic elements when tested in granulocyte smears.

COMPOUNDS: ECHINACEA PALLIDA HERBA

Volatile oil (under 0.1%)

Flavonoids: in particular rutin

Caffeic acid derivatives: Cichoriic acid, chlorogenic acid, isochlorogenic acid, verbascoside

Alkamides: including dodeca-2E,4E-8Z,10E-tetracetyliso-butylamide

EFFECTS: ECHINACEA PALLIDA HERBA

In the carbon-clearance test conducted in animals, alcoholic root extracts as well as extracts of the above-ground herb show a rate increase in elimination of carbon particles. In vitro, alcoholic root extracts show a 23% increase in phagocytic elements when tested in granulocyte smears.

COMPOUNDS: ECHINACEA PALLIDA RADIX

Water-soluble immunstimulating polysaccharides (arabino-rhamnogalactans)

Volatile oil (0.2 - 2%): chief components: pentadeca-8Z-en-2-on, pentadeca-1,8Z-dien, 1-pentadecan

Caffeic acid derivatives: echinacoside

Alkamides: including isomeric dodeca-2E,4E-8Z,10E/Z-tet-racetylliso- butylamide

Polyynes: including trideca-1-en-3,5,7,9,11-pentain, pontica epoxide

EFFECTS: ECHINACEA PALLIDA RADIX

In animal studies, a carbon clearance test using alcohol root extracts showed an increase in the elimination of carbon particles by a factor of 2.2. In vitro, a 23% increase in phagocytic elements was noted when the drug was tested in granulocyte smears at a concentration of 10^{-4} to 10^{-2} mg/ml. A virostatic effect was demonstrated in a placebo-controlled monocentric clinical study. A rapid improvement of an influenza infection was observed.

COMPOUNDS: ECHINACEA ANGUSTIFOLIA HERBA ET RADIX

Volatile oil (under 0.1%): typical components epishyobunol, beta-farnesene, alpha- and beta-pinenes, myrcene, carvomen-thene, caryophyllene

Flavonoids

Caffeic acid derivatives: cichoriic acid, chlorogenic acid, isochlorogenic acid, verbascoside, echinacoside

Alkamides: including dodeca-2E,4E-8Z,10E-tetracetyliso-butylamide

Polyynes: including trideca-1-en-3,5,7,9,11-pentaine, pontica epoxide

Water-soluble immunostimulating polysaccharides (rhamno-arabinogalactans)

Non alkylatingly effective pyrrolizidine alkaloids: tussilag-ine, isotussilagine

EFFECTS: ECHINACEA ANGUSTIFOLIA HERBA ET RADIX

In vitro, a 23% increase in phagocytic elements was noted when an alcoholic root extract was tested in granulocyte smears. The immune system is unspecifically stimulated. The drug possesses an antibacterial and biostatic effect. In animal experiments the drug is a tumor inhibitor and has an anti-edemic effect on induced rat paw edemas.

INDICATIONS

ECHINACEA PURPUREA HERBA

- Common cold
- Cough/bronchitis
- Fevers and colds
- Infections of the urinary tract
- Inflammation of the mouth and pharynx
- Tendency to infection
- Wounds and burns

Echinacea purpurea herba is used internally as supportive therapy for colds and chronic infections of the respiratory tract and lower urinary tract. It can be applied locally to poorly healing wounds and chronic ulcerations.

ECHINACEA PURPUREA RADIX

Echinacea purpurea radix is also used for acute and chronic respiratory tract infections (of viral and bacterial origin); increased susceptibility to infection due to temporarily lowered resistance, treatment of leukopenia following radio and cytostatic therapy and in support of anti-infectious chemotherapy.

ECHINACEA PALLIDA HERBA

- Common cold
- Cough/bronchitis
- Fevers
- Inflammation of the mouth and pharynx
- Tendency to infection

Echinacea pallida herba is also used to support and promote the natural powers of resistance of the body, especially in infectious conditions (influenza and colds, etc.).

ECHINACEA PALLIDA RADIX

- Fevers and colds

Echinacea pallida radix is used as a supportive therapy for influenza-like infections.

ECHINACEA ANGUSTIFOLIA HERBA ET RADIX

Preparations of Echinacea angustifolia are used to support and promote the natural immune system of the body, especially in infectious conditions (influenza and colds, etc.) of the nose and throat, inflammatory and purulent wounds, abscesses, furuncles, herpes simplex, inflammation of con-nective tissue, wounds, headaches, metabolic disturbances. In folk medicine the drug is employed much more widely: for wounds, burns, swelling of the lymph nodes, insect bites, gastric spasms, measles, gonorrhea and as a snake bite antidote.

The efficacy of these uses is not proven.

CONTRAINDICATIONS

ALL VARIETIES AND FORMS

Because of a conceivable activation of autoimmune aggressions and other overreactive immune responses, the drug should not be administered in the presence of multiple sclerosis, leukoses, collagenoses, AIDS or tuberculosis. Parenteral administration should not be used in patients with tendencies to allergies, especially allergies to members of the composite family (Asteraceae), as well as in pregnancy.

PRECAUTIONS AND ADVERSE REACTIONS

ALL VARIETIES AND FORMS

General: Health risks or side effects following the proper administration of designated therapeutic dosages are not recorded. When used parenterally, dose-dependent short-term fever reactions, nausea and vomiting can occur. In individual cases, allergic reactions of the immediate type are possible. Caution should be exercised if the drug is administered parenterally to people with diabetes.

Pregnancy: Parenteral administration should be avoided during pregnancy.

DOSAGE

ECHINACEA PURPUREA HERBA

Mode of Administration: Pressed juice and galenic preparations for internal and external use.

Preparation: The pressed juice is prepared in a concentration of 2.5:1 and is stabilized with 22% alcohol. Other complicated methods are known.

Daily Dosage: When used internally, the recommended dosage is 6 to 9 ml of the expressed juice. The recommended dosage for parenteral administration should be individualized, depending on the seriousness of the condition as well as the specific nature of the respective preparation. Parenteral application requires a gradation of dosage, especially for children. The manufacturer is required to show this information for the respective preparation. When used externally, semi-solid preparations containing at least 15% pressed juice are used for a maximum of 8 weeks.

ECHINACEA PURPUREA RADIX

Mode of Administration: Comminuted drug for decoctions and galenic preparations.

Daily Dosage: When using the tincture, 30 to 60 drops should be taken three times a day.

Storage: Must be protected from light sources, and, if possible be uncomminuted.

ECHINACEA PALLIDA HERBA AND RADIX

Mode of Administration: As a liquid preparation for oral use.

Preparation: A 1:5 tincture is made using 50% (V/V) ethanol and native dried extract (50% ethanol in a 7 to 11:1 proportion)

Daily Dosage: The daily dose is 900 mg of drug. The drug should be used for a maximum of 8 weeks.

Storage: Protect from light sources. If possible, store uncomminuted.

ECHINACEA ANGUSTIFOLIA HERBA ET RADIX

Mode of Administration: Since the efficacy in the claimed areas of application has not been documented, therapeutic application cannot be recommended. Because of the risks, the use of parenteral preparations is not justified.

Preparation: The root tea is prepared using 1/2 teaspoonful comminuted drug with boiling water. Strain after 10 minutes.

Daily Dosage: For colds, drink 1 cup freshly made tea several times daily.

Storage: Protect from light sources. If possible, store uncomminuted.

LITERATURE

ECHINACEA PURPUREA HERBA

Bauer R, Arzneipflanzenporträt: Echinacea- welche Inhaltsstoffe wirken immunmodulierend? In: DAZ 132(23):1233. 1992.

Bauer R, Echinacea. In: PM 59(6):94. 1992.

Bauer R, Jurcic K, Puhlmann J, Wagner H, Immunologische in vivo- und in vitro Untersuchnugnen mit Echinacea-Extrakten. In: Arzneim Forsch 38:276-281. 1988.

Bauer R, Neues von ''immunmodulierenden Drogen'' und ''Drogen mit antiallergischer und antiinflammatorischer Wirkung''. In: ZPT 14(1):23-24. 1993.

Bauer R, Remiger P, Jurcic K, Wagner H, Beeinflussung der Phagozytoseaktivität durch Echinacea-Extrakte. In: ZPT 10:43-48. 1989.

Bauer R, Remiger P, Wagner H, Echinacea-Vergleichende DC- und HPLC-Analyse der Herba-Drogen von Echinacea purpurea, Echinacea pallida und Echinacea angustifolia. In: DAZ 128:174-180. 1988.

Bauer R, Wagner H, Echinacea - Der Sonnenhut - Stand der Forschung. In: ZPT 9(8):151. 1988.

Bauer R, Wagner H, Echinacea-Drogen - Who is who? In: ZPT 9(6):191. 1988.

Bauer R, Wagner H, Echinacea. Wissenschaftliche Verlagsgesellschaft mbH Stuttgart 1990.

Bauer, R et al., (1985) Helv Chim Acta 68:2355.

Bauer, R et al., (1987) Phytochemistry 26(4):1198.

Becker H, (1982) Dtsch Apoth Ztg 122(45):2320.

Beuscher N, Scheit KH, Bodinet C, Egert D, Modulation der körpereigenen Immunabwehr durch polymere Substanzen aus Baptisia tinctoria und Echinacea purpurea. In:

Immunotherapeutic prospects of infectious diseases, Hrsg. Masihi KN, Lange W. Springer, Heidel.

Beuscher N, Über die medikamentöse Beeinflussung zellulärer Resistenzmechanismen im Tierversuch. Aktivierung von Peritonealmakrophagen der Maus durch pflanzliche Reizkörper. In: Arzneim Forsch 32(I):134-138. 1977.

Bohlmann F, Hoffman H, (1983) Phytochemistry 22(5):1173.

Büsing KH, Hyaluronidasehemmung durch Echinacin. In: Arzneim Forsch 2:467-469. 1952.

Coeugniet EG, Elek E, Immunmodulation with Viscum album and Echinacea purpurea Extracts. In: Beilage zur Onkologie 27-33. 1987.

Die Chemie der Pflanze (Standard, Wirksamkeit). In: Symbiose 4(3):11. 1992.

Dorn M, (1989) Milderung grippaler Effekte durch ein pflanzliches Immunstimulans. Natur- und Ganzheitsmedizin 2:314-319.

Forth H, Beuscher N, Beeinflussung der Häufigkeit banaler Erkältungsinfekte durch Esberitox. In: Z Allgemeinmed 57:2272-2275. 1981.

Harnischfeger G, Stolze H, (1980) Notabene Medici 10:484.

Jacobson M, (1967) J Org Chem 32:1646.

Jurcic K, Melchart D, Holzmann M, Martin P, Bauer R, Doenecke A, Wagner H, Zwei Probandenstudien zur Stimulierung der Granulozytenphagozytose durch Echinacea-Extrakt-haltige Präparate. In: ZPT 10(2):67-70. 1989.

Kinkel HJ, Plate M, Tüllner HU, Objektivierbare Wirkung von Echinacin-Salbe auf die Wundheilung. In: Med Klinik 79:580-583. 1984.

May G, Willuhn G, (1978) Arzneim Forsch 28:1.

Melchart D, Linde K, Worku F, Bauer R, Wagner H, (1994) Immunomodulation with Echinacea - a systematic review of controlled clinical trials. Phytomedicine 1:245-254.

Mose JR, (1983) Med Welt 34:51.

Parnham MJ, Benefit-risk assessment of the squeezed sap of the purple coneflower (Echinacea purpurea) for long-term oral immunostimulation. In: Phytomedicine 3(1):95-102. 1996.

Proksch A, (1982) Über ein immunstimulierendes Wirkprinzip aus Echinacea purpurea. Dissertation, Ludwig-Maximilians-Universität, München.

Samochowie CE et al., (1979) Wiad Parazyt. 25(1) 77.

Schulte KE et al., (1967) Arzneim Forsch 17:825.

Schulte KE, Rücker G, Perlick J, Das Vorkommen von Polyacetylen-Verbindungen in Echinacea purpurea MOENCH und Echinacea angustifolia DC. In: Arzneim-Forsch 17:825-829. 1967.

Stimpel M et al., (1984) Infect Immunol 46(3):845.

Stimpel M, Proksch A, Wagner H et al., (1984) Macrophage activation and induction of macrophage cytotoxicity by purified polysaccaride fractions from the plant Echinacea purpurea. Infect Immunity 46:845-849.

Stimpel M, Proksch A, Wagner H, Lohmann-Matthes ML, Macrophage activation and induction of macrophage cytotoxicity by purified polysccharide fraction from plant Echinacea purpurea. In: Infect Immun 46:845-849. 1984.

Vergin H, Wolter R, Untersuchungen zur Phagozytose-Aktivität der isoliert perfundierten Rattenleber mit Echinacea purpurea-haltigen Präparaten. In: Natura med 1/2:27-29. 1988.

Vömel Th, (1985) Arzneim Forsch 35II(9):1437.

Von Röder E et al., (1984) Dtsch Apoth Ztg 124(45):2316.

Wacker A, Hilbig W, (1978) Planta Med 33:89.

Wacker A, Hilbig W, Virushemmung mit Echinacea purpurea. In: PM 33:89-102. 1978.

Wagner H et al., (1984) Arzneim Forsch 34:659.

Wagner H, Stuppner H, Puhlmann J, Brümmer B, Deppe K, Zenk MH, Gewinnung von immunologisch aktiven Polysacchariden aus Echinacea-Drogen und - Gewebekulturen. In: ZPT 10(2):35. 1989.

Further information in:

Hänsel R, Keller K, Rimpler H, Schneider G (Hrsg.), Hagers Handbuch der Pharmazeutischen Praxis, 5. Aufl., Bde 4-6 (Drogen), Springer Verlag Berlin, Heidelberg, New York, 1992-1994.

Schulz R, Hänsel R, Rationale Phytotherapie, Springer Verlag Heidelberg 1996.

Steinegger E, Hänsel R, Pharmakognosie, 5. Aufl., Springer Verlag Heidelberg 1992.

Teuscher E, Lindequist U, Biogene Gifte - Biologie, Chemie, Pharmakologie, 2. Aufl., Fischer Verlag Stuttgart 1994.

Teuscher E, Biogene Arzneimittel, 5. Aufl., Wiss. Verlagsges. mbH Stuttgart 1997.

Wagner H, Wiesenauer M, Phytotherapie. Phytopharmaka und pflanzliche Homöopathika, Fischer-Verlag, Stuttgart, Jena, New York 1995.

ECHINACEA PURPUREA RADIX

Bauer R et al., (1985) Helv Chim Acta 68:2355.

Bauer R et al., (1987) Phytochemistry 26(4):1198.

Bauer R, Arzneipflanzenporträt: Echinacea- welche Inhaltsstoffe wirken immunmodulierend? In: DAZ 132(23):1233. 1992.

Bauer R, Echinacea. In: PM 59(6):94. 1992.

Bauer R, Jurcic K, Puhlmann J, Wagner H, Immunologische in vivo- und in vitro Untersuchnugnen mit Echinacea-Extrakten. In: Arzneim Forsch 38:276-281. 1988.

Bauer R, Remiger P, Jurcic K, Wagner H, Beeinflussung der Phagozytoseaktivität durch Echinacea-Extrakte. In: ZPT 10:43-48. 1989.

Bauer R, Neues von ''immunmodulierenden Drogen'' und ''Drogen mit antiallergischer und antiinflammatorischer Wirkung''. In: ZPT 14(1):23-24. 1993.

Bauer R, Remiger P, Wagner H, Echinacea-Vergleichende DC- und HPLC-Analyse der Herba-Drogen von Echinacea purpurea,

Echinacea pallida und Echinacea angustifolia. In: DAZ 128:174-180. 1988.

Bauer R, Wagner H, Echinacea - Der Sonnenhut - Stand der Forschung. In: ZPT 9(8):151. 1988.

Bauer R, Wagner H, Echinacea-Drogen - Who is who? In: ZPT 9(6):191. 1988.

Bauer R, Wagner H, Echinacea. Wissenschaftliche Verlagsgesellschaft mbH Stuttgart 1990.

Becker H, (1982) Dtsch Apoth Ztg 122(45):2320.

Bodinet C, Beuscher N, Antiviral and immunological activity of glykoproteins from the root of Echinacea purpurea. In: PM, Abstracts of the 39th Annual Congress of Medicinal Plant Research. 1991.

Bohlmann F, Hoffman H, (1983) Phytochemistry 22(5):1173.

Bräunig B, Dorn M, Knick E, Echinaceae purpureae radix: zur Stärkung der körpereigenen Abwehr bei grippalem Infekten. In: ZPT 13(1):7. 1992.

Die Chemie der Pflanze (Standard, Wirksamkeit). In: Symbiose 4(3):11. 1992.

Dorn M, (1989) Milderung grippaler Effekte durch ein pflanzliches Immunstimulans. Natur- und Ganzheitsmedizin 2:314-319.

Harnischfeger G, Stolze, H, (1980) Notabene Medici 10:484.

Jacobson M, (1967) J Org Chem 32:1646.

May G, Willuhn G, (1978) Arzneim Forsch 28:1.

Melchart D, Linde K, Worku F, Bauer R, Wagner H, (1994) Immunomodulation with Echinacea - a systematic review of controlled clinical trials. Phytomedicine 1:245-254.

Mose JR, (1983) Med Welt 34:51.

Proksch A, (1982) Über ein immunstimulierendes Wirkprinzip aus Echinacea purpurea. Dissertation, Ludwig-Maximilians-Universität, München.

Samochowie CE et al., (1979) Wiad Parazyt 25(1)77.

Schulte KE et al., (1967) Arzneim Forsch 17:825.

Stimpel M et al., (1984) Infect Immunol 46(3):845.

Stimpel M, Proksch A, Wager H et al., (1984) Macrophage activation and induction of macrophage cytotoxicity by purified polysaccaride fractions from the plant Echinacea purpurea. Infect Immunity 46:845-849.

Vömel, Th, (1985) Arzneim Forsch 35II(9):1437.

Von Röder, E et al., (1984) Dtsch Apoth Ztg 124(45):2316.

Wacker A, Hilbig W, (1978) Planta Med 33:89.

Wagner H et al., (1984) Arzneim Forsch 34:659.

Further information in:

Hänsel R, Keller K, Rimpler H, Schneider G (Hrsg.), Hagers Handbuch der Pharmazeutischen Praxis, 5. Aufl., Bde 4-6 (Drogen), Springer Verlag Berlin, Heidelberg, New York, 1992-1994.

Wagner H, Wiesenauer M, Phytotherapie. Phytopharmaka und pflanzliche Homöopathika, Fischer-Verlag, Stuttgart, Jena, New York 1995.

ECHINACEA PALLIDA HERBA

Bauer R et al., (1985) Helv Chim Acta 68:2355.

Bauer R et al., (1987) Phytochemistry 26(4):1198.

Bauer R, Arzneipflanzenporträt: Echinacea- welche Inhaltsstoffe wirken immunmodulierend? In: DAZ 132(23):1233. 1992.

Bauer R, Jurcic K, Puhlmann J, Wagner H, Immunologische in vivo- und in vitro Untersuchnugnen mit Echinacea-Extrakten. In: Arzneim Forsch 38:276-281. 1988.

Bauer R, Neues von ''immunmodulierenden Drogen'' und ''Drogen mit antiallergischer und antiinflammatorischer Wirkung''. In: ZPT 14(1):23-24. 1993.

Bauer R, Remiger P, Jurcic K, Wagner H, Beeinflussung der Phagozytoseaktivität durch Echinacea-Extrakte. In: ZPT 10:43-48. 1989.

Bauer R, Remiger P, Wagner H, Echinacea-Vergleichende DC- und HPLC-Analyse der Herba-Drogen von Echinacea purpurea, Echinacea pallida und Echinacea angustifolia. In: DAZ 128:174-180. 1988.

Bauer R, Wagner H, Echinacea - Der Sonnenhut - Stand der Forschung. In: ZPT 9(8):151. 1988.

Bauer R, Wagner H, Echinacea-Drogen - Who is who? In: ZPT 9(6):191. 1988.

Bauer R, Wagner H, Echinacea. Wissenschaftliche Verlagsgesellschaft mbH Stuttgart 1990.

Becker H, (1982) Dtsch Apoth Ztg 122(45):2320.

Bohlmann F, Hoffman H, (1983) Phytochemistry 22(5):1173.

Die Chemie der Pflanze (Standard, Wirksamkeit). In: Symbiose 4(3):11. 1992.

Harnischfeger G, Stolze H, (1980) Notabene Medici 10:484.

Jacobson M, (1967) J Org Chem 32:1646.

May G, Willuhn G, (1978) Arzneim Forsch 28:1-7.

Mose JR, (1983) Med Welt 34:51.

Samochowie CE et al., (1979) Wiad Parazyt. 25(1)77.

Von Röder E et al., (1984) Dtsch Apoth Ztg 124(45):2316.

Wacker A, Hilbig W, (1978) Planta Med 33:89.

Wagner H et al., (1984) Arzneim Forsch 34:659.

Further information in:

Hänsel R, Keller K, Rimpler H, Schneider G (Hrsg.), Hagers Handbuch der Pharmazeutischen Praxis, 5. Aufl., Bde 4-6 (Drogen), Springer Verlag Berlin, Heidelberg, New York, 1992-1994.

Teuscher E, Biogene Arzneimittel, 5. Aufl., Wiss. Verlagsges. mbH Stuttgart 1997.

ECHINACEA PALLIDA RADIX

Bauer R et al., (1985) Helv Chim Acta 68:2355.

Bauer R et al., (1987) Phytochemistry 26(4):1198.

Bauer R, Arzneipflanzenporträt: E0chinacea- welche Inhaltsstoffe wirken immunmodulierend? In: DAZ 132(23):1233. 1992.

Bauer R, Jurcic K, Puhlmann J, Wagner H, Immunologische in vivo- und in vitro Untersuchnugnen mit Echinacea-Extrakten. In: Arzneim Forsch 38:276-281. 1988.

Bauer R, Neues von ''immunmodulierenden Drogen'' und ''Drogen mit antiallergischer und antiinflammatorischer Wirkung''. In: ZPT 14(1):23-24. 1993.

Bauer R, Remiger P, Jurcic K, Wagner H, Beeinflussung der Phagozytoseaktivität durch Echinacea-Extrakte. In: ZPT 10: 43-48. 1989.

Bauer R, Remiger P, Wagner H, Echinacea-Vergleichende DC- und HPLC-Analyse der Herba-Drogen von Echinacea purpurea, Echinacea pallida und Echinacea angustifolia. In: DAZ 128:174-180. 1988.

Bauer R, Wagner H, Echinacea - Der Sonnenhut - Stand der Forschung. In: ZPT 9(8):151. 1988.

Bauer R, Wagner H, Echinacea-Drogen - Who is who? In: ZPT 9(6):191. 1988.

Bauer R, Wagner H: Echinacea. Wissenschaftliche Verlagsgesellschaft mbH Stuttgart 1990

Becker H, (1982) Dtsch Apoth Ztg 122(45):2320.

Bohlmann F, Hoffman H, (1983) Phytochemistry 22(5):1173.

Cheminat A, Zawatzky R, Becker H, Brouillard R, Caffeoylconjugates from Echinacea Species: Structure and biological activity. In: PH 27(9):2787-2794. 1988.

Die Chemie der Pflanze (Standard, Wirksamkeit). In: Symbiose 4(3):11. 1992.

Harnischfeger G, Stolze H, (1980) Notabene Medici 10:484.

Jacobson M, (1967) J Org Chem 32:1646.

May G, Willuhn G, (1978) Arzneim Forsch 28:1-7.

Mose JR, (1983) Med Welt 34:51.

Samochowie CE et al., (1979) Wiad Parazyt. 25(1)77.

Von Röder E et al., (1984) Dtsch Apoth Ztg 124(45):2316.

Wacker A, Hilbig W, (1978) Planta Med 33:89.

Wagner H et al., (1984) Arzneim Forsch 34:659.

Further information in:

Hänsel R, Keller K, Rimpler H, Schneider G (Hrsg.), Hagers Handbuch der Pharmazeutischen Praxis, 5. Aufl., Bde 4-6 (Drogen), Springer Verlag Berlin, Heidelberg, New York, 1992-1994.

Schulz R, Hänsel R, Rationale Phytotherapie, Springer Verlag Heidelberg 1996.

Teuscher E, Biogene Arzneimittel, 5. Aufl., Wiss. Verlagsges. mbH Stuttgart 1997.

Wagner H, Wiesenauer M, Phytotherapie. Phytopharmaka und pflanzliche Homöopathika, Fischer-Verlag, Stuttgart, Jena, New York 1995.

Wichtl M (Hrsg.), Teedrogen, 4. Aufl., Wiss. Verlagsges. Stuttgart 1997.

ECHINACEA ANGUSTIFOLIA HERBA ET RADIX

Bauer R et al., (1985) Helv Chim Acta 68:2355.

Bauer R et al., (1987) Phytochemistry 26(4):1198.

Bauer R, Arzneipflanzenporträt: Echinacea- welche Inhaltsstoffe wirken immunmodulierend? In: DAZ 132(23):1233. 1992.

Bauer R, Jurcic K, Puhlmann J, Wagner H, Immunologische in vivo- und in vitro Untersuchnugnen mit Echinacea-Extrakten. In: Arzneim Forsch 38:276-281. 1988.

Bauer R, Neues von ''immunmodulierenden Drogen'' und ''Drogen mit antiallergischer und antiinflammatorischer Wirkung''. In: ZPT 14(1):23-24. 1993.

Bauer R, Remiger P, Jurcic K, Wagner H, Beeinflussung der Phagozytoseaktivität durch Echinacea-Extrakte. In: ZPT 10: 43-48. 1989.

Bauer R, Remiger P, Wagner H, Echinacea-Vergleichende DC- und HPLC-Analyse der Herba-Drogen von Echinacea purpurea, Echinacea pallida und Echinacea angustifolia. In: DAZ 128:174-180. 1988.

Bauer R, Wagner H, Echinacea - Der Sonnenhut - Stand der Forschung. In: ZPT 9(8):151. 1988.

Bauer R, Wagner H, Echinacea-Drogen - Who is who? In: ZPT 9(6):191. 1988.

Bauer R, Wagner H, Echinacea. Wissenschaftliche Verlagsgesellschaft mbH Stuttgart 1990.

Becker H, (1982) Dtsch Apoth Ztg 122(45):2320.

Bohlmann F, Hoffman H, (1983) Phytochemistry 22(5):1173.

Die Chemie der Pflanze (Standard., Wirksamkeit). In: Symbiose 4(3):11. 1992.

Harnischfeger G, Stolze H, (1980) Notabene Medici 10:484.

Jacobson M, (1967) J Org Chem 32:1646.

May G, Willuhn G, (1978) Arzneim Forsch 28:1.

Mose JR, (1983) Med Welt 34:51.

Samochowie CE et al., (1979) Wiad Parazyt. 25(1)77.

Schulte KE et al., (1967) Arzneim Forsch 17:825.

Schumacher A, Echinacea angustifolia und die spezifische und unspezifische zelluläre Immunantwort der Maus. In: Dissertation Heidelberg. 1989.

Stimpel M et al., (1984) Infect. Immunol 46(3):845.

Vömel Th, (1985) Arzneim Forsch 35II(9):1437.

Von Röder E et al., (1984) Dtsch Apoth Ztg 124(45):2316.

Wacker A, Hilbig W, (1978) Planta Med 33:89.

Wagner H et al., (1984) Arzneim Forsch 34:659.

Further information in:

Hänsel R, Keller K, Rimpler H, Schneider G (Hrsg.), Hagers Handbuch der Pharmazeutischen Praxis, 5. Aufl., Bde 4-6 (Drogen), Springer Verlag Berlin, Heidelberg, New York, 1992-1994.

Steinegger E, Hänsel R, Pharmakognosie, 5. Aufl., Springer Verlag Heidelberg 1992.

Teuscher E, Lindequist U, Biogene Gifte - Biologie, Chemie, Pharmakologie, 2. Aufl., Fischer Verlag Stuttgart 1994.

Wagner H, Wiesenauer M, Phytotherapie. Phytopharmaka und pflanzliche Homöopathika, Fischer-Verlag, Stuttgart, Jena, New York 1995.

Elecampane

See Inula Helenium

Elettaria Cardamomum

Cardamom

DESCRIPTION

Medicinal Parts: The medicinal parts are the oil extracted from the seeds and fruit plus seeds harvested shortly after ripening.

Flower and Fruit: The flowering shoots grow on the stem very close to the ground. The panicle branches can grow up to 8 cm. The flowers are alternate and covered by sheath-like bracts before opening. The calyx is slightly wider above, finely striped, obtusely 3-tipped and does not droop. The corolla is greenish white. The lobes are rounded, somewhat curly, white with a yellowish border with blue veins and lines in the center. The only fertile stamen is set into the edge of the petals. The sterile stamens are arranged beside the styles on the receptacle. The pollen is globular and prickly. The ovary is inferior, oblong, obovate with 3 valves each with 12 horizontal ovules. The fruit is 6 to 18 mm long, 6 to 10 mm thick, short-stemmed, ovate or elliptical to oblong. The seeds are light brown, gray or dark red brownish, very roughly wrinkled, 4 to 5 mm, long irregular edged and the whole seed is surrounded by an almost colorless seed coat. Mysore and Malabar cardamoms are usually blanched pale, and have a smooth surface. They are sold commercially less often than the Green Aleppy or Ceylon varieties.

Leaves, Stem and Root: Elettaria cardamomum is a perennial with a thick, tuberous rhizome and numerous long roots. There are up to 30 erect, glabrous, green stems, 2 to 3 m high. The leaves are in 2 rows with a leaf membrane at the end of soft-haired sheath. The leaf surface is lanceolate, clearly acuminate up to 60 cm long, entire-margined, downy above, silky-haired beneath and punctuated by numerous small oil cells. All samples should be whole, containing seeds which are about 4 mm diameter and dark-reddish-brown.

Characteristics: The odor is highly aromatic and pleasant; the taste is aromatic and pungent.

Habitat: The plant is indigenous in southern India and Sri Lanka and is cultivated in tropical regions in southeast Asia and Guatamala.

Production: Cardamom consists of the dried, almost ripe, greenish to yellow-gray fruit of Elettaria cardamomum. Medicinal use is made only of the seed removed from its fruit capsule.

ACTIONS AND PHARMACOLOGY

COMPOUNDS

Volatile oil: composition varying according to the specific strain, chief components cineol, alpha-terpinyl acetate, linalyl acetate

Fatty oil

Starch

EFFECTS

The drug is reported to be a cholagogue and to have virustatic properties.

INDICATIONS AND USAGE

- Common cold
- Cough/bronchitis
- Fevers and colds
- Inflammation of the mouth and pharynx
- Liver and gallbladder complaints
- Loss of appetite
- Tendency to infection

Cardamom is also used for dyspepsia.

PRECAUTIONS AND ADVERSE REACTIONS

No health hazards or side effects are known in conjunction with the proper administration of designated therapeutic dosages. The drug can trigger gallstone colic, due to its motility-enhancing effect.

DOSAGE

Mode of Administration: Ground seeds, as well as galenic preparations for internal use.

Daily Dosage: The average daily dosage is 1.5 gm of drug. When using a tincture, the dosage range is 1 to 2 gm.

LITERATURE

Haginiwa H et al., (1963) Yakagaku Zasshi 83:623.

Lewis YS, Nambuduri ES, Philip T, Perfum Essent Oli Res 57:623-628. 1966.

Further information in:

Fenaroli's Handbook of Flavor Ingredients, Vol. 1, 2nd Ed., CRC Press 1975.

Hänsel R, Keller K, Rimpler H, Schneider G (Hrsg.), Hagers Handbuch der Pharmazeutischen Praxis, 5. Aufl., Bde 4-6 (Drogen), Springer Verlag Berlin, Heidelberg, New York, 1992-1994.

Leung AY, Encyclopedia of Common Natural Ingredients Used in Food Drugs and Cosmetics, John Wiley & Sons Inc., New York 1980.

Teuscher E, Biogene Arzneimittel, 5. Aufl., Wiss. Verlagsges. mbH Stuttgart 1997.

Wagner H, Wiesenauer M, Phytotherapie. Phytopharmaka und pflanzliche Homöopathika, Fischer-Verlag, Stuttgart, Jena, New York 1995.

Eleutherococcus Senticosus

Siberian Ginseng

DESCRIPTION

Medicinal Parts: The medicinal parts are the pulverized root rind, the pulverized root and an alcoholic fluid extract of the rhizome and the roots.

Flower and Fruit: The flowers are in umbels. The central umbel is on a long, thick peduncle. The style is fused into a column to the tip and has 5 small stigma lobes.

Leaves, Stem and Root: Siberian Ginseng is a 1 to 3 m high shrub whose branches are thickly covered with pale, thorny bristles pointing downwards at an angle. The leaves are in groups of 5 and are thorny-serrate. The petiole is covered in fine bristles.

Habitat: Siberian Ginseng grows in Siberia, northern China, Korea and Japan.

Production: Siberian Ginseng consists of the dried roots and/or rhizome of Eleutherococcus senticosus as well as their preparations in effective dosage.

ACTIONS AND PHARMACOLOGY

COMPOUNDS

Polysaccharides: immunstimulatingly effective polysaccharides (eleutherane A-G)

Triterpene saponins: eleutheroside I, eleutheroside K (beta-hederin), eleutheroside L, eleutheroside M (hederasaponin B), for all of these aglycone oleanolic acid

Steroid glycosides: eleutheroside A (daucosterol, beta-stigmasterol-3-O-beta-D-glucoside)

Hydroxycoumarins: isofraxidin

Phenylacrylic acid derivatives: eleutheroside B (syringin)

Lignans: sesamine, eleutheroside D (epimeric diglucosides of syringaresinols)

EFFECTS

In various stress models, e.g., immobilization test and coldness test, the endurance of rodents was enhanced. With healthy volunteers, the lymphocyte count, especially that of T-lymphocytes, increased following intake of liquid extracts.

CONTRAINDICATIONS

The drug should not be administered in the presence of high blood pressure.

INDICATIONS AND USAGE

■ Tendency to infection

Siberian Ginseng is used as a tonic for invigoration and fortification in times of fatigue and debility or declining capacity for work and concentration, and during convalescence.

PRECAUTIONS AND ADVERSE REACTIONS

Health risks or side effects following the proper administration of designated therapeutic dosages are not recorded.

DOSAGE

Mode of Administration: Powdered or cut root for teas, as well as aqueous-alcoholic extracts for internal use.

Daily Dosage: The average daily dosage is 2 to 3 gm of root.

LITERATURE

Bauer R, Neues von ''immunmodulierenden Drogen'' und ''Drogen mit antiallergischer und antiinflammatorischer Wirkung''. In: ZPT 14(1):23-24. 1993.

Bladt S, Wagner H, Woo WS, (1990) Taiga-Wurzel. Dtsch Apoth Ztg 27:1499-1508.

Bohn B, Nebe Cr, Birr C, (1987) Flow-cytometric studies with Eleutherococcus senticosus extract as an immunomodulatory agent. Arzneim Forsch (Drug Res) 37:1193-1196.

Kaemmerer K, Fink J, (1980) Untersuchungen von Eleutherococcus-Extrakt auf trophanabole Wirkungen bei Ratten. Der Praktische Tierarzt 61:748-753.

Koch HP, Eidler S, (1988) Eleutherococcus Senticosus. Sibirischer Ginseng. Wissenschaftlicher Bericht. Kooperation Phytopharmaka, Köln Bonn Frankfurt Bad Homburg.

Obermeier A, (1980) Zur Analytik der Ginseng-und Eteutherococcusdroge. Dissertation Ludwig-Maximilians-Universität München.

Sprecher E, Pflanzliche Geriatrika. In: ZPT 9(2):40. 1988.

Wagner H, Nörr H, Winterhoff H, Drogen mit ''Adaptogenwirkung'' zur Stärkung der Widerstandskräfte. In: ZPT 13(2):42. 1992.

Wagner H, Pflanzliche Immunstimulanzien. In: DAZ 131(4):117. 1991.

Weber R, Eleutherococcus senticosus. In: PTA 4(11):558. 1990.

Wichtl M, Pflanzliche Geriatrika. In: DAZ 132(30):1576. 1992.

Zorikov PS, Lyapustina TA, (1974) Change in a concentration of protein and nitrogen in the reproductive organs of hens under the effect of Eleutherococcus extract. Deposited DOC VIN1:732-774, 58-63: ref Chem Abstracts 86 (1977) 119732.

Further information in:

Schulz R, Hänsel R, Rationale Phytotherapie, Springer Verlag Heidelberg 1996.

Steinegger E, Hänsel R, Pharmakognosie, 5. Aufl., Springer Verlag Heidelberg 1992.

Tang W, Eisenbrand G, Chinese Drugs of Plant Origin, Springer Verlag Heidelberg 1992.

Teuscher E, Biogene Arzneimittel, 5. Aufl., Wiss. Verlagsges. mbH Stuttgart 1997.

Wagner H, Wiesenauer M, Phytotherapie. Phytopharmaka und pflanzliche Homöopathika, Fischer-Verlag, Stuttgart, Jena, New York 1995.

Elm Bark

See Ulmus Minor

Elymus Repens

Couch Grass

DESCRIPTION

Medicinal Parts: The medicinal part is the rhizome collected in spring or autumn.

Flower and Fruit: Five to 7 flowered spikelets in groups of 20 form a 10 cm long ear. The ears are usually short, upright and usually dense green and inconspicuous grass with 5 veined, lanceolate, sharply keeled glume. The spike stem is glabrous. The glume is 8 to 11 mm long, acuminate or awned. The anthers are 5 to 6 mm. The fruit is 6 to 7 mm long, flat to the front with 1 groove.

Leaves, Stem and Root: Couch grass is a 0.2 to 1.5 m perennial plant with a hardy creeping rhizome with long white runners, segmented and hollow. The leaves are thin, flat, grass green or gray-green, upper surface rough often covered in solitary long hairs.

Characteristics: Spikelets have their broad side turned towards the wave-like curved main axis; odorless, taste sweetish.

Habitat: Indigenous to the temperate regions of the northern Hemisphere. Introduced to Greenland, South America, Australia, and New Zealand.

Production: The rhizomes are collected after the fields are harrowed and are then cleaned, washed, and dried at approximately 35°C.

Not To Be Confused With: The rhizomes of Cynodon dactylon, Poaceae and Carex species (a frequent occurrence).

Other Names: Quitch grass, Witch Grass, Twitch-grass, Scotch Quelch, Dog-grass, Quickgrass, Cutch, Durfa Grass, Quack Grass, Triticum

ACTIONS AND PHARMACOLOGY

COMPOUNDS

Mucilages

Triticin (polyfructosan)

Sugar alcohols

Soluble silicic acid

Volatile oil: including carvacrol and carvone-containing P-hydroxyalkyl cinnamic acid alkyl ester

EFFECTS

The essential oil has an antimicrobial effect, however, there is no exact description available.

INDICATIONS AND USAGE

- Common cold
- Cough/bronchitis
- Fevers and colds
- Infections of the urinary tract
- Inflammation of the mouth and pharynx
- Tendency to infection

Couch Grass is also used for flushing-out therapy for inflammatory diseases of the urinary tract and for the prevention of kidney gravel.

In folk medicine, the drug is applied for cystitis, nephrolithiasis, gout, rheumatic pain, and chronic skin disorders.

Due to the high mucus content, the drug is used as a cough remedy. The infusion is used for constipation. The drug is also used for diabetes as a dietetic.

Folk medicinal uses are unproven.

CONTRAINDICATIONS

No flushing-out therapy if edema is present due to cardiac or renal insufficiency.

PRECAUTIONS AND ADVERSE REACTIONS

No health hazards or side effects are known in conjunction with the proper administration of designated therapeutic dosages.

DOSAGE

Mode of Administration: Comminuted herb decoctions and other galenic preparations for internal use.

Preparation: Liquid extract: 1:1; Tincture: 1:5; Tea: Pour boiling water over the drug and strain after 10 minutes.

Daily Dosage: The average single dose is 3 to 10 gm of drug in 1 cup of boiling water; average daily dose is 6 to 9 gm of drug.

For flushing-out therapy, ensure copious fluid intake.

Storage: The drug must be kept in sealed containers and be protected from light and moisture.

LITERATURE

Bell EA, Jansen DH, (1971) Nature 229:136.

Boesel R, Schilcher H, PM 55:399-400. 1989.

Kiesewetter R, Müller M, (1958) Pharmazie 13:777.

Koetter U et al., Isolierung und Strukturaufklärung von p-Hydroxyzimtsäurealkylesterverbindungen aus dem Rhizom von Agropyron repens, 2. Mitt. In: PM 60(5):488. 1994.

Koetter U, Kaloga M, Schilcher H, Isolierung und Strukturaufklärung von p-Hydroxyzimtsäurealkylester-Verbindungen aus dem Rhizom von Agropyron repens; 1. Mitt. In: PM 59(3):279. 1993.

Paslawska S, Piekos R, (1976) Planta Med 30:216.

Racz-Kotilla E and Mozes E, (1971) Rev Med 17:82.

Schilcher H, Boesel R, Effenberger ST, Segebrecht S, Neuere Untersuchungsergebnisse mit aquaretisch, antibakteriell und prostatotrop wirksamen Arzneipflanzen. In: ZPT 10(3):77. 1989.

Further information in:

Hänsel R, Keller K, Rimpler H, Schneider G (Hrsg.), Hagers Handbuch der Pharmazeutischen Praxis, 5. Aufl., Bde 4 - 6 (Drogen), Springer Verlag Berlin, Heidelberg, New York, 1992-1994.

Wagner H, Wiesenauer M, Phytotherapie. Phytopharmaka und pflanzliche Homöopathika, Fischer-Verlag, Stuttgart, Jena, New York 1995.

Wichtl M (Hrsg.), Teedrogen, 4. Aufl., Wiss. Verlagsges. Stuttgart 1997.

English Adder's Tongue

See Ophioglossum Vulgatum

English Horsemint

See Mentha Longifolia

English Ivy

See Hedera Helix

Ephedra Sinica

Ma-Huang

DESCRIPTION

Medicinal Parts: The medicinal parts are the young canes collected in autumn and the dried rhizome with roots.

Flower and Fruit: The flowers are small and occasionally reduced to acuminate scales. They are fused in pairs at the base. They are unisexual, usually dioecious and sometimes monoecious. The male inflorescences consist of 2 to 24 blooms. The involucre is 2-lobed and fused to a tube. The fruit is a red, berry-like false fruit formed from the upper bract.

Leaves, Stem and Root: The plant is a 30 cm high lightly branched subshrub with lengthened, cylindrical branches 1 to 2 mm in diameter. It is similar in appearance to Horsetail, and is sometimes twining and often has underground runners. The stem and branches are round with numerous vertical grooves of gray-green or bright green coloring. Very small leaves are occasionally reduced to pointed scales and are almost always fused at the base to form a sheath. They are reddish brown.

Habitat: Ephedra sinica grows mainly in Mongolia and the bordering area of China, Ephedra gerardiana is from India.

Production: Ma-Huang consists of the dried, young branchlets, harvested in the fall, of Ephedra sinica, Ephedra shennungiana, or other equivalent Ephedra species. It is mostly cultivated. The plant is harvested as late as possible after the last rain, but before the winter frost and is air-dried in the sun.

Not To Be Confused With: Many similar species

Other Names: Desert Herb, Ephedrine

ACTIONS AND PHARMACOLOGY

COMPOUNDS

Alkaloids of the 2-aminophenylpropane type: main alkaloids L-(-)-ephedrine (1R,2S-(-)- ephedrine) and D-pseudoephedrine (1S,2S-(+)- ephedrine); lesser alkaloids L-norephedrine, D- norpseudoephedrine.

EFFECTS

The level of the active principles can fluctuate so drastically that dose-related statements must take this into account. Ephedrine acts by indirectly stimulating the sympathomimetic and central nervous system. It is bacteriostatic, positively inotropic and positively chronotropic. In animal tests ephedrine acts as an antitussive.

INDICATIONS AND USAGE

■ Cough/bronchitis

Ma-Huang is used for diseases of the respiratory tract with mild bronchospasms in adults and children over the age of six. Various indications include: asthma, cardiovascular stimulation and as a stimulant.

CONTRAINDICATIONS

Contraindications include states of anxiety and restlessness, high blood pressure, angle-closure glaucoma, cerebral perfusions, prostate adenoma with residual urine volume, pheochromocytoma and thyrotoxicosis.

PRECAUTIONS AND ADVERSE REACTIONS

General: Health risks following the proper administration of designated therapeutic dosages are not recorded. The following side effects could occur: headache, irritability, motor restlessness, nausea, sleeplessness, tachycardias, urinary disorders, vomiting, and with higher dosages strong rise in blood pressure and cardiac rhythm disorders.

Dependence upon the drug can develop with extended intake. Because of the danger of the development of tachyphylaxis and of dependence, the drug should only be administered for short periods. Ephedrine and the drug itself are considered doping substances.

Drug Interactions: Numerous reciprocal actions with other medications have been observed.

- Heart glycosides or halothane: disturbance of heart rhythm.
- Guanethidine: enhancement of the sympathomimetic effect.
- MAO-inhibitors: potentiate the sympathomimetic action of ephedrine.
- Secale alkaloid derivatives or oxytocin: development of high blood pressure.

OVERDOSAGE

Life-threatening poisonings are only conceivable with very high dosages of the drug (over 100 gm, lethal dosage with oral administration corresponding to approximately 1 to 2 gm L-ephedrine). Symptoms of poisoning include severe outbreaks of sweating, enlarged pupils, spasms and elevated body temperature, with death following through heart failure and asphyxiation. Following stomach emptying (gastric lavage with burgundy-colored potassium permaganate solution), therapy consists of the administration of activated charcoal and prophylaxis against shock. Spasms should be treated with diazepam, electrolyte substitution should be employed, and sodium bicarbonate infusions should be used to prevent acidosis. Intubation and oxygen respiration are also on occasion necessary.

DOSAGE

Mode of Administration: Ma-Huang is administered as a comminuted herb, as well as other galenic preparations for internal use.

Daily Dosage: For adults, the average single dose is 15 to 30 mg total alkaloid, calculated as ephedrine, for a total dose of 300 mg per day. When used in children, single doses of herb preparations corresponding to 0.5 mg total alkaloid per kg of body weight are employed. The recommended daily dosage for children is 2 mg.

Tea: 1 to 4 gm 3 times daily.

Tinctura Ephedrae (1:1): medium single dose 5 gm.

Extractum Ephedrae: 1 to 3 ml 3 times daily.

Tinctura Ephedrae (1:4): 6 to 8 ml 3 times daily.

Storage: Ma-Huang must be protected from light.

LITERATURE

Gazaliev AM, Fazilov SD, Zhurinov MZ, Khim Prorod Soed 23:862-864. 1987.

Harada M, Nishimura M, J Pharm Dyn 4:691-699. 1981.

Further information in:

Hänsel R, Keller K, Rimpler H, Schneider G (Hrsg.), Hagers Handbuch der Pharmazeutischen Praxis, 5. Aufl., Bde 4-6 (Drogen), Springer Verlag Berlin, Heidelberg, New York, 1992-1994.

Madaus G, Lehrbuch der Biologischen Arzneimittel, Bde 1-3, Nachdruck, Georg Olms Verlag Hildesheim 1979.

Roth L, Daunderer M, Kormann K, Giftpflanzen, Pflanzengifte, 4. Aufl., Ecomed Fachverlag Landsberg Lech 1993.

Schulz R, Hänsel R, Rationale Phytotherapie, Springer Verlag Heidelberg 1996.

Steinegger E, Hänsel R, Pharmakognosie, 5. Aufl., Springer Verlag Heidelberg 1992.

Tang W, Eisenbrand G, Chinese Drugs of Plant Origin, Springer Verlag Heidelberg 1992.

Teuscher E, Lindequist U, Biogene Gifte - Biologie, Chemie, Pharmakologie, 2. Aufl., Fischer Verlag Stuttgart 1994.

Teuscher E, Biogene Arzneimittel, 5. Aufl., Wiss. Verlagsges. mbH Stuttgart 1997.

Wagner H, Wiesenauer M, Phytotherapie. Phytopharmaka und pflanzliche Homöopathika, Fischer-Verlag, Stuttgart, Jena, New York 1995.

Epigae Repens

Trailing Arbutus

DESCRIPTION

Medicinal Parts: The medicinal parts are the fresh or dried leaves.

Flower and Fruit: The flowers are in apical dense racemes. They are white with a reddish tinge and are very fragrant. They are divided at the tip into 5 segments which open in a star shape.

Leaves, Stem and Root: The plant is a fragrant, prostrate, evergreen branching shrub with rust-colored, pubescent, round stems. Roots develop at the stem nodes, which spread quickly. The leaves are petioled, broadly ovate, 2.5 to 4 cm long and about 2 cm wide, coriaceous, entire-margined, reticulate, with a cordate base and short pointed apex and short hairs on the undersurface. The branches, petioles and leaf nerves are very pubescent.

Characteristics: The plant has a similar action to Buchu on the urinary system.

Habitat: Indigenous to North America, established as an ornamental plant in Europe.

Production: Trailing Arbutus is the aerial part of Epigaea repens.

Other Names: Gravel Plant, Ground Laurel, Mountain Pink, Water Pink, Winter Pink

ACTIONS AND PHARMACOLOGY

COMPOUNDS

Arbutin (hydroquinone glucoside)

Tannins

EFFECTS

Trailing Arbutus has astringent and diuretic properties.

INDICATIONS AND USAGE

Trailing Arbutus is used for urinary tract conditions.

PRECAUTIONS AND ADVERSE REACTIONS

Health risks or side effects following the proper administration of designated therapeutic dosages are not recorded. Nausea and vomiting can also occur with stomach sensitivity in children. Liver damage, cachexia, hemolytic anemia and depigmentation of the hair are conceivable with long-term use of the drug.

OVERDOSAGE

Overdosages could lead to inflammatory reactions of the mucous membranes of the bladder and urinary passages, accompanied by strangury and possible blood in the urine.

DOSAGE

Mode of Administration: As an infusion or extract for internal use.

LITERATURE

Kern W, List PH, Hörhammer L (Hrsg.), Hagers Handbuch der Pharmazeutischen Praxis, 4. Aufl., Bde. 1-8, Springer Verlag Berlin, Heidelberg, New York, 1969.

Epilobium Species

Willow Herb

DESCRIPTION

Medicinal Parts: The medicinal parts are the herb and the roots of the drug containing Epilobium varieties.

Flower and Fruit: The flowers are arranged in long clusters of crimson flowers. The receptacle extends over the ovary. There are 4 sepals which are often colored and 8 stamens. The petals are purple to pink, seldom white or yellow. The style is erect or curved downwards. The stigma is capitual or club-like and has 4 grooves or is divided into 4. The fruit is long, linear capsule-like, quadrangular, 4-valved and opens with 4 bending valves. The seeds are numerous and smooth or they may be covered in tiny warts with a white, often short-stemmed, tuft of hair.

Leaves, Stem and Root: The species includes perennial herbs and occasionally up to 2 m high subshrubs with an underground creeping rhizome. The stems are erect, glabrous or covered with simple hairs or glandular hairs. The leaves are entire-margined or dentate, alternate or opposite in whorls of 3, flat or occasionally with a turned-back border.

Habitat: The plant is found all over Europe, Asia apart from the tropical islands, Africa and America, Australia, Tasmania and New Zealand.

Production: Willow Herb is the aerial part of Epilobium parviflorum and other small-blossomed Willow Herbs. The herb is dried in the open air in the shade.

Other Names: Blood Vine, Blooming Sally, Rose Bay Willow Herb, Willow-Herb

ACTIONS AND PHARMACOLOGY

COMPOUNDS : EPILOBIUM ANGUSTIFOLIUM

Flavonoids: in particular myricitrin, isoquercitrin, quercitrin, guaiaverin, quercetin-3-O-beta-D-glucuronide

Steroids: in particular beta-sitosterol and its ester, including among others beta-sitosterol caproate

Palmitate

Tannins

EFFECTS: EPILOBIUM ANGUSTIFOLIUM
Willow Herb is reported to have antiphlogistic and antiexsudative effects: a watery infusion revealed a significant inhibitory effect on edemas in rat paws. The methanol infusion had a distinctly weaker effect.

Antimicrobial effects have also been demonstrated. A suspension of the fresh drug in ethanol stunts the growth of the bacteria of *Pseudomonas pyocyanea.* Tincture and the liquid extract work antimicrobially against *Candida albicans, Staphylococcus albus* and *Staphylococcus aureus.* The dried residue of a maceration, which is fixed on filter paper, shows a weak effect against *Bacillus subtilis, Escherichia coli, Mycobacterium smegmatis, Shigella flexneri, Shigella sonnei* and *Staphylococcus aureus.* An extra fraction of the drug (insufficiently chemically defined) showed a tumor-inhibiting effect on transplanted tumors in mice and rats. Furthermore, the drug was apparently protective and curative in benign prostate hyperplasia and certain micturition disorders for Epilobium angustifolium were antiphlogistic.

COMPOUNDS: EPILOBIUM HIRSUTUM
Flavonoids: in particular guaiaverin, hyperoside, myricitrin, quercetin-3-O-beta-D-glucuronide,quercetin-3-O-alpha-L-arabinofuranoside

Steroids: in particular beta-sitosterol

Tannins

EFFECTS: EPILOBIUM HIRSUTUM
Willow Herb is reported to have antiphlogistic and antiexudative effects: a watery infusion revealed a significant inhibitory effect on edemas in rat paws. The methanol infusion had a distinctly weaker effect.

Antimicrobial effects have also been demonstrated. A suspension of the fresh drug in ethanol stunts the growth of the bacteria of *Pseudomonas pyocyanea.* Tincture and the liquid extract work antimicrobially against *Candida albicans, Staphylococcus albus* and *Staphylococcus aureus.* The dried residue of a maceration, which is fixed on filter paper, shows a weak effect against *Bacillus subtilis, Escherichia coli, Mycobacterium smegmatis, Shigella flexneri, Shigella sonnei* and *Staphylococcus aureus.* An extra fraction of the drug (insufficiently chemically defined) showed a tumor-inhibiting effect on transplanted tumors in mice and rats. Furthermore, the drug was apparently protective and curative in benign prostate hyperplasia.

COMPOUNDS: EPILOBIUM PARVIFLORUM
Flavonoids: in particular guaiaverin, quercetin-3-O-beta-D-glucuronide, quercitrin

Steroids: in particular beta-sitosterol and its ester, including among others beta-sitosterol caproate

Palmitate

Tannins

EFFECTS: EPILOBIUM PARVIFLORUM
Willow Herb is reported to have antiphlogistic and antiexudative effects: a watery infusion revealed a significant inhibitory effect on edemas in rat paws. The methanol infusion had a distinctly weaker effect.

Antimicrobial effects have also been demonstrated. A suspension of the fresh drug in ethanol stunts the growth of the bacteria of *Pseudomonas pyocyanea.* Tincture and the liquid extract work antimicrobially against *Candida albicans, Staphylococcus albus* and *Staphylococcus aureus.* The dried residue of a maceration, which is fixed on filter paper, shows a weak effect against *Bacillus subtilis, Escherichia coli, Mycobacterium smegmatis, Shigella flexneri, Shigella sonnei* and *Staphylococcus aureus.* An extra fraction of the drug (insufficiently chemically defined) showed a tumor-inhibiting effect on transplanted tumors in mice and rats. Furthermore, the drug was apparently protective and curative in benign prostate hyperplasia.

INDICATIONS AND USAGE
Willow Herb is used internally for prostate disorders, as an infusion for gastrointestinal disorders and mucous membrane lesions of the mouth. Indians use the drug for rectal bleeding; the Chinese for menstrual disorders. The watery extract is used externally to improve the healing of wounds.

Efficacy has not been proven to date.

PRECAUTIONS AND ADVERSE REACTIONS
Health risks or side effects following the proper administration of designated therapeutic dosages are not recorded.

DOSAGE
Mode of Administration: The drug is not available as a ready made medicinal preparation; only as a tea, watery extract or as a vegetable.

LITERATURE
Ducrey B et al., Inhibition of 5alpha-Reduktase and aromatase by ellagitannins oenothein A and eonothein B from Epilobium species. In: PM 63(2):111-114. 1997.

Hiemann A, Mayr K, Sci Pharm 53:39. 1985.

Hiermann A, Sci Pharm 63:135. 1995.

Lesuisse D et al., Determination of Oenothein B as the active 5-alpha-reductase-inhibiting principles of the folk medicine Epilobium parvifloruam. In: JNP 59(5):490-492. 1996.

Slacanin I et al., J Chromatogr 557:391. 1991.

Further information in:

Hänsel R, Keller K, Rimpler H, Schneider G (Hrsg.), Hagers Handbuch der Pharmazeutischen Praxis, 5. Aufl., Bde 4-6

(Drogen), Springer Verlag Berlin, Heidelberg, New York, 1992-1994.

Wichtl M (Hrsg.), Teedrogen, 4. Aufl., Wiss. Verlagsges. Stuttgart 1997.

Equisetum Arvense

Horsetail

DESCRIPTION

Medicinal Parts: The medicinal parts are the dried green, sterile shoots and fresh sterile shoots.

Flower and Fruit: Horsetail appears in two forms during the year: in March to April the red-brown to straw yellow, 20 cm high, simple stem develops with leaves arranged in a number of levels on the stem in whorls; the leaves are brown, fused to a sheath at the lower level with black-tipped, dry sporangia cones at the tip sprinkling greenish spore powder. In May and June the sterile summer form with 10 to 14 cm high stems and numerous branches arranged in whorls at the nodes; stem and branches are deeply grooved, usually square, rough.

Habitat: Horsetail grows throughout all of Europe, in Asia southwards as far as Turkey, Iran, the Himalayas, central and north China as well as Japan. It grows in North America from Greenland and Alaska to Texas.

Production: Horsetail consists of the fresh or dried, green, sterile stems of Equisetum arvense.

Not To Be Confused With: Other Equisetum species.

Other Names: Bottle-brush, Corn Horsetail, Dutch Rushes, Field Horsetail, Horse Willow, Horsetail Grass, Horsetail Rush, Paddock-pipes, Pewterwort, Scouring Rush, Shave Grass, Toadpipe

ACTIONS AND PHARMACOLOGY

COMPOUNDS

Flavonoids: in particular quercetin-, kaempferol-, luteolin-, genkwanin-3-O-glucosides, 5-O-,7-O-glucosides and diglucosides

Caffeic acid ester: including chlorogenic acid, dicoffeoyl-meso-tartaric acid

Silicic acid: to some extent water-soluble

Styrolpyrone glucoside: equisetumpyron

Pyridine alkaloids: nicotine (traces)

EFFECTS

Horsetail has a mild diuretic action.

INDICATIONS AND USAGE

- Infections of the urinary tract
- Kidney and bladder stones
- Wounds and burns

Internal preparations are used for post-traumatic and static edema, flushing-out therapy for bacterial and inflammatory diseases of the lower urinary tract and renal gravel.

It is used externally as a supportive treatment for poorly healing wounds.

In folk medicine, Equisetum arvense is used for tuberculosis, as a catarrh in the kidney and bladder regions, as a hematostatic for profuse menstruation, nasal, pulmonary and gastric hemorrhages, for brittle finger nails and loss of hair, for rheumatic diseases, gout, poorly healing wounds and ulcers, swelling and fractures and for frostbite, although this use is not proven.

CONTRAINDICATIONS

Horsetail is contraindicated in patients who have edema due to impaired heart and kidney function.

PRECAUTIONS AND ADVERSE REACTIONS

Health risks or side effects following the proper administration of designated therapeutic dosages are not recorded.

A doctor should be consulted when the drug is utilized as a bath additive in cases of major skin lesions, acute skin lesions of unknown origin, major feverish and infectious diseases, cardiac insufficiency and hypertonia.

DOSAGE

Mode of Administration: Comminuted herb for infusions and other galenic preparations are available for oral administration. Comminuted herb for decoctions and other galenic preparations are used externally.

Preparations: To make a tea, pour boiling water over 2 to 3 gm drug and boil for 5 minutes. Strain after 10 to 15 minutes. To make an infusion, use 1.5 gm drug per 1 cup water. A liquid extract is prepared in a 1:1 ratio in 25% alcohol.

Daily Dosage: For internal use, the average daily dosage of herb is 6 gm. Observe ample intake of liquid. When using an infusion, the dosage is 2 to 4 gm. The dosage for a liquid extract is 1 to 4 ml three times daily. The tea is drunk repeatedly during the day between meals. For external use, the recommended dosage is 10 gm of herb per liter of water for use in compresses.

Storage: The drug must be protected from light in well-sealed containers.

LITERATURE

Beckert C, Veit M, Styrylpyrone im Schachtelhalm. In: DAZ 137(28):2474-2475. 1997.

Eugster C, Heterocycles 4:51. 1976.

Gibelli C (1931) Arch Int Pharmacodyn 41:419.

Hiller K, Pharmazeutische Bewertung ausgewählter Teedrogen. In: DAZ 135(16):1425-1440. 1995.

Karrer P et al., Helv Chim Acta 32:2397-2399. 1949.

Pohl RW, (1955) Am Fern J 45:95.

Sökeland J, Phytotherapie in der Urologie. In: ZPT 10(1):8. 1989.

Veit M, Problem bei der Bewertung pflanzlicher Diuretika. Als Beispiel Schachtelhalmkraut DAB 10 (Equiseti herba). In: ZPT 15(6):331-341. 1994.

Veit M et al., Flavonoids of the Equisetum hybrids in the subgenus Equisetum. In: PM 58(7):A697. 1992.

Further information in:

Hänsel R, Keller K, Rimpler H, Schneider G (Hrsg.), Hagers Handbuch der Pharmazeutischen Praxis, 5. Aufl., Bde 4-6 (Drogen), Springer Verlag Berlin, Heidelberg, New York, 1992-1994.

Madaus G, Lehrbuch der Biologischen Arzneimittel, Bde 1-3, Nachdruck, Georg Olms Verlag Hildesheim 1979.

Steinegger E, Hänsel R, Pharmakognosie, 5. Aufl., Springer Verlag Heidelberg 1992.

Teuscher E, Biogene Arzneimittel, 5. Aufl., Wiss. Verlagsges. mbH Stuttgart 1997.

Wagner H, Wiesenauer M, Phytotherapie. Phytopharmaka und pflanzliche Homöopathika, Fischer-Verlag, Stuttgart, Jena, New York 1995.

Wichtl M (Hrsg.), Teedrogen, 4. Aufl., Wiss. Verlagsges. Stuttgart 1997.

Ergot

See Claviceps Purpurea

Erigeron Canadensis

Canadian Fleabane

DESCRIPTION

Medicinal Parts: The medicinal parts are the dried aerial parts of the plant and the fresh aerial parts of the flowering plant.

Flower and Fruit: Very small yellowish-white composite flowers in long, terminal, branched panicle-like inflorescences. The involucre is in a number of rows. The composite head has numerous florets. The ray florets are linguiform, female, white or reddish. The disc florets are tubular and androgynous. The stamens are fused. The fruit is an achaene, 1.2 to 1.5 mm long, brownish and has short appressed hair.

Leaves, Stem and Root: Erigeron canadensis is an annual or biennial 30 to 100 cm high. The root is thin and fusiform, the stem erect, roundish, slightly ribbed, greenish with paler ribs and is covered in scattered patent hairs. It is branched from the peduncle. The leaves are alternate, pointed, ciliate, narrowly lanceolate and up to 10 cm wide and tapering to the petiole.

Habitat: The plant is indigenous to America but is found globally today.

Production: Canadian Trailing Arbutus is the flowering plant and seeds (without the root) of Erigeron canadensis.

Other Names: Coltstail, Flea Wort, Horseweed, Prideweed

ACTION AND PHARMACOLOGY

COMPOUNDS

Volatile oil: including mit (+)-limonene, alpha-cis-bergamots, beta-trans-farnesene, beta-pinenes, myrcene, cis, cis-matricariamethyl ester (polyyne)

Tannins

EFFECTS

The drug is reported to be antiphlogistic.

INDICATIONS AND USAGE

The drug is used for diarrhea, as an antithelmintic, a mild hemostyptic, for uterine bleeding, dysentery, dropsy, tumors and bronchitis. In African folk medicine, it is used in the treatment of granuloma annulare, sore throats, urinary tract infections and for medicinal baths.

PRECAUTIONS AND ADVERSE REACTIONS

Health risks or side effects following the proper administration of designated therapeutic dosages are not recorded.

DOSAGE

Mode of Administration: The drug is used topically and in alcoholic extracts.

LITERATURE

Grancia D et al., (1985) Ceskoslov Farm 34(6):209.

Lasser B et al., (1983) Naturwissenschaften 70:95.

Further information in:

Hänsel R, Keller K, Rimpler H, Schneider G (Hrsg.), Hagers Handbuch der Pharmazeutischen Praxis, 5. Aufl., Bde 4-6 (Drogen), Springer Verlag Berlin, Heidelberg, New York, 1992-1994 (unter Conyza).

Madaus G, Lehrbuch der Biologischen Arzneimittel, Bde 1-3, Nachdruck, Georg Olms Verlag Hildesheim 1979.

Wagner H, Wiesenauer M, Phytotherapie. Phytopharmaka und pflanzliche Homöopathika, Fischer-Verlag, Stuttgart, Jena, New York 1995.

Eriodictyon Californicum

Yerba Santa

DESCRIPTION

Medicinal Parts: The medicinal parts are the dried leaves.

Flower and Fruit: The flowers are tubular to funnel-shaped, lavender or white and clustered at the top of the plant. The calyx is ciliate. The fruit is a small, oval, grayish-brown seed capsule containing shriveled, almost black seeds.

Leaves, Stem and Root: The plant is a 2.5 m high, sticky, evergreen shrub, with woody rhizomes. The trunk is smooth and usually branched near the ground. It is completely covered in sticky resin. The leaves are up to 15 cm long and about 2 cm broad, thick, coriaceous, glabrous, greenish white, lanceolate, irregularly dentate at the margins. The upper surface appears to be varnished with resin, the lower surface is reticulate and tomentose.

Characteristics: The taste is balsamic and the odor, pleasant and aromatic.

Habitat: The plant grows in California, Oregon and parts of Mexico.

Production: Yerba Santa is the aerial part of Eriodictyon Californicum.

Other Names: Bear's Weed, Consumptive's Weed, Eriodictyon, Gum Bush, Holy Herb, Mountain Balm, Sacred Herb, Tarweed

ACTIONS AND PHARMACOLOGY

COMPOUNDS

Flavonoids: including eriodictyonin, eriodictyol, chrysoeriodictyol, xanthoeriodictyol

Volatile oil (very little)

Resinous substances: made up of flavonone and flavone aglycones

Tannins

EFFECTS

Yerba Santa is mildly diuretic and masks bitter tastes.

INDICATIONS AND USAGE

The drug is used as a constituent of antiasthmatic treatments and application by brush (painted on) to counteract bitter tastes.

PRECAUTIONS AND ADVERSE REACTIONS

Health risks or side effects following the proper administration of designated therapeutic dosages are not recorded.

DOSAGE

Mode of Administration: As an additive to mask bitter flavors and for painting on as Tinctura Eriodictyonis.

LITERATURE

Johnson ND, Biochem Syst Ecol 11:211. 1983.

Liu YL, Ho DK, Cassady JM, Isolation of potential cancer chemopreventive agents from Eriodictyon californicum. In: JNP 55(3):357-363. 1992.

Further information in:

Kern W, List PH, Hörhammer L (Hrsg.), Hagers Handbuch der Pharmazeutischen Praxis, 4. Aufl., Bde 1-8, Springer Verlag Berlin, Heidelberg, New York, 1969.

Eryngium Campestre

Eryngo

DESCRIPTION

Medicinal Parts: The medicinal parts are the dried leaves and flowers and roots.

Flower and Fruit: The plant bears small terminal cymes on oval to globular capitula on sweeping inflorescences. The linear-lanceolate to awl-shaped bracts terminate in sharp thorns. The sepals are lanceolate and terminate in thorny tips and are twice as long as the white or gray-green petals. The fruit is compressed obovate with lanceolate pointed scales.

Leaves, Stem and Root: The plant is 15 to 60 cm high, perennial, with a whitish or yellow-green color. The bifurcated stem is erect, thick, grooved and spare. The stem forms a round bush with the branches. The leaves are tough, short-petioled or sessile. The upper leaves are clasping, double pinnatesect and thorny dentate. The root is cylindrical, thick, brown and woody.

Characteristics: The root is spicy.

Habitat: The plant grows in most parts of Europe and northern Africa and has been introduced into North America.

Production: Erngo root is the root of Eryngium campestre, which is gathered and dried in the Spring and Autumn. It is gathered in uncultivated regions. The roots are halved and air-dried. Eryngo herb is the dried leaves and blossoms of Eryngium campestre.

Other Names: Eringo, Sea Holly, Sea Holme, Sea Hulver

ACTIONS AND PHARMACOLOGY

COMPOUNDS: ERYNGII RADIX

Triterpene saponins

Procoumarins

Pyranocoumarins: (to date only demonstrated when the source is E. campestre), including aegelinol and its ester agasyllin, grandivetin

Monoterpene glycosides of the cyclohexenol-type: (to date only demonstrated when the source is E. campestre)

Caffeic acid ester: chlorogenic acid, rosmaric acid

*Oligosaccharides:*1-kestose

EFFECTS: ERYNGII RADIX

The root is mildly expectorant and spasmolytic.

COMPOUNDS: ERYNGII HERBA

Triterpene saponins

Caffeic acid ester: chlorogenic acid, rosmaric acid

Flavonoids

EFFECTS: ERYNGII HERBA

The herb is a mild diuretic.

INDICATIONS AND USAGE

ERYNGII RADIX

The root is used in the treatment of bladder and kidney stones, renal colic, kidney and urinary tract inflammation, urinary retention and edema. It is also used for coughs, bronchitis, skin and respiratory disorders. Its efficacy has not been proven.

ERYNGII HERBA

The herb is used in the treatment of urinary tract infections and as an adjuvant to treat inflammation of the efferent urinary tract, prostatitis and bronchial catarrh. Its efficacy has not been proven.

PRECAUTIONS AND ADVERSE REACTIONS

ERYNGII RADIX AND HERBA

Health risks or side effects following the proper administration of designated therapeutic dosages are not recorded.

DOSAGE

ERYNGII RADIX

Mode of Administration: The drug is contained in tea mixtures, extracts, decoctions, liquids, tinctures and homeopathic dilutions (from E. yuccifolium).

Preparation: To make a tea, use 1 level teaspoonful of the ground root per cup of boiling water (30 to 40 gm per liter boiling water). Allow to draw until cold. To make a decoction, boil 4 teaspoonfuls of the ground root in 1 liter of water for 10 minutes and allow to draw for 15 minutes. The tincture is prepared by soaking 20 gm ground drug in 80 gm of 60% alcohol for 10 days.

Daily Dosage: The daily dosage is 3 to 4 cups of the tea; 2 to 3 cups of the decoction; 50 to 60 drops of the tincture in 3 or 4 divided doses; or 2 to 3 gm of the liquid extract.

ERYNGII HERBA

Mode of Administration: The drug is administered as an extract.

LITERATURE

ERYNGII RADIX

Bhargava SK, Dixit VP, (1985) Plant Med Phytother 19(1):29.

Erdelmeier CAJ, Sticher O, (1985) Planta Med 51(5):407.

Gracza L et al., (1985) Arch Pharm 312(12):1090.

Hiller K, In "The Biology and Chemistry of the Umbelliferae". Ed. V. N. Heywood, Academic Press London 1971.

Hiller K, Linzer B, PA 22:321. 1967.

Kartnig T, Wolf J, Flavonoide aus den oberirdischen Teilen von Eryngium campestre. In: PM 59(3):285. 1993.

Lisciani R et al., (1984) J Ethnopharmacol 12(39):263.

Further information in:

Hänsel R, Keller K, Rimpler H, Schneider G (Hrsg.), Hagers Handbuch der Pharmazeutischen Praxis, 5. Aufl., Bde 4-6 (Drogen), Springer Verlag Berlin, Heidelberg, New York, 1992-1994.

Madaus G, Lehrbuch der Biologischen Arzneimittel, Bde 1-3, Nachdruck, Georg Olms Verlag Hildesheim 1979.

Steinegger E, Hänsel R, Pharmakognosie, 5. Aufl., Springer Verlag Heidelberg 1992.

ERYNGII HERBA

Bhargava SK, Dixit VP, (1985) Plant Med Phytother 19(1):29.

Erdelmeier CAJ, Sticher O, (1985) Planta Med 51(5):407-409.

Gracza L et al., (1985) Arch Pharm 312(12):1090.

Hiller K, In "The Biology and Chemistry of the Umbelliferae". Ed. V. N. Heywood, Academic Press London 1971.

Hiller K, Linzer B, PA 22:321. 1967.

Kartnig T, Wolf J, Flavonoide aus den oberirdischen Teilen von Eryngium campestre. In: PM 59(3):285. 1993.

Lisciani R et al., (1984) J Ethnopharmacol 12(39):263.

Further information in:

Hänsel R, Keller K, Rimpler H, Schneider G (Hrsg.), Hagers Handbuch der Pharmazeutischen Praxis, 5. Aufl., Bde 4-6 (Drogen), Springer Verlag Berlin, Heidelberg, New York, 1992-1994.

Madaus G, Lehrbuch der Biologischen Arzneimittel, Bde 1-3, Nachdruck, Georg Olms Verlag Hildesheim 1979.

Steinegger E, Hänsel R, Pharmakognosie, 5. Aufl., Springer Verlag Heidelberg 1992.

Eryngo

See Eryngium Campestre

Erythronium Americanum

American Adder's Tongue

DESCRIPTION

Medicinal Parts: The medicinal parts are the leaves and tubers.

Flower and Fruit: The flowers are terminal, large, hanging, lily-like and are 2.5 cm in diameter. The bracts of the involucre are sharply revolute, bright yellow and often tinged purple and sprinkled at the base. There are 6 stamens. The fruit is a fusiform nodule about 2 cm long.

Leaves, Stem and Root: The plant grows from a small, ovate fern-colored corm to between 2 and 2.5 cm long. It is perennial with a bulbous light brown root. The stem is thin and about 25 cm high. There are only 2 leaves, lanceolate, pale green with purplish or brownish spots, about 6 cm long by 2 to 3 cm wide, minutely wrinkled and with parallel veins. The petioles are 5 to 7.5 cm long.

Characteristics: The fresh leaves have emollient and anti-scrofulous properties when applied as a poultice.

Habitat: The plant grows in the eastern U.S. as far south as Florida and westward as far as Ontario and Arkansas.

Production: American Adder's Tongue leaves are the fresh leaves of Erythronium americanum.

Other Names: Dog's Tooth Violet, Erythronium, Lamb's Tongue, Rattlesnake Violet, Serpent's Tongue, Snake Leaf, Yellow Snakeleaf, Yellow Snowdrop

ACTION AND PHARMACOLOGY

COMPOUNDS

Alpha-methylene-gamma-butyrolactones: tuliposides

EFFECTS

When used internally, the drug is emetic. Externally it is an emollient.

INDICATIONS AND USAGE

It is used externally for ulcers.

PRECAUTIONS AND ADVERSE REACTIONS

The plant has a strongly sensitizing effect. Reciprocal reactions occur with tulip, fritallaria, lily, alstroemeria and Bomarea species. Nothing is known regarding health hazards or side effects in connection with the administration of the drug.

DOSAGE

Mode of Administration: Fresh leaves are applied topically as a poultice or administered internally as an infusion.

LITERATURE

Cavallito CJ, Haskell TH, (1946) J Am Chem Soc 66:2332.

Further information in:

Hausen B, Allergiepflanzen, Pflanzenallergene, ecomed Verlagsgesellsch. mbH, Landsberg 1988.

Kern W, List PH, Hörhammer L (Hrsg.), Hagers Handbuch der Pharmazeutischen Praxis, 4. Aufl., Bde 1-8, Springer Verlag Berlin, Heidelberg, New York, 1969.

Teuscher E, Lindequist U, Biogene Gifte - Biologie, Chemie, Pharmakologie, 2. Aufl., Fischer Verlag Stuttgart 1994.

Erythroxylum Coca

Coca

DESCRIPTION

Medicinal Parts: The medicinal parts are the leaves of the coca bush.

Flower and Fruit: The flowers are small and greenish white. They are in axillary clusters. The fruit is a red almost 1 cm long drupe with 1 seed.

Leaves, Stem and Root: Erythroxylum Coca is a small shrub-like tree up to 5 m tall. The leaves are brownish-green, oval, thin but tough, up to 5 cm long and 2.5 cm wide with two lines on the surface parallel to the midrib. The margins are entire, the apex rounded. There are 2 faint projecting lines on the upper surface parallel to the midrib which stiffen the leaf. There are small stipules in the leaf axils, which later become brown and hard.

Habitat: The plant is indigenous to the Andes region of South America; it is cultivated in Indonesia, India and Sri Lanka.

Production: Coca leaves are the dried leaves of Erythroxylum coca.

Other Names: Bolivian Coca, Cocaine, Cuca, Peruvian Coca

ACTIONS AND PHARMACOLOGY

COMPOUNDS

Tropane alkaloids: main alkaloid (-)-cocaine, including, among others, cis-cinnamoyl cocaine, trans-cinnamoyl cocaine, also including alpha-truxillin, beta-truxillin, benzoylecgonin

EFFECTS

The leaves act as a local anesthetic and stimulate the central nervous system. In high doses, it causes paralysis of motor neuron fibers.

INDICATIONS AND USAGE

The drug is used in the manufacture of cocaine chloride as a local anaesthetic. It is a model for synthetic local anesthetics. It is no longer itself in use, except occasionally in ophthalmology.

PRECAUTIONS AND ADVERSE REACTIONS

General: Chewing an excessively large quantity of the leaves can bring about psychic disturbances and hallucinations. Dangerous poisonings are not possible with the drug (though the opposite is certainly true with cocaine or cocoa paste). Chronic use can lead to poor nutritional states and disinterest in work, due to the suppression of feelings of hunger and the resulting reduction in food intake. The enhanced vulnerability to illness and the reduced life expectancy are also conditioned by the immunosupressive effect of the drug. Beyond that, the drug is probably carcinogenic in effect, embryotoxic and sensitizing. The observed dependence on the drug (cocoaism) is mainly psychically conditioned, although withdrawal symptoms are also known (need for sleep, bulimia, anxiety, irritability, tremor). For the toxicology of cocaine, consult publications (Lewin, Teuscher).

Pregnancy: Cocaine passes into the embryo or fetus and is embryotoxic.

Nursing Mothers: Cocaine passes into the mother's milk.

DOSAGE

Mode of Administration: Use of Erythroxylum coca is obsolete except for use in 2% eyedrops.

LITERATURE

Aynilian G et al., (1974) J Pharm Sci 63:1938.

Brustschmerzen und Atherosklerose durch Cocain. In: DAZ 130(49):2723. 1990.

Chen GJ, Pillai R, Erickson JR, Martinez F, Estrada ALÖ, Watso RR, Cocaine immunotoxicity - abnormal cytokine production in hispanic drug users. In: Toxicol Lett 59(1-3):81. 1991.

Evans WC, ETH 3:265. 1981.

Grieb G, Mißbildungen: Schädigt Cocain menschliche Spermien? In: DAZ 132(12):578. 1992.

Homstedt B et al., (1977) Phytochemistry 16:1753.

Moore JM et al., 1-Hydroxytropacocaine: an abundant alkaloid of Erythroxylum novogranatense var. novogranatense and var. truxillense. In: PH 36(2):357. 1994.

Novak M, Salemink C, (1987) Planta Med 53(1):113.

Novak M, Salemink CA, Khan I, ETH 10:261. 1984.

Sukrasno N, Yeoman MM, Phenylpropanoid metabolism during growth and development of Capsicum frutescens fruits. In: PH 32:839. 1993.

Tuerner CE, Ma C, Elsohly MA, ETH 3:293. 1981.

Wiggins RC, Pharmacokinetics of Cocaine in pregnancy and effects on fetal maturation. In: Clinical Pharmacokinetics 22(2):85. 1992.

Further information in:

Hänsel R, Keller K, Rimpler H, Schneider G (Hrsg.), Hagers Handbuch der Pharmazeutischen Praxis, 5. Aufl., Bde 4-6 (Drogen), Springer Verlag Berlin, Heidelberg, New York, 1992-1994.

Leung AY, Encyclopedia of Common Natural Ingredients Used in Food Drugs and Cosmetics, John Wiley & Sons Inc., New York 1980.

Lewin L, Gifte und Vergiftungen, 6. Aufl., Nachdruck, Haug Verlag, Heidelberg 1992.

Roth L, Daunderer M, Kormann K, Giftpflanzen, Pflanzengifte, 4. Aufl., Ecomed Fachverlag Landsberg Lech 1993.

Steinegger E, Hänsel R, Pharmakognosie, 5. Aufl., Springer Verlag Heidelberg 1992.

Teuscher E, Lindequist U, Biogene Gifte - Biologie, Chemie, Pharmakologie, 2. Aufl., Fischer Verlag Stuttgart 1994.

Teuscher E, Biogene Arzneimittel, 5. Aufl., Wiss. Verlagsges. mbH Stuttgart 1997.

Eschscholtzia Californica

California Poppy

DESCRIPTION

Medicinal Parts: The medicinal parts of Eschscholtzia californica are the aerial parts collected during the flowering season and dried.

Flower and Fruit: The bright yellow-to-orange flowers are solitary, axillary and long-pedicled. They are 2.5 to 4 cm in diameter with a cup-shaped receptacle. The sepals are fused. Four crenate petals, orange-red at the base, form an open dish. The stigma is thread-like. There are numerous yellow stamens. The fruit is an oblong, 4 to 6 cm pod-like exploding capsule which spreads small globular seeds.

Leaves, Stem and Root: Eschscholtzia californica is a bluish-green annual to perennial that grows 30 to 60 cm high. The leaves are sparse. Strongly pinnatifid leaves with linear sections taper to a thin tip.

Habitat: The plant grows in California and is cultivated in central Europe and southern France.

Production: The Californian Poppy herb consists of the aerial parts of Eschscholtzia californica.

ACTIONS AND PHARMACOLOGY

COMPOUNDS

Isoquinoline alkaloids: The main alkaloid is californidin. Included are others, such as eschscholzine (escholzine), protopine, alpha-allocryptopine, beta-allocryptopine.

Cyanogenic glycosides (in the freshly-harvested plant)

EFFECTS

In mice, a hot water extract was sleep-inducing.

INDICATIONS AND USAGE

Preparations of the drug are used for insomnia, aches, nervous agitation, enuresis nocturna in children, diseases of the bladder and liver, reactive agitative and masked depressions, melancholia, neurasthenia, neuropathy, organic neuroses, vegetative-dystonic disorders, mood swings, weather sensitivity, vasomotoric dysfunctions, vegetative-endocrine syndrome, constitutional weakness of the nervous system and vasomotoric cephalgia. The tea is used as a sedative.

PRECAUTIONS AND ADVERSE REACTIONS

Health risks or side effects following the proper administration of designated therapeutic dosages are not recorded. Older scientific literature (Lewin) speaks of the drug having the effect of ''bringing about a condition of sleep''.

DOSAGE

Mode of Administration: The drug is rarely prescribed, yet is a component of some standardized preparations in combination with plant sedatives. Medical or clinical documentation and other experimental material about phytotherapeutic application of the Californian Poppy herb is unavailable. As the efficacy of the claimed uses has not been documented, a therapeutic application cannot be justified.

Preparation: The tea is prepared using 2 gm herb per 150 ml water. The liquid extract (Extractum Eschscholziae) should be prepared according to the German Pharmacopoeia (DAB)10.

Daily Dosage: The tea is taken as a drink. The average single dose for the liquid extract is 1 to 2 ml.

LITERATURE

Jain L et al., Alkaloids of Eschscholtzia californica. In: PM 62(2):188. 1997.

Sturm S, Stuppner H, Mulinacci N, Vincieri F, Capillary zone electrophoretic analysis of the main alkaloids from Eschscholtzia californica. In: PM 59(7):A625. 1993.

Weischer ML, Okpanyi SN, Pharmakologie eines pflanzlichen Schlafmittels. In: ZPT 15(5):257-262. 1994.

Further information in:

Hänsel R, Keller K, Rimpler H, Schneider G (Hrsg.), Hagers Handbuch der Pharmazeutischen Praxis, 5. Aufl., Bde 4-6 (Drogen), Springer Verlag Berlin, Heidelberg, New York, 1992-1994.

Lewin L, Gifte und Vergiftungen, 6. Aufl., Nachdruck, Haug Verlag, Heidelberg 1992.

Roth L, Daunderer M, Kormann K, Giftpflanzen, Pflanzengifte, 4. Aufl., Ecomed Fachverlag Landsberg Lech 1993.

Teuscher E, Lindequist U, Biogene Gifte - Biologie, Chemie, Pharmakologie, 2. Aufl., Fischer Verlag Stuttgart 1994.

Eucalyptus Globulus

Eucalyptus

DESCRIPTION

Medicinal Parts: The medicinal parts are the oil extracted from the fresh leaves and branch tips as well as the dried leaves.

Flower and Fruit: The flowers are solitary on short pedicles. They have a somewhat pointed, but low operculum stretching over the surface of the stamens. There are no sepals but there are numerous long stamens turned inwards, which open along the whole length in 2 splits. The fruit is 10 to 15 by 15 to 30 mm and is a depressed-globose, somewhat tapering towards the base, with 4 main ribs.

Leaves, Stem and Root: Eucalyptus is a deciduous tree up to 40 m with silver-gray bark which has scattered warts. The trunk is twisted. The juvenile leaves are 7 to 16 by 4 to 9 cm, ovate to broadly lanceolate, cordate, very glaucus. The mature leaves are 10 to 13 by 3 to 4 cm, lanceolate to falcate-lanceolate, acuminate, asymmetrical rounded and glossy green.

Habitat: Eucalyptus is indigenous to Australia and Tasmania. It is cultivated today in some subtropical regions of southern Europe, Africa, Asia and America.

Production: Eucalyptus oil consists of the volatile oil from various cineol-rich species of Eucalyptus, such as Eucalyptus globulus, Eucalyptu fructicetorum (syn. Eucalyptus polybractea) and/or Eucalyptus smithii. The oil is obtained by steam distillation, followed by rectification of the fresh leaves and branch tops. Eucalyptus leaf (Eucalypti folium) consists of the dried, mature leaves from older trees of Eucalyptus globulus. To harvest eucalyptus, the trees are cut down; drying follows in the shade.

Not To Be Confused With: Camphor oil and by-products of turpentine manufacture; the oil is also blended with other expensive oils, such as rosemary and thyme. The properties of Eucalyptus leaves vary from species to species.

Other Names: Blue Gum, Fever Tree, Gum Tree, Red Gum, Stringy Bark Tree

ACTIONS AND PHARMACOLOGY

COMPOUNDS: EUCALYPTUS GLOBULUS

Chief constituent of the rectified volatile oil: 1,8-cineol (over 80%), furthermore p-cymene, alpha-pinenes, limonene, geraniol, camphene

EFFECTS: EUCALYPTUS GLOBULUS

Some of the subsequent properties mentioned refer to isolated cineole. As the standardized commodity, the drug contains 80 to 90% cineole.

In vitro, eucalyptus oil has an antibacterial and fungicidal effect. The drug inhibits prostaglandin biosynthesis and has a mild hyperemic, expectorant and secretolytic motor effect when used topically. In animal experiments eucalyptus was demonstrably cough-relieving and displayed a surfactant effect. In vitro, the oil was enzyme inducing and improved pulmonary compliance. It is secretolytic, expectorant, mildly antispasmodic, and a mild local hyperemic.

COMPOUNDS: EUCALYPTI FOLIUM

Volatile oil: chief constituent 1,8-cineol (45-75%), in additions myrtenol, alpha-pinenes, beta-pinenes, pinocarvon, gamma-terpenes, aliphatic aldehydes (butyr-, capron-, valerenaldehyde)

Euglobale: macrocarpale (with acylphloroglucinol-monoterpene or else sesquiterpene- parent substances)

Flavonoids: rutin, hyperoside, quercitrin

EFFECTS: EUCALYPTI FOLIUM

The drug has been shown to be secretolytic, expectorant, weakly antispasmodic, deodorizing, cooling and diuretic. In animal experiments the blood-sugar level of uninfluenced plasma insulin was reduced. The euglobulin is said to have an anti-inflammatory and antiproliferative effect in animal experiments and inhibits in vitro TPA-induced EBV-EA activity.

INDICATIONS AND USAGE

EUCALYPTUS GLOBULUS

- Cough/bronchitis
- Rheumatism

Eucalyptus globulus is used internally and externally for catarrh of the respiratory tract and externally for rheumatic complaints. In folk medicine, it is used for asthma, coughs, diseases of the frontal sinuses, fever, flu, gastric complaints, hoarseness, incipient scarlet fever and measles, worm infestation and as an intestinal antiseptic. These applications are undocumented.

EUCALYPTI FOLIUM

- Cough/bronchitis

Eucalyptus folium is used as a catarrh of the respiratory tract. In folk medicine, it is used for the treatment of acne, asthma, bleeding gums, bladder diseases, diabetes, fever, flu, gonorrhea, liver and gallbladder complaints, loss of appetite, neuralgia, poorly healing ulcers, rheumatism, stomatitis, ulalgia, whooping cough, wounds, and as a gastrointestinal remedy. These popular applications are not sufficiently documented.

PRECAUTIONS AND ADVERSE REACTIONS

EUCALYPTUS GLOBULUS

General: The administration of the drug leads in rare cases to nausea, vomiting and diarrhea. It should not be taken internally with inflammation of the gastrointestinal area and the biliary ducts or with severe illnesses of the liver.

Pediatric Use: Infants and small children should not have preparations containing the oil applied to their faces as this practice can lead to glottal spasm or bronchial spasms through asthma-like attacks or even death by asphyxiation.

EUCALYPTI FOLIUM

General: The administration of the drug leads in rare cases to nausea, vomiting and diarrhea. It should not be taken internally with inflammation of the gastrointestinal area and the biliary ducts or with severe illnesses of the liver. Poisonings occur with the volatile oil but are hardly conceivable with administration of the leaf drug.

Pediatric Use: Infants and small children should not have preparations containing the oil applied to their faces as this practice can lead to glottal spasm or bronchial spasms through asthma-like attacks or even death by asphyxiation.

OVERDOSAGE

EUCALYPTUS GLOBULUS

Overdosages can lead to life-threatening poisonings. Severe poisonings are possible for children after a few drops; poisonings have been known in adults with 4 to 5 ml. Symptoms include drop in blood pressure, circulatory disorders, collapse and asphyxiation. Because of the danger of aspiration, vomiting should not be induced. Following the administration of activated charcoal, therapy consists of diazepam for spasms, atropine for colic, electrolyte replenishment and sodium bicarbonate infusions for any acidosis that may arise. Intubation and oxygen respiration may also be necessary.

DOSAGE

EUCALYPTUS GLOBULUS

Mode of Administration: Essential oil and other galenic preparations are available for internal and external application.

Preparation: 1,8-cineole is recovered through a renewed fractional distillation of the oil.

Daily Dosage: For internal use, the average daily dose is 0.3 to 0.6 gm eucalyptus oil. When used externally, the concentration is 5 to 20% in oil and semi-solid preparations and 5 to 10% in aqueous-alcoholic preparations. If the essential oil is used, several drops may be rubbed into the skin.

Storage: Eucalyptus must be kept in appropriate, tightly-sealed containers; different consignments must be stored separately.

EUCALYPTI FOLIUM

Mode of Administration: Eucalypti folium is administered as the comminuted leaf for infusions and other galenic preparations for internal and external application. The drug may also be administered by inhalation.

Daily Dosage: The average daily dose is 4 to 16 gm of drug, divided up every 3 to 4 hours. The average dose for the tincture is 3 to 4 gm. An infusion of Eucalypti folium may be taken several times a day.

Storage: Eucalyptus must be kept in appropriate, tightly-sealed containers; different consignments must be stored separately.

LITERATURE

EUCALYPTUS GLOBULUS

Anonym, Phytotherapie:Pflanzliche Antirheumatika - was bringen sie? In: DAZ 136(45):4012-4015. 1996.

Boland B, In: Eucalyptus leaf oils. Boland DJ, Brophy JJ, House APN (Eds.). Inkata Press, Melbourne, XII + 252 pp. 1992.

Boland DJ, Brophy JJ, House APN, Eucalyptus leave oils. In: Inkata Press Melbourne. 1991.

Boukef K et al., (1976) Plant Med Phytother 10:24, 30:119.

Burrow A, Eccles R, Jones AS, (1983) The effects of camphor, eucalyptus and menthol vapor on nasal resistance to airflow and nasal sensation. Acta Otolaryng (Stockholm) 96:157-161.

Fox N, (1977) Effect of Camphor, Eucalyptol and Menthol on the vascular state of the mucos membrane. Arch Otolaryngol 6: 112-122.

Göbel H, Schmidt G, (1995a) Effekt von Pfefferminz- und Eukalyptusölpräparationen in experimentellen Kopfschmerzmodellen. Z Phytother 16:23-33.

Göbel H, Schmidt G, Dworschak M, Stolze H, Heuss D, (1995) Essential plant oils and headache mechanisms. Phytomedicine 2: 93-102.

Göbel H, Schmidt G, Dworschak M, Stolze H, Heuss D, (1995) Essential plant oils and headache mechanisms. Phytomedicine 2: 93-103.

Göbel H, Schmidt G, Soyka D, (1994) Effect of peppermint and eucalyptus oil preparations on neurophysiological and experimental algesimetric headache parameters. Cephalalgia 14: 228-234.

Göbel H, Stolze H, Dworschak M, Heinze A, (1995) Oleum menthae piperitae, Wirkmechanismen und klinische Effektivität bei Kopfschmerz vom Spannungstyp. In: Loew D, Rietbrock N (Hrsg) Phytopharmaka in Forschung und klinischer Anwendung. Steinkopff Verlag, Darmstadt, S. 177-184.

Gräfe AK, Besonderheiten der Arzneimitteltherapie im Säuglings- und Kindesalter. In: PZ 140(30):2659-2667. 1995.

Ikeda RM et al., (1962) J Food Sci 27:455.

Linsenmann P, Hermat H, Swoboda M, (1989) Therapeutischer Wert ätherischer Öle bei chronisch-abstruktiver Bronchitis. Atemw Lungenkrankh 15:152-156.

Linsenmann P, Swoboda M, (1986) Therapeutische Wirksamkeit ätherischer Öle bei chronisch-obstruktiver Bronchitis. Therapiewoche 36:1161-1166.

Osawa K et al., Macrocarpals H, I, and J from the leaves of Eucalyptus globulus. In: JNP 59(9):824-827. 1996.

Patel S, Wiggins J, (1980) Eucalyptus oil poisoning. Arch Dis Childh 55:405-406.

Römmelt H, Schnizer W, Swoboda M, Senn E, (1988) Pharmakokinetik ätherischer Öle nach Inhalation mit einer terpenhaltigen Salbe. Z Phytother 9:14-16.

Zänker KS, Blümel G, (1983) Terpene-induced lowering of surface tension in vitro. In: A rationale for surfactant substitution. Resp Exp Med 182:33-38.

Zänker KS, Blümel G, Probst J, Reiterer W, (1984) Theoretical and experimental evidence for the action of terpens as modulators in lung function. Prog Resp Res 18:302-304.

Further information in:

Fenaroli's Handbook of Flavor Ingredients, Vol. 1, 2nd Ed., CRC Press 1975.

Frohne D, Pfänder HJ, Giftpflanzen - Ein Handbuch für Apotheker, Toxikologen und Biologen, 4. Aufl., Wiss. Verlagsges. mbH Stuttgart 1997.

Hänsel R, Keller K, Rimpler H, Schneider G (Hrsg.), Hagers Handbuch der Pharmazeutischen Praxis, 5. Aufl., Bde 4-6 (Drogen), Springer Verlag Berlin, Heidelberg, New York, 1992-1994.

Leung AY, Encyclopedia of Common Natural Ingredients Used in Food Drugs and Cosmetics, John Wiley & Sons Inc., New York 1980.

Lewin L, Gifte und Vergiftungen, 6. Aufl., Nachdruck, Haug Verlag, Heidelberg 1992.

Madaus G, Lehrbuch der Biologischen Arzneimittel, Bde 1-3, Nachdruck, Georg Olms Verlag Hildesheim 1979.

Roth L, Daunderer M, Kormann K, Giftpflanzen, Pflanzengifte, 4. Aufl., Ecomed Fachverlag Landsberg Lech 1993.

Schulz R, Hänsel R, Rationale Phytotherapie, Springer Verlag Heidelberg 1996.

Steinegger E, Hänsel R, Pharmakognosie, 5. Aufl., Springer Verlag Heidelberg 1992.

Teuscher E, Biogene Arzneimittel, 5. Aufl., Wiss. Verlagsges. mbH Stuttgart 1997.

Wagner H, Wiesenauer M, Phytotherapie. Phytopharmaka und pflanzliche Homöopathika, Fischer-Verlag, Stuttgart, Jena, New York 1995.

Wichtl M (Hrsg.), Teedrogen, 4. Aufl., Wiss. Verlagsges. Stuttgart 1997.

EUCALYPTI FOLIUM

Anonym, Phytotherapie:Pflanzliche Antirheumatika - was bringen sie? In: DAZ 136(45):4012-4015. 1996.

Boland B, In: Eucalyptus leaf oils. Boland DJ, Brophy JJ, House APN (Eds.). Inkata Press, Melbourne, XII + 252 pp. 1992.

Boland DJ, Brophy JJ, House APN, Eucalyptus leave oils. In: Inkata Press Melbourne. 1991.

Boukef K et al., (1976) Plant Med Phytother 10:24, 30:119.

Burrow A, Eccles R, Jones AS, (1983) The effects of camphor, eucalyptus and menthol vapor on nasal resistance to airflow and nasal sensation. Acta Otolaryng (Stockholm) 96:157-161.

Fox N, (1977) Effect of Camphor, Eucalyptol and Menthol on the vascular state of the mucos membrane. Arch Otolaryngol 6: 112-122.

Göbel H, Schmidt G, (1995a) Effekt von Pfefferminz- und Eukalyptusölpräparationen in experimentellen Kopfschmerzmodellen. Z Phytother 16:23-33.

Göbel H, Schmidt G, Dworschak M, Stolze H, Heuss D, (1995) Essential plant oils and headache mechanisms. Phytomedicine 2:93-102.

Göbel H, Schmidt G, Dworschak M, Stolze H, Heuss D, (1995) Essential plant oils and headache mechanisms. Phytomedicine 2:93-103.

Göbel H, Schmidt G, Soyka D, (1994) Effect of peppermint and eucalyptus oil preparations on neurophysiological and experimental algesimetric headache parameters. Cephalalgia 14: 228-234.

Göbel H, Stolze H, Dworschak M, Heinze A, (1995) Oleum menthae piperitae, Wirkmechanismen und klinische Effektivität bei Kopfschmerz vom Spannungstyp. In: Loew D, Rietbrock N (Hrsg) Phytopharmaka in Forschung und klinischer Anwendung. Steinkopff Verlag, Darmstadt, S. 177-184.

Gräfe AK, Besonderheiten der Arzneimitteltherapie im Säuglings- und Kindesalter. In: PZ 140(30):2659-2667. 1995.

Ikeda RM et al., (1962) J Food Sci 27:455.

Linsenmann P, Hermat H, Swoboda M, (1989) Therapeutischer Wert ätherischer Öle bei chronisch-abstruktiver Bronchitis. Atemw Lungenkrankh 15:152-156.

Linsenmann P, Swoboda M, (1986) Therapeutische Wirksamkeit ätherischer Öle bei chronisch-obstruktiver Bronchitis. Therapiewoche 36:1161-1166.

Osawa K et al., Macrocarpals H, I, and J from the leaves of Eucalyptus globulus. In: JNP 59(9):824-827. 1996.

Patel S, Wiggins J, (1980) Eucalyptus oil poisoning. Arch Dis Childh 55:405-406.

Römmelt H, Schnizer W, Swoboda M, Senn E, (1988) Pharmakokinetik ätherischer Öle nach Inhalation mit einer terpenhaltigen Salbe. Z Phytother 9:14-16.

Zänker KS, Blümel G, (1983) Terpene-induced lowering of surface tension in vitro. In: A rationale for surfactant substitution. Resp Exp Med 182:33-38.

Zänker KS, Blümel G, Probst J, Reiterer W, (1984) Theoretical and experimental evidence for the action of terpens as modulators in lung function. Prog Resp Res 18:302-304.

Further information in:

Fenaroli's Handbook of Flavor Ingredients, Vol. 1, 2nd Ed., CRC Press 1975.

Frohne D, Pfänder HJ, Giftpflanzen - Ein Handbuch für Apotheker, Toxikologen und Biologen, 4. Aufl., Wiss. Verlagsges. mbH Stuttgart 1997.

Hänsel R, Keller K, Rimpler H, Schneider G (Hrsg.), Hagers Handbuch der Pharmazeutischen Praxis, 5. Aufl., Bde 4-6 (Drogen), Springer Verlag Berlin, Heidelberg, New York, 1992-1994.

Leung AY, Encyclopedia of Common Natural Ingredients Used in Food Drugs and Cosmetics, John Wiley & Sons Inc., New York 1980.

Lewin L, Gifte und Vergiftungen, 6. Aufl., Nachdruck, Haug Verlag, Heidelberg 1992.

Madaus G, Lehrbuch der Biologischen Arzneimittel, Bde 1-3, Nachdruck, Georg Olms Verlag Hildesheim 1979.

Roth L, Daunderer M, Kormann K, Giftpflanzen, Pflanzengifte, 4. Aufl., Ecomed Fachverlag Landsberg Lech 1993.

Schulz R, Hänsel R, Rationale Phytotherapie, Springer Verlag Heidelberg 1996.

Steinegger E, Hänsel R, Pharmakognosie, 5. Aufl., Springer Verlag Heidelberg 1992.

Teuscher E, Biogene Arzneimittel, 5. Aufl., Wiss. Verlagsges. mbH Stuttgart 1997.

Wagner H, Wiesenauer M, Phytotherapie. Phytopharmaka und pflanzliche Homöopathika, Fischer-Verlag, Stuttgart, Jena, New York 1995.

Wichtl M (Hrsg.), Teedrogen, 4. Aufl., Wiss. Verlagsges. Stuttgart 1997.

Eugenia Chequen

Cheken

DESCRIPTION

Medicinal Parts: The medicinal parts are the dried leaves.

Flower and Fruit: The flowers are usually solitary, occasionally in threes. The receptacle is top-shaped and pubescent.

There are 4 pubescent or ciliate sepals. The petals are white, oval and 5 to 8 mm long. The stamens are numerous but small. The ovary is glabrous. The fruit is a red or black-violet, glabrous, globular berry, 6 to 8 mm in diameter. It has 2 to 3 seeds which are dark, lentil-shaped and are about 4 mm in diameter.

Leaves, Stem and Root: The plant is an evergreen tree, which grows up to 15 m high and sometimes looks like a shrub. The leaves are coriaceous, ovate, about 1 to 1.5 cm long, 0.5 to 1 cm wide, entire-margined, very shortly petioled with numerous minute, round, translucent oil-cells.

Characteristics: The leaves have a bitter taste that is astringent and aromatic, reminiscent of bay leaves. The odor is slight and they contain an essential oil.

Habitat: Eugenia chequen grows in Chile.

Production: Cheken leaves are the leaves of Eugenia chequen.

Other Names: Arryan, Myrtus Chekan

ACTIONS AND PHARMACOLOGY

COMPOUNDS

Unknown

EFFECTS

The ethanol extract inhibits xanthinoxydasis. The essential oil has a similar effect on germinating salad seeds such as auxin. An antibacterial and antimycotic effect has also been demonstrated. In the agar diffusion test, the leaf oil was effective against *Pseudomonas acruginsosa, Trichophyton mentagrophytes* and *Asperigillus niger.* It also affects fat metabolism: the oil is used against hyperlipoproteinemia. It is used as a tonic, a diuretic and an expectorant.

INDICATIONS AND USAGE

In South American folk medicine, a decoction of the leaves is used in the treatment of diarrhea, fever, gout, and as a tonic, a diuretic, an antihypertensive and a digestive. Its efficacy has not been proven.

PRECAUTIONS AND ADVERSE REACTIONS

Health risks or side effects following the proper administration of designated therapeutic dosages are not recorded.

DOSAGE

Mode of Administration: As a decoction and as a liquid extract.

LITERATURE

No literature references.

Euonymus Atropurpureus

Wahoo Root Bark

DESCRIPTION

Medicinal Parts: The medicinal parts are the trunk and root bark and the fruit.

Flower and Fruit: The flowers are yellowish-green, small and flat in double cymes with few blossoms. There are 4 sepals, 4 petals, 4 stamens and 4 styles on a glandular disc, which surrounds the ovary. The fruit is a 4-lobed, obtuse, pink capsule which bursts open at the tip showing the seeds covered in an orange-yellow skin.

Leaves, Stem and Root: The plant is an unwieldy shrub up to 3 m high with green rectangular young branches. The older branches are light gray. The leaves are opposite, oblong-lanceolate or elliptical, acuminate, finely serrate, glabrous.

Characteristics: The seeds are poisonous.

Habitat: The plant grows in the Eastern and Central U.S. and Canada.

Production: Wahoo root bark is the bark of the root and young branches of Euonymus atropurpuraeus.

Other Names: Burning Bush, Fusanum, Fusoria, Gadrose, Gatten, Gatter, Indian Arrowroot, Pigwood, Prickwood, Skewerwood, Spindle Tree

ACTION AND PHARMACOLOGY

COMPOUNDS: EUONYMUS ATROPURPUREUS

Cardioactive steroids (cardenolides) in the root: including euatroside, euatromonoside

EFFECTS: EUONYMUS ATROPURPUREUS

The drug is reported to be a laxative and a choleretic. Larger doses have an effect on the heart.

COMPOUNDS: EUONYMUS EUROPAEUS

Cardioactive steroids (cardenolides) in the seeds: including evonoside, evobioside, evomonoside, evolonoside, glucoevonoloside, glucoevonogenin

Alkaloids: polyester from a sesquiterpene polyol with pyrridine carbon acids (for example, evonine)

Peptide alkaloids: including frangula amine, franganin, frangufolin

1-benzyl-tetrahydro-isoquinoline alkaloids

Purine alkaloids: caffeine, theobromine

EFFECTS: EUONYMUS EUROPAEUS

The drug is reported to be a laxative and a choleretic. Larger doses have an effect on the heart.

INDICATIONS AND USAGE

In the past, the drug was used as a cholagogue, laxative, diuretic and tonic, and for dyspepsia.

Its efficacy has not been scientifically proven.

PRECAUTIONS AND ADVERSE REACTIONS

Poisonings caused by the berries have been recorded. Thirty-six berries of Eunymus europaeus are said to be enough to kill a person. After a latency period of several hours, the following appear: intestinal colic; severe, sometimes bloody diarrhea; elevation of body temperature; shortness of breath; circulatory disorders; signs of collapse; elevation of cerebrospinal pressure; meningism; increasing stupor all the way to unconsciousness, alternating with motoric restlessness; severe tonic-clonic spasms with trismus and coma. The first measures to be taken with poisonings are gastric lavage, intestinal emptying, the instillation of activated charcoal and shock prophylaxis (which includes quiet, heat and the possible administration of a plasma volume expander). All other measures depend upon the symptoms: for loss of potassium, careful replenishment of potassium; with ectopic irritation build-up in the ventricle, administration of phenytoin as an antiarrhythmatic; lidocaine for ventricular extrasystole; atropine for partial atrioventricular block. For elimination of the glycosides hemoperfusion is possible, as is the administration of cholestyramine for interrupting the enterohepatic circulation. Intubation and oxygen respiration may also be necessary in cases of asphyxiation.

DOSAGE

Mode of Administration: Wahoo root bark is not recommended for use, as it is considered too dangerous.

LITERATURE

Bishay DW et al., PH 12:693. 1973.

Bliss CA, Ramstad E, J Am Pharm Assoc 46:423. 1957.

Brüning R, Wagner H, PH 17:1821. 1978.

Kislichenko SG et al., Khim Prir Soedin 386. 1969.

Kislichenko SG et al., Khim Prir Soedin 193 et 241. 1967.

Tschesche R, Wirtz S, Snatzke G, Chem Ber 88:1619. 1955.

Further information in:

Frohne D, Pfänder HJ, Giftpflanzen - Ein Handbuch für Apotheker, Toxikologen und Biologen, 4. Aufl., Wiss. Verlagsges. mbH Stuttgart 1997.

Kern W, List PH, Hörhammer L (Hrsg.), Hagers Handbuch der Pharmazeutischen Praxis, 4. Aufl., Bde. 1-8, Springer Verlag Berlin, Heidelberg, New York, 1969.

Lewin L, Gifte und Vergiftungen, 6. Aufl., Nachdruck, Haug Verlag, Heidelberg 1992.

Madaus G, Lehrbuch der Biologischen Arzneimittel, Bde 1-3, Nachdruck, Georg Olms Verlag Hildesheim 1979.

Roth L, Daunderer M, Kormann K, Giftpflanzen, Pflanzengifte, 4. Aufl., Ecomed Fachverlag Landsberg Lech 1993.

Teuscher E, Biogene Arzneimittel, 5. Aufl., Wiss. Verlagsges. mbH Stuttgart 1997.

Eupatorium Cannabinum

Hemp Agrimony

DESCRIPTION

Medicinal Parts: The medicinal part is the flowering herb.

Flower and Fruit: The flowers are in compact, terminal, umbrella-like umbels. They are small dull pink tubular androgynous flowers whose corolla tube has a 5-tipped edge. The epicalyx is cylindrical and consists of a few bracts. The edge of the calyx consists of yellowish hairs. The style is divided in two parts and shows above the flower. The corolla is covered in resinous spots. The angular fruit bears a crown of hair and is dirty white.

Leaves, Stem and Root: The plant is a small perennial herb 75 to 150 cm high. The rhizome is woody and has stems growing from it, which have short axillary branches. The stems are erect, reddish, pubescent and resinous below. The root leaves are long-petioled. The opposite cauline leaves are short-petioled, trifoliate and serrate and covered in resinous spots.

Habitat: Hemp Agrimony grows in damp regions of Europe.

Production: Hemp Agrimony is the flowering herb of Eupatorium cannabium.

Other Names: Holy Rope, St. John's Herb, Sweet-smelling Trefoil, Water Maudlin

ACTIONS AND PHARMACOLOGY

COMPOUNDS

Sesquiterpene lactones: including eupatoriopicrin, eupatolid

Pyrrolizidine alkaloids: including echinatine, supinine, eucanecine, amabiline, lycopsamin, intermedin

Immunostimulating polysaccharides (heteroxylans)

Caffeic acid ester: chlorogenic acid

EFFECTS

The eupatorin is said to be cytotoxic. It is also a bitter and a tannic acid.

INDICATIONS AND USAGE

The herb is used for disorders of the liver and gallbladder and for fevers.

PRECAUTIONS AND ADVERSE REACTIONS

Because of the pyrrolizidine alkaloid content with 1,2-unsaturated necic parent substances, hepatotoxicity and carcinogenicity are to be assumed. The drug should therefore not be taken internally. Sensitization through skin contact with the plant also seems possible.

DOSAGE

Mode of Administration: The herb is used topically as an alcoholic extract, as a tea, and as an inhalation for the treatment of colds.

LITERATURE

Anonym, Positive Auswirkungen von Olivenöl auf den Blutdruck. In: ZPT 12(1):13. 1991.

Antibiotika und Immunabwehr. In: Symbiose 4(2):20. 1992.

Elsässer-Beile U, Willenbacher W, Bartsch HH, Gallati H, Schulte Mönting J, Kleist von S et al., Cytokine production in leukocyte cultures during therapy with echinacea extract. In: J Clin Lab Analysis 10(6):441-445. 1996.

Hendriks H et al., (1983) Pharm Weekblad 5:281.

Pederson E (1975) Phytochemistry 14:2086.

Röder E, Pyrrolizidinhaltige Arzneipflanzen. In: DAZ 132(45):2427-2435. 1992.

Vollmar A et al., (1986) Phytochemistry 25(2):377.

Winterhoff H, Gumbinger HG, Pharmakologische Untersuchungen mit Pflanzenextrakten. Probleme und Lösungsmöglichkeit. In: DAZ 130(49):2668. 1990.

Woerdenbag HJ et al., (1987) Phytother Res 2(2):76.

Further information in:

Kern W, List PH, Hörhammer L (Hrsg.), Hagers Handbuch der Pharmazeutischen Praxis, 4. Aufl., Bde 1-8, Springer Verlag Berlin, Heidelberg, New York, 1969.

Madaus G, Lehrbuch der Biologischen Arzneimittel, Bde 1-3, Nachdruck, Georg Olms Verlag Hildesheim 1979.

Roth L, Daunderer M, Kormann K, Giftpflanzen, Pflanzengifte, 4. Aufl., Ecomed Fachverlag Landsberg Lech 1993.

Teuscher E, Lindequist U, Biogene Gifte - Biologie, Chemie, Pharmakologie, 2. Aufl., Fischer Verlag Stuttgart 1994.

Wagner H, Wiesenauer M, Phytotherapie. Phytopharmaka und pflanzliche Homöopathika, Fischer-Verlag, Stuttgart, Jena, New York 1995.

Eupatorium Perfoliatum

Boneset

DESCRIPTION

Medicinal Parts: The medicinal part is the herb after flowering.

Flower and Fruit: There are numerous flower heads in terminal, large and slightly convex cymose-paniculate inflorescences. They consist of 10 to 12 white, inconspicuous florets with bristly pappus whose hairs are arranged in a single row. The fruit is a tufted achene.

Leaves, Stem and Root: Eupatorium perfoliatum is a perennial herb with a horizontal hairy rootstock. The stems are rough-haired and grow to about 1.5 m. The leaves are opposite, 10 to 15 cm long, lanceolate, crenate, tapering to narrow point and fused at the base. They have shiny yellow points due to the resin glands, which are visible on the undersurface.

Characteristics: The taste is astringent and persistently bitter.

Habitat: The herb is indigenous to the eastern U.S.

Production: Boneset is the complete aerial part of Eupatorium perfoliatum.

Other Names: Agueweed, Crosswort, Feverwort, Indian Sage, Sweating Plant, Teasel, Thoroughwort, Vegetable Antimony

ACTIONS AND PHARMACOLOGY

COMPOUNDS

Flavonoids: including eupatorin, astragalin, rutin, hyperoside

Sesquiterpene lactones: including eupafolin, euperfolitin, eufoliatin, eufoliatorin, euperfolide

Immunostimulating polysaccharides (heteroxylans)

EFFECTS

The herb acts as an antiphlogistic, a diaphoretic and a bitter, in addition to stimulating the body's immune system. In a comparative study of the homeopathic preparation Eupatorium D2 with aspirin in the treatment of feverish catarrh, a similar positive tendency was observed. In vitro, the phagocytic action of granulocytes was increased.

INDICATIONS AND USAGE

Boneset is used in homeopathy as a treatment for flu and febrile diseases.

On rare occasions, it is used in folk medicine.

PRECAUTIONS AND ADVERSE REACTIONS

Health risks or side effects following the proper administration of designated therapeutic dosages are not recorded. Sensitization through skin contact with the plant is possible. Older scientific literature (Lewin) calls attention to the fact that the drug can lead to enhanced outbreaks of sweat and diarrhea in therapeutic use.

DOSAGE

Mode of Administration: Boneset is used in homeopathic preparations and dilutions. On rare occasions, it is used in folk medicine.

LITERATURE

Antibiotika und Immunabwehr. In: Symbiose 4(2):20. 1992.

Benoit PS et al., (1976) Lloydia 39:160.

Bohlmann F et al., (1977) Phytochemistry 16:1973.

Elsässer-Beile U, Willenbacher W, Bartsch HH, Gallati H, Schulte Mönting J, Kleist von S et al., Cytokine production in leukocyte cultures during therapy with echinacea extract. In: J Clin Lab Analysis 10(6):441-445. 1996.

Herz W et al., (1977) J Org Chem 42(13):2264.

Vollmar A et al., (1986) Phytochemistry 25:377.

Wagner H (1972) Phytochemistry 11:1504.

Röder E, Pyrrolizidinhaltige Arzneipflanzen. In: DAZ 132(45):2427-2435. 1992.

Woerdenbag HJ, Eupatorium perfoliatum L.- der ''durchwachsene'' Wasserhanf. In: ZPT 13(4):134-139. 1992.

Further information in:

Chan, EH et al., (Eds), Advances in Chinese Medicinal Materials Research, World Scientific Pub. Co. Singapore 1985.

Kern W, List PH, Hörhammer L (Hrsg.), Hagers Handbuch der Pharmazeutischen Praxis, 4. Aufl., Bde. 1-8, Springer Verlag Berlin, Heidelberg, New York, 1969.

Leung AY, Encyclopedia of Common Natural Ingredients Used in Food Drugs and Cosmetics, John Wiley & Sons Inc., New York 1980.

Lewin L, Gifte und Vergiftungen, 6. Aufl., Nachdruck, Haug Verlag, Heidelberg 1992.

Madaus G, Lehrbuch der Biologischen Arzneimittel, Bde 1-3, Nachdruck, Georg Olms Verlag Hildesheim 1979.

Roth L, Daunderer M, Kormann K, Giftpflanzen, Pflanzengifte, 4. Aufl., Ecomed Fachverlag Landsberg Lech 1993.

Wagner H, Wiesenauer M, Phytotherapie. Phytopharmaka und pflanzliche Homöopathika, Fischer-Verlag, Stuttgart, Jena, New York 1995.

Euphorbia Cyparissias

Cypress Spurge

DESCRIPTION

Medicinal Parts: The medicinal part of the plant is the flowering plant with the root.

Flower and Fruit: The flowers are in terminal cymes. They are yellow-green but usually red after flowering. What appear to be flowers are in fact inflorescences. In the jug-shaped invulucres there is 1 hanging pistil with a 3 valved ovary and 3 styles each with 2 stigmas and numerous stamens. Four half-moon-shaped nectaries are at the edge. The fruit is covered in small papilla.

Leaves, Stem and Root: The plant is about 15 to 30 cm high. The stem is erect, unbranched, and glabrous. The leaves are alternate, sessile, linear, entire-margined and very narrow on the non-flowering branches.

Characteristics: The entire plant contains white latex, which is poisonous.

Habitat: Indigenous to Europe and Mediterranean.

Production: Cypress Spurge herb and root is the whole plant in flower and root of Euphorbia cyparissias.

ACTIONS AND PHARMACOLOGY

COMPOUNDS

Diterpenes: ingenan-di- and triester, for example 13-hydroxy-ingenol-3-(2,3-dimethylbutyryl)-13- dodecanoate, 13-hydroxy-ingenol-5-(2,3-dimethylbutyryl)-13-dodecanoate, 13-hydroxy- ingenol-3-(2,3-dimethylbutyryl)-13-decanoate

Triterpenes

EFFECTS

No information available

INDICATIONS AND USAGE

Used in homeopathy for diseases of the respiratory organs, diarrhea, and skin diseases.

PRECAUTIONS AND ADVERSE REACTIONS

The Ingenan esters are severely inflammatory in their effect and cocarcinogenic. Any administration of the drug must be ruled out because of the cocarcinogenenic effect.

A particular danger exists with the chyle of the freshly harvested plant, but the ingenan ester retains its efficacy even after drying, which means that the drug also contains acute toxicity. If it gets on the skin, the chyle causes reddening, itching, burning and after a time blisters.

In the eye, the chyle leads to swelling of the lids, conjunctiva inflammation and corneal defects. If taken internally, the chyle of the drug causes burning in the mouth and vomiting, with very high dosages pupil enlargement, dizziness, stupor, painful bowel movements, cardiac rhythm disorders and ultimately collapse. Skin contact with the chyle requires thorough cleaning, in cases of contact with the eye thorough rinsing with water. Following stomach and intestinal emptying, the treatment of poisonings can only be carried out symptomatically.

DOSAGE

Mode of Administration: Cypress Spurge is used only in homeopathic dilutions.

LITERATURE

Öksüz S et al., Biological active compounds. In: PM 60(6):594-596. 1994.

Ott HH, Hecker E, Experientia 37:88. 1981.

Further information in:

Frohne D, Pfänder HJ, Giftpflanzen - Ein Handbuch für Apotheker, Toxikologen und Biologen, 4. Aufl., Wiss. Verlagsges. mbH Stuttgart 1997.

Kern W, List PH, Hörhammer L (Hrsg.), Hagers Handbuch der Pharmazeutischen Praxis, 4. Aufl., Bde. 1-8, Springer Verlag Berlin, Heidelberg, New York, 1969.

Lewin L, Gifte und Vergiftungen, 6. Aufl., Nachdruck, Haug Verlag, Heidelberg 1992.

Madaus G, Lehrbuch der Biologischen Arzneimittel, Bde 1-3, Nachdruck, Georg Olms Verlag Hildesheim 1979.

Roth L, Daunderer M, Kormann K, Giftpflanzen, Pflanzengifte, 4. Aufl., Ecomed Fachverlag Landsberg Lech 1993.

Teuscher E, Lindequist U, Biogene Gifte - Biologie, Chemie, Pharmakologie, 2. Aufl., Fischer Verlag Stuttgart 1994.

Euphrasia Officinalis

Eyebright

DESCRIPTION

Medicinal Parts: The medicinal part is the flowering plant.

Flower and Fruit: White, bluish or reddish-violet flowers are in spike-like inflorescence in the axils of the upper leaves. The calyx has 4 tips and is glabrous to short bristly. The corolla is bilabiate and is 8 to 12 mm long. The upper lip is domed, helmet-like and revolute at the tips. The lower lip has 9 dark violet long stripes. There are 4 stamens and 1 superior ovary. The fruit is a narrow, oblong capsule with a ciliate edge. The seeds are numerous and grooved.

Leaves, Stem and Root: The plant is about 30 cm high. It is annual. The stem is rigid, erect, lightly branched below. The leaves are opposite, sessile, grass-green, ovate or oblong-ovate and twice as long as wide, dentate and glabrous. The involucral bracts have 4 to 7 teeth.

Characteristics: Eyebright is odorless and has a bitter and salty taste. It is semi-parasitic.

Habitat: Europe.

Production: Eyebright consists of the whole plant of Euphrasia officinalis gathered during flowering season. Eyebright herb consists of the fresh or dried, above-ground parts of Euphrasia officinalis.

Other Names: Euphrasia

ACTIONS AND PHARMACOLOGY

COMPOUNDS

Iridoide monoterpenes: aucubin, catalpol, euphroside, ixoroside, veronicoside, verproside, mussaenoside, ladroside

Lignans: dehydrodiconiferyl-4-beta-D-glucoside

Flavonoids

Tannins

EFFECTS

No documentation available.

INDICATIONS AND USAGE

Eyebright preparations are used externally as lotions, poultices, and eye-baths, for eye complaints associated with disorders and inflammation of the blood vessels, inflammation of the eyelids and conjunctiva, as a preventive measure against mucus and catarrh of the eyes.

In folk medicine, Eyebright is used for blepharitis, conjunctivitis, styes, eye fatigue symptoms, functional eye disorders of muscular and nervous origin, coughs and hoarseness.

The efficacy of the herb for its claimed uses is not documented.

PRECAUTIONS AND ADVERSE REACTIONS

Health risks or side effects following the proper administration of designated therapeutic dosages are not recorded.

DOSAGE

Mode of Administration: Since the efficacy of the claimed uses is undocumented, and external eye application is not absolutely hygienic, therapeutic use cannot be recommended.

Preparation: Tea: 2 to 3 gm of finely cut drug with boiling water; strain after 5 to 10 minutes.

Decoction: 2%.

Daily Dosage: A decoction is used 3 to 4 times daily for eye rinses.

LITERATURE

Harkiss KJ, Timmins P, (1973) Planta Med 23:342.

Luczak S, Swiatek L, Plantes Med Phytothér 24:66. 1990.

Salama O et al., PH 20:2603. 1981.

Salama O, Sticher O, (1983) Planta Med 47:90.

Sicher O, Salama O, PM 39:269. 1980.

Sicher O, Salama O, PM 42:122. 1981.

Further information in:

Kern W, List PH, Hörhammer L (Hrsg.), Hagers Handbuch der Pharmazeutischen Praxis, 4. Aufl., Bde 1-8, Springer Verlag Berlin, Heidelberg, New York, 1969.

Madaus G, Lehrbuch der Biologischen Arzneimittel, Bde 1-3, Nachdruck, Georg Olms Verlag Hildesheim 1979.

Wagner H, Wiesenauer M, Phytotherapie. Phytopharmaka und pflanzliche Homöopathika, Fischer-Verlag, Stuttgart, Jena, New York 1995.

Wichtl M (Hrsg.), Teedrogen, 4. Aufl., Wiss. Verlagsges. Stuttgart 1997.

European Five-Finger Grass

See Potentilla Reptans

European Water Hemlock

See Cicuta Virosa

Evening Primrose

See Oenothera Biennis

Eyebright

See Euphrasia Officinalis

Fagopyrum Esculentum

Buckwheat

DESCRIPTION

Medicinal Parts: The medicinal parts are the leaves and flowers collected during the flowering season and later dried and the fresh aerial part.

Flower and Fruit: Short compact, long peduncled thryses form in the leaf axils and at the end of the branches. The involucre is 3 to 4 mm long, has 5 bracts and is pink or white and usually green at the base. The floret has 8 stamens with golden yellow nectaries at the base. The fruit is a sharply triangular achaene.

Leaves, Stem and Root: Buckwheat is an annual 15 to 60 cm high plant with an erect, usually red stem covered in alternating, sagittate, and sessile leaves. The lobes are obtuse or rounded with sweeping borders. The lower leaves are petioled, the upper ones less so. The root is fusiform. Tatar buckwheat (Fagopyrum tataricum), which is used in the pharmaceutical industry is easily distinguishable from Fagopyrum esculentum by its green flowers, usually green stems and curved, dentated, and squat achaenes.

Habitat: The plant is indigenous to northern and central Asia; cultivated in China and U.S.

Production: Buckwheat herb is the aerial part of Fagopyrum esculentum or Fagopyrum tataricum. The harvest takes place 50 to 60 days after sewing and before the fruit forms. There is a slight or small loss of rutin if quickly dried at high temperatures.

ACTIONS AND PHARMACOLOGY

COMPOUNDS

Flavonoids: rutin (up to 8% in the leaves), quercitrin, hyperoside

Anthracene derivatives (naphthadianthrones, chiefly in the blossoms): fagopyrin, frotofagopyrin

EFFECTS

Buckwheat increases the venous tone (antiedematic, capillary sealing).

INDICATIONS AND USAGE

In folk medicine, the drug is used as a venous and capillary tonic and as a prophylaxis to prevent general hardening of the arteries. The drug alleviates venous stasis and varicose veins.

Efficacy has not been proven.

PRECAUTIONS AND ADVERSE REACTIONS

Health risks or side effects following the proper administration of designated therapeutic dosages are not recorded.

OVERDOSAGE

The intake of large quantities of the buckwheat plant leads to phototoxicoses in animals due to the photosensitizing effect of the naphthadianthrones. There are no dangers for humans in the application of therapeutic dosages.

DOSAGE

Mode of Administration: Buckwheat is taken orally in teas, and as an extract.

Preparation: Buckwheat tea and tablets are commercially available.

LITERATURE

Adamek B, Drozdzik M, Samochowiec L, Wojcicki J, Clinical effect of buckwheat herb, Ruscus extract and troxerutin on retinopathy and lipids in diabetic patients. In: Phytotherapy Res 10(8):659-662. 1996.

Anonym, Nicht-Brotgetreidearten: Alternative Körner unter der Lupe. In: DAZ 136(38):3229-2330. 1996.

Bässler R, PA 12:758-772 et 834-841. 1985.

Couch JF, Naghski J, Krewson CF, Science 103:197-198. 1974.

Gaidies I, Buchweizen, eine Venenhilfe. In: PTA 6(7):439. 1992.

Hagels H et al., Two anthraquinones and a bianthraquinone from Fagopyrum tataricum. In: PM 62, Abstracts of the 44th Ann Congress of GA, 125. 1996.

Ihme N et al., Leg oedema protection from a buckwheat herb tea in patients with chronic venous insufficiency: A single centre, randomised, double blind, placebo controlled clinical trial. In: European J Clin Pharmacol 50(6)443-447. 1996.

Koscielny J, Radtke H, Hoffmann KH, Jung F, Müller A, Grützner KI, Kiesewetter H, Fagorutin-Tee bei chronisch venöser Insuffizienz (CVI). In: ZPT 17(3):145-159. 1996.

Samel D, de Witte P, Fagopyrins from Fagopyrum esculentum and their PTK inhibitory activity. In: PM 61(Abstracts of 43rd Ann Congr):67. 1995.

Further information in:

Hänsel R, Keller K, Rimpler H, Schneider G (Hrsg.), Hagers Handbuch der Pharmazeutischen Praxis, 5. Aufl., Bde 4-6 (Drogen): Springer Verlag Berlin, Heidelberg, New York, 1992-1994.

Lewin L, Gifte und Vergiftungen, 6. Aufl., Nachdruck, Haug Verlag, Heidelberg 1992. (unter Buchweizen).

Roth L, Daunderer M, Kormann K, Giftpflanzen, Pflanzengifte, 4. Aufl., Ecomed Fachverlag Landsberg Lech 1993.

Teuscher E, Lindequist U, Biogene Gifte - Biologie, Chemie, Pharmakologie, 2. Aufl., Fischer Verlag Stuttgart 1994.

Wagner H, Wiesenauer M, Phytotherapie. Phytopharmaka und pflanzliche Homöopathika, Fischer-Verlag, Stuttgart, Jena, New York 1995.

False Unicorn Root

See Veratrum Luteum

Fennel

See Foeniculum Vulgare

Fenugreek

See Trigonella Foenum-Graecum

Ferula Foetida

Asa Foetida

DESCRIPTION

Medicinal Parts: The medicinal part is oily gum-resin extracted from the plant.

Flower and Fruit: The flowers appear after 5 years in yellow umbels on a 10 cm thick naked stem. They are numerous, pale greenish-yellow to white. The fruit is ovate, flat, thin, flaky, reddish-brown with distinct oil marks.

Leaves, Stem and Root: The plant is a herbaceous monoecious perennial, 1.5 to 2 m high with a large, fleshy rhizome, which is 14 cm thick at the crown. The leaves are large, bipinnate, and radical.

Characteristics: The fruit has milky juice and a strong smell.

Habitat: Afghanistan and eastern Iran.

Production: Asafoetida is the gum resin of Ferula foetida.

Other Names: Devil's Dung, Food of the Gods, Gum Asafoetida

ACTIONS AND PHARMACOLOGY

COMPOUNDS

Volatile oil: chief constituent is sec-propenyl-isobutyl disulphide

Gum resin: consisting mainly of ferulic acid esters, farnesiferol A, B, C and bassorin-like mucilage

Sesquiterpenoide coumarins: including asafoetida

EFFECTS

Asafoetida has a mild intestinal disinfectant effect; its sedative effect is uncertain.

INDICATIONS AND USAGE

The drug is used for chronic gastritis, dyspepsia and irritable colon.

PRECAUTIONS AND ADVERSE REACTIONS

No health hazards or side effects are known in conjunction with the proper administration of designated therapeutic dosages. The intake of larger dosages can lead to swelling of the lips, digestive complaints (belching, flatulence, diarrhea), discomfort and headache, as well as to convulsions in susceptible individuals. Swelling of the genital organs has been observed following external administration on the abdomen.

DOSAGE

Mode of Administration: The drug is available as an extract.

Preparation: Gum-resin is obtained by incising the roots, which contain a fetid juice, this solidifies to a brown resin, sometimes with a pinkish tint, in sticky lumps with a pungent, acrid, persistent, alliaceous odor.

Daily Dosage: Tincture: 20 drops as a single dose.

LITERATURE

Buddrus J et al., (1985) Phytochemistry 24(4):869.

Naimie H et al., (1972) Collect Czec Chem Commun 37:1166.

Rajanikanth B et al., (1984) Phytochemistry 23(4):899.

Further information in:

Kern W, List PH, Hörhammer L (Hrsg.), Hagers Handbuch der Pharmazeutischen Praxis, 4. Aufl., Bde 1-8, Springer Verlag Berlin, Heidelberg, New York, 1969.

Lewin L, Gifte und Vergiftungen, 6. Aufl., Nachdruck, Haug Verlag, Heidelberg 1992.

Madaus G, Lehrbuch der Biologischen Arzneimittel, Bde 1-3, Nachdruck, Georg Olms Verlag Hildesheim 1979.

Roth L, Daunderer M, Kormann K, Giftpflanzen, Pflanzengifte, 4. Aufl., Ecomed Fachverlag Landsberg Lech 1993.

Ferula Gummosa

Galbanum

DESCRIPTION

Medicinal Parts: The medicinal part is the oily gum-resin.

Two types of Galbanum are used: Levant or Soft Galbanum is more viscous and often contains small root pieces. Persian or Hard Galbanum sometimes contains pieces of stem and is friable in texture.

Flower and Fruit: The plant bears yellowish-white flowers in a few flat umbels. The fruit is thin and flat. The seeds are glossy.

Leaves, Stem and Root: Ferula gummosa is a perennial plant with a firm, smooth and hollow stem up to 1.75 m tall. The leaflets are glossy, ovate, wedge-shaped and have sharply serrate margins.

Characteristics: The gum-resin occurs in translucent, yellowish or bluish-green masses of tears. Soft Galbanum (Levant) is more viscous and may contain small pieces of root. Hard Galbanum (Persian) is friable and may contain pieces of stem. The odor is rather like musk or turpentine.

Habitat: The plant is found in central Asia, Iran, the Mediterranean region and also at the Cape of Good Hope.

Production: Galbanum is the resin from the roots and trunk of Ferula gummosa (Boiss.) and other related varieties.

ACTIONS AND PHARMACOLOGY

COMPOUNDS

Resinous substances (60%): chiefly galbaresenic acid and galbanic acid

Mucilages (40%)

Volatile oil (10-20%): including among others alpha-pinenes, beta-pinenes, myrcene, cadinenes, guaiazulene, aroma bearer undecatriene

EFFECTS

Acts as stimulant, expectorant, and vulnerary.

INDICATIONS AND USAGE

Internally used for digestive disorders and flatulence; externally it is used in the treatment of wounds.

PRECAUTIONS AND ADVERSE REACTIONS

Health risks or side effects following the proper administration of designated therapeutic dosages are not recorded.

DOSAGE

Mode of Administration: Preparations for internal and external use.

LITERATURE

Kern W, List PH, Hörhammer L (Hrsg.), Hagers Handbuch der Pharmazeutischen Praxis, 4. Aufl., Bde 1-8, Springer Verlag Berlin, Heidelberg, New York, 1969.

Ferula Sumbul

Sumbul

DESCRIPTION

Medicinal Parts: The medicinal part is the rhizome with the roots.

Leaves, Stem and Root: The plant is a 2.5 m tall shrub. It has a solid, cylindrical, thin stem, which produces about 12 branches. The fern-like leaflets are blue-gray. The basal leaves are about 50 cm long and triangular while the cauline leaves reduce gradually in size until they are little more than sheath leaves. The roots are 2.5 to 7.5 cm thick. They are covered on the outside with a blackish-brown, paper-like, horizontally folded cork, which is sometimes fibrous. The fracture is spongy and roughly fibrous with white spots and resin drops.

Characteristics: The odor is strong and musk-like, the taste is bitter and aromatic.

Habitat: The plant is found in some parts of Russia, Turkestan, and northern India.

Production: Sumbul or Musk root is the root of Ferula moschata (Reinsch, Kozo) or Ferula sumbul.

Other Names: Ferula, Musk root

ACTIONS AND PHARMACOLOGY

COMPOUNDS

Volatile oil (0.3-0.5%): musk like odor

Resins

Bitter substances

Hydroxycoumarins: including among others umbelliferone

Short-chained acids: butyric acid, angelic acid, methylcrotonic acid, and valeric acid

EFFECTS

The active agents include essential oil, resin, angelic acid, umbelliferon.

The effects are unclear; and sedative effect is questionable.

INDICATIONS AND USAGE

Antispasmodic. Formerly used in the treatment of asthma and bronchitis.

PRECAUTIONS AND ADVERSE REACTIONS

No health hazards or side effects are known in conjunction with the proper administration of designated therapeutic dosages.

DOSAGE

Mode of Administration: Sambul is used as liquid extract or tincture.

LITERATURE

Kern W, List PH, Hörhammer L (Hrsg.), Hagers Handbuch der Pharmazeutischen Praxis, 4. Aufl., Bde. 1-8: Springer Verlag Berlin, Heidelberg, New York, 1969.

Madaus G, Lehrbuch der Biologischen Arzneimittel, Bde 1-3, Nachdruck, Georg Olms Verlag Hildesheim 1979.

Fever Bark

See Alstonia Constricta

Feverfew

See Tanacetum Parthenium

Ficus Carica

Figs

DESCRIPTION

Medicinal Parts: The medicinal parts are the fruit and the latex.

Flower and Fruit: In its known form, the fig is neither a fruit nor a flower. It is a hollow, fleshy receptacle enclosing numerous flowers, which are never exposed to sunlight, but nevertheless develop fully and produce seeds. The inflorescence is hidden in the body of the fruit. The edge of the pear-shaped receptacle is curved inwards forming an almost closed hollow space. The numerous fertile and sterile florets are on the inner surface. When it ripens, the receptacle enlarges and the one-seeded fruit becomes embedded in it. The whole appears as a single purple-brown fruit.

Leaves, Stem and Root: Ficus Carica is a deciduous, heavily branched tree growing to 4 m or more. The leaves are 10 to 20 cm long, broad-ovate to orbicular with 3 to 5 deep lobes and downy beneath.

Habitat: Indigenous to Asia Minor, Syria and Iran. It is cultivated or grows wild in many subtropical regions.

Production: Figs consists of the dried fruits of Ficus carica.

ACTIONS AND PHARMACOLOGY

COMPOUNDS

Inverted sugar (50%)

Mucilages

Fruit acids: citric acid, malic acid

EFFECTS

No information available.

INDICATIONS AND USAGE

Fig preparations are used as a laxative. The claimed efficacy has not been sufficiently documented.

PRECAUTIONS AND ADVERSE REACTIONS

No health hazards or side effects are known in conjunction with the proper administration of designated therapeutic dosages.

LITERATURE

Siewek F et al. (1985) Z NaturForsch 40 (1/2): 8.

Further information in:

Kern W, List PH, Hörhammer L (Hrsg.), Hagers Handbuch der Pharmazeutischen Praxis, 4. Aufl., Bde. 1-8, Springer Verlag Berlin, Heidelberg, New York, 1969.

Teuscher E, Biogene Arzneimittel, 5. Aufl., Wiss. Verlagsges. mbH Stuttgart 1997.

Field Scabious

See Knautia Arvensis

Figs

See Ficus Carica

Figwort

See Scrophularia Nodosa

Filipendula Ulmaria

Meadowsweet

DESCRIPTION

Medicinal Parts: The medicinal parts are the dried flowers, dried aerial parts of the flowering plant, and the fresh underground and aerial parts of the flowering plant.

Flower and Fruit: The radial flowers are in terminal compound, loose cymes arranged with erect, very irregular branches. The 5 to 6 free sepals are triangular, pointed, 1 mm long, downy on the outside and fused to the flat receptacle at the base. The 5 to 6 petals are obviate, narrowed to a short stem, yellowish white and 2 to 5 mm long. The ovaries are glabrous or downy and have a flattened-stigma-bearing style under 1 mm. The one-seeded indehiscent fruit twine in a spiral.

Leaves, Stem and Root: The plant is perennial and grows to about 50 to 200 cm high. The stem is erect, simple or branched above, woody below, angular, usually glabrous or occasionally tomentose. The leaves are alternate, long-petioled to almost sessile, irregularly odd-pinnate with paired opposite pinna. These are ovate, rounded at the base or short-wedge-shaped, double serrate to dentate. The pinna is dark green and usually glabrous above and gray to white tomentose beneath and only pubescent on the ribs.

Characteristics: The leaves smell very different from the flowers, having a pleasant, almond-like fragrance.

Habitat: The plant is found in northern and southern Europe, North America and northern Asia.

Production: Meadowsweet flower consists of the dried flower of Filipendula ulmaria Maximowicz (syn. Spiraea ulmaria), as well as its preparations. Meadowsweet herb consists of the dried above-ground parts of Filipendula ulmaria Maximowicz, harvested during flowering season, as well as its preparations.

Other Names: Bridewort, Dolloff, Meadsweet, Meadow Queen, Meadow-wort, Queen of the Meadow, Lady of the Meadow, Spireaea ulmaria

ACTIONS AND PHARMACOLOGY

COMPOUNDS

Volatile oil (0.2%): chief components salicylaldehyde and methyl salicylate (yielded through dehydration from monotropitin - salicylaldehyde primveroside - and spiraeine - salicylic acid ester primveroside), further, a little vanillin and heliotropine

Flavonoids: chief components - spiraeoside (quercetin-4′-O-glucosides, 3-4%), further including among others kaempferol-4′-O-glucosides, hyperoside, rutin

Tannins: ellagic tannins

EFFECTS

Meadowsweet has antiphlogistic and astringent effects.

INDICATIONS AND USAGE

- Cough
- Bronchitis

Meadowsweet is used as supportive therapy for colds.

In folk medicine: Used as diuretic, for rheumatism of the joints and muscles, and for gout.

CONTRAINDICATIONS

Preparations are contraindicated when sensitivity to salicylate exists.

PRECAUTIONS AND ADVERSE REACTIONS

No health hazards or side effects are known in conjunction with the proper administration of designated therapeutic dosages.

OVERDOSAGE

Overdosage can lead to queasiness and stomach complaints.

DOSAGE

Mode of Administration: Comminuted drug and other galenic preparations for infusions. Meadowsweet flower is contained in various tea mixtures for the flu indications, rheumatism, kidney and bladder inflammations.

Preparation: A prepare an infusion, pour boiling water over 3 to 6 gm cut drug, steam for 10 minutes and then strain.

Daily Dosage: 2.5 to 3.5 gm of Meadowsweet flower or 4 to 5 gm Meadowsweet herb. Infusion dosage is 1 cup several times a day (1 tsp. = 1.4 gm drug).

LITERATURE

Barnaulov OD, (1978) Rastit Resur 14(4):573.

Barnaulov OD et al., (1977) Rastit Resur 13(4):661.

Barnaulov OD, Denisenko P, (19809 Farmakol Toksicol 43(6):700.

Csedö K et al., The antibiotic activity of Filipendula ulmaria. 1988. In: PM 59(7):A675. 1993.

Genig AY et al., (1977) Mater S'ezola Farm B SSR 3:162.

Gräfe AK, Besonderheiten der Arzneimitteltherapie im Säuglings- und Kindesalter. In: PZ 140(30):2659-2667. 1995.

Haslam E et al., (1985) Ann Proc Phytochemistry Soc Eur 25: 252.

Hörhammer L et al., Arch Pharm 61:133. 1956.

Kasarnovski LS, (1962) Tr Khar'kovsk Farmats Inst 2:23.

Lindeman A et al., (1982) Lebensm Wiss Technol. 15(5):286.

Thieme H, (1965) Pharmazie 20:113.

Valle MG et al., PM 54:181.

Further information in:

Hänsel R, Keller K, Rimpler H, Schneider G (Hrsg.), Hagers Handbuch der Pharmazeutischen Praxis, 5. Aufl., Bde 4-6 (Drogen): Springer Verlag Berlin, Heidelberg, New York, 1992-1994.

Madaus G, Lehrbuch der Biologischen Arzneimittel, Bde 1-3, Nachdruck, Georg Olms Verlag Hildesheim 1979.

Steinegger E, Hänsel R, Pharmakognosie, 5. Aufl., Springer Verlag Heidelberg 1992.

Wichtl M (Hrsg.), Teedrogen, 4. Aufl., Wiss. Verlagsges. Stuttgart 1997.

Flaxseed

See Linum Usitatissimum

Foeniculum Vulgare

Fennel

DESCRIPTION

Medicinal Parts: The medicinal parts are the fennel oil extracted from the ripe fruit and the dried ripe fruit of Foeniculum vulgare; also the fennel seed, which consists of Foeniculum vulgare.

Flower and Fruit: The inflorescence is fairly large umbels almost 15 cm across on very irregular rays. The flowers are fairly small and usually androgynous. The petals are a rich yellow, broadly ovate and have an involute lobe at the tip. The style is very short and almost wart-like. The fruit is glabrous, brownish or greenish-gray, 6 to 10 mm long, somewhat cylindrical with blunt ribs and is strongly domed.

Leaves, Stem and Fruit: The plant is biennial to perennial, about 80 to 150 cm high, glabrous, sea-green to glaucus and has a strong spicy smell. The stem is erect, round, glabrous, smooth and filled with latex. The lower leaves are petiolate and have long sheaths with the upper of these sitting on the sheaths, 3 or more pinnate and with a hair-like tip.

Characteristics: Spicy aroma.

Habitat: Indigenous to the Mediterranean region, spread to England, Germany, South Tyrol and Argentina. Fennel is also found today in Iran, India and China.

Production: Fennel oil is the essential oil obtained from the dried, ripe fruits of the Foeniculum vulgare by steam distillation. Fennel seed consists of the dried, ripe fruits of Foeniculum vulgare.

Other Names: Large fennel, Sweet fennel, Wild fennel, Fenkel, Bitter Fennel

ACTIONS AND PHARMACOLOGY

COMPOUNDS: FENNEL OIL

When extracted from bitter fennel the chief components are:

Trans-anethols (50-75%)

Fenchone (12-33%)

Estragole (2-5%)

Additional components are - alpha-pinenes, camphene, p-cymene, myrcene, limonene, alpha- and beta-phellandrene, gamma-terpenes, terpinols, cis-ocimene

When extracted from sweet fennel the chief components are:

Trans-anethole (80-90%)

Fenchone (1-10%)

Estragole (3-10%)

Additional components are - alpha-pinenes, camphene, p-cymene, myrcene, limonene, alpha- and beta-phellandrene, gamma-terpenes, terpinols, gamma-fenchen

EFFECTS: FENNEL OIL

Stimulation of gastrointestinal motility; in higher concentrations, antispasmodic; experimentally, anethole and fenchone have shown a secretolytic action on the respiratory tract. In vitro, it is antimicrobial.

COMPOUNDS: FENNEL SEED

Volatile oil

With bitter fennel the chief components are:

Trans-anethole (50-75%)

Fenchon (12-33%)

Estragole (2-5%)

Additional components - alpha-pinenes, camphene, p-cymene, myrcene, limonene, alpha- and beta-phellandrene, gamma-terpenes, terpinols cis-ocimene

With sweet fennel the chief components are:

Trans-anethole (80-90%)

Fenchon (1-10%)

Estragole (3-10%)

Additional components - alpha-pinenes, camphene, p-cymene, myrcene, limonene, alpha- and beta-phellandrene, gamma-terpenes, terpinols, gamma-fenchen

Hydroxycoumarins (traces): umbelliferone, scopoletine, osthenol, scoparin, Furocoumarins traces) including bergapten, columbianetin, psoralen, xanthotoxin

Pyranocoumarins

Flavonoids

Fatty oil

EFFECTS: FENNEL SEED

Promotes gastrointestinal motility; in higher concentrations acts as an antispasmodic. Experimentally, anethole and fenchone have been shown to have a secretolytic effect in the respiratory tract in frogs, and aqueous fennel extracts raised the mucociliary activity of the ciliary epithelium.

INDICATIONS AND USAGE

FENNEL OIL

- Cough
- Bronchitis

Peptic discomforts, such as mild, spastic disorders of the gastrointestinal tract, feeling of fullness, flatulence; catarrh of the upper respiratory tract. Fennel honey is used for catarrh of the upper respiratory tract in children.

FENNEL SEED

- Cough
- Bronchitis

Dyspepsias such as mild, spastic gastrointestinal ailments, fullness, flatulence; catarrh of the upper respiratory tract. Fennel syrup and fennel honey are used for catarrh of the upper respiratory tract in children.

PRECAUTIONS AND ADVERSE REACTIONS

General: Health risks or side effects following the proper administration of designated therapeutic dosages are not recorded. Allergic reactions following intake of fennel have been only very rarely observed. Reciprocal reactions among patients with celery allergy appear to be possible.

Pregnancy: Preparations, excluding the drug itself and tea infusions are not to be administered during pregnancy.

Pediatric Use: Preparations, excluding the drug itself and tea infusions are not to be administered to small children.

DOSAGE

FENNEL OIL

Mode of Administration: Essential oil and galenic preparations for internal use.

Note: Diabetics must check the sugar content.

Daily Dosage: 0.1 to 0.6 ml of fennel oil

Duration of administration: Maximum of 2 weeks.

FENNEL SEED

Mode of Administration: Crushed or ground seeds for teas, tea-like products, as well as other galenic preparations for internal use.

Daily Dosage: 5 to 7 gm of drug

LITERATURE

FENNEL OIL

Albert-Puleo M, (1980) J Ethnopharmacol 2:337.

Betts TJ, J Pharm Pharmacol 20:469-472 et 61S-64S. 1968.

Czygan FC, ZPT 8:82. 1987.

El-Khrisy EAM et al., (1980) Fitoterapia 51:273.

Forster HB et al., (1980) Planta Med 40(4):309.

Gershbein LL, (1977) Food Cosmet Toxicol 15(3):173.

Harborne JB, Williams CE, (1972) Phytochemistry 11:1741.

Harries N et al., (1978) J Clin Pharm 2:171.

Hiller K, Pharmazeutische Bewertung ausgewählter Teedrogen. In: DAZ 135(16):1425-1440. 1995.

Karlsen J et al., (1969) Planta Med 17:281.

Karlsen J et al., PM 17:281-293. 1969.

Kunzemann J, Hermann K, (1977) Z Lebensm Unters Forsch 164:194.

Massoud H, Study on the essential oil in seeds of some fennel cultivars under egyptian environmental conditions. In: PM 58(7):A681. 1992.

Parzinger R, Fenchel. In: DAZ 136(7):529-530. 1996.

Rothbacher H, Kraus A, (1970) Pharmazie 25:566.

Shah CS et al., PM 18:285-295. 1970.

Stahl E, (1980) Dtsch Apoth Ztg 45:2324.

Trenkle K, PA 27:319-324. 1972.

Further information in:

Hänsel R, Keller K, Rimpler H, Schneider G (Hrsg.), Hagers Handbuch der Pharmazeutischen Praxis, 5. Aufl., Bde 4-6 (Drogen), Springer Verlag Berlin, Heidelberg, New York, 1992-1994.

Leung AY, Encyclopedia of Common Natural Ingredients Used in Food Drugs and Cosmetics, John Wiley & Sons Inc., New York 1980.

Madaus G, Lehrbuch der Biologischen Arzneimittel, Bde 1-3, Nachdruck, Georg Olms Verlag Hildesheim 1979.

Schulz R, Hänsel R, Rationale Phytotherapie, Springer Verlag Heidelberg 1996.

Steinegger E, Hänsel R, Pharmakognosie, 5. Aufl., Springer Verlag Heidelberg 1992.

Teuscher E, Biogene Arzneimittel, 5. Aufl., Wiss. Verlagsges. mbH Stuttgart 1997.

Wagner H, Wiesenauer M, Phytotherapie. Phytopharmaka und pflanzliche Homöopathika, Fischer-Verlag, Stuttgart, Jena, New York 1995.

FENNEL SEED

Albert-Puleo M, (1980) J Ethnopharmacol 2:337.

Betts TJ, J Pharm Pharmacol 20:469-472 et 61S-64S. 1968.

Czygan FC, ZPT 8:82. 1987.

El-Khrisy EAM et al., (1980) Fitoterapia 51:273.

Forster HB et al., (1980) Planta Med 40(4):309.

Gershbein LL, (1977) Food Cosmet Toxicol 15(3):173.

Harborne JB, Williams CE, (1972) Phytochemistry 11:1741.

Harries N et al., (1978) J Clin Pharm 2:171.

Hiller K, Pharmazeutische Bewertung ausgewählter Teedrogen. In: DAZ 135(16):1425-1440. 1995.

Karlsen J et al., (1969) Planta Med 17:281.

Karlsen J et al., PM 17:281-293. 1969.

Kunzemann J, Hermann K, (1977) Z Lebensm Unters Forsch 164:194.

Massoud H, Study on the essential oil in seeds of some fennel cultivars under egyptian environmental conditions. In: PM 58(7):A681. 1992.

Parzinger R, Fenchel. In: DAZ 136(7):529-530. 1996.

Rothbacher H, Kraus A, (1970) Pharmazie 25:566.

Shah CS et al., PM 18:285-295. 1970.

Stahl E, (1980) Dtsch Apoth Ztg 45:2324.

Trenkle K, PA 27:319-324. 1972.

Further information in:

Hänsel R, Keller K, Rimpler H, Schneider G (Hrsg.), Hagers Handbuch der Pharmazeutischen Praxis, 5. Aufl., Bde 4-6 (Drogen), Springer Verlag Berlin, Heidelberg, New York, 1992-1994.

Leung AY, Encyclopedia of Common Natural Ingredients Used in Food Drugs and Cosmetics, John Wiley & Sons Inc., New York 1980.

Madaus G, Lehrbuch der Biologischen Arzneimittel, Bde 1-3, Nachdruck, Georg Olms Verlag Hildesheim 1979.

Schulz R, Hänsel R, Rationale Phytotherapie, Springer Verlag Heidelberg 1996.

Steinegger E, Hänsel R, Pharmakognosie, 5. Aufl., Springer Verlag Heidelberg 1992.

Teuscher E, Biogene Arzneimittel, 5. Aufl., Wiss. Verlagsges. mbH Stuttgart 1997.

Wagner H, Wiesenauer M, Phytotherapie. Phytopharmaka und pflanzliche Homöopathika, Fischer-Verlag, Stuttgart, Jena, New York 1995.

Wichtl M (Hrsg.), Teedrogen, 4. Aufl., Wiss. Verlagsges. Stuttgart 1997

Fool's Parsley

See Aethusa Cynapium

Forget-Me-Not

See Myosotis Arvensis

Foxglove

See Digitalis Purpurea

Fragaria Vesca

Strawberry leaf

DESCRIPTION

Medicinal Parts: The medicinal parts are dried leaves collected during the flowering season, the dried rhizome and ripe fruit.

Flower and Fruit: The small white flowers are arranged on a repeatedly bifurcated pedicle. They are usually androgynous. There are 5 sepals and 5 petals. The sepals are triangular, pointed or briefly acuminate appressed pubescent. The petals are oribicular or ovate, glabrous and pure white. There are 20 stamens and numerous ovate, glabrous carpels and a style at the side. After flowering the receptacle turns into a fleshy false fruit. The receptacle is 2 cm long, ovate, globular or clavate, carmine red when ripe. The nutlets are ovate, 0.8 to 1.5 mm long, brown and matte.

Leaves, Stem and Root: The perennial, herbaceous plant grows from 20 to 30 cm high. The rhizome is cylindrical, horizontal or crooked and thickly covered with the residual died off leaves and stipules. Long runners grow from the axils of the basal leaves. The stem is erect and is slightly longer than the basal leaves. The cauline leaves are trifoliate and roughly serrate from the first quarter upwards. The petioles are very long and, like the stem have patent hairs. The stipules are lanceolate, long-acuminate, entire-margined, reddish brown, glabrous above and hairy beneath.

Habitat: Found in almost all of the temperate zones of Europe and Asia.

Production: Strawberry leaf consists of the dried leaf of Fragaria species, mainly Fragaria vesca.

Not To Be Confused With: Other Fragaria species, although they have the same value.

Other Names: Wild Strawberry, Mountain Strawberry, Wood Strawberry

ACTIONS AND PHARMACOLOGY

COMPOUNDS

Tannins: ellagic acid tannins, oligomeric proanthocyanidins

Flavonoids: including rutin, quercetin

EFFECTS

Strawberry leaf has astringent and diuretic properties; but no studies are available.

INDICATIONS AND USAGE

Preparations of strawberry leaf are used externally as compresses for rashes, and internally for catarrhs of the gastrointestinal tract, diarrhea, intestinal sluggishness, liver disease, jaundice, catarrhs of the respiratory tract, gout, rheumatoid arthritis, nervous tension, kidney ailments involving gravel and stones, as a diuretic.

PRECAUTIONS AND ADVERSE REACTIONS

Health risks or side effects following the proper administration of designated therapeutic dosages are not recorded. The drug is not to be taken in presence of strawberry allergy.

DOSAGE

Mode of Administration: Strawberry leaves are only used occasionally in folk medicine, the berries are used more commonly.

Preparation: Pour boiling water over 1 gm of comminuted drug and strain after 5 to 10 minutes.

Daily Dosage: Tea: As an antidiarrheal agent, several cups per day.

LITERATURE

Henning W (1981) Z Lebensm Unters Forsch 173:180.

Haddock EA et al., PH 21:1049. 1982.

Lund K, Dissertation Universität Freiburg i. Br. 1986.

Further information in:

Hänsel R, Keller K, Rimpler H, Schneider G (Hrsg.), Hagers Handbuch der Pharmazeutischen Praxis, 5. Aufl., Bde 4-6 (Drogen), Springer Verlag Berlin, Heidelberg, New York, 1992-1994.

Teuscher E, Biogene Arzneimittel, 5. Aufl., Wiss. Verlagsges. mbH Stuttgart 1997.

Wichtl M (Hrsg.), Teedrogen, 4. Aufl., Wiss. Verlagsges. Stuttgart 1997.

Frankincense

See Boswellia Carteri

Fraxinus Excelsior

Ash

DESCRIPTION

Medicinal Parts: The medicinal parts are the dried leaves, the fresh bark, the branch bark, and the fresh leaves.

Flower and Fruit: The flowers are in richly blossomed panicles, the terminal ones appearing on the new flowering branches. They are usually androgynous, occasionally male, polygamous or dioecious. They have no calyx or corolla. The anthers of the male flowers are dark purple and are on short filaments. The female flowers consist of 1 inferior ovary with a 2-lobed stigma and 2 split staminoids. The fruit is a narrow lanceolate to oblong-obovate nutlet hanging on a thin stem. The fruit is 25 to 50 mm long and 7 to 10 mm wide, glossy brown, 1-seeded with a veined winged border.

Leaves, Stem and Root: The ash is an impressive 15 to 30 m tall tree with a gray-brown, smooth, later fissured and wrinkled bark and large, black-brown, pubescent buds. The leaves are entire-margined, opposite and odd pinnate. There are 9 to 15 leaflets. The leaflets are sessile, usually 5 to 11 cm long by 1 to 3 cm wide, oblong-ovate to lanceolate, long acuminate, finely and sharply serrate. They are glabrous above, rich green, loosely tomentose or almost glabrous, and greenish brown beneath.

Habitat: The plant is distributed in most parts of Europe except the northern, southern and eastern edges.

Production: Ash bark consists of the bark of young branches of Fraxinus excelsior. Ash leaf consists of the leaf of Fraxinus excelsior. The leaves are harvested in spring and air-dried.

Other Names: Bird's Tongue, European Ash, Common Ash, Weeping Ash

ACTIONS AND PHARMACOLOGY

COMPOUNDS: FRAXINUS EXCELSIOR LEAF

Flavonoids: including rutin (0.1-0.9%)

Tannins

Mucilages (10-20%)

Mannitol (16-28%)

Triterpenes, phytosterols

Iridoide monoterpenes: including syringoxide, deoxysyringoxidin

COMPOUNDS: FRAXINUS EXCELSIOR BARK
Hydroxycoumarins: aesculin, fraxin, aesculetin, fraxetin, fraxidin, isofraxidin, fraxinol, scopoletine

Tannins

Iridoide monoterpenes: including 10-hydroxyligstroside

EFFECTS: FRAXINUS EXCELSIOR BARK
Preparations of fresh ash bark showed an analgesic, antioxidative, and antiphlogistic action.

INDICATIONS AND USAGE

FRAXINUS EXCELSIOR LEAF
Preparations of ash leaf are used for arthritis, gout, bladder complaints, as well as a laxative and diuretic.

FRAXINUS EXCELSIOR BARK
Preparations of ash bark are used for fever and as a tonic.

PRECAUTIONS AND ADVERSE REACTIONS

Health risks or side effects following the proper administration of designated therapeutic dosages are not recorded.

DOSAGE

Mode of Administration: Since the efficacy for the claimed applications has not been documented, therapeutic application cannot be recommended. The efficacy of Ash in fixed combinations must be verified specifically for each preparation.

LITERATURE

Carnat A, Lamaison JL, Dubnand F, Plant Méd Phytothér 24:145-151. 1990.

Genius OB, DAZ 120:1505-1506. 1980.

Jensen SR, Nielsen BJ, PH 15:221-223. 1976.

Marekov N et al., Khim Ind 58:132-135. 1986.

Tissut M, Ravane P, PH 19:2077-2081. 1980.

Yamagami I, Suzuki Y, Koichiro I, Pharmacological studies on the components of Fraxinus japonica. In: Nippon Yakurigaku Zasshi 64(6):714-729 (jap.). 1968.

Further information in:

Hänsel R, Keller K, Rimpler H, Schneider G (Hrsg.), Hagers Handbuch der Pharmazeutischen Praxis, 5. Aufl., Bde 4-6 (Drogen), Springer Verlag Berlin, Heidelberg, New York, 1992-1994.

Madaus G, Lehrbuch der Biologischen Arzneimittel, Bde 1-3, Nachdruck, Georg Olms Verlag Hildesheim 1979.

Poisonous Plants in Britain and their Effects on Animals and Man, Ministry of Agriculture Fisheries and Food, HMSO UK 1984.

Fraxinus Ornus

Manna

DESCRIPTION

Medicinal Parts: The medicinal part is the juice extracted from the bark starting from the 8th to the 10th year. This tree yields from its bark a sugary sap known in pharmacy as Manna.

Flower and Fruit: The inflorescence is upright, later hanging, feathery panicles. The sepals are very short. The petals are fused at the base in pairs, they are linear to narrowly linguiform and white. The 2 stamens have very long filaments. The fruit is a nutlet. It is hanging, linguiform, 3 to 4 mm long, 7 to 10 mm wide. It is rounded at the base or narrowed wedge-shaped, glossy dark brown, flat, longitudinally striped. The seeds are ovate, 15 to 20 mm by 4 to 5 mm, broad, flat, longitudinally striped and brown.

Leaves, Stem and Root: Fraxinus ornus is a tree growing up to 8 m tall with gray, crust-embossed bark. The new-year's branchlets are olive-green or browny gray-green, somewhat glossy, with numerous, light-brown lenticels. The long shoots are downy to the tip, the short shoots are awned at the base. The terminal and lateral buds are orbicular and 4-scaled. The leaflets are elliptical-ovate-lanceolate or ovate, tapering to a tip, crenate-serrate. The upper surface is rich green and the underside lighter green with pink veins. The nerves are pink-tomentose.

Habitat: The tree is indigenous to southern Europe, extending to the southern borders of the Alps and as far as European Turkey. The tree is cultivated in Italy.

Production: Manna consists of the dried sap generated from the slit bark of trunk and branches of Fraxinus ornus, as well as its preparations in effective dosage.

Other Names: Flowering Ash, Manna Ash, Flake Manna

ACTIONS AND PHARMACOLOGY

COMPOUNDS
Mannitol (70-90%)

Stachyose (10-15%)

Mannotriose, glucose, fructose

EFFECTS
Acts as a laxative.

INDICATIONS AND USAGE

■ Constipation

Used in Constipation. Manna is also used for ailments where an easier elimination and a soft stool is desirable, such as anal fissures, hemorrhoids, and post-rectal/anal surgery.

CONTRAINDICATIONS

The drug is not to be used in the presence of ileus.

PRECAUTIONS AND ADVERSE REACTIONS

No health hazards or side effects are known in conjunction with the proper administration of designated therapeutic dosages. Susceptible persons could experience flatulence and nausea.

DOSAGE

Mode of Administration: Comminuted herb and other galenic preparations for internal use.

Daily Dosage: For adults, 20 to 30 gm of drug; For children, 2 to 16 gm of drug. Manna, like other laxatives, should not be used for an extended period of time.

LITERATURE

Hänsel R, Keller K, Rimpler H, Schneider G (Hrsg.), Hagers Handbuch der Pharmazeutischen Praxis, 5. Aufl., Bde 4-6 (Drogen), Springer Verlag Berlin, Heidelberg, New York, 1992-1994 (unter Fraxinus ornus).

Fringetree

See Chionanthus Virginicus

Frostwort

See Helianthemum Canadense

Fucus Vesiculosus

Bladderwrack

DESCRIPTION

Medicinal Parts: The medicinal parts are the dried thallus and the fresh thallus of the bladderwrack.

Flower and Fruit: Some thallus ends look grainy and it is here that the reproductive organs are found. The fructifications consisting of 3 cm long ovoid receptacles are found in the tips of these thalli. They are either cordate or ovately flattened with grainy bladders.

Leaves, Stem and Root: The plant is often over 1 m long, olive green when fresh, black brown when dry. The stem of the thallus is flat, repeatedly bifurcated and has a midrib along the whole length. Beside this midrib there are often scattered pores and numerous air-filled bladders.

Habitat: The plant is found on the North Sea coast, the western Baltic coast, and on the Atlantic and Pacific coasts.

Production: Bladderwrack consists of the dried thallus of Fucus vesiculosus, of Ascophyllum nodosum Le Jolis, or of both species, as well as preparations of same.

Other Names: Seawrack, Kelpware, Black-tang, Bladder Fucus, Cutweed, Fucus, Quercus marina, Sea-Wrack, Kelp-Ware

ACTIONS AND PHARMACOLOGY

COMPOUNDS

Inorganic iodine salts

Organically-bound iodine: in particular in proteins and lipids, also present as diiodothyrosine

Polysaccharides: including alginic acid, fucane, fucoidine (strongly sulfated)

Polyphenold: Phlorotannins

EFFECTS

No information available.

INDICATIONS

Preparations of Bladderwrack are used for disease of the thyroid, obesity, overweight, arteriosclerosis and digestive disorders.

The effectiveness for the claimed applications is not verified.

PRECAUTIONS AND ADVERSE REACTIONS

Dosages above 150 g iodide/day carry with them the danger of induction or worsening of a hyperthyroidism. For that reason, the drug should no longer be administered, due to its variable iodide content (0.03 - 1%). Allergic reactions have been known to occur.

LITERATURE

Béress A, Wassermann O, Bruhn T, Béress L, A new procedure for the isolation of anti-HIV compounds (polysaccharides and polyphenols) from the marine alga Fucus vesiculosus. In: JNP 56(4):478-488. 1993.

Criado MT et al., (1983) IRC Med Sci 11(3):286.

Curro F et al., (1976) Arch Med Interna 28(1):19.

Frohne D, Phytotherapeutika und Schilddrüse. In: Intern Praxis 32(1)158. 1992.

Glombitza KW et al., (1977) Planta Med 32(1):33.

Glombitza KW, Lentz G (1981) Tetrahedron 37(22):3861.

Phillips DJH (1979) Environ Pollut 18(1):31.

Quang-Liem P, Laur MH (1974) Biochimie 56(6/7):925.

Quang-Liem P, Laur MH (1976) Biochimie 58(11/12):1367.

Stahl E et al., DAZ 115:1893. 1975.

Further information in:

Hänsel R, Keller K, Rimpler H, Schneider G (Hrsg.), Hagers Handbuch der Pharmazeutischen Praxis, 5. Aufl., Bde 4-6 (Drogen), Springer Verlag Berlin, Heidelberg, New York, 1992-1994.

Madaus G, Lehrbuch der Biologischen Arzneimittel, Bde 1-3, Nachdruck, Georg Olms Verlag Hildesheim 1979.

Steinegger E, Hänsel R, Pharmakognosie, 5. Aufl., Springer Verlag Heidelberg 1992.

Teuscher E, Biogene Arzneimittel, 5. Aufl., Wiss. Verlagsges. mbH Stuttgart 1997.

Wichtl M (Hrsg.), Teedrogen, 4. Aufl., Wiss. Verlagsges. Stuttgart 1997.

Fumaria Officinalis

Fumitory

DESCRIPTION

Medicinal Parts: The medicinal parts are the dried herb and the aerial parts of the fresh flowering plant.

Flower and Fruit: The short pedicled flowers are in erect, dense, terminal racemes opposite the leaves and are 5 to 8 mm long. The outer petals are rounded at the front and are crimson to pink. But like the inner petals they are dark-red to black at the tip and have a green keel. The fruit, which appears in the flowering season, is nut-like, globular, slightly flattened at the side, green and has a dent in the top.

Leaves, Stem and Root: The plant is 10 to 50 cm high and has a tender, erect, angular, branched hollow and glabrous stem which, like the leaves, is bluish green. The leaves are alternate and divided into 3-pinnate sections. They are petiolate, double pinnate, soft with petioled palmate or pinnatifid pinna.

Characteristics: The herb has a bitter, salty taste.

Habitat: The plant is indigenous to the Mediterranean region to northern Africa and in all of Europe and Siberia. The herb has been introduced into North and South America.

Production: Common fumitory herb consists of the dried, above ground parts of Fumaria officinalis, gathered during the flowering season.

Not To Be Confused With: The very similar species F. vaillanti and F. schleicheri Soy-Vill.

Other Names: Earth Smoke, Hedge Fumitory, Beggary, Fumus, Vapor, Wax Dolls

ACTIONS AND PHARMACOLOGY

COMPOUNDS

Isoquinoline alkaloids: some of them include -

Protoberberine-type: including (-)-scoulerine

Protopine-type: including protopine; main alkaloid

Spirobenzylisoquinoline-type: fumaricine, (+)-fumariline

Indenobenzazepine-type: including fumaritine, fumarofine

Flavonoids: including rutin

Organic acids: fumaric acid

Hydroxycinnamic acid derivatives: including caffeoylmalic acid

EFFECTS

Fumitory has a light, antispasmodic effect on the bile ducts and the gastrointestinal tract. It is also amphicholeretic.

INDICATIONS AND USAGE

■ Liver and gallbladder complaints

Spastic discomfort in the area of the gallbladder and bile ducts, as well as the gastrointestinal tract.

In folk medicine, the herb has been used for skin diseases, cystitis, atherosclerosis, rheumatism, arthritis, as a blood purifier, hypoglycemia and for infections.

PRECAUTIONS AND ADVERSE REACTIONS

Health risks or side effects following the proper administration of designated therapeutic dosages are not recorded.

DOSAGE

Mode of Administration: Comminuted drug and its galenic preparations for internal use.

Preparation: To prepare an infusion, pour boiling water over 2 to 3 gm drug and strain after 20 minutes.

Daily Dosage: 6 gm of drug. Infusion for gallbladder complaints, warm, and drink 1 cup before meals.

Storage: Protect from light and moisture.

LITERATURE

Duke JA (1985) Die amphocholeretische Wirkung der Fumaria officinalis. Z Allg Med 34: 1819.

Hahn R, Nahrstedt A, High Content of Hydroxycinnamic Acids Esterified with (+)-D-Malic-Acid in the Upper Parts of Fumaria officinalis. In: PM 59(2):189. 1993.

Mardirossian ZH et al., PH 22:759. 1983.

Willaman JJ, Hui-Li L (1970) Lloydia 33 (3A): 1.

Further information in:

Hänsel R, Keller K, Rimpler H, Schneider G (Hrsg.), Hagers Handbuch der Pharmazeutischen Praxis, 5. Aufl., Bde 4-6 (Drogen), Springer Verlag Berlin, Heidelberg, New York, 1992-1994.

Madaus G, Lehrbuch der Biologischen Arzneimittel, Bde 1-3, Nachdruck, Georg Olms Verlag Hildesheim 1979.

Roth L, Daunderer M, Kormann K, Giftpflanzen, Pflanzengifte, 4. Aufl., Ecomed Fachverlag Landsberg Lech 1993.

Teuscher E, Lindequist U, Biogene Gifte - Biologie, Chemie, Pharmakologie, 2. Aufl., Fischer Verlag Stuttgart 1994.

Wichtl M (Hrsg.), Teedrogen, 4. Aufl., Wiss. Verlagsges. Stuttgart 1997.

Fumitory

See Fumaria Officinalis

Galangal

See Alpinia Officinarum

Galbanum

See Ferula Gummosa

Galega Officinalis

Goat's Rue

DESCRIPTION

Medicinal Parts: The medicinal parts are the leaves collected at the beginning of the flowering season and dried, as well as the tips of the flowering branches.

Flower and Fruit: Long-peduncled, axillary racemes made up of 1 cm long slightly inclined florets. The petals are bluish white and short-stemmed. All the filaments are fused. The fruit is a 2 to 3 cm long and 2 to 3 mm thick, round, many-seeded, indented pod.

Leaves, Stem and Root: Strong, bright green shrub with numerous, 40 cm to 1 m high, erect, branched, hollow stems. It has a divided rhizome with brown fibers sprouting numerous erect, corrugated, round, tall stems. The leaves are odd-pinnate; the leaflets are 1.5 to 4 cm long and 4 to 16 mm wide elliptical to lanceolate and thorny-tipped with a rich green upper surface and a lighter undersurface.

Characteristics: The plant is without odor unless bruised, whereupon it emits a disagreeable smell, which probably gave rise to the common name Goat's Rue.

Habitat: Grows wild in Europe and Asia.

Production: Goat's Rue herb consists of the dried, above ground parts of Galega officinalis, harvested during the flowering season.

Other Names: Italian Fitch, French Lilac

ACTIONS AND PHARMACOLOGY

COMPOUNDS

Guanidine derivatives: galegine, 4-hydroxygalegine

Quinazoline alkaloids: (+)-peganine

Lectins

Flavonoids

EFFECTS

The herb contains galegin, which affects blood sugar. The blood sugar-lowering effect of Goat's Rue herb has not been documented.

INDICATIONS AND USAGE

Preparations of Goat's Rue herb are used as a diuretic, as well as supportive therapy for diabetes.

The efficacy for the claimed applications is not documented.

PRECAUTIONS AND ADVERSE REACTIONS

Health risks or side effects following the proper administration of designated therapeutic dosages are not recorded.

Poisonings have only been observed in animals, and then following the intake of large quantities of the plant (in sheep salivation, spasms, paralyses, death through asphyxiation).

DOSAGE

Mode of Administration: Since the efficacy for the claimed uses is not documented, therapeutic application cannot be recommended. Goat's Rue cannot be justified for diabetes mellitus because of the severity of the disease and the availability of effective therapeutic alternatives.

Preparation: To prepare an infusion, pour boiling water over 2 gm of comminuted drug and strain after 5 to 10 minutes.

LITERATURE

Barthel A, Reuter G, PA 23:26. 1968.

Reuter G, Flora 154:136. 1964.

Schreiber K, Pufahl K, Bräuninger H, Liebigs Ann Chem 671:142. 1964.

Further information in:

Frohne D, Pfänder HJ, Giftpflanzen - Ein Handbuch für Apotheker, Toxikologen und Biologen, 4. Aufl., Wiss. Verlagsges. mbH Stuttgart 1997.

Kern W, List PH, Hörhammer L (Hrsg.), Hagers Handbuch der Pharmazeutischen Praxis, 4. Aufl., Bde. 1-8, Springer Verlag Berlin, Heidelberg, New York, 1969.

Lewin L, Gifte und Vergiftungen, 6. Aufl., Nachdruck, Haug Verlag, Heidelberg 1992.

Madaus G, Lehrbuch der Biologischen Arzneimittel, Bde 1-3, Nachdruck, Georg Olms Verlag Hildesheim 1979.

Poisonous Plants in Britain and their effects on Animals and Man, Ministry of Agriculture Fisheries and Food, HMSO, UK 1984.

Roth L, Daunderer M, Kormann K, Giftpflanzen, Pflanzengifte, 4. Aufl., Ecomed Fachverlag Landsberg Lech 1993.

Steinegger E, Hänsel R, Pharmakognosie, 5. Aufl., Springer Verlag Heidelberg 1992.

Teuscher E, Lindequist U, Biogene Gifte - Biologie, Chemie, Pharmakologie, 2. Aufl., Fischer Verlag Stuttgart 1994.

Galeopsis Segetum

Hempnettle

DESCRIPTION

Medicinal Parts: The medicinal part is the flowering herb.

Flower and Fruit: The large pale yellow bilabiate flowers are in false whorls on the branch ends. The calyx is evenly 5-dentate and covered in patent glandular hairs. The upper lip of the corolla is domed, finely dentate and pubescent. The lateral tips of the 3-lobed lower lip are obtuse and have 1 hollow erect tooth at either side of the base. The stamen halves are horizontal. The fruit is smooth.

Leaves, Stem and Root: The herb grows to 15 to 100 cm high. The stem is erect, heavily branched, and downy with unthickened nodes. The leaves are ovate, serrate, the lower ones long petioled, the upper ones short petioled.

Habitat: Southern and central Europe.

Production: Hempnettle consists of the above ground parts of Galeopsis segetum Necker (synonym Galeopsis ochroleuca Lamarck) and is gathered during the flowering season.

ACTIONS AND PHARMACOLOGY

COMPOUNDS

Iridoide monoterpenes: including harpagide, 8-O-acetylharpagide, antirrinoside, 5-O-glucosylantirrinoside

Silicic acid: to some extent water-soluble

Tannins

Flavonoids

EFFECTS

Astringent, expectorant.

INDICATIONS AND USAGE

- Cough
- Bronchitis

In folk medicine, the herb is used for pulmonary afflictions and as a diuretic.

PRECAUTIONS AND ADVERSE REACTIONS

Health risks or side effects following the proper administration of designated therapeutic dosages are not recorded.

DOSAGE

Mode of Administration: Comminuted herb for teas and other galenic preparations for internal use.

Preparation: To prepare an infusion, pour boiling water over 2 gm of comminuted drug, strain after 5 minutes.

Standardized preparations that contain the drug extract are Pertussin and Tussiflorin.

Daily Dosage: Average daily dose: 6 gm drug. The infusion may be taken repeatedly daily and may be sweetened with honey.

LITERATURE

Junod-Busch U, Dissertation ETH Zürich. 1976.

Tomas-Barberan FA et al., PH 30:3311. 1991.

Further information in:

Kern W, List PH, Hörhammer L (Hrsg.), Hagers Handbuch der Pharmazeutischen Praxis, 4. Aufl., Bde. 1-8, Springer Verlag Berlin, Heidelberg, New York, 1969.

Madaus G, Lehrbuch der Biologischen Arzneimittel, Bde 1-3, Nachdruck, Georg Olms Verlag Hildesheim 1979.

Steinegger E, Hänsel R, Pharmakognosie, 5. Aufl., Springer Verlag Heidelberg 1992.

Wichtl M (Hrsg.), Teedrogen, 4. Aufl., Wiss. Verlagsges. Stuttgart 1997.

Galipea Officinalis

Angostura

DESCRIPTION

Medicinal Parts: The medicinal part is the dried bark of the tree.

Flower and Fruit: The strongly scented flowers are in terminal, peduncled, and closed racemes. The fruit is a 5-valved capsule, of which 2 or 3 are often sterile. There are 2 seeds in each capsule. They are round and black and usually only one of them fertile.

Leaves, Stem and Root: Galipea officinalis is a small 4 to 5 m high tree, which is 7.5 to 12.5 cm in diameter and has a straight trunk and irregular branches. The bark is smooth and gray. It is slightly curved or quilled. The inner surface is yellowish-gray. The outer layer is sometimes soft and spongy. The transverse section is dark brown. The bright green leaves are smooth, glossy, alternate, and petiolate. They sometimes have white spots. The 3 leaflets are oblong, pointed, and 4 cm long.

Habitat: Angostura is indigenous to Venezuela and tropical regions of South America.

Production: Angostura is the whole or ground bark of Galipea officinalis.

Other Names: Cusparia Bark, True Angostura

ACTIONS AND PHARMACOLOGY

COMPOUNDS

Volatile oil

Quinolin alkaloids: including cusparine

Angustorine (bitter iridoid glycoside)

EFFECTS

Angostura is a stimulant, a bittering substance, and a tonic. In larger doses, the drug also has an emetic and strong laxative effect.

INDICATIONS AND USAGE

The drug is used for diarrhea and also as a febrifuge.

PRECAUTIONS AND ADVERSE REACTIONS

No health hazards or side effects are known in conjunction with the proper administration of designated therapeutic dosages. The administration of larger doses can lead to nausea and vomiting.

LITERATURE

Brieskorn CH, Beck V, (1971) Phytochemistry 10:3205.

Further information in:

Hoppe HA, (1975-1987) Drogenkunde, 8. Aufl., Bde 1-3, W. de Gruyter Verlag, Berlin, New York.

Kern W, List PH, Hörhammer L (Hrsg.), Hagers Handbuch der Pharmazeutischen Praxis, 4. Aufl., Bde 1-8, Springer Verlag Berlin, Heidelberg, New York, 1969.

Leung AY, Encyclopedia of Common Natural Ingredients used in Food Drugs and Cosmetics, John Wiley & Sons Inc. New York 1980.

Madaus G, Lehrbuch der Biologischen Arzneimittel, Bde 1-3, Nachdruck, Georg Olms Verlag Hildesheim 1979.

Roth L, Daunderer M, Kormann K, Giftpflanzen, Pflanzengifte, 4. Aufl., Ecomed Fachverlag Landsberg Lech 1993.

Galium Aparine

Clivers

DESCRIPTION

Medicinal Parts: The medicinal parts are the aerial parts collected during the flowering season and dried, as well as the fresh, flowering herb or the fresh or dried whole plant.

Flower and Fruit: There are a few small white or greenish flowers in axillary, peduncled cymes. The corolla is about 1.5 to 1.7 mm long and has a pointed tip. The pedicles do not turn back before the fruit ripens. The 4 to 7 mm-long mericarps are covered in barbed bristles.

Leaves, Stem and Root: The plant is 60 to 150 cm high. The stem is decumbent or climbing, sharply quadrangular even to the point of being winged and branched. There are long cauline leaves. The margins and midrib of the leaves are thorny. The foliage leaves are arranged in false whorls of 6 or 8. They are lanceolate from a wedge-shaped base, 30 to 60 mm long and 3 to 8 mm wide, obtuse, and thorny tipped.

Habitat: A common wild plant throughout Europe, Asia from Siberia to the Himalayas, and in North and South America.

Production: Clivers is the flowering herb of the aerial part of Galium aparine, which is gathered and then dried.

Other Names: Cleavers, Goosegrass, Barweed, Hedgeheriff, Hayriffe, Eriffe, Grip Grass, Hayruff, Catchweed, Scratweed, Mutton Chops, Robin-run-in-the-Grass, Love-man, Goosebill, Everlasting Friendship, Bedstraw, Coachweed, Cleaverwort, Goose Grass, Gosling Weed, Hedge-burs, Stick-a-back, Sweethearts

ACTIONS AND PHARMACOLOGY

COMPOUNDS

Iridoide monoterpenes: asperuloside

Benzyl isoquinoline alkaloids: including protopine

Beta-carbolin alkaloids: harmine

Quinazoline alkaloids: 1-hydroxydesoxypeganin, 8-hydroxy-2,3-dehydrodesoxypeganin

Flavonoids

EFFECTS

No information is available.

INDICATIONS AND USAGE

The drug is used internally as well as externally for ulcers, festering glands, lumps in the breast, and skin rashes. It is also used for lithuresis and calculosis and as a diuretic for dropsy, bladder catarrh, and retention of urine (ischuria).

Efficacy has not been proven.

PRECAUTIONS AND ADVERSE REACTIONS

Health risks or side effects following the proper administration of designated therapeutic dosages are not recorded.

DOSAGE

Mode of Administration: Used topically in alcoholic extracts. Internally as a tea and juice.

Daily Dosage: As a tea, add 4 teaspoonfuls (3.3 to 4.4 gm) of the drug to 2 glasses of hot water. Drink in sips during the course of the day.

LITERATURE

Berkowitz, WF et al., (1982) J Org Chem 47:824.

Bhan MK et al., (1976) Ind J Chem 14:475.

Buckova et al., (1970) Acta Fac Pharm Univ Comeniana 19:7.

Burnett AR, Thomsom RH, (1968) J Clin Soc (6):854.

Corrigan D et al., (1978) Phytochemistry 17:1131.

Inouye H et al., (1974) Planta Med 25:285.

Further information in:

Hänsel R, Keller K, Rimpler H, Schneider G (Hrsg.), Hagers Handbuch der Pharmazeutischen Praxis, 5. Aufl., Bde 4-6 (Drogen), Springer Verlag Berlin, Heidelberg, New York, 1992-1994.

Hegnauer R, Chemotaxonomie der Pflanzen, Bde 1-11, Birkhäuser Verlag Basel, Boston, Berlin 1962-1997.

Madaus G, Lehrbuch der Biologischen Arzneimittel, Bde 1-3, Nachdruck, Georg Olms Verlag Hildesheim 1979.

Galium Odorata

Woodruff

DESCRIPTION

Medicinal Parts: The medicinal parts are the dried or fresh aerial parts collected during or shortly before the flowering season.

Flower and Fruit: The flowers are in loose terminal cymes. The petals are fused to a funnel-shaped, white, 1.5 mm long tube. The border of the tube is divided in 4 and is 2 to 3.5 mm long. The 4 stamens are fused with the corolla. The involucre bracts are small, lanceolate or almost bristle-like. The 2-seeded indehiscent fruit is globular, 2 to 3 mm long and thickly covered with white barbed bristles.

Leaves, Stem and Root: Woodruff is a 10 to 35 cm herbaceous perennial with a thin cylindrical circular rhizome. The stem is erect, quadrangular, smooth and apart from the bristly nodes, glabrous and glossy. The leaves are in false whorls of 6 to 9, the lower ones are obovate-oblong, the middle and upper ones are lanceolate to oblong-lanceolate. They are entire-margined, thorny tipped, glabrous and rough-edged.

Characteristics: Woodruff is aromatic when dried; the taste is bitter and tangy.

Habitat: The plant grows in northern and central Europe, and Siberian and northern Africa.

Production: Woodruff herb is the fresh or dried aerial part of Galium odoratum. It is gathered during or shortly before flowering, must be turned regularly while being dried.

Not To Be Confused With: Gallium mollugo or Gallium sylvaticum.

Other Names: Master of the Wood, Woodwrad

ACTIONS AND PHARMACOLOGY

COMPOUNDS

Iridoide monoterpenes: asperuloside, monotropein, scandoside in the freshly-harvested plant

O-hydroxycinnamic acidglucoside: melilotosidin of the dried plant

Coumarin

EFFECTS

The coumarin content may impart antiphlogistic, antiedematic, spasmolytic and lymphokinetic properties. However, due to the low level of coumarin, the therapeutic effect is doubtful.

INDICATIONS AND USAGE

Woodruff is occasionally used as a diuretic and as an aid in treating edema. It is generally used for nervous agitation, cardiac irregularity, sleeplessness, hysteria, and nervous menstrual disorders.

PRECAUTIONS AND ADVERSE REACTIONS

The freshly-harvested plant contains melilotoside as glycosidic precursor of coumarins. In the process of dehydration, coumarin is released (content up to 1% coumarin in freshly-dried drug). Health risks or side effects following the proper administration of designated therapeutic dosages are not recorded. Headache and stupor can occur with the administration of higher dosages of the drug. Susceptible patients could experience liver damage following long-term administration. This effect is reversible following discontinuation of the drug. Liver enzyme values should be monitored.

DOSAGE

Mode of Administration: The herb is obsolete as drug in many countries, and since 1981 is not allowed to be used in the manufacture of aroma or flavoring in German speaking countries.

Preparation: To make a tea, place 2 teaspoonfuls (1.8 gm drug) in one glass water.

Daily Dosage: The average single dose is 1.0 gm drug. The tea can be taken during the day or shortly before going to bed.

Storage: The drug should be protected from light sources to avoid brown coloring.

LITERATURE

Anonym, Cumarin (1,2-b-Benzopyron) - Neue Erkenntnisse zur Tumortherapie. In: Med Welt 45(5):62-63. 1994.

Anonym, Leberschäden durch Cumarin? In: DAZ 134(15):1372. 1994.

Berkowitz WF et al., (1982) J Org Chem 47:824.

Böjthe-Horvath K et al., PH 21:2917-2919. 1982.

Burnett AR, Thomsom RH, (1968) J Clin Soc (6):854.

Casley-Smith JR, Casley-Smith JR, Effects of varying doses of 7-hydroxy-coumarin and coumarin in acute lymphoedema and other high-protein oedemas. In: Progress in Lymphology, X, Adelaide, 1985: 194-196. 1985.

Cox D, O'Kennedy R, Thornes RD, The rarity of liver toxicity in patients treated with coumarine (1,2-Benzopyrone). In: Human Toxikol 8:501-506. 1989.

Egan D, O'Kennedy R, Moran E, Cox D, Prosser E, Thornes RD, The pharmacology, metabolism, analysis, and applications of coumarin and coumarin-related compounds. In: Drug Metabolism Reviews 22(5):503-529. 1990.

Ellinger A, Zur pharmako-dynamischen Charakterisierung des Cumarins. In: Schmiedebergs Arch exp Pathol Pharmakol Suppl. Festschrift, S.150-163. 1908.

Fentem JH, Fry JR, Thomas NW, Species differences in the hepatotoxicity of coumarin - a comparision of rat and Mongolian gerbil. In: Toxicology 71(1-2):129. 1992.

Hardt TJ, Ritschel WA, The effect of coumarin and 7-hydroxycoumarin on in vitro macrophage phagocytosis of latex particles. In: Methods Find Exp Clin Pharmacol 5(1):39-43. 1983.

Hausen BM, Schmieder M, The sensitizing capacity of coumarins. In: Contact Dermatitis 15(3):157-163. 1986.

Hazleton LW, Tusing TW, Zeitlin BR, Thiesen R, Murer HK, Toxicity of coumarin. In: J Pharmacol Exp Ther 116:348-358. 1956.

Inouye H et al., (1974) Planta Med 25:285.

Kooiman P, Acta Bot Neerl 18:124-137. 1966.

Laub E, Olszowski W, Woller R, Waldmeister und Maibowle. Pharmazeutisch und lebensmittelchemische Aspekte. In: Dtsch Apoth Ztg 125:848-850. 1985.

Mascolo N et al., (1987) Phytother Res 1 (1):28.

Rosskopf F, Kraus J, Franz G, Immunological and antitumor effects of coumarin and some derivatives. In: PA 47(2):139-142. 1992.

Sporn A, Toxicity of coumarin as a flavoring agent. In: Igenia (Bucharest)9:121-126. 1960.

Sticher O et al., (1971) Dtsch Apoth Ztg 111:1795.

Wüstenberg, P, Baumann G, Verdacht der Toxizität von Cumarin nicht bestätigt. In: PZ 139(13):1058. 1994.

Further information in:

Frohne D, Pfänder HJ: Giftpflanzen - Ein Handbuch für Apotheker, Toxikologen und Biologen, 4. Aufl., Wiss. Verlagsges. mbH Stuttgart 1997.

Hänsel R, Keller K, Rimpler H, Schneider G (Hrsg.), Hagers Handbuch der Pharmazeutischen Praxis, 5. Aufl., Bde 4-6 (Drogen), Springer Verlag Berlin, Heidelberg, New York, 1992-1994.

Leung AY, Encyclopedia of Common Natural Ingredients Used in Food Drugs and Cosmetics, John Wiley & Sons Inc., New York 1980.

Madaus G, Lehrbuch der Biologischen Arzneimittel, Bde 1-3, Nachdruck, Georg Olms Verlag Hildesheim 1979.

Roth L, Daunderer M, Kormann K, Giftpflanzen, Pflanzengifte, 4. Aufl., Ecomed Fachverlag Landsberg Lech 1993.

Steinegger E, Hänsel R, Pharmakognosie, 5. Aufl., Springer Verlag Heidelberg 1992.

Teuscher E, Lindequist U, Biogene Gifte - Biologie, Chemie, Pharmakologie, 2. Aufl., Fischer Verlag Stuttgart 1994.

Teuscher E, Biogene Arzneimittel, 5. Aufl., Wiss. Verlagsges. mbH Stuttgart 1997.

Galium Verum

Lady's Beadstraw

DESCRIPTION

Medicinal Parts: The medicinal part is the herb collected during the flowering season and dried.

Flower and Fruit: The small lemon-yellow flowers are in dense terminal panicles. The peduncle is very downy. The corolla is 2 to 3 mm wide, usually golden yellow and smells strongly of honey. The border of the calyx is pointed and the ovaries are bivalvular and inferior. The fruit is smooth, indehiscent, 1.5 mm long, glabrous, and eventually black.

Leaves, Stem and Root: The true plant is a 30 to 100 cm high herbaceous perennial with a cylindrical, creeping rhizome which spouts runners. The stem is ascending or erect, bluntly quadrangular with 4 vertical lines, downy or glabrous and rough. The leaves are in false whorls of 8 to 12. They are linear, dark green above, and short-haired gray beneath.

Characteristics: The flowers have a strong honey fragrance.

Habitat: The plant grows all over Europe except Lapland and arctic Russia as well as in Asia Minor, Iran, and Syria.

Other Names: Yellow Galium, Cheese Rennet, Curdwort, Maid's Hair, Yellow Cleavers, Petty Mugget, Cheese Renning

ACTIONS AND PHARMACOLOGY

COMPOUNDS

Iridoide monoterpenes: asperuloside, monotropein, scandoside, desacetylasperulosidic acid, asperulosidic acid, ginipo-sidic acid, daphylloside

Rennin

Flavonoids, including rutin, isorutin, palustroside, cynaroside

Anthracene derivatives

Caffeic acid ester: chlorogenic acid

EFFECTS

No information is available.

INDICATIONS AND USAGE

Internally, the drug is used for swollen ankles and as a diuretic for bladder and kidney catarrh. Externally, the drug is used for poorly healing wounds.

The efficacy of this drug has not been proven.

PRECAUTIONS AND ADVERSE REACTIONS

Health risks or side effects following the proper administration of designated therapeutic dosages are not recorded.

DOSAGE

Mode of Administration: Currently obsolete but formerly the drug was used internally as a tea, and topically, in alcoholic extracts.

Preparation: To prepare moist poultices, pour 250 ml of cold water over 2 heaping teaspoonfuls of the drug, bring to simmering point, simmer for 2 minutes, and then allow to draw.

Daily Dosage: Internally, 2 to 3 cups of drug daily. Externally, as a moist poultice.

LITERATURE

Böjthe-Horvath K et al., PH 21:2917-2919. 1982.

Borisov MI et al., Rastit Resur 11:351. 1975.

Burnett AR, Thomsom RH, (1968) J Clin Soc (6):854.

Corrigan D et al., (1978) Phytochemistry 17:1131.

Mathé I et al., (1982) Planta Med 45:158.

Raynaud J, Mnajed H, (1972) C R Acad Sci Paris 274:1746.

Further information in:

Hänsel R, Keller K, Rimpler H, Schneider G (Hrsg.), Hagers Handbuch der Pharmazeutischen Praxis, 5. Aufl., Bde 4-6 (Drogen), Springer Verlag Berlin, Heidelberg, New York, 1992-1994.

Wichtl M (Hrsg.), Teedrogen, 4. Aufl., Wiss. Verlagsges. Stuttgart 1997.

Gamboge

See Garcinia Hanburyi

Garcinia Hanburyi

Gamboge

DESCRIPTION

Medicinal Parts: The medicinal part is the resin extracted from the plant.

Leaves, Stem and Root: The tree grows to about 15 m and has a diameter of about 30 cm. The bark is usually in the form of cylindrical sticks, deep orange-brown and opaque. The transverse fracture should be smooth and conchoidal.

Characteristics: The taste is innocuous at first becoming very acrid. The powder is highly sternutatory.

Habitat: The plant is indigenous to Indochina and Sri Lanka.

Production: Gamboge is the gum-resin from the trunk of Garcinia hanburyi.

Other Names: Camboge, Gutta Cambodia, Gutta Gamba, Gummigutta, Tom Rong, Gambodia

ACTIONS AND PHARMACOLOGY

COMPOUNDS

Resins (70-75%): consisting mainly of yellow or red-colored benzophenones and xanthones, including morellic acid, isomorellic acid, alpha-gambogic acid

Mucilages (25-30%)

EFFECTS

The drug has a strong laxative effect.

INDICATIONS AND USAGE

Gamboge is used for the treatment of digestive disorders, in particular constipation, generally used in combination with other laxatives.

PRECAUTIONS AND ADVERSE REACTIONS

As little as 0.2 gm of the drug can lead to abdominal pain and vomiting.

OVERDOSAGE

Fatalities have been observed with administration of 4 gm.

DOSAGE

Preparation: The ground drug is used.

LITERATURE

Lu GB et al., (1984) Yao Hsueh Husueh Pao 19 (8): 636.

Further information in:

Hegnauer R, Chemotaxonomie der Pflanzen, Bde 1-11, Birkhäuser Verlag Basel, Boston, Berlin 1962-1997.

Kern W, List PH, Hörhammer L (Hrsg.), Hagers Handbuch der Pharmazeutischen Praxis, 4. Aufl., Bde. 1-8, Springer Verlag Berlin, Heidelberg, New York, 1969.

Lewin L, Gifte und Vergiftungen, 6. Aufl., Nachdruck, Haug Verlag, Heidelberg 1992.

Wagner H, Wiesenauer M, Phytotherapie. Phytopharmaka und pflanzliche Homöopathika, Fischer-Verlag, Stuttgart, Jena, New York 1995.

Garden Cress

See Lepidium Sativum

Garden Violet

See Viola Odorata

Garlic

See Allium Sativum

Gaultheria Procumbens

Wintergreen

DESCRIPTION

Medicinal Parts: The medicinal parts are the leaves or the oil extracted from them as well as the fruit.

Flower and Fruit: The 7.5 mm long, solitary, hanging flowers grow from the base of the leaves. They are white or pale pink and campanulate. The fruit is the enlarged calyx. They are scarlet berries, dull red and about 0.5 cm in diameter when dried. They are globular, bilocular, containing numerous whitish, ovoid flattened seeds.

Leaves, Stem and Root: Gaultheria procumbens is an evergreen bushy plant with procumbent stems and upright rigid branches up to 15 cm high which grows preferably under trees and shrubs. The branches bear clusters of leaves at their tips. The leaves are coriaceous, oval, 3 to 5 cm long, glabrous and glossy above, paler beneath, long, and solitary.

Characteristics: Wintergreen has an aromatic odor; the taste of the whole plant is astringent.

Habitat: Indigenous to North America and Canada.

Production: Wintergreen leaves are the dried leaves of Gaultheria procumbens.

Other Names: Canada Tea, Checkerberry, Deerberry, Ground Berry, Hillberry, Mountain Tea, Partridge Berry, Spiceberry, Wax Cluster, Boxberry, Teaberry

ACTIONS AND PHARMACOLOGY

COMPOUNDS: FRESHLY-HARVESTED PLANT

Monotropitoside (Gaultherin): changing over into methyl salicylate when the plant is dried.

COMPOUNDS: DRIED PLANT

Volatile oil: chief components - methyl salicylate (96-98%), additionally, oenanthic alcohol (n-heptan-1-ol) and its ester (which contributes to the odor of the volatile oil)

EFFECTS

The essential oil has a rubefacient effect.

INDICATIONS AND USAGE

Wintergreen was previously used as a carminative, tonic, antiseptic, and aromatic. The drug was also used for neuralgia, particularly sciatica, gastralgias, pleurisy, pleurodynia, especially for medium stage pain, for ovarialgia, orchitis, epidydimitis, diaphragmitis, uratic arthritis, and dysmenorrhea.

In folk medicine, the drug is also considered as effective against asthma and as an antiseptic.

The drug is administered externally in the treatment of rheumatoid arthritis and related conditions.

PRECAUTIONS AND ADVERSE REACTIONS

Health risks or side effects following the proper administration of designated therapeutic dosages are not recorded. The drug and its volatile oil can trigger contact allergies.

OVERDOSAGE

Signs of poisoning appear with overdosage of the drug (severe stomach and kidney irritation). Fatal poisonings can occur through peroral but also through percutaneous administration of the pure volatile oil (signs in the central nervous system, lung edema, collapse). Poisonings with fatal results have been observed following the peroral intake of as little as 4 to 6 gm of the volatile oil.

DOSAGE

The drug is seldom used today. The active ingredient, methyl salicylate, is produced synthetically at a lower cost. Methyl salicylate is a constituent of liniments and bath additives.

LITERATURE

Friedrich H, Krüger, N, (1974) Planta Med 26:327.

Further information in:

Frohne D, Pfänder HJ, Giftpflanzen - Ein Handbuch für Apotheker, Toxikologen und Biologen, 4. Aufl., Wiss. Verlagsges. mbH Stuttgart 1997.

Kern W, List PH, Hörhammer L (Hrsg.), Hagers Handbuch der Pharmazeutischen Praxis, 4. Aufl., Bde. 1-8, Springer Verlag Berlin, Heidelberg, New York, 1969.

Leung AY, Encyclopedia of Common Natural Ingredients Used in Food Drugs and Cosmetics, John Wiley & Sons Inc., New York 1980.

Lewin L, Gifte und Vergiftungen, 6. Aufl., Nachdruck, Haug Verlag, Heidelberg 1992.

Madaus G, Lehrbuch der Biologischen Arzneimittel, Bde 1-3, Nachdruck, Georg Olms Verlag Hildesheim 1979.

Roth L, Daunderer M, Kormann K, Giftpflanzen, Pflanzengifte, 4. Aufl., Ecomed Fachverlag Landsberg Lech 1993.

Steinegger E, Hänsel R, Pharmakognosie, 5. Aufl., Springer Verlag Heidelberg 1992.

Gelidium Amansii

Agar

DESCRIPTION

Medicinal Parts: The medicinal part is the seaweed extract known as Agar.

Flower and Fruit: The perennial seaweed is up to 1 m long. The thallus sprouts from a permanent base every year and is heavily branched. It is cylindrical or flattened, pinnately subdivided and tough. It is brownish white, translucent, and has prickly appendages on the branchings. The fruit is spherical.

Characteristics: Agar is colorless and tasteless and capable of absorbing up to 200 times its volume of water to form a jelly.

Habitat: The plant is indigenous to the Pacific coasts of Japan and China, Sri Lanka and the South African coast.

Production: Agar, or Agar-agar, having been dried out and cut into sutures (threads), is the purified and bleached gel derived from algae mucilage of the Rhodophyceae Gelidium amansii (Lamour). An aqueous extract is obtained from the algae, through autoclaving (pressure-cooking) using overheated steam. It is then left to cool in ice cells into ice-blocks, which are crushed and thawed. Water separates from the gel in the thawing process. The gel mass is dried by warm air.

Other Names: Agar-Agar, Japanese Isinglass

ACTIONS AND PHARMACOLOGY

COMPOUNDS

Heteropolysaccharides: made up of D-galactose- and 3,6-anhydro-L-galactose- components, partially bearing sulfate or pyruvic acid residues, low-sulfate fraction designated agarose

EFFECTS

The drug has a laxative effect due to its ability to swell in the intestine and the resulting expansion stimulus on the intestinal muscles, and it aids peristalsis. The mucilaginous substances cause an increase in the bulk of the content of the intestine and stimulate peristalsis.

INDICATIONS AND USAGE

The drug is used as a mild laxative.

PRECAUTIONS AND ADVERSE REACTIONS

No health hazards or side effects are known in conjunction with the proper administration of designated therapeutic dosages.

DOSAGE

Mode of Administration: The drug is used internally.

Daily Dosage: Laxative: take 1 to 2 teaspoons of the powder with some liquid, fruit, or jam before meals, 1 to 3 times daily.

Never take dry!

Storage: The dried drug can be kept for up to 5 years without being checked, however, once it has been checked it should not be stored for more than 10 years.

LITERATURE

Ataki C, Chem Soc Japan 29:543. 1956.

Franz G (Hrsg.), Polysaccharide. Springer Verlag Berlin, Heidelberg, New York 1991.

Murano E et al., Pyruvate-rich agarose from the red alga Gracilaria dura. In: PM 58(Suppl. 7):A588. 1992.

Schmid OJ, Marina (Hamburg) 1:54. 1959.

Vessal M, Mehrani HA, Omrani GH, Effects of an aqueous extract of Physalis alkekengi fruit on estrus cycle, reproduction and uterine craetive kinase BB-isoenzyme in rats. In: ETH 34(1):69-78. 1991.

Further information in:

Kern W, List PH, Hörhammer L (Hrsg.), Hagers Handbuch der Pharmazeutischen Praxis, 4. Aufl., Bde. 1-8, Springer Verlag Berlin, Heidelberg, New York, 1969.

Steinegger E, Hänsel R, Pharmakognosie, 5. Aufl., Springer Verlag Heidelberg 1992.

Teuscher E, Biogene Arzneimittel, 5. Aufl., Wiss. Verlagsges. Stuttgart 1997.

Gelsemium Sempervirens

Yellow Jessamine

DESCRIPTION

Medicinal Parts: The medicinal part is the dried rhizome with the roots.

Flower and Fruit: Yellow, strongly perfumed, 2.5 to 4 cm, funnel-shaped, long flowers in axillary or terminal cymes of 2 to 5 blooms. The fruit consists of 2 separable, connected pods containing numerous flat-winged seeds.

Leaves, Stem and Root: The plant is a perennial evergreen vine on a tortuous, smooth root with a thin bark and woody center, showing broad, medullary rays. The stem is slender, woody and up to 6 m high. The leaves are opposite, lanceolate to ovate-lanceolate, short-stemmed, entire-margined, 2.5 to 10 cm long, dark green above, and paler beneath.

Habitat: The plant is indigenous to North America, along the coast from Virginia to Florida and Mexico.

Production: Gelsemium root, consisting of the rhizome and roots of Gelsemium sempervirens.

Not To Be Confused With: The plant should not be confused with the yellow flowering Jasmine.

Other Names: Gelsemin, Woodbine, Yellow Jasmine, False Jasmin

ACTIONS AND PHARMACOLOGY

COMPOUNDS

Indole alkaloids: main alkaloid gelsemin, including among others gelsemicin, gelsidin, gelsevirin, sempervirin

Hydroxycoumarins: including scopoletine (gelseminic acid)

EFFECTS

Gelsemium-tincture/liquid extract: vasodilatory, hypotensive, and bronchodilatory. These effects have been documented in animal tests.

INDICATIONS AND USAGE

The drug is used for neuralgia, headache, gastric disorders, nervous stomach, feelings of fullness, and heartburn.

PRECAUTIONS AND ADVERSE REACTIONS

Health risks following the proper administration of designated therapeutic dosages are not recorded. The following side effects could appear: heaviness of the eyelids, inhibition of movement of the eyeball, double vision, hypocyclosis, dryness of the mouth, and vomiting. Particular dangers lie with administration in the presence of cardiac weakness.

OVERDOSAGE

Poisonings through overdosages, sometimes with fatal outcome, are possible (extracts, corresponding to approximately 0.5 gm of the drug can kill a child, 2 to 3 gm an adult). Symptoms of poisoning include headache, dizziness, loss of speech ability, vision weakness or double vision, pupil enlargement, dryness of the mouth, trembling of the limbs, paralysis or stiffening of the muscles, cyanosis, dyspnea, and coma.

The therapy for poisonings, following stomach emptying (gastric lavage with burgundy-colored potassium permanganate solution), consists of prophylaxis for shock, diazepam for spasms, electrolyte replenishment and sodium bicarbonate infusions for any acidosis that may arise. Intubation and oxygen respiration may also be necessary.

DOSAGE

Medicinal preparations are obsolete. Currently used in homeopathic dilutions only.

LITERATURE

Jensen SR et al., (1987) Phytochemistry 26(6):1725.

Wenkert E et al., (1971) Experientia 28:377.

Further information in:

Frohne D, Pfänder HJ, Giftpflanzen - Ein Handbuch für Apotheker, Toxikologen und Biologen, 4. Aufl., Wiss. Verlagsges. mbH Stuttgart 1997.

Kern W, List PH, Hörhammer L (Hrsg.), Hagers Handbuch der Pharmazeutischen Praxis, 4. Aufl., Bde 1-8, Springer Verlag Berlin, Heidelberg, New York, 1969.

Leung AY, Encyclopedia of Common Natural Ingredients Used in Food Drugs and Cosmetics, John Wiley & Sons Inc., New York 1980.

Lewin L, Gifte und Vergiftungen, 6. Aufl., Nachdruck, Haug Verlag, Heidelberg 1992.

Madaus G, Lehrbuch der Biologischen Arzneimittel, Bde 1-3, Nachdruck, Georg Olms Verlag Hildesheim 1979.

Roth L, Daunderer M, Kormann K, Giftpflanzen, Pflanzengifte, 4. Aufl., Ecomed Fachverlag Landsberg Lech 1993.

Wagner H, Wiesenauer M, Phytotherapie. Phytopharmaka und pflanzliche Homöopathika, Fischer-Verlag, Stuttgart, Jena, New York 1995.

Genista Tinctoria

Dyer's Broom

DESCRIPTION

Medicinal Parts: The medicinal part is the whole plant.

Flower and Fruit: The flowers are in short, terminal racemes. They are golden yellow and bean-shaped, 1.5 to 2

cm and are on pedicles, which are shorter than the calyx. The petal stems of the 4 lower petals are initially straight, but in moments of tension, when for instance, they are touched by an insect, they curl down suddenly and the flower opens. The fruit is a smooth pod 2.5 to 3.5 cm long. It is compressed at the sides, brown, and contains 5 to 10 seeds.

Leaves, Stem and Root: The plant is a 30 to 60 cm high, always thornless subshrub with a creeping, woody rhizome. The florescent green stems are smooth and produce fairly rigid, smooth or pubescent forked branches. The leaves are lanceolate alternate, glabrous, entire-margined, 1.25 to 2.5 cm long, nearly sessile, and with a ciliate margin. There are linear-awl-shaped stipules.

Habitat: Found in the Mediterranean region, on the Canaries, in Europe, western Asia, and cultivated elsewhere including the eastern U.S.

Other Names: Dyer's Weed, Dyer's Greenwood, Dyer's Whin, Furze, Green Broom, Greenweed, Wood Waxen

ACTIONS AND PHARMACOLOGY

COMPOUNDS

Quinolizidine alkaloids: main alkaloids - methylcytisine, anagyrine, including, among others, isosparteine, lupanine, tinctorin, cytisine

Flavonoids: in particular luteolin glycosides

Isoflavonoids: genistein, genistin

Lectins

EFFECTS

The drug acts as a purifier, cathartic, diuretic, purgative and emetic. It increases heart rate, strengthens the walls of blood vessels, stimulates kidney blood circulation, and effects metabolism.

INDICATIONS AND USAGE

Formerly, the drug was used as a purgative and to remove bladder stones, as well as for digestive disorders and gout. Once an infusion has been taken, breathing deepens and pain in the lumbar and pelvic region is alleviated.

PRECAUTIONS AND ADVERSE REACTIONS

Health risks or side effects following the proper administration of designated therapeutic dosages are not recorded. Overdosage can lead to diarrhea.

DOSAGE

Mode of Administration: The drug is used internally as an infusion.

Preparations: To prepare an infusion, use 1 teaspoonful of the ground drug per cup of water.

Daily Dosage: Drink 1 to 2 cups of infusion daily.

LITERATURE

Atkinson JE et al., (1969) Tetrahedron 25:1507.

Bricout J, (1974) Phytochemistry 13:2819.

Harborne JB, (1969) Phytochemistry 8:1449.

Hrochova V, Sitaniova H, Farm Obz 51:131. 1982.

Inouye H et al., (1968) Tetrahedron Letters 4429.

Inouye H et al., (1970) Chem Pharm Bull 18:1856.

Lewis JR, Gupta P, (1971) J Chem Soc Chem Comm 4:629.

Rulko F, (1976) Pr Nauk Akád. Med Wroclawin 8:3.

Sadritdinov F, (1971) Farmakol Alkaloidov Serdechnykh Glikozidov 146.

Swietek L, Dombrowicz E, (1984) Farm Pol 40(12):729.

Ulubelen A et al., (1971) Lloydia 34(2):258.

Further information in:

Chan, EH et al. (Eds), Advances in Chinese Medicinal Materials Research, World Scientific Pub. Co. Singapore 1985.

Kern W, List PH, Hörhammer L (Hrsg.), Hagers Handbuch der Pharmazeutischen Praxis, 4. Aufl., Bde. 1-8, Springer Verlag Berlin, Heidelberg, New York, 1969.

Leung AY, Encyclopedia of Common Natural Ingredients Used in Food Drugs and Cosmetics, John Wiley & Sons Inc., New York 1980.

Lewin L, Gifte und Vergiftungen, 6. Aufl., Nachdruck, Haug Verlag, Heidelberg 1992.

Madaus G, Lehrbuch der Biologischen Arzneimittel, Bde 1-3, Nachdruck, Georg Olms Verlag Hildesheim 1979.

Roth L, Daunderer M, Kormann K, Giftpflanzen, Pflanzengifte, 4. Aufl., Ecomed Fachverlag Landsberg Lech 1993.

Teuscher E, Lindequist U, Biogene Gifte - Biologie, Chemie, Pharmakologie, 2. Aufl., Fischer Verlag Stuttgart 1994.

Wichtl M (Hrsg.), Teedrogen, 4. Aufl., Wiss. Verlagsges. Stuttgart 1997.

Gentiana Lutea

Yellow Gentian

DESCRIPTION

Medicinal Parts: The medicinal parts are the dried, underground plant organs or the fresh aerial parts.

Flower and Fruit: The flowers are yellow, terminal, pedicled, in cyme-like false whorls. The calyx is deeply divided in 2. The corolla is rotate and is divided almost to the base into lanceolate tips. There are 5 stamens with 8 mm long anthers and there is 1 superior ovary. The fruit is 6 cm and capsule shaped. The numerous seeds are flat, oblong or round, with a membranous edge.

Leaves, Stem and Root: The plant is perennial, up to 140 cm high and completely glabrous. The rhizome has a number of heads and the top of it can have the thickness of an arm. The main root is a tap root which grows to 1 m. The stem is round, unbranched, hollow and grooved in the upper region to finger thickness. The leaves are elliptical, bluish green, have strongly curved ribs and are up 30 cm long and 15 cm wide.

Characteristics: The drug has a weak sweetish odor, tastes metallic sweet at first then bitter.

Habitat: The plant is indigenous to central and southern European mountainous regions. It is also cultivated in other regions.

Production: The roots are collected from spring into the autumn, cleaned, and swiftly dried; longer drying causes the roots to ferment; roots become brittle through drying, swollen and spongy through contact with moisture.

Not To Be Confused With: The roots of Rumex alpinus or Gentiana asclepiadea.

Other Names: Bitter Root, Bitterwort, Gentian Root, Pale Gentian

ACTIONS AND PHARMACOLOGY

COMPOUNDS

Iridoide monoterpenes (bitter principles): amarogentin (determines the value), gentiopricroside, swertiamarine, sweroside

Sugars: saccharose, gentianose (somewhat bitter), gentiobiose (bitter)

Pyrridine alkaloids

Xanthone derivatives (colored yellow): including gentisin, gentisein, isogentisin, 1,3,7-trimethoxyxanthone

Volatile oil (traces)

EFFECTS

The essential active principles are the bitter substances contained in the herb. These bring about a reflex stimulation of the taste receptors, leading to increased secretion of saliva and the digestive juices. Gentian root is therefore considered to be not simply a pure bitter, but also a roborant and tonic.

INDICATIONS AND USAGE

- Dyspeptic complaints
- Loss of appetite

The drug is used for digestive disorders, such as loss of appetite, fullness, and flatulence.

PRECAUTIONS AND ADVERSE REACTIONS

Health risks or side effects following the proper administration of designated therapeutic dosages are not recorded. The drug's stimulation of gastric juice secretion rules out its administration in the presence of stomach or duodenal ulcers.

DOSAGE

Mode of Administration: Comminuted drug and dried extracts for infusions, bitter-tasting forms of medications for oral administration.

Preparation: Tea is prepared by pouring boiling water over 1/2 tsp. of the drug (1 to 2 gm) and allowing it to steep for 5 to 10 minutes. The tea may be sweetened with honey to alleviate the bitter taste.

Daily Dosage: The average single dose is 1 gm of the drug; daily dose is 2 to 4 gm. The average daily dose of tincture is 1 to 3 gm; liquid extract: 2 to 4 gm; root: 2 to 4 gm.

Storage: The drug must be stored away from light sources.

LITERATURE

Chialva F et al., Z Lebensm Unters Forsch 182:212. 1986.

Hayashi T, Yamagishi T, PH 27:3696. 1988.

Schultze J, Dissertation T.U. München. 1980.

Wagner H, Münzing-Vasirian K, DAZ 115:1233. 1975.

Further information in:

Hänsel R, Keller K, Rimpler H, Schneider G (Hrsg.), Hagers Handbuch der Pharmazeutischen Praxis, 5. Aufl., Bde 4-6 (Drogen), Springer Verlag Berlin, Heidelberg, New York, 1992-1994.

Madaus G, Lehrbuch der Biologischen Arzneimittel, Bde 1-3, Nachdruck, Georg Olms Verlag Hildesheim 1979.

Schulz R, Hänsel R, Rationale Phytotherapie, Springer Verlag Heidelberg 1996.

Steinegger E, Hänsel R, Pharmakognosie, 5. Aufl., Springer Verlag Heidelberg 1992.

Teuscher E, Biogene Arzneimittel, 5. Aufl., Wiss. Verlagsges. mbH Stuttgart 1997.

Wagner H, Wiesenauer M, Phytotherapie. Phytopharmaka und pflanzliche Homöopathika, Fischer-Verlag, Stuttgart, Jena, New York 1995.

Wichtl M (Hrsg.), Teedrogen, 4. Aufl., Wiss. Verlagsges. Stuttgart 1997.

Geranium Robertianum

Herb Robert

DESCRIPTION

Medicinal Parts: The medicinal parts are the dried aerial parts collected during the flowering season, the fresh aerial parts collected during the flowering season, and the whole fresh or dried plant.

Flower and Fruit: The peduncles are usually distinctly longer than the bracts and the 2.2 to 7 mm long, permanently erect pedicles. The flowers are longer than their pedicles. There are 5 separate sepals and 5 petals. The sepals are erect when they are first in bloom and hang when the fruit matures. The petals have long stems. There are 10 stamens, 5 ovaries with long styles, which dissolve in an upward curve when mature. The fruit is circular, 2 cm long and has a 3 mm long protruding, reticulate, upwards horizontally wrinkled, glabrous or pubescent fruit lobes which permanently enclose the smooth, finely spotted seeds. The fruit lobes burst off from the central column without the awn.

Leaves, Stem and Root: Geranium robertianum is a 20 to 40 cm high annual or hardy annual with a weak, branched tap root, and a long hypocotyl. The stems are heavily branched, usually red, and glandular-haired. The leaves are 3 to 5 sectioned compound leaves with petiolate, entire-margined to double pinnasect leaflets.

Characteristics: Herb Robert has an unpleasant smell of goats or bugs.

Habitat: The plant is indigenous to Europe, China, Japan; to Africa southwards as far as Uganda and to the Atlantic North and temperate South America.

Production: The aerial parts are gathered between May and October in uncultivated regions, dried in the open air in the shade.

Not To Be Confused With: As an adulteration, the herbs of Geranium palustre and Geranium pratense are frequently found on the market.

Other Names: Dragon's Blood, Storkbill, Wild Crane's-bill

ACTIONS AND PHARMACOLOGY

COMPOUNDS

Flavonoids: including rutin, quercetin-3-O-rhamnogalactoside, kaempferol-3-O-rhamnoglucoside, hyperoside

Tannins: geraniin, isogeraniin, beta-penta-O-galloylglucose

EFFECTS

The drug has the following effects:

Antiviral: A crystalline fraction derived from the ether extract protects the tobacco plant from particular plant pathogenic viruses. The extract of the fresh herb, including rhizome, has been shown to have a mild antiviral effect against the *vesicular stomatitis virus.* In another study, however, the aqueous solution of the ethanol extract was not shown to have an antiviral effect against the *polio virus Type 1, measles, coxsachie-B2, adeno-* or *Semliki forest virus.*

Antimicrobial: The fraction of an extract produced with 80% ethanol was shown to have an inhibitory effect on the growth of *Escherichia coli, Pseudomonas aeruginosa,* and *Staphylococcus aureus.* In the serial dilution test, growth of *Microsporum canis* and *Trichophyton mentagrophytes* was completely stunted.

Hypotensive effect: Only described in general reviews.

INDICATIONS AND USAGE

The drug is used internally for diarrhea, poor functioning of liver and gallbladder, functional impairment of the liver and gallbladder, inflammatory conditions of gallbladder and its ducts, inflammation of the kidney and bladder, and calculosis.

Externally, it is used as an infusion or decoction to be used as mouthwashes or gargle; the washed, fresh leaves are chewed for inflammation of the oral cavity.

Efficacy has not been sufficiently proven to date.

PRECAUTIONS AND ADVERSE REACTIONS

Health risks or side effects following the proper administration of designated therapeutic dosages are not recorded.

DOSAGE

Mode of Administration: The drug is used internally and as well as externally.

Daily Dosage: Internally, the average single dose of the drug is 1.5 gm; put 1 dessertspoonful into 1/2 liter of cold water. Bring to a boil and leave to draw; drink 2 to 3 cups daily, between meals.

Externally, as an infusion or decoction for mouthwashes or gargles; fresh leaves are chewed to ease inflammation of the oral cavity.

LITERATURE

Haddock EA et al., J Chem Soc Perkin Trans 1:2535-2545. 1982.

Karnig T, Bucar-Stachel J, PM 57:292-293. 1991.

Further information in:

Hänsel R, Keller K, Rimpler H, Schneider G (Hrsg.), Hagers Handbuch der Pharmazeutischen Praxis, 5. Aufl., Bde 4-6 (Drogen), Springer Verlag Berlin, Heidelberg, New York, 1992-1994.

Madaus G, Lehrbuch der Biologischen Arzneimittel, Bde 1-3, Nachdruck, Georg Olms Verlag Hildesheim 1979.

German Ipecac

See Cynanchum Vincetoxicum

German Sarsaparilla

See Carex Arenaria

Germander

See Teucrium Chamaedrys

Geum Rivale

Water Avens

DESCRIPTION

Medicinal Parts: The medicinal parts are the dried, underground parts of the plant, the fresh, flowering plant and the roots.

Flower and Fruit: The flowering peduncle usually sprouts singly from the axils of the rosette leaves, rarely from the ends of the stems. It is often tinged red-brown and is downy. The flowers and subinflorescences are on long, dense and glandular-haired pedicles. The 5 sepals are red-brown. The 5 petals are pale yellow and tinged dirty-pink. The flower remains attached long after flowering. The carpel axis is stemmed, villous, and stretches when mature. The fruit is hooked at the tip.

Leaves, Stem and Root: The plant is a 30 to 100 cm high semi-rosette shrub with the primary root replaced by adventitious roots. The rhizome is simple, thick, cylindrical, and crooked with a terminal rosette. The rosette leaves are long-petioled, irregularly lyre-shaped, and pinnate. The upper surface is glandular and hairy. The underside is heavily ciliated along the veins.

Habitat: The plant is found in Europe, temperate Asia, and North America.

Other Names: Cure All, Water Flower, Indian Chocolate, Chocolate Root, Throat Root, Water Chisch

ACTIONS AND PHARMACOLOGY

COMPOUNDS: IN THE FRESHLY-HARVESTED RHIZOME

Gein (eugenol-vicianose): transformed through drying or size reduction into eugenol

Tannins

COMPOUNDS: IN THE DRIED RHIZOME AND ROOT

Volatile oil (traces): chief components eugenol

EFFECTS

See Geum urbanum, very weak action.

INDICATIONS AND USAGE

Uses are the same in folk medicine as Geum urbanum.

PRECAUTIONS AND ADVERSE REACTIONS

Health risks or side effects following the proper administration of designated therapeutic dosages are not recorded.

DOSAGE

No information is available.

LITERATURE

Hegnauer R, Pharm Weekblad 87:641-646. 1952.

Further information in:

Hänsel R, Keller K, Rimpler H, Schneider G (Hrsg.), Hagers Handbuch der Pharmazeutischen Praxis, 5. Aufl., Bde 4-6 (Drogen). Springer Verlag Berlin, Heidelberg, New York, 1992-1994.

Madaus G, Lehrbuch der Biologischen Arzneimittel, Bde 1-3, Nachdruck, Georg Olms Verlag Hildesheim 1979.

Geum Urbanum

Bennet's Root

DESCRIPTION

Medicinal Parts: The medicinal parts are the dried flowering herb, the dried underground parts, the fresh underground parts, and the roots.

Flower and Fruit: The inflorescence is a loose panicled, umbelled cyme with few flowers. The flowers are terminal and erect. The pedicles are short-haired. The sepals are 3 to 8 cm long with long tips, pubescent on the outside, glabrous on the inside except for a tomentose border. The epicalyx bracts are half as long as the sepals, pubescent on both sides, and narrowly lanceolate. The petals are 3 to 7 mm long, slightly stemmed, and drop easily. The style is jointed and the stigma flat. The small fruit have no stems and are pubescent.

Leaves, Stem and Root: The plant is a semi-rosette shrub with adventitious roots, which die off early and are replaced by primary roots. The rhizome is simple, thick, cylindrical, and crooked. The stem is erect, soft-haired, 15 to 70 cm high, and sprouts from the basal rosette. The basal leaves are rosette-like and pinnate. The cauline leaves are trifoliate to tri-pinnate and the stipules are small, fused with the stem in the lower part, and ovate-lanceolate roughly dentate to pinnatesect.

Characteristics: The root has a scent of cloves.

Habitat: Widespread in central and southern Europe, central Asia, and North America.

Production: Gei urbani herba is the aerial part of Geum urbanum. Gei urbani radix is the root of Geum urbanum.

Other Names: Avens Root, Colewort, Herb Bennet, City Avens, Wild Rye, Way Bennet, Goldy Star, Geum, European Avens, Blessed Herb, Star of the Earth, Yellow Avens

ACTIONS AND PHARMACOLOGY

COMPOUNDS: GEI URBANI HERBA

Tannins

EFFECTS: GEI URBANI HERBA

The drug has an astringent effect.

COMPOUNDS: GEI URBANI RADIX

In the freshly harvested rhizome:

Tannins

Gein (eugenol-vicianose): transformed through drying or size reduction into eugenol

In the dried rhizome and the roots:

Volatile oil (traces): chief components - eugenol, additionally cis- and trans-myrtanal, cis- and trans-myrtanol

EFFECTS: GEI URBANI RADIX

The drug has an astringent effect.

INDICATIONS AND USAGE

The drug is used for digestive complaints and diarrhea.

PRECAUTIONS AND ADVERSE REACTIONS

Health risks or side effects following the proper administration of designated therapeutic dosages are not recorded.

DOSAGE

The herb is rarely used medicinally today. It is found in some pharmaceutical preparations.

LITERATURE

GEI URBANI HERBA

Hänsel R, Keller K, Rimpler H, Schneider G (Hrsg.), Hagers Handbuch der Pharmazeutischen Praxis, 5. Aufl., Bde 4-6 (Drogen), Springer Verlag Berlin, Heidelberg, New York, 1992-1994.

Madaus G, Lehrbuch der Biologischen Arzneimittel, Bde 1-3, Nachdruck, Georg Olms Verlag Hildesheim 1979.

Psenák M et al., (1970) Planta Med 19(2):154.

Vollmann C, Schultze W, Nelkenwurz. In: DAZ 135(14):1238-1248. 1995.

Vollmann C, Untersuchung der Nelkenwurz. In: DAZ 131(40):2081. 1991.

GEI URBANI RADIX

Psenák M et al., (1970) Planta Med 19(2):154.

Vollmann C, Schultze W, Nelkenwurz. In: DAZ 135(14):1238-1248. 1995.

Vollmann C, Untersuchung der Nelkenwurz. In: DAZ 131(40):2081. 1991.

Further information in:

Hänsel R, Keller K, Rimpler H, Schneider G (Hrsg.), Hagers Handbuch der Pharmazeutischen Praxis, 5. Aufl., Bde 4-6 (Drogen), Springer Verlag Berlin, Heidelberg, New York, 1992-1994.

Madaus G, Lehrbuch der Biologischen Arzneimittel, Bde 1-3, Nachdruck, Georg Olms Verlag Hildesheim 1979.

Wichtl M (Hrsg.), Teedrogen, 4. Aufl., Wiss. Verlagsges. Stuttgart 1997.

Gillenia Trifoliata

Indian Physic

DESCRIPTION

Medicinal Parts: The medicinal part is the dried and pulverized root bark.

Flower and Fruit: The flowers are white and tinged with red. They are arranged in a few loose, terminal panicles.

Leaves, Stem and Root: The plant is a perennial herb. The irregular, cylindrical roots are usually transversely grooved and up to 15 cm long. The external surface is blackish, and the transverse section shows a thick, reddish bark, which easily separates from the white woody center. A number of stems sprout from the root, which are 60 to 90 cm high and have very long and thin fibers. The leaves and leaflets have various forms.

Characteristics: The taste is pleasantly bitter; it is odorless.

Habitat: The plant is indigenous to eastern U.S. cultivated in Europe and elsewhere.

Other Names: Indian Hippo, Bowman's Root, American Ipecacuanha, Gillenia

ACTIONS AND PHARMACOLOGY

COMPOUNDS

Resins

Gillein (Gillenin)

The constituents of the drug have not been fully investigated.

EFFECTS

The drug is an expectorant, emetic, and a ''blood purifier.''

INDICATIONS AND USAGE

The drug is used in the treatment of digestive disorders and in all cases where an emetic is required.

PRECAUTIONS AND ADVERSE REACTIONS

Health risks or side effects following the proper administration of designated therapeutic dosages are not recorded.

DOSAGE

Mode of Administration: The drug is available as a powder, an infusion, or as a tonic.

LITERATURE

Kern W, List PH, Hörhammer L (Hrsg.), Hagers Handbuch der Pharmazeutischen Praxis, 4. Aufl., Bde 1-8, Springer Verlag Berlin, Heidelberg, New York, 1969.

Ginger

See Zingiber Officinale

Ginkgo Biloba

Ginkgo

DESCRIPTION

Medicinal Parts: The medicinal parts are the dried leaves, the seeds separated from their fleshy outer layer, and the fresh leaves.

Flower and Fruit: The tree flowers for the first time when it is between 20 to 30 years old. The flowers are dioecious. They are in the axils of the lower leaves of the annual growth short shoots. The male flowering parts are attached to short catkins. The female flowers have longer pedicles and are at the end of a leafless branch. Fertilization occurs months after pollination by spermatozoids, although usually only one ovule is fully formed. The seeds, incorrectly called fruit, later become fleshy and plum-like round, light green or yellow. They have a diameter of 2.5 to 3 cm and contain a two-edged edible nut. They smell like butyric, capric, or valeric acid when ripe.

Leaves, Stem and Root: Ginkgo biloba is a 30 to 40 m high dioecious tree with a girth of about 4 m. The trees can live for hundreds of years. The bark is light to dark brown with rough grooves and reticulate fissures. The leaves are fan-shaped with bifurcated ribs and glabrous. They are fresh green to golden yellow in autumn. The female trees are pointed and pyramid-shaped; the male trees are broad and sparer.

Habitat: Indigenous to China, Japan, and Korea.

Production: A dry extract from the dried leaf of Ginkgo biloba is manufactured using acetone/water and subsequent purification steps without addition of concentrates or isolated ingredients.

Other Names: Maidenhair-Tree

ACTIONS AND PHARMACOLOGY

COMPOUNDS

Flavonoids: including monosides, biosides and triosides of quercetin, isorhamnetins, 3′-O- methylmyristicins, kaempferol, to some extent estered with p-cumaric acid

Biflavonoides: for example amentoflavone, bilobetin, 5-methoxybilobetin, ginkgetin, isoginkgetin

Proanthocyanidins

Trilactonic diterpenes: ginkgolide A, B, C

Trilactonic sesquiterpene: bilabolide

EFFECTS

Inhibition of the development of traumatically or toxically induced cerebral edema and acceleration of its regression; reduction of retinal edema and of cellular lesions in the retina; inhibition in age-related reduction of muscarinergic cholinoceptors as well as stimulation of choline uptake in the hippocampus.

Clinical double-blind studies have been carried out for both standard preparations. In animal experiment, improvement of hypoxic tolerance, improvement of glucose utilization, membrane stabilizing, and reduction of blood viscosity have been noted.

INDICATIONS AND USAGE

- Organic brain dysfunction, symptomatic relief of
- Intermittent claudication
- Vertigo (vascular origin)
- Tinnitus (vascular origin)

The Commission E approvals listed are limited to special standard extracts of Ginkgo.

The drug is used for disturbed brain functions, which result in dizziness, tinnitus, and headache with emotional lability and anxiety. Ginkgo has also been demonstrated to improve concentration and memory deficits as a result of peripheral arterial occlusive disease.

CONTRAINDICATIONS

The drug is contraindicated in patients known to be hypersensitive to Ginkgo biloba preparations.

PRECAUTIONS AND ADVERSE REACTIONS

General: Health risks or side effects following the proper administration of designated therapeutic dosages are not recorded. Mild gastrointestinal complaints could occur as side effects. Allergic skin reactions have been observed on extremely rare occasions. The possible hypersensitivity reactions are: occurrence of spasms and cramps and, in cases of acute toxicity, atonia and adynamia.

Drug Interactions: The ginkgolide B component has a potent inhibitory effect on the platelet-activating factor (PAF) by displacing PAF from receptor binding sites. For this reason, extracts of Ginkgo biloba have the potential to interact with antithrombotic therapy.

DOSAGE

Mode of Administration: Ginkgo is available in liquid or solid pharmaceutical forms, for oral intake.

Daily Dosage: The average daily dose is 120 mg of dried extract in 2 or 3 doses orally (in clinical studies up to 240 mg were used as a daily dose); parenteral daily dose is 50 to 100 mg of the drug.

In traditional Chinese medicine, the daily dose is 3 to 6 gm of leaves as an infusion.

Storage: Ginkgo must be protected from light and moisture.

LITERATURE

American Psychiatric Association (Ed.), DSM-IV. Diagnostic and Statistical Manual of Mental Disorders, 4th Ed. R. R. Donnelly & Sons Company 1994.

Amling R, Phytotherapeutika in der Neurologie. In: ZPT 12(1):9. 1991.

Anonym, Ginkgo und Crataegus. In: DAZ 137(20):1751-1753. 1997.

Anonym, Phytopharmaka für ältere Menschen: Ginkgo, Kava, Hypericum und Crataegus. In: DAZ 135(5):400-402. 1995.

Anonym, Psycho-Phytos: Ginkgo, Johanniskraut und Kava-Kava. In: DAZ 135(18):1632-1634. 1995.

Bach D, Behandlung der benignen Prostatahypertrophie. In: ZPT 17(4):209-218. 1996.

Bauer R, Zschocke S, Medizinische Anwendung von Ginkgo biloba Geschichtliche Entwicklung. In: ZPT 17(5):275-283. 1996.

Beske F, Kunczik T, (1991) Frühzeitige Therapie kann Milliarden sparen. Der Kassenarzt 42:36-42.

Blaha L, (1989) Differentialdiagnose der zerebralen Insuffizienz in der Praxis. Geriatrie und Rehabilitation 2,1:23-28.

Braquet P (Ed.), Ginkgolides. Chemistry, Biology, Pharmacology and Clinical Perspectives. Vol I. JR Prous Science, Barcelona 1988.

Braquet P (Ed.), Ginkgolides. Chemistry, Biology, Pharmacology and Clinical Perspectives. Vol II, JR Prous Science, Barcelona 1989.

Brüchert E, Heinrich SE, Ruf-Kohler P, (1991) Wirksamkeit von LI 1370 bei älteren Patienten mit Hirnleistungsschwäche. Münch Med Wschr 133(Suppl 1):9-14.

Bundesgesundheitsamt, (1991) Empfehlungen zum Wirksamkeitsnachweis von Nootropika im Indikationsbereich ''Demenz'' (Phase III). Bundesgesundheitsblatt 7:342-350.

Burkard G, Lehrl S, (1991) Verhältnis von Demenzen vom Multiinfarkt- und vom Alzheimertyp in ärztlichen Praxen. Münch Med Wschr 133(Supp. 1):38-43.

Caesar W, Alles über Ginkgo. In: DAZ 134(44):4363. 1994.

Della Loggia R, Sosa S, Tubaro A, Bombardelli E, Anti-inflammatory activity of Ginkgo biloba flavonoids. In: PM 59(7):A588. 1992.

Deutsches Institut für medizinische Dokumentation und Information (Hrsg.), ICD-10. Internationale und statistische Klassifikation der Krankheiten und verwandter Gesundheitsprobleme. 10. Revision. Bd 1. Urban & Schwarzenberg, München Wien Baltimore 1994.

Dfeudis FV, Ginkgo biloba extract (EGb 761): Pharmacological activities and clinical applications. In: Elsevier Editions Scientifiques Paris. 1991.

Dingermann T, Phytopharmaka im Alter: Crataegus, Ginkgo, Hypericum und Kava- Kava. In: PZ 140(23):2017-2024. 1995.

Dorn M, Bräunig B, Gross HD, Ginkgo-Dragees bei zerebraler Leistungsschwäche. In: ZPT 12(6):180. 1991.

Ermini-Fünfschilling D, (1992) Möglichkeiten und Grenzen eines Gedächtnistrainings mit Patienten bei beginnender Demenz. Z Moderne Geriatrie 12:459-456.

Gräßel E, (1989) Vergleich zweier Personengruppen bezüglich der Auswirkungen des mentalen Trainings (''Gehirn-Jogging'') auf die Selbsteinschätzung der Leistungsfähigkeit in Abhängigkeit von der Trainingszeit (Tageszeit der Trainingsdurchführung). Geriatrie & Rehabilitation 2,1:44-46.

Hartmann A, Schulz V (Hrsg.), (1991) Ginkgo biloba, Aktuelle Forschungsergebnisse 1990/91. Münch Med Wschr 133:1-64.

Hopfenmüller W, (1994) Nachweis der therapeutischen Wirksamkeit eines Ginkgo biloba-Spezialextraktes. Metaanalyse von 11 klinischen Studien bei Patienten mit Hirnleistungsstörungen im Alter Arzneim Forsch/Drug Res 44:1005-1013.

Israel L, Dell'Accio E, Martin G, Hugonot R, (1987) Extrait de Ginkgo biloba et exerciçes d'entra nement de la memoire. Evaluation comparative chez personnes (gées ambulatoiRes Psychologie Médicinale 19(8):1431-1439.

Joyeux M et al., Comparative antilipoperoxidant, antinecrotic and scavenging properties of terpenes and biflavones from Ginkgo and some flavonoids. In: PM 61(2):126-129. 1995.

Kanowski S, (1991) Klinischer Wirksamkeitsnachweis bei Nootropika. Münch Med Wschr 133:5-8.

Kanowski S, Herrmann WM, Stephan K, Wierich W, Hörr R, (1995) Proof of efficacy of the ginkgo biloba special extract Egb 761 in outpatients suffering from primary degenerative dementia of the Alzheimer type and multi-infarct dementia. Pharmacopsychiatry 4:149-158

Kleijnen J, Knipschild P, (1992a) Ginkgo biloba for cerebral insufficiency. Br J Clin Pharmac 35:352-358.

Kleijnen J, Knipschild P, (1992b) Ginkgo biloba. Lancet, 1136-1139.

Koalik F et al., (1992) Kombinierte Anwendung von nootroper Therapie und kognitivem Training bei chronischen organischen Psychosyndromen. Neuropsychiatrie 6:47-52.

Krieglstein J, Neuroprotective properties of Ginkgo biloba-constituents. In: ZPT 15(2):92-96. 1994.

Kurz A, Ginkgo biloba bei Demenzerkrankungen. In: Loew D, Rietbrock N (Hrsg.), Phytopharmaka. Steinkopff Verlag, Darmstadt 1995, S 145-149.

Nieder M, (1991) Pharmakokinetik der Ginkgo-Flavonole im Plasma. Münch Med Wschr 133:61-62.

Oberpichler-Schwenk H, Krieglstein J, (1992) Pharmakologische Wirkungen von Ginkgo-biloba-Extrakt und -Inhaltsstoffen. Pharmazie in unserer Zeit 21:224-235.

Pfister-Hotz G, Phytotherapie in der Geriatrie. In: ZPT 18(3):165-162. 1997.

Riederer P, Laux G, Pöldinger W (Hrsg.), Neuropsychopharmaka. Band 5: Parkinsonmittel und Nootropika. Springer Verlag, Wien Noew York 1992, S. 161-324.

Rosenblatt M, Mindel J, Spontaneous bilateral hyphema associated with ingestion of ginkgo biloba extract. N Engl J Med, April 10, 1997:1108.

Rupalla K, Oberpichler-Schwenk H, Krieglstein J, Neuroprotektive Wirkungen des Ginkgo-biloba-Extrakts und seiner Inhaltsstofe. In: Loew D, Rietbrock N (Hrsg.) Phytopharmaka in Forschung und klinischer Anwendung. Steinkopff Verlag, Darmstadt 1995, S 17-27.

Schilcher H, Ginkgo biloba L. In: ZPT 9(4):119. 1988.

Schmid M, Schmoll H (Hrsg.), Ginkgo. Wissenschaftliche Verlagsgesellschaft mbH Stuttgart 1994.

Schmid B, In: Schmid, Schmoll gen. Eisenwert: Ginkgo, Ur-Baum und Arzneipflanze, Mythos, Dichtung und Kunst. 1994.

Schwabe U, Paffrath D (Hrsg.), Arzneiverordnungsreport '95. Gustav Fischer Verlag, Stuttgart Jena 1995, S 214-224, 373-374.

Sowers S, Weary PE, Collins OD, Cnoley EP, Ginkgo tree dermatitis. In: Arch Dermatol 81:452-456. 1965.

Spegg H, Ginkgo biloba - ein Baum aus Urzeiten, ein Phytopharmakon mit Zukunft. In: PTA 4(12):576. 1990.

Sprecher E, Pflanzliche Geriatrika. In: ZPT 9(2):40. 1988.

Sticher O, (1993) Ginkgo biloba - Ein modernes pflanzliches Arzneimittel. Vierteljahresschrift der Naturforschenden Gesellschaft in Zürich 138/3:125-168.

Sticher O, Hasler A, Meier B, Ginkgo biloba - Eine Standortbestimmung. In: DAZ 131(36):1827. 1991.

Sticher O, Quality of Ginkgo preparations. In: PM 59(1):2-11. 1993.

Vesper J, Hänsgen KD, (1994) Efficacy of Ginkgo biloba in 90 Outpatients with Cerebral Insufficiency Caused by Old Age. Phytomedicine 1:9-16.

Volz HP, Hänsel R, (1994) Ginkgo biloba - Grundlagen und Anwendung in der Psychiatrie. Psychopharmakotherapie 1:70-76.

Volz HP, Hänsel R, (1994) Kava-Kava und Kavain in der Psychopharmakotherapie. Psychopharmakotherapie 1:33-39.

Vorberg G, Schenk N, Schmidt U, (1989) Wirksamkeit eines neuen Ginkgo-biloba- Extraktes bei 100 Patienten mit zerebraler Insuffizien. Z Herz + Gefäße 9:396-401.

Wichtl M, Pflanzliche Geriatrika. In: DAZ 132(30):1576. 1992.

Woerdenberg HJ, Van Beek T.A. Ginkgo biloba. In: DeSmet PAGM, Keller K, Hansel R, Chandler RF, ed. Adverse Effects of Herbal Drugs. Springer-Verlag Berlin Heidelberg 1997; 3:51-66.

Further information in:

Hänsel R, Keller K, Rimpler H, Schneider G (Hrsg.), Hagers Handbuch der Pharmazeutischen Praxis, 5. Aufl., Bde 4-6 (Drogen), Springer Verlag Berlin, Heidelberg, New York, 1992-1994.

Madaus G, Lehrbuch der Biologischen Arzneimittel, Bde 1-3, Nachdruck, Georg Olms Verlag Hildesheim 1979.

Schulz R, Hänsel R, Rationale Phytotherapie, Springer Verlag Heidelberg 1996.

Steinegger E, Hänsel R, Pharmakognosie, 5. Aufl., Springer Verlag Heidelberg 1992.

Tang W, Eisenbrand G, Chinese Drugs of Plant Origin, Springer Verlag Heidelberg 1992.

Teuscher E, Biogene Arzneimittel, 5. Aufl., Wiss. Verlagsges. mbH Stuttgart 1997.

Wagner H, Wiesenauer M, Phytotherapie. Phytopharmaka und pflanzliche Homöopathika, Fischer-Verlag, Stuttgart, Jena, New York 1995.

Wichtl M (Hrsg.), Teedrogen, 4. Aufl., Wiss. Verlagsges. Stuttgart 1997.

Ginseng

See Panax Ginseng

Glechoma Hederacea

Ground Ivy

DESCRIPTION

Medicinal Parts: The medicinal parts are the herb collected during the flowering season and dried, the fresh aerial parts collected during the flowering season, and the whole plant.

Flower and Fruit: The flowers are in 2 to 6 blossomed false whorls in the axils of the foliage leaves. The individual flowers are 1 to 2 cm long with distinct pedicles and with short, 1 to 1.5 mm long bracteoles. The calyx is bilabiate, tubular, and has 5 tips. The corolla is 15 to 22 mm long, bilabiate, blue-violet, occasionally red-violet or white. The fruit is a nut of about 2 mm.

Leaves, Stem and Root: The plant is a perennial herb 15 to 60 cm high, with a creeping main stem, which roots at the lower nodes and keeps its leaves in winter. The stem is quadrangular up to 2 mm thick and often tinged with blue-violet as are the petioles. The leaves are crossed opposite, long-petioled, reniform to broadly cordate, crenate, and dark green above and paler green beneath.

Characteristics: The plant has a mild unpleasant smell; taste is hot and bitter.

Habitat: Ground Ivy is a common wild plant in Europe.

Production: The plant is air-dried in the shade, in order to keep loss of the essential oil to a minimum.

Other Names: Alehoof, Gill-go-over-the-Ground, Lizzy-run-up-the-Hedge, Gill-go-by-the-Hedge, Robin-run-in-the-Hedge, Catsfoot, Hedgemaids, Tun-hoof, Haymaids, Turnhoof, Creeping Charlie, Cat's-paw

ACTIONS AND PHARMACOLOGY

COMPOUNDS

Volatile oil (traces): chief components (-)-pinocarvone, (-)-menthone, (+)-pulegone

Sesquiterpenes: glechomafuran, glechomanolide

Hydroxy fatty acid: 9-hydroxy-10-trans, 12-cis-octadeca-diendic acid

Caffeic acid derivatives: rosmaric acid

Flavonoids: including cymaroside, cosmosyin, hypersoside

EFFECTS

The drug is said to be an anti-inflammatory, which is believed to be due to the tripterpen content.

No detailed information is available.

INDICATIONS AND USAGE

In folk medicine, the drug is used for gastrointestinal catarrh and diarrhea. Ground Ivy is also used for mild respiratory complaints of the upper bronchia; in the symptomatic treatment of coughs, and as a diuretic in cases of bladder and kidney stones. Externally, the drug is used for the treatment of poorly healing wounds, ulcers, and other skin diseases.

In Chinese medicine, it is used to treat irregular menstruation. In Italy, it is used for arthritis and rheumatism. Efficacy has not, however, been documented.

PRECAUTIONS AND ADVERSE REACTIONS

Health risks or side effects following the proper administration of designated therapeutic dosages are not recorded. Fatal poisonings were observed among horses following intake of large quantities of the fresh plant. Mice who were fed solely on the plant died after 3 to 4 days.

DOSAGE

Mode of Administration: The drug is used internally as well as externally.

Preparations: The liquid extract (1:1) is prepared by using 25% ethanol.

Daily Dosage: The normal single daily dose of the dried drug is 2 to 4 gm internally; externally, crushed leaves are placed on the affected areas.

Storage: Keep away from light.

LITERATURE

Barberan FAT, (1986) Fitoterapia 57(2):67.

Bohinc P, Korbar-Smid J, Cicerov-Cergol M, Über die kardiotonischen Substanzen des Gnadenkrautes - Gratiola officinalis. In: Sci Pharm 47:108-113. 1979.

Mascolo N et al., (1987) Phytother Res 1(1):28.

Further information in:

Hänsel R, Keller K, Rimpler H, Schneider G (Hrsg.), Hagers Handbuch der Pharmazeutischen Praxis, 5. Aufl., Bde 4-6 (Drogen), Springer Verlag Berlin, Heidelberg, New York, 1992-1994.

Lewin L, Gifte und Vergiftungen, 6. Aufl., Nachdruck, Haug Verlag, Heidelberg 1992.

Madaus G, Lehrbuch der Biologischen Arzneimittel, Bde 1-3, Nachdruck, Georg Olms Verlag Hildesheim 1979.

Roth L, Daunderer M, Kormann K, Giftpflanzen, Pflanzengifte, 4. Aufl., Ecomed Fachverlag Landsberg Lech 1993.

Globe Flower

See Trollius Europaeus

Glycine Soja

Soybean

DESCRIPTION

Medicinal Parts: The medicinal parts are the soya lecithin extracted from the soya bean, the soya oil, and the soya seed.

Flower and Fruit: The flowers are small, inconspicuous, short pedicled, upright, axillary, and in 3 to 8 blossomed clusters. The sepals are campanulate or tubular-campanulate and somewhat bilabiate. The corolla is usually purple, exceeding the calyx only slightly or not at all. The stamens are diadelphous or monodelphous. The style is glabrous. The pod is linear or oblong and constricted between the seeds. The pod is septate and dehiscent. There are 2 to 4 seeds, which are oblong-ovate, white, yellow or black-brown.

Leaves, Stem and Root: The soya plant is an erect or twining annual bushy plant. The stem and leaves are thickly villous. The leaves are trifoliate, the leaflets are large, ovate, entire-margined, and, particularly on the margins and on the ribs of the lower surface, pubescent.

Habitat: The soya plant is indigenous to east Asia but has never been found in the wild. The wild form Glycine soya is found in the Amur-Ussuri delta, northern China, Taiwan, Korea and Japan.

Production: Lecithin is extracted from glycine enriched soybean extract with 73 to 79% 3-sn-phosphatidylcholine. Also present are phosphatidylethanolamine (maximum 7%), phosphatidylinositic acid (<0.5%), oil (2 - 6%), vitamine (0.2 to 0.5%). The range given includes production and analytical variances.

ACTIONS AND PHARMACOLOGY

COMPOUNDS

Phospholipids (45-60%): in particular phosphatidylcholine, phosphatidylethanolamine, phosphatidylinositol

Fatty oil (30-35%)

EFFECTS

Phospholipids are degraded to lyso-phosphatidylcholine in the intestine and absorbed primarily in this form. In the gut wall, phospholipids are in part re-synthesized, then circulated through the lymphatic system. In part the resynthesized phosphatidylcholine is processed in the liver to form fatty acids, choline, and glycerine-3-phosphate. In plasma, phosphatidylcholine and other phosphoglycerides are tightly bound to lipoproteins and/or albumin.

INDICATIONS AND USAGE

■ Raised levels of cholesterol

Soybean is used for less severe forms of hypercholesterolemia, improvement of subjective complaints, such as loss of appetite and feeling of pressure in the liver, in toxic/nutritional liver disease and chronic hepatitis.

PRECAUTIONS AND ADVERSE REACTIONS

No health hazards or side effects are known in conjunction with the proper administration of designated therapeutic dosages. Side effects include occasional gastrointestinal effects, such as stomach pain, loose stool, and diarrhea.

DOSAGE

Mode of Administration: Preparations for oral administration.

Daily Dosage: The average daily dose is 1.5 to 3.5 gm of phospholipids from Soyabean with 73 to 79% 3-sn-phosphatidylcholine in a single dose.

LITERATURE

Hänsel R, Keller K, Rimpler H, Schneider G (Hrsg.), Hagers Handbuch der Pharmazeutischen Praxis, 5. Aufl., Bde 4-6 (Drogen): Springer Verlag Berlin, Heidelberg, New York, 1992-1994 (unter Glycine).

Steinegger E, Hänsel R: Pharmakognosie, 5. Aufl., Springer Verlag Heidelberg 1992.

Teuscher E, Biogene Arzneimittel, 5. Aufl., Wiss. Verlagsges. Stuttgart 1997.

Glycyrrhiza Glabra

Licorice

DESCRIPTION

Medicinal Parts: The medicinal parts are the unpeeled, dried roots and the runners, the dried roots, and the rhizome with the roots.

Flower and Fruit: The inflorescences are axillary. They are upright, spike-like and 10 to 15 cm long. The individual flowers are 1 to 1.5 cm long, bluish to pale violet and short-pedicled. The calyx is short-campanulate and glandular-haired. The tips of the calyx are longer than the tube, and are pointed lanceolate. The petals are narrow, the carina petals are not fused, and they are pointed but not beaked. The fruit is a pod, 1.5 to 2.5 cm long, and 4 to 6 mm wide. It is erect and splayed, flat with thick sutures, glabrous, somewhat reticulate-pitted, and usually has 3 to 5 brown, reniform seeds.

Leaves, Stem and Root: The plant is a herbaceous perennial. It is 1 to 2 m high on a long sturdy primary taproot. The taproot is 15 cm long and subdivides into 3 to 5 subsidiary roots, 1.25 m in length, and several horizontal woody stolons which may reach 8 m. New stems are produced every year. They are sturdy, erect, branched either from the base or from further up, and are generally rough at the top. The foliage leaves are alternate, odd pinnate and 10 to 20 cm long. The leaflets are in 3 to 8 pairs. The stipules are very small and drooping.

Habitat: The individual varieties are found in different regions. Glycyrrhiza glanulifera is found in southeastern Europe and western Asia. Glycyrrhiza pallida and violocea are found in Iraq. Glycyrrhiza tyica is indigenous to southern Europe and southwest Asia.

Production: Licorice root consists of the peeled and un-peeled, dried roots and stolons of Glycyrrhiza glabra. Licorice juice is the extract of Glycyrrhiza glabra.

Other Names: Sweet Root

ACTIONS AND PHARMACOLOGY

COMPOUNDS: LIQUIRITIAE RADIX

Triterpene saponins (3-15%): chief components are glycyrrhetic acid (sweet-tasting, aglycone 18 beta-glycyrrhetic acid, salts termed glycyrrhetic)

Flavonoids: aglycones including, among others, liquiritigenin, isoliquiritigenin (its chalcone), isolicoflavonol

Isoflavonoids: aglycones formononetin, glabrene, glabridin, glabrol, 3-hydroxyglabrol, glycyrrhisoflavone

Cumestan derivatives: glycyrol, isoglycyrol, liqcoumarin

Hydroxycoumarins: including, among others, herniarin, umbelliferone, glycycoumarin, licopyranocumarin

Sterols: including, among others, beta-sitosterol, stigmasterol

Volatile oil (very little 0.05%): with anethole, estragole, eugenol, hexanoic acid

EFFECTS: LIQUIRITIAE RADIX

According to controlled clinical studies, glycyrrhizic acid and the aglycone of glycyrrhizic acid accelerate the healing of gastric ulcers. Secretolytic and expectorant effects have been confirmed in tests on rabbits. In the isolated rabbit ileum, an antispasmodic action has been observed at concentrations of 1:2500 to 1:5000.

COMPOUNDS: LIQUIRITIAE SUCCUS

Triterpene saponins: (according to DAB 1996, 4-6 % in the adjusted liquorice extract, according to DAC 1995, 5-7% in the dry liquorice extract): chief components glycyrrhetic acid (sweet-tasting, aglycone 18beta-glycyrrhetic acid, salts termed glycyrrhetic)

Flavonoids: aglycones including, among others, liquiritigenin, isoliquiritigenin (its chalcone), isolicoflavonol

Isoflavonoids: aglycones formononetin, glabren, glabridin, glabrol, 3-hydroxyglabrol, glycyrrhisoflavone

Cumestan derivatives: glycyrol, isoglycyrol, liquocoumarin

Hydroxycoumarins: including, among others, herniarin, umbelliferone, glycycumarin, licopyranocumarin

Sterols: including, among others, beta-sitosterol, stigmasterol

The drug contains considerably more free flavonoid and isoflavonoid aglycones than the rhizome drug does, due to the hydrolysis that takes place during the extraction procedure.

EFFECTS: LIQUIRITIAE SUCCUS

The drug is an expectorant. It is also antiphlogistic, which accounts for its effectiveness in treating gastritis and gastric ulcers and its use in ulcer prophylaxis (a mineral corticoidal effect). Glycyrrhizine acid is used in the treatment of viral liver inflammation (also post-hepatital liver cirrhosis). The juice may work as an antiviral agent by means of interferon induction.

INDICATIONS AND USAGE

LIQUIRITIAE RADIX

- Cough/bronchitis
- Gastritis

The drug is used for catarrh of the upper respiratory tract as well as for gastric/duodenal ulcers.

LIQUIRITIAE SUCCUS

The drug is used for gastritis, gastric (stomach) ulcers, ulcer prophylaxis, and viral liver inflammation.

CONTRAINDICATIONS

LIQUIRITIAE RADIX AND SUCCUS

Contraindications include chronic hepatitis, cholestatic diseases of the liver, cirrhosis of the liver, severe renal insufficiency, hypertonia, hypokalemia, and pregnancy.

PRECAUTIONS AND ADVERSE REACTIONS

LIQUIRITIAE RADIX

General: No health hazards or side effects are known in conjunction with the proper administration of designated therapeutic dosages.

Drug Interactions: Potassium loss occurs due to other drugs, e.g., thiazide diuretics; with potassium loss, sensitivity to digitalis glycosides increases.

LIQUIRITIAE SUCCUS

General: No health hazards or side effects are known in conjunction with the proper administration of designated therapeutic dosages.

Drug Interactions: Due to the intervention of glycyrrhetine acid in the metabolism of corticosteroids, the half-life of cortisol is prolonged. This leads to symptoms such as hypokalemia, high blood pressure and edema.

OVERDOSAGE

LIQUIRITIAE RADIX

The intake of higher dosages (above 50 gm per day) over an extended period of time will lead to hypernatremia, edema, hypertension and cardiac complaints. In rare cases, myoglobinemia, due to the aldosterone-like effect of the saponins has been seen. Preparations from the drug should for that reason not be administered for longer than 6 weeks. The complaints disappear after discontinuing the drug.

LIQUIRITIAE SUCCUS

The intake of higher dosages (above 50 gm per day) over an extended period of time will lead to hypokalemia, hypernatremia, edemas, hypertension, and cardiac complaints, in rare cases to myoglobinemia, due to the mineralcorticomimetische (aldosterone-like) effect of the saponins.

Preparations from the drug should for that reason not be administered for longer than 6 weeks. This sort of poisoning occurs in particular through unrestrainted consumption of liquorices (containing 5 to 30% liquorice extract). The complaints disappear after discontinuing the drug.

DOSAGE

LIQUIRITIAE RADIX

Mode of Administration: Comminuted drug, drug powder, dry extracts for infusions, decoctions, liquid or solid forms for internal use. Various teas contain extracts of the drug, for example, bronchial teas, gastric teas, and laxative teas.

The drug should not be administered for more than 6 weeks (see side effects).

Preparation: To prepare an infusion, use 1 to 1.5 gm of finely comminuted drug and put in cold water. Bring to a boil, or pour the boiling water over the drug and allow to draw for 10 to 15 minutes and then strain (1 teaspoonful = 3 gm drug).

Daily Dosage: The average daily dose is 5 to 15 gm of the root, equivalent to 200 to 600 mg of glycyrrhizin; succus liquiritiae, 0.5 to 1 gm for catarrhs of the upper respiratory tract, 1.5 to 3.0 gm for gastric/duodenal ulcers.

LIQUIRITIAE SUCCUS

Mode of Administration: The drug is widely available in medicinal preparations or as tea or in drop form; the juice of liquorice is found in liquorice edible goods and preparations.

Preparation: For preparation of tea, pour a cup of boiling water over 1 teaspoon of juice, leave to draw for 5 minutes.

Daily Dosage: Drink one cup of tea after each meal. The dosage for the drop form is 25 drops to be taken 4 times daily.

LITERATURE

LIQUIRITIAE RADIX

Aikawa Y, Yoshiike T, Ogawa H, Effect of glycyrrhizin pain and HLA-DR antigen expression on CD8-positive cells in peripheral blood of herpes zoster patients in comparsion with other antiviral agents. In: Skin Pharmacol 3:268-271. 1990.

Amagaya S et al., J Pharmacobiodynamics 7 (12):923.

Anderson J, Smith WG, (1961) The antitussive activity of glycyrrhetinic acid and its derivatives. J Pharm Pharmacol 13:396-404.

Baba M, Shigeta S, Antiviral activity of glycyrrhizin against varicella-zoster virus in vitro. In: Antiviral Res 7:99-106. 1987.

Bardhan KD et al., (1978) Gut 19:779.

Bhardwaj DK et al., (1977) Phytochemistry 15:352.

Bhardwaj DK et al., (1977) Phytochemistry 16:401.

Bhardwaj DK, Singh R, (1977) Curr Sci 46:753.

Christensen SB et al., An antileishmanial chalcone from chinese licorice roots. In: PM 60(2):121. 1994.

Epstein MT et al., (1977) Brit Med J 19:488.

Fintelmann V, Moderne Phytotherapie am Beispiel gastroenterologischer Erkrankungen. In: ZPT 11(5):161. 1990.

Hattori T, Ikematsu Sh, Koito A, Matsushita Sh, Maeda Y, Hada M, Fujimaki M, Takatsuki K, Preliminary evidence for inhibitory effects of glycyrrhizin on HIV replication in patients with AIDS. In: Antiviral Res 11:255-262. 1989.

Hayashi H et al., Distribution patterns of saponine in different organs of Glycyrrhiza glabra. In: PM 59(4):351. 1993.

Hayashi Y et al., (1979) Yakuri to Chiryo 7:3861.

Inoue H, Saito K, Koshihara Y, Murota S, (1986) Inhibitory effect of glyzyrrhetinic acid derivatives of lipoxygenase and prostaglandin synthetase. Chem Pharm Bull 34:897.

Ito M, Nakashima H, Baba M, Pauwels R, De Clercq E, Shigeta S, Yamamoto N, Inhibitory effect of glycyrrhizin on the in vitro infectivity and cytopathic activity of the human immunodeficiency virus (HIV (HTLV-III/LAV). In: Antiviral Res 7:127-137. 1987.

Khaksa G et al., Anti-inflammatory and anti-nociceptive activity of disodium glycyrrhetinic acid hemiphthalate. In: PM 62(4):326-328. 1996.

Killacky J et al., (1976) Planta Med 30:310.

Kinoshita T et al., (1978) Chem Pharm Bull 26: 141 et 135.

Kiso Y et al., (1984) Planta Med 50:298.

Kumagai A, Takata M, (1978) Proc Symp Wakan-Yaku 11:73.

Miething H, Speicher-Brinker A, Hänsel R, Hochdruckflüssigchromatographische Untersuchungen der Flavonoidfraktion in Süβholzwurzeln und deren pharmazeutischen Zubereitungen. In: PZW 135(6)253. 1990.

Neilsen I, Pedersen RS, (1984) Lancet 1: 8389.

Nose M et al., A comparision of the antihepatotoxic activity between glycyrrhizin and glycerrhetinic acid. In: PM 60(2):136. 1994.

Numuzaki K, Umetsu M, Chiba S, Effects of glycyrrhizin in children with liver dysfunction assiciated with cytomegalovirus infections. In: Tohoku J Exp Med 172:147-153. 1994.

Rees WDW et al., (1979) Scand. J Gastroenterol. 14:605.

Saitoh T et al., (1976) Chem Pharm Bull 24:991.

Saitoh T et al., (1978) Chem Pharm Bull 26:752.

Saitoh T et al., (1976) Chem Pharm Bull 24:752 et 1242.

Segal R et al., (1985) J Pharm Sci 74 (1):79.

Suzuki H, Ohta Y, Takino T, Fujisawa K, Hirayama C, Effect of glycyrrhizin on biochemical test in patients with chronic hepatitis. Double blind trial. In: Asian Med J 26:423-438. 1983.

Takechi M, Tanaka Y, Structure-activity relationships of the synthetic methyl glycyrrhetate glycosides. In: PH 32:1173. 1993.

Tamura Y, Nishikawa T, Yamada K, Yamamoto M, Kumagai A, (1979) Effects of glyzyrrhetinic acid and ist derivatives on Delta5-reductase in rat liver. Arzneimittel Forsch/Drug Res 29: 647.

Tanaka S et al., (1987) Planta Med 53 (1):5.

Van Hulle C, (1970) Pharmazie 25:620.

Veit M, Wirkungen der Glycyrrhetinsäure auf den Steroidstoffwechsel. In: ZPT 14(1):43. 1993.

Watanabe Y, Watanabe K, (1980) Proc Symp Wakan-Yaku 13:16.

Yagura T et al., (1978) Proc Symp Wakan-Yaku 11:79.

Yamamura Y, Kawakami J, Santa T, Kotaki H, Uchino K, Sawada Y, Tanaka N, Iga T, Pharmacokinetic profile of glycyrrhizin in healthy volunteers by a new high-performance liquid chromatographic method. In: J Pharm Sci 81(10):1042-1046. 1992.

Further information in:

Chang EH et al., (Eds), Advances in Chinese Medicinal Materials Research, World Scientific Pub. Co. Singapore 1985.

Frohne D, Pfänder HJ, Giftpflanzen - Ein Handbuch für Apotheker, Toxikologen und Biologen, 4. Aufl., Wiss. Verlags-Ges Stuttgart 1997.

Hänsel R, Keller K, Rimpler H, Schneider G (Hrsg.), Hagers Handbuch der Pharmazeutischen Praxis, 5. Aufl., Bde 4-6 (Drogen): Springer Verlag Berlin, Heidelberg, New York, 1992-1994.

Hikino H, Economic and Medicinal Plant Research, Vol I., Academic Press UK 1985.

Leung AY, Encyclopedia of Common Natural Ingredients Used in Food Drugs and Cosmetics, John Wiley & Sons Inc., New York 1980.

Madaus G, Lehrbuch der Biologischen Arzneimittel, Bde 1-3, Nachdruck, Georg Olms Verlag Hildesheim 1979.

Roth L, Daunderer M, Kormann K, Giftpflanzen, Pflanzengifte, 4. Aufl., Ecomed Fachverlag Landsberg Lech 1993.

Schulz R, Hänsel R, Rationale Phytotherapie, Springer Verlag Heidelberg 1996.

Steinegger E, Hänsel R, Pharmakognosie, 5. Aufl., Springer Verlag Heidelberg 1992.

Tang W, Eisenbrand G, Chinese Drugs of Plant Origin, Springer Verlag Heidelberg 1992.

Teuscher E, Lindequist U, Biogene Gifte - Biologie, Chemie, Pharmakologie, 2. Aufl., Fischer Verlag Stuttgart 1994.

Wagner H, Wiesenauer M, Phytotherapie. Phytopharmaka und pflanzliche Homöopathika, Fischer-Verlag, Stuttgart, Jena, New York 1995.

Wichtl M (Hrsg.), Teedrogen, 4. Aufl., Wiss. Verlagsges. Stuttgart 1997.

LIQUIRITIAE SUCCUS

Aikawa Y, Yoshiike T, Ogawa H, Effect of glycyrrhizin pain and HLA-DR antigen expression on CD8-positive cells in peripheral blood of herpes zoster patients in comparsion with other antiviral agents. In: Skin Pharmacol 3:268-271. 1990.

Amagaya S et al., J Pharmacobiodynamics 7 (12):923.

Anderson J, Smith WG, (1961) The antitussive activity of glycyrrhetinic acid and its derivatives. J Pharm Pharmacol 13:396-404.

Baba M, Shigeta S, Antiviral activity of glycyrrhizin against varicella-zoster virus in vitro. In: Antiviral Res 7:99-106. 1987.

Bardhan KD et al., (1978) Gut 19:779.

Bhardwaj DK et al., (1977) Phytochemistry 15:352.

Bhardwaj DK et al., (1977) Phytochemistry 16:401.

Bhardwaj DK, Singh R (1977) Curr Sci 46:753.

Christensen SB et al., An antileishmanial chalcone from chinese licorice roots. In: PM 60(2):121. 1994.

Epstein MT et al., (1977) Brit Med J 19:488.

Fintelmann V, Moderne Phytotherapie am Beispiel gastroenterologischer Erkrankungen. In: ZPT 11(5):161. 1990.

Hattori T, Ikematsu Sh, Koito A, Matsushita Sh, Maeda Y, Hada M, Fujimaki M, Takatsuki K, Preliminary evidence for inhibitory effects of glycyrrhizin on HIV replication in patients with AIDS. In: Antiviral Res 11:255-262. 1989.

Hayashi H et al., Distribution patterns of saponine in different organs of Glycyrrhiza glabra. In: PM 59(4):351. 1993.

Hayashi Y et al., (1979) Yakuri to Chiryo 7:3861.

Inoue H, Saito K, Koshihara Y, Murota S (1986) Inhibitory effect of glyzyrrhetinic acid derivatives of lipoxygenase and prostaglandin synthetase. Chem Pharm Bull 34:897.

Ito M, Nakashima H, Baba M, Pauwels R, De Clercq E, Shigeta S, Yamamoto N, Inhibitory effect of glycyrrhizin on the in vitro infectivity and cytopathic activity of the human immunodeficiency virus HIV (HTLV-III/LAV). In: Antiviral Res 7:127-137. 1987.

Khaksa G et al., Anti-inflammatory and anti-nociceptive activity of disodium glycyrrhetinic acid hemiphthalate. In: PM 62(4):326-328. 1996.

Killacky J et al., (1976) Planta Med 30:310.

Kinoshita T et al., (1978) Chem Pharm Bull 26:141 et 135.

Kiso Y et al., (1984) Planta Med 50:298.

Kumagai A, Takata M, (1978) Proc Symp. Wakan-Yaku 11:73.

Miething H, Speicher-Brinker A, Hänsel R, Hochdruckflüssigchromatographische Untersuchungen der Flavonoidfraktion in Süβholzwurzeln und deren pharmazeutischen Zubereitungen. In: PZW 135(6)253. 1990.

Neilsen I, Pedersen RS, (1984) Lancet 1:8389.

Nose M et al., A comparision of the antihepatotoxic activity between glycyrrhizin and glycerrhetinic acid. In: PM 60(2):136. 1994.

Numuzaki K, Umetsu M, Chiba S, Effects of glycyrrhizin in children with liver dysfunction assiciated with cytomegalovirus infections. In: Tohoku J Exp Med 172:147-153. 1994.

Rees WDW et al., (1979) Scand. J Gastroenterol. 14:605.

Saitoh T et al., (1976) Chem Pharm Bull 24:991.

Saitoh T et al., (1978) Chem Pharm Bull 26:752.

Saitoh T et al., (1976) Chem Pharm Bull 24:752 et 1242.

Segal R et al., (1985) J Pharm Sci 74 (1):79.

Suzuki H, Ohta Y, Takino T, Fujisawa K, Hirayama C, Effect of glycyrrhizin on biochemical test in patients with chronic hepatitis. Double blind trial. In: Asian Med J 26:423-438. 1983.

Takechi M, Tanaka Y, Structure-activity relationships of the synthetic methyl glycyrrhetate glycosides. In: PH 32:1173. 1993.

Tamura Y, Nishikawa T, Yamada K, Yamamoto M, Kumagai A, (1979) Effects of glyzyrrhetinic acid and ist derivatives on Delta5-reductase in rat liver. Arzneimittel Forsch/Drug Res 29:647.

Tanaka S et al., (1987) Planta Med 53 (1):5.

Van Hulle C, (1970) Pharmazie 25:620.

Veit M, Wirkungen der Glycyrrhetinsäure auf den Steroidstoffwechsel. In: ZPT 14(1):43. 1993.

Watanabe Y, Watanabe K (1980) Proc Symp Wakan-Yaku 13:16.

Yagura T et al., (1978) Proc Symp Wakan-Yaku 11:79.

Yamamura Y, Kawakami J, Santa T, Kotaki H, Uchino K, Sawada Y, Tanaka N, Iga T, Pharmacokinetic profile of glycyrrhizin in healthy volunteers by a new high-performance liquid chromatographic method. In: J Pharm Sci 81(10):1042-1046. 1992.

Further information in:

Chang EH et al., (Eds), Advances in Chinese Medicinal Materials Research, World Scientific Pub. Co. Singapore 1985.

Frohne D, Pfänder HJ, Giftpflanzen - Ein Handbuch für Apotheker, Toxikologen und Biologen, 4. Aufl., Wiss. Verlags-Ges Stuttgart 1997.

Hänsel R, Keller K, Rimpler H, Schneider G (Hrsg.), Hagers Handbuch der Pharmazeutischen Praxis, 5. Aufl., Bde 4-6 (Drogen): Springer Verlag Berlin, Heidelberg, New York, 1992-1994.

Hikino H, Economic and Medicinal Plant Research, Vol I., Academic Press UK 1985.

Leung AY, Encyclopedia of Common Natural Ingredients Used in Food Drugs and Cosmetics, John Wiley & Sons Inc., New York 1980.

Madaus G, Lehrbuch der Biologischen Arzneimittel, Bde 1-3, Nachdruck, Georg Olms Verlag Hildesheim 1979.

Roth L, Daunderer M, Kormann K, Giftpflanzen, Pflanzengifte, 4 Aufl., Ecomed Fachverlag Landsberg Lech 1993.

Schulz R, Hänsel R, Rationale Phytotherapie, Springer Verlag Heidelberg 1996.

Steinegger E, Hänsel R, Pharmakognosie, 5. Aufl., Springer Verlag Heidelberg 1992.

Tang W, Eisenbrand G, Chinese Drugs of Plant Origin, Springer Verlag Heidelberg 1992.

Teuscher E, Lindequist U, Biogene Gifte - Biologie, Chemie, Pharmakologie, 2. Aufl., Fischer Verlag Stuttgart 1994.

Wagner H, Wiesenauer M, Phytotherapie. Phytopharmaka und pflanzliche Homöopathika, Fischer-Verlag, Stuttgart, Jena, New York 1995.

Wichtl M (Hrsg.), Teedrogen, 4. Aufl., Wiss. Verlagsges. Stuttgart 1997.

Gnaphalium Uliginosum

Cudweed

DESCRIPTION

Medicinal Parts: The medicinal parts are the aerial parts of the plant.

Flower and Fruit: The composite flower heads are 3 to 4 by 5 mm, sessile, in terminal racemes of 3 to 10. They are shorter than the leaves growing from the leaf axil. The involucral bracts are oblong to linear and brownish. There are 50 to 150 female florets, 5 to 8 hermaphrodite florets. The achaene is 0.5 mm, oblong-cylindrical. The pappus is 1.5 mm.

Leaves, Stem and Root: The stems are 5 to 20 cm high and branched. The leaves are 10 to 50 mm by 2 to 5 mm, linear, and lanceolate to oblong-obovate. They are downy and greenish above, and whitish more downy beneath.

Habitat: The plant is found in many parts of Europe, in the Caucasus, and west Asia. It has been introduced into America.

Production: Cudweed is the aerial part of Gnaphalium uglinosum.

Other Names: Cotton Weed, Dysentery Weed, Everlasting, Mouse Ear, Wartwort, Cotton Dawes

ACTIONS AND PHARMACOLOGY

COMPOUNDS

Volatile oil

Tannins

The constituents of the drug have been investigated minimally.

EFFECTS

Cudweed is an astringent and a stomachic. According to unconfirmed sources, the drug also has antidepressive, aphrodisiac, and hypotensive effects.

INDICATIONS AND USAGE

The drug is used as a gargle and rinse in the treatment of diseases of the mouth and throat.

PRECAUTIONS AND ADVERSE REACTIONS

Health risks or side effects following the proper administration of designated therapeutic dosages are not recorded.

LITERATURE

Shcheptoin BM et al., (1984) Vrach Delo 6:18.

Further information in:

Kern W, List PH, Hörhammer L (Hrsg.), Hagers Handbuch der Pharmazeutischen Praxis, 4. Aufl., Bde. 1-8, Springer Verlag Berlin, Heidelberg, New York, 1969.

Goa Powder

See Andira Araroba

Goat's Rue

See Galega Officinalis

Golden Rod

See Solidago Species

Golden Seal

See Hydrastis Canadensis

Goldthread

See Coptis Trifolia

Gossypium Herbaceum

Cotton

DESCRIPTION

Medicinal Parts: The medicinal parts are the fresh, inner root bark, the root bark, and the seeds.

Flower and Fruit: The flowers are yellow and have a dark red spot at the base of the petals. The calyx is 2 to 2.5 cm long. The bracts are broadly deltate-ovate to semicircular, usually at least as wide as long. The margins have acute or shortly acuminate teeth, usually less than 3 times as long as wide. The fruit is short-beaked 2 to 3.5 cm, subglobose, up to 18 mm long and has 3 to 4 chambers. The seeds which are embedded in the hairs are square and gray-haired.

Leaves, Stem and Root: Gossypium herbaceum is an evergreen shrub 2 m high and 1 to 1.5 m wide. The few branches are sparse-haired and foliated. The leaves are broadly cordate, coriaceous, reticulate, pubescent with undulate margins, short tip, and a narrow base.

Habitat: The variety is indigenous to Asia and Africa. Mainly cultivated today in Egypt, China, India, Anatolia, and the southern U.S.

Other Names: Cotton Root

ACTIONS AND PHARMACOLOGY

COMPOUNDS

Volatile oil (traces): including with beta-bisabolol

Resinous substance: containing, among others, salicylic acid and 2,3-dihydroxybenzoic acid

Dimeric sesquiterpenes: (+)-gossypol, (+) -gossypol, in some breeds p-hemigossypol (presumably in very low quantities)

The drug has not been investigated in recent times.

EFFECTS

A histamine releasing effect has been observed in vitro, in the lung tissue of pigs. The drug also has emmenagogic, oxytocic, and contraceptive (male) effects.

INDICATIONS AND USAGE

The drug has many indications: amenorrhea, dysmenorrhea, irregular menstruation, nausea, fever, headache, diarrhea and dysentery; as an oxytoxic, to expel the afterbirth, for urethritis, nerve inflammation, poor lactation, metrorrhagia, hemorrhage, menorrhagia and atonic amenorrhea, painful menstruation, climateric complaints; it is used in China as a male contraceptive.

PRECAUTIONS AND ADVERSE REACTIONS

Health risks or side effects following the proper administration of designated therapeutic dosages are not recorded. Numerous poisonings, some of them fatal, have been observed following long-term feeding of animals with large quantities of cotton-seed press cakes.

DOSAGE

Mode of Administration: The drug is used as a decoction, liquid extract, and tincture, as well as in combination with secale, hydrastis, chaemaelirium, and leonurus.

Preparations: Tincture and liquid extract of 2 to 4 ml, liquid extract 20 to 40 drops per single dose.

Daily Dosage: The standard single dose of the drug to be taken internally is 2 or 10 gm of 20% decoction, i.e. 1 tsp. for a single dose decoction. The dosage of the liquid extract administered during labor is a single dose of 1 to 2 level teaspoonfuls; 1 to 2 level teaspoonfuls are given 2 to 4 times daily as a post-natal styptic.

LITERATURE

Dai RX et al., (1978) Acta Biol Exp Sinica 11:27.

Dorsett PH et al., (1975) J Pharm Sci 64:1073.

Hamasaki Y, Tae HH, (1985) Biochim Biophys Acta 843(1):37.

Liu ZQ et al., In: Recent Advances in Fertility Regulation. Beijing 1980, Eds. C. C. Fen et al. Pub. S. A. Atar, Geneva 1981.

Qian SZ et al., (1980) Chin Med J 93:477.

Stipanovic RD et al., (1975) Phytochemistry 14:1077.

Further information in:

Hänsel R, Keller K, Rimpler H, Schneider G (Hrsg.), Hagers Handbuch der Pharmazeutischen Praxis, 5. Aufl., Bde 4-6 (Drogen), Springer Verlag Berlin, Heidelberg, New York, 1992-1994.

Hausen B, Allergiepflanzen, Pflanzenallergene, ecomed Verlagsgesellsch. mbH, Landsberg 1988.

Lewin L, Gifte und Vergiftungen, 6. Aufl., Nachdruck, Haug Verlag, Heidelberg 1992.

Madaus G, Lehrbuch der Biologischen Arzneimittel, Bde 1-3, Nachdruck, Georg Olms Verlag Hildesheim 1979.

Oliver-Bever B (Ed.), Medicinal Plants of Tropical West Africa, Cambridge University Press Cambridge, London 1986.

Roth L, Daunderer M, Kormann K, Giftpflanzen, Pflanzengifte, 4. Aufl., Ecomed Fachverlag Landsberg Lech 1993.

Teuscher E, Lindequist U, Biogene Gifte - Biologie, Chemie, Pharmakologie, 2. Aufl., Fischer Verlag Stuttgart 1994.

Gotu Kola

See Centella Asiatica

Goutweed

See Aegopodium Podagraria

Grains of Paradise

See Aframomum Melegueta

Grape

See Vitis Vinifera

Gratiola Officinalis

Hedge-Hyssop

DESCRIPTION

Medicinal Parts: The medicinal parts are the herb and roots. In contrast to what its name suggests, Hedge Hyssop is not a member of the Hyssop family, but the bitter taste is rather similar.

Flower and Fruit: The flowers are arranged singly in the axils of the upper leaf pair. They are pale-reddish or yellowish-white and pedicled. The calyx is only fused at the base and has 5 tips. The corolla has a distinct tube and a bilabiate border. The upper lip is margined and the lower lip is divided into 3. There are 4 stamens, 2 sterile and 2 fertile. There is 1 superior ovary. The fruit has 4 lids, which burst open.

Leaves, Stem and Root: The plant is a perennial up to 15 to 30 cm high. The stem grows from a creeping scaly rhizome, is erect, glabrous and quadrangular higher up. The leaves are opposite, lanceolate, weakly serrate, smooth and pale green.

Characteristics: It has a bitter taste and is poisonous.

Habitat: The herb is indigenous to southern Europe.

Production: Hedge-Hyssop is the herb, which is harvested shortly before flowering, of Gratiola officinalis. The upper portion of the stem is mown and then dried in thin layers, in the shade, at temperatures not exceeding 45°C.

Other Names: Gratiola

ACTIONS AND PHARMACOLOGY

COMPOUNDS

Cucurbitacins: gratiogenin, 16-hydroxygratiogenin, cucurbitacins E, I, the glycosides gratiogenin-3beta-D-glucoside, gratioside (gratiolin, gratiogenindiglucoside), elaterinide, desacetylelaterinide

Saponins

Lignans

Flavonoids

EFFECTS

The glycosides are said to be cardiotonic. The drug is a strong purgative; it eliminates intestinal parasites and increases micturation.

INDICATIONS AND USAGE

The herb was formerly used as a purgative and for treating the liver. In folk medicine, it is used as purgative and emetic. The drug is only to be taken under medical supervision of a doctor.

PRECAUTIONS AND ADVERSE REACTIONS

Health risks or side effects following the proper administration of designated therapeutic dosages are not recorded. The drug is extremely poisonous. It is irritating to mucous membranes due to the cucurbitacin glycosides and cucurbitacin content, out of which cucurbitacins are released in watery environments.

OVERDOSAGE

The intake of toxic dosages leads to vomiting, bloody diarrhea, colic, kidney irritation and initially to elevated diuresis then to anuria. Very high dosages lead to spasm, paralysis and circulatory collapse. Fatalities are seen only rarely. Following gastric lavage, the treatment for poisonings should proceed symptomatically.

DOSAGE

Mode of Administration: It is most effective in alcoholic extracts, otherwise, it is used in infusions or in homeopathic dilutions. Today, it is rarely used in folk medicine.

LITERATURE

Bohinc P, Korbar-Smid J, Cicerov-Cergol M, Über die kardiotonischen Substanzen des Gnadenkrautes - Gratiola officinalis. In: Sci Pharm 47:108-113. 1979.

Müller A, Wichtl M, Herzwirsamkeit des Gnadenkrautes (Gratiola officinalis). In: Pharm Ztg 124(37):1761-1766. 1979.

Further information in:

Kern W, List PH, Hörhammer L (Hrsg.), Hagers Handbuch der Pharmazeutischen Praxis, 4. Aufl., Bde. 1-8, Springer Verlag Berlin, Heidelberg, New York, 1969.

Lewin L, Gifte und Vergiftungen, 6. Aufl., Nachdruck, Haug Verlag, Heidelberg 1992.

Madaus G, Lehrbuch der Biologischen Arzneimittel, Bde 1-3, Nachdruck, Georg Olms Verlag Hildesheim 1979.

Roth L, Daunderer M, Kormann K, Giftpflanzen, Pflanzengifte, 4. Aufl., Ecomed Fachverlag Landsberg Lech 1993.

Teuscher E, Lindequist U, Biogene Gifte - Biologie, Chemie, Pharmakologie, 2. Aufl., Fischer Verlag Stuttgart 1994.

Great Burnet

See Sanguisorba Officinalis

Greater Bindweed

See Calystegia Sepium

Green Tea

See Camellia Sinensis

Grindelia Camporum

Gumweed

DESCRIPTION

Medicinal Parts: The medicinal parts are the flowering branches.

Flower and Fruit: There are a number of individual composite heads with a diameter of 2 to 3 cm at the end of leafy stems. There are 3 to 8 involucral bracts 0.5 to 1 mm, with cylindrical, squarrose-deflected apex, very viscid. The ligules are 7 to 15 mm, yellow to orange-yellow, sometimes absent. The inner florets are yellow. The achaenes are 2 to 3 mm, oblong, and brown. The 2 to 8 pappus-awns are 3 to 5 mm long and usually finely serrulate.

Leaves, Stem and Root: The plant is an erect biennial or perennial herb or small bush up to 1 m high, often branched above. The alternate leaves are 3 to 7 cm long, triangular to ovate-oblong, clasping, resinous-punctate, serrate-crenate or entire-margined and light green. They break off easily when dry.

Habitat: Southwest U.S. and Mexico.

Production: Gumweed herb consists of the dried tops and leaves of Grindelia robusta and/or Grindelia squarrosa gathered during flowering season.

Other Names: August Flower, Grindelia, Rosin Weed, Tar Weed

ACTIONS AND PHARMACOLOGY

COMPOUNDS

Diterpene acids: grindelic acid, hydroxygrindelic acid, 6-oxogrindelic acid. 7alpha,8alpha-epoxygrindelic acid

Volatile oil: including, among others, borneol

Polyynes: including matricarianol, matricarianolacetate

Saponins

Tannins

EFFECTS

Antibacterial effects have been demonstrated in vitro.

INDICATIONS AND USAGE

- Cough
- Bronchitis

Gumweed is also used for catarrh of the upper respiratory tract.

PRECAUTIONS AND ADVERSE REACTIONS

Health risks following the proper administration of designated therapeutic dosages are not recorded. Side effects listed in older scientific literature (Lewin) include gastric irritation and diarrhea. Large dosages are said to have a poisonous effect.

DOSAGE

Mode of Administration: Comminuted herb for teas and other galenic preparations for internal use.

Preparation: The tincture is prepared in a 1:10 or 1:5 concentration with 60%-80% ethanol (v/v).

Daily Dosage: The recommended dosage is as follows: 4 to 6 gm of drug can be taken or 3 to 6 gm Grindelia liquid extract. If using the tincture, the dosage is 1.5 to 3 ml.

LITERATURE

Mascolo, N et al., (1987) Phytother Res 1(1):28.

Schimmer O, Egersdörfer S, Grindelia-Arten - Die Grindelie. In: ZPT 9(3):86. 1988.

Timmermann B et al., (1985) Phytochemistry 24(5):1031.

Further information in:

Hegnauer R, Chemotaxonomie der Pflanzen, Bde 1-11, Birkhäuser Verlag Basel, Boston, Berlin 1962-1997.

Kern W, List PH, Hörhammer L (Hrsg.), Hagers Handbuch der Pharmazeutischen Praxis, 4. Aufl., Bde. 1-8, Springer Verlag Berlin, Heidelberg, New York, 1969.

Lewin L, Gifte und Vergiftungen, 6. Aufl., Nachdruck, Haug Verlag, Heidelberg 1992.

Madaus G, Lehrbuch der Biologischen Arzneimittel, Bde 1-3, Nachdruck, Georg Olms Verlag Hildesheim 1979.

Wagner H, Wiesenauer M, Phytotherapie. Phytopharmaka und pflanzliche Homöopathika, Fischer-Verlag, Stuttgart, Jena, New York 1995.

Ground Ivy

See Glechoma Hederacea

Ground Pine

See Ajuga Chamaepitys

Groundsel

See Senecio Vulgaris

Guaiac

See Guaiacum Officinale

Guaiacum Officinale

Guaiac

DESCRIPTION

Medicinal Parts: The medicinal parts are the wood and the various preparations of the resin of the heartwood. The resin is used more in medicine than the wood.

Flower and Fruit: The pale blue star-shaped flowers are in false umbels with 6 to 10 blooms that have 2 cm long pedicles. There are 5 sepals and 5 petals. There are 10 stamens and a bilocular ovary. The fruit is a bilocular, cordate capsule compressed at the side containing a seed in each chamber, which is hard and long.

Leaves, Stem and Root: Guaiacum officinale is an evergreen tree up to 13 m high that has a greenish-brown, almost always twisted trunk with furrowed bark. The heartwood is greenish brown, heavier than water and has an aromatic taste. The opposite leaves are short-petioled, coriaceous, di- to tri-pinnate. The leaflets are ovate or oblong, obtuse and entire-margined.

Characteristics: The shavings turn green on exposure to the air and blue-green in the presence of nitrogen.

Habitat: The plant grows in Florida, on the Antilles, in Guayana, Venezuela and Columbia. It is closely related to Guaiacum sanctum which grows in the Bahamas and southern Florida.

Production: Guaiac wood consists of the heartwood and sapwood of Guaiacum officinale and/or Guaiacum sanctum.

Other Names: Guaiacum, Lignum Vitae, Pockwood

ACTION AND PHARMACOLOGY

COMPOUNDS

Triterpene saponins: aglycone oleanolic acid

Resin: containing, among others, the lignans (-)-guajaretic acid, dihydroguajaretic acid, guajacin

Isoguajacin: alpha-guajaconic acid, tetrofuroguajacine A and B

Volatile oil: chief components sesquiterpene alcohols; such as guajole with steam distillate changing over into guajazulene

EFFECTS

Guaiacum officinale is fungistatic.

INDICATIONS AND USAGE

■ Rheumatism

Guaiac is used as supportive therapy for rheumatic complaints. In folk medicine, it is used for respiratory complaints, skin disorders and syphilis.

PRECAUTIONS AND ADVERSE REACTIONS

Health risks or side effects following the proper administration of designated therapeutic dosages are not recorded. High dosages of the drug can lead to diarrhea, gastroenteritis and intestinal colic. Skin rashes have also been observed following intake of the drug.

DOSAGE

Mode of Administration: Guaiacum officinale is used as an additive to mouth washes to retard bacterial growth. The comminuted wood is used for decoctions and other galenic preparations for internal use. The essential oil, known as guaiac wood oil, must be evaluated separately.

Preparation: To make an infusion, use 1.5 gm drug in 1 cup cold water (150ml). Slowly bring to a boil and strain after 15 minutes.

Daily Dosage: The average daily dose is 4 to 5 gm drug. When using a tincture (Guajaci Ligni Tinctura), 20 to 40 drops make a single dose.

LITERATURE

Ahmad VU, Bano N, Bano S, PH 23:2612-2616. 1984.

Ahmad VU, Bano N, Bano S, PH 25:951-952. 1986.

King FE, Wilson JG, (1964) J Chem Soc:4011-4024.

King FE, Wilson JG, J Chem Soc:1572-1580. 1965.

Kratochvil JF et al., (1971) Phytochem 10:2529.

Majuinder PL, Bhattacharya M, (1974) Chem Ind 77.

Schrecker AW, (1957) J Am Chem Soc 79:3823.

Further information in:

Hänsel R, Keller K, Rimpler H, Schneider G (Hrsg.), Hagers Handbuch der Pharmazeutischen Praxis, 5. Aufl., Bde 4-6 (Drogen), Springer Verlag Berlin, Heidelberg, New York, 1992-1994.

Lewin L, Gifte und Vergiftungen, 6. Aufl., Nachdruck, Haug Verlag, Heidelberg 1992.

Madaus G, Lehrbuch der Biologischen Arzneimittel, Bde 1-3, Nachdruck, Georg Olms Verlag Hildesheim 1979.

Roth L, Daunderer M, Kormann K, Giftpflanzen, Pflanzengifte, 4. Aufl., Ecomed Fachverlag Landsberg Lech 1993.

Teuscher E, Biogene Arzneimittel, 5. Aufl., Wiss. Verlagsges. mbH Stuttgart 1997.

Guarana

See Paullinia Cupana

Gumweed

See Grindelia Camporum

Haematoxylon Campechianum

Logwood

DESCRIPTION

Medicinal Parts: The medicinal part is the unfermented heartwood.

Flower and Fruit: The flowers are small and yellow and grow in axillary racemes. There are 5 petals. The fruit is a flat, usually 1-seeded pod.

Leaves, Stem and Root: Haematoxylon campechianum is a small, 10 to 12 m high tree with twisted branches. They are thorny and the bark is rough and dark. The leaves have 4 pairs of small, smooth and cordate stipules whose tips point to the small trunk.

Habitat: The plant comes from the tropical regions of America and is cultivated in the Caribbean and other regions.

Production: Logwood is the wood from Haematoxylon campechianum.

Other Names: Bloodwood, H. Lignum, Peachwood

ACTIONS AND PHARMACOLOGY

COMPOUNDS

Haematoxylon (neoflavane derivatives): to some extent in glycosidic bonds, changing over into the intensively red-colored, quinoide haematein through oxidation

Tannins

EFFECTS

Haematoxylon campechianum has astringent properties.

INDICATIONS AND USAGE

Logwood was formerly used for diarrhea and hemorrhage.

PRECAUTIONS AND ADVERSE REACTIONS

Health risks or side effects following the proper administration of designated therapeutic dosages are not recorded.

DOSAGE

Mode of Administration: The drug is administered as an infusion and a liquid extract.

LITERATURE

Kern W, List PH, Hörhammer L (Hrsg.), Hagers Handbuch der Pharmazeutischen Praxis, 4. Aufl., Bde. 1-8, Springer Verlag Berlin, Heidelberg, New York, 1969.

Hagenia Abyssinica

Kousso

DESCRIPTION

Medicinal Parts: The medicinal parts are the leaves, the unripe fruit and the dried panicles of female flowers.

Flower and Fruit: The small flowers are large branched, thickly glandular-haired panicles up to 0.5 m long. They are androgynous, male or female. The male flowers are greenish and have fertile stamens and hairy bracts. The female flowers are dark-red.

Leaves, Stem and Root: Hagenia abyssinica is tree that grows up to 20 m high with tuft-like erect pinnatifid leaves.

Habitat: The plant is indigenous to northeast Africa and is cultivated in Ethiopia.

Production: Kousso flowers are the flowers of Hagenia abyssinica.

Other Names: Cossoo, Kooso, Kosso

ACTION AND PHARMACOLOGY

COMPOUNDS

Acylphloroglucinols (kosotoxine): monomeric, dimeric, trimeric compounds, such as protocosin (trimeric)

Tannins

EFFECTS

Kousso is a vermifuge and acts a typical muscle poison for lower class animals.

INDICATIONS AND USAGE

The drug was formerly used to treat tapeworm infestation. Its efficacy depends on the composition of the drug.

PRECAUTIONS AND ADVERSE REACTIONS

Side effects include irritation of the gastrointestinal tract, salivation, nausea and diarrhea. A tendency towards fainting spells, headache and general weakness has been connected with the use of the drug as a tapeworm cure. The drug should no longer be administered.

OVERDOSAGE

Conditions of collapse and vision disorders have been observed with overdosages. The treatment of poisoning consists of gastrointestinal emptying (inducement of vomiting, gastric lavage with burgundy-colored potassium permanganate solution, sodium sulphate), installation of activated charcoal and shock prophylaxis (quiet, warmth). Diazepam (i.v.) should be used to treat spasms. Atropine should be used to treat colic, and electrolyte substitution should be employed. Possible cases of acidosis should be countered with sodium bicarbonate infusions. In case of shock, plasma volume expanders should be administered. Monitoring of kidney function is essential. Intubation and oxygen respiration may also be necessary.

DOSAGE

Mode of Administration: The drug is obsolete in most countries.

LITERATURE

Metzner J et al., Antispastische Wirkung von Hagenia abyssinica. In: PM 47(4):240-241. 1983.

Schiemenz GP, Schroeder JM, Z Naturforsch 40B(5):669-680. 1985.

Further information in:

Kern W, List PH, Hörhammer L (Hrsg.), Hagers Handbuch der harmazeutischen Praxis, 4. Aufl., Bde. 1-8, Springer Verlag Berlin, Heidelberg, New York, 1969.

Lewin L, Gifte und Vergiftungen, 6. Aufl., Nachdruck, Haug Verlag, Heidelberg 1992.

Madaus G, Lehrbuch der Biologischen Arzneimittel, Bde 1-3, Nachdruck, Georg Olms Verlag Hildesheim 1979.

Roth L, Daunderer M, Kormann K, Giftpflanzen, Pflanzengifte, 4. Aufl., Ecomed Fachverlag Landsberg Lech 1993.

Teuscher E, Lindequist U, Biogene Gifte - Biologie, Chemie, Pharmakologie, 2. Aufl., Fischer Verlag Stuttgart 1994.

Hamamelis Virginiana

Witch Hazel

DESCRIPTION

Medicinal Parts: The medicinal parts are the hamamelis water which is distilled from hamamelis bark, the leaves which are collected in autumn and dried, the fresh bark of the roots and branches, the dried bark of the trunk and branches, and the fresh leaves and preparations from various plant parts.

Flower and Fruit: The androgynous and unisexual flowers are in light to golden yellow, short-stemmed clusters on the trees before the leaves come out. The inflorescence is a small, head-like spike in the axils of the dropping leaves, with 5 to 8 flowers. The 4 sepals are ovate or triangular, curved outwards, yellow-brown to brown on the inside. The petals are bright yellow, long, narrow-linear, rolled to a spiral in the bud and crushed like tissue paper when open.

The ovary is villous, bivalvlar with 2 anatropic ovules. Fertilization takes place the following spring, 5 to 7 months after pollination. The fruit capsule is woody, ovate, sectioned and divided, hazelnut-like, 12 to 15 mm long and thickly pubescent. It bursts so dramatically in autumn that the 2 dark seeds are thrown up to 4 m away.

Leaves, Stem and Root: The plant is a tree-like deciduous bush that grows 2 to 3 m high or sometimes up to 10 m high with a trunk diameter of 40 cm. The bark is thin, brown on the outside, reddish on the inside. The older branches are bushy, divided and silver-gray to gray brown. The younger branches are yellowish brown with hairs. The leaves are alternate. There are stipules. The leaf margin is roughly crenate, bluntly indented to irregularly sweeping.

Habitat: The tree is from the deciduous forest of Atlantic North America. It grows in Europe in gardens and parks and is cultivated in subtropical countries.

Production: Witch Hazel leaf consists of the dried leaf of Hamamelis virginiana. Witch Hazel bark consists of the dried bark of the trunk and branches of Hamamelis virginiana.

Not To Be Confused With: Hazelnut bark to which it bears a resemblance or the leaves of Corylus avellana (hazelnut leaves).

Other Names: Hamamelis, Hazel Nut, Snapping Hazel, Spotted Alder, Striped Alder, Tobacco Wood, Winterbloom

ACTIONS AND PHARMACOLOGY

COMPOUNDS

Tannins: including hamamelitannin (2,5-di-O-galloyl-D-hamamelose), monogalloylhamameloses, oligomeric procyanidins

Volatile oil: consisting chiefly in steam distillate out of aliphatic carbonyl compounds, for example hex-2-en-1-al, 6-methyl-hepta-3,5-dien-2-on, aliphatic alcohols, aliphatic esters

EFFECTS

Witch Hazel is astringent, anti-inflammatory and locally hemostatic.

INDICATIONS AND USAGE

- Hemorrhoids
- Inflammation of the mouth and pharynx
- Inflammation of the skin
- Venous conditions
- Wounds and burns

The leaf is used in folk medicine for non-specific diarrheic ailments and for menstrual complaints. The bark is used for minor injuries of the skin, local inflammation of skin and mucous membranes, hemorrhoids and varicose veins. It is also used in folk medicine for inflammation of the mucosa of the colon, hematemesis, and hemoptysis. It is used externally for locally inflamed swelling.

PRECAUTIONS AND ADVERSE REACTIONS

Health risks following the proper administration of designated therapeutic dosages are not recorded. If taken internally, the tannin content of the drug can lead to digestive complaints. In rare cases liver damage is conceivable following long-term administration.

DOSAGE

Mode of Administration: Witch hazel leaves and bark are available as comminuted drug or extracts for internal and external use as galenic preparations. A steam distillate of the fresh leaves and bark is used for internal and external application.

Preparation: Various formulations of Hamamelis virginiana are prepared as follows:

- External: aqueous steam distillate (Witch Hazel water) undiluted, or diluted 1:3 with water.
- For poultices: 20 to 30% in semi-solid preparations.
- Extract preparations: semi-solid and liquid preparations, corresponding to 5 to 10% drug.
- Decoctions of 5 to 10 gm of herb per cup (250 ml) of water for compresses and rinses.
- Ointment/Gel: 5 gm witch hazel extract in 100 gm ointment base.
- Suppositories: Use 0.1 to 1 gm drug.

Daily Dosage: Suppositories can be used 1 to 3 times a day.

LITERATURE

Bernard P et al. J Pharm Belg 26: 661.

Dorsch W, Neues über antientzündliche Drogen. In: ZPT 14(1):26. 1993.

Erdelmeier CAJ et al., Antiviral and antiphlogistic activities of Hamamelis virginiana bark. In: PM 62(3):241-245. 1996.

Friedrich H, Krüger N (1974) Planta Med 25: 138.

Haberland C, Kolodziej H, Novel galloylhamamelose from Hamamelis virginiana. In: PM 59(7)08. 1993.

Hartisch C et al., Dual inhibitory activities of tannins from Hamamelis virginiana and related polyphenols on 5-lipoxygenase and Lyso-PAF: Acetyl-CoA-Acetyltransferase. In: PM 63(2):106-110. 1997.

Hartisch C et al., Proanthocyanidin pattern in Hamamelis virginiana. In: PM 62, Abstracts of the 44th Ann Congress of GA, 119. 1996.

Hartisch C et al., Study on the localisation and composition of the volatile fraction of Hamamelis virginiana. In: PM 62, Abstracts of the 44th Ann Congress of GA, 133. 1996.

Knoch HG, (1991) Hämorrhoiden I. Grades, Wirksamkeit einer Salbe auf pflanzlicher Basis. Münch Med Wschr 31/32: 481-484.

Knoch HG, Klug W, Hübner WD (1992) Salbenbehandlung von Hämorrhoiden ersten Grades. Wirksamkeitsvergleich eines Präparates auf pflanzlicher Grundlage mit zwei nur synthetische Wirkstoffe enthaltenen Salben. Fortschr Med. 110: 135-138.

Korting HC, Schüfer-Korting M, Hart H, Laux P, Schmid M (1993) Anti-inflammatory activity of hamamelis distillate applied topically to the skin. Influence of vehicle and dose. Eur J Clin Pharmacol 44: 315-318.

Laux P, Oschmann R (1993) Die Zaubernuβ - Hamamelis virginiana L. Z Phytother 14: 155-166.

Mennet-von Eiff M, Meier B, Phytotherapie in der Dermatologie. In: ZPT 16(4):201-210. 1995.

Messerschmidt W (1967) Arch Pharm 300: 550.

Messerschmidt W (1968) Arzneim Forsch 18: 1618.

Sorkin B, (1980) Hametum-Salbe, eine kortikoidfreie antiinflammatorische Salbe. Phys Med Rehab 21: 53-57.

Further information in:

Hänsel R, Keller K, Rimpler H, Schneider G (Hrsg.), Hagers Handbuch der Pharmazeutischen Praxis, 5. Aufl., Bde 4-6 (Drogen), Springer Verlag Berlin, Heidelberg, New York, 1992-1994.

Leung AY, Encyclopedia of Common Natural Ingredients Used in Food Drugs and Cosmetics, John Wiley & Sons Inc., New York 1980.

Madaus G, Lehrbuch der Biologischen Arzneimittel, Bde 1-3, Nachdruck, Georg Olms Verlag Hildesheim 1979.

Schulz R, Hänsel R, Rationale Phytotherapie, Springer Verlag Heidelberg 1996.

Steinegger E, Hänsel R, Pharmakognosie, 5. Aufl., Springer Verlag Heidelberg 1992.

Teuscher E, Biogene Arzneimittel, 5. Aufl., Wiss. Verlagsges. mbH Stuttgart 1997.

Wagner H, Wiesenauer M, Phytotherapie. Phytopharmaka und pflanzliche Homöopathika, Fischer-Verlag, Stuttgart, Jena, New York 1995.

Wichtl M (Hrsg.), Teedrogen, 4. Aufl., Wiss. Verlagsges. Stuttgart 1997.

Haronga Madagascariensis

Haronga

DESCRIPTION

Medicinal Parts: The medicinal parts are the leaves and bark.

Flower and Fruit: The inflorescences are richly blossomed, terminal, umbel-like and have a diameter of about 20 cm. The flowers are small and white, have 5 sepals and petals, 4 stamens, and a fanned ovary with 2 ovules per section. The fruit is a roundish, reddish drupe. There are 10 seeds which are cylindrical and have black glandular hairs and a reticulate surface structure.

Leaves, Stem and Root: Harungana madagascariensis is a small evergreen tree up to 8 m high with a heavily branched crown. It has opposite, elliptical-oval leaves which are rounded to cordate at the base and are dotted black. The upper surface is dark green. The lower surface has red-brown hairs.

Habitat: The plant comes from Madagascar and east Africa and is widely distributed in tropical Africa.

Production: Haronga bark with dried leaves consists of the bark and leaves of Harungana madagascariensis, as well as its preparations. The leaves are collected and then air-dried in their entirety; the bark is peeled and also air-dried.

ACTION AND PHARMACOLOGY

COMPOUNDS

Anthracene derivatives: including harunganin, madagascin, madagascinanthrone, haronginanthrone, chrysophanol, physcione, hypericin, pseudohypericin, madagascarine

Volatile oil (traces)

Oligomeric procyanidins

EFFECTS

Haronga has a digestion regulatory effect. It stimulates the excretory function of the pancreas and gastric juice secretion. It is a cholagogue and a cholecystokinetic. It also has an antihepatoxic effect. A protective effect for the liver was observed in animal experiments. An antimicrobial effect has also been observed.

INDICATIONS AND USAGE

- Dyspeptic complaints
- Liver and gallbladder complaints
- Loss of appetite

Haronga is also used for mild exocrine pancreatic insufficiency.

CONTRAINDICATIONS

The drug is not to be used in patients with acute pancreatitis, severe liver function disorders, gallstone illnesses, obstruction of the biliary ducts, gallbladder empyema or ileus.

PRECAUTIONS AND ADVERSE REACTIONS

Health risks or side effects following the proper administration of designated therapeutic dosages are not recorded. A phototoxic effect is conceivable, but due to the small size of therapeutic dosages, is unlikely.

DOSAGE

Mode of Administration: As comminuted Haronga bark with leaves for decoctions, extracts and other preparations.

Daily Dosage: The average daily dose is 7.5 to 15 mg of an aqueous-alcoholic dry extract corresponding to 25 to 50 mg drug.

LITERATURE

Baldi A et al., Polyphenols from Harungana madagascarienis. In: PM 58(7):A691. 1992.

Buckley DG et al., Aust J Chem 25:843-855. 1972.

Fisel J et al., DAZ 106:1053-1060. 1966.

Gehrmann B, Analytische Studie an Harungana madagascariensis Lam. ex Poir. In: Dissertation Universität Hamburg. 1989.

Messerschmidt W, DAZ 106:1209-1211. 1966.

Further information in:

Hänsel R, Keller K, Rimpler H, Schneider G (Hrsg.), Hagers Handbuch der Pharmazeutischen Praxis, 5. Aufl., Bde 4-6 (Drogen), Springer Verlag Berlin, Heidelberg, New York, 1992-1994.

Steinegger E, Hänsel R, Pharmakognosie, 5. Aufl., Springer Verlag Heidelberg 1992.

Harpagophytum Procumbens

Devil's Claw

DESCRIPTION

Medicinal Parts: The medicinal parts are the dried tubular secondary roots cut into slices or pieces or pulverized, and the macerated thick lateral tubers before they are dry. These are very difficult to cut or pulverize when dry.

Flower and Fruit: The flowers are solitary, large and foxglove-like on short pedicles in the leaf axils. The petals are pale-pink to crimson. The seed capsules are bivalvular, compressed at the sides and ovate. They are 7 to 20 cm long, 6 cm in diameter, very woody with longitudinally striped rind. They have a double row of elastic, arm-like, branched appendages with an anchor-like hook. The capsules contain about 50 oblong, dark seeds with a rough surface.

Leaves, Stem and Root: The plant is perennial, leafy, and has a branched root system and branched, prostrate shoots 1 to 1.5 m long. The leaves are petiolate and lobed and may be opposite or alternate. The aerial parts die down in the dry season. The tuber roots are formed from the main and lateral roots. The main roots have an obtuse, quadrangular, 10 to 20 cm long and 30 to 60 cm thick upright sections which are covered in a fissured cork layer. The nodes of the lateral roots are up to 60 mm thick and 20 cm long. They are light-brown to red-brown on the outside. They are found in a area of about 150 cm around the plant and grow down to a depth of 30 to 60 cm.

Characteristics: The dried, pulverized secondary tubers and roots are yellowish-gray to bright pink, hard, horn-like, and have a bitter taste.

Habitat: The plant grows in South Africa and Namibia. It is spread throughout the Savannas and the Kalahari.

Production: Devil's Claw root consists of the dried, secondary tubers of Harpagophytum procumbens, as well as their preparations.

Other Names: Grapple Plant, Wood Spider

ACTION AND PHARMACOLOGY

COMPOUNDS

Liridoide monoterpenes: including harpagoside (extremely bitter), harpagide, procumbide

Phenylethanol derivatives: including acteoside (verbascoside); isoacteoside

Oligosaccharides: stachyose

Harpagoquinones (traces)

EFFECTS

Harpagophytum procumbens is an appetite stimulant and has choleretic, antiphlogistic, and mild analgesic effects. The constraints cinnamylic acid and terpene may have allergic effects.

INDICATIONS AND USAGE

- Dyspeptic complaints
- Liver and gallbladder complaints
- Loss of appetite
- Rheumatism

Devil's Claw is also used for supportive therapy of degenerative disorders of the locomotor system.

In folk medicine, the root is used as an ointment for skin injuries and disorders; the dried root for pain relief and for pregnancy complaints.

CONTRAINDICATIONS

The drug should not be used in the presence of stomach or duodenal ulcers, due to the drug's stimulation of gastric juice secretion.

PRECAUTIONS AND ADVERSE REACTIONS

Health risks or side effects following the proper administration of designated therapeutic dosages are not recorded. The drug has a sensitizing effect.

DOSAGE

Mode of Administration: As comminuted drug for infusions and other preparations for internal use.

Preparation: To make an infusion, use 1 teaspoonful (equivalent to 4.5 gm) comminuted drug with 300 ml boiling water. Steep for 8 hours and strain.

Daily Dosage: For loss of appetite, the recommended dosage is 1.5 gm of drug; otherwise 4.5 gm of drug is used. The infusion can be taken 3 times a day.

LITERATURE

Abramowitz M, (1979) Med Letters 21:30.

Amling R, Phytotherapeutika in der Neurologie. In: ZPT 12(1):9. 1991.

Anonym, Phytotherapie:Pflanzliche Antirheumatika - was bringen sie? In: DAZ 136(45):4012-4015. 1996.

Baghdikian B et al., An analyticyl study, anti-inflammatory and analgesic effects of Harpagophytum procumbens and Harpagophytum zeyheri. In: PM 63(2):171-176. 1997.

Carle R, Pflanzliche Antiphlogistika und Spasmolytika. In: ZPT 9(3):67. 1988.

Circosta C et al., (1984) J Ethnopharmacol 11:259.

Eichler O, Koch C, (1970) Arzneim Forsch 20(1):107.

Erdos A et al., (1978) Planta Med 34:97.

Haag-Berrurier, M et al., (1978) Plant Med Phytother 12(3):197.

Kreymeier J, Rheumatherapie mit Phytopharmaka. In: DAZ 137(8):611-613. 1997.

Lichti H, Von Wartburg A, (1964) Tetrahedron Letters 15:835.

Sticher O, (1977) Dtsch Apoth Ztg 32:1279.

Tunmann P, Stierstorfer N, Tetrahedron Letters 15:1697.

Wenzel P, Wegener T, (1995) Teufelskralle. Ein pflanzliches Antirheumatikum. Dtsch Apoth Ztg 135(13):1131-1144.

Wolf E, Teufelskralle hat Entzündungen im Griff. In: PZ 142(14):1122. 1997.

Further information in:

Hänsel R, Keller K, Rimpler H, Schneider G (Hrsg.), Hagers Handbuch der Pharmazeutischen Praxis, 5. Aufl., Bde 4-6 (Drogen), Springer Verlag Berlin, Heidelberg, New York, 1992-1994.

Schulz R, Hänsel R, Rationale Phytotherapie, Springer Verlag Heidelberg 1996.

Steinegger E, Hänsel R, Pharmakognosie, 5. Aufl., Springer Verlag Heidelberg 1992.

Teuscher E, Biogene Arzneimittel, 5. Aufl., Wiss. Verlagsges. mbH Stuttgart 1997.

Wagner H, Wiesenauer M, Phytotherapie. Phytopharmaka und pflanzliche Homöopathika, Fischer-Verlag, Stuttgart, Jena, New York 1995.

Wichtl M (Hrsg.), Teedrogen, 4. Aufl., Wiss. Verlagsges. Stuttgart 1997.

Hartstongue

See Scolopendrium Vulgare

Hawthorn

See Crataegus Species

Heartsease

See Viola Tricolor

Heather

See Calluna Vulgaris

Hedera Helix

English Ivy

DESCRIPTION

Medicinal Parts: The medicinal parts are the leaves.

Flower and Fruit: The inflorescences are greenish-yellow umbels, which form dense, semi-globular clusters. The calyx tips are short, almost triangular, tomentose and drooping. The 5 petals are oblong and slightly involute. There are 5 stamens, 1 inferior ovary with 5 valves. The style is fused into a column. The fruit is a globular, usually 5-valved berry, which becomes black and ripens in spring. It contains 3 to 5 seeds, which are reddish violet when young, later dark brown and finally black.

Leaves, Stem and Root: The plant is a 3 to 15 m creeping or, by means of adventitious roots, climbing woody, evergreen perennial. The stem is branched, the leaves are alternate, petioled, glabrous, glossy, coriaceous; the younger ones 5 lobed. The leaves of older flowering plants are ovate-rhomboid.

Characteristics: The berries and leaves have a bitter taste.

Habitat: Hendera helix grows in Britain, the temperate regions of Europe and North and Central Asia. It is cultivated in the USA as English Ivy.

Production: Ivy leaf consists of the dried leaves of Hedera helix.

Other Names: Gum Ivy, True Ivy, Woodbind

ACTIONS AND PHARMACOLOGY

COMPOUNDS

Triterpene saponins: chief components hederosaponin C (hederacoside C, slightly transforming into alpha-hederin, aglycone hederagenin), additionally hederosaponin B (hederacoside B)

Volatile oil: among others with methylethylketone, methylisobutylketone

Polyynes: including falcarinol, 11,12-didehydrofalcarinol

Sterols: including beta-sitosterol, campesterol

EFFECTS

English Ivy is an expectorant and antispasmodic and an irritant to the skin and mucosa.

INDICATIONS AND USAGE

- Cough
- Bronchitis

Hendera helix is a respiratory catarrh used for the symptomatic treatment of chronic inflammatory bronchial conditions.

In folk medicine, English Ivy is used internally for liver, spleen, and gallbladder disorders and for gout, rheumatism and scrofulosis. Externally, it is used for burn wounds, calluses, cellulitis, inflammations, neuralgia, parasitic disorders, ulcers, rheumatic complaints and for phlebitis.

The folk medicine uses listed have not been clinically proven.

PRECAUTIONS AND ADVERSE REACTIONS

Health risks or side effects following the proper administration of designated therapeutic dosages are not recorded. The drug has a medium potential for sensitization through skin contact.

DOSAGE

Mode of Administration: English Ivy is available as comminuted drug and other galenic preparations for internal use.

Preparation: To make an infusion, use 1 heaping teaspoonful drug with one-quarter cup boiling water and steep for 10 minutes.

Daily Dosage: The infusion can be taken internally 3 times daily. The average daily dose is 0.3 to 0.8 gm of drug. When used externally, fresh leaves may be laid upon festering wounds and burns; a decoction of fresh leaves (200gm/liter water) may be used for rheumatism.

LITERATURE

Balansard G et al., (1980) Planta Med 39:234.

Czygan FC, Hedera helix L. - Der Efeu. In: ZPT 11(4):133. 1990.

Elias R et al., JNP 54:98-103. 1991.

Gladtke E, Zur Wirksamkeit eines Efeublätterpräparates (Prospan). In: Intern Praxis 32(1)187. 1992.

Hansen L, Boll PM, (1986) Phytochemistry 25(2):285.

Julien J et al., (1985) Planta Med (3):205.

Mahran GH et al., (1975) Planta Med 29:127.

Trute A, Gross J, Mutschler E, Nahrstedt A, In vitro antispasmodic compounds of the dry extract obtained from Hedera helix. In: PM 63(2):125-129. 1997.

Trute A, Nahrstedt A, Identification and quantitative analysis of phenolic dry extracts of Hedera helix. In: PM 63(2):177-179. 1997.

Tschesche R, Schmidt R, Wulff G, Z Naturforsch 20B:708-709. 1965.

Wulff G, DAZ 108:797-807. 1968.

Further information in:

Frohne D, Pfänder HJ, Giftpflanzen - Ein Handbuch für Apotheker, Toxikologen und Biologen, 4. Aufl., Wiss. Verlagsges. mbH Stuttgart 1997.

Hänsel R, Keller K, Rimpler H, Schneider G (Hrsg.), Hagers Handbuch der Pharmazeutischen Praxis, 5. Aufl., Bde 4-6 (Drogen), Springer Verlag Berlin, Heidelberg, New York, 1992-1994.

Hausen B, Allergiepflanzen, Pflanzenallergene, ecomed Verlagsgesellsch. mbH, Landsberg 1988.

Lewin L, Gifte und Vergiftungen, 6. Aufl., Nachdruck, Haug Verlag, Heidelberg 1992.

Madaus G, Lehrbuch der Biologischen Arzneimittel, Bde 1-3, Nachdruck, Georg Olms Verlag Hildesheim 1979.

Roth L, Daunderer M, Kormann K, Giftpflanzen, Pflanzengifte, 4. Aufl., Ecomed Fachverlag Landsberg Lech 1993.

Schulz R, Hänsel R, Rationale Phytotherapie, Springer Verlag Heidelberg 1996.

Steinegger E, Hänsel R, Pharmakognosie, 5. Aufl., Springer Verlag Heidelberg 1992.

Teuscher E, Biogene Arzneimittel, 5. Aufl., Wiss. Verlagsges. mbH Stuttgart 1997.

Teuscher E, Lindequist U, Biogene Gifte - Biologie, Chemie, Pharmakologie, 2. Aufl., Fischer Verlag Stuttgart 1994.

Wagner H, Wiesenauer M, Phytotherapie. Phytopharmaka und pflanzliche Homöopathika, Fischer-Verlag, Stuttgart, Jena, New York 1995.

Wichtl M (Hrsg.), Teedrogen, 4. Aufl., Wiss. Verlagsges. Stuttgart 1997.

Hedge Mustard

See Sisymbrium Officinale

Hedge-Hyssop

See Gratiola Officinalis

Helianthemum Canadense

Frostwort

DESCRIPTION

Medicinal Parts: The medicinal part is the herb.

Flower and Fruit: The plant flowers twice per season. The first flowers are bright yellow with large petals. The second flowers are apetalous in small axillary clusters.

Leaves, Stem and Root: The plant is a perennial with an unbranched white stem. The twigs are slender, purplish-green, with opposite leaf scars. The leaves are linear, up to 1.5 cm long, grayish-green and downy.

Characteristics: The taste is astringent and bitter. It is odorless.

Habitat: Helianthemum canadense is originally from the eastern U.S. and is now found in Europe.

Production: Frostwort is the aerial part of Helianthemum canadense.

Other Names: Frost Plant, Frostweed, Rock-rose, Sun Rose

ACTIONS AND PHARMACOLOGY

COMPOUNDS

Tannins

Glycoside: helianthinin

The constituents of the drug have not been fully investigated.

EFFECTS

Frostwort is astringent and tonic.

INDICATIONS AND USAGE

The herb is used internally for digestive disorders and externally for ulcers.

PRECAUTIONS AND ADVERSE REACTIONS

Health risks or side effects following the proper administration of designated therapeutic dosages are not recorded.

DOSAGE

Mode of Administration: Frostwort is administered as a liquid extract.

LITERATURE

Further information in:

Kern W, List PH, Hörhammer L (Hrsg.), Hagers Handbuch der Pharmazeutischen Praxis, 4. Aufl., Bde. 1-8, Springer Verlag Berlin, Heidelberg, New York, 1969.

Madaus G, Lehrbuch der Biologischen Arzneimittel, Bde 1-3, Nachdruck, Georg Olms Verlag Hildesheim 1979.

Wagner H, Wiesenauer M, Phytotherapie. Phytopharmaka und pflanzliche Homopathika, Fischer-Verlag, Stuttgart, Jena, New York 1995.

Helianthus Annuus

Sunflower

DESCRIPTION

Medicinal Parts: The medicinal parts are the ray florets collected at the beginning of the flowering season, the leaves collected at the same time, the ripe fruit, the oil extracted from the seeds and the mature flower heads.

Flower and Fruit: The very large, composite flowers are solitary or in small clusters, usually nodding and 10 to 40 cm wide, on the stems. The bracts in a number of rows are leaf-like, ovate, acute and sparsely bristly. There are 20 to 70 asexual, linguiform golden-yellow, 3 to 10 cm long and 1 to 3 cm wide ray florets and numerous tubular, brown, purple or yellow, disc florets with black or purple anthers. There are 3 pointed bracts on the receptacle. The fruit is compressed at the sides, obovate to almost wedge-shaped, and is an achaene. It is densely appressed downy, whitish, straw yellow or gray to black.

Leaves, Stem and Root: The sunflower is a 1 to 3 m high annual plant with a long primary root and numerous lateral roots. The stem is erect, branched higher up, densely covered in hairs, filled with thin white pith. The leaves are alternate, cordate-triangular, long-petioled, irregularly crenately serrate and covered with short bristles on both sides.

Habitat: Helianthus annuus is indigenous to central and eastern North America and is cultivated worldwide.

Production: Sunflower oil is the fatty oil of the achenes of Helianthus annuus, which is recovered from the fruits (excluding the shell), by cold pressing. The mother tincture is extracted from the Jerusalem artichokes Helianthus tuberosus.

Other Names: Corona Solis, Marigold of Peru

ACTIONS AND PHARMACOLOGY

COMPOUNDS: HELIANTHI ANNUI OLEUM

Triglycerides: chief fatty acids linoleic acid (35-62%), oleic acid (25-42%), palmitic acid (4-7%)

Sterols: including campesterol, cholesterol, beta-sitosterol

EFFECTS: HELIANTHI ANNUI OLEUM

Useful as a dietary supplement

COMPOUNDS: HELIANTHI TUBEROSI TINCTURA

Polysaccharides: in particular inulin (fructosan)

Diterpene acids

Volatile oil: including some containing beta-bisabolen

EFFECTS: HELIANTHI TUBEROSI TINCTURA

No information is available.

INDICATIONS AND USAGE

HELIANTHI ANNUI OLEUM

Sunflower oil is used internally to alleviate constipation (as a lubricant). It is used externally as a massage oil, for poorly healing wounds (as an oil dressing), and in the treatment of skin lesions, psoriasis and rheumatism. Sufficient information on the efficacy of the drug is not available.

HELIANTHI TUBEROSI TINCTURA

In homeopathy, it is used for constipation, obesity and as a therapeutic aid in treating diabetes mellitus.

PRECAUTIONS AND ADVERSE REACTIONS

HELIANTHI ANNUI OLEUM

Health risks or side effects following the proper administration of designated therapeutic dosages are not recorded.

HELIANTHI TUBEROSI TINCTURA

Health risks following the proper administration of designated therapeutic dosages are not recorded. Flatulence and/or meteorism are possible following intake of the drug or the pressed must. Intakes of larger quantities of the partially hydrolyzed pressed must (which has a high fructose content) can lead to elevated serum triglyceride levels in men.

DOSAGE

HELIANTHI ANNUI OLEUM

Mode of Administration: In folk medicine, the drug is mainly for external use. In other areas, it is used as an inactive ingredient in pharmaceutical preparations.

Storage: Keep protected from light, in tightly-sealed containers. Oils from different deliveries should not be mixed.

HELIANTHI TUBEROSI TINCTURA

Mode of Administration: The tincture is administered as a homoeopathic dilution (D1) in drops, tonics and tablets.

Daily Dosage: Quantities that correspond to 50 gm fructose per day should not be exceeded, particularly in the presence of hypertriglyceridaemia or kidney insufficiency.

LITERATURE

HELIANTHI ANNUI OLEUM

Huesa Lope J et al., Grasas Aceites 25:350-353 via CA 82:135733. 1974.

Matsumoto T, Nagakawa M, Itoh T, PH 23:921-923. 1984.

Further information in:

Hänsel R, Keller K, Rimpler H, Schneider G (Hrsg.), Hagers Handbuch der Pharmazeutischen Praxis, 5. Aufl., Bde 4-6 (Drogen), Springer Verlag Berlin, Heidelberg, New York, 1992-1994.

Madaus G, Lehrbuch der Biologischen Arzneimittel, Bde 1-3, Nachdruck, Georg Olms Verlag Hildesheim 1979.

Teuscher E, Biogene Arzneimittel, 5. Aufl., Wiss. Verlagsges. mbH Stuttgart 1997.

HELIANTHI TUBEROSI TINCTURA

Laube H, Dtsch Med Wochenschr 113:1534. 1988.

Further information in:

Hänsel R, Keller K, Rimpler H, Schneider G (Hrsg.), Hagers Handbuch der Pharmazeutischen Praxis, 5. Aufl., Bde 4-6 (Drogen), Springer Verlag Berlin, Heidelberg, New York, 1992-1994.

Helichrysum Arenarium

Immortelle

DESCRIPTION

Medicinal Parts: The medicinal parts are the composite heads or the whole of the flowering plant.

Flower and Fruit: The flowers are in dense clustered cymes. They are small and orange. The bracts are dry-membranous and usually lemon-yellow. All the florets are tubular and funnel-shaped. The fruit is pentangular with a tuft of hair.

Leaves, Stem and Root: The plant grows from 10 to 30 cm high. The stem is erect, unbranched, gray-tomentose. The leaves are alternate, the lower ones are spatulate, the upper ones lanceolate, acute and as gray-tomentose as the stem.

Characteristics: Immortelle has a weak aroma; the plant is a protected species

Habitat: The plant grows in Europe and the U.S.

Production: Immortelle consists of the dried flowers of Helichrysum arenarium gathered shortly before fully unfolding.

Not To Be Confused With: The capitula of Helichrysum stoechas and Helichrysum augustifolium.

Other Names: Common Shrubby Everlasting, Eternal Flower, Goldilocks, Yellow Chaste Weed

ACTIONS AND PHARMACOLOGY

COMPOUNDS

Flavonoids: in particular isosalipurposide (intensive yellow chalcone glycoside), naringenin-5-glucosyl-glucoside, helichrysin A and B (C-2-enantiomeric narigenin-5-O-glucosides, B-salipurposide)

Phthalides: including 5-methoxy-7-hydroxy-phthalides and their monoglucoside

Alpha-pyrone derivatives: arenole, homoarenole

Sesquiterpene bitter principles

Volatile oil (traces)

Caffeic acid derivatives

EFFECTS

The drug has antibacterial principles. It is mildly choleretic and mildly spasmolytic.

INDICATIONS AND USAGE

- Liver and gallbladder complaints
- Loss of appetite

The drug is used for dyspepsia and as an adjunct in the treatment of chronic cholecystitis and gallbladder complaints with accompanying cramps. In folk medicine, it is used as a diuretic.

CONTRAINDICATIONS

Because of the bile-stimulating effect of the drug, it is not to be administered when there is biliary obstruction.

PRECAUTIONS AND ADVERSE REACTIONS

Health risks or side effects following the proper administration of designated therapeutic dosages are not recorded. The presence of gallstone illnesses can lead to colic.

DOSAGE

Mode of Administration: Comminuted herb for infusions and other galenic preparations for internal use. Pharmaceutical cholagogues contain extracts of the drug. It is an inactive ingredient in many tea specialties.

Preparation: To make an infusion, pour boiling water over 2 teaspoonfuls drug (3 to 4 gm). Allow to stand for 10 minutes and then strain. Drink throughout the day and make fresh each time.

Daily Dosage: The average daily dose is 3 gm of drug.

Storage: Protect from light and moisture.

LITERATURE

Derkach AI et al., Chem Nat Comp 6:722. 1986.

Mericli AH et al., Sci Pharm 54:363. 1986.

Further information in:

Kern W, List PH, Hörhammer L (Hrsg.), Hagers Handbuch der Pharmazeutischen Praxis, 4. Aufl., Bde. 1-8, Springer Verlag Berlin, Heidelberg, New York, 1969.

Leung AY, Encyclopedia of Common Natural Ingredients Used in Food Drugs and Cosmetics, John Wiley & Sons Inc., New York 1980.

Madaus G, Lehrbuch der Biologischen Arzneimittel, Bde 1-3, Nachdruck, Georg Olms Verlag Hildesheim 1979.

Teuscher E, Biogene Arzneimittel, 5. Aufl., Wiss. Verlagsges. mbH Stuttgart 1997.

Wichtl M (Hrsg.), Teedrogen, 4. Aufl., Wiss. Verlagsges. Stuttgart 1997.

Helleborus Niger

Black Hellebore

DESCRIPTION

Medicinal Parts: The medicinal parts of the plant are the dried rhizome with or without roots and the fresh underground parts.

Flower and Fruit: The flower is white with a greenish margin, reddish on the outside. It is hanging and splayed. There are 5 broadly ovate, campanualate bracts with red-brown borders, which tend towards each other. The petals are altered to nectaries. There are numerous yellow stamens. The fruit is a pod-like, many-seeded follicle with a curved beak and horizontal stripes. The seeds are matte black, ovate and have a long swelling on them.

Leaves, Stem and Root: The plant is a perennial subshrub up to 50 cm high. The stem is erect, glabrous, branched, woody at the base and almost leafless. The basal leaves are long-petioled, thickish, coriaceous, glabrous, dark green above, underside lighter. The stem is unbranched and leafless, with 2 to 3 ovate bracts.

Characteristics: Poisonous, rhizome is black-brown.

Habitat: The plant is indigenous to the forests of southern and central Europe.

Production: Black Hellebore root is the root of Helleborus niger.

Not To Be Confused With: Helleboris foetidus, Helleborus niger and Helleborus viridis are different plants with different active compounds. They may be confused with the subterranean parts of Trollius eurpaeus, Aconitum napellus, Astrantia major; Actaea spicata and Adonis vernalis.

Other Names: Christe Herbe, Christmas Rose, Melampode

ACTIONS AND PHARMACOLOGY

COMPOUNDS: HELLEBORUS FOETIDUS

Steroid saponins: mixture known as helleborin

COMPOUNDS: HELLEBORUS NIGER

Steroid saponins: mixture known as helleborin

Cardioactive steroid glycosides (bufadienolide): including hellebrin, desglucohellebrin (only traces)

Alkaloids: celliamine, sprintillamine

COMPOUNDS: HELLEBORUS VIRIDIS

Steroid saponins: mixture known as helleborin

Cardioactive steroid glycosides (bufadienolide): including hellebrin, desglucohellebrin

Alkaloids: celliamine, sprintillamine, sprintillin

EFFECTS: ALL SPECIES

The plant is said to have a typical saponin effect (irritates mucous membranes). Note that other varieties of Helleborus also contain hellebrin with a digitalis-like effect.

INDICATIONS AND USAGE

In folk medicine, Black Hellebore is used as a laxative, for nausea, worm infestation, to regulate menstruation and as an abortifacient, as well as for acute nephritis. Also used in the treatment of head colds.

Efficacy has not been proven for these indications.

PRECAUTIONS AND ADVERSE REACTIONS

General: The mucous membrane-irritating saponine effect of the drug is the chief focus in cases of poisoning. Symptoms include scratchy feeling in mouth and throat, salivation, nausea, vomiting, diarrhea, dizziness, shortness of breath, possible spasm and asphyxiation. Disorders of cardiac function (cardiac arrhythmias) are to be expected with large intakes of the rhizome of Helleborus viridis. Poisonings are recorded among the animals that feed on the plant. Following stomach and intestinal emptying (gastric lavage, sodium sulphate) and the administration of activated charcoal, therapy for poisonings consists of diazepam for spasm and electrolyte replenishment and sodium bicarbonate infusions for any acidosis that may arise. Intubation and oxygen respiration may also be necessary.

Pregnancy: In folk medicine, it is used as an abortifacient.

DOSAGE

Mode of Administration: Black Hellebore is obsolete and dangerous as a drug.

Daily Dosage: The average dose is 0.05 gm; the maximum single dose is 0.2 gm; the largest daily dose is 1.0 gm. A powder with a medium content of 10% is used for head colds.

LITERATURE

Glombitza KW et al., Do roots of Helleborus niger contain cardioactive substances. In: PM 55:107. 1989.

Petricic J et al., Acta Pharm Jugosl 27:127. 1977.

Petricic J, Acta Pharm Jugosl 24:179. 1974.

Wiβner W, Kating H, Botanische und phytochemische Untersuchung an europäischen und kleinasiatischen Arten der Gattung Helleborus. In: PM 26:128-143, 228-249, 364-374. 1974.

Further information in:

Frohne D, Pfänder HJ, Giftpflanzen - Ein Handbuch für Apotheker, Toxikologen und Biologen, 4. Aufl., Wiss. Verlagsges. mbH Stuttgart 1997.

Hänsel R, Keller K, Rimpler H, Schneider G (Hrsg.), Hagers Handbuch der Pharmazeutischen Praxis, 5. Aufl., Bde 4-6 (Drogen), Springer Verlag Berlin, Heidelberg, New York, 1992-1994.

Lewin L, Gifte und Vergiftungen, 6. Aufl., Nachdruck, Haug Verlag, Heidelberg 1992.

Madaus G, Lehrbuch der Biologischen Arzneimittel, Bde 1-3, Nachdruck, Georg Olms Verlag Hildesheim 1979.

Poisonous Plants in Britain and their effects on Animals and Man, Ministry of Agriculture Fisheries and Food, Pub; HMSO, UK 1984.

Roth L, Daunderer M, Kormann K, Giftpflanzen, Pflanzengifte, 4. Aufl., Ecomed Fachverlag Landsberg Lech 1993.

Teuscher E, Lindequist U, Biogene Gifte - Biologie, Chemie, Pharmakologie, 2. Aufl., Fischer Verlag Stuttgart 1994.

Hemlock

See Conium Maculatum

Hemp Agrimony

See Eupatorium Cannabinum

Hempnettle

See Galeopsis Segetum

Henbane

See Hyoscyamus Niger

Henna

See Lawsonia Inermis

Heracleum Sphondylium

Masterwort

DESCRIPTION

Medicinal Parts: The medicinal parts are the dried roots, the herb collected in the flowering season and dried, the fruit, the fresh herb, and the whole fresh flowering plant.

Flower and Fruit: The flowers are 15 to 30 rayed, flat umbels with no involucre. The numerous epicalyx leaves are lanceolate and densely pubescent. The petals have a cordate margin with indented lobes. They are irregular, often pubescent on the outside, whitish or greenish, green-yellow or yellowish and sometimes pink. The fruit is compressed, flat, 8 mm long and 5 mm wide, roundish-oval and brownish yellow. The fruit has 10 ribs and oil grooves.

Leaves, Stem and Root: The plant grows from 80 to 150 cm high, is biennial to perennial and has a strong tuberous, whitish-yellow root. The stem is erect, angular, grooved, hollow, stiff-haired, and branched above. The leaves are large, odd-pinnate, with 1 to 3 pairs of leaflets. The leaflets are large, ovate, and lobed to pinnate. There is a 3-lobed terminal leaflet. The basal leaves are very large and have grooved petioles, which gradually merge into leaf sheaths. The basal and stem foliage are clasping.

Characteristics: There is hot, yellow latex in the stem. The leaf umbel is fragrant.

Habitat: Heracleum sphondylium is found in most of Europe and in western and northern Asia, as well as northern Africa. Subspecies are found mainly in northwest Europe, east and central Europe, and in the Mediterranean region.

ACTIONS AND PHARMACOLOGY

COMPOUNDS

Furocoumarins: in particular bergapten, isopimpinellin, pimpinellin, isobergapten, sphondin

Volatile oil: including ones containing n-octylacetate

EFFECTS

Masterwort is a mild expectorant, however, this has not been scientifically proven.

INDICATIONS AND USAGE

In folk medicine, the drug is used to relieve muscle cramps, stomach disorders, digestion problems, diarrhea, gastrointestinal catarrh, and diarrhea following a cold. The furocoumarin methoxsalin is used in the treatment of psoriasis.

Efficacy has not been proven.

PRECAUTIONS AND ADVERSE REACTIONS

Phototoxic effects must be avoided following intake of the drug due to its furocoumarin content. For that reason, UV-radiation and solaria should be avoided after its administration. The same danger exists following contact with the freshly-bruised plant.

DOSAGE

Mode of Administration: The decoction is used internally in isolated cases.

Preparation: For stomach disorders, add 3 teaspoonfuls of the herb to 2 glasses of water and allow to draw for 8 hours.

Daily Dosage: The preparation is to be drunk during the course of the day.

LITERATURE

Baerheim Svendsen A et al., PM 7:113-117. 1959.

Ognyanov I et al., PM 14:19-21. 1966.

Further information in:

Frohne D, Pfänder HJ: Giftpflanzen - Ein Handbuch für Apotheker, Toxikologen und Biologen, 4. Aufl., Wiss. Verlagsges. mbH Stuttgart 1997.

Hänsel R, Keller K, Rimpler H, Schneider G (Hrsg.), Hagers Handbuch der Pharmazeutischen Praxis, 5. Aufl., Bde 4-6 (Drogen), Springer Verlag Berlin, Heidelberg, New York, 1992-1994.

Madaus G: Lehrbuch der Biologischen Arzneimittel, Bde 1-3, Nachdruck, Georg Olms Verlag Hildesheim 1979.

Roth L, Daunderer M, Kormann K: Giftpflanzen, Pflanzengifte, 4.Aufl., Ecomed Fachverlag Landsberg Lech 1993.

Teuscher E, Lindequist U: Biogene Gifte - Biologie, Chemie, Pharmakologie, 2. Aufl., Fischer Verlag Stuttgart 1994.

Herb Paris

See Paris Quadrifolia

Herb Robert

See Geranium Robertianum

Herniaria Glabra

Rupturewort

DESCRIPTION

Medicinal Parts: The medicinal part is the fresh flowering plant.

Flower and Fruit: The flowers are in flat clusters of 7 to 10 in the leaf axils or opposite the leaves along the stem. They are yellow-white and very small. The fruit is a membranous capsule covered by the calyx. It contains 1 seed.

Leaves, Stem and Root: The plant is an annual small shrub of about 15 cm. The stem tends to be decumbent. It is round and branched. The leaves are sessile, entire-margined, elliptical, and opposite. If there is no flower cluster opposite the leaf. The leaves are alternate.

Characteristics: The plant is yellow-green and glabrous and creates suds when rubbed under water.

Habitat: The plant is found in the temperate and southern regions of Europe and in Asian Russia.

Production: Rupturewort is the complete aerial part of Hernaria glabra or Hernaria hirsuta.

Other Names: Flax Weed, Herniary

ACTIONS AND PHARMACOLOGY

COMPOUNDS

Triterpene saponins: herniaria saponins I-VII (aglycones medicagen, gypsogen, 16-hydroxy-medicagen)

Flavonoids: including hyperoside

Hydroxycoumarins: umbelliferone, herniarin

EFFECTS

The main active principles (saponines, flavonoids, coumarins and small amounts of tannins) are reported to have mild spasmolytic and diuretic effects, which have not been scientifically proven.

INDICATIONS AND USAGE

Hernaria glabra is used for disorders of the efferent urinary tract, inflammatory disorders of the kidneys and bladder, respiratory disorders, nerve inflammation, gout, rheumatism, and as a blood purifier.

PRECAUTIONS AND ADVERSE REACTIONS

Health risks or side effects following the proper administration of designated therapeutic dosages are not recorded.

DOSAGE

Mode of Administration: The drug is administered as an infusion and in tea mixtures, as an extract in drops and in urological pharmaceutical preparations.

Preparation: Put 1.5 gm comminuted drug (1 teaspoonful = 1.4 gm) in cold water and bring briefly to a boil. Strain after 5 minutes.

Daily Dosage: Drink 1 cup 2 to 3 times daily as a diuretic.

LITERATURE

Cart J, Reznicek G, Korhammer S, Haslinger E, Jurenitsch J, Kubelka W, The first spectroscopically confirmed saponin from Herniaria glabra. In: PM 58(7):A709. 1992.

Franck HP, (1975) Dtsch. Apoth Ztg 115:1206.

Freiler M et al., A new triterpenesaponin from Herniaria glabra. In: PM 61(Abstracts of 43rd Ann Congr):66. 1995.

Freiler M et al., Sci Pharm 64:359. 1996.

Krolikowska M, Wolbis M, (1979) Acta Pol Pharm 36:469.

Reznicek G et al., PA 48:450. 1993.

Tama M et al., (1981) Clujul Med 54(1):73 (via CA 96:149036).

Zoz et al., (1976) Rastit Resur 12(3):411 (via CA 85:174257).

Further information in:

Kern W, List PH, Hörhammer L (Hrsg.), Hagers Handbuch der Pharmazeutischen Praxis, 4. Aufl., Bde. 1-8, Springer Verlag Berlin, Heidelberg, New York, 1969.

Madaus G, Lehrbuch der Biologischen Arzneimittel, Bde 1-3, Nachdruck, Georg Olms Verlag Hildesheim 1979.

Steinegger E, Hänsel R, Pharmakognosie, 5. Aufl., Springer Verlag Heidelberg 1992.

Teuscher E, Biogene Arzneimittel, 5. Aufl., Wiss. Verlagsges. mbH Stuttgart 1997.

Wichtl M (Hrsg.), Teedrogen, 4. Aufl., Wiss. Verlagsges. Stuttgart 1997.

Hibiscus Abelmoschus

Muskmallow

DESCRIPTION

Medicinal Parts: The medicinal parts are the seeds of the plant and the oil extracted from them.

Flower and Fruit: The flowers are solitary and axillary. They have 5 to 7 pubescent, linear and about 1.5 cm long epicalyx leaves. The sepals are about 3 cm long. The corolla has a diameter of 7.5 cm. The petals are sulfur yellow with a crimson spot at the base. The petals are ovate and lightly pubescent. The fruit is a 5 to 8 cm long capsule, which is shaped like a pentagonal pyramid and filled with numerous large seeds. The seeds are kidney-shaped, compressed and about 3 mm in diameter. They are grayish-brown, with numerous striations which are concentric around the hilum.

Leaves, Stem and Root: The plant is an annual erect herb about 1 to 2 m high with star-shaped, pubescent stem, stalks and leaves. The leaves are 15 to 25 cm long, cordate to round with 3 to 7 lobes, which taper to a point. The petioles are as long or longer than the leaves. The stipules are oblong and pubescent.

Characteristics: The seeds have a strong, musky smell and the taste is oily. The seed pods have an aromatic flavor and are used in some parts of the Middle East to mix with and flavor coffee.

Habitat: The plant is indigenous to Africa, India, Java and South America and is cultivated in all tropical regions.

Production: Musk-Mallow seeds are the dried seeds of Hibiscus abelmoschus. The seeds are dried in the open-air.

Not To Be Confused With: Foenugraeci semen.

Other Names: Muskseed, Ambrette Seed, Abelmosk, Ambretta, Egyptian Alcée, Target-leaved Hibiscus, Okra

ACTION AND PHARMACOLOGY

COMPOUNDS

Fatty oil and chief fatty acids: palmitic acid, linoleic acid, stearic acid

Volatile oil: ambrette oil, chief components farnesylacetate, macrocyclic lactones as carriers of the musk smell such as hexadec-7-en-16-olide (ambrettolide), tetradec-5-en-14-olide

Sterols: including beta-sitosterin, beta-sitosterin-beta-D-glucoside

EFFECTS

Muskmallow is said to be an aromatic, stimulant and carminative. Efficacy has not been proven.

INDICATIONS AND USAGE

The various preparations are used for snake bite, cramps, stomach and intestinal disorders with cramps, loss of appetite and headache.

Efficacy has not been proven.

PRECAUTIONS AND ADVERSE REACTIONS

Health risks or side effects following the proper administration of designated therapeutic dosages are not recorded.

DOSAGE

Mode of Administration: Muskmallow is used as a tea or tincture, and is administered both internally and externally.

LITERATURE

Maurer B, Greider A, (1977) Helv Chim Acta 60:1155.

Srivastava KC, Rastogi SC, (1969) Planta Med 17:189.

Further information in:

Hänsel R, Keller K, Rimpler H, Schneider G (Hrsg.), Hagers Handbuch der Pharmazeutischen Praxis, 5. Aufl., Bde 4-6 (Drogen), Springer Verlag Berlin, Heidelberg, New York, 1992-1994 (unter Abelmoschus moschatus).

Hibiscus Sabdariffa

Hibiscus Flowers

DESCRIPTION

Medicinal Parts: The medicinal parts of the plant are the flowers.

Flower and Fruit: The flowers are solitary, axillary and almost sessile. The calyx is red, the corolla yellow, and the anthers blood red. The fruit is a 2 cm long, ovoid, many seeded capsule.

Leaves, Stem and Root: Hibiscus is a 0.15 to 1 m bushy annual that is branched from the base. The stems are reddish, almost glabrous. The basal leaves are undivided and ovate; the cauline leaves are 3-lobed and 7.5 to 10 cm wide. The lobes are 2.5 cm wide and crenate.

Habitat: Hibiscus sabdariffa originally came from the area around the source of the Niger. It grows worldwide in the tropics and is cultivated in Europe.

Production: Hibiscus flowers consists of the calyces of Hibiscus sabdariffa (sabdariffa ruber variety).

Other Names: Guinea Sorrel, Jamaica Sorrel, Red Sorrel, Roselle

ACTION AND PHARMACOLOGY

COMPOUNDS

Fruit acids (15-30%): in particular hibiscus ((+)-allohydroxy citric acid lacton), additionally lemons, malic acid, tartaric acid

Anthocyans (intensive red): including delphinidin-3-xyloglucoside, delphinidin-3-glucoside, cyanidin-3-xyloglucoside

Flavonoids: including gossypetin

Mucilages: rhamnogalacturonans, arabinogalactans, arabinans

EFFECTS

Hibiscus tea has a laxative effect due to the high content of poorly absorbable fruit acids.

Aqueous extracts of hibiscus leaves effect a relaxation of the uterus musculature and have a hypotensive effect.

INDICATIONS AND USAGE

Hibiscus flowers are used for loss of appetite, for colds that affect the respiratory tract and stomach, to dissolve phlegm, as a gentle laxative, diuretic, and for disorders of circulation.

The claimed efficacies have not been substantiated.

PRECAUTIONS AND ADVERSE REACTIONS

Health risks or side effects following the proper administration of designated therapeutic dosages are not recorded.

DOSAGE

Mode of Administration: Hibiscus sabdariffa is available as a tea preparation.

Preparation: To make a tea, pour boiling water over 1.5 gm comminuted drug and strain after 5 to 10 minutes.

LITERATURE

Franz M, Franz G, Hibiscus sabdariffa - Hibiscusblüten. In: ZPT 9(2):63. 1988.

Menβen HG, Staesche K, DAZ 114:1211. 1974.

Müller BM, Franz G, PM 58:60. 1992.

Further information in:

Kern W, List PH, Hörhammer L (Hrsg.), Hagers Handbuch der Pharmazeutischen Praxis, 4. Aufl., Bde. 1-8, Springer Verlag Berlin, Heidelberg, New York, 1969.

Steinegger E, Hänsel R, Pharmakognosie, 5. Aufl., Springer Verlag Heidelberg 1992.

Teuscher E, Biogene Arzneimittel, 5. Aufl., Wiss. Verlagsges. mbH Stuttgart 1997.

Wichtl M (Hrsg.), Teedrogen, 4. Aufl., Wiss. Verlagsges. Stuttgart 1997.

Hippophaë Rhamnoides

Sea Buckthorn

DESCRIPTION

Medicinal Parts: The medicinal parts are the ripe, yellow-red berries.

Flower and Fruit: The plant is dioecious and has greenish-yellow, insignificant flowers in numerous, sturdy clusters in the axils of scales with 2 bracts and a simple calyx. The male calyx is divided in 2 down to the base, with brown-spotted ovate sepals and has 4 stamens attached to the base. The female calyx is a tight tube clasping the ovary with erect, inward-inclined tips. The fruit is a bright orange, globular, ellipsoid false berry.

Leaves, Stem and Root: The plant is an angular, thorny 1.5 to 4.5 m high shrub with numerous, thorn-tipped and thorny branches. The leaves are 5 to 8 cm long, linear-lanceolate, short-petioled, glabrous above, tomentose beneath. The plant spreads by underground runners.

Habitat: Hippophaë rhamnoides is indigenous to Europe and some northern regions of Asia.

Production: Sea Buckthorn berries are the false fruit of Hippophaë rhamnoides. The fatty oil is extracted from both the seeds and the fruit flesh. The harvest is from August to December, until the first snow. As soon as the fruit has been picked it is immediately processed. The juice is produced without having any contact with metal substances.

Other Names: Sallow Thorn

ACTIONS AND PHARMACOLOGY

COMPOUNDS

Fruit acids: chiefly malic acid, additionally acetic acid, quinic acid

Ascorbic acid (Vitamin C): 0.2-1.4%

Flavonoids: in particular kaempferol, isorhamnetin-as well as quercetin tri- and tetra-glycosides

Carotinoids: beta-carotine, gamma-carotine, lycopene

Fatty oil (in the seeds 12%): chief fatty acids oleic acid, isolinol acid, linolenic acid, stearic acid

Sugar alcohols: mannitol, quebrachit

EFFECTS

The Vitamin C constituent encourages the healing of wounds and epithelization. It strengthens sight and inhibits sclerosis and the aging process.

INDICATIONS AND USAGE

The drug is used as an infection prophylaxis, in particular during the time just before spring and during periods of convalescence. It is used externally as a treatment for radiation damage, such as x-ray damage and sunburn and as a fatty oil for the treatment of wounds.

PRECAUTIONS AND ADVERSE REACTIONS

No health hazards or side effects are known in conjunction with the proper administration of designated therapeutic dosages.

DOSAGE

Mode of Administration: Buckthorn is not used as a drug in German-speaking countries. It is found as an extract constituent in various Vitamin C concentrates and juices.

Daily Dosage: The recommended daily dose is 5 to 10 gm of one of the Buckthorn products.

LITERATURE

Kern W, List PH, Hörhammer L (Hrsg.), Hagers Handbuch der Pharmazeutischen Praxis, 4. Aufl., Bde. 1-8, Springer Verlag Berlin, Heidelberg, New York, 1969.

Holly

See Ilex Aquifolium

Hollyhock

See Alcea Rosea

Honeysuckle

See Lonicera Caprifolium

Hops

See Humulus Lupulus

Hordeum Distychum

Barley

DESCRIPTION

Medicinal Parts: The medicinal part is the grain.

Flower and Fruit: The spike is 7 to 15 cm long. The long form is nodding and the shorter one erect and compressed at the side that does not bear spikelets. The spike spindle is tough and loosens the spikelets when ripe. The lateral spikelets are unbearded, male or sexless. The middle spikelet is seed-bearing with a beard up to 15 cm long.

Leaves, Stem and Root: The plant is an annual, 60 to 130 cm high cereal. It has a long hollow stalk and lanceolate leaves. The leaflets are very wide, long and glabrous.

Habitat: Barley is cultivated worldwide.

Production: Barley seeds are the seeds of Hordeum distychum.

Other Names: Pearl Barley, Pot Barley, Scotch Barley

ACTIONS AND PHARMACOLOGY

COMPOUNDS

Polysaccharides: starch (50%), fructans

Mono- and oligosaccharides: saccharose, raffinose, glucodi-fructose, glucose, fructose

Proteins (10%): including, among others, prolamines: horde-in- glutelins: hordenine (not to be confused with the amine of the same name, see below)- albumins and globulins

Fatty oil (2%): chief fatty acids linoleic and oleic acid

Vitamins: Vitamin E, nicotinic acid, pantothenic acid, Vitamins B6, B2, folic acid

Hydroxycoumarins (only in the stalks): including, among others, umbelliferone, scopoletin, herniarin, aesculetin (in the sprouts amines: tyramine, hordenine (dimethyltyramine), gramine also with certain strains (dimethy-laminomethylindol)

EFFECTS

Barley is soothing on the alimentary tract.

INDICATIONS AND USAGE

Barley is used for convalescents and in the treatment of diarrhea, gastritis and inflammatory bowel conditions.

PRECAUTIONS AND ADVERSE REACTIONS

No health hazards or side effects are known in conjunction with the proper administration of designated therapeutic dosages.

DOSAGE

Mode of Administration: Barley is used as a malt extract, in preparations and in combinations.

LITERATURE

Dhar ML et al., (1968) Indian J Exp Biol 6:232.

Labbe M, (1936) J Canad Med Assoc 34:141.

Further information in:

Kern W, List PH, Hörhammer L (Hrsg.), Hagers Handbuch der Pharmazeutischen Praxis, 4. Aufl., Bde. 1-8, Springer Verlag Berlin, Heidelberg, New York, 1969.

Oliver-Bever B (Ed.), Medicinal Plants of Tropical West Africa, Cambridge University Press, Cambrigde 1986.

Horehound

See Ballota Nigra

Horse Chestnut

See Aesculus Hippocastanum

Horsemint

See Monarda Punctata

Horseradish

See Armoracia Rusticana

Horsetail

See Equisetum Arvense

Hound's Tongue

See Cynoglossum Officinale

Houseleek

See Sempervivum Tectorum

Humulus Lupulus

Hops

DESCRIPTION

Medicinal Parts: The medicinal parts are the glandular hairs separated from the infructescence, the whole dried female flowers, the fresh (preferably with few seeds) cones collected before the seeds ripen and the fresh or dried female inflorescences.

Flower and Fruit: The male flowers are yellowish-greenish, inconspicuous, and about 5 mm in diameter. The female flowers are in richly blossomed, heavily branched inflorescences. The ovary, which has 2 long downy stigma, is surrounded at the base by a round compressed nutlet. A yellowish fruit cone grows from the female flower. The inside of the bracts is covered with small, glossy, light yellow glandular scales, which contain hop bitter (Lupulin).

Leaves, Stem and Root: The hop plant is a perennial. The annual shoots reach a height of 6 m (12 m when cultivated). The stems are pencil-thick, green and do not turn woody. They are covered in 6 rows of climbing barbs. The leaves are 3 to 5 lobed, serrate and opposite.

Characteristics: Lupulin has a very strong odor and an extremely bitter taste.

Habitat: Indigenous to Europe, cultivated in Asia, U.S., and elsewhere.

Production: Hop cones consist of the whole dried female inflorescences of Humulus lupulus.

ACTION AND PHARMACOLOGY

COMPOUNDS

Acylphloroglucinols (10%)

Alpha-bitter acids: including, among others, humulone, cohumulone, adhumulone

Beta-bitter acids: including, among others, lupulone, colupulone, adlupulone

Volatile oil (0.3-1.0%): very complex in makeup, chief components myrcene, humulene, beta-caryophyllene, undecane-2-on, furthermore 2-methyl-but-3-en-ol (particularly following storage, as breakdown product of the acylphloroglucinols)

Resins

Phenolic acid: including, among others, ferulic acid, caffeic acid and their derivatives, for example, chlorogenic acid

Tannins: oligomeric proanthocyanidines

Flavonoids: including, among others, xanthohumole

EFFECTS

Sedative and therefore sleep inducing.

INDICATIONS AND USAGE

■ Nervousness and insomnia

Useful as a sleeping aid and for restlessness and anxiety. As a bitter and stomachic to stimulate the appetite and increase the secretion of gastric juices.

PRECAUTIONS AND ADVERSE REACTIONS

No health hazards or side effects are known in conjunction with the proper administration of designated therapeutic dosages. The fresh plant has a sensitizing effect (hop-picker's disease), which may occur, more rarely, with the dust of the drug as well.

DOSAGE

Mode of Administration: Comminuted drug, powdered drug or dry extract powder for infusions or decoctions or other preparations; liquid and solid preparations for internal use and externally for bath additives.

Note: combinations with other sedatives can be beneficial.

Preparation: To prepare an infusion, boiling water is poured over the ground hop cones and left to draw for 10 to 15 minutes (1 teaspoonful = 0.4 g drug).

Daily Dosage: The single dose is 0.5 g.

Storage: Protect from light and moisture.

LITERATURE

Bravo L et al., (1974) Boll Chim Farm:306.

Caujolle F et al., (1969) Agressologie 10:405.

Field JA et al., Determination of essential oils in hops by headspace solid- phase microextraktion. In: J Agric Food Chem 44(7):1768-1772. 1996.

Fintelmann V, Klinisch-ärztliche Bedeutung des Hopfens. In: ZPT 13(5):165. 1992.

Ganzer BM, Hopfen: nicht nur für die Bierbrauerei. In: PZ 137(38):2824. 1992.

Hänsel R et al., (1982) Planta Med 45(4):224.

Hänsel R, Pflanzliche Beruhigungsmittel Möglichkeiten und Grenzen der Selbstmedikation. In: DAZ 135(32):2935-2943. 1995.

Hänsel R, Wagener HH, (1967) Versuche, sedativ-hypnotische Wirkstoffe im Hopfen nachzuweisen. Arzneim Forsch/Drug Res 17:79-81.

Hartley RD, (1968) Phytochemistry 7:1641.

Hartley RD, Fawcett CH, (1968) Phytochemistry 7:1395.

Hölzl J, Inhaltsstoffe des Hopfens (Humulus lupulus L.). In: ZPT 13(5):155. 1992.

Kumai A, Okamoto R, (1984) Toxicol Lett 21(2):203.

Moir M et al., (1980) Phytochemistry 19(10):2201.

Orth-Wagner S, Ressin WJ, Friedrich I, Phytosedativum gegen Schlafstörungen. In: ZPT 16(3):147-156. 1995.

Schmalreck AF et al., (1975) Can J Microbiol 21:205.

Schulz V, Hübner WD, Ploch M, Klinische Studien mit Psycho-Phytopharmaka. In: ZPT 18(3):141-154. 1997.

Stevens JF, Ivancic M, Hsu VL, Deinzer ML, Prenylflavonoids from Humulus lupulus. In: PH 44(8):1575-1585. 1997.

Stocker HR, (1967) Sedative und hypnogene Wirkung des Hopfens. Schweizer Brauerei Rundschau 78:80-89.

Tobe H, Muraki Y, Kitamura K, Komiyama O, Sato Y, Sugioka T, Maruyama HB, Matsuda E, Nagai M, Bone resorption inhibitors from hope extract. In: Biosc Biotech Biochem 61(1):158-159. 1997.

Wohlfart R, (1983) Dtsch Apoth Ztg 123:1637.

Wohlfart R, Hänsel R, Schmidt H, (1983) Nachweis sedativ-hypnotischer Wirkstoffe im Hopfen. 4. Mittlg. Die Pharmakologie des Hopfeninhaltsstoffes 2-Methyl-3-buten-2-ol. Planta Med 48:120-123.

Wohlfart R, Wurm G, Hänsel R, Schmidt H, (1983) Der Abbau der Bittersäuren zum 2-Methyl-3-buten-2-ol, einem Hopfeninhaltsstoff mit sedativ-hypnotischer Wirkung. Arch Pharmaz 315:132-137.

Further information in:

Hänsel R, Keller K, Rimpler H, Schneider G (Hrsg.), Hagers Handbuch der Pharmazeutischen Praxis, 5. Aufl., Bde 4-6 (Drogen), Springer Verlag Berlin, Heidelberg, New York, 1992-1994.

Lewin L, Gifte und Vergiftungen, 6. Aufl., Nachdruck, Haug Verlag, Heidelberg 1992.

Madaus G, Lehrbuch der Biologischen Arzneimittel, Bde 1-3, Nachdruck, Georg Olms Verlag Hildesheim 1979.

Roth L, Daunderer M, Kormann K, Giftpflanzen, Pflanzengifte, 4. Aufl., Ecomed Fachverlag Landsberg Lech 1993.

Schulz R, Hänsel R, Rationale Phytotherapie, Springer Verlag Heidelberg 1996.

Steinegger E, Hänsel R, Pharmakognosie, 5. Aufl., Springer Verlag Heidelberg 1992.

Teuscher E, Biogene Arzneimittel, 5. Aufl., Wiss. Verlagsges. Stuttgart 1997

Wagner H, Wiesenauer M, Phytotherapie. Phytopharmaka und pflanzliche Homöopathika, Fischer-Verlag, Stuttgart, Jena, New York 1995.

Wichtl M (Hrsg.), Teedrogen, 4. Aufl., Wiss. Verlagsges. Stuttgart 1997.

Hydnocarpus Species

Chaulmoogra

DESCRIPTION

Medicinal Parts: Any of the named species can be found in Chaulmoogra. The expressed oil is known as Gynocardia oil in Britain and Oleum Chaulmoograe in the U.S.

Flower and Fruit: The seeds grayish, about 2 to 3 cm long and 1.5 cm in diameter. They are irregularly angular with rounded ends. The kernel is oily and encloses two thin, heart-shaped, three-veined cotyledons and a straight radical.

Characteristics: The taste is acrid and the odor disagreeable.

Habitat: Malaysia, Indian subcontinent.

Production: Chaulmoogra seeds are the seeds of various Hydnocarpus varieties. Chaulmoogra oil is the fatty oil extracted from the seeds.

Other Names: Hydnocarpus

ACTION AND PHARMACOLOGY

COMPOUNDS: HYDNOCARPUS SPECIES SEMEN

Fatty oil (30-40%, bitter-type consistency)

Proteins (25%)

Cyanogenic glycosides

Flavolignans

COMPOUNDS: HYDNOCARPUS SPECIES OLEUM

Triglycerides: chief fatty acids D-hydnocarpic acid, D-chaulmoogric acid, D-gorli acid (cyclopentene fatty acids)

EFFECTS

The drug has sedative, febrifuge and dermatic effects.

INDICATIONS AND USAGE

Externally, preparations of Hydnocarpus are used in the treatment of various skin conditions such as psoriasis and eczema. It is also used as an injection in the treatment of leprosy.

PRECAUTIONS AND ADVERSE REACTIONS

Coughing, dyspnea, laryngospasms, kidney damage, visual disorders, head and muscle pain and central paralyses are side effects following intake of the oil. It is severely irritating in local application.

OVERDOSAGE

Following stomach and intestinal emptying (inducement of vomiting, gastric lavage with burgundy-colored potassium permanganate solution, sodium sulfate), the treatment for poisonings consists of the instillation of activated charcoal and shock prophylaxis (quiet, warmth), and of electrolyte substitution and the countering of any acidosis imbalance that may appear through sodium bicarbonate infusions. In the event of shock, plasma volume expanders should be infused. Monitoring of kidney function is necessary. Intubation and oxygen respiration may also be required.

The seeds are severely poisonous due to their cynagenic glycoside content. Injections of solutions of Dicobalt-EDTA or of thiosulphates, or administration of methemoglobin-forming agents, such as amyl nitrite, are recommended as antidotes. The triggering of vomiting and gastric lavage should be carried out in a parallel fashion. Circulatory support measures and artificial respiration may be required.

Mode of Administration: The seeds and oil in various preparations, as powder, oil, emulsion and ointments.

LITERATURE

Lefort D et al., (1969) Planta Med 17:261.

Sleumer, (1947) Pharm Ztg 83:165.

Further information in:

Kern W, List PH, Hörhammer L (Hrsg.), Hagers Handbuch der Pharmazeutischen Praxis, 4. Aufl., Bde 1-8, Springer Verlag Berlin, Heidelberg, New York, 1969.

Madaus G, Lehrbuch der Biologischen Arzneimittel, Bde 1-3, Nachdruck, Georg Olms Verlag Hildesheim 1979.

Roth L, Daunderer M, Kormann K, Giftpflanzen, Pflanzengifte, 4. Aufl., Ecomed Fachverlag Landsberg Lech 1993.

Teuscher E, Biogene Arzneimittel, 5. Aufl., Wiss. Verlagsges. Stuttgart 1997.

Hydrangea Arborescens

Hydrangea

DESCRIPTION

Medicinal Parts: The medicinal parts are the dried rhizome and the roots.

Flower and Fruit: The inflorescences are flat cymes of umbels with creamy white flowers. They are androgynous or completely sexless and have inferior ovaries. The fruit is a schizocarp or capsule.

Leaves, Stem and Root: Hydrangea is a marsh plant, a bush up to 3 m high whose leaves are only pubescent on the veins of the undersides. The petiole is 2 to 5 cm long. The leaves are simple or lobed and opposite. There are no stipules. The bark is rough and tends to peel off. The roots are of various lengths and widths. They are pale gray on the outside and solid with a slight splitting structure and white inside.

Habitat: Indigenous to the eastern U.S. as far south as Florida.

Production: Hydrangea root is the root of Hydrangea arborescens.

Other Names: Seven Barks

ACTION AND PHARMACOLOGY

COMPOUNDS

Saponins

Flavonolids: including, among others, rutin

Etheric oil

Isocoumarine derivatives: including, among others, hydrangenol

EFFECTS

The drug has a diuretic effect.

INDICATIONS AND USAGE

Hydrangea is used in the treatment of conditions of the urinary tract, in particular, bladder and kidney stones.

PRECAUTIONS AND ADVERSE REACTIONS

No health hazards or side effects are known in conjunction with the proper administration of designated therapeutic dosages. According to information in older medical literature, the intake of larger dosages can lead to dizziness, feelings of constriction in the chest and to central disorders. The plant has a weak potential for sensitization (chief allergen hydrangenol).

DOSAGE

Mode of Administration: Liquid extract, in preparations.

LITERATURE

Bate-Smith EC, (1978) Phytochemistry 17:267.

Der Mardirossian A et al., (1976) J Toxicol Environ Health 1: 939.

Further information in:

Frohne D, Pfänder HJ, Giftpflanzen - Ein Handbuch für Apotheker, Toxikologen und Biologen, 4. Aufl., Wiss. Verlags-Ges. Stuttgart 1997.

Hausen B, Allergiepflanzen, Pflanzenallergene, ecomed Verlagsgesellsch. mbH, Landsberg 1988.

Kern W, List PH, Hörhammer L (Hrsg.), Hagers Handbuch der Pharmazeutischen Praxis, 4. Aufl., Bde 1-8, Springer Verlag Berlin, Heidelberg, New York, 1969.

Leung AY, Encyclopedia of Common Natural Ingredients Used in Food Drugs and Cosmetics, John Wiley & Sons Inc., New York 1980.

Lewin L, Gifte und Vergiftungen, 6. Aufl., Nachdruck, Haug Verlag, Heidelberg 1992.

Madaus G, Lehrbuch der Biologischen Arzneimittel, Bde 1-3, Nachdruck, Georg Olms Verlag Hildesheim 1979.

Roth L, Daunderer M, Kormann K, Giftpflanzen, Pflanzengifte, 4. Aufl., Ecomed Fachverlag Landsberg Lech 1993.

Hydrastis Canadensis

Golden Seal

DESCRIPTION

Medicinal Parts: The medicinal parts are the air-dried rhizome with the root fibers.

Flower and Fruit: The flower is small, solitary, terminal and erect. It has 3 small greenish white petals which drop as soon as they come out. The fruit is a group of small, fleshy, oblong carmine berries with 1 or 2 hard, black and glossy seeds. The fruit is similar to the raspberry but is not edible.

Leaves, Stem and Root: The plant is a low herbaceous perennial about 30 cm high. It has a horizontal bright yellow, knotty and twisted rhizome about 0.6 to 1.8 cm thick out of which the root fibers grow. It is folded longitudinally and encircled by old leaf scars. The fracture is short and shows a dark, yellow cut surface, thick bark, large pith and broad medullary rays. The flowering stem appears in spring and is erect, cylindrical, downward pubescent, 15 to 30 cm tall and has a few short brown scales at the base. It bears 2 clearly ribbed, dark green and pubescent, cauline leaves. The lower one is sessile the upper one petiolate, round and divided into 7 lobes and finely serrate. There is also a root leaf on a long petiole, which is similar to the cauline leaves but larger.

Characteristics: The taste is very bitter, the smell is strong, characteristic and disagreeable.

Habitat: Indigenous to the U.S., cultivated elsewhere.

Production: Golden Seal root is the rhizome of hydrastis canadensis. The root is dug up in the autumn and dried.

Other Names: Orange Root, Yellow Root, Yellow Puccoon, Ground Raspberry, Wild Curcuma, Turmeric Root, Indian Dye, Eye Root, Eye Balm, Indian Paint, Jaundice Root, Warnera, Indian Plant

ACTION AND PHARMACOLOGY

COMPOUNDS

Isoquinoline alkaloids: chief alkaloids hydrastine, berberine, (-)-canadine

Starch

EFFECTS

The drug is oxytocic. It is also a mild laxative and anti-inflammatory as well as a vasoconstrictor and hypertensive.

INDICATIONS AND USAGE

Golden Seal is used externally on wounds and herpes labialis.

PRECAUTIONS AND ADVERSE REACTIONS

If taken over an extended period, the drug can bring about digestive disorders, constipation, excitatory states, hallucinations and occasionally deliria.

OVERDOSAGE

High dosages lead to vomiting, difficulty in breathing, bradycardia, spasms, eventually to central paralysis. Following stomach and intestinal emptying (inducement of vomiting, gastric lavage with burgundy-colored potassium permanganate solution, sodium sulfate) the treatment for poisonings consists of the instillation of activated charcoal and shock prophylaxis (quiet, warmth). The treatment of spasms with diazepam (I.V.), electrolyte substitution and the countering of any acidosis imbalance that may appear with sodium bicarbonate infusions may be necessary. In the event of shock, plasma volume expanders should be infused. Intubation and oxygen respiration may also be required.

DOSAGE

Mode of Administration: The drug is no longer in used externally as a fluid extract but is used in homeopathic dilutions for internal administration.

LITERATURE

Galefi C et al., Canadinic acid: an alkaloid from Hydrastis canadensis. In: PM 63(2):194. 1997.

Gleye J et al., (1974) Phytochemistry 13:675.

Haginiwa J, Harada M, (1962) Yakugaku Zasshi 82:726.

Further information in:

Kern W, List PH, Hörhammer L (Hrsg.), Hagers Handbuch der Pharmazeutischen Praxis, 4. Aufl., Bde 1-8, Springer Verlag Berlin, Heidelberg, New York, 1969.

Leung AY, Encyclopedia of Common Natural Ingredients Used in Food Drugs and Cosmetics, John Wiley & Sons Inc., New York 1980.

Lewin L, Gifte und Vergiftungen, 6. Aufl., Nachdruck, Haug Verlag, Heidelberg 1992.

Madaus G, Lehrbuch der Biologischen Arzneimittel, Bde 1-3, Nachdruck, Georg Olms Verlag Hildesheim 1979.

Roth L, Daunderer M, Kormann K, Giftpflanzen, Pflanzengifte, 4. Aufl., Ecomed Fachverlag Landsberg Lech 1993.

Steinegger E, Hänsel R, Pharmakognosie, 5. Aufl., Springer Verlag Heidelberg 1992.

Wagner H, Wiesenauer M, Phytotherapie. Phytopharmaka und pflanzliche Homöopathika, Fischer-Verlag, Stuttgart, Jena, New York 1995.

Hyoscyamus Niger

Henbane

DESCRIPTION

Medicinal Parts: The medicinal parts are the dried leaves or the dried leaves with the flowering branches, the dried seeds and the whole fresh flowering plant.

Flower and Fruit: The flowers are in almost sessile terminal, one-sided leafy and revolute spikes. The calyx is jug-shaped, 5-tipped and does not drop. The corolla is funnel-shaped, 5-lobed, dirty yellow with violet veins and dark violet in the tube. The flower has 1 superior ovary and 5 stamens. The fruit is a swollen pixidium with up to 200 seeds. The seeds are gray-brown, pitted, slightly reniform, compressed, 1 to 1.3 mm long and 1 mm wide.

Leaves, Stem and Root: The plant is an erect up to 80 cm high herb with simple leaves. The root is fusiform and turnip-like at the top. The stem is erect and sticky-villous. The leaves are oblong, roughly crenate-dentate and gray-green. The basal leaves are petiolate and the cauline leaves are stem-clasping.

Characteristics: The odor is numbing. It is poisonous.

Habitat: The plant is indigenous to Europe and western and northern Asia and northern Africa. It has been introduced to eastern Asia, North America and Australia.

Production: Henbane leaf consists of the dried leaves or the dried leaves and flowering tops of Hyoscyamus niger, harvested from cultures or in the wild when in bloom and dried mechanically or in the sun. Henbane seeds are the seeds of Hyoscyamus niger.

Other Names: Devil's Eye, Fetid Nightshade, Stinking Nightshade, Hen Bell, Hogbean, Jupiter's Bean, Poison Tobacco

ACTION AND PHARMACOLOGY

COMPOUNDS: HYOSCYAMI FOLIUM

Tropane alkaloids (0.05- 0.28%): chief alkaloid (-)-hyoscyamine, under storage conditions changing over to some extent into atropine, and scopolamine

Flavonoids: including, among others, rutin

COMPOUNDS: HYOSCYAMI SEMEN

Tropane alkaloids (0.05-0.3%): chief alkaloid (-)-hyoscyamine, under storage conditions changing to some extent into atropine, and scopolamine

Fatty oil

EFFECTS: HYOSCYAMI FOLIUM AND SEMEN

Main active agents: Alkaloids, flavonids. Henbane preparations produce a parasympatholytic or anticholinergic effect by competitive inhibition of acetylcholine. This inhibition affects the muscarinic action of acetylcholine but not its nicotine-like effects on ganglia and motor end-plates.

Henbane preparations exert peripheral actions on the autonomic nervous system and on smooth muscle, as well as the central nervous system. Because of their parasympatholytic properties, they cause relaxation of organs containing smooth muscle, particularly in the region of the gastrointestinal tract. Furthermore, they relieve muscular tremors of central nervous origin.

The spectrum of actions of Hyoscyamus niger additionally includes a sedative effect.

INDICATIONS AND USAGE

HYOSCYAMI FOLIUM

Spasms of the gastrointestinal tract; preparations of henbane oil are used for the treatment of scar tissue.

CONTRAINDICATIONS

HYOSCYAMI FOLIUM AND SEMEN

Tachycardiac arrhythmias, prostatic adenoma, angle-closure glaucoma, acute pulmonary edema, mechanical stenoses in the area of the gastrointestinal tract, megacolon.

PRECAUTIONS AND ADVERSE REACTIONS

HYOSCYAMI FOLIUM AND SEMEN

General: No health hazards are known in conjunction with the proper administration of designated therapeutic dosages. Skin reddening, dryness of the mouth, tachycardiac arrhythmias, mydriasis (the 4 early warning symptoms of a poisoning), accomodation disorders, heat build-up through decline in sweat secretion, miction disorders and obstipation can occur as side effects, particularly with overdosages.

Drug Interactions: Enhancement of anticholinergic action by tricyclic antidepressants, amantadine, antihistamines, phenothiazines, procainamide and quinidine.

OVERDOSAGE

Because of the high content of scopolamine in the drug, poisonings lead at first to somnolence, but then also, after the intake of very high dosages, to central excitation (restlessness, hallucinations, deliria, manic episodes), followed by exhaustion and sleep. Lethal dosages carry with them the danger of asphyxiation (for adults starting at 100 mg atropine, with an alkaloid-rich drug at 30, considerably less for children). Severe poisonings are particularly conceivable in connection with the misuse of the drug as an intoxicant. Treatment for poisonings include gastric lavage, temperature-lowering measures with wet cloths (no antipyretics!), oxygen respiration for respiratory distress, intubation, parenteral physostigmine salts as an antidote, diazepam for spasms, and chlorpromazine for severe excitation.

DOSAGE

HYOSCYAMI FOLIUM

Mode of Administration: Standardized henbane powder and galenic preparations for internal application.

Daily Dosage: The average single dose is 0.5 g of standardized henbane powder corresponding to 0.25 to 0.35 mg total alkaloid. Maximum daily dose is 3.0 g of standardized henbane powder corresponding to 1.5 to 2.1 mg total alkaloid, calculated as hyoscyamine.

HYOSCYAMI SEMEN

Mode of Administration: The drug is available as an emulsion or powder.

LITERATURE

HYOSCYAMI FOLIUM

Kraft K, Europäische Rauschdrogen. In: ZPT 17(6):343-355. 1996.

Sharova EG et al., Khim Prir Soedin (1):126. 1977.

Wellen BJ, Zur Geschichte des Bilsenkrautes. Eine pharmaziehistorische Untersuchung besonders zu Hyoscyamus niger L. In: Dissertation Universität Marburg. 1986.

Further information in:

Frohne D, Pfänder HJ, Giftpflanzen - Ein Handbuch für Apotheker, Toxikologen und Biologen, 4. Aufl., Wiss. Verlags-Ges. Stuttgart 1997.

Hänsel R, Keller K, Rimpler H, Schneider G (Hrsg.), Hagers Handbuch der Pharmazeutischen Praxis, 5. Aufl., Bde 4-6 (Drogen), Springer Verlag Berlin, Heidelberg, New York, 1992-1994.

Lewin L, Gifte und Vergiftungen, 6. Aufl., Nachdruck, Haug Verlag, Heidelberg 1992.

Madaus G, Lehrbuch der Biologischen Arzneimittel, Bde 1-3, Nachdruck, Georg Olms Verlag Hildesheim 1979.

Roth L, Daunderer M, Kormann K, Giftpflanzen, Pflanzengifte, 4. Aufl., Ecomed Fachverlag Landsberg Lech 1993.

Steinegger E, Hänsel R, Pharmakognosie, 5. Aufl., Springer Verlag Heidelberg 1992.

Teuscher E, Lindequist U, Biogene Gifte - Biologie, Chemie, Pharmakologie, 2. Aufl., Fischer Verlag Stuttgart 1994.

Teuscher E, Biogene Arzneimittel, 5. Aufl., Wiss. Verlagsges. Stuttgart 1997.

Wagner H, Wiesenauer M, Phytotherapie. Phytopharmaka und pflanzliche Homöopathika, Fischer-Verlag, Stuttgart, Jena, New York 1995.

HYOSCYAMI SEMEN

Tattje DHE et al., Zusammensetzung der etherischen Öle von Laurus nobilis, L. nobilis var. angustifolia und L. azorica. In: PM 44(2):116-119. 1982.

Further information in:

Frohne D, Pfänder HJ, Giftpflanzen - Ein Handbuch für Apotheker, Toxikologen und Biologen, 4. Aufl., Wiss. Verlags-Ges. Stuttgart 1997.

Hänsel R, Keller K, Rimpler H, Schneider G (Hrsg.), Hagers Handbuch der Pharmazeutischen Praxis, 5. Aufl., Bde 4-6 (Drogen), Springer Verlag Berlin, Heidelberg, New York, 1992-1994.

Lewin L, Gifte und Vergiftungen, 6. Aufl., Nachdruck, Haug Verlag, Heidelberg 1992.

Madaus G, Lehrbuch der Biologischen Arzneimittel, Bde 1-3, Nachdruck, Georg Olms Verlag Hildesheim 1979.

Roth L, Daunderer M, Kormann K, Giftpflanzen, Pflanzengifte, 4. Aufl., Ecomed Fachverlag Landsberg Lech 1993.

Teuscher E, Lindequist U, Biogene Gifte - Biologie, Chemie, Pharmakologie, 2. Aufl., Fischer Verlag Stuttgart 1994.

Hypericum Perforatum

St. John's Wort

DESCRIPTION

Medicinal Parts: The medicinal parts include the fresh buds and flowers separated from the inflorescences, the aerial parts collected during the flowering season and dried, and the whole fresh flowering plant.

Flower and Fruit: The golden yellow flowers are in sparsely-blossomed terminal cymes. The 5 sepals are ovate-lanceolate to lanceolate, very pointed, entire-margined or serrate at the tip, glabrous and marked by many light and dark glands. The 5 petals and numerous stamens are fused into 3 bundles. The ovary is broad to narrowly ovate. The fruit is an ovate, triangular, 3-valvular capsule. The seeds are cylindrical, shortly pointed at both ends and covered in small warts. The seeds are 1 to 3 mm long, black or dark brown.

Leaves, Stem and Root: The plant is a perennial with a long-living, fusiform, branched root and branched rhizome. The stem is erect with 2 raised edges, reddish tinged and 100 cm high. The leaves are oval-oblong, entire-margined, opposite, translucent punctate, sessile and often covered in black glands.

Characteristics: When squeezed the flowers release a red juice which colors violet. It is odorless and the taste is weakly bitter, scratchy.

Habitat: The plant is indigenous to all of Europe, western Asia, and northern Africa. It has been introduced to eastern Asia, Australia, New Zealand. It is cultivated elsewhere.

Production: St. John's Wort consists of the dried above-ground parts of Hypericum perforatum gathered during flowering season. The herb is cut at the start of the flowering season and dried in bunches. It should be dried quickly (in warm weather in a drying room), in order to preserve oil and secreted contents.

Not To Be Confused With: Other Hypericum species, such as Hypericum barbatum, Hypericum hirsutum, Hypericum maculatum, Hypericum montanum and Hypericum tetrapterum.

Other Names: Hardhay, Amber, Goatweed, Klamath Weed, Tipton Weed

ACTION AND PHARMACOLOGY

COMPOUNDS

Anthracene derivatives (0.1-0.15%): favoring naphthadihydrodianthrones, in particular hypericin, pseudohypericin

Flavonoids (2-4%): in particular hyperoside, quercitrin, rutin, isoquercitrin, also biflavonolids, including, among others, amentoflavone

Xanthones: 1,3,6,7-tetrahydroxy-xanthone

Acylphloroglucinols: hyperforin with small quantities of adhhyperforin

Volatile oil: chief components aliphatic hydrocarbons, including, among others, 2- methyloctane, undecane, furthermore dodecanol, mono- and sesquiterpenes: including, among others, alpha-pinene, caryophyllene, additionally also 2-methyl-3-but-3-en-2-ol

Oligomeric procyanidines

Catechin tannins

Caffeic acid derivatives: including, among others, chlorogenic acid

EFFECTS

A mild antidepressant, sedative and anxiolytic action of the herb and its preparations has been observed and reported by numerous doctors. Studies have demonstrated that the antidepressive effect may be due to the presence of a monoamine oxidase inhibiting function in the active agents. More recent studies have indicated that the antidepressive effect may be largely due to the ability of the herb to inhibit the reuptake of serotonin. Oily hypericum preparations demonstrate an anti-inflammatory action due to their high flavonoid content.

INDICATIONS

- Anxiety
- Depressive moods
- Inflammation of the skin
- Blunt injuries
- Wounds and burns

Internally, the drug is used for psychovegetative disturbances, depressive moods, anxiety, or nervous unrest. Oily hypericum preparations are used for dyspeptic complaints. Externally, oily hypericum preparations are used for treatment and post-therapy of acute and contused injuries, myalgia and first-degree burns.

PRECAUTIONS AND ADVERSE REACTIONS

No health hazards are known in conjunction with the proper administration of designated therapeutic dosages. The tannin content of the drug can lead to digestive complaints, such as feeling of fullness or constipation. Photosensitization has been observed in animals following intakes of large quantities of the drug (starting at 3 g per kg body weight, which would be 150 g for a person weighing 50 kg) (hypericismus). However, such a reaction is unlikely with administration of therapeutic dosages.

DOSAGE

Mode of Administration: Comminuted drug, herb powder, liquid and solid preparations for internal use; liquid and semi-solid preparations for external use; preparations made with fatty oils for external and internal use.

Preparation: To prepare an infusion, use 2 teaspoonfuls of drug in 150 ml boiling water and steep for 10 minutes.

Daily Dosage: The average daily dose for internal use is 2 to 4 g of drug or 0.2 to 1.0 mg of total hypericin in other forms of drug application.

For depressive moods an intake over a duration of 4 to 6 weeks is recommended; if no improvement is apparent, another therapy should be used (response quotient 60-80%).

LITERATURE

Araya OS, Ford EJH, (1981) An investigation of the type of photosensitization caused by the ingestion of St. John's Wort (hypericum perforatum) by calves. J Comp Pathol 91:135-141.

Baldt S, Wagner H, (1994) Inhibition of MAO by Fractions and Constiuents of Hypericum Extract. J Geriatr Psychiatry Neurol 7(Suppl 1):57-59.

Borsini F, Meli A, (1988) Is the forced swimming test a suitable model for revealing antidepressant activity? Psychopharmacology 94:147-160.

Butterweck V et al., Isolation by MLCCC and NMR spectroscopy of hypericin, pseudohypericin and I3,II8-biapigenin from Hypericum perforatum. In: PM 62, Abstracts of the 44th Ann Congress of GA, 119. 1996.

Butterweck V, Winterhoff H, Schulz V, Nahrstedt A, Pharmacological in vivo testing of fractions obtained from Hypericum perforatum L. In: PM 62, Abstracts of the 44th Ann Congress of GA, 65. 1996.

Carpenter S, Kraus GA, Photosensitization required for inactivation of equine infectious anaemia virus by hypericin. In: Photochem Photobiol 53:169-174. 1991.

Czygan FC, (1993) Kulturgeschichte und Mystik des Johanniskrautes. Z Phytother 14:276-281.

Danie K, (1939) Inhaltsstoffe und Prüfmethoden homöopathisch verwendeter Arzneipflanzen. Hippokrates 10:5-6.

Decoaterd LA, Hoffmann E, Kyburz D, Bray D, Hostettmann K, A new phloroglucinol derivative from Hypericum-calycinum with antifungal and in vitro antimalarial activity. In: PM 57:548. 1991.

Dingermann T, Phytopharmaka im Alter: Crataegus, Ginkgo, Hypericum und Kava-Kava. In: PZ 140(23):2017-2024. 1995.

Engelhardt A, (1962) Justinus Kerner und das Johanniskraut. Apotheker-Dienst Roche 3:51-55.

Ernst E, (1959) St. John's Wort, an anti-depressant? A systematic, criteria-based overview. Phytomedicine 2:67-71.

Freytag WE, (1984) Dtsch Apoth Ztg 124(46):2383.

Giese AC, (1980) Hypericism. Photochem Photobiol Rev 5:229-255.

Hänsel R, Keller K, Rimpler H, Schneider G, (Hrsg.), (1993) Hagers Handbuch der Pharmazeutischen Praxis, 5. Auflage, Drogen E-O. Springer Verlag, Berlin Heidelberg New York, S 268-292.

Hänsgen KD, Vesper J, (1996) Antidepressive Wirksamkeit eines hochdosierten Hypericum-Extraktes. Münch Med Wschr 138:29-33.

Harrer G, Payk TR, Schulz V, (Hrsg) Hypericum als pflanzliches Antidepressivum. Nervenheilkunde 12:268-366.

Harrer G, Schulz V, (1993) Zur Prüfung der antidepressiven Wirksamkeit von Hypericum. Nervenheilkunde 12:271-273.

Harrer G, Sommer H, Treatment of mild/moderate depressions with Hypericum. In: Phytomedicine 1:3-8. 1994.

Hiller KO, Rahlfs V, Therapeutische Äquivalenz eines hochdosierten Phytopharmakons mit Amytriptylin bei ängstlich-depressiven Versimmungen - Reanalyse einer randomisierten Studie unter besonderer Beachtung biometrischer und klinischer Aspekte. In: Forsch.

Hölzl J, Inhaltsstoffe und Wirkungsmechanismen des Johanniskrautes. In: ZPT 14(5):255. 1993.

Hölzl J, Ostrowski E, (1986) Planta Med 6:62P.

Hölzl J, Sattler S, Schütt H, Johanniskraut: eine Alternative zu synthetischen Antidepressiva. In: PZ 139(46):3959. 1994.

Jenike MA, (ed) (1994) Hypericum: A Novel Antidepressant. J Geriatr Psychiatry Neurol 7:S1-S68.

Kil KS, Yum YN, Seo SH, Antitumor activities of hypericin as a protein tyrosine kinase blocker. In: Arch Pharmacal Res 19(6):490-496. 1996.

Kitanov G et al., (1984) Khim Prir Soedin 2:269.

Koren H, Schenk GM, Jindra RH, Alth G, Ebermann R, Kubin A, Koderhold G, Kreitner M, Hypericin in phototherapy. In: J Photochem Photobiol B - Biology 36(2):113-119. 1996.

Laux G, (1995) Kontrollierte Vergleichsstudien mit Moclobemid in der Depressionsbehandlung. Münch Med Wschr 137:296-300.

Leuschner J, (1995) Gutachten zur experimentellen Toxikologie von Hypericum-Extrakt LI 160. Lichtwer Pharma GmbH, Berlin.

Linde K et al., St John's wort for depression - An overview and meta-analysis of randomized clinical trials. In: Brit Med J 313(7052):253-258. 1996.

Lopez-Bazzocchi I, Hudson JB, Towers GHN, Antiviral activity of the photoactive plant pigment hypericin. In: Photochem Photobiol 54:95-98. 1991.

Maisenbacher P, Johanniskrautöl. In: DAZ 132(6):281. 1992.

Mathic C, Ourrison G, (1964) Phytochemistry 3:115, 133, 377, 379.

Müller WE, Schäfer C, Johanniskraut In-vitro-Studie über Hypericum-Extrakt, Hypericin und Kämpferol. In: DAZ 136(13):1015-1022. 1996.

Müller WEG, Rossol R, (1994) Effects of Hypericum Extract on the Expression of Serotonin Receptors. J Geriatr Psychiatry Neurol 7(Suppl 1):63-64.

Muldner H, Zoller M, (1984) Arzneim Forsch. 34II(8):918.

Niesel S, (1992) Untersuchungen zum Freisetzungsverhalten und zur Stabilität ausgewählter wertbestimmender Pflanzeninhaltsstoffe unter besonderer Berücksichtigung moderner phytochemischer Analysenverfahren. Inaugural-Dissertation. Freie Universität Berlin.

Popovic M et al., Biochemical and pharmacodynamic study of Hypericum perforatum. In: PM 62, Abstracts of the 44th Ann Congress of GA, 67. 1996.

Rammert K, Phytopharmaka: Johanniskraut als Antidepressivum. In: DAZ 136(46):4131-4132. 1996.

Reuter HD, Hypericum als pflanzliches Antidepressivum. In: ZPT 14(5):239. 1993.

Roth L, Hypericum - Hypericin: Botanik, Inhaltsstoffe, Wirkung. In: ZPT 13(5):174. 1992.

Roth L, Hypericum. In: Roth L: Hypericum Hypericin, Botanik, Inhaltsstoffe, Wirkung. 1990.

Saller R, Hellenbrecht D, Johanniskraut (Hypericum perforatum). In: Tägl Praxis 33(3):689. 1992.

Sparenberg B, Demisch L, Hölzl J, Untersuchungen über antidepressive Wirkstoffe von Johanniskraut. In: PZW 138(2)50. 1993.

Suzuki O et al., (1984) Planta Med 3:272.

Thiele, B, Brink I, Ploch M, (1993) Modulation der Zytkokin-Expression durch Hypericum-Extrakt. Mervemjeoölimde 12:353-356.

Volz HP, Hänsel R, (1995) Hypericum (Johanniskraut) als pflanzliches Antidepressivum. Psychopharmakotherapie 2:1-9.

Wagner H, Bladt S, (1993) Pharmazeutische Qualität der Hypericum-Extrakte. Nervenheilkunde 12:362-366.

Willner P, (1984) The validity of animal models of depression. Psychopharmacology 83:1-16.

Winterhoff H, Butterweck V, Nahrstedt A, Gumbinger HG, Schulz V, Erping S, Boßhammer F, Wieligmann A, (1995) Pharmakologische Untersuchungen zur antidepressiven Wirkung von Hypericum perforatum L. In: Loew D, Rietbrock N (Hrsg.) Phytopharmaka in Forschung und klinischer Anwendung. Steinkopff Verlag, Darmstadt, S 39-56.

Winterhoff H, Hambrügge M, Vahlensieck W, (1993) Testung von Hypericum perforatum L. im Tierexperiment. Nervenheilkunde 12:341-345.

Further information in:

Frohne D, Pfänder HJ, Giftpflanzen - Ein Handbuch für Apotheker, Toxikologen und Biologen, 4. Aufl., Wiss. Verlags-Ges. Stuttgart 1997.

Hänsel R, Keller K, Rimpler H, Schneider G (Hrsg.), Hagers Handbuch der Pharmazeutischen Praxis, 5. Aufl., Bde 4-6 (Drogen), Springer Verlag Berlin, Heidelberg, New York, 1992-1994.

Lewin L, Gifte und Vergiftungen, 6. Aufl., Nachdruck, Haug Verlag, Heidelberg 1992.

Madaus G, Lehrbuch der Biologischen Arzneimittel, Bde 1-3, Nachdruck, Georg Olms Verlag Hildesheim 1979.

Roth L, Daunderer M, Kormann K, Giftpflanzen, Pflanzengifte, 4. Aufl., Ecomed Fachverlag Landsberg Lech 1993.

Schulz R, Hänsel R, Rationale Phytotherapie, Springer Verlag Heidelberg 1996.

Steinegger E, Hänsel R, Pharmakognosie, 5. Aufl., Springer Verlag Heidelberg 1992.

Teuscher E, Lindequist U, Biogene Gifte - Biologie, Chemie, Pharmakologie, 2. Aufl., Fischer Verlag Stuttgart 1994.

Teuscher E, Biogene Arzneimittel, 5. Aufl., Wiss. Verlagsges. Stuttgart 1997.

Wagner H, Wiesenauer M, Phytotherapie. Phytopharmaka und pflanzliche Homöopathika, Fischer-Verlag, Stuttgart, Jena, New York 1995.

Wichtl M (Hrsg.), Teedrogen, 4. Aufl., Wiss. Verlagsges. Stuttgart 1997.

Hyssopus Officinalis

Hyssop

DESCRIPTION

Medicinal Parts: The medicinal parts are the leaves, the flower tips and the essential oil.

Flower and Fruit: The dark-blue bilabiate flowers are medium-sized false whorls in one-sided, terminal leafy racemes. The calyx is downy, 5-tiped and glabrous inside. There are 4 stamens, which are turned away from each other and extend far above the perianth. The style is very long.

Leaves, Stem and Root: The plant is an evergreen subshrub about 60 cm high. The stem is erect, quadrangular, shrubby and branched. The leaves are sessile, lanceolate, acute, entire-margined, punctate, glabrous, dark green and paler beneath.

Characteristics: The plant has a weak sweetish smell. The taste is bitter.

Habitat: The plant is indigenous to southern Europe and grows wild in the Mediterranean region. It is cultivated elsewhere.

Production: Hyssop herb consists of the fresh or dried above-ground parts of Hyssopus officinalis. Hyssop oil consists of the essential oil of Hyssopus officinalis, obtained by steam distillation.

ACTION AND PHARMACOLOGY

COMPOUNDS

In the foliage:

Volatile oil

Tannins

Bitter principles: including, among others, marubiin

Flavonoids: glycosides of hesperidin and diosmetin in the volatile oil

Chief components: pinocamphone, alpha- and beta-pinene

EFFECTS

No information is available.

INDICATIONS AND USAGE

- Fevers and colds
- Liver and gallbladder complaints

Preparations of Hyssop herb are used for the gentle stimulation of circulation, for intestinal catarrhs, for diseases of the respiratory tract, colds, chest and lung ailments.

The effectiveness for the claimed applications is not documented.

PRECAUTIONS AND ADVERSE REACTIONS

No health hazards are known in conjunction with the proper administration of designated therapeutic dosages. Isolated cases of tonic-clonic spasms have been observed among adults after intakes of 10 to 30 drops of the volatile oil over a number of days (2 to 3 drops for children).

DOSAGE

No information is available.

LITERATURE

Joulain D, (1979) Riv Ital Ess Prof Piante Off Ar Sap Cosm 48:479.

Opdyke DLJ, (1978) Food Cosmet Toxicol 16 (Suppl. 1):787.

Further information in:

Kern W, List PH, Hörhammer L (Hrsg.), Hagers Handbuch der Pharmazeutischen Praxis, 4. Aufl., Bde. 1-8, Springer Verlag Berlin, Heidelberg, New York, 1969.

Leung AY, Encyclopedia of Common Natural Ingredients Used in Food Drugs and Cosmetics, John Wiley & Sons Inc., New York 1980.

Madaus G, Lehrbuch der Biologischen Arzneimittel, Bde 1-3, Nachdruck, Georg Olms Verlag Hildesheim 1979.

Iceland Moss

See Cetraria Islandica

Ignatius Beans

See Strychnos Ignatii

Ilex Aquifolium

Holly

DESCRIPTION

Medicinal Parts: The medicinal parts are the dried foliage leaves, the fresh leaves, the young leafy branches with the ripe berries and the flowers of the branch tips with the leaves.

Flower and Fruit: Because of the shrinking of the one sex, the flowers are usually dioecious. The inflorescence is a 1 to 3 flowered axillary cyme. They are white. The calyx is small and has 4 to 5 tips. The 5-petalled corolla is rotate. The ovary is superior. There are 4 to 5 stamens. The coral red fruit is a 4-sectioned, sessile, berry-like, pea-sized drupe with 4 to 5 seeds.

Leaves, Stem and Root: The plant is a 10 m high evergreen bush or tree smooth dark gray-brown bark. The bark on the younger branches is green and glossy. The branches and foliage are glabrous. The leaves are alternate, coriaceous, stiff, ovate or elliptical and acute. The lower ones are thorny denate, the upper ones entire-margined.

Characteristics: The flowers have a weak pleasant scent. The berries are poisonous to children.

Habitat: The plant is found in central Europe, North America and eastern Asia.

Production: Holly leaves and fruit are the leaves and fruit of Ilex aquifolium.

Other Names: Hulver Bush, Holm, Hulm, Holme Chase, Holy Tree, Christ's Thorn, Hulver Tree.

ACTION AND PHARMACOLOGY

COMPOUNDS

Saponins

Nitrile glycosides: menisdaurin, not cyanogenic

Flavonoids: including, among others, rutin, kaempferol and quercetin glycosides

Caffeic acid derivatives: chlorogenic acid

Sterols: beta-sitosterol, stigmasterol

Triterpenes: alpha-amyrin, alpha-amyrinester, beta-amyrin, ursolic acid

Purine alkaloids: only traces of theobromine

EFFECTS

No information is available.

INDICATIONS AND USAGE

Holly is used as a diuretic. Also used for coughs, digestive disorders and jaundice.

PRECAUTIONS AND ADVERSE REACTIONS

No health hazards or side effects are known in conjunction with the proper administration of designated therapeutic dosages.

OVERDOSAGE

The intake of more than 5 berries can lead to nausea, vomiting and diarrhea. Fatal gastrointestinal inflammation is said to have taken place following the ingestion of very large quantities (20 to 30 berries) (Lewin). Stomach emptying and the administration of activated charcoal should therefore be carried out with the intake of more than 10 berries. Further treatment should proceed according to symptoms. Poisonings have not been reported in recent times.

DOSAGE

Mode of Administration: As a tea and alcoholic extract.

LITERATURE

Lassere B et al., (1983) Naturwissenschaft 70:95.

Catalano S, Marsili A, Morelli J, Pistelli L, Constituents of the leaves of Ilex aquifolium. In: PM 33:416. 1978.

Further information in:

Frohne D, Pfänder HJ, Giftpflanzen - Ein Handbuch für Apotheker, Toxikologen und Biologen, 4. Aufl., Wiss. Verlags-Ges Stuttgart 1997.

Hänsel R, Keller K, Rimpler H, Schneider G (Hrsg.), Hagers Handbuch der Pharmazeutischen Praxis, 5. Aufl., Bde 4-6 (Drogen), Springer Verlag Berlin, Heidelberg, New York, 1992-1994 (unter Ilex paraguariensis).

Lewin L, Gifte und Vergiftungen, 6. Aufl., Nachdruck, Haug Verlag, Heidelberg 1992.

Madaus G, Lehrbuch der Biologischen Arzneimittel, Bde 1-3, Nachdruck, Georg Olms Verlag Hildesheim 1979.

Poisonous Plants in Britain and their effects on Animals and Man, Ministry of Agriculture Fisheries and Food, Pub; HMSO UK 1984.

Roth L, Daunderer M, Kormann K, Giftpflanzen, Pflanzengifte, 4. Aufl., Ecomed Fachverlag Landsberg Lech 1993.

Teuscher E, Lindequist U, Biogene Gifte - Biologie, Chemie, Pharmakologie, 2. Aufl., Fischer Verlag Stuttgart 1994.

Ilex Paraguariensis

Maté

DESCRIPTION

Medicinal Parts: The medicinal parts are the dried or roasted leaves.

Flower and Fruit: The white flowers are axillary and are in clusters of 40 to 50. They have a 4 to 5 sepaled calyx and 4 to 5 petalled corolla, are unisexual and dioecious. The fruit is a globoid reddish drupe with 5 to 8 seeds.

Leaves, Stem and Root: The plant is an evergreen shrub or tree up to 20 m tall with pale bark and an oblong-oval crown. The leaves are alternate, obovate, acuminate with a crenate or serrate margin. They are dark green above and pale green beneath and are tough, coriaceous and 6 to 20 cm long and 3 to 9 cm wide.

Characteristics: The taste is astringent and bitter. The odor is characteristic and aromatic.

Habitat: The plant is only found in South America between the 20th and 30th parallel.

Production: Maté consists of the dried leaf and leaf stem of Ilex paraguariensis.

Other Names: Yerba Maté, Jesuit's Tea, Paraguay Tea

ACTION AND PHARMACOLOGY

COMPOUNDS

Purine alkaloids: chief alkaloids caffeine (0.4-2.4%) and theobromine (0.3-0.5%)

Caffeic acid derivatives: including among others chlorogenic acid, neochlorogenic acid, cryptochlorogenic acid

Flavonoids: including among others rutin, isoquercitrin, kaempferol glycosides

Triterpene saponins (mate saponins)

Nitrile glycosides: menisdaurin, not cyanogenic

EFFECTS

The main active principles are caffeine in varying amounts, tannins and small amounts of essential oil. The drug stimulates the CNS, is analeptic, diuretic, positively inotropic, positively chronotropic, glycogenolytic and lipolytic.

INDICATIONS AND USAGE

- Infections of the urinary tract
- Cardiac insufficiency NYHA I and II
- Arrhythmia
- Lack of stamina
- Nervous heart complaints
- Kidney and bladder stones

Maté is used for mental and physical fatigue and as a diuretic.

PRECAUTIONS AND ADVERSE REACTIONS

No health hazards or side effects are known in conjunction with the proper administration of designated therapeutic dosages. For a statement regarding toxicology, see Coffea semen.

DOSAGE

Mode of Administration: Maté is available as comminuted herb for infusions, herb powder, and as galenic preparations for internal use. The drug is available as filter teas in mono tea form and in various tea combinations such as bladder and kidney teas.

Preparation: To prepare an infusion, pour water which has just been brought to boil over 1 teaspoonful drug (2 g) and leave to draw for 5 to 10 minutes, strain. The briefly infused drink is more stimulating, less astringent and tastes better (caffeine dissolves more quickly than the tannins).

Daily dosage: 3 g drug.

LITERATURE

Baltassat F et al., (1985) Plant Med Phytother 18(4):194.

Gosmann G et al., Triterpenoid saponins from Ilex paraguariensis. In: JNP 58(3):438-441. 1995.

Kraemer KH et al., A new polar saponin from Ilex paraguariensis. In: PM 61 (Abstracts of 43rd Ann Congr):62. 1995.

Further information in:

Fenaroli's Handbook of Flavor Ingredients, Vol. 1, 2nd Ed., CRC Press Boca Raton 1975.

Hänsel R, Keller K, Rimpler H, Schneider G (Hrsg.), Hagers Handbuch der Pharmazeutischen Praxis, 5. Aufl., Bde 4-6

(Drogen), Springer Verlag Berlin, Heidelberg, New York, 1992-1994 (unter Ilex paraguariensis).

Roth L, Daunderer M, Kormann K, Giftpflanzen, Pflanzengifte, 4. Aufl., Ecomed Fachverlag Landsberg Lech 1993.

Teuscher E, Lindequist U, Biogene Gifte - Biologie, Chemie, Pharmakologie, 2. Aufl., Fischer Verlag Stuttgart 1994.

Teuscher E, Biogene Arzneimittel, 5. Aufl., Wiss. Verlagsges. Stuttgart 1997.

Wichtl M (Hrsg.),Teedrogen, 4. Aufl., Wiss. Verlagsges. Stuttgart 1997.

Illicium Verum

Star Anise

DESCRIPTION

Medicinal Parts: The medicinal parts are the oil extracted from the ripe fruit, the whole dried fruit and the seeds.

Flower and Fruit: The flowers are yellowish or reddish white. The follicles have a diameter of about 2 cm. They are star-like and formed from eight cybiform carpels. The follicles open when ripe, each containing one smooth, polished brown seed. The pericarp of the seed is brown and wrinkled below.

Leaves, Stem and Root: The plant is an evergreen tree up to 10 m tall with white, birch-like bark. The leaves are 7.5 cm long, entire-margined, glossy, elliptic-lanceolate and acuminate.

Habitat: The plant is only known in its cultivated form. It is cultivated in China and Vietnam.

Production: Star anise consists of the ripe syncarp of Illicium verum.

Not To Be Confused With: Should not be confused with the smaller Japanese star anise (I. lanceolatum or I. religiosum) which is poisonous.

Other Names: Aniseed Stars, Badiana

ACTION AND PHARMACOLOGY

COMPOUNDS

Volatile oil: chief constituent trans-anethol, chavicol methyl ether (estragole), d-limonene, l-limonene, d-fenchone, d-pinene, dl-limonene, anisaldehyde

Fatty oil

Flavonoids

Tannins

EFFECTS

Bronchial expectorant, antispasmodic for the gastrointestinal tract.

INDICATIONS AND USAGE

- Loss of appetite
- Cough/bronchitis

Star Anise is used for catarrhs of the respiratory tract, peptic discomfort.

PRECAUTIONS AND ADVERSE REACTIONS

No health hazards or side effects are known in conjunction with the proper administration of designated therapeutic dosages. Sensitization has occurred very rarely in cases of repeated administration. The very similar berries of Illicium anisatum contain spasmogenic sesquiterpene lactones; confusions with star anis have been observed.

DOSAGE

Mode of Administration: Herb, ground fresh just prior to use, and other galenic preparations for internal use.

Daily Dosage: 3.0 g of drug or 0.3 g essential oil.

LITERATURE

Kubeczka KH, DAZ 122:2309. 1982.

Zänglein A, Schultze W, Illicium verum - Sternanis. In: ZPT 10(6):191. 1989.

Further information in:

Frohne D, Pfänder HJ, Giftpflanzen - Ein Handbuch für Apotheker, Toxikologen und Biologen, 4. Aufl., Wiss. Verlags-Ges Stuttgart 1997.

Hänsel R, Keller K, Rimpler H, Schneider G (Hrsg.), Hagers Handbuch der Pharmazeutischen Praxis, 5. Aufl., Bde 4-6 (Drogen), Springer Verlag Berlin, Heidelberg, New York, 1992-1994.

Leung AY, Encyclopedia of Common Natural Ingredients Used in Food Drugs and Cosmetics, John Wiley & Sons Inc., New York 1980.

Schulz R, Hänsel R, Rationale Phytotherapie, Springer Verlag Heidelberg 1996.

Steinegger E, Hänsel R, Pharmakognosie, 5. Aufl., Springer Verlag Heidelberg 1992.

Teuscher E, Lindequist U, Biogene Gifte - Biologie, Chemie, Pharmakologie, 2. Aufl., Fischer Verlag Stuttgart 1994.

Teuscher E, Biogene Arzneimittel, 5. Aufl., Wiss. Verlagsges. Stuttgart 1997.

Wichtl M (Hrsg.), Teedrogen, 4. Aufl., Wiss. Verlagsges. Stuttgart 1997.

Immortelle

See Helichrysum Arenarium

Impatiens Biflora

Jewel Weed

DESCRIPTION

Medicinal Parts: The medicinal part is the herb.

Flower and Fruit: The axillary flowers are orange-yellow with large reddish-brown spots. They have an irregular form. The sepal sac abruptly contracts to a spur of about 5 to 9 mm. The spur is bent 180 degrees to lie parallel with the sac. The fruit is an oblong capsule which, when ripe, bursts open at the slightest touch and spreads the seeds over large distances.

Leaves, Stem and Root: The plant is a glabrous, fleshy annual 20 to 180 cm high. The stems are simple or branched and have swollen nodes. The leaves are thin, ovate, with 5 to 12 (up to 14) teeth on each side and are often undulate. They are rich green.

Habitat: Impatiens is common in the temperate regions and in South Africa but grows mostly in the mountainous, tropical regions of Asia and Africa.

Production: Jewel Weed is the aerial part of Impatiens biflora.

Other Names: Wild Balsam, Balsam-weed, Spotted Touch-me-not, Slipperweed, Silverweed, Wild Lady's Slipper, Speckled Jewels, Wild Celandine, Quick-in-the-hand

ACTION AND PHARMACOLOGY

COMPOUNDS

Naphthacene derivatives: 1.4-naphthoquinone, in particular lawsone (2-hydroxy-1,4- naphthoquinone), yielding from the precursor through drying of the leaves 1,2,4-trihydroxy-naphthalene-4-beta-D-glucoside

EFFECTS

Digestive, diuretic.

INDICATIONS AND USAGE

Jewel Weed is used for mild digestive disorders.

PRECAUTIONS AND ADVERSE REACTIONS

No health hazards or side effects are known in conjunction with the proper administration of designated therapeutic dosages.

DOSAGE

Mode of Administration: Administered as the ground drug and as an infusion.

LITERATURE

Hegnauer R, Chemotaxonomie der Pflanzen, Bde 1-11, Birkhäuser Verlag Basel, Boston, Berlin 1962-1997.

Indian Physic

See Gillenia Trifoliata

Inula Helenium

Elecampane

DESCRIPTION

Medicinal Parts: The medicinal part is the dried or fresh rhizome.

Flower and Fruit: The inflorescences are yellow composite flowers in loose, terminal, panicled cymes. They are 7 to 8 cm in diameter. The involucre is imbricate and cup-shaped. The inner bracts are dry at the tip and splayed, the outer ones are like leaves and ovate. The female lateral florets are narrowly linguiform. The androgynous disc florets are tubular. The receptacle is flat, slightly pitted and glabrous. The flowers are a bright yellow. The achaenes are cylindrical, 4 to 5 mm long, brown, glabrous and have 4 tips. The pappus is 8 to 10 mm long and consists of brownish, fine, rough, brittle bristles.

Leaves, Stem and Root: The plant is perennial and 80 to 180 cm high. The rhizome is short with compact branches. It is tuberous and has sturdy, 1 cm thick and 50 cm long roots. The stem is erect, branched above and villous. The leaves are large, tomentose beneath and irregularly dentate. The cauline leaves are cordate acute. The basal leaves are oblong and petiolate.

Characteristics: The rhizome has a strong odor, the taste is pungent, bitter and tangy.

Habitat: Indigenous to Europe and temperate Asia, introduced to the U.S. and China.

Production: Elecampane root is the root of Inula helenium.

Other Names: Elfdock, Elfwort, Horse-Elder, Horseheal, Scabwort, Wild Sunflower, Velvet Dock

ACTION AND PHARMACOLOGY

COMPOUNDS

Volatile oil: chief components alantolactone, isoalantolactone, 11,13- dihydroisoalantolactone, 11,13- dihydroalantolactone (the mixture of alantolactone derivatives is also known as helenalin or elecampane camphor)

Polyynes

Polysaccharides: above all inulin (fructosan)

EFFECTS

The main active principles are alantolacton, isoalantolacton and other sesquiterpenlactones. Compounds of this kind have an antiphlogostic and antibiotic effect. Antifungal activity was also demonstrated. The plant is mildly antiseptic and has expectorant properties.

INDICATIONS AND USAGE

Preparations of the rhizome are used to treat bronchitis, whooping cough and bronchial catarrh. In folk medicine, Elecampane is used as a stomachic, diuretic, carminative, cholagogue as well as for menstrual complaints.

PRECAUTIONS AND ADVERSE REACTIONS

The drug is severely irritating to mucous membranes and strongly sensitizing.

OVERDOSAGE

Larger administrations of the drug lead to vomiting, diarrhea, spasms and signs of paralysis. Following gastric lavage, intestinal emptying (sodium sulfate) and the administration of activated charcoal powder, poisonings are treated with the antimetic trifluopromazine.

DOSAGE

Mode of Administration: The comminuted drug is used in tea mixtures. The extract is used as a constituent in numerous pharmaceutical preparations, including gastrointestinal remedies, alterants, gout remedies, diuretics, as well as in numerous expectorants.

Preparation: To prepare an infusion, boiling water is poured over 1 g of ground drug and left to draw for 10 to 15 minutes after which time it is strained through a tea strainer (1 teaspoonful corresponds to about 4 g drug).

Daily Dosage: Drink 1 cup of the infusion 3 to 4 times daily as an expectorant; may be sweetened with honey.

Storage: Store cool, protected from light, not in plastic containers.

LITERATURE

Kerimov SS, Chishov OS, (1974) Khim Prir Soed 10:254.

Khvorost PP, Komissarenko NF, (1976) Khim Prir Soed 6:820.

Kiesewetter R, Müller M, (1958) Pharmazie 13:777.

Rosik GH et al., Khim Farm Zh 21:632-634. 1987.

Vishnakova SA et al., (1977) Rastit Resur 13:428.

Zinchenko V et al., Rastit Res 19:544-548. 1983.

Further information in:

Hänsel R, Keller K, Rimpler H, Schneider G (Hrsg.), Hagers Handbuch der Pharmazeutischen Praxis, 5. Aufl., Bde 4-6 (Drogen), Springer Verlag Berlin, Heidelberg, New York, 1992-1994.

Hausen B, Allergiepflanzen, Pflanzenallergene, ecomed Verlagsgesellsch. mbH, Landsberg 1988.

Leung AY, Encyclopedia of Common Natural Ingredients Used in Food Drugs and Cosmetics, John Wiley & Sons Inc., New York 1980.

Madaus G, Lehrbuch der Biologischen Arzneimittel, Bde 1-3, Nachdruck, Georg Olms Verlag Hildesheim 1979.

Roth L, Daunderer M, Kormann K, Giftpflanzen, Pflanzengifte, 4. Aufl., Ecomed Fachverlag Landsberg Lech 1993.

Tang W, Eisenbrand G, Chinese Drugs of Plant Origin, Springer Verlag Heidelberg 1992.

Teuscher E, Lindequist U, Biogene Gifte - Biologie, Chemie, Pharmakologie, 2. Aufl., Fischer Verlag Stuttgart 1994.

Wagner H, Wiesenauer M, Phytotherapie. Phytopharmaka und pflanzliche Homöopathika, Fischer-Verlag, Stuttgart, Jena, New York 1995.

Wichtl M (Hrsg.), Teedrogen, 4. Aufl., Wiss. Verlagsges. Stuttgart 1997.

Ipecac

See Cephaelis Ipecacuanha

Ipomoea Orizabensis

Jalap

DESCRIPTION

Medicinal Parts: The medicinal parts are the dried roots and the steamed, ethanol extract from the roots.

Flower and Fruit: The plant has reddish purple, campanulate flowers.

Leaves, Stem and Root: False jalap is a twinning plant with large cordate leaves. The root tuber is about 18 to 25 cm long and 9 to 10 cm wide and cylindrical-fusiform. It is grayish-brown to brownish black and wrinkled externally. Inside the section shows irregular concentric rings and scattered resin glands, resembling jalap.

Characteristics: The taste is acrid and resinous. The odor is slight.

Habitat: Mexico.

Production: Mexican Jalep is the root extracted from Ipomoea orizabensis. Both the root and the yielded resin are effective as drugs.

Other Names: Mexican Scammony Root, Ipomoea

ACTION AND PHARMACOLOGY

COMPOUNDS

Glycoretines (12-15%, resinous): polymeric ester glycosides

EFFECTS

The drug has a strong laxative effect on the small and large intestines caused by Resin (Resina Scammoniae) combined with esterglycoside.

INDICATIONS AND USAGE

Drastic purgative.

CONTRAINDICATIONS

The drug is contraindicated in pregnancy.

PRECAUTIONS AND ADVERSE REACTIONS

General: No health hazards are known in conjunction with the proper administration of designated therapeutic dosages. Intestinal colic occurs frequently as a side effect.

Pregnancy: Absolutely contraindicated.

OVERDOSAGE

Overdosages cause vomiting. The drug is to be rejected as a purgative for that reason.

DOSAGE

Mode of Administration: Obsolete as a drug many countries. Used on rare occasions in combination preparations. The same applies to other Ipomoea varieties e.g., I. turpethum, I. operculata.

LITERATURE

Noda N et al., Tetrahedron 43:3889. 1987.

Shellard EJ, PM 9:146-152. 1961.

Singh S, Stacey BE, (1973) Phytochemistry 12:1701.

Wagner H, (1973) In ''Chemistry in Biochemical Classification'', Nobel Symposium (1973).

Further information in:

Hänsel R, Keller K, Rimpler H, Schneider G (Hrsg.), Hagers Handbuch der Pharmazeutischen Praxis, 5. Aufl., Bde 4-6 (Drogen): Springer Verlag Berlin, Heidelberg, New York, 1992-1994.

Lewin L, Gifte und Vergiftungen, 6. Aufl., Nachdruck, Haug Verlag, Heidelberg 1992.

Madaus G, Lehrbuch der Biologischen Arzneimittel, Bde 1-3, Nachdruck, Georg Olms Verlag Hildesheim 1979.

Roth L, Daunderer M, Kormann K, Giftpflanzen, Pflanzengifte, 4. Aufl., Ecomed Fachverlag Landsberg Lech 1993.

Steinegger E, Hänsel R, Pharmakognosie, 5. Aufl., Springer Verlag Heidelberg 1992.

Iris Species

Orris Root

DESCRIPTION

Medicinal Parts: The medicinal part is the rhizome with the roots.

Flower and Fruit: The flowers are long-pedicled and perfumed. The tepals are white or slightly blue. The outer ones are darker with a yellow beard. The anthers are as big as the filaments. The upper lip of the stigma branch is inclined forward. The fruit is a large capsule with a number of sections in which the brown seeds are lined up like rolls of coins.

Leaves, Stem and Root: The plants are perennial, 30 to 100 cm high. The rhizome is thick and short. The strong flower-bearing stem is branched from the middle. The leaves are broad, sword-shaped, usually curved and gray-green.

Habitat: Indigenous to southern Europe.

Production: Orris root is the root of Iris germanica and other varieties, in homeopathy, in particular, Iris versicolor.

Other Names: Iris, Florentine Orris, White Flag Root, Blue Flag, Flag Lily, Liver Lily, Poison Flag, Snake Lily, Water Flag, Wild Iris, Yellow Flag, Yellow Iris, Dragon Flower, Myrtle Flower, Fliggers, Flaggon, Sheggs, Segg, Daggers, Jacob's Sword, Gladyne

ACTION AND PHARMACOLOGY

COMPOUNDS

Volatile oil: chief constituents irone, in particular alpha-, beta- and gamma-irone (odor resembling violets)

Triterpenes: Iridale (mono-, bi- and spirocyclic compounds, precursors of the irones), including among others irigermanal

Isoflavonoids: including, among others, irilon, irisolone, irigenine, tectoridine

Flavonoids

Xanthones: C-glucosylxanthones

Starch

EFFECTS

Mildly expectorant.

INDICATIONS AND USAGE

Disorders of the respiratory system.

PRECAUTIONS AND ADVERSE REACTIONS

No health hazards or side effects are known in conjunction with the proper administration of designated therapeutic dosages. The juice of the fresh plant has a severely irritating effect upon skin and mucous membranes. If taken internally, it can lead to vomiting, abdominal pain and bloody diarrhea. Severe inflammation occurs following mucous membrane contact.

DOSAGE

Mode of Administration: Iris is available in homeopathic dilutions, as a constituent of various combination preparations, and in various tea mixtures.

LITERATURE

Bambhole VD, Jiddewar GG, (1985) Sach Ayurveda 37(9):557.

El Moghazy AM et al., (1980) Fitoterapia 5:237.

Krick W et al., (1983) Z Naturforsch Sect C Biosci 38 (9/10): 689.

Morita N et al., (1973) Chem Pharm Bull 21, 600.

Tsukida K et al., (1973) Phytochemistry 12:2318.

Further information in:

Duke JA, A Handbook of Medicinal Herbs, Pub. CRC Press Boca Raton 1985.

Frohne D, Pfänder HJ, Giftpflanzen - Ein Handbuch für Apotheker, Toxikologen und Biologen, 4. Aufl., Wiss. Verlags-Ges Stuttgart 1997.

Kern W, List PH, Hörhammer L (Hrsg.), Hagers Handbuch der Pharmazeutischen Praxis, 4. Aufl., Bde. 1-8, Springer Verlag Berlin, Heidelberg, New York, 1969.

Lewin L, Gifte und Vergiftungen, 6. Aufl., Nachdruck, Haug Verlag, Heidelberg 1992.

Madaus G, Lehrbuch der Biologischen Arzneimittel, Bde 1-3, Nachdruck, Georg Olms Verlag Hildesheim 1979.

Poisonous Plants in Britain and their effects on Animals and Man, Ministry of Agriculture Fisheries and Food, Pub; HMSO UK 1984.

Steinegger E, Hänsel R, Pharmakognosie, 5. Aufl., Springer Verlag Heidelberg 1992.

Teuscher E, Lindequist U, Biogene Gifte - Biologie, Chemie, Pharmakologie, 2. Aufl., Fischer Verlag Stuttgart 1994.

Wagner H, Wiesenauer M, Phytotherapie. Phytopharmaka und pflanzliche Homöopathika, Fischer-Verlag, Stuttgart, Jena, New York 1995.

Wichtl M (Hrsg.), Teedrogen, 4. Aufl., Wiss. Verlagsges. Stuttgart 1997.

Jaborandi

See Pilocarpus Microphyllus

Jacob's Ladder

See Polemonium Coeruleum

Jalap

See Ipomoea Orizabensis

Jamaica Dogwood

See Piscidia Piscipula

Jambolan

See Syzygium Cumini

Japanese Mint

See Mentha Arvensis Var Piperascens

Jateorhiza Palmata

Colombo

DESCRIPTION

Medicinal Parts: The medicinal parts of the plant are the roots cut in slices when fresh and then dried.

Flower and Fruit: The plant is dioecious. The male inflorescences are 40 cm long and have green sepals, which are 2.7 to 3.2 mm long and 1.2 to 1.6 mm wide. The stamens are free and are fused at the base with the involuted margins of the petals. The female inflorescences are 8 to 10 cm long and have a 1 to 1.5 mm rust-red, pubescent ovary. The fruit is a 2 to 2.5 cm long and 1.5 to 2 cm wide globose drupe containing a moon-shaped stone.

Leaves, Stem and Root: The plant is a woody, branched liane, which can climb to tree height. The liane is initially downy, then bristly to villous. The leaves are opposite and have an 18 to 25 cm long petiole. The leaf blades are 15 to 35 cm long and 18 to 40 cm wide. They are bristly haired on both surfaces, broadly rounded, deeply cordate at the base and usually have 5 broad-ovate lobes. The root has a diameter of 3 to 8 cm. It is greenish-black. The root has a floury consistency, an indented center and a thick bark. The transverse section is yellowish, with vascular bundles in radiating lines.

Characteristics: The taste is mucilaginous and very bitter, the odor is slight.

Habitat: Indigenous to Mozambique, east Africa and Madagascar. It is cultivated elsewhere.

Production: Columbo root is the root of Jatrorrhiza palmata, which has been sliced horizontally and dried. The tuber roots, stemming from the rhizome, are dug up in March, washed and thinly sliced and then dried quickly in the shade to avoid decomposition.

Other Names: Calumba

ACTION AND PHARMACOLOGY

COMPOUNDS

Isoquinoline alkaloids: main alkaloid palmatine, additionally jatrorrhizines (jateorhizine), columbamine, bisjatrorrhizines

Diterpene bitter principles: including palmarin, chasmanthin and their glucosides (palmatoside A and B), columbin, jateorin and their glucosides (palmatoside D and E)

EFFECTS

The drug is no longer used as a bitter (amarum). The alkaloids have a narcotic effect. They act similarly to morphine, increasing resting muscle tone in the smooth muscle of the intestinal tract. Colombo alkaloids are said to act as a CNS paralyzing agent in frogs and palmatin has the same effect on mammals. No further information is available.

INDICATIONS AND USAGE

For subacidic gastritis, dyspeptic disorders and chronic enterocolitis.

PRECAUTIONS AND ADVERSE REACTIONS

Health risks or side effects following the proper administration of designated therapeutic dosages are not recorded. Higher dosages of the drug may trigger vomiting and pains in the epigastrium.

OVERDOSAGE

According to older sources, very high dosages can also lead to signs of paralysis and unconsciousness (Lewin).

DOSAGE

Mode of Administration: Due to its morphine-type action its use as an antidiarrheal agent is limited. Otherwise, the chopped root is used (no preparations known).

Preparation: Extractum Columbo Fluidum is prepared with diluted ethanol according to the German pharmacopoeia. Columbo wine is prepared using 100 parts coarsely powdered drug and 1000 parts xeres wine. The extract is pressed out after 8 days and filtered.

Daily Dosage: The dose of the decoction is 1 dessertspoonful hourly. The liquid extract standard single dose is 20 drops. Tincture of columbo standard single dose is 2.5 g. Columbo wine standard single dose is 5 g.

Storage: Must be kept dry at all times.

LITERATURE

Overton KH, Wier NG, Wylie A, J Chem Soc 1482-1490. 1966.

Further information in:

Chan, EH et al., (Eds), Advances in Chinese Medicinal Materials Research, World Scientific Pub. Co. Singapore 1985.

Fenaroli's Handbook of Flavor Ingredients, Vol. 1, 2nd Ed., CRC Press 1975.

Hänsel R, Keller K, Rimpler H, Schneider G (Hrsg.), Hagers Handbuch der Pharmazeutischen Praxis, 5. Aufl., Bde 4-6 (Drogen), Springer Verlag Berlin, Heidelberg, New York, 1992-1994.

Lewin L, Gifte und Vergiftungen, 6. Aufl., Nachdruck, Haug Verlag, Heidelberg 1992.

Steinegger E, Hänsel R, Pharmakognosie, 5. Aufl., Springer Verlag Heidelberg 1992.

Java Tea

See Orthosiphon Spicatus

Jequirity

See Abrus Precatorius

Jewel Weed

See Impatiens Biflora

Jimson Weed

See Datura Stramonium

Jojoba

See Simmondsia Chinesis

Juglans Cinerea

Butternut

DESCRIPTION

Medicinal Parts: The medicinal parts are the bark of the tree and root.

Flower and Fruit: The tree has male catkins and female flowers. The male catkins are 5 to 8 cm long. The fruit is 4 to 6.5 cm and ovoid-oblong. The fruit is pubescent, viscid and strong smelling. The hard nut is ovoid-oblong with 4 prominent and 4 less prominent sharp ridges and many broken grooves between them.

Leaves, Stem and Root: Butternut tree is up to 30 m tall. The bark is gray and deeply fissured. The leaf scars have a prominent pubescent band on their upper edge. The 6 to 12 cm long leaflets are oblong-lanceolate, accuminate and appressed-serrate. They are finely pubescent above, glandular and pubescent beneath.

Habitat: Butternut is indigenous to the forests of the U.S.

Production: Butternut bark is the inner rind of Juglans cinerea.

Other Names: White Walnut, Oil Nut, Lemon Walnut, Black Walnut

ACTION AND PHARMACOLOGY

COMPOUNDS

Fatty oil

Tannins

Juglone

Juglandis folium

EFFECTS

Vermifuge, laxative, tonic.

INDICATIONS AND USAGE

Preparations of the bark are used for disorders of the gallbladder, for hemorrhoids and in the treatment of skin diseases. Juglone has antimicrobial, antineoplastic and antiparasitic properties as well as being a gentle laxative.

PRECAUTIONS AND ADVERSE REACTIONS

No health hazards or side effects are known in conjunction with the proper administration of designated therapeutic dosages.

DOSAGE

Mode of Administration: Available preparations include liquid and dry extracts that are used internally and externally.

LITERATURE

Hegnauer R, Chemotaxonomie der Pflanzen, Bde 1-11, Birkhäuser Verlag Basel, Boston, Berlin 1962-1997.

Kern W, List PH, Hörhammer L (Hrsg.), Hagers Handbuch der Pharmazeutischen Praxis, 4. Aufl., Bde. 1-8, Springer Verlag Berlin, Heidelberg, New York, 1969.

Madaus G, Lehrbuch der Biologischen Arzneimittel, Bde 1-3, Nachdruck, Georg Olms Verlag Hildesheim 1979.

Juglans Regia

Walnut

DESCRIPTION

Flower and Fruit: The flowers are green and appear before the leaves. They are monoecious. The male flowers are 10 cm long, sessile, globular-cylindrical, limp, hanging catkins. The female ones are in groups of 1 to 3 at the tip of annual growth. They are greenish with a glandular pubescent calyx and 2 large, curved, warty, reddish stigmas. The fruit is globular or oblong-globular with a smooth, green, white-spotted outer shell and a wooden, wrinkled inner shell.

Leaves, Stem and Root: The plant grows to 25 m and has a broad, loose-branched crown. The bark is smooth and ash gray at first; later dark and fissured. The leaves are large, long-petioled, odd-pinnate with 7 to 9 oblong or ovate, entire-margined leaflets. The leaflets are spotted with glands when young. The terminal leaflet is the largest and is petiolate.

Characteristics: The leaves are aromatic when rubbed. The taste is bitter.

Habitat: The walnut is indigenous to the Middle East and Iran. Today, it is cultivated in many regions.

Production: Walnut leaf consists of the dried leaf of Juglans regia.

ACTION AND PHARMACOLOGY

COMPOUNDS

Tannins (galloylglucose, ellagitannins)

Naphthalene derivatives: The fresh leaves and the fruit peels contain 1,4,5- trihydroxynaphthalene-4-beta-D-glucoside, which is transformed into juglone through bruising or drying. Juglone polymerizes readily into yellow or brown products (that stain the skin), so there can be hardly any juglone present in the drug itself.

Flavonoids: including, among others, hyperoside, quercitrin

EFFECTS

The main active principles are the tannins and juglon. There is an astringent effect because of the tannins. The antifungal effect comes from the juglon content and the essential oil.

INDICATIONS AND USAGE

- Inflammation of the skin
- Excessive perspiration

Externally, Walnut is used for mild, superficial inflammation of the skin and excessive perspiration. Internally, the drug is used for gastrointestinal catarrh and as an anthelmintic (so-called blood purifier).

PRECAUTIONS AND ADVERSE REACTIONS

No health hazards or side effects are known in conjunction with the proper administration of designated therapeutic dosages.

DOSAGE

Mode of Administration: Comminuted drug for decoctions and other galenic preparations for external use.

Preparation: To prepare a decoction, soak 2 teaspoonfuls of drug in 1 cup of water, boil and strain. An infusion is prepared by using 1.5 g of finely cut drug, soak in cold water, bring to simmer and strain after 3 to 5 minutes.

Daily Dosage: The average daily dose for external use 3 to 6 g of drug.

LITERATURE

Nahrstedt A et al., (1981) Planta Med 42(4):313.

Willuhn G, Pflanzliche Dermatika. Eine kritische Übersicht.. In: DAZ 132(37):1873. 1992.

Further information in:

Hegnauer R, Chemotaxonomie der Pflanzen, Bde 1-11, Birkhäuser Verlag Basel, Boston, Berlin 1962-1997.

Madaus G, Lehrbuch der Biologischen Arzneimittel, Bde 1-3, Nachdruck, Georg Olms Verlag Hildesheim 1979.

Teuscher E, Lindequist U, Biogene Gifte - Biologie, Chemie, Pharmakologie, 2. Aufl., Fischer Verlag Stuttgart 1994.

Teuscher E, Biogene Arzneimittel, 5. Aufl., Wiss. Verlagsges. Stuttgart 1997.

Thomson RH, Naturally Occuring Quinones, 2nd Ed., Academic Press New York 1971.

Wagner H, Wiesenauer M, Phytotherapie. Phytopharmaka und pflanzliche Homöopathika, Fischer-Verlag, Stuttgart, Jena, New York 1995.

Jujube

See Zyzyphus Jujube

Juniper

See Juniperus Communis

Juniperus Communis

Juniper

DESCRIPTION

Medicinal Parts: The medicinal parts are the essential oil from the berry cones, the ripe, dried berry cones, the ripe fresh berry cones, the fresh or dried pseudo fruit or berry and the ripe berry.

Flower and Fruit: The plant is usually dioecious, occasionally monoecious and occasionally bears androgynous flowers. The yellowish male flowers are in elliptical catkins consisting of numerous stamens in 3-segmented whorls in the leaf axils of young shoots. The greenish female flowers are almost ovoid and consist of 3 carpels. The carpels become fleshy and in the second year when ripe form pea-sized, globular, dark-brown to violet, blue-frosted juniper berries. The berries ripen for 2 or 3 years so that blue (ripe) and green (unripe) berries are found on the same tree. The seeds are light brown, oblong-triangular. They are somewhat warty between the edges and have a hard shell.

Leaves, Stem and Root: Juniperus Communis is a tree or shrub found in varying forms from 2 to 10 m in height. The bark is smooth and yellow-brown at first, later fissured, gray-black and peeling. The buds are covered in scale-like needles which can be distinguished from the foliage needles by their length. The leaves are needles in whorls of 3 spreading from the branchlets. They are evergreen, stiff, pointed, prickly and sea green. The outer and inner membranes have thickened cell walls.

Characteristics: The berries have a tangy smell. The taste is tangy-sweet, then resinous and bitter.

Habitat: Europe, northern Africa, north Asia, North America.

Production: Juniper Berry is the ripe, fresh or dried spherical ovulate cone (berry) of Juniper communis as well as its preparations.

Other Names: Juniper Berry, Ginepro, Enebro

ACTION AND PHARMACOLOGY

COMPOUNDS

Volatile oil (1-2%): make-up is very dependent upon the source of the drug, chief components monoterpene hydrocarbons, for example alpha-pinene, beta-myrcene, gamma-muurolen, sabinene, additionally including among others limonene, beta-elemene, beta-caryophyllene, beta-pinene, gamma-cadinene, terpinene-4-ol

Diterpenes

Catechin tannins

Inverted sugar (20-30%)

Flavonoids

EFFECTS

The attributed diuretic effect is a so-called ''water diuresis'' that is a result of the essential oil content; the drug works to lower blood pressure and as an antidiabetic. Animal tests have shown an increase in urine excretion as well as a direct effect on smooth muscle contraction.

INDICATIONS AND USAGE

- Loss of appetite
- Infections of the urinary tract
- Kidney and bladder stones

Juniper is used for dyspeptic disorders and for digestive disorders such as eructation, heartburn and bloating. The drug is also used as flushing out therapy for inflammatory diseases of the lower urinary tract.

CONTRAINDICATIONS

Contraindications for internal administration include pregnancy and inflammatory renal diseases.

PRECAUTIONS AND ADVERSE REACTIONS

No health hazards or side effects are known in conjunction with the proper administration of designated therapeutic dosages. Long-term internal administration or overdosage can bring about kidney irritation and kidney damage. External administration for large skin wounds, acute skin diseases, feverish diseases, cardiac insufficiency or hypertonia should only take place under the supervision of a doctor.

DOSAGE

Mode of Administration: Whole, crushed, or powdered drug for infusions and decoctions, alcohol extracts, and in wine. Essential oil is used for oral application in liquid and solid medicinal forms. Combinations with other plant drugs in bladder and kidney teas and similar preparations may be useful. Juniper berry is also used as bath salts in the treatment of rheumatism.

Daily Dosage: The daily dose is 2 to 10 g of the drug, corresponding to 20 to 100 mg of the essential oil. The duration of use should be limited to a maximum of 6 weeks. A 1:20 dilution infusion (0.5 g in 1 teacup) may be taken 3 times daily.

LITERATURE

Chatzopoulou PS, Katsiotis ST, Study of the Essential Oil from Juniperus communis ''Berries'' (Cones)Growing in Greece. In: PM 59(6):554. 1993.

De Pascuale Teresa J, (1977) An Quim. 73(3):463.

Freidrich H, Engelshowe R, (1978) Planta Med 33:251.

Lamer-Zarawska E, Phytochemical studies on flavonoids and other compounds of juniper fruits (Juniperus communsi L.). In: Pol J Chem 54(2):213-219. 1980.

Mascolo N et al., (1987) Phytother Res 1(1):28.

Ramic S, Murko D, Chemical composition of fruit of Juniperus species. In: Archiv Farm 33(1):15-20. 1983.

Schilcher H, Boesel R, Effenberger ST Segebrecht S, Neuere Untersuchungsergebnisse mit aquaretisch, antibakteriell und prostatotrop wirksamen Arzneipflanzen. In: ZPT 10(3):77. 1989.

Schilcher H, Emmrich D, Koehler C, Gaschromatographischer Vergleich von ätherischen Wacholderölen und deren toxikologische Bedeutung. In: PZW 138(3/4)85. 1993.

Schilcher H, Heil BM, Nierentoxizität von Wacholderbeerzubereitungen. In: ZPT 15(4):205-213. 1994.

Schmidt M, Wacholderzubereitungen. Muβ die Monographie umgeschrieben werden? In: DAZ 135(14):1260-1264. 1995.

Sökeland J, Phytotherapie in der Urologie. In: ZPT 10(1):8. 1989.

Thomas AF, (1972) Helv Chim Acta 55:2429.

Thomas AF, (1972) Helv Chim. Acta 56:1800.

Further information in:

Frohne D, Pfänder HJ, Giftpflanzen - Ein Handbuch für Apotheker, Toxikologen und Biologen, 4. Aufl., Wiss. Verlags-Ges Stuttgart 1997.

Hänsel R, Keller K, Rimpler H, Schneider G (Hrsg.), Hagers Handbuch der Pharmazeutischen Praxis, 5. Aufl., Bde 4-6 (Drogen), Springer Verlag Berlin, Heidelberg, New York, 1992-1994.

Leung AY, Encyclopedia of Common Natural Ingredients Used in Food Drugs and Cosmetics, John Wiley & Sons Inc., New York 1980.

Madaus G, Lehrbuch der Biologischen Arzneimittel, Bde 1-3, Nachdruck, Georg Olms Verlag Hildesheim 1979.

Roth L, Daunderer M, Kormann K, Giftpflanzen, Pflanzengifte, 4. Aufl., Ecomed Fachverlag Landsberg Lech 1993.

Steinegger E, Hänsel R, Pharmakognosie, 5. Aufl., Springer Verlag Heidelberg 1992.

Teuscher E, Biogene Arzneimittel, 5. Aufl., Wiss. Verlagsges. Stuttgart 1997.

Teuscher E, Lindequist U, Biogene Gifte-Biologie, Chemie, Pharmakologie, 2. Aufl., Fischer Verlag Stuttgart 1994.

Wagner H, Wiesenauer M, Phytotherapie. Phytopharmaka und pflanzliche Homöopathika, Fischer-Verlag, Stuttgart, Jena, New York 1995.

Wichtl M (Hrsg.), Teedrogen, 4. Aufl., Wiss. Verlagsges. Stuttgart 1997.

Juniperus Sabina

Savin Tops

DESCRIPTION

Medicinal Parts: The medicinal parts are the essential oil of the leaves and branch tips; the dried leafy branch tips; the fresh, youngest non-woody branch tips with leaves; and the branches and leaves.

Flower and Fruit: The male and female flowers are at the end of the twigs which are covered in leaf-scales. The male flowers are up to 2 mm wide and oblong to ovate. The female flowering branch bears the flowers erect when in bloom, later curved inwards. The flowers have 4 carpels which develop into pea-sized berry-cones with 4 ovate seeds. The seeds are ovate and striped with numerous edges.

Leaves, Stem and Root: It is generally a 4.5 m high, dioecious, evergreen shrub with either an erect trunk and an irregular crown or numerous low-lying branches with erect tips. The bark of the young branches are light brown, of more mature branches red-brown and peeling. The young plants up to 10 years have only needle-like 4 mm long, blue-green leaves whose tips stand out. Mature plants have triangular, scale-like, imbricate leaves.

Habitat: Found in southern and central Europe, the Caucasus, the southern mountains of Asian Russia and also in the northern U.S.

Production: Savin Tops is the young shoots and twig tips of Juniperus sabina.

Other Names: Savin, Savine

ACTION AND PHARMACOLOGY

COMPOUNDS

Volatile oil (3-5%): chief components sabinyl acetate, sabinene, further including among others beta-myrcene, terpin-4-ol, gamma-terpinene, alpha-pinene, limonene

Lignans: including among others deoxypodorhizone, deoxypodophyllotoxin, junaphtoinsäure, deoxypicropodophyllotoxin, dehydropodophyllotoxin

Hydroxycoumarins: including among others cumarsabine, 8-methoxycumarsabine, siderin, 4-methoxy-5-methylcoumarin- propiophenone

Derivatives: including among others 2-hydroxy-3,4-dimethoxy-6-methyl-propiophenone

EFFECTS

Internal: strong hyperaematic of the lower abdominal organs.

External: severe irritation of the skin and mucous membrane.

Lignans are also said to have antineoplastic and antiviral properties: The main substance is 3 to 5% essential oil with thujon acting as the principal ingredient, along with containing podophyllotoxine and other Lignans.

INDICATIONS AND USAGE

For external use only, in the treatment of fig warts.

PRECAUTIONS AND ADVERSE REACTIONS

External administration, in particular of the volatile oil, can lead to severe skin irritation, blister formation, necroses and resorbent poisonings.

OVERDOSAGE

One is cautioned against internal administration of the drug and of the volatile oil. Fatal poisonings have occurred repeatedly following administration of the drug in either powder form or infusion as an abortient. Symptoms include, among others, queasiness, cardiac rhythm disorders, spasm, kidney damage and hematuria. Death finds the patient in a state of central paralysis and deep unconsciousness. The internal administration of 6 drops of the volatile oil is life-threatening for humans.

Following gastrointestinal emptying, (inducement of vomiting, gastric lavage, sodium sulfate) and instillation of activated charcoal, the therapy for poisonings consists of treating spasms with diazepam (I.V.), colic with atropine, electrolyte substitution and treating possible cases of acidosis with sodium bicarbonate infusions. Monitoring of kidney function, blood coagulation and liver values is essential. Intubation and oxygen respiration may also be necessary. The level of danger depends upon the age of the drug of the volatile oil, as the toxicity probably develops chiefly through the formation of terpene peroxides during storage. The fresh tips of the branches contain presumably very little toxicity.

DOSAGE

Mode of Administration: For external use, as a powdered drug.

Daily Dosage: Savin Tops powder - Powder twice daily, put bandages into the folds of skin.

The drug is severely toxic.

LITERATURE

Feliciano AS, Del Corral JMM, Gordaliza M, Castro A, Acid and phenolic lignans from Juniperus sabina. In: PH 30: 3483-3485. 1991.

Fournier G et al., PM 57:392-393. 1991.

Fournier G et al., Pharm Belg 45:293. 1990.

Hartwell, JL et al. (1953) J Chem Soc 75: 235.

Further information in:

Frohne D, Pfänder HJ, Giftpflanzen - Ein Handbuch für Apotheker, Toxikologen und Biologen, 4. Aufl., Wiss. Verlags-Ges. Stuttgart 1997.

Hänsel R, Keller K, Rimpler H, Schneider G (Hrsg.), Hagers Handbuch der Pharmazeutischen Praxis, 5. Aufl., Bde 4-6 (Drogen): Springer Verlag Berlin, Heidelberg, New York, 1992-1994.

Lewin L, Gifte und Vergiftungen, 6. Aufl., Nachdruck, Haug Verlag, Heidelberg 1992.

Madaus G, Lehrbuch der Biologischen Arzneimittel, Bde 1-3, Nachdruck, Georg Olms Verlag Hildesheim 1979.

Roth L, Daunderer M, Kormann K, Giftpflanzen, Pflanzengifte, 4. Aufl., Ecomed Fachverlag Landsberg Lech 1993.

Steinegger E, Hänsel R, Pharmakognosie, 5. Aufl., Springer Verlag Heidelberg 1992.

Teuscher E, Lindequist U, Biogene Gifte - Biologie, Chemie, Pharmakologie, 2. Aufl., Fischer Verlag Stuttgart 1994.

Justicia Adhatoda

Malabar Nut

DESCRIPTION

Medicinal Parts: The medicinal parts are the dried foliage leaves, the flower collected in the flowering season, the dried bark of the trunk, branches and roots and the fresh leaves.

Flower and Fruit: The flowers are in dense, 2.5 to 7.5 cm long peduncled, axillary spikes. The bracts are elliptical and the bracteoles are oblong-lanceolate. The calyx is 1.5 cm long, glabrous or black pubescent, has 5 sections with regular lanceolate segments. The corolla is white with red to purple bands. The corolla tube is 1.3 cm long and is cylindrical and pubescent inside of the lower half. The upper lip is convexly domed. The anthers are arrow-shaped and sometimes spurred at the base. The ovary is bivalvular with a 2-lobed stigma. The fruit is a 4-seeded, short-haired, longitudinally grooved capsule. The seeds are orbicular, glabrous, slightly bumpy-warty and 5 to 7 mm across.

Leaves, Stem and Root: The plant is an evergreen, unpleasant smelling shrub 2.5 m high with numerous, usually opposite branches. The bark is yellow. The leaves are 8 to 25 cm long, 2.5 to 8 cm wide, short-stalked, opposite, lanceolate to elliptical, tapering to an acute apex with entire margins. The leaf blade and petiole are finely pubescent.

Characteristics: The taste is bitter and the odor tea-like.

Habitat: Originally indigenous to northern India, the plant is now found in all the areas of Ayurveda medicine in India, Sri Lanka and the Maylan archipelago.

Production: Vasaca leaves are the leaves of Justicia adhatoda.

Other Names: Arusa, Adulsa

ACTIONS AND PHARMACOLOGY

COMPOUNDS

Quinazoline alkaloids: including vasicine and vasicinone

Volatile oil

EFFECTS

Mildly spasmolytic, bronchodilatory and expectorant.

INDICATIONS AND USAGE

Vasicin was formerly used as the starting substance for the development of the mucolytics Bromhexin® and Ambroxol®. It is used in Indian medicine as an expectorant and secretory agent.

CONTRAINDICATIONS

The drug is contraindicated in pregnancy.

PRECAUTIONS AND ADVERSE REACTIONS

General: No health hazards or side effects are known in conjunction with the proper administration of designated therapeutic dosages. Because of the vasicine content, the administration of large dosages can lead to excitatory states.

Pregnancy: Administration during pregnancy is to be avoided.

DOSAGE

Mode of Administration: Today, the extract of the leaves is only found in some combination preparations.

LITERATURE

Brain KR, Thapa BB, J Chromatogr 258:183-188. 1988.

Cooper-Driver G, Swain T, Bot J Linn Soc 74:1-21. 1977.

Further information in:

Hänsel R, Keller K, Rimpler H, Schneider G (Hrsg.), Hagers Handbuch der Pharmazeutischen Praxis, 5. Aufl., Bde 4-6 (Drogen), Springer Verlag Berlin, Heidelberg, New York, 1992-1994.

Madaus G, Lehrbuch der Biologischen Arzneimittel, Bde 1-3, Nachdruck, Georg Olms Verlag Hildesheim 1979.

Kalmia Latifolia

Mountain Laurel

DESCRIPTION

Medicinal Parts: The medicinal parts are the fresh or dried leaves.

Flower and Fruit: The inflorescence is a compound umbelled-raceme with numerous flowers. The flowers are red, whitish or purple-brown to chocolate brown; solitary on long glandular-hairy pedicles in the axils of the bracts and 2 lateral, brown bracteoles. The bud has 10 folds and spreads out in a bowl shape. There are 10 stamens, red anthers without appendages that burst open at irregular holes. The fruit is an erect, orbicular, 5-to-7-valvular capsule. The numerous seeds are flat, oblong, 1 mm long and fly easily.

Leaves, Stem and Root: The plant is a heavily branched shrub or tree about 4 m high with reddish brown or gray branches. The evergreen, laurel-like, ovate-lanceolate acuminate, glabrous leaves are alternate, 4 to 12 cm long and have a 1 to 3 cm long petiole. They are red-brown on the lower surface, have numerous glandular hairs and a distinct midrib. The upper surface is dark green.

Habitat: Eastern U.S.

Production: Mountain Laurel leaves are the leaves (fresh or dried) of Kalmia latifolia.

Other Names: Broad-leafed Laurel, Calico Bush, Spoonwood, Sheep Laurel, Rose Laurel, Laurel, Lambkill, Mountain Ivy

ACTION AND PHARMACOLOGY

COMPOUNDS

Diterpenes (andromedan- derivatives): including among others grayanotoxin I (andromedotoxin, asebotoxin, acetylandromedol, rhodotoxin), grayanotoxin II, III, XVIII, lyonol A, leucothol A, kalmiatoxine

Acylphloroglucinols: including among others 2',6'-dihydroxy-4'-methoxy-acetophenone, phloretin

Flavonoids: including among others asebotin, hyperoside

EFFECTS

According to earlier sources (which are questionable), the drug is antiphlogistic and mildly diuretic.

INDICATIONS AND USAGE

Today, the drug is only used in homeopathic dilutions. In the past it was used as a decoction in the treatment of tinea capitis and to treat psoriasis, herpes and secondary syphilis. Efficacy has not been proven.

PRECAUTIONS AND ADVERSE REACTIONS

The andromedan derivatives of the drug prevent the closure of the excitable cells of the sodium channels and thereby prevent conduction. Painful mucous membranes in the mouth and in the stomach, increased salivation, cold sweat, nausea, vomiting, diarrhea and paresthesias are experienced following intake of the drug. Dizziness, headache, fever attacks as well as intoxicated states with temporary loss of vision follow later. Muscle weakness, coordination disorders and spasms can also occur. Bradycardia, cardiac arrhythmias, drop in blood pressure, eventual cardiac arrest and respiratory failure can lead to death.

OVERDOSAGE

Following gastrointestinal emptying, (inducement of vomiting, gastric lavage with burgundy-colored potassium permanganate solution, sodium sulfate) and instillation of activated charcoal, the treatment of poisoning consists of electrolyte replacement, countering of acidosis with sodium bicarbonate, plasma volume expanders if required, diazepam (I.V.) in case of spasms, and oxygen in case of respiratory failure.

DOSAGE

Mode of Administration: Available in homeopathic preparations.

LITERATURE

Wolters B, Zierpflanzen aus Nordamerika. In: DAZ 137(26):2253-2261. 1997.

Further information in:

Frohne D, Pfänder HJ, Giftpflanzen - Ein Handbuch für Apotheker, Toxikologen und Biologen, 4. Aufl., Wiss. Verlags-Ges Stuttgart 1997.

Hänsel R, Keller K, Rimpler H, Schneider G (Hrsg.), Hagers Handbuch der Pharmazeutischen Praxis, 5. Aufl., Bde 4-6 (Drogen), Springer Verlag Berlin, Heidelberg, New York, 1992-1994.

Lewin L, Gifte und Vergiftungen, 6. Aufl., Nachdruck, Haug Verlag, Heidelberg 1992.

Madaus G, Lehrbuch der Biologischen Arzneimittel, Bde 1-3, Nachdruck, Georg Olms Verlag Hildesheim 1979.

Roth L, Daunderer M, Kormann K, Giftpflanzen, Pflanzengifte, 4. Aufl., Ecomed Fachverlag Landsberg Lech 1993.

Teuscher E, Lindequist U, Biogene Gifte - Biologie, Chemie, Pharmakologie, 2. Aufl., Fischer Verlag Stuttgart 1994.

Wagner H, Wiesenauer M, Phytotherapie. Phytopharmaka und pflanzliche Homöopathika, Fischer-Verlag, Stuttgart, Jena, New York 1995.

Kamala

See Mallotus Philippinensis

Kava-Kava

See Piper Methysticum

Knautia Arvensis

Field Scabious

DESCRIPTION

Medicinal Parts: The medicinal parts are the leafy stem including the flower heads and the fresh aerial parts of the flowering plant.

Flower and Fruit: The flat domed, composite flowers are on long, pubescent, glandular or non-glandular pedicles. The androgynous heads are 2 to 4 cm in diameter and contain 85 to 100 florets. The female capitula are smaller and contain 55 to 60 florets. The florets are blue-lilac, occasionally red-lilac or yellowish white to pure white. The lateral florets are ray-like. The 2 to 3-rowed involucre bracts are lanceolate, compressed and long-haired. The edge of the calyx has 8 to 16 bristles. The corolla is fused and 4 tipped. There are 4 stamens and 1 inferior ovary. The fruit is a nutlet 5 to 6 mm long and about 2 mm wide. The fruit is thickly covered in vertical hairs

Leaves, Stem and Root: The plant is perennial and 30 to 150 cm high. The rhizome is branched and has a strong taproot. The rhizome produces a flowering stem from the leaf rosette which survives the winter. The stem is erect, lightly branched and has short gray hairs. The leaves are opposite, gray-green and matte. The lower ones are petioled, oblong and entire-margined. The upper leaves are sessile, pinnatisect and have lanceolate tips.

Habitat: The plant is found all over Europe except the arctic. It is also found in the Caucasus and western Siberia.

Production: Field scabious herb consists of the leafy stems and flower heads and also occasionally the root of Knautia arvensis.

ACTIONS AND PHARMACOLOGY

COMPOUNDS

Triterpene saponins: knautioside, knautioside A and B

Iridoide monoterpenes: including among others dipsacan

Flavonoids

Tannins

EFFECTS

The drug is said to have an astringent, antiseptic, expectorant and even purgative effect. None of these effects have been proven.

INDICATIONS AND USAGE

The drug is used for chronic skin diseases, eczema, anal fissures, pruritis ani, urticaria, scabies and favus. Other uses include cleansing and healing of ulcers, for contusions and inflammation, also for coughs and throat complaints, as well as cystitis.

Efficacy has not been proven.

PRECAUTIONS AND ADVERSE REACTIONS

No health hazards or side effects are known in conjunction with the proper administration of designated therapeutic dosages.

DOSAGE

Mode of Administration: Decoction and infusion preparations are used both internally and externally. The drug is also available as an alcoholic extract and tea.

Preparation: For preparation of the drug, use approximately 30 gm infusion or decoction, add to 1 liter of hot water, strain and cool.

Daily Dosage: For chronic eczema, add 4 teaspoonfuls to 2 glasses of water, leave to draw for 10 minutes and drink during the course of the day.

LITERATURE

Hänsel R, Keller K, Rimpler H, Schneider G (Hrsg.), Hagers Handbuch der Pharmazeutischen Praxis, 5. Aufl., Bde 4-6 (Drogen), Springer Verlag Berlin, Heidelberg, New York, 1992-1994.

Madaus G, Lehrbuch der Biologischen Arzneimittel, Bde 1-3, Nachdruck, Georg Olms Verlag Hildesheim 1979.

Knotweed

See Polygonum Aviculare

Kousso

See Hagenia Abyssinica

Krameria Triandra

Rhatany

DESCRIPTION

Medicinal Parts: The medicinal part is the root.

Flower and Fruit: The 7 to 12 mm-long flowers are spare terminal racemes. The calyx is petaloid, the sepals are splayed, lanceolate, dark red, silky haired on the outside. The petals are irregular, with 2 glands, wedge-shaped, 3 to 5 mm wide, crimson and spatulate. The flower has 3 stamens. The ovary is ovate, covered in bristly hairs with a thick glabrous style. The fruit is solitary angular and bristled. It is ovate and has numerous red-black bristly thorns.

Leaves, Stem and Root: The plant is a 0.3 to 1 m high subshrub whose long, 3 cm thick root is covered in a brown-red, smooth, peeling bark. The younger branches are dark green, silky to bristly haired, the older ones are black and often gnarled. The leaves are entire-margined, ovate, 6 to 15 mm long and 2 to 6 mm wide and silver-gray pubescent.

Habitat: Generally found in the central Andes but mostly in Peru. There are only a few areas in countries bordering Peru where it is found.

Production: Rhatany root consists of the dried root of Krameria triandra Ruiz et Pavon as well as its preparations.

Not To Be Confused With: Roots of other Krameria species.

Other Names: Rhatania, Krameria Root, Mapato

ACTION AND PHARMACOLOGY

COMPOUNDS

Tannins (10-15%): oligomeric proanthocyanidins

Tanner's reds (phlobaphenes): polymeric, insoluble oxydation products of the tannins

Neolignans: including among others rhatany phenols I-III (0.3%)

EFFECTS

Astringent.

INDICATIONS AND USAGE

■ Inflammation of the mouth and pharynx

External: topical treatment of mild inflammation of the oral and pharyngeal mucosa and inflammation of the gums.

Internal: as an antidiarrheal agent for enteritis.

PRECAUTIONS AND ADVERSE REACTIONS

No health hazards or side effects are known in conjunction with the proper administration of designated therapeutic dosages. Internal administration can lead to digestive complaints because of the secretion-inhibiting efficacy. Allergic mucus membrane reactions have been observed in rare cases.

DOSAGE

Mode of Administration: Comminuted herb for decoctions and other galenic preparations for topical application, especially in oral and pharyngeal areas.

The drug is a component of various standardized preparations of pharyngeal remedies.

Preparation: 1.5 to 2 g coarsely powdered drug in boiling water, strain after 10 to 15 minutes. (1 teaspoonful = approx. 3 g drug)

Daily Dosage: About 1 g comminuted drug in 1 cup of water as decoction or 5-10 drops of rhatany tincture in 1 glass of water, 2 to 3 times daily.

Undiluted rhatany tincture painted on the affected surface 2 to 3 times daily.

LITERATURE

Scholz E, Rimpler H, Österr Apoth Ztg 48:138. 1994.

Scholz E, Rimpler H, PM 55:379. 1098.

Scholz R, Rimpler H, (1986) Planta Med (6):58P.

Williams V et al., (1983) Phytochemistry 22:569.

Further information in:

Hänsel R, Keller K, Rimpler H, Schneider G (Hrsg.), Hagers Handbuch der Pharmazeutischen Praxis, 5. Aufl., Bde 4-6 (Drogen): Springer Verlag Berlin, Heidelberg, New York, 1992-1994.

Madaus G, Lehrbuch der Biologischen Arzneimittel, Bde 1-3, Nachdruck, Georg Olms Verlag Hildesheim 1979.

Steinegger E, Hänsel R, Pharmakognosie, 5. Aufl., Springer Verlag Heidelberg 1992.

Teuscher E, Biogene Arzneimittel, 5. Aufl., Wiss. Verlagsges. Stuttgart 1997.

Wichtl M (Hrsg.), Teedrogen, 4. Aufl., Wiss. Verlagsges. Stuttgart 1997.

Labrador Tea

See Ledum Latifolium

Laburnum

See Cytisus Laburnum

Lactuca Virosa

Wild Lettuce

DESCRIPTION

Medicinal Parts: The medicinal parts are the dried latex and the leaves.

Flower and Fruit: The composite flowers are in pyramid-shaped panicles. The capitula have a few florets. They are androgynous pale yellow lingual florets. The bracts are imbricate. The fruit is 4-lipped and black with a broad edge. It is glabrous at the tip. It has a whitish beak which is as long as the fruit, making the hair tuft look as if it was stemmed.

Leaves, Stem and Root: The plant is biennial, up to 1.2 m high with a fusiform, pale root which produces the erect, branched and hollow stem. It is smooth, light green and sometimes has purple spots. The leaves are oblong to obovate, narrowed at the base, clasping usually simple, thorny-tipped, lie horizontally and is thorny on the underside of the midrib.

Characteristics: The whole plant contains milky latex.

Habitat: The plant is indigenous to western and southern Europe and is cultivated in Germany, Austria, France and Scotland.

Production: Wild Lettuce leaves are the leaves of the aerial part of Lactuca virosa. They are gathered when in flower and then dried.

Not To Be Confused With: L.sativa, L.serriola, L.quercina and Sonchus oleraceus.

Other Names: Prickly Lettuce, Strong-scented Lettuce, Green Endive, Lettuce Opium, Acrid Lettuce, Poison Lettuce, Lactucarium

ACTION AND PHARMACOLOGY

COMPOUNDS

Sesquiterpene lactones: lactucin, lactucopicrin (lactupictin, intybin)

Triterpenes: including among others taraxasterol, beta-amyrin

EFFECTS

The herb is supposed to have a narcotic effect. It is an analgesic and spasmolytic and is said to act as a tranquilizer.

INDICATIONS AND USAGE

Medicines containing Wild Lettuce are used to treat whooping cough attacks. The drug is used for bronchial catarrh, asthma and urinary tract diseases. The oil of the seeds is used for arteriosclerosis and was also used as wheat germ oil.

PRECAUTIONS AND ADVERSE REACTIONS

No health hazards or side effects are known in conjunction with the proper administration of designated therapeutic dosages. The drug possesses a low potential for sensitization.

OVERDOSAGE

The following signs of poisoning can occur through overdosage or following intake of the fresh leaves, as in salads: outbreaks of sweating, acceleration of breathing, tachycardia, pupil dilation, dizziness, ringing in the ears, vision disorders, pressure in the head, somnolence, on occasion also excitatory states. The toxicity is however relatively low. Following gastrointestinal emptying (inducement of vomiting, gastric lavage with burgundy-colored potassium permanganate solution, sodium sulfate), as well as instillation of activated charcoal, the treatment of poisonings should proceed symptomatically.

DOSAGE

Mode of Administration: Due to its poison content, the drug is only administered under medical supervision. It is ground and used as an alcoholic extract and further processed in the pharmaceutical industry.

LITERATURE

Huang ZJ et al., (1982) J Pharm Sci 71(2):270.

Marquardt P et al., (1976) Planta Med 30:68.

Rees S, Harborne J, (1984) Bot J Linn Soc 89(4):313.

Ruban G et al., (1978) Acta Crystalogr Sect B 34(4):1163.

Further information in:

Frohne D, Pfänder HJ, Giftpflanzen - Ein Handbuch für Apotheker, Toxikologen und Biologen, 4. Aufl., Wiss. Verlags-Ges Stuttgart 1997.

Kern W, List PH, Hörhammer L (Hrsg.), Hagers Handbuch der Pharmazeutischen Praxis, 4. Aufl., Bde. 1-8, Springer Verlag Berlin, Heidelberg, New York, 1969.

Lewin L, Gifte und Vergiftungen, 6. Aufl., Nachdruck, Haug Verlag, Heidelberg 1992.

Madaus G, Lehrbuch der Biologischen Arzneimittel, Bde 1-3, Nachdruck, Georg Olms Verlag Hildesheim 1979.

Roth L, Daunderer M, Kormann K, Giftpflanzen, Pflanzengifte, 4. Aufl., Ecomed Fachverlag Landsberg Lech 1993.

Teuscher E, Lindequist U, Biogene Gifte - Biologie, Chemie, Pharmakologie, 2. Aufl., Fischer Verlag Stuttgart 1994.

Lady Fern

See Athyrium Filix-Femina

Lady's Beadstraw

See Galium Verum

Lady's Mantle

See Alchemilla Vulgaris

Laminaria Hyperborea

Laminaria

DESCRIPTION

Medicinal Parts: The medicinal part is the stem-like part of the thallus.

Flower and Fruit: The plant fits the general description of brown algae. It is unsegmented or heavily segmented and can grow into plants many meters in length. The thallus is reminiscent of root, leaf or stem-like organs (in the case of L. hyperborea stem-like). The color is greenish to brown to reddish.

Habitat: The plant grows on the North Atlantic coast.

Production: Kelp consists of the dried, stem-like parts of the thallus of Laminaria hyperborea (syn. Laminaria cloustonii).

ACTIONS AND PHARMACOLOGY

COMPOUNDS

Salts of alginic acid

Iodine: to some extent organically-bound (0.3-0.45%)

Reserve carbohydrates: laminarin, fucoidin, mannitol, mannitolglucoside

EFFECTS

No information is available.

INDICATIONS AND USAGE

Preparations of kelp are used for the regulation of thyroid function as well as in combination for goiter. The effectiveness for the claimed applications is not verified.

PRECAUTIONS AND ADVERSE REACTIONS

No health hazards or side effects are known in conjunction with the proper administration of designated therapeutic dosages. The danger of induction or worsening of a hyperthyroidism following internal administration of the drug exists with dosages above 150 g iodide/day. In rare cases, it can lead to severe allergic reactions.

DOSAGE

No information is available.

LITERATURE

Kern W, List PH, Hörhammer L (Hrsg.), Hagers Handbuch der Pharmazeutischen Praxis, 4. Aufl., Bde. 1-8, Springer Verlag Berlin, Heidelberg, New York, 1969.

Lamium Album

White Dead Nettle

DESCRIPTION

Medicinal Parts: The medicinal parts are the flowers and leaves.

Flower and Fruit: The white, fairly large bilabiate flowers are in axillary false whorls of 6 to 16 flowers. The campanulate calyx is green and has 5 tips. The tube of the corolla is bent like a knee and the upper lip is curved like a helmet with a ciliate margin. The lower lip is gordate. The tube has 1 large and 1 small tip at the edge. There are 2 long and 2 short stamens under the upper lip. The calyx remains after flowering and protects the small nut. When the nut is ripe, slight pressure is sufficient to fling out the seeds.

Leaves, Stem and Root: The plant is 30 to 50 cm high with an underground creeping stem from which the aerial stems grow. These are erect, quadrangular, grooved, hollow and noded. The leaves are crossed opposite, petiolate, ovate to cordate, acuminate, serrate. The plant has no nettle hairs. The plant is similar to the stinging nettle but has different stem.

Characteristics: The flowers have a weak honey-like fragrance and a slimy-sweet taste.

Habitat: The plant is common in Europe and central and northern Asia.

Production: White dead nettle flower consists of the dried petal with attached stamens of Lamium album as well as its preparations.

Other Names: Blind Nettle, Dumb Nettle, Deaf Nettle, Bee Nettle, Archangel, Stingless Nettle, White Archangel

ACTION AND PHARMACOLOGY

COMPOUNDS

Iridoide monoterpenes: including among others lamalbide, caryoptoside, alboside A and B

Triterpene saponins

Caffeic acid derivatives: including among others rosmaric acid, chlorogenic acid

Flavonoids: including among others kaempferol glycosides

Mucilages

EFFECTS

Expectorant, astringent.

INDICATIONS AND USAGE

- Inflammation of the skin
- Cough/bronchitis
- Inflammation of the mouth and pharynx

Internally: catarrh of the upper respiratory passages, gastrointestinal disorders such as gastritis, sensation of bloating and flatulence.

Externally: mild inflammation of the mucous membranes of the mouth and throat, non-specific fluor albus (leukorrhea) mild, superficial inflammation of the skin.

PRECAUTIONS AND ADVERSE REACTIONS

No health hazards or side effects are known in conjunction with the proper administration of designated therapeutic dosages.

DOSAGE

Mode of Administration: Comminuted drug for infusions and other galenic preparations for internal applications, rinses, baths and moist compresses; occasionally used as a constituent of sedative teas and bronchial teas.

Preparation: Infusion - Pour one cup of water over 1 g drug, leave to draw for 5 minutes and strain.

Extract for poultices - Scald 50 g of flowers with water, draw for 5 minutes and strain.

Daily Dosage: For internal use, the average daily dose is 3 g drug. For external use, 5 g drug is added to a bath.

LITERATURE

Damtoft S, Iridoid glucosides from Lamium album. In: PH 31(1):175. 1992.

Gora J et al., Chemical comparative studies of the herb and flowers of Lamium album L. In: Acta Pol Pharm 40(3):389-393. 1983.

Kooiman P, (1972) Acta Bot Neerl 21(4)417.

Skrypczak L et al., Phenylpropanoid esters and flavonoids in taxonomy of Lamium species. In: PM 61(Abstracts of 43rd Ann Congr):70. 1995.

Further information in:

Kern W, List PH, Hörhammer L (Hrsg.), Hagers Handbuch der Pharmazeutischen Praxis, 4. Aufl., Bde. 1-8, Springer Verlag Berlin, Heidelberg, New York, 1969.

Madaus G, Lehrbuch der Biologischen Arzneimittel, Bde 1-3, Nachdruck, Georg Olms Verlag Hildesheim 1979.

Wichtl M (Hrsg.), Teedrogen, 4. Aufl., Wiss. Verlagsges. Stuttgart 1997.

Larch

See Larix Decidua

Larix Decidua

Larch

DESCRIPTION

Medicinal Parts: The medicinal part is the outer bark.

Flower and Fruit: The female flowers are cone-shaped, erect, 2 cm long, short-pedicled, round-ovate and encircled by scales at the base. The covering scales turn dark red when in bloom. The male catkins are sessile about 1.5 cm long, sulfur-yellow, ovoid-globular. The seeds are light brown, glossy with 13 mm long and 5 mm wide wings.

Leaves, Stem and Root: The larch is a deciduous, up to 54 m high tree stunted at high altitudes with a straight trunk, brown-red bark and pyramid-shaped, sparsely foliated crown. The main branches are horizontal and turned up at the tips. The secondary branches are hanging. The foliage is light green with delicate needles, arranged singly in spiral rows on long shoots and in bushels on short ones. They fall in autumn.

Habitat: The plant is indigenous to central Europe, cultivated in North America. It was first introduced to England in 1639.

Production: The balsam of Larix decidua is obtained by drilling into the trunks. The balsam contains up to 20% essential oil.

Other Names: European larch, Common Larch

ACTION AND PHARMACOLOGY

COMPOUNDS

Volatile oil (14-15%): chief components: (-)-alpha-pinene (70%), Delta3-carene (10%) (-)-beta-pinene (6.5%), beta-pyrones (3%)

Resins: including among others oleoresin acids (50-65%): including among others laricinolic acid, alpha- and beta-laricinolic acid

EFFECTS

Hyperaemic, antiseptic.

INDICATIONS AND USAGE

- Fevers and colds
- Cough/bronchitis
- Tendency for infections
- Blood pressure problems
- Inflammation of the mouth and pharynx
- Rheumatism
- Common cold

Rheumatic and neuralgic discomforts, catarrhal diseases of the respiratory tract, furuncles.

CONTRAINDICATIONS

Inhalation may cause acute inflammation of the airway passages.

PRECAUTIONS AND ADVERSE REACTIONS

General: No health hazards or side effects are known in conjunction with the proper external administration of designated therapeutic dosages.

OVERDOSAGE

Resorptive poisonings, such as kidney and central nervous system damage, are possible with large-area administration. Kidney damage is conceivable with internal administration.

DOSAGE

Mode of Administration: Embrocations in form of ointments, gels, emulsions and oils.

Preparation: Liquid and semi-solid preparations 10 to 20%.

LITERATURE

Freudenberg K, Weinges K, (1959) Tetrahedron Letters 17:19.

Further information in:

Kern W, List PH, Hörhammer L (Hrsg.), Hagers Handbuch der Pharmazeutischen Praxis, 4. Aufl., Bde. 1-8: Springer Verlag Berlin, Heidelberg, New York, 1969.

Larkspur

See Delphinium Consolida

Laurel

See Laurus Nobilis

Laurus Nobilis

Laurel

DESCRIPTION

Medicinal Parts: The medicinal parts are the leaves, the fruit and the oil.

Flower and Fruit: The flowers are in axillary bushy umbels or short racemous panicles. They are dioecious, whitish-green with 4 petals fused at the base. The male flower usually has 10 to 12 stamens; the female has 4 staminoids. The ovary is short-stemmed with one chamber with a hanging ovule, a short style and a triangular obtuse stigma. The fruit develops on the stem into deep-black 2 cm long ovate berries.

Leaves, Stem and Root: Laurel is an evergreen shrub or up to 10 m high tree with smooth, olive green to black bark. The dark-green bay leaves are lanceolate and alternate, about 10 cm long and acuminate at both ends. They are short petioled and their margins are often sinuate and coriaceous.

Habitat: The laurel is indigenous to Mediterranean countries.

Production: Bay leaves are the leaves of Laurus nobilis. Bay berries are the fruits of Laurus nobilis.

Other Names: Sweet Bay, True Laurel, Bay, Roman Laurel, Noble Laurel, Daphne, Bay Laurel, Bay Tree, Grecian Laurel

ACTION AND PHARMACOLOGY

COMPOUNDS: LAURI FOLIUM

Volatile oil (1-3%): chief components 1,8-cineol

Sesquiterpene lactones: dehydrocostuslactone, costunolide, furthermore eremanthin, laurenbiolide

Isoquinoline alkaloids: including, among others, reticulin

COMPOUNDS: LAURI FRUCTUS

Volatile oil (1-4%): including, among others, 1,8-cineol, alpha- and beta-pinene, citral, methylcinnamat

Sesquiterpene lactones: dehydrocostuslactone, costunolid, furthermore eremanthin, laurenbiolide

Fatty oil (25-55%): chief fatty acids lauric, palmitic, oleic acid The green salve-like laurel oil is gained by pressing or cooking the berries. Besides fatty oil, it contains the components of the volatile oil and a large percentage of sesquiterpene lactones.

EFFECTS

Rubefacient.

INDICATIONS AND USAGE

Both forms are used as a skin stimulant (rubefacient) and for rheumatic conditions.

PRECAUTIONS AND ADVERSE REACTIONS

No health hazards or side effects are known in conjunction with the proper administration of designated therapeutic dosages. The drug possess medium potential for sensitization.

DOSAGE

LAURI FOLIUM

Mode of Administration: The essential oil is used in ointments and soaps.

LAURI FRUCTUS

Mode of Administration: The mixture of essential and fatty oils, extracted through pressing, were formerly used in the treatment of furuncles; today Laurel is used externally in veterinary medicine, as an udder ointment.

LITERATURE

LAURI FOLIUM

Hogg JW et al., (1974) Phytochemistry 13:868.

Novak M, (1985) Phytochemistry 24(4):585.

Tada H et al., (1976) Chem Pharm Bull 24:667.

Tori K et al., (1976) Tetrahedron Lett 5:387.

Further information in:

Hausen B, Allergiepflanzen, Pflanzenallergene, ecomed erlagsgesellsch. mbH, Landsberg 1988.

Hegnauer R, Chemotaxonomie der Pflanzen, Bde 1-11, Birkhäuser Verlag Basel, Boston, Berlin 1962-1997.

Kern W, List PH, Hörhammer L (Hrsg.), Hagers Handbuch der Pharmazeutischen Praxis, 4. Aufl., Bde 1-8, Springer Verlag Berlin, Heidelberg, New York, 1969.

Roth L, Daunderer M, Kormann K, Giftpflanzen, Pflanzengifte, 4. Aufl., Ecomed Fachverlag Landsberg Lech 1993.

Steinegger E, Hänsel R, Pharmakognosie, 5. Aufl., Springer Verlag Heidelberg 1992.

Teuscher E, Lindequist U, Biogene Gifte - Biologie, Chemie, Pharmakologie, 2. Aufl., Fischer Verlag Stuttgart 1994.

LAURI FRUCTUS

Hogg JW et al., (1974) Phytochemistry 13:868.

Novak M, (1985) Phytochemistry 24(4):585.

Tada H et al., (1976) Chem Pharm Bull 24:667.

Tori K et al., (1976) Tetrahedron Lett 5:387.

Further information in:

Hausen B, Allergiepflanzen, Pflanzenallergene, ecomed Verlagsgesellsch. mbH, Landsberg 1988.

Kern W, List PH, Hörhammer L (Hrsg.), Hagers Handbuch der Pharmazeutischen Praxis, 4. Aufl., Bde 1-8, Springer Verlag Berlin, Heidelberg, New York, 1969.

Roth L, Daunderer M, Kormann K, Giftpflanzen, Pflanzengifte, 4. Aufl., Ecomed Fachverlag Landsberg Lech 1993.

Steinegger E, Hänsel R, Pharmakognosie, 5. Aufl., Springer Verlag Heidelberg 1992.

Teuscher E, Lindequist U, Biogene Gifte - Biologie, Chemie, Pharmakologie, 2. Aufl., Fischer Verlag Stuttgart 1994.

Lavandula Angustifolia

Lavender

DESCRIPTION

Medicinal Parts: The medicinal parts are the essential oil extracted from the fresh flowers and/or the inflorescences, the flowers collected just before opening and dried, the fresh flowers and the dried flowers.

Flower and Fruit: The flowers are in false whorls of 6 to 10 blossoms forming interrupted terminal spikes. The pedicles are 10 to 15 cm long downy stems. The bracts are 5 mm long, ovate to broadly triangular, often brown and brown-violet or violet-tinged. The tubular calyx has 5 uneven tips, it is amethyst-colored, tomentose and after flowering it is closed by a lidlike appendage of its upper tip. The corolla is longer with a cylindrically fused base, the lips are flat, and the upper lip is larger with 2 lobes. The lower lip is 3-lobed with even tips. The stamens are enclosed in the tube. The ovary consists of 4 carpels and has a nectary below it. The fruit is a glossy brown nutlet.

Leaves, Stem and Root: Lavender is a 60 cm high subshrub and is heavily branched with leafy, erect, rod-like, gray-green, young branches. The leaves are sessile, oblong-lanceolate, entire-margined, involute, gray, later green with glandular spots beneath.

Characteristics: The flowers have a fresh aromatic fragrance.

Habitat: The plant is indigenous to the Mediterranean region but is common in most of southern Europe and is cultivated extensively.

Production: Lavender flower consists of the dried flower of Lavandula angustifolia, gathered shortly before fully unfolding, as well as its preparations. Flowering shoots are harvested when the middle section of the spike is flowering; it is cut 10 cm beneath the insertion of the spike. The most valuable part is the receptacle.

Not To Be Confused With: Other varieties of lavender such as Lavendula intermedia (Lavendin) and Lavendula latifolia. The varieties are often mixed commercially. When the drug material has a high proportion of stem and leaf material, it is considered less valuable.

ACTION AND PHARMACOLOGY

COMPOUNDS

Volatile oil (1-3%): chief components (-)-linalool (making up 20-50%) and linalyl acetate (30-40%), furthermore, including among others, cis-ocimene, terpinene-4-ol, beta-caryophyllene, lavandulyl acetate

Hydroxycoumarins: including, among others, umbelliferone, herniarin

Tannins

Caffeic acid derivatives: including, among others, rosmaric acid

EFFECTS

Lavender has choleretic and cholagogic effects. Internally, it is mildly sedative, antiflatulent and a cholagogue. Externally, Lavender is rubefacient.

INDICATIONS AND USAGE

- Loss of appetite
- Nervousness and insomnia

Internally, Lavender is used for mood disturbances such as restlessness or insomnia, functional abdominal complaints (nervous stomach irritations, Roehmheld syndrome, meteorism, nervous intestinal discomfort).

Externally, Lavender is used in balneotherapy for treatment of functional circulatory disorders.

PRECAUTIONS AND ADVERSE REACTIONS

No health hazards or side effects are known in conjunction with the proper administration of designated therapeutic dosages. The volatile oil possesses a weak potential for sensitization.

DOSAGE

Mode of Administration: The whole drug is used for infusions, as an extract and as bath additive. Combinations with other sedative and/or carminative herbs may be beneficial.

Preparation: An infusion is prepared by adding 5 to 10 ml of drug per cup of hot water (150ml), draw for 10 minutes, and strain. For external use as bath additive, 100 g of drug is scalded or boiled with 2 liters of water and added to the bath.

Daily Dosage: 3 to 5 g of the drug. One to 4 drops of Lavender oil may be placed on a sugar cube.

LITERATURE

Atanassova-Shopova S, Roussinow KS, (1970) On certain central neurotropic effects of lavender essential oil. Bull Inst Physiol 8:69-76.

Buchbauer G, Jirovet L, Jäger W, Dietrich H, Plank C, Karamat E, (1991) Aromatherapy: Evidence for Sedative Effects of the Essential Oil of Lavender after Inhalation. Z Naturforsch 46c:1067-1072.

Guillemain J, Rousseau A, Delaveau P, (1989) Effets neurodépresseurs de l'huile essentielle de Lavandula angustifolia Mill. Ann Pharmaceutiques Francaises 47:337-343.

Herisset A et al., (1971) Plant Med Phytother 5:305.

Ianova LG et al., (1977) Khim Prir Soedin 1:111.

Kaiser R, Lamparsky D, (1977) Tetrahedron Lett 7:665.

Meyer A, Der Duft des Monats:Lavendel. In: DAZ 133(40):3667. 1993.

Mukherjee BD, Trenkle RW, (1973) J Agric Food Chem 21:298.

Schilcher H, Pflanzliche Psychopharmaka. Eine neue Klassifizierung nach Indikationsgruppen. In: DAZ 135(20):1811-1822. 1995.

Schulz V, Hübner WD, Ploch M, Klinische Studien mit Psycho-Phytopharmaka. In: ZPT 18(3):141-154. 1997.

Ter Heide R et al., (1970) J Chromatography 50:127.

Timiner R et al., (1975) J Agric Food Chem 23:53.

Further information in:

Hänsel R, Keller K, Rimpler H, Schneider G (Hrsg.), Hagers Handbuch der Pharmazeutischen Praxis, 5. Aufl., Bde 4-6 (Drogen): Springer Verlag Berlin, Heidelberg, New York, 1992-1994.

Hausen B, Allergiepflanzen, Pflanzenallergene, ecomed Verlagsgesellsch. mbH, Landsberg 1988.

Madaus G, Lehrbuch der Biologischen Arzneimittel, Bde 1-3, Nachdruck, Georg Olms Verlag Hildesheim 1979.

Roth L, Daunderer M, Kormann K, Giftpflanzen, Pflanzengifte, 4. Aufl., Ecomed Fachverlag Landsberg Lech 1993.

Schulz R, Hänsel R, Rationale Phytotherapie, Springer Verlag Heidelberg 1996.

Steinegger E, Hänsel R, Pharmakognosie, 5. Aufl., Springer Verlag Heidelberg 1992.

Teuscher E, Biogene Arzneimittel, 5. Aufl., Wiss. Verlagsges. Stuttgart 1997.

Wagner H, Wiesenauer M, Phytotherapie. Phytopharmaka und pflanzliche Homöopathika, Fischer-Verlag, Stuttgart, Jena, New York 1995.

Wichtl M (Hrsg.), Teedrogen, 4. Aufl., Wiss. Verlagsges. Stuttgart 1997.

Lavender

See Lavandula Angustifolia

Lavender Cotton

See Santolina Chamaecyparissias

Lawsonia Inermis

Henna

DESCRIPTION

Medicinal Parts: The medicinal parts are the pulverized leaves, the fruit and the bark.

Flower and Fruit: The flowers are in small impressive groups of 4 panicles and yellowy-white to brick-red. The calyx is top-shaped, later bowl-shaped without appendages. The petals are thick, very wrinkled, yellowy-white to brick-red. The stamens are arranged in pairs. The fruit is an indehiscent or a fibrously torn berry. The seeds are small and angular and the seed skin is spongy at the tip.

Leaves, Stem and Root: Henna is a deciduous, 2 to 6 m high shrub with partly thorny, short shoots and opposite paired, narrowly acuminate lanceolate leaves.

Habitat: Found in Egypt, India, the Middle East, Kurdistan and Iran.

Production: Henna is the aerial part of Lawsonia inermis.

Other Names: Alcanna, Egyptian Privet, Jamaica Mignonette, Mignonette Tree, Reseda, Henne, Mehndi, Mendee, Smooth Lawsonia

ACTION AND PHARMACOLOGY

COMPOUNDS

Naphthalene derivatives (1,4-naphthaquinones): in particular lawsone (2-hydroxy-1,4-naphthaquinone), arising during dehydration of the leaves out of the precursor 1,2,4-trihydroxy-naphthalen-4-beta-D-glucoside

Tannins

EFFECTS

The drug is an astringent and a diuretic, and has an antibacterial effect.

INDICATIONS AND USAGE

The drug is used externally for eczemas, scabies, fungal infections and ulcers. It is also used for amebic dysentery and gastrointestinal ulcers. The drug is also contained in face and hair lotions and is used to treat dandruff.

PRECAUTIONS AND ADVERSE REACTIONS

Health risks or side effects following the proper administration of designated therapeutic dosages are not recorded. Stomach complaints are possible due to the tannin content.

DOSAGE

Mode of Administration: Henna is used rarely for internal use in ground form or as an infusion.

Daily Dosage: For internal use, 3 g of powder leaves to be taken daily, for amoebiasis and ulcers.

LITERATURE

Bardwaj DK et al., (1978) Phytochemistry 17:1440.

Karawya MS et al., (1969) Lloydia 32:76.

Mahmood ZF et al., (1983) Fitoterapia 4:153.

Further information in:

Kern W, List PH, Hörhammer L (Hrsg.), Hagers Handbuch der Pharmazeutischen Praxis, 4. Aufl., Bde. 1-8, Springer Verlag Berlin, Heidelberg, New York, 1969.

Teuscher E, Biogene Arzneimittel, 5. Aufl., Wiss. Verlagsges. mbH Stuttgart 1997.

Wichtl M (Hrsg.), Teedrogen, 4. Aufl., Wiss. Verlagsges. mbH Stuttgart 1997.

Ledum Latifolium

Labrador Tea

DESCRIPTION

Medicinal Parts: The medicinal parts are the leaves and the flowering shoots.

Flower and Fruit: The flowers are in flat, terminal umbels. The calyx is small and has 5 tips. The 5-petalled corolla is white. The 10 stamens grow from the edge of a honey ring. The ovary is superior. The fruit is a 5-valvular capsule.

Leaves, Stem and Root: The evergreen, branched shrub grows to about 1.5 m. The young branches are gray or rust-colored. The 1.25 to 2.5 cm long leaves are alternate, short-petioled, entire-margined, linear, have revolute margins, are stiff, coriaceous, dark green above, rust-colored and woolly-downy underneath. L. palustre is larger, more regularly formed and has larger leaves.

Characteristics: It has a numbing, tangy aroma and is poisonous. It is a protected species.

Habitat: The plant grows in Greenland, Canada and the U.S. The very similar variety L. palustre is more common in northern Europe and northern Asia.

Production: Labrador herb is the aerial part of Ledum latifolium and L. palustre.

Other Names: St. James's Tea, Marsh Tea, Wild Rosemary

ACTION AND PHARMACOLOGY

COMPOUNDS

Volatile oil (0.9-2.6%): chief components sesquiterpenes, in particular ledol (ledum camphor, porst camphor) and palustrol, Japanese sources also yield ascaridol

Catechin tannins

Flavonoids: including among others hyperoside

Arbutin

EFFECTS

Internally mildly expectorant.

Externally antiphlogistic (neither proven).

INDICATIONS AND USAGE

Respiratory conditions. Externally for skin inflammations.

CONTRAINDICATIONS

The drug is contraindicated in pregnancy.

PRECAUTIONS AND ADVERSE REACTIONS

General: Initially, the drug causes severe gastrointestinal irritation (vomiting, gastroenteritis, diarrhea), due to its ledol content; leading, following resorption, to severe central excitation, observed in intoxicated states. This may be accompanied by spasms, and later by paralysis.

Pregnancy: Contraindicated. Poisonings in earlier times were particularly seen in connection with its misuse for purposes of abortion.

OVERDOSAGE

Following gastrointestinal emptying (inducement of vomiting, gastric lavage with burgundy-colored potassium permanganate solution, sodium sulfate), and instillation of activated charcoal, the treatment of poisonings consists of treating spasms with diazepam (I.V.) and colic with atropine; electrolyte substitution and treating possible cases of acidosis with sodium bicarbonate infusions. Monitoring of kidney function is essential. Intubation and oxygen respiration may also be necessary.

DOSAGE

Mode of Administration: Labrador Tea is obsolete as a drug. It has been used as an extract in some bath additives and is also contained in homeopathic preparations.

LITERATURE

Belleau F, Collin G, Composition of the essential oil of Ledum groenlandicum. In: PH 33:117. 1993.

Further information in:

Frohne D, Pfänder HJ, Giftpflanzen - Ein Handbuch für Apotheker, Toxikologen und Biologen, 4. Aufl., Wiss. Verlags-Ges. Stuttgart 1997.

Kern W, List PH, Hörhammer L (Hrsg.), Hagers Handbuch der Pharmazeutischen Praxis, 4. Aufl., Bde. 1-8, Springer Verlag Berlin, Heidelberg, New York, 1969.

Lewin L, Gifte und Vergiftungen, 6. Aufl., Nachdruck, Haug Verlag, Heidelberg 1992.

Madaus G, Lehrbuch der Biologischen Arzneimittel, Bde 1-3, Nachdruck, Georg Olms Verlag Hildesheim 1979.

Roth L, Daunderer M, Kormann K, Giftpflanzen, Pflanzengifte, 4. Aufl., Ecomed Fachverlag Landsberg Lech 1993.

Teuscher E, Lindequist U, Biogene Gifte - Biologie, Chemie, Pharmakologie, 2. Aufl., Fischer Verlag Stuttgart 1994.

Wagner H, Wiesenauer M, Phytotherapie. Phytopharmaka und pflanzliche Homöopathika, Fischer-Verlag, Stuttgart, Jena, New York 1995.

Lemna Minor

Duckweed

DESCRIPTION

Medicinal Parts: The medicinal part is the whole fresh plant.

Flower and Fruit: The plant flowers infrequently. The tiny inconspicuous flowers have 2 unevenly-sized stamens and 1 pistil. A delicate membranous bract surrounds 3 flowers, which are located on the edge of the stem. The fruit is tubular with 1 ovule. The seeds have longitudinal ribs.

Leaves, Stem and Root: Lemna minor is a swimming plant and has 2 to 6 mm long leaf-like organs. These are flat, have 3 to 5 ribs and are sometimes pigmented with red. Two to 6 leaf-like shoots stick together and each bears a root with a rounded root cover.

Characteristics: The plant has leaf-like shoots with 1 root per leaf.

Habitat: The plant is found worldwide in cooler, oceanic climates. The plant is not found in east Asia and South Africa.

ACTIONS AND PHARMACOLOGY

COMPOUNDS

Flavonoids: in particular C-glucosyl-flavone, including, among others, orientin, isoorientin, vitexin, isovitexin, lutonarin, vicenin-1, also O-glycosides, including, among others, apigenin-7-O-glucoside

Cyclopentane fatty acids with structure resembling prostaglandin

Polysaccharides: apiogalacturonans

Cardiac steroids (cardenolides)

EFFECTS

No information is available.

INDICATIONS AND USAGE

Duckweed is used for inflammation of the upper respiratory tract, jaundice, and rheumatism.

PRECAUTIONS AND ADVERSE REACTIONS

No health hazards or side effects are known in conjunction with the proper administration of designated therapeutic dosages.

DOSAGE

Mode of Administration: The plant is available in powder form and as an extract.

LITERATURE

Hänsel R, Keller K, Rimpler H, Schneider G (Hrsg.), Hagers Handbuch der Pharmazeutischen Praxis, 5. Aufl., Bde 4-6 (Drogen), Springer Verlag Berlin, Heidelberg, New York, 1992-1994.

Madaus G. Lehrbuch der Biologischen Arzneimittel, Bde 1-3, Nachdruck, Georg Olms Verlag Hildesheim 1979.

Lemon

See Citrus Limon

Lemon Balm

See Melissa Officinalis

Lemon Verbena

See Aloysia Triphylla

Leonurus Cardiaca

Motherwort

DESCRIPTION

Medicinal Parts: The medicinal parts are the fresh aerial parts collected during the flowering season.

Flower and Fruit: Small, bright red bilabiate flowers are in dense false whorls in the upper leaf axils. The calyx is funnel-shaped with 5 rigid, awned tips, which are bent outwards. The corolla is densely villous on the outside and longer than the calyx. The stamens stretch out longer than the flower. The fruit is a brown, triangular, 2.5 to 3 mm long nutlet with a tuft of hair at the tip.

Leaves, Stem and Root: The plant is perennial and has a short woody rhizome. It grows to about 120 cm. The stem is erect, quadrangular, grooved, hollow, often red-violet and usually hairy. The leaves are long-petioled, pubescent or glabrous. The lower leaves are palmate and cordate at the base. The upper leaves are 3-lobed. The upper surface is dark green the lower surface light green.

Characteristics: Motherwort has an unpleasant smell.

Habitat: The plant is indigenous to central Europe and Scandinavia through temperate Russia to central Asia. It was introduced to North America and has become established in the wild there.

Production: Motherwort herb consists of the above-ground parts of Leonurus cardiaca, gathered during flowering season, as well as their preparations.

Other Names: Lion's Tail, Lion's Ear, Throw-wort

ACTION AND PHARMACOLOGY

COMPOUNDS

Diterpene bitter principles: leocardin

Iridoide monoterpenes: ajugoside (leonuride), ajugol, galiridoside, reptoside

Flavonoids: including, among others, rutin, quercitrin, isoquercitrin, hyperoside, genkwanin

Leonurin: (syringa acid esters of 4-guanidino-butane-1-ols)

Betaine: stachydrine (N-dimethyl-L-proline)

Caffeic acid derivatives: caffeic acid-4-O-rutinoside

Tannins

Volatile oil: (traces)

EFFECTS

Mildly negatively chronotropic, hypotonic, sedative.

INDICATIONS AND USAGE

- Cardiac insufficiency NYHA I and II
- Arrhythmia
- Nervous heart complaints

Nervous cardiac disorders, thyroid hyperfunction, flatulence.

PRECAUTIONS AND ADVERSE REACTIONS

No health hazards or side effects are known in conjunction with the proper administration of designated therapeutic dosages.

DOSAGE

Mode of Administration: Comminuted herb for infusions and other galenic preparations for internal use.

Daily Dosage: 4.5 g herb.

Acute states - regular use (every 30 to 60 minutes), 5 drops, 1 tablet, 10 pellets or a knife tip.

Chronic states - 1 to 3 times daily, 5 drops, 1 tablet, 10 pellets or a knife tip.

LITERATURE

Buzogany K, Cucu V, Accumulation, distribution and conservation dynamics of iridoids in Leonurus cardiaca L. and L. villosus Desf. In: Farmacia (Bukarest): 34(3):173-176. 1986.

Chang CF, Li CZ, (1986) Chung I Chieh Ho Tsa Chih 6(1):39.

Kartnig T et al., (1985) J Nat Prod 48(3):494.

Kooiman P, (1972) Acta Bot Neerl. 21(4) 417.

Malakov P et al., (1985) Phytochemistry 24(10):2341.

Peng Y, (1983) Bull Chin. Mat Med 8:41.

Reuter G, Diehl H.J, (1970) Pharmazie 25:586.

Schilling G et al., (1975) Liebigs Ann Chem:230.

Tschesche R et al., (1980) Phytochemistry 19:2783.

Weischer ML, Okpanyi SN, Pharmakologie eines pflanzlichen Schlafmittels. In: ZPT 15(5):257-262. 1994.

Xia XX, (1983) J Trad Chin Med 3:185.

Further information in:

Hänsel R, Keller K, Rimpler H, Schneider G (Hrsg.), Hagers Handbuch der Pharmazeutischen Praxis, 5. Aufl., Bde 4-6 (Drogen), Springer Verlag Berlin, Heidelberg, New York, 1992-1994.

Madaus G, Lehrbuch der Biologischen Arzneimittel, Bde 1-3, Nachdruck, Georg Olms Verlag Hildesheim 1979.

Steinegger E, Hänsel R, Pharmakognosie, 5. Aufl., Springer Verlag Heidelberg 1992.

Teuscher E, Biogene Arzneimittel, 5. Aufl., Wiss. Verlagsges. Stuttgart 1997.

Wagner H, Wiesenauer M, Phytotherapie. Phytopharmaka und pflanzliche Homöopathika, Fischer-Verlag, Stuttgart, Jena, New York 1995.

Wichtl M (Hrsg.), Teedrogen, 4. Aufl., Wiss. Verlagsges. Stuttgart 1997.

Lepidium Sativum

Garden Cress

DESCRIPTION

Medicinal Parts: The medicinal part is the fresh or dried herb harvested during or shortly after the flowering season.

Flower and Fruit: The racemes are terminal or axillary. The sepals are elliptical, 1 to 1.5 mm long and bristly downy. The petals are longer than the calyx, white or reddish, oblong-spatulate and indistinctly stemmed. The anthers are often violet. The fruit is a compressed, orbicular-ovate, 5 to 6 mm long, clearly winged small pod on an erect stem. The seeds are ovate, almost smooth and red-brown.

Leaves, Stem and Root: Garden cress is a 20 to 40 cm high herb with a glabrous bluish bloom. The stem is erect, round and branched. The leaves are light green and thin. The basal leaves are usually lyrate-pinatesect. The lower cauline leaves are usually doubly or singly pinnatesect. All leaves have dentate to prickly segments.

Characteristics: Garden Cress has a radish-like taste. The seeds have a slimy skin and swell in water.

Habitat: The herb is grown worldwide.

Production: Garden Cress is the fresh plant (aerial part) of Lepidium sativum, harvested during the flowering season or shortly afterwards. The fresh herb has a spicy odor. It is rarely dried, naturally or artificially, since the fresh plant is used more often.

Not To Be Confused With: Adulterations rarely occur, since it is usually cultivated.

ACTIONS AND PHARMACOLOGY

COMPOUNDS

Glucosinolates: chief components glucotropaeolin, yielding benzyl cyanide when the plant is bruised

Ascorbic acid (Vitamin C) and B vitamins in the seeds

Cucurbitacins

Cardiac steroids (cardenolides)

EFFECTS

The antibacterial action of cress has been demonstrated in various tests. It was completely inhibitory in the case of 3 microorganisms, although the antibacterial characteristics depended largely on the age of the plants used. An antiviral effect against the encephalitis virus *Columbia SH*, was demonstrated in tests on mice. Its diuretic action has not been proven through experiments.

INDICATIONS AND USAGE

The herb is used for coughs and Vitamin C deficiency. In folk medicine, it is used for constipation, as a diuretic, and for poor immunity.

PRECAUTIONS AND ADVERSE REACTIONS

No health hazards or side effects are known in conjunction with the proper administration of designated therapeutic dosages. The administration of higher dosages of the freshly-harvested plant can lead to mucous membrane irritation of the gastrointestinal tract.

DOSAGE

Mode of Administration: As a freshly cut herb in oral preparations.

LITERATURE

Hänsel R, Keller K, Rimpler H, Schneider G (Hrsg.), Hagers Handbuch der Pharmazeutischen Praxis, 5. Aufl., Bde 4-6 (Drogen), Springer Verlag Berlin, Heidelberg, New York, 1992-1994.

Leptandra Virginica

Black Root

DESCRIPTION

Medicinal Parts: The medicinal part is the dried rhizome with the roots. The roots have a very different action according to whether they are used fresh or dry. The dried root is milder.

Flower and Fruit: The stems end in terminal, 15 to 25 cm long spikes of white flowers.

Leaves, Stem and Root: The plant is a perennial herb, which grows to about 120 cm high. The rhizome is horizontal, cylindrical, branched and dark red to dark purple-brown on the outside. The simple, erect stems grow in intervals of 1.2 to 3.2 cm from the rhizome. They are smooth and finely downy. The leaves are whorled (4 to 7 in one whorl), lanceolate, on short petioles, pointed and finely serrate.

Habitat: Indigenous to the eastern U.S. but grows elsewhere.

Production: Black root and rhizome are the complete underground parts of Leptandra virginica.

Other Names: Bowman's Root, Physic Root, Hini, Oxadoddy, Tall Speedwell, Tall Veronica, Whorlywort, Culveris Root

ACTIONS AND PHARMACOLOGY

COMPOUNDS

Volatile oil: composition unknown

Cinnamic acid derivatives: including, among others, 4-methoxycinnamic acid, 3,4-dimethoxycinnamic acid and their esters

Tannins

The constituents of the drug have not been fully investigated.

EFFECTS

Diaphoretic, carminative, cholagogue, cathartic and laxative.

INDICATIONS AND USAGE

Black Root is used for chronic constipation, liver and gallbladder disorders.

PRECAUTIONS AND ADVERSE REACTIONS

No health hazards are known in conjunction with the proper administration of designated therapeutic dosages. The emetic and laxative effects of the drug are used therapeutically.

DOSAGE

Mode of Administration: As a powder in various preparations and combinations

LITERATURE

Hänsel R, Keller K, Rimpler H, Schneider G (Hrsg.), Hagers Handbuch der Pharmazeutischen Praxis, 5. Aufl., Bde 4-6 (Drogen), Springer Verlag Berlin, Heidelberg, New York, 1992-1994 (unter Veronica virginica).

Lewin L, Gifte und Vergiftungen, 6. Aufl., Nachdruck, Haug Verlag, Heidelberg 1992.

Madaus G, Lehrbuch der Biologischen Arzneimittel, Bde 1-3, Nachdruck, Georg Olms Verlag Hildesheim 1979.

Wagner H, Wiesenauer M, Phytotherapie. Phytopharmaka und pflanzliche Homöopathika, Fischer-Verlag, Stuttgart, Jena, New York 1995.

Lesser Celandine

See Ranunculus Ficaria

Levisticum Officinale

Lovage

DESCRIPTION

Medicinal Parts: The medicinal parts are the dried rhizome and roots, the cut, dried herb and the dried fruit.

Flower and Fruit: The flowers are in 8 to 20 rayed compound umbels. There is an involucre and epicalyx. There is no calyx. The orbicular petals are pale yellow and involute. The fruit is yellow-brown, 5 to 7 mm long, compressed, and has sharply keeled to winged ribs.

Leaves, Stem and Root: The plant is a sturdy perennial. It has a thick, spindle-shaped, branched root, which is brownish-yellow on the outside and whitish on the inside. The stem is erect, round, hollow, finely grooved, glabrous, and up to 4 cm thick at the base. The leaves are rich green, glossy, coriaceous; the lower ones double-pinnate, the upper ones simple-pinnate. The leaflets are broad and obovate.

Characteristics: The rubbed leaves give off an aromatic scent. The fruit is very fragrant.

Habitat: Lovage is indigenous to the Mediterranean region, it grows wild in the Balkans and northern Greece, and is cultivated elsewhere.

Production: Lovage root consists of the dried rhizomes and roots of Levisticum officinale, as well as their preparations. Roots of 2-year-old plants are collected in autumn. It is important that the roots are not damaged during the drying process since this would result in a loss of the essential oil.

Not To Be Confused With: Angelicae radix, Pastinacae radix or Pimpinellae radix.

Other Names: Lavose, Sea Parsley

ACTION AND PHARMACOLOGY

COMPOUNDS

Volatile oil (0.35-1.7%): chief components alkylphthalides (aroma-bearers), including among others 3-butylphthalide, ligusticumlactone (E- and Z-butylidenphthalides), E- and Z-ligustilide furthermore, including among others, alpha- and beta-pinene, beta-phellandrene, citronellal

Hydroxycoumarins: umbelliferone

Coumarin

Furocoumarins: bergaptene, apterin

Polyynes: including among others, falcarindiol (probably only in the fresh rhizome)

EFFECTS

Diuretic, sedative, antimicrobial, cholinergic.

The ligustilide-containing essential oil has an antispasmodic effect on smooth muscle.

The folk use for gastric complaints is probably based on the specific odor caused by phthalide as well as on the bitter taste, which increases saliva and gastric secretions.

INDICATIONS AND USAGE

- Infections of the urinary tract
- Kidney and bladder stones

Flushing-out therapy for inflammation of the lower urinary tract and flushing-out therapy for prevention of kidney gravel.

The folk medicine uses include dyspeptic complaints such as indigestion, heartburn, feelings of fullness, flatulence, menstrual complaints. Lovage is also used as a secretolytic for respiratory catarrh.

CONTRAINDICATIONS

Because of the irritating effect of the volatile oil, the drug should not be administered in the presence of inflammation of the kidneys or of the urinary drainage passages, nor with reduced kidney function. No irrigation therapy is to be carried out in the presence of edema resulting from reduced cardiac and kidney function.

PRECAUTIONS AND ADVERSE REACTIONS

No health hazards or side effects are known in conjunction with the proper administration of designated therapeutic dosages. The drug possesses a low potential for sensitization. An elevation of UV-sensitivity among light-skinned people is possible (phototoxic effect of the furocoumarins).

DOSAGE

Mode of Administration: Comminuted herb and other galenic preparations for internal use.

Daily Dosage: 4 to 8 g drug. Ample intake of liquid is essential.

Storage: Protect from light and insects in well sealed containers. The whole drug should be stored not longer than 18 months; the powdered drug, not longer than 24 hours.

LITERATURE

Albulescu D et al., (1975) Farmacia 23:159.

Bjeldanes LF, Kim I, (1977) J Org Chem 42:2333.

Fischer FC, Svendson AB, (1976) Phytochemistry 15:1079.

Gijbels MJ et al., (1981) Chromatographia 14(8):451.

Gijbels MJ et al., (1982) Planta Med 44:207.

Lawrence BM, (1980) Perf Flav 5:29.

Vollmann C, Levisticum officinale - Der Liebstöckel. In: ZPT 9(4):128. 1988.

Yu SR, You SQ, (1984) Yao Hsueh Hsueh Pao 19(8):566.

Further information in:

Hänsel R, Keller K, Rimpler H, Schneider G (Hrsg.), Hagers Handbuch der Pharmazeutischen Praxis, 5. Aufl., Bde 4-6 (Drogen), Springer Verlag Berlin, Heidelberg, New York, 1992-1994.

Leung AY, Encyclopedia of Common Natural Ingredients Used in Food Drugs and Cosmetics, John Wiley & Sons Inc., New York 1980.

Madaus G, Lehrbuch der Biologischen Arzneimittel, Bde 1-3, Nachdruck, Georg Olms Verlag Hildesheim 1979.

Steinegger E, Hänsel R, Pharmakognosie, 5. Aufl., Springer Verlag Heidelberg 1992.

Teuscher E, Biogene Arzneimittel, 5. Aufl., Wiss. Verlagsges. Stuttgart 1997.

Teuscher E, Lindequist U, Biogene Gifte - Biologie, Chemie, Pharmakologie, 2. Aufl., Fischer Verlag Stuttgart 1994.

Wichtl M (Hrsg.), Teedrogen, 4. Aufl., Wiss. Verlagsges. Stuttgart 1997.

Liatris Spicata

Marsh Blazing Star

DESCRIPTION

Medicinal Parts: The medicinal parts are the roots.

Flower and Fruit: The inflorescences are compound spikes of carmine red flowers, 4 to 8 mm in diameter.

Leaves, Stem and Root: The plant is a perennial and has an erect, leafy stem up 2 m. The leaves are opposite, up to 30 cm long and 1 cm wide. The rhizome is 1 cm or more in diameter. It is gnarled with several cup-shaped scars. The rhizome is brownish and slightly wrinkled on the outside. Inside it is whitish with dark gray spots.

Characteristics: The root is very solid. The taste is bitter and the odor is faintly aromatic, resembling cedar.

Habitat: U.S. cultivated in parts of Europe.

Other Names: Button Snakeroot, Gay-feather, Backache Root, Colic Root, Devil's Bite

ACTION AND PHARMACOLOGY

COMPOUNDS

Coumarin

EFFECTS

Main active principle: Coumarin.

INDICATIONS AND USAGE

Marsh Blazing Star has been used for disorders of the kidney, dysmenorrhea, as a diuretic, and as a gonorrhea treatment.

PRECAUTIONS AND ADVERSE REACTIONS

No health hazards or side effects are known in conjunction with the proper administration of designated therapeutic dosages.

DOSAGE

Mode of Administration: Ground drug as an infusion.

LITERATURE

Lowry JB, (1973) Nature 241:61.

Seshadri TF, (1972) Phytochemistry 11:881.

Further information in:

Kern W, List PH, Hörhammer L (Hrsg.), Hagers Handbuch der Pharmazeutischen Praxis, 4. Aufl., Bde. 1-8, Springer Verlag Berlin, Heidelberg, New York, 1969.

Madaus G, Lehrbuch der Biologischen Arzneimittel, Bde 1-3, Nachdruck, Georg Olms Verlag Hildesheim 1979.

Licorice

See Glycyrrhiza Glabra

Life Root

See Senecio Aureus; Senecio Nemorensis

Lilium Candidium

White Lily

DESCRIPTION

Medicinal Parts: The medicinal part is the fresh and dried bulb.

Flower and Fruit: The inflorescence has 5 to 20 blossoms. The flowers are white, occasionally striped crimson or spotted and very fragrant. They are on erect pedicles, the lower ones nodding. The tepals are obtuse, the anthers yellow. The style is as long as the sepals. The fruit is obovate and is seldom developed.

Leaves, Stem and Root: The plant is perennial, 60 to 150 cm high. It has a broad, ovate, scaled and yellow bulb. The stem is rigid, erect and leafy. The leaves are oblong to linear-lanceolate and glabrous. The leaves survive winter, as does the rest of the plant, which is hardy. The bulb consists of imbricate, fleshy, lanceolate and bent scales, which are 3.25 cm long and 2.5 cm wide at the broadest point.

Characteristics: The bulbs are odorless and have a mildly bitter and unpleasant flavor.

Habitat: The plant is indigenous to Mediterranean regions and is cultivated in many other regions.

Production: Baurenlilien (Farmer's Lily) root is the subterranean part (onion) of Lilium candidum.

Other Names: Meadow Lily, Madonna Lily

ACTION AND PHARMACOLOGY

COMPOUNDS

Soluble polysaccharides: glucomannans

Starch

Gamma-methylene glutamic acid

Tuliposide

The constituents of the drug have not been investigated extensively.

EFFECTS

Active agents: Plant mucous, tannin, sterine and glycoside.

Astringent, anti-inflammatory, softener, pain reliever, diuretic, hemorrhagic blood conditions and expectorant properties.

INDICATIONS AND USAGE

Internally: For gynecological disorders.

Externally: For ulcers, inflammation, furuncles, finger ulcers, reddened skin, burns and injuries.

PRECAUTIONS AND ADVERSE REACTIONS

No health hazards or side effects are known in conjunction with the proper administration of designated therapeutic dosages.

DOSAGE

Mode of Administration: An infusion made from the ground drug is used internally. The drug is also used externally as a wet compress (paste).

Daily Dosage: Apply a thick paste, made from fresh or cooked onions, in the middle of a compress or poultice, to the affected area. This should be done several times during the day.

LITERATURE

Delaveau P et al., (1980) Planta Med 40:49.

Masterova I et al., (1987) Phytochemistry 26(6):1844.

Nagy E et al., (1984) Z Naturforsch 39B(12):1813.

Further information in:

Kern W, List PH, Hörhammer L (Hrsg.), Hagers Handbuch der Pharmazeutischen Praxis, 4. Aufl., Bde. 1-8, Springer Verlag Berlin, Heidelberg, New York, 1969.

Lilium Martagon

Martagon

DESCRIPTION

Medicinal Parts: The medicinal parts are the leaves, stem, and flowers, which are collected when the plant is completely mature.

Flower and Fruit: The inflorescence is terminal and racemous with 3 to 10 inclined flowers. The flower buds are globose or oblong-ovate. The tepal petals are 3 to 3.5 cm long, involute, orange with dark spots, and contain a ciliate mauve honey gland. The anthers are red. The fruit is a 2-winged capsule with an erect fruit stem. The seeds are flat, light brown, and 6 to 8 mm long. Since the seeds do not ripen in northern regions, propagation takes place by means of bulbils, which occur at the leaf axils. Flowers are produced during the third year of growth.

Leaves, Stem and Root: The plant is a perennial, 30 to 60 cm high or higher. The bulb is golden yellow, ovate, and about 5 cm long. The stem is erect, round, glabrous or with short rough hairs on the upper section. The stem is green or spotted red and leafy in the middle. The leaves are 7 to 11 ribbed, oblong-spatulate, shortly ciliated, and are up to 15 cm long.

Habitat: The plant comes from China and Japan but is also found today in central and southern Europe.

Other Names: Purple Turk's Cap Lily, Turk's Cap

ACTIONS AND PHARMACOLOGY

COMPOUNDS

Soluble polysaccharides

Starch

Gamma-methylene glutamic acid

Tuliposide

The constituents of the drug have not been fully investigated.

EFFECTS

No information is available.

INDICATIONS AND USAGE

The drug is used as a diuretic and in the treatment of dysmenorrhea. It is used externally for ulcers. The most common use is in homeopathy.

PRECAUTIONS AND ADVERSE REACTIONS

No health hazards or side effects are known in conjunction with the proper administration of designated therapeutic dosages.

DOSAGE

Mode of Administration: The drug is available in the powdered form as an infusion and for poultices. Homeopathic dilutions are also available.

LITERATURE

No literature is available.

Lily-of-the-Valley

See Convallaria Majalis

Lime

See Citrus Aurantifolia

Linaria Vulgaris

Yellow Toadflax

DESCRIPTION

Medicinal Parts: The medicinal part is the fresh or dried herb.

Flower and Fruit: The flowers are in terminal dense racemes. They are sulfur-yellow and remain closed until a bee gains entry. The calyx is only fused at the base and is 5-tipped. The corolla has a long sharp spur and is bilabiate with orange edges. There are 2 large and 2 small stamens and 1 superior ovary. The fruit is an orbicular, dry capsule with some chambers, which open when ripe, flinging out the seeds. The seeds are flattened and are in the middle of a circular wing.

Leaves, Stem and Root: A number of slim, glabrous, erect, simple stems 30 to 60 cm high grow from a perennial creeping root. The numerous leaves are alternate, sessile, very long and narrow. The leaves and stems are pale-blue and completely glabrous.

Habitat: The plant is indigenous to the northern hemisphere and the southwest U.S.

Production: True toadflax is the flowering herb of Linaria vulgaris.

Other Names: Fluellin, Pattens and Clogs, Flaxweed, Ramsted, Snapdragon, Churnstaff, Dragon-bushes, Brideweed, Toadpipe, Yellow Rod, Larkspur Lion's Mouth, Devil's Ribbon, Eggs and Collops, Devil's Head, Pedlar's Basket, Gallwort, Rabbits, Doggies, Calves' Snout, Eggs and Bacon, Buttered Haycocks, Monkey Flower, Butter and Eggs, Pennywort

ACTION AND PHARMACOLOGY

COMPOUNDS

Iridoide monoterpenes: chief component - antirrhinoside

Flavonoids: including among others linarin, pectolinarin, linariin (pectolinarigenin-7-rhamnoglucoside- acetate)

Aurones: including among others aureusin, bracteatin-6-O-glucoside

Quinazoline alkaloids: peganine (vasicin)

EFFECTS

The main active agents are the flavon glycosides linarin und pectolinarin, pectin, Phytosterol, tannic acid and Vitamin C.

Diaphoretic and diuretic effects have been documented.

Anti-inflammatory.

INDICATIONS AND USAGE

Internally: To aid digestion problems and urinary tract disorders.

Externally: For hemorrhoids, ablution of festering wounds, skin rashes, ulcus cruris.

PRECAUTIONS AND ADVERSE REACTIONS

No health hazards or side effects are known in conjunction with the proper administration of designated therapeutic dosages.

DOSAGE

Mode of Administration: The powdered form and the extract are used as a diuretic and a mild laxative (tea).

Externally the herb is used in poultices.

Preparation: Tea infusion is prepared from 1 to 2 teaspoonfuls of the drug and 2 to 4 cups of boiling water left to draw for 18 minutes.

Daily Dosage: Drink the tea during the course of the day.

LITERATURE

Ilieva E et al., 5-O-Allosylantirrinoside from Linaria species. In: PH 32:1068. 1993.

Further information in:

Hegnauer R, Chemotaxonomie der Pflanzen, Bde 1-11, Birkhäuser Verlag Basel, Boston, Berlin 1962-1997.

Kern W, List PH, Hörhammer L (Hrsg.), Hagers Handbuch der Pharmazeutischen Praxis, 4. Aufl., Bde. 1-8, Springer Verlag Berlin, Heidelberg, New York, 1969.

Madaus G, Lehrbuch der Biologischen Arzneimittel, Bde 1-3, Nachdruck, Georg Olms Verlag Hildesheim 1979.

Linden

See Tilia Species

Linum Catharticum

Mountain Flax

DESCRIPTION

Medicinal Parts: The medicinal parts are the herb, the fresh flowering plant and the whole plant.

Flower and Fruit: The flowers are on loose, panicled-branched, sparsely leafed twining stems on long peduncles in the leaf axils. They hang before flowering. The sepals are elliptically acuminate, 2 to 2.5 mm long with ciliate glands. The 5 petals are up to 5 mm long, white, and yellow at the base. There are 5 stamens fused at the base and 1 ovary with 5 headed stigma on long thin styles. The fruit is erect, globular, 2 to 3 cm long and incomplete 10-valved with long, pubescent dividing membranes. The seeds are elliptical, 1 to 1.5 mm long, flat, smooth and light brown.

Leaves, Stem and Root: The plant is an inconspicuous annual (occasionally perennial) which grows up to 30 cm. It has a long erect or ascending stem, which is undivided or dividing into the flowering branches. The leaves are opposite or alternate, entire-margined, sessile and have a partly ciliate margin.

Habitat: Found in central Europe as far as the British Isles and southwards as far as the Mediterranean countries, the Caucasus, Iran and northern Africa.

Production: Mountain Flax is the flowering plant (aerial part) of Linum catharticum and is collected in the wild.

Other Names: Purging Flax, Dwarf Flax, Fairy Flax, Mill Mountain

ACTION AND PHARMACOLOGY

COMPOUNDS

Lignans: achromatin (bitter), presumably present in the fresh plant as a glycoside

Tannins

Volatile oil

The constituents of the drug have not been extensively investigated.

EFFECTS

Mountain Flax has a laxative effect in therapeutic doses of up to 0.5 g.

INDICATIONS AND USAGE

As a purgative and emetic.

PRECAUTIONS AND ADVERSE REACTIONS

No health hazards or side effects are known in conjunction with the proper administration of designated therapeutic dosages. The drug can lead to vomiting, inflammations of the gastrointestinal tract and diarrhea. The emetic and laxative effects are used therapeutically.

DOSAGE

Mode of Administration: Ground and as an extract.

Preparation: To prepare an infusion, add 2.5 g to 1 cup of hot water.

Dosage: 2.0 g powder as a single dose.

LITERATURE

Hänsel R, Keller K, Rimpler H, Schneider G (Hrsg.), Hagers Handbuch der Pharmazeutischen Praxis, 5. Aufl., Bde 4-6

(Drogen), Springer Verlag Berlin, Heidelberg, New York, 1992-1994.

Madaus G, Lehrbuch der Biologischen Arzneimittel, Bde 1-3, Nachdruck, Georg Olms Verlag Hildesheim 1979.

Linum Usitatissimum

Flaxseed

DESCRIPTION

Medicinal Parts: The medicinal parts are the stem as a sterile linen thread, the oil extracted from the seeds, the dry ripe seeds, the linseed cakes and the fresh flowering plant.

Flower and Fruit: The flowers are panicle-like loose cymes on long peduncles in the leaf axils of the upper part of the stem. They have 5 ovate, acuminate, finely ciliate sepals and 5 obovate petals, which are sky blue and longer than the sepals. There are 5 stamens fused at the base and 1 ovary. The fruit is an almost globular, 6 to 8 mm long capsule on an erect or slightly bent stem. The seeds are flat, brown and glossy.

Leaves, Stem and Root: The plant is an annual and grows from 20 to 150 cm high. The root is short, fusiform and light yellow. The stem is unbranched, erect or ascending in short curves. The leaves are smooth edged, gray-green, sessile and almost awn-like acuminate.

Characteristics: The plant flowers only in the morning.

Habitat: The plant is cultivated in temperate and tropical regions the world over.

Production: Flaxseed consists of the dried, ripe seed of the collective variations of Linum usitatissimum as well as its preparations. The various cultivars of Linum usitatissimum are equally acceptable for the indications listed. The plant is cultivated. The ripe seeds are recovered from the capsules by threshing.

Not To Be Confused With: Lolium temulentum and weed seeds.

Other Names: Flax, Lint Bells, Winterlien, Linseed

ACTION AND PHARMACOLOGY

COMPOUNDS

Mucilages (3-10%, in the epidermis, high swelling capacity)

Cyanogenic glycosides (0.05-0.1%): linustatin and neolinustatin (yielding under optimal conditions 30-50 mg HCN per 100 g)

Fatty oil (30-45%): chief fatty acids linolenic acid (40-70%), linoleic acid (10-25%), oleic acid (13-30%)

Proteins (20-27%)

Ballast, (25%)

Lignans: secoisolariciresinol-diglucoside

Phenylpropane derivatives: including among others, linusitamarine

EFFECTS

Laxative, lipid-reducing, sugar-reducing, anticarcinogenic effects have been demonstrated in various studies and animal tests; swelling agent stimulates intestinal peristalsis causing the laxative effect.

INDICATIONS AND USAGE

■ Constipation

Internally: Used for chronic constipation, for colons damaged by abuse of laxatives, irritable colon, diverticulitis and as mucilage for gastritis and enteritis. A decoction is used for bladder catarrh and inflammation, gastritis.

Externally: For removing foreign bodies from the eye a single linseed is moistened and placed under the eyelid, the foreign body should stick to the mucous secretion of the seed; as cataplasm for local skin inflammation.

CONTRAINDICATIONS

Flaxseed is contraindicated in the following conditions: ileus, stricture of the esophagus and in the gastrointestinal area, acute inflammatory illnesses of the intestine, of the esophagus and of the stomach entrance.

PRECAUTIONS AND ADVERSE REACTIONS

General: No health hazards or side effects are known in conjunction with the proper administration of designated therapeutic dosages. The use of large quantities of the drug as a laxative with too little fluid intake can lead to ileus. The cyanogenic glycosides present no danger with the intake of therapeutic dosages; the glycosides are broken down only to a limited extent in the body. An elevation in the concentration of cyanide ions and of the detoxification product thiocyanic acid in the blood could not be demonstrated.

Drug Interactions: The absorption of other drugs taken simultaneously may be delayed.

DOSAGE

Mode of Administration: Internally, the cracked or coarsely ground seed, in which only the cuticle and mucilage epidermis are damaged is used. Linseed gruel and other galenic preparations are also available for internal use.

Externally: as linseed meal or linseed expellent.

Daily Dosage: Internal - 1 tablespoon of whole or bruised (not ground) seed with 150 ml of liquid 2 to 3 times daily for gastritis and enteritis: 2 to 4 tablespoons of milled linseed for the preparation of linseed gruel.

External - 30 to 50g Flaxseed flour for a hot moist cataplasm or compress.

LITERATURE

Anonym, Leinöl als diätetisches Adjuvans. In: DAZ 135(16):1501. 1995.

Anonym, Leinsamen (Semen Lini) ist ungiftig. In: ZPT 5:770. 1984.

Anonym, Pharmaceutical Care:''Den Miβbrauch von Laxanzien vermeiden helfen''. In: DAZ 135(20):1867-1868. 1995.

Curry CE, (1982) Laxative products. In: Handbook of Nonprescription Drugs, Am Pharmac Assoc, Washington, S 69-92.

Ecker-Schlipf B, Östrogensubstitution mit Leinsamen und Sojamehl. In: DAZ 131(19):953. 1991.

Hiller K, Pharmazeutische Bewertung ausgewählter Teedrogen. In: DAZ 135(16):1425-1440. 1995.

Schiebel-Schlosser G, Leinsamen - die richtige Wahl. In: PTA 8(4):300. 1994.

Schulz V, (1984) Clinical Pharmacokinetics of Nitroprusside, Cyanide, Thiosulphate and Thiocyanate. Clinical Pharmacokinetics 9:239-251.

Schulz V, Löffler A, Gheorghiu Th, (1983) Resorption von Blausäure aus Leinsamen. Leber Magen Darm 13:10-14.

Sewing KFR, (1986) Obstipation. In: Fülgraff G, Palm D (Hrsg) Pharmakotherapie, Klinische Pharmakologie, 6. Auflage. Fischer, Stuttgart, S 162-168.

Further information in:

Frohne D, Pfänder HJ, Giftpflanzen - Ein Handbuch für potheker, Toxikologen und Biologen, 4. Aufl., Wiss. Verlags-Ges Stuttgart 1997.

Hänsel R, Keller K, Rimpler H, Schneider G (Hrsg.), Hagers Handbuch der Pharmazeutischen Praxis, 5. Aufl., Bde 4-6 (Drogen), Springer Verlag Berlin, Heidelberg, New York, 1992-1994.

Lewin L, Gifte und Vergiftungen, 6. Aufl., Nachdruck, Haug Verlag, Heidelberg 1992.

Madaus G, Lehrbuch der Biologischen Arzneimittel, Bde 1-3, Nachdruck, Georg Olms Verlag Hildesheim 1979.

Roth L, Daunderer M, Kormann K, Giftpflanzen, Pflanzengifte, 4. Aufl., Ecomed Fachverlag Landsberg Lech 1993.

Schulz R, Hänsel R, Rationale Phytotherapie, Springer Verlag Heidelberg 1996.

Steinegger E, Hänsel R, Pharmakognosie, 5. Aufl., Springer Verlag Heidelberg 1992.

Teuscher E, Biogene Arzneimittel, 5. Aufl., Wiss. Verlagsges. Stuttgart 1997.

Teuscher E, Lindequist U, Biogene Gifte - Biologie, Chemie, Pharmakologie, 2. Aufl., Fischer Verlag Stuttgart 1994.

Wagner H, Wiesenauer M, Phytotherapie. Phytopharmaka und pflanzliche Homöopathika, Fischer-Verlag, Stuttgart, Jena, New York, 1995.

Wichtl M (Hrsg.), Teedrogen, 4. Aufl., Wiss. Verlagsges. Stuttgart 1997.

Liquidambar Orientalis

Storax

DESCRIPTION

Medicinal Parts: The medicinal part is the balsam from the trunk and the inner bark.

Flower and Fruit: The flowers and inflorescences are unisexual, monoecious and arranged in small, round solitary capitula. The flowers are yellow. The male flowers show no signs of a calyx or corolla. The female flowers have tiny scaly sepals and the floret tubes are fused. There are numerous stamens and the ovary is semi-inferior. The fruit is a hard globular schizocarp.

Leaves, Stem and Root: Liquidambar orientalis is a deciduous tree about 12 m tall with many branches and a thick reddish-gray bark. It has alternate, usually 5-lobed leaves. The leaf blades are usually roughly-toothed.

Characteristics: Raw storax is a thick, viscous, sticky, aromatic and somewhat bitter tasting gray-brown mass. When stored, the drug becomes clearer, an effect caused by a reduction in the water content.

Habitat: The tree is indigenous from Asia Minor to Syria.

Not To Be Confused With: Fir resin, turpentine, colophony, olive oil.

Production: Storax (amber tree balm) is extracted from Liquidambar orientalis. To extract the balsam, the trunk is beaten, causing the bark to soak up the exuding resin. The bark is then boiled and the resulting decoction is further refined.

Other Names: Balsam Styracis, Sweet Gum, Copalm, Gum Tree, Liquid Amber, Opossum Tree, Red Gum, White Gum

ACTIONS AND PHARMACOLOGY

COMPOUNDS

Cinnamic acid (up to 30%): cinnamic acid esters, including among others cinnamylcinnamate (styracine), cinnamic acid ethyl esters

Vanillin

Styrene

Aromatic alcohols: phenylpropyl-, cinnamic-, benzyl alcohol

Triterpenes: oleanolic acid, 3-epioleanolic acid (resin fraction)

EFFECTS

Storax has anti-inflammatory, diaphoretic, and stimulant effects.

INDICATIONS AND USAGE

Storax is used for coughs and bronchitis as an inhalation, externally for wounds and ulcers.

PRECAUTIONS AND ADVERSE REACTIONS

No health hazards are known in conjunction with the proper administration of designated therapeutic dosages. Internal administration of the drug occasionally leads to diarrhea. Storax can also trigger contact allergies.

OVERDOSAGE

External administration over large areas can lead to absorptive poisonings that are characterized by kidney damage (albuminuria, hemorrhagic nephritis).

DOSAGE

Mode of Administration: Storax is used in combination preparations for coughs and bronchitis as an inhalation, externally for wounds and ulcers.

LITERATURE

Huneck S, (1968) Tetrahedron 19: 479.

Further information in:

Hänsel R, Keller K, Rimpler H, Schneider G (Hrsg.), Hagers Handbuch der Pharmazeutischen Praxis, 5. Aufl., Bde 4-6 (Drogen), Springer Verlag Berlin, Heidelberg, New York, 1992-1994.

Leung AY, Encyclopedia of Common Natural Ingredients Used in Food Drugs and Cosmetics, John Wiley & Sons Inc., New York 1980.

Lewin L, Gifte und Vergiftungen, 6. Aufl., Nachdruck, Haug Verlag, Heidelberg 1992.

Liverwort

See Anemone Hepatica

Lobaria Pulmonaria

Lungmoss

DESCRIPTION

Medicinal Parts: The medicinal part is the lichen.

Flower and Fruit: Lobaria pulmonaria is a lichen, with deeply pinnatisect lobes from 1.5 cm up to hand size with indented tips. It is found on the trunks of old woodland trees, is browinsh-green or red-brown with a reticulate, punctate structure. It is tomentose and whitish-brown beneath and is covered with glabrous white spots on the margin and on the reticulate ridges.

Habitat: Lungmoss is found throughout Europe.

Production: Lungmoss is the whole lichen tissue of Lobaria pulmonaria. The lichen is gathered throughout the entire year. The minute roots in the subterranean part, along with any possible earth, are cleaned off (do not gather dry lichen, as they are mostly found on dead plants, and therefore, are no longer effective).

Not To Be Confused With: Common Lungwort, which is a plant.

Other Names: Oak Lungs, Lungwort

ACTIONS AND PHARMACOLOGY

COMPOUNDS

Lichen acids: including among others stictictic, norstictic, thelophoric acid, gyrophoric acid

Mucilages

EFFECTS

The drug has diaphoretic, expectorant, anti-inflammatory, and antimicrobial effects.

The active agents exhibiting the antimicrobial effects are as of yet, unknown.

INDICATIONS AND USAGE

As a result of the relaxing effect of lungmoss on the respiratory tract, the drug is used for all chronic respiratory tract illnesses: bronchitis, coughs, asthma, and for irritable coughs and smoker's cough.

PRECAUTIONS AND ADVERSE REACTIONS

No health hazards or side effects are known in conjunction with the proper administration of designated therapeutic dosages.

DOSAGE

Mode of Administration: Lungmoss is available as dried lichen as a liquid extract for internal use. Lichen preparations can be bought as sweets, syrups or pastilles.

Storage: The drug should be stored in glass or porcelain containers, protected from light.

LITERATURE

Catalano S et al., (1976) Phytochemistry 15:22.

Further information in:

Kern W, List PH, Hörhammer L (Hrsg.), Hagers Handbuch der Pharmazeutischen Praxis, 4. Aufl., Bde. 1-8, Springer Verlag Berlin, Heidelberg, New York, 1969.

Madaus G, Lehrbuch der Biologischen Arzneimittel, Bde 1-3, Nachdruck, Georg Olms Verlag Hildesheim 1979.

Wagner H, Wiesenauer M, Phytotherapie. Phytopharmaka und pflanzliche Homöopathika, Fischer-Verlag, Stuttgart, Jena, New York 1995.

Lobelia Inflata

Lobelia

DESCRIPTION

Medicinal Parts: The medicinal parts are the fresh and dried herb and the seeds.

Flower and Fruit: The flowers are on long pedicles in the leaf axils. They are pale violet-blue and lightly tinged with pale yellow. The fruit consists of an ovoid or flattened bilocular capsule containing numerous small, brown, and reticulate seeds.

Leaves, Stem and Root: The plant is an erect annual or biennial herb 30 to 60 cm high. The stem is pubescent, angular, branching near the top, and contains an acrid latex. The leaves are pale green or yellowish, the lower ones are petiolate, the upper ones are sessile. They are alternate, ovate-lanceolate, 3 to 8 cm long, with a dentate margin and a finely pubescent lamina.

Characteristics: After chewing the leaves, the taste is similar to tobacco. The taste is acrid, the odor faintly irritant.

Habitat: The plant is indigenous to the regions in the north of U.S., Canada, Kamchatka, and is cultivated elsewhere.

Production: Lobelia is the aerial part of Lebelia inflata.

Other Names: Indian Tobacco, Pukeweed, Asthma Weed, Gagroot, Vomitwort, Bladderpod, Eyebright, Emetic Herb, Emetic Weed, Wild Tobacco, Vomitroot

ACTIONS AND PHARMACOLOGY

COMPOUNDS

Piperidine alkaloids (6%): chief alkaloids L-lobeline (alpha-lobeline); companion alkaloids including among others lobelanine, lobelanidine, norlobelanine, isolobinine

EFFECTS

The drug has a stimulating effect on the respiratory center but it is broken down too quickly in the body to be used as a respiratory analeptic.

INDICATIONS AND USAGE

The drug is used only in homeopathy as an asthma treatment and also as an aid in curing addiction to smoking.

PRECAUTIONS AND ADVERSE REACTIONS

No health hazards or side effects are known in conjunction with the proper administration of designated therapeutic dosages.

OVERDOSAGE

Overdosage leads to dryness of the mouth, nausea, vomiting, diarrhea, abdominal pain, burning in the urinary passages, feelings of anxiety, dizziness, headache, shivering, respiratory difficulties, paraesthesias, outbreak of sweating, bradycardia, cardiac arrhythmias, somnolence, and muscle twitchings; death can occur through respiratory failure, accompanied by convulsions.

0.6 to 1 gm of the leaves are said to be toxic, 4 gm fatal.

Following gastrointestinal emptying (inducement of vomiting, gastric lavage with burgundy-colored potassium permanganate solution, sodium sulfate), instillation of activated charcoal, and shock prophylaxis (quiet, warmth), the therapy for poisonings consists of treating spasms with diazepam (i.v.), children with chloral hydrate (rectal); administration von orciprenaline (i.v.), monitoring of ECG. Cardiac massage and artificial respiration may also be required.

DOSAGE

The drug is no longer used. In homeopathic dilutions, it is a constituent in some preparations.

LITERATURE

Gross D, (1971) Fortschr Chem Org Naturst 29:1.

Karawya MS et al., (1971) J Ass Off Ann Chem 54(6):1423.

Schwarz HD, 100 Jahre Lobelin. In: ZPT 11(5):159. 1990.

Further information in:

Chang, EH et al., (Eds): Advances in Chinese Medicinal Materials Research, World Scientific Pub. Co. Singapore 1985.

Kern W, List PH, Hörhammer L (Hrsg.), Hagers Handbuch der Pharmazeutischen Praxis, 4. Aufl., Bde. 1-8, Springer Verlag Berlin, Heidelberg, New York, 1969.

Leung AY, Encyclopedia of Common Natural Ingredients Used in Food Drugs and Cosmetics, John Wiley & Sons Inc., New York, 1980.

Lewin L, Gifte und Vergiftungen, 6. Aufl., Nachdruck, Haug Verlag, Heidelberg 1992.

Madaus G, Lehrbuch der Biologischen Arzneimittel, Bde 1-3, Nachdruck, Georg Olms Verlag Hildesheim 1979.

Roth L, Daunderer M, Kormann K, Giftpflanzen, Pflanzengifte, 4. Aufl., Ecomed Fachverlag Landsberg Lech 1993.

Wagner H, Wiesenauer M, Phytotherapie. Phytopharmaka und pflanzliche Homöopathika, Fischer-Verlag, Stuttgart, Jena, New York, 1995.

Logwood

See Haematoxylon Campechianum

Lolium Temulentum

Taumelloolch

DESCRIPTION

Medicinal Parts: The medicinal part of the plant is the ripe seeds.

Flower and Fruit: The spikes are uninterrupted, 30 cm long and green. The 5 to 7 spikelets form the ear. The glume is longer than the spikelet, which has 7 ribs and no awn. The husk is cartilaginous, has 5 ribs and a stiff, straight awn.

Leaves, Stem and Root: The stalk is rigid and erect. The leaf sheaths are rough and weakly bulbous on the upper leaves.

Characteristics: The spikelets have their narrow sides turned towards the main axis, (in contrast to the couch grass). A parasitic fungus, which is often present on the plant, forms an alkaloid, making the plant poisonous.

Habitat: The plant grows in Europe and Mediterranean region.

Production: Taumellolch seeds are the ripe seeds of Lolium temulentum.

Other Names: Bearded Darnel, Cheat, Drake, Ray-grass, Tare

ACTIONS AND PHARMACOLOGY

COMPOUNDS

The active ingredients are not known. However, the toxicity of Lolium rigidum is caused by bacterial toxins, the so-called kidney toxins, which are unusual nucleosides with uracil as the base.

EFFECTS

The active agents are temulentin, temultin acid, free fatty acids, tannin, and glycoside. The lolch fruit has been suspected of poisoning for some time, however the toxic principle generally remains unexplained. The drug's ability to relieve gastroenteritis can possibly be attributed to the free fatty acids.

INDICATIONS AND USAGE

Taumelloolch is used for dizziness, nerve pain, nose bleeds, sleeplessness and stomach cramps.

PRECAUTIONS AND ADVERSE REACTIONS

The drug can be toxic. In earlier times, poisonings were frequently caused by the presence of the berries of the plant in grain. No cases of poisoning are known in recent times. The plant has now become extremely rare through intensive seed-corn purification.

OVERDOSAGE

Symptoms of poisoning include dizziness, headache, colic, confusion, staggering, vision and speech disorders, somnolence, and, in rare cases, death through respiratory failure. The treatment of poisoning consists of gastrointestinal emptying, (inducement of vomiting, gastric lavage with burgundy-colored potassium permanganate solution, sodium sulphate), administration of activated charcoal and shock prophylaxis (quiet, warmth). Further management consists of treating spasms with careful administration of diazepam (i.v.) and icepacks for fever. Phenothiazines and analeptics should be not be administered. Intubation and oxygen therapy may be required.

DOSAGE

Mode of Administration: The plant is administered ground and as a liquid extract.

LITERATURE

Frohne D, Pfänder HJ, Giftpflanzen - Ein Handbuch für Apotheker, Toxikologen und Biologen, 4. Aufl., Wiss. Verlags-Ges Stuttgart 1997.

Kern W, List PH, Hörhammer L, (Hrsg.), Hagers Handbuch der Pharmazeutischen Praxis, 4. Aufl., Bde 1-8, Springer Verlag Berlin, Heidelberg, New York, 1969.

Lewin L, Gifte und Vergiftungen, 6. Aufl., Nachdruck, Haug Verlag, Heidelberg 1992.

Madaus G, Lehrbuch der Biologischen Arzneimittel, Bde 1-3, Nachdruck, Georg Olms Verlag Hildesheim 1979.

Roth L, Daunderer M, Kormann K, Giftpflanzen, Pflanzengifte, 4. Aufl., Ecomed Fachverlag Landsberg Lech 1993.

Teuscher E, Lindequist U, Biogene Gifte - Biologie, Chemie, Pharmakologie, 2. Aufl., Fischer Verlag Stuttgart 1994.

Lonicera Caprifolium

Honeysuckle

DESCRIPTION

Medicinal Parts: The medicinal parts are the flowers, the seeds, and the leaves.

Flower and Fruit: The flowers are in sixes directly on the upper leaf pair. There are sometimes whorls of 6 in the next 1 or 2 leaf pairs. The corolla has a tight, 25 to 28 mm-long tube, and a bilabiate margin. It is yellowish-white, often red-tinged, glabrous inside, and glandular outside. The ovary is jug-shaped. The fruit is a berry. They are ellipsoid, 8 mm-long, and coral red. The seeds are ellipsoid, flattened, longitudinally grooved, and 4 mm-long.

Leaves, Stem and Root: Honeysuckle is an up to 4 m high, deciduous, clockwise climbing shrub. The foliage leaves are short-petioled, elliptical or obovate, blunt, entire, glabrous, blue-green beneath and 4 to 10 cm by 3.5 to 6 cm. The leaves are shortly fused in pairs but the upper ones are fused to an oval or circular leaf through which the stem grows. They are short-petioled and elliptical. The lower leaves are paired.

Habitat: The plant grows in the northern temperate zones as far as the northern edges of the subtropics and is cultivated extensively.

Other Names: Goat's Leaf, Woodbine

ACTIONS AND PHARMACOLOGY

COMPOUNDS

Saponins

Further constituents are largely unknown; iridoide monoterpenes have been demonstrated in the rind, including among others loganin (extremely bitter), that possibly also occur in the drug.

EFFECTS

The main active principles are saponin and luteolin. The drug has a laxative and diaphoretic effect.

INDICATIONS AND USAGE

The drug is used for digestive disorders, malignant tumors, and also as a diaphoretic agent.

Rarely used.

PRECAUTIONS AND ADVERSE REACTIONS

No health hazards or side effects are known in conjunction with the proper administration of designated therapeutic dosages.

OVERDOSAGE

Because of the saponin content, irritation of the gastrointestinal tract and possibly of the kidneys, urinary passages, and urinary bladder are possible in the event of overdosage. Case studies are not known.

DOSAGE

The drug is obsolete.

LITERATURE

Frohne D, Pfänder HJ, Giftpflanzen - Ein Handbuch für Apotheker, Toxikologen und Biologen, 4. Aufl., Wiss. Verlags-Ges Stuttgart 1997.

Kern W, List PH, Hörhammer L (Hrsg.), Hagers Handbuch der Pharmazeutischen Praxis, 4. Aufl., Bde. 1-8, Springer Verlag Berlin, Heidelberg, New York, 1969.

Roth L, Daunderer M, Kormann K, Giftpflanzen, Pflanzengifte, 4. Aufl., Ecomed Fachverlag Landsberg Lech 1993.

Teuscher E, Lindequist U, Biogene Gifte - Biologie, Chemie, Pharmakologie, 2. Aufl., Fischer Verlag Stuttgart 1994.

Loosestrife

See Lysimachia Vulgaris

Lophophora Williamsii

Peyote

DESCRIPTION

Medicinal Parts: The medicinal parts are the pin cushion-like, aerial, transversely cut and dried, tough-corky shoot, and the fresh plant.

Flower and Fruit: The flowers grow from the center of the cactus head. They are 1 to 2.5 cm long, and 1 to 2.2 cm across. The outer petals are green with a darker middle stripe and have green-pink or white margins. The filaments are white with yellow anthers. The ovary is glabrous. The fruit is a 15 to 20 mm-long berry, which is 2 to 3.5 mm across, sturdy, clavate, initially fleshy, glabrous, and red. It turns brown-white and dries out when ripe. The seeds are black, rough, 1 to 1.5 mm long, and 1 mm wide.

Leaves, Stem and Root: The plant is a succulent, spineless globular or top-shaped, bluish-green cactus with up to 13 distinct vertical ribs and grows to 20 cm. From one rhizome side shoots are produced to create a cactus formation of 1.5 m across. The roots are tuberous and 8 to 11 cm long. The aerial part has a diameter of 4 to 12 cm, and the pressed-in top is filled with gray, woolly bushels of hair. The head is divided into irregular flat warts by horizontal grooves. Roundish aeroles of paintbrush-like yellowish or whitish tufts of hair grow from the tip of the warts.

Habitat: The plant grows in northern Mexico and bordering southern Texas.

Production: The root and hair tuft of the peyote plant are cut off. The particularly mescalin and chlorophyll-rich center is dried as a slice. This slice is referred to as the mescalin button.

Other Names: Pellote, Mescal Buttons, Devil's Root, Dumpling Cactus, Sacred Mushroom

ACTIONS AND PHARMACOLOGY

COMPOUNDS

Alkaloids of the phenylethylamine type: chief among them mescaline (up to 7%), hordenine- tetrahydroisoquinoline type: including among others pellotin, anhalonidine, anhalamine

EFFECTS

Peyote has an emetic and a hallucinogenic effect. The psychotropic effects of peyote consumption are mainly due to the mescaline content. Controlled pharmacological studies on the peyote cactus are unknown. Mescal beans cause visual, auditory, taste, kinesthetic, and synesthetic hallucinations.

INDICATIONS AND USAGE

Peyote is rarely used as a medicinal preparation. In folk medicine, peyote is one of the oldest hallucinogens.

PRECAUTIONS AND ADVERSE REACTIONS

Due to its mescaline content, the drug causes chiefly visual, but also aural, kinesthetic, and synesthetic hallucinations when taken in dosages of between 4 and 12 dried slices of the sprout (so-called mescal buttons: diameter 3 to 4.5 cm, thickness 0.5 cm).

DOSAGE

Mode of Administration: Peyote is obsolete as a drug, it is often ingested illegally for its hallucinogenic effect.

LITERATURE

Kapadia GJ, Fayez MB (1970) J Pharm Sci 59:1699.

Seeger R, Mescalin. In: DAZ 133(2):24. 1993.

Willaman JJ, Hui-Li L, (1970) Lloydia 33(3A):1.

Further information in:

Hänsel R, Keller K, Rimpler H, Schneider G (Hrsg.), Hagers Handbuch der Pharmazeutischen Praxis, 5. Aufl., Bde 4-6 (Drogen), Springer Verlag Berlin, Heidelberg, New York, 1992-1994.

Madaus G, Lehrbuch der Biologischen Arzneimittel, Bde 1-3, Nachdruck, Georg Olms Verlag Hildesheim 1979 (unter Anhalonium).

Roth L, Daunderer M, Kormann K, Giftpflanzen, Pflanzengifte, 4. Aufl., Ecomed Fachverlag Landsberg Lech 1993.

Steinegger E, Hänsel R, Pharmakognosie, 5. Aufl., Springer Verlag Heidelberg 1992.

Teuscher E, Lindequist U, Biogene Gifte - Biologie, Chemie, Pharmakologie, 2. Aufl., Fischer Verlag Stuttgart 1994.

Lotus

See Nelumbo Nucifera

Lovage

See Levisticum Officinale

Luffa Aegyptica

Luffa

DESCRIPTION

Medicinal Parts: The medicinal part is the dried network of vascular bundles of the ripe cucumber-like plant. When dried, the dense net of vascular bundles which makes up the fruit becomes the Loofah, used to scrub and soften the skin.

Flower and Fruit: The plant bears solitary, yellow, female flowers which are 5 to 10 cm wide and have an oblong, clavate calyx tube. The fruit is cylindrical or oblong-clavate. It is not ribbed, prickly or sharp-edged. It is somewhat tomentose, up to 40 cm long and 5 to 15 cm thick. The seeds are blackish, smooth and winged.

Leaves, Stem and Root: The plant is an annual climbing plant which grows from 3 to 6 m high. The stems are thin and pentangular. The leaves are cordate-indented, 15 to 30 cm long and wide and 3- to 7-lobed.

Habitat: The plant probably originated in India and was brought to Egypt in the Middle Ages. Today, it is cultivated in the tropical regions of the world.

Production: Luffa sponge consists of the dried fiber structure of the ripe cucumber-like fruits of Luffa aegyptiaca. The ripe fruit is freed of soft material by banging and washing.

ACTIONS AND PHARMACOLOGY

COMPOUNDS

The fresh fruit contains:

Triterpene saponins: including, among others, lucyoside A-M (aglycones including among others oleanolic acid, hederagenin 21-hydroxy-hederagenin, gypsogenine, arjunol acid)

Cucurbitacins (the young fruits are eaten as salad)

The luffa fungus (luffa, Luffa aegyptica), is likely to be mostly free of soluble constituents and to consist chiefly of cellulose, hemicellulose and pectins.

EFFECTS

No information is available.

INDICATIONS AND USAGE

Preparations of luffa sponge are used as a preventive for infections or colds, as a remedy for colds and nasal catarrhs, as well as sinusitis and suppuration of the sinus. The efficacy for the claimed applications is not documented.

PRECAUTIONS AND ADVERSE REACTIONS

No health hazards or side effects are known in conjunction with the proper administration of designated therapeutic dosages.

DOSAGE
No information is available.

LITERATURE
Hänsel R, Keller K, Rimpler H, Schneider G (Hrsg.), Hagers Handbuch der Pharmazeutischen Praxis, 5. Aufl., Bde 4-6 (Drogen), Springer Verlag Berlin, Heidelberg, New York, 1992-1994.

Lungmoss

See Lobaria Pulmonaria

Lungwort

See Pulmonaria Officinalis

Lupinus Luteus

Yellow Lupin

DESCRIPTION
Medicinal Parts: The medicinal parts are the seeds and the aerial parts of the plant.

Flower and Fruit: The terminal flowers are almost sessile. They are arranged in numerous, distinct whorls. They have dropping, silky haired bracts. The corolla is bright yellow with a blunted boat-shaped tip. The fruit is an oblong-lanceolate, 5 to 7 cm by 1 cm, densely pubescent pod with nodes. It contains 4 to 7 yellowish, reddish-white, black or dark violet marbled seeds 5.5 to 6.5 mm long.

Leaves, Stem and Root: The plant is an annual with up to a 1 m long taproot, which contains numerous lateral roots. The stem is light green and pubescent with numerous side shoots. The 5 to 10 leaves are oblong-obovate to lanceolate, 4 to 8 cm long, acuminate, and pubescent on both sides.

Habitat: The plant is indigenous to Europe, Asia, and North and South America.

ACTIONS AND PHARMACOLOGY
COMPOUNDS: IN THE FOLIAGE
Quinolizidine alkaloids (0.6-1.6%): sparteine, 13-hydroxylupanine, lupinines, p-cumaroyllupinine

COMPOUNDS: IN THE SEEDS
Quinolizidine alkaloid (0.4-3.3%): lupinines, sparteine, in some cultivated strains gramine.

Fatty oil

Carbohydrates

Proteins

Flavonoids

EFFECTS
The drug has anthelmintic and diuretic effects.

There has been no recent research on the effects of the drug.

INDICATIONS AND USAGE
Yellow Lupin is used externally for ulcers. It is used internally for urinary tract disorders and worm infestation.

PRECAUTIONS AND ADVERSE REACTIONS
See **OVERDOSAGE** section.

OVERDOSAGE
Symptoms of poisoning include salivation, vomiting, dysphagia, cardiac rhythm disorders, ascending paralysis, and possible death through respiratory failure. The lupinosis seen in animals is caused by mycotoxins that are formed from the fungus Phomopsis leptostromiformis, which can live as an endophyte in lupins. Vomiting should be induced following intake of more than one capsule of the plant. Following gastrointestinal emptying, (inducement of vomiting, gastric lavage with burgundy-colored potassium permanganate solution, sodium sulfate) and installation of activated charcoal, the therapy for severe poisonings (that are, in fact, very unlikely) consists of electrolyte substitution, treating possible cases of acidosis with sodium bicarbonate infusions and administering orciprenaline or lidocaine for cardiac rhythm disorders. In case of shock, plasma volume expanders should be administered. Intubation and oxygen respiration may also be necessary.

DOSAGE
Mode of Administration: The drug is used internally as an infusion, and externally in poultices.

LITERATURE
Plakhota VA, Berezyuk NK, Oleinik GV, Boiko VP, Poisoning of animals with lupins. In: Veterinariya, Moscow, USSR, No. 8, 79-81. 1966.

Schmeller Th et al., Binding of quinolizidine alkaloids to nicotinic and muscarinic acetylcholine receptors. In: JNP 57(9):1316-1319. 1994.

Seeger R, Lupanin und Anagyrin. In: DAZ 133(17):35. 1993.

Further information in:

Frohne D, Pfänder HJ, Giftpflanzen - Ein Handbuch für Apotheker, Toxikologen und Biologen, 4. Aufl., Wiss. Verlags-Ges Stuttgart 1997.

Kern W, List PH, Hörhammer L (Hrsg.), Hagers Handbuch der Pharmazeutischen Praxis, 4. Aufl., Bde 1-8, Springer Verlag Berlin, Heidelberg, New York, 1969.

Lewin L, Gifte und Vergiftungen, 6. Aufl., Nachdruck, Haug Verlag, Heidelberg 1992.

Roth L, Daunderer M, Kormann K, Giftpflanzen, Pflanzengifte, 4. Aufl., Ecomed Fachverlag Landsberg Lech 1993.

Teuscher E, Lindequist U, Biogene Gifte - Biologie, Chemie, Pharmakologie, 2. Aufl., Fischer Verlag Stuttgart 1994.

Lycoperdon Species

Puff Ball

DESCRIPTION

Medicinal Parts: The medicinal parts are the aerial parts and the mature spores of the fungus.

Flower and Fruit: The giant form of this fungus attains a diameter of 20 to 50 cm and a weight of 9 kg. The outer covering is at first whitish, smooth and downy. It later turns gray-yellow or ochre, develops grooves and patches and starts to break off from above. The now-visible inner section bursts at the vertex and disintegrates. The content is composed of a whitish mass, which turns yellow and mushy and finally breaks down into greenish-brown spore dust. A cup-shaped receptacle with torn edges remains.

Habitat: Lycoperdon species are indigenous to Europe.

Other Names: Bovista, Hart's Truffle, Deer Balls

ACTIONS AND PHARMACOLOGY

COMPOUNDS

Calvacin (mucoprotein)

Urea

The active ingredients are unknown.

EFFECTS

The main active agents are various amino acids, glucosamine, sterol, enzymes and approximately 3% urea.

INDICATIONS AND USAGE

The drug is used for dysmenorrhea, nose bleeds, and skin disorders.

PRECAUTIONS AND ADVERSE REACTIONS

No health hazards or side effects are known in conjunction with the proper administration of designated therapeutic dosages. The young mushroom is edible.

DOSAGE

Preparation: Puff Ball is available ground or in alcoholic extracts.

LITERATURE

Gasco A et al., (1974) Tetrahedron Lett 38:3431.

Further information in:

Kern W, List PH, Hörhammer L (Hrsg.), Hagers Handbuch der Pharmazeutischen Praxis, 4. Aufl., Bde. 1-8, Springer Verlag Berlin, Heidelberg, New York, 1969.

Madaus G, Lehrbuch der Biologischen Arzneimittel, Bde 1-3, Nachdruck, Georg Olms Verlag Hildesheim 1979.

Lycopersicon Esculentum

Tomato

DESCRIPTION

Medicinal Parts: The medicinal parts are the fresh leaves, the fresh herb collected during the flowering season or the whole plant.

Flower and Fruit: The flowers are in lateral, cyme-like coils. The tips of the calyx are linear-lanceolate. The corolla is yellow, as long as the calyx and has a very short tube. It is divided into pointed, lanceolate lobes. The stamens are fused to the tube. The stigma is greenish and capitular. The fruit is a large, juicy, smooth, round to ovoid berry with a short, obtuse tip. It is scarlet, occasionally yellow or whitish with a diameter of 2 to 10 cm. The seeds are reniform, flattened, whitish-gray-yellow, and villous-tomentose.

Leaves, Stem and Root: The tomato plant is an annual with a fusiform, fibrous root. The stem grows to 120 cm is leafy, heavily-branched, and glandular-haired. The leaves are broad-petiolate, odd-pinnate, petiolate, ovate-lanceolate, pinnatifid, dentate and slightly involute leaflets. The leaves have a gray-green underside.

Habitat: The plant probably originated in southern or central America, today it is only cultivated.

Production: Tomato tincture is the homeopathic mother tincture of the whole plant Lycopersicon esculentum.

Other Names: Love Apple

ACTIONS AND PHARMACOLOGY

COMPOUNDS

Steroid alkaloid glycosides: chief alkaloid alpha-tomatine

EFFECTS

No information is available.

INDICATIONS AND USAGE

Tomato is used in homeopathy to treat rheumatic conditions, colds, chills, and digestive disorders.

PRECAUTIONS AND ADVERSE REACTIONS

No health hazards or side effects are known in conjunction with the proper administration of designated therapeutic dosages.

OVERDOSAGE

Signs of poisoning are not to be expected with less than 100 gm of the fresh leaves (or green tomatoes) and for that reason is unlikely. Symptoms would be severe mucous membrane irritation (vomiting, diarrhea, colic). Following absorption, dizziness, stupor, headache, bradycardia, respiratory disturbances, mild spasms, and in very severe cases death through respiratory failure could occur.

Case studies are not known.

DOSAGE

Mode of Administration: The drug is commonly used in homeopathic dilutions.

Preparation: The mother tincture is produced by maceration or percolation of the fresh or dried drug, with an ethanol content of 45%.

LITERATURE

Tomaten als Krebsschutz. In: DAZ 134(6):485. 1994.

Further information in:

Hänsel R, Keller K, Rimpler H, Schneider G (Hrsg.), Hagers Handbuch der Pharmazeutischen Praxis, 5. Aufl., Bde 4-6 (Drogen), Springer Verlag Berlin, Heidelberg, New York, 1992-1994.

Lycopodium Clavatum

Club Moss

DESCRIPTION

Medicinal Parts: The medicinal parts are the spores and the fresh plant.

Flower and Fruit: Sulfur yellow, minute spores, carried in large numbers in 2 to 3 cylindrical yellow-green cones, develop in August at the ends of leafy, 15 cm high stalks extending from aerial branches.

Leaves, Stem and Root: The plant has 1 m long, procumbent stem with only a few roots. It is covered with yellowish-green leaves, densely arranged in spirals, which are entire-margined, linear, smooth, and end in a long, white, upwardly bent hair tip. There are numerous erect, circular, 5 cm high branches on the mainstem.

Habitat: The plant is found worldwide.

Other Names: Stags Horn, Witch Meal, Wolfs Claw, Vegetable Sulfur

ACTIONS AND PHARMACOLOGY

COMPOUNDS

Alkaloids (0.2%): including among others those of the lycopodine- and lycodan-types (derived from piperidine alkaloids), chief alkaloids lycopodine and dihydrolycopodine, in traces also nicotine

Flavonoids: including among others chrysoeriol, luteolin

EFFECTS

Club Moss has a diuretic effect.

INDICATIONS AND USAGE

In folk medicine, the drug is used for bladder and kidney complaints.

PRECAUTIONS AND ADVERSE REACTIONS

No health hazards or side effects are known in conjunction with the proper administration of designated therapeutic dosages. Irritations should be expected with extended used of the drug.

OVERDOSAGE

Despite the toxicity of the alkaloids, no poisonings have been recorded.

DOSAGE

Mode of Administration: In folk medicine, chopped drug is used in teas.

LITERATURE

Blumenkopf TA, Heathcock CH, The Alkaloids, Vol. 5, Ed. SW Pelletier, John Wiley 1985.

Leete E, The Alkaloids, Vol. 1, Ed. SW Pelletier, John Wiley 1983.

Further information in:

Kern W, List PH, Hörhammer L (Hrsg.), Hagers Handbuch der Pharmazeutischen Praxis, 4. Aufl., Bde. 1-8, Springer Verlag Berlin, Heidelberg, New York, 1969.

Madaus G, Lehrbuch der Biologischen Arzneimittel, Bde 1-3, Nachdruck, Georg Olms Verlag Hildesheim 1979.

Wichtl M (Hrsg.), Teedrogen, 4. Aufl., Wiss. Verlagsges. Stuttgart 1997.

Lycopus Virginicus

Bugleweed

DESCRIPTION

Medicinal Parts: The medicinal part is the fresh or dried herb collected during the flowering season.

Flower and Fruit: The flowers are small, almost radial in dense axillary whorls. The calyx is campanulate with a glabrous tube and 4 or 5 regular usually erect tips. The corolla is whitish with the tube only partly showing and a few uneven lobes. The epicalyx and calyx sepals are shorter than in the European variety. There are only 2 fertile stamens with initially parallel, later spreading pollen sacs. The upper stamens are reduced to staminoids or completely disappear. The fruit is a flattened, rectangular, stunted, and smooth nutlet.

Leaves, Stem and Root: The plant is a herbaceous perennial with runners. The quadrangular, 60 cm high smooth stems grow from the perennial creeping root. The stems bear pairs of opposite, short-petioled leaves. The upper ones are dentate and pointed; the lower ones wedge-shaped to entire-margined. They are glabrous and glandular-punctate on the lower surface.

Habitat: The plant grows in North America. Lycopus europaeus, Gypsywort, is a close European relative.

Production: Bugle weed consists of the fresh or dried, above-ground parts of Lycopus europaeus and/or Lycopus virginicus, as well as their preparations in effective dosage.

Other Names: Sweet Bugle, Water Bugle, Virginia Water Horehound, Gypsywort

ACTIONS AND PHARMACOLOGY

COMPOUNDS

Caffeic acid derivatives: rosmaric acid, lithospermic acid and their oligomerics created through oxydation

Flavonoids

EFFECTS

Bugleweed has antigonadotropic and antithyrotropic effects. It inhibits the peripheral deiodination of T4 and also lowers the prolactin levels.

INDICATIONS AND USAGE

- Nervousness and insomnia
- Premenstrual syndrome (PMS)

Bugleweed is used for mild thyroid hyperfunction associated with disturbances of the autonomic nervous system. It is also used for tension and pain in the breast (mastodynia).

CONTRAINDICATIONS

The drug is contraindicated in hypofunction of the thyroid and thyroid gland enlargement without function disturbance. There should not be any simultaneous administration of thyroid hormone preparations.

PRECAUTIONS AND ADVERSE REACTIONS

General: No health hazards or side effects are known in conjunction with the proper administration of designated therapeutic dosages. Enlargement of the thyroid gland is possible only through administration of the drug in very high-dosage. Sudden discontinuation of Lycopus preparation can lead to worsening of the complaint.

Drug Interactions: No simultaneous administration of thyroid preparations. Administration of Lycopus preparations disturbs the administration of diagnostic procedures with radioactive isotopes.

DOSAGE

Mode of Administration: Comminuted herb, freshly pressed juice, and other galenic preparations for internal use.

Daily Dosage: The average daily dose is 1 to 2 gm of the drug for teas; and water-ethanol extracts containing the equivalent of 20 mg of the drug.

Each patient has his own individual optimal level of thyroid hormone. Only rough estimations of dosage are possible for thyroid disorders, in which age and weight must be considered.

LITERATURE

Auf'mkolk M, (1985) Endocrinology 116(5):1687.

Bucar R et al., Flavonoid glycosides from Lycopus europaeus. In: PM 61(5):489. 1995.

Frömbling-Borges A, (1987) Intrathyreoidale Wirkung von Lycopus europaeus, Pflanzensäuren, Tyrosinen, Thyroninen und Lithiumchlorid. Darstellung einer Schilddrüsensekretionsblockade. Inauguraldissertation. Westfälische Wilhelms- Universtität Münster.

Frömbling-Borges A, Intrathyreoidale Wirkung von Lycopus europaeus, Pflanzensäuren, Kaliumjodid und Lithiumchlorid. In: ZPT 10(1):1. 1990.

Gumbinger HG et al., (1981) Contraception 23(6):661.

Hegnauer R, Kooiman P (1978) Planta Med 33(1):13.

Jeremic D et al., (1985) Tetrahedron 41(2):357.

John M, Gumbinger HG, Winterhoff H, The oxidation of caffeic acid derivatives as model reaction for the formation of potent gonadotropin inhibitors in plant extracts. In: PM 59(3):195. 1993.

Jung F, Kiesewetter H, Mrowietz C, Pindur G, Heiden M, Miyashita C, Wenzel E, Akutwirkungen eines zusammengesetzten Knoblauchpräparates auf die Fließfähigkeit des Blutes. In: ZPT 10(3):87. 1989.

Kartnig T, Lycopus europaeus L. - Wolfsfuß oder Wolfstrapp. In: ZPT 10(1):31. 1989.

Kooiman P, (1972) Acta Bot Neerl 21(4)417.

Sourgens H et al., (1982) Planta Med 45:78.

Further information in:

Kern W, List PH, Hörhammer L (Hrsg.), Hagers Handbuch der Pharmazeutischen Praxis, 4. Aufl., Bde. 1-8, Springer Verlag Berlin, Heidelberg, New York, 1969.

Schulz R, Hänsel R, Rationale Phytotherapie, Springer Verlag Heidelberg 1996.

Teuscher E, Biogene Arzneimittel, 5. Aufl., Wiss. Verlagsges. Stuttgart 1997.

Wagner H, Wiesenauer M, Phytotherapie. Phytopharmaka und pflanzliche Homöopathika, Fischer-Verlag, Stuttgart, Jena, New York 1995.

Lysimachia Nummularia

Moneywort

DESCRIPTION

Medicinal Parts: The medicinal parts are the fresh or dried whole flowering plant.

Fruit and Flower: The flowers are solitary or in pairs. The leaf axils have 5 free, almost cordate sepals. The corolla is rotate, divided into 5 and fused at the base. It is rich yellow and spotted with dark red glands on the inside. There are 5 glandular-haired stamens fused at the base and 1 ovary. The fruit is a 4 to 5 mm long globular capsule. The seeds are triangular, blackish-brown, warty and 1.5 mm long.

Leaves, Stem and Root: The plant is a perennial. The stem is a runner-like creeper, is lightly branched, quadrangular, glabrous to slightly pubescent and roots at the nodes. It grows from 10 to 45 cm. The leaves are entire-margined, crossed-opposite, short-petioled, red-glandular punctate and orbicular elliptical.

Habitat: The plant is indigenous to all of Europe and the Caucasus and has been introduced into America and Japan.

Production: Moneywort is the aerial part of Lysimachia nummularia. The whole flowering plant, including the root, is collected, cleaned, and dried in the sun.

Other Names: Creeping Jenny, Creeping Joan, Herb Two-pence, Meadow Runagates, Running Jenny, Serpentaria, String of Sovereigns, Twopenny Grass, Wandering Jenny, Wandering Tailor

ACTIONS AND PHARMACOLOGY

COMPOUNDS

Flavonoids: including, among others, glycosides of myricetins, kaempferols and quercetins, including, among others, rutin, hyperosides

Tannins

Triterpene saponins

The constituents of the drug have not been fully investigated.

EFFECTS

Moneywort is mildly astringent and expectorant. Extracts of the aerial plant parts are said to be antibacterial in vitro, however, scientific results are not available.

INDICATIONS AND USAGE

It is a constituent of gels, ointments and drops for dermatological preparations. Moneywort is used externally as a vulnerary and for acute and chronic eczema. It is used internally for diarrhea, to increase salivation, and as an expectorant for coughs.

PRECAUTIONS AND ADVERSE REACTIONS

No health hazards or side effects are known in conjunction with the proper administration of designated therapeutic dosages.

DOSAGE

Preparation: To make a tea, pour 250 ml boiling water over 2 heaping teaspoonfuls drug and leave to draw for 5 minutes.

Daily Dosage: For the treatment of coughs, drink 1 cup of tea, 2 to 3 times daily with honey if desired.

LITERATURE

Prum N et al., PA 38:494. 1083.

Further information in:

Hänsel R, Keller K, Rimpler H, Schneider G (Hrsg.), Hagers Handbuch der Pharmazeutischen Praxis, 5. Aufl., Bde 4-6 (Drogen), Springer Verlag Berlin, Heidelberg, New York, 1992-1994.

Madaus G, Lehrbuch der Biologischen Arzneimittel, Bde 1-3, Nachdruck, Georg Olms Verlag Hildesheim 1979.

Lysimachia Vulgaris

Loosestrife

DESCRIPTION

Medicinal Parts: The medicinal part is the dried herb.

Flower and Fruit: The flowers grow in long peduncled racemes in the axils of the upper stem and in terminal panicled inflorescences. The pedicle is about 1 cm long, downy, and glandular-haired. The calyx is split almost to the base. The filaments are glandular-haired, usually fused to the middle with each other and in a tube containing the ovary. The seeds are triangular, covered thickly in long warts, whitish, and 1.5 mm long.

Leaves, Stem and Root: The plant is a perennial and has underground runners, which produce new buds. The stem is erect, up to 1.5 m tall, branched, obtusely angular, leafy and thickly downy. The leaves are slightly downy with glandular hairs. The leaves are in whorls or opposite, rarely spiralled, up to 14 cm long and 3.5 cm wide, short-petioled, tightly reticulate and red-glandular punctate.

Habitat: The plant is found in the temperate regions of Europe and Asia.

Other Names: Yellow Willowherb

ACTIONS AND PHARMACOLOGY

COMPOUNDS

Flavonoids: glycosides of the myricetin, kaempferol and quercetin, including among others rutin

The constituents of the drug have not been extensively investigated.

EFFECTS

Loosestrife has an astringent effect. The main active principle is rutin.

INDICATIONS AND USAGE

Loosestrife is used for scurvy, diarrhea and dysentery as well as hemorrhages (nose bleeds and heavy menstrual blood flow) and wounds.

PRECAUTIONS AND ADVERSE REACTIONS

No health hazards or side effects are known in conjunction with the proper administration of designated therapeutic dosages.

DOSAGE

Mode of Administration: The herb is used externally in the powdered form.

LITERATURE

Hänsel R, Keller K, Rimpler H, Schneider G (Hrsg.), Hagers Handbuch der Pharmazeutischen Praxis, 5. Aufl., Bde 4-6 (Drogen), Springer Verlag Berlin, Heidelberg, New York, 1992-1994.

Lythrum Salicaria

Purple Loosestrife

DESCRIPTION

Medicinal Parts: The medicinal parts are the flowering plant without the roots and flowering branch tips.

Flower and Fruit: The purple flowers are in axillary whorls and form terminal spikes. There are 6 small sepals, 6 long thin tips, 6 free petals, 12 stamens, and 1 half-superior ovary. There are flowers with long, short, or medium-long styles, and similar stamens.

Leaves, Stem and Root: The plant is an annual and grows from 60 to 120 cm high. It has a creeping rhizome with 4 to 6 unbranched, erect, 6-sided, and reddish brown pubescent stems. The leaves are simple lanceolate 7.5 to 15 cm long, sometimes opposite and sometimes clasping whorls.

Habitat: The plant is indigenous to Europe including Russia, Central Asia, Australia, and North America.

Production: The flowering plants, before the seeds form, are cut and gathered during the blossoming period, which occurs from June to August. The material is bound into small bundles. It is hung in an open-air, shaded area to dry.

Other Names: Loosestrife, Lythrum, Purple Willow-herb, Long Purples, Milk Willow-herb, Rainbow Weed, Soldiers, Spiked Loosestrife, Spiked, Willow Sage, Salicaire, Flowering Sally, Blooming Sally

ACTIONS AND PHARMACOLOGY

COMPOUNDS

Tannins (ellagitannins = lythrartannin, condensed tannins)

Flavonoids: including, among others, vitexin, orientin

Phthalides: diisobutyl-, butyl-, isobutyl-, dibutylphthalides

EFFECTS

The active agents are tannin, pectin, resins, cholin, and salicarin.

The drug has an anti-inflammatory, astringent, and antibiotic effect. The astringent properties of the Purple Loosestrife is attributed to not just the tannin content, but also to the glycoside salcarin, which has a special antimicrobial effect on various bacteria in the intestinal tract.

INDICATIONS AND USAGE

The drug is used internally for diarrhea, chronic intestinal catarrh, and menstrual complaints; externally, in the treatment of varicose veins, bleeding of the gums, hemorrhoids, and eczema.

PRECAUTIONS AND ADVERSE REACTIONS

No health hazards or side effects are known in conjunction with the proper administration of designated therapeutic dosages.

DOSAGE

Mode of Administration: The drug is used internally as well as externally.

Preparation: For internal use, an infusion is made from 3 gm of the drug added to 100 ml of water. To prepare a tincture, add 20 gm of the drug to 100 ml of 20% alcohol (leave to set for 5 days).

Daily Dosage: Two to 3 cups of an infusion are to be taken per day. Two to 3 teaspoons of the tincture should be taken per day.

Storage: Keep wrapped in paper or in cloth sacks.

LITERATURE

Kern W, List PH, Hörhammer L (Hrsg.), Hagers Handbuch der Pharmazeutischen Praxis, 4. Aufl., Bde. 1-8, Springer Verlag Berlin, Heidelberg, New York, 1969.

Madaus G, Lehrbuch der Biologischen Arzneimittel, Bde 1-3, Nachdruck, Georg Olms Verlag Hildesheim 1979.

Madder

See Rubia Tinctorum

Magnolia Glauca

Magnolia

DESCRIPTION

Medicinal Parts: The bark is the medicinal part.

Leaves, Stem and Root: The inner bark occurs in long, fibrous strips. The outer surface is rough, almost granular and pitted. The inner surface is striated but almost smooth. The fracture is short with the inner part tough and fibrous.

Habitat: The plant is indigenous to North America.

Other Names: White Laurel, Beaver Tree, Swamp Sassafras, White Bay, Sweet Bay, Holly Bay, Indian Bark, Red Bay, Swamp Laurel

ACTIONS AND PHARMACOLOGY

COMPOUNDS

Neolignans: magnolol

The constituents of the drug have not been widely investigated.

EFFECTS

Magnolia has diaphoretic, anti-inflammatory, and stimulant effects. It is also a tonic.

INDICATIONS AND USAGE

The preparations are used for digestive disorders; used rarely, except in oriental medicine.

PRECAUTIONS AND ADVERSE REACTIONS

No health hazards or side effects are known in conjunction with the proper administration of designated therapeutic dosages.

DOSAGE

Mode of Administration: Magnolia has been used internally as a powder or liquid extract.

LITERATURE

Yajara S, Nishiyori T, Kohda A, Nohra T, Nishioka I, Isolation and characterization of phenolic compounds from Magnolia cortex produced in China. In: Chem Pharm Bull Tokyo 39:2024. 1991.

Further information in:

Hegnauer R, Chemotaxonomie der Pflanzen, Bde 1-11, Birkhäuser Verlag Basel, Boston, Berlin 1962-1997.

Kern W, List PH, Hörhammer L (Hrsg.), Hagers Handbuch der Pharmazeutischen Praxis, 4. Aufl., Bde. 1-8, Springer Verlag Berlin, Heidelberg, New York, 1969.

Mahonia Aquifolium

Mountain Grape

DESCRIPTION

Medicinal Parts: The medicinal parts are the dried rhizome and the roots, the dried branch and twig bark as well as the root bark.

Flower and Fruit: The heavily scented flowers are either in dense 5 to 8 cm panicles or in twos or threes in erect 5 to 8 cm racemes in the leaf axils. The flowers are yellow and have 9 sepals, 6 petals and 6 stamens, which are about 8 cm long. The pedicles are 5 to 10 mm long. The fruit is a globose, purple-blue, frosted berry with red juice. The 2 to 5 seeds are glossy brown.

Leaves, Stem and Root: The plant is a fast-growing, evergreen, stoloniferous shrub about 50 to 150 cm high with stout stems, sparingly branched. The leaves are odd-pinnate, 10 to 20 cm long with 3 to 6 pairs of leaflets. The leaflets are 4 to 8 by 2 to 4 cm, ovate, distally spinose dentate, coriaceous, dark and shining green.

Habitat: Indigenous to the pacific U.S.; ornamental or cultivated in Europe.

Production: Mountain Grape bark consists of the branch and twig bark as well as the twig tips of Mahonia aquifolium.

Other Names: Holly-leaved Berberis

ACTIONS AND PHARMACOLOGY

COMPOUNDS

Isoquinoline alkaloids (2.4-4.5%) of the- benzyl isoquinoline type: including among others berberine- bisbenzylisoquinoline-type: including among others berbamine, oxyacanthine-aporphine-type: including among others isocorydin

EFFECTS

The plant has an antiprolific effect caused by the alkaloid content, special Barberry (Berberin). It is an antipsoriatic when used externally.

INDICATIONS AND USAGE

In homeopathy for dry skin rashes (for dandruff between the acute phases) and in the treatment of psoriasis.

PRECAUTIONS AND ADVERSE REACTIONS

No health hazards or side effects are known in conjunction with the proper administration of designated therapeutic dosages.

DOSAGE

Mode of Administration: In homeopathic dilutions and ointments with a partially higher concentration of Mother Tincture.

Storage: Protect from light.

LITERATURE

Anonym, Ein Lichtblick in der Psoriasistherapie. In: DAZ 134(8):646. 1994.

Augustin M, Mahonia aquifolium bei Psoriasis. In: ZPT 17(1):44. 1996.

Galle K, Bladt S, Wagner H, Mahonia. In: DAZ 134(49):4883. 1994.

Mennet-von Eiff M, Meier B, Phytotherapie in der Dermatologie. In: ZPT 16(4):201-210. 1995.

Misik V et al., Lipoxygenase inhibition and antioxidant properties of protoberberine and aporphine alkaloids isolated from Mahonia aquifolium. In: PM 61(4):372-373. 1995.

Müller K, Ziereis K, Gawlik I, The antipsoriatic Mahonia aquifolium and its active constituents II: Antiproliferative activity against cell growth of human keratinocytes. In: PM 61(1):74-75. 1995.

Müller K, Ziereis K, The antisporiatic Mahonia aquifolium and its active constitutents; Pro- and antioxidant properties and inhibition of 5-lipoxygenase. In: PM 60(5):421. 1994.

Niedner R, Wiesnauer M, Dermatologie: Mahonia aquifolium - ein Phytopharmakon in der Psoriasistherapie. In: DAZ 132(37)1890. 1992.

Petersen-Lehmann J, Homöopathische Salbe gegen Schuppenflechte. In: PZ 137(38):2892. 1992.

Willaman JJ, Hui-Li L, (1970) Lloydia 33(3A):1.

Further information in:

Frohne D, Pfänder HJ: Giftpflanzen - Ein Handbuch für Apotheker, Toxikologen und Biologen, 4. Aufl., Wiss. Verlags-Ges. Stuttgart 1997.

Hänsel R, Keller K, Rimpler H, Schneider G (Hrsg.), Hagers Handbuch der Pharmazeutischen Praxis, 5. Aufl., Bde 4-6 (Drogen), Springer Verlag Berlin, Heidelberg, New York, 1992-1994.

Madaus G, Lehrbuch der Biologischen Arzneimittel, Bde 1-3, Nachdruck, Georg Olms Verlag Hildesheim 1979 (unter Berberis aquifolium).

Roth L, Daunderer M, Kormann K, Giftpflanzen, Pflanzengifte, 4. Aufl., Ecomed Fachverlag Landsberg Lech 1993.

Teuscher E, Lindequist U, Biogene Gifte - Biologie, Chemie, Pharmakologie, 2. Aufl., Fischer Verlag Stuttgart 1994.

Wagner H, Wiesenauer M, Phytotherapie. Phytopharmaka und pflanzliche Homöopathika, Fischer-Verlag, Stuttgart, Jena, New York 1995.

Ma-Huang

See Ephedra Sinica

Maidenhair

See Adiantum Capillus-Veneris

Maize

See Zea Mays

Malabar Nut

See Justicia Adhatoda

Male Fern

See Dryopteris Filix-Mas

Mallotus Philippinensis

Kamala

DESCRIPTION

Medicinal Parts: The medicinal parts are the glands and hairs covering the fruit.

Flower and Fruit: The tree has dioecious flowers. The male flowers are in threes in the axils of the bracts, while the female flowers are on longer, heavily branched lateral boughs. Both flowers are covered by rust-red matted hairs. The fruit is a 3-lobed, pea-sized capsule from which a red, mealy powder is obtained which consists of minute glands and hairs.

Leaves, Stem and Root: Mallotus philippinensis is an 8 to 10 m high tree with a diameter of 90 to 120 cm. The bark of the slender branches is pale and the younger ones are covered in rust-red matted hairs. The leaves are alternate and have articulate petioles which are 2.5 to 5 cm long. The leaf blade is rusty tomentose, 8 to 15 cm long, ovate with two inconspicuous basal glands. It is entire-margined, coriaceous, and glabrous above with very prominent ribs below.

Habitat: The plant is indigenous to India, Ethiopia, Saudi Arabia, China, and Australia.

Production: Kamala fruit skins are from the fruit skins of philippinensis, covered in hairs and glands.

Other Names: Kameela, Kamcela, Spoonwood, Röttlera tinctoria

ACTIONS AND PHARMACOLOGY

COMPOUNDS

Bergenin

Tannins

EFFECTS

The drug has an anthelmintic and purgative effect.

INDICATIONS AND USAGE

The drug is used to treat tape worm infestation (especially in India).

PRECAUTIONS AND ADVERSE REACTIONS

No health hazards or side effects are known in conjunction with the proper administration of designated therapeutic dosages.

DOSAGE

The drug is used orally as a powder or liquid extract.

LITERATURE

Lounasmaa M et al., (1975) Planta Med 28:16.

Widen CF, Puri HS, (1980) Planta Med 40:284.

Further information in:

Kern W, List PH, Hörhammer L (Hrsg.), Hagers Handbuch der Pharmazeutischen Praxis, 4. Aufl., Bde. 1-8, Springer Verlag Berlin, Heidelberg, New York, 1969.

Mallow

See Malva Sylvestris

Malus Domestica

Apple Tree

DESCRIPTION

Medicinal Parts: The medicinal parts are the fresh false fruit, the fruit peels, and the inflorescences with their leaves and solid peduncles.

Flower and Fruit: The flowers are umbelled racemes with only a few blossoms. The petals are obovate, up to 2.5 cm long, stemmed, white, pink or pink on the outside and white on the inside. The carpels are fused with the false fruit.

Leaves, Stem and Root: The plant is a 6 to 10 m high tree or shrub. Boughs and branches are initially villous-haired, later becoming glabrous. The leaves are alternate, ovate, usually shortly acuminate, and finely crenate-serrate.

Habitat: The plant is cultivated in the temperate regions of the Northern Hemisphere, and occasionally grows wild.

ACTIONS AND PHARMACOLOGY

COMPOUNDS: IN THE FRUIT PULP

Fruit acids: chief acid, malic acid, in unripe apples quinic acid, citric acid, succinic acid, lactic acid

Caffeic acid derivatives: including, among others, 5-coffeoylchina acid

Aromatic substances: in particular 2-trans-hexenal, 3-cis-hexenal, 2-trans-hexenol, 3-cis-hexenol, beta-damascenone, butyric acid ethyl ester, methyl butyric acid hexylester, with some strains, 1-methoxy-4-(2-propenyl)benzole

Pectins

Vitamins: in particular ascorbic acid (3 to 30 mg/100 gm)

COMPOUNDS: IN THE SEEDS

Cyanogenic glycoside: amygdalin (0.5 to 1.5%, corresponding to 30 to 90 mg HCN/100 gm)

Fatty oil

EFFECTS

Medicinal and pharmaceutical preparations of apples come in liquid and dried pectin. The source material is the apple residue with 10 to 20% pectin in the dried mass. The residue is extracted at pH 1.5 to 3 and 60° to 100°C. Pectin is a swelling agent. Apple pectins have a mild binding effect.

INDICATIONS AND USAGE

Finely ground fruit or preparations which contain liquid or dry pectin are used for milder forms of dyspepsia and diarrhea and digestive complaints, especially in children.

Efficacy has not been scientifically proven.

PRECAUTIONS AND ADVERSE REACTIONS

No health hazards or side effects are known in conjunction with the proper administration of designated therapeutic dosages.

DOSAGE

Mode of Administration: The fruit is available for oral use in the grated or chopped form. The skin peel can be used in teas.

LITERATURE

Belitz HD, Grosch W, Lehrbuch der Lebensmittelchemie, 4. Aufl., Springer Verlag Berlin, Heidelberg, New York 1992.

Hänsel R, Keller K, Rimpler H, Schneider G (Hrsg.), Hagers Handbuch der Pharmazeutischen Praxis, 5. Aufl., Bde 4-6 (Drogen), Springer Verlag Berlin, Heidelberg, New York, 1992-1994.

Kern W, List PH, Hörhammer L (Hrsg.), Hagers Handbuch der Pharmazeutischen Praxis, 4. Aufl., Bde. 1-8, Springer Verlag Berlin, Heidelberg, New York, 1969.

Madaus G, Lehrbuch der Biologischen Arzneimittel, Bde 1-3, Nachdruck, Georg Olms Verlag Hildesheim 1979.

Roth L, Daunderer M, Kormann K, Giftpflanzen, Pflanzengifte, 4. Aufl., Ecomed Fachverlag Landsberg Lech 1993.

Teuscher E, Lindequist U, Biogene Gifte - Biologie, Chemie, Pharmakologie, 2. Aufl., Fischer Verlag Stuttgart 1994.

Malva Sylvestris

Mallow

DESCRIPTION

Medicinal Parts: The medicinal parts are the dried flowers, the dried leaves, and the whole of the flowering fresh plant.

Flower and Fruit: The bright purple flowers with long dark stripes are clustered in leaf axils. They have 3 epicalyx leaves, 5 sepals, 5 petals which are much longer than the calyx and have a deep margin. The numerous stamens are fused to a 10 to 12 mm column. The fruit stems are erect or slanted to one side. The ovaries are made up of a ring of 9 to 11 carpels. The fruit is a 7 to 9 mm wide and 2 mm thick disc, which breaks up into mericarps. These are glabrous or covered in a few scattered hairs, sharply angular, and punctate.

Leaves, Stem and Root: Malva sylvestris is a biennial or perennial leafy herb 0.3 to 1.2 m high. The stems are branched, prostrate to curved, ascending, slightly woody, and roughly pubescent. The leaves are alternate, long-petioled, reniform-orbicular, 5-lobed, and crenate-serrate.

Characteristics: Mallow has a 3-leaved epicalyx (compare with Althaea officinalis).

Habitat: Probably originated in southern European-Asia region. Today the tree can be found in subtropical and temperate latitudes of both hemispheres.

Production: Mallow leaves are harvested from June to the beginning of September and dried in thin layers in the shade. Mallow flowers are harvested without the pedicles from the end of June to October and are dried in layers in the shade.

Not To Be Confused With: Other varieties of Malvae, the leaves of Althaea officinalis.

Other Names: Blue Mallow, Mauls, Cheeseflower

ACTIONS AND PHARMACOLOGY

COMPOUNDS: MALVAE FOLIUM

Mucilages: 6-8% (galacturonorhamane and arabinogalactans)

Flavonoids: including, among others, hypolaetin-3-glucoside, gossypetin-3-glucoside; also flavonoid sulfates including among others gossypetin-8-O-beta-D-glucuronide-3-sulfate

COMPOUNDS: MALVAE FLOS

Mucilages: 10% (galacturonorhamane and arabinogalactane)

Anthocyans: including, among others, malvin

EFFECTS: MALVAE FOLIUM AND MALVAE FLOS

The drug has a mucous membrane protective effect; relieves irritation because of the high level of muculaginous material.

INDICATIONS AND USAGE

MALVAE FLOS

- Cough
- Bronchitis

The flowers are used for irritations of the oral and pharyngeal mucosa; dry, irritative coughs.

In folk medicine, the drug is used internally for bronchial catarrh, gastroenteritis, bladder complaints, and externally for wounds. Externally, it is used as a poultice and bath additive for wound treatment.

PRECAUTIONS AND ADVERSE REACTIONS

No health hazards or side effects are known in conjunction with the proper administration of designated therapeutic dosages.

DOSAGE

MALVAE FLOS

Mode of Administration: Mallow flowers are in various tea mixtures as an inactive ingredient.

Preparation: To prepare an infusion, 1.5 to 2 gm of comminuted drug is added to cold water and boiled or scalded and strained after 10 minutes.

Daily Dosage: The average daily dose is 5 gm of the drug.

Storage: The drug should be protected from light, moisture, and insects.

MALVAE FOLIUM

Mode of Administration: Comminuted herb for teas and other preparations are for internal use.

Daily Dosage: The average daily dose is 5 gm of the drug.

Preparation: To prepare an infusion, pour 150 ml of boiling water over 3 to 5 gm of the drug (about 2 teaspoonfuls) and leave to draw for 2 to 3 hours; stir occasionally.

Storage: The drug should be protected from light, moisture, and insects.

LITERATURE

Classen B, Amelunxen F, Blaschek W, Analytical and structural investigations of the mucilage of Malva species. In: PM 59(7):A614. 1993.

Classen B, Amelunxen F, Blaschek W, Malva sylvestris - Mikroskopische Untersuchungen zur Entstehung von Schleimbehältern. In: DAZ 134(38):3597. 1994.

Papageorgiou VP, (1980) Planta Med 38 (3):193.

Schneider K, Ullmann V, Kubelka W, Malvaceen-Schleimdrogen. Zur Bestimmung des Quellungsfaktors. In: DAZ 130(42):2303. 1990.

Further information in:

Hänsel R, Keller K, Rimpler H, Schneider G (Hrsg.), Hagers Handbuch der Pharmazeutischen Praxis, 5. Aufl., Bde 4-6 (Drogen), Springer Verlag Berlin, Heidelberg, New York, 1992-1994.

Madaus G, Lehrbuch der Biologischen Arzneimittel, Bde 1-3, Nachdruck, Georg Olms Verlag Hildesheim 1979.

Steinegger E, Hänsel R, Pharmakognosie, 5. Aufl., Springer Verlag Heidelberg 1992.

Teuscher E, Biogene Arzneimittel, 5. Aufl., Wiss. Verlagsges. Stuttgart 1997.

Wagner H, Wiesenauer M, Phytotherapie. Phytopharmaka und pflanzliche Homöopathika, Fischer-Verlag, Stuttgart, Jena, New York, 1995.

Wichtl M (Hrsg.), Teedrogen, 4. Aufl., Wiss. Verlagsges. Stuttgart 1997.

Manaca

See Brunfelsia Hopeana

Mandragora Vernalis

Mandrake

DESCRIPTION

Medicinal Parts: The medicinal parts are the dried underground part, the fresh herb, and the root.

Flower and Fruit: The numerous flowers are on light green pedicles. They are glabrous on the outside. The corolla is light green to yellow. The calyx is lanceolate with a pointed tip, half as long as the 3 cm corolla. The hairs on the outside of the corolla have heads which consist of 15 cells and sit on a tiny stem of 2 to 3 cm. The fruit is yellow, globular, and extends with a diameter of 2 to 3 cm well beyond the calyx.

Leaves, Stem and Root: The plant has a thick, tuberous root and is almost stemless. The root is light brown on the outside, simple or branched, and up to 60 cm deep. The leaves are all the same size, pubescent, short petiolate, ovate-lanceolate, and have a disgusting smell.

Habitat: The plant is indigenous to the Mediterranean region and bordering frost-free regions.

Production: The plant is gathered in uncultivated regions.

Not To Be Confused With: The roots of Atropa belladona, whose alkaloid pattern is similar.

Other Names: Mandragora, Satan's Apple

ACTIONS AND PHARMACOLOGY

COMPOUNDS: MANDRAGORA RADIX

Tropane alkaloids (0.4%): chief alkaloids (-)-hyoscyamine, under storage conditions changing over to some extent into atropine, and scopolamine

COMPOUNDS: MANDRAGORA HERB

The leaves have hardly been investigated, but in view of the demonstrated toxicity, the same alkaloid mixture is to be assumed.

EFFECTS: MANDRAGORA RADIX AND HERB

The action of the drug is due mainly to the anticholinergic effect of the main alkaloid.

INDICATIONS AND USAGE

Mandragora is one of the oldest of the medicinal plants. In folk medicine, a tincture of Mandragora radix was used for stomach ulcers, colic, asthma, hay fever, and whooping cough. Today, Mandrake is only used in homeopathy.

PRECAUTIONS AND ADVERSE REACTIONS

No health hazards are known in conjunction with the proper administration of designated therapeutic dosages. Skin reddening, dryness of the mouth, tachycardiac arrhythmias, mydriasis (the 4 early warning symptoms of a poisoning), accommodation disorders, heat build-up through decline in sweat secretion, micturition disorders and obstipation can occur as side effects, particularly with overdosages.

OVERDOSAGE

Because of the high content of scopolamine in the drug, poisonings lead at first to somnolence, but then also, after the intake of very high dosages, to central excitation (restlessness, hallucinations, delirium, manic episodes), followed by exhaustion and sleep. Lethal dosages (for adults starting at 100 mg atropine, considerably less for children) carry with them the danger of respiratory failure. Severe poisonings are particularly conceivable in connection with the misuse of the drug as an intoxicant.

The treatment for poisonings include stomach emptying; temperature-lowering measures with wet cloths (no antipyretics!); oxygen respiration for respiratory distress; intubation; parenteral physostigmine salts as antidote; diazepam for spasms while monitoring respiratory function; catheter for cystoparalysis.

DOSAGE

Mode of Administration: The drug is now obsolete and is only rarely used in medicinal preparations. In homeopathy, dilutions from the fresh herb are used.

LITERATURE

Al-Khali S, Alkofahi A, The chemical constituents of Mandragora autumnalis. In: PM 62, Abstracts of the 44th Ann Congress of GA, 149. 1996.

Jackson BP, Berry MI, Hydroxytropane tigliates in the roots of Mandragora species. In: PH 12(5):1165-1166. 1973.

Kraft K, Europäische Rauschdrogen. In: ZPT 17(6):343-355. 1996.

Scholz E, Alraunenfrüchte - ein biblisches Aphrodisiakum. In: ZPT 16(2):109-110. 1995.

Further information in:

Frohne D, Pfänder HJ, Giftpflanzen - Ein Handbuch für Apotheker, Toxikologen und Biologen, 4. Aufl., Wiss. Verlags-Ges. Stuttgart 1997.

Hänsel R, Keller K, Rimpler H, Schneider G (Hrsg.), Hagers Handbuch der Pharmazeutischen Praxis, 5. Aufl., Bde 4-6 (Drogen), Springer Verlag Berlin, Heidelberg, New York, 1992-1994.

Lewin L, Gifte und Vergiftungen, 6. Aufl., Nachdruck, Haug Verlag, Heidelberg 1992.

Madaus G, Lehrbuch der Biologischen Arzneimittel, Bde 1-3, Nachdruck, Georg Olms Verlag Hildesheim 1979.

Roth L, Daunderer M, Kormann K, Giftpflanzen, Pflanzengifte, 4. Aufl., Ecomed Fachverlag Landsberg Lech 1993.

Teuscher E, Lindequist U, Biogene Gifte - Biologie, Chemie, Pharmakologie, 2. Aufl., Fischer Verlag Stuttgart 1994.

Wagner H, Wiesenauer M, Phytotherapie. Phytopharmaka und pflanzliche Homöopathika, Fischer-Verlag, Stuttgart, Jena, New York 1995.

Mandrake

See Mandragora Vernalis

Manna

See Fraxinus Ornus

Maranta Arundinaceae

Arrowroot

DESCRIPTION

Medicinal Parts: The medicinal parts are the starch from the rhizome tubers and the dried rhizome.

Flower and Fruit: The flowers are in pairs, 3.5 cm long and pedicled. They have 3 green, lanceolate sepals and a white, tubular fused corolla with 1 hanging and two erect tips. The stamens are in 2 circles; the first consists of 2 petal-like staminoids, the second of 1 hood-like. There is 1 thickened stamen partly developed like a petal. The ovary is inferior and 3-sectioned. Only 1 carpel is developed. The fruit is 1-valved and has 1 seed.

Leaves, Stem and Root: The plant is a herbaceous perennial, 1 to 2 m high with thin, reed-like, branched, and cane-like stems. The rhizome produces, along with the usual root, a sturdy, fusiform, swollen, up to 8 cm thick and 35 cm long tuber. The tuber is thickly covered with whitish, scaly stipules. The leaves are obovate, light green, lightly pubescent, and short-petioled. They have long sheaths and up to 13 cm long and 6 cm ovate-lanceolate leaf blades.

Habitat: The plant is indigenous to Central America and is found today in all tropical regions around the world.

Production: Arrowroot is the rhizome of Maranta arundinaceae. The drug istself is a white powder extracted from the rhizome. The rhizome is washed, peeled, macerated, and the starch is then extracted, using water in a process of elutriation. The resulting starch mass is purified by repeated sieving and dried in the sun.

Not To Be Confused With: Cheaper starches, such as potato, maize, wheat, or rice starch. These are often used as replacements (substitutes).

Other Names: Maranta

ACTIONS AND PHARMACOLOGY

COMPOUNDS

Starch (25-27%, with respect to the fresh bulbs): as Marantae amylum, maranta starch, medicinal arrowroot

Other constituent elements are not known.

EFFECTS

Animal tests: in rats that received a Marantae-rich diet, a reduction in the increase of the cholesterin levels in the aorta and heart muscle was reported. The effect was put down to an increased elimination of bile acids.

In humans, the drug is a demulcent and soothing agent.

INDICATIONS AND USAGE

Arrowroot is used as a nutritive (nutritional food stuff) for infants and convalescents, a dietary aid in gastrointestinal disorders, and also for acute diarrhea.

PRECAUTIONS AND ADVERSE REACTIONS

No health hazards or side effects are known in conjunction with the proper administration of designated therapeutic dosages.

DOSAGE

Mode of Administration: The powder is boiled with water.

LITERATURE

Hänsel R, Keller K, Rimpler H, Schneider G (Hrsg.), Hagers Handbuch der Pharmazeutischen Praxis, 5. Aufl., Bde 4-6 (Drogen), Springer Verlag Berlin, Heidelberg, New York, 1992-1994.

Marigold

See Calendula Officinalis

Marijuana

See Cannabis Sativa

Marjoram

See Origanum Majorana

Marrubium Vulgare

White Horehound

DESCRIPTION

Medicinal Parts: The medicinal parts are the dried flowering branches, the fresh aerial parts of the flowering plant, and the whole plant.

Flower and Fruit: The small, white 5 to 7 mm long, labiate globular flowers are sessile. There are 6 to 8 richly flowered false whorls that are 1.5 to 2 cm long on each stem. The calyx is tubular, white and tomentose with 10 awl-shaped tips, which are curved back in a hook. The corolla is white and downy. The fruit is an ovate, 1.5 to 2 mm long, obtusely triangular, smooth, gray-brown with darker marbling or light brown nut.

Leaves, Stem and Root: The plant is a perennial herb with a fusiform root and a multi-headed, often woody root crown. The stems are erect, branched, obtusely quadrangular, and about 40 to 60 cm high and 7 mm thick at the base. The branches are curved, spreading out, obtusely quadrangular, and loosely downy, like the leaves. The leaves are tomentose-downy, petiolate, orbicular, unevenly crenate, have distinct veins on the underside, and are wrinkled.

Characteristics: The leaves smell tangy when rubbed, and contain musk juice, which taste bitter and hot.

Habitat: The plant is indigenous to the Mediterranean region to central Asia. It has become established in central Europe; introduced to America, South Africa, and Australia.

Production: The plant is harvested during the flowering season from June to August, fast drying is recommended.

Other Names: Houndsbane, Marrubium

ACTIONS AND PHARMACOLOGY

COMPOUNDS

Diterpene bitter principles: chief components marrubiin (0.1-1.0%), premarrubiin (0.1%)

Caffeic acid derivatives: including among others chlorogenic acid, cryptochlorogenic acid

Flavonoids: including among others chrysoeriol, vicenin II, lactoyl flavones, for example luteolin-7-lactate, apigenin-7-lactate

Volatile oil (traces): including among others camphene, p-cymene, fenchene

EFFECTS

The bitter ingredients act as a gastric juice stimulant; marrubinic acid acts as a choleretic.

INDICATIONS AND USAGE

- Cough/bronchitis
- Dyspeptic complaints
- Liver and gallbladder complaints
- Loss of appetite

The drug is used for dyspepsia, loss of appetite, bloating and flatulence, and respiratory catarrh.

Folk uses: Internally, White Horehound is used for acute and chronic bronchitis, whooping cough, asthma, tuberculosis, pulmonary catarrh, respiratory infections, diarrhea, jaundice, debility, painful menstruation, and as a laxative in higher doses; externally for skin damage, ulcers, and wounds.

PRECAUTIONS AND ADVERSE REACTIONS

No health hazards or side effects are known in conjunction with the proper administration of designated therapeutic dosages.

DOSAGE

Mode of Administration: Comminuted herb, freshly pressed plant juice, and other galenic preparations for internal use.

Preparation: To prepare an infusion, pour boiling water over 1 to 2 gm of the drug; strain after 10 minutes. For a liquid extract, prepare as a (1:1) dilution with ethanol (20%).

Daily Dosage: The average daily dose is 4.5 gm of the drug; 30 to 60 ml pressed juice.

The infusion dosage is 1 to 2 gm of the drug taken up to 3 times daily. The liquid extract dosage is 2 to 4 ml 3 times daily.

LITERATURE

Bartarelli IM, (1966) Boll Chim Farm 105:787.

Brieskorn CH, Feilner K, (1968) Phytochemistry 7:485.

Busby MC et al., (1983) Proc R IR Acad Sect B 83:1.

Cahen R, (1970) C R Soc Biol 164:1467.

Henderson MS, McCrindle R, (1969) J Chem Soc Chem Comm 15:2014.

Karryev MO et al., (1976) Izv Akad Nauk Turkm Ser Biol 3:86.

Mascolo N et al., (1987) Phytother Res 1(1):28.

Nicholas HJ, (1964) J Pharm Sci 53:895.

Pandler WW, Wagner S, (1963) Chem Ind 42:1693.

Popa DP et al., (1968) Khim Prir Soedin 4(6):345.

Popa DP et al., (1974) Rastit Resur 10(3):365.

Popa DP, Salei LA, (1973) Rastit Resur 9(3):384.

Further information in:

Hänsel R, Keller K, Rimpler H, Schneider G (Hrsg.), Hagers Handbuch der Pharmazeutischen Praxis, 5. Aufl., Bde 4-6 (Drogen), Springer Verlag Berlin, Heidelberg, New York, 1992-1994.

Leung AY, Encyclopedia of Common Natural Ingredients Used in Food Drugs and Cosmetics, John Wiley & Sons Inc., New York 1980.

Madaus G, Lehrbuch der Biologischen Arzneimittel, Bde 1-3, Nachdruck, Georg Olms Verlag Hildesheim 1979.

Roth L, Daunderer M, Kormann K, Giftpflanzen, Pflanzengifte, 4. Aufl., Ecomed Fachverlag Landsberg Lech 1993.

Steinegger E, Hänsel R, Pharmakognosie, 5. Aufl., Springer Verlag Heidelberg 1992.

Teuscher E, Biogene Arzneimittel, 5. Aufl., Wiss. Verlagsges. Stuttgart 1997.

Wichtl M (Hrsg.), Teedrogen, 4. Aufl., Wiss. Verlagsges. Stuttgart 1997.

Marsdenia Cundurango

Condurango

DESCRIPTION

Medicinal Parts: The medicinal part is the dried bark of the branches and trunks.

Flower and Fruit: The flowers are in umbel-like inflorescences. The calyx and the campanulate to funnel-shaped corolla have 5 sepals and petals. Pollination is only possible by insects. The fruit is a follicle containing the seeds, with a tuft of hair.

Leaves, Stem and Root: The plant is a climbing shrub with pubescent shoots. The trunk can have a diameter of 10 cm. The transverse section shows granular, yellowish-white, scattered, fine and silky fibers. The outer surface is brownish-gray, often warty, with patches of lichen. The tough, ovate, 8 to 11 cm long and 5 to 8 cm wide leaves are very pubescent. They are crossed opposite.

Characteristics: The taste is bitter and acrid. The odor is faintly aromatic.

Habitat: The plant grows on the western slopes of the Andes in Ecuador, Peru, and Columbia.

Production: Condurango bark consists of the dried bark of branches and trunk of Marsedenia condurango.

Not To Be Confused With: Asclepias umbellata or Elcomarrhiza amylacea

Other Names: Eagle Vine

ACTIONS AND PHARMACOLOGY

COMPOUNDS

Pregnane- and pregn-5-ene glycosides (mixture known as condurangin): including condurango glycosides A, A0, A1, B0, C, C1, D0, E0, E2

Caffeic acid derivatives: including chlorogenic acid

EFFECTS

The drug stimulates the secretion of saliva and gastric juices. It has an antitumoral effect in animals.

INDICATIONS AND USAGE

- Dyspeptic complaints
- Loss of appetite

Condurango is used for loss of appetite; formerly used for stomach cancer.

PRECAUTIONS AND ADVERSE REACTIONS

Health risks or side effects following the proper administration of designated therapeutic dosages are not recorded.

DOSAGE

Mode of Administration: Comminuted drug for infusions and other bitter-tasting preparations for internal use.

Preparation: An infusion is prepared by adding 1.5 gm comminuted drug to cold water and bringing to a boil; strain when cold. The drug is also added to wine. 50 to 100 gm of the drug per liter.

Daily Dosage: The average daily dose of aqueous extract is 0.2 to 0.5 gm; tincture, 2 to 5 gm; liquid extract, 2 to 4 gm; bark, 2 to 4 gm.

Infusion and wine: 1 cup or 1 liquor glass 30 minutes before meals.

LITERATURE

Berger S et al., Arch Pharm 320:924. 1987.

Berger S et al., PH 27:1451. 1988.

Hayashi K et al., (1980) Chem Pharm Bull 28:1954.

Hayashi K et al., (1981) Chem Pharm Bull 29:2725.

Steinegger E, Koch H, Pharm Acta Helv 56:244 et 57:211. 1982.

Takase M et al., (1982) Chem Pharm Bull 30:2429.

Tschesche R, Kohl H, Tetrahedron 24:4359. 1968.

Further information in:

Hänsel R, Keller K, Rimpler H, Schneider G (Hrsg.), Hagers Handbuch der Pharmazeutischen Praxis, 5. Aufl., Bde 4-6 (Drogen): Springer Verlag Berlin, Heidelberg, New York, 1992-1994.

Madaus G, Lehrbuch der Biologischen Arzneimittel, Bde 1-3, Nachdruck, Georg Olms Verlag Hildesheim 1979.

Steinegger E, Hänsel R, Pharmakognosie, 5. Aufl., Springer Verlag Heidelberg 1992.

Teuscher E, Biogene Arzneimittel, 5. Aufl., Wiss. Verlagsges. mbH Stuttgart 1997.

Wichtl M (Hrsg.), Teedrogen, 4. Aufl., Wiss. Verlagsges. Stuttgart 1997.

Marsh Blazing Star

See Liatris Spicata

Marsh Marigold

See Caltha Palustris

Marshmallow

See Althaea Officinalis

Martagon

See Lilium Martagon

Masterwort

See Heracleum Sphondylium; Peucedanum Ostruthium

Mastic Tree

See Pistacia Lentiscus

Maté

See Ilex Paraguariensis

Matricaria Chamomilla

Chamomile

DESCRIPTION

Medicinal Parts: The medicinal parts are the whole flowering herb or only the flowers.

Flower and Fruit: The composite flower is white with a yellow center. The flower heads are terminal and long-pedicled. The bracts are obtuse with a membranous margin. The ray florets are white, linguiform, female and 3-toothed. The disc florets are tubular, androgynous, 5-toothed, with a hollow receptacle.

Leaves, Stem and Root: The plant is a 20 to 40 cm high herb with an erect, glabrous stem, which is branched above. The leaves are 2 to 3 pinnatisect and have a narrow thorny tip.

Characteristic: The receptacle of the compound head of the true camomile is hollow which distinguishes it from other types of camomile.

Habitat: True camomile is indigenous to Europe and northwest Asia, naturalized in North America and elsewhere.

Production: Camomile consists of the fresh or dried flower heads of Matricaria recutita and their preparations.

Other Names: Pin Heads, Chamomilla

ACTIONS AND PHARMACOLOGY

COMPOUNDS

Volatile oil (0.4-1.5%): chief components (-)-alpha-bisabolol (levomenol), bisabolol oxide A, bisabolol oxide B, bisabolol oxide C, beta-trans-farnesene, trans-en-yn-dicycloether (polyyne spiroether, adjoining cis-en-yn-dicycloether), chamazulene (blue in color, arising from the non-volatile proazulene matricine after steam distillation)

Flavonoids: flavone glycosides; aglycones apigenin, lureolin, chrysoeriol, chief glycosides apigenin-7-O-glucoside, apigenine glucoside acetate, - flavonol glycosides, aglycones including among others quercetin, isorhamnetin, patuletin, for example rutin, hyperoside - freely present highly methoxylised flavonoids, for example jaceidine

Hydroxycoumarins: including among others umbelliferone, herniarin

Mucilages: (10%, fructans, rhamanogalacturonane)

EFFECTS

The main active principles are flavonoids and essential oils. The drug has antiphlogistic, antispasmodic, and antibacterial effects. It also promotes wound healing. The anti-inflammatory effect is caused by the camomile flavones.

INDICATIONS AND USAGE

- Common cold
- Cough/bronchitis
- Fevers and colds
- Inflammation of the skin
- Inflammation of the mouth and pharynx
- Liver and gallbladder complaints
- Loss of appetite
- Tendency to infection
- Wounds and burns

Chamomile is used internally for inflammatory diseases of the gastrointestinal tract with gastrointestinal spasms. Externally, the drug is used for skin and mucous membrane inflammations, pulpitis, gingivitis, respiratory catarrh, and ano-genital inflammation.

PRECAUTIONS AND ADVERSE REACTIONS

No health hazards or side effects are known in conjunction with the proper administration of designated therapeutic dosages. The drug possesses a very weak potential for sensitization.

DOSAGE

Mode of Administration: Liquid and solid preparations are available for external and internal application.

Preparation: An infusion for internal use is prepared by pouring boiling water (150 ml) over 3 gm of camomile, cover for 5 to 10 minutes and strain. (1 teaspoonful = 1 gm drug).

An infusion for external poultice application is prepared by pouring one and one-half cups of hot water over 2 dessert spoons of the drug, cover, leave to draw for 15 minutes and then strain. Ointments and gels are available in strengths of 3 to 10%. As a bath additive, 50 g is added to 1 Liter of water.

Daily Dosage: The average daily internal dose of the drug is 10 to 15 gm.

LITERATURE

Achterrath-Tuckerman U et al., (1980) Planta Med 39(1):38.

Aertgeerts P, Albring M, Klaschka F, Nasemann T, Patzelt-Wenczler R, Rauhut K, Weigl B, (1985) Vergleichende Prüfung von Kamillosan(Creme gegenüber steroidalen (0,25 % Hydrocortison, 0,75 % Bluocortinbutylester) und nichtsteroidalen (5 % Bufexamac) Externa in der Erhaltungstherapie von Ekzemerkrankungen. Z Hautkr 60:270-277.

Albring M, Albrecht H, Alcorn G, Lücker PW, (1983) The measuring of the antiinflammatory effect of a compound of the skin of volunteers. Meth Find Exp Clin Pharmacol 5:75-77.

Ammon HPT, Kaul R, (1992) Pharmakologie der Kamille und ihrer Inhaltsstoffe. Dtsch Apoth Z 132(SuppI 27):3-26.

Dorsch W, Neues über antientzündliche Drogen. In: ZPT 14(1):26. 1993.

Füller E et al., Anti-inflammatory activity of Chamomilla polysaccharides. In: PM 59(7):A666. 1993.

Füller E, Franz G, Neues von den Kamillenpolysacchariden. In: DAZ 133(45):4224. 1993.

Gasic O et al., (1983) Fitoterapia 2:51.

Habersang S, (1979) Planta Med 37(2):115.

Hausen HM, Busker E, Carle R, (1984) Über das Sensibilierungsvermögen von Compositenarten. VII. Experimentelle Untersuchungen mit Auszügen und Inhaltsstoffen von Chamomilla recutita L. Rauschert und Anthemis cotula L. Planta Med 50:229-234.

Heilmann J, Kamillenflavonoide: Nur Aglyka dringen in die Haut ein. In: DAZ 133(37):3296. 1993.

Isaac D, (1980) Die Kamillentherapie - Erfolg und Bestätigung. Dtsch Apoth Ztg 120:567-570.

Isaac O, (1979) Planta Med 35(2):3, 118.

Jakovlev V et al., (1979) Planta Med 35(2):3.

Jakovlev V et al., (1983) Planta Med 49(2):67.

Jakovlev V, Isaac O, Flaskamp E, (1983) Pharmakologische Untersuchungen von Kamillen-Inhaltsstoffen. VI. Untersuchungen zur antiphlogistischen Wirkung von Chamazulen und Matricin. Planta Med 49:67-73.

Jakovlev V, Isaac O, Flaskamp E, Pharmakologische Untersuchungen von Kamilleninhaltsstoffen VI. Untersuchungen zur antiphlogistischen Wirkung von Chamazulen und Matricin. In: PM 49:67. 1983.

Jenss H, (1985) Zur Problematik funktioneller Magen-Darm-Krankheiten am Beispiel des Colon irritabile. In: Oepen I (Hrsg) An den Grenzen der Schulmedizin, eine Analyse umstrittener Methoden. Deutscher Ärzte-Verlag Köln, S 197-212.

Maiche AG, Gröhn P, Mäki-Hokkonen H, (1991) Effect of chamomile cream and almond ointment of acute radiation skin reaction. Acta Oncol 30:395-396.

Miller Th, Wittstock U, Lindequist U, Teuscher E, Effects of some components of the essential oil of chamomile, Chamomilla recutita, on Histamine release from mast cells. In: PM 62(1):60-61. 1997.

Nissen HP, Blitz H, Kreysel HW, (1988) Profilometrie, eine Methode zur Beurteilung der therapeutischen Wirksamkeit von Kamillosan-Salbe. Z Hautkr 63:184-190.

Redaelli C et al., (1981) J Chrom. 209:110.

Redaelli C et al., (1981) Plant Med 42:288.

Safayhi H et al., Chamazulene: an antioxydant-type inhibitor of leukotriene B4 formation. In: PM 60(5):410. 1994.

Schilcher H, (1987) Die Kamille. Handbuch für Ärzte, Apotheker und andere Naturwissenschaftler. Wissenschaftliche Verlagsgesellschaft, Stuttgart Ammon HPT, Sabieraj J, Kaul R, Kamille - Mechanismus der antiphlogistischen Wirkung von Kamillenextrakten und -inhaltsstoffen. In: DAZ 136(22):1821-1834. 1996.

Sorkin B, Untersuchungen zur Wirksamkeit von Kamille am Menschen. In: Seifen, Öle, Fette, Wachse 108(1):9-10. 1982.

Szelenyi I et al., (1979) Planta Med 35(3):218.

Vilagines P et al., (1985) C R Acad Sci (III)301(6):289.

Further information in:

Hänsel R, Keller K, Rimpler H, Schneider G (Hrsg.), Hagers Handbuch der Pharmazeutischen Praxis, 5. Aufl., Bde 4-6 (Drogen), Springer Verlag Berlin, Heidelberg, New York, 1992-1994 (unter Chamomilla recutita).

Hausen B, Allergiepflanzen, Pflanzenallergene, ecomed Verlagsgesellsch. mbH, Landsberg 1988 (unter Chamomilla recutita).

Leung AY, Encyclopedia of Common Natural Ingredients Used in Food Drugs and Cosmetics, John Wiley & Sons Inc., New York 1980.

Madaus G, Lehrbuch der Biologischen Arzneimittel, Bde 1-3, Nachdruck, Georg Olms Verlag Hildesheim 1979.

Schulz R, Hänsel R, Rationale Phytotherapie, Springer Verlag Heidelberg 1996.

Steinegger E, Hänsel R, Pharmakognosie, 5. Aufl., Springer Verlag Heidelberg 1992.

Teuscher E, Biogene Arzneimittel, 5. Aufl., Wiss. Verlagsges. Stuttgart 1997.

Wagner H, Wiesenauer M, Phytotherapie. Phytopharmaka und pflanzliche Homöopathika, Fischer-Verlag, Stuttgart, Jena, New York 1995.

Wichtl M (Hrsg.), Teedrogen, 4. Aufl., Wiss. Verlagsges. Stuttgart 1997.

Mayapple

See Podophyllum Peltatum

Meadowsweet

See Filipendula Ulmaria

Medicago Sativa

Alfalfa

DESCRIPTION

Medicinal Parts: The medicinal parts are the whole flowering plant or the germinating seeds.

Flower and Fruit: The clover-like flowers can be yellow to violet-blue. They are 9 to 10 mm long in oblong, many-blossomed racemes. The fruit is a spiralled pod with 2 or 3 twists; the center is hollow and not thorny.

Leaves, Stem and Root: The annual, succulent plant grows from 45 to 100 cm high. The stems are erect, smooth and sharply angled and bear upright branches. The leaves are trifoliate, petiolate, and alternate. The leaflets are thorny-tipped, dentate toward the front, obovate, and villous beneath. The stipules are ovate, lanceolate, slightly dentate, and acuminate.

Characteristics: The taste is unpleasantly salty, bitter and dry.

Habitat: The plant is indigenous to the Mediterranean region and has been widely cultivated elsewhere for centuries.

Other Names: Lucerne, Purple Medick, Purple Medicle, Buffalo Herb, Purple Medic

ACTIONS AND PHARMACOLOGY

COMPOUNDS: IN THE FOLIAGE

Carotinoids: including, among others, lutein

Triterpene saponins: sojasapogenols A-E aglycones medicagenic acid, hederagenin

Isoflavonoids: including, among others, formononetin glycosides, genistein, daidzein

Coumarins; coumestrol, 3′-methoxy coumestrol, lucernol, sativol, trifoliol

Triterpenes: including, among others, stigmasterol, spinasterol

Cyanogenic glycosides: (corresponding to less than 80 mg HCN/100 g)

COMPOUNDS: IN THE SEEDS

L-canavaine

Betaine: stachydrine, homostachydrine

Trigonelline

Fatty oil

EFFECTS

The saponin contents act on the cardiovascular, nervous, and digestive systems.

INDICATIONS AND USAGE

In folk medicine, the drug is used in the treatment of diabetes and malfunctioning of the thyroid gland.

Alfalfa has isolated use as a diuretic and aromatic.

PRECAUTIONS AND ADVERSE REACTIONS

No health hazards or side effects are known in conjunction with the proper administration of designated therapeutic dosages.

LITERATURE

Berrang B, (1974) Phytochemistry 13:2253.

Gestetner B, (1974) Phytochemistry 10:2221.

Keeler RF, (1975) Lloydia 38:56.

Larher F et al., (1983) Plant Sci Lett 29(2/3):315.

Malinow MR et al., (1977) Steroids 29:105.

Morton JF, (1975) Morris Arbor Bull 26:24.

Nowacki E et al., (1976) Biochem. Physiol Pflanz. 169:183.

Tapper BA et al., (1975) J Sci Food Agric 26:277.

Further information in:

Hegnauer R, Chemotaxonomie der Pflanzen, Bde 1-11, Birkhäuser Verlag Basel, Boston, Berlin 1962-1997.

Kern W, List PH, Hörhammer L (Hrsg.), Hagers Handbuch der Pharmazeutischen Praxis, 4. Aufl., Bde. 1-8, Springer Verlag Berlin, Heidelberg, New York, 1969.

Leung AY, Encyclopedia of Common Natural Ingredients Used in Food Drugs and Cosmetics, John Wiley & Sons Inc., New York 1980.

Madaus G, Lehrbuch der Biologischen Arzneimittel, Bde 1-3, Nachdruck, Georg Olms Verlag Hildesheim 1979.

Teuscher E, Lindequist U, Biogene Gifte - Biologie, Chemie, Pharmakologie, 2. Aufl., Fischer Verlag Stuttgart 1994.

Wagner H, Wiesenauer M, Phytotherapie. Phytopharmaka und pflanzliche Homöopathika, Fischer-Verlag, Stuttgart, Jena, New York 1995.

Melaleuca Leucadendron

Cajuput

DESCRIPTION

Medicinal Parts: The medicinal part is the oil distilled from the fresh leaves and twigs.

Flower and Fruit: The tree has racemes of small sessile, creamy white flowers on long terminal spikes up to 15 cm long, which themselves terminate in a tuft of leaves. The flowers have numerous stamens extending to 15 mm.

Leaves, Stem and Root: Melaleuca leucadendron is a large tree up to 40 m tall with a flexible trunk and irregular pendulous branches. The tree is covered in a pale, lamellate bark, which is soft and spongy and occasionally peels off its layers. The leaves are alternate, entire-margined, oblong-lanceolate, tapering, ash-colored and on short-petioles.

Characteristic: It has an odor reminiscent of camphor and eucalyptus.

Habitat: The plant is indigenous to southeast Asia and the tropical regions of Australia. It is cultivated elsewhere.

Production: Cajuput oil, consisting of the essential oil of Melaleuca leucodendra, is extracted from the fresh leaves and twig tips of a number of varieties through steam distillation.

Other Names: White Tea Tree, Swamp Tea Tree, Paperbark Tree, White Wood

ACTIONS AND PHARMACOLOGY

COMPOUNDS

Chief constituents: cineol, (+)-alpha-terpineol, (-)-alpha-terpineol, (+)-alpha-terpineol valerate, (-)- alpha-terpineol valerate, furthermore alpha-pinenes and bicyclic sesquiterpenes, non-rectified oils also contain 3,5-dimethyl-4,6-di-O-methyl-phloroacetophenone

EFFECTS

In vitro, the drug has an antimicrobial and a rubefacient effect.

INDICATIONS AND USAGE

■ Rheumatism

The drug is used for painful muscles and joints in rheumatic disorders, sciatica, lumbago, slipped disk and low back pain. Cajuput is also used for muscular tension and pain following sports injuries such as sprains, bruising, and pulled muscles or ligaments.

PRECAUTIONS AND ADVERSE REACTIONS

General: No health hazards or side effects are known in conjunction with the proper administration of designated therapeutic dosages, however, contact dermatitis is possible.

Pediatric Use: The drug should not be applied to the facial area, in particular not around the nose, of infants and small children (glottal spasms could occur).

DOSAGE

Mode of Administration: Cajuput oil is used externally.

LITERATURE

Lowry JB, (1973) Nature 241:61.

Opdyke DLJ, (1976) Food Cosmet Toxicol:14.

Further information in:

Fenaroli's Handbook of Flavor Ingredients, Vol. 1. 2nd Ed., CRC Press 1975.

Kern W, List PH, Hörhammer L (Hrsg.), Hagers Handbuch der Pharmazeutischen Praxis, 4. Aufl., Bde 1-8, Springer Verlag Berlin, Heidelberg, New York, 1969.

Leung AY, Encyclopedia of Common Natural Ingredients Used in Food Drugs and Cosmetics, John Wiley & Sons Inc., New York 1980.

Steinegger E, Hänsel R, Pharmakognosie, 5. Aufl., Springer Verlag Heidelberg 1992.

Teuscher E, Biogene Arzneimittel, 5. Aufl., Wiss. Verlagsges. Stuttgart 1997.

Melaleucea Viridiflora

Niauli

DESCRIPTION

Medicinal Parts: The medicinal parts are the young or shrubby plants.

Flower and Fruit: The plant grows up to 15 m.

Characteristics: The presence of traces of copper in the Niauli oil make it slightly greenish. The aromatic odor is reminiscent of camphor.

Habitat: The plant grows in tropical parts of southeast Asia and Australia.

Production: Caje oil consists of the essential oil from the leaves of Melaleuca viridiflora, obtained by water distillation.

ACTION AND PHARMACOLOGY

COMPOUNDS

Chief components: 1,8-cineol (35-65%), (+)-alpha-terpineol and (-)-alpha-terpineol as well as their valeric acid esters, additionally alpha-pinene, Viridiflorol

EFFECTS

In vitro, the drug is antibacterial, stimulatory to circulation.

INDICATIONS AND USAGE

■ Cough/bronchitis

Niauli is used for catarrhs of the upper respiratory tract.

CONTRAINDICATIONS

Contraindications to internal use include inflammatory illnesses of the gastrointestinal area or of the biliary ducts, and severe liver diseases.

PRECAUTIONS AND ADVERSE REACTIONS

General: No health hazards or side effects are known in conjunction with the proper administration of designated therapeutic dosages. The internal administration of the Niauli oil as a drug leads, in rare cases to nausea, vomiting and diarrhea.

Drug Interactions: Caje oil contains 35 - 60% cineol. Cineol causes the induction of the enzymes involved in the detoxification of the liver. The effect of other drugs can, therefore, be reduced and/or shortened.

Pediatric Use: Preparations containing the oil should not be applied to the faces of infants or small children since glottal spasm, bronchial spasm and asthma-like attacks are possible, as is respiratory failure.

OVERDOSAGE

Overdosages of niauli oil (more than 10 gm), can lead to life-threatening poisonings, due to the high cineol content. Symptoms include, among others, fall in blood pressure, circulatory disorders, collapse and respiratory failure. In case of poisoning, vomiting should not be induced because of the danger of aspiration. Following administration of activated charcoal, the therapy for poisonings consists of treating spasms with diazepam (i.v.), treating colics with atropine, electrolyte substitution and treating possible cases of acidosis with sodium bicarbonate infusions. Intubation and oxygen respiration may also be necessary.

DOSAGE

Mode of Administration: The oil and other galenic preparations are for internal and external application.

Preparation: Oily nose drops are prepared in a 2 to 5% concentration in vegetable oil. For external use, preparations contain 10 to 30% active ingredient in oil.

Daily Dosage: For internal use, the single dose is 0.2 gm, with the daily dosage ranging from 0.2 to 2.0 gm.

LITERATURE

Kern W, List PH, Hörhammer L (Hrsg.), Hagers Handbuch der Pharmazeutischen Praxis, 4. Aufl., Bde. 1-8, Springer Verlag Berlin, Heidelberg, New York, 1969.

Steinegger E, Hänsel R, Pharmakognosie, 5. Aufl., Springer Verlag Heidelberg 1992.

Teuscher E, Biogene Arzneimittel, 5. Aufl., Wiss. Verlagsges. Stuttgart 1997.

Melilotus Officinalis

Sweet Clover

DESCRIPTION

Medicinal Parts: The medicinal part is the flowering herb.

Flower and Fruit: The small yellow flowers are in many-blossomed, long peduncled racemes. The standard and wings are the same length, but longer than the carina. Of the 10 stamens, 9 are fused. The fruit is an obtuse, glabrous, light brown to black, thorny-tipped, horizontally wrinkled, and usually one-seeded pod.

Leaves, Stem and Root: The plant is perennial and 60 to 120 cm high. The smooth ascending or decumbent stems are heavily branched. The leaves are alternate, glabrous, trifoliate, and long-petioled. The leaflets are obovate and dentate. The stipules are awl-like bristly.

Characteristics: The plant has a fragrance of woodruff or hay.

Habitat: The plant is found all over Europe, Australia, and North America as well as in temperate regions of Asia.

Production: Sweet Clover consists of the dried or fresh leaf and flowering branches of Melilotus officinalis, and/or Melilotus altissimus.

Other Names: Melilot, King's Clover, Yellow Sweet Clover, Hay Flowers, Sweet Lucerne, Wild Laburnum, Hart's Tree

ACTIONS AND PHARMACOLOGY

COMPOUNDS: IN THE FRESH PLANT

Coumarinic acids

COMPOUNDS: IN THE DEHYDRATED DRUG

Free coumarin (0.4-0.9%): formed from the coumarinic acids during dehydration, furthermore 3,4-dihydrocoumarin, melilotol, melilotin

Hydroxycoumarins: including among others umbelliferone, scopoletin, herniarin, fraxidin

Flavonoids: including among others kaempferol- and quercetin glycosides

Triterpene saponins

COMPOUNDS: IN THE SEEDS

Canavanin

Trigonelline

EFFECTS

The drug has anti-edematous properties, which explain its use for inflammatory and congestive edema. It increases venous reflux and improves lymphatic kinetics.

Animal experiments showed an increase in healing wounds.

INDICATIONS AND USAGE

- Blunt injuries
- Hemorrhoids
- Venous conditions

The drug is used internally for problems arising from chronic venous insufficiency, such as pain and heaviness in legs, night cramps in the legs, itching, and swelling; for the supportive treatment of thrombophlebitis, postthrombotic syndromes, hemorrhoids, and lymphatic congestion. Externally, the drug is used for contusions and superficial effusions of blood.

In folk medicine, Sweet Clover is also utilized as a diuretic.

PRECAUTIONS AND ADVERSE REACTIONS

No health hazards or side effects are known in conjunction with the proper administration of designated therapeutic dosages. Administration of the drug in higher dosages can lead to headache and stupor, transitory liver damage is possible for a very small number of particularly susceptible patients. Elevation of liver enzyme values usually disappears following discontinuance of the drug. (Monitoring of the liver enzyme values is recommended.)

DOSAGE

Mode of Administration: Comminuted drug for infusions and other galenic preparations for oral use; liquid forms of medication for parenteral application; ointments, liniments, cataplasms, and herbal sachets for external use; ointments and suppositories for rectal use.

Preparation: To prepare an infusion, pour boiling water over 1 to 2 teaspoonfuls of comminuted, cut drug, strain after 5 to 10 minutes.

Daily Dosage: The average daily dose of the herb or preparation in amounts corresponding to 3 to 30 mg of coumarin; parenteral application corresponding to 1.0 to 7.5 mg of coumarin.

Infusion: As a therapy for varicose veins, 2 to 3 cups daily.

External: As a poultice for hemorrhoids.

Storage: The drug must be stored away from light in sealed containers to prevent loss of coumarin.

LITERATURE

Abou-Donia AHA, (1976) Ph. D. Thesis, Faculty of Pharmacy, University of Alexandria, Egypt.

Bos R et al., Analysis of coumarin in Melilotus officinalis. In: PM 61(Abstracts of 43rd Ann Congr):68. 1995.

Földi M, Kovach AGB, Varga L, Zoltan ÖT, Die Wirkung des Melilotus-Präparates Esberiven R auf die Lymphströmung. In: Ärztl Forsch 16:99. 1962.

Földi M, Zoltán ÖT, Obál F, Experimentelle lymphostatische Encephalopathie als Folgeerscheinung einer cervikalen Lymphangiothrombophlebitis und deren Therapie mit Cumarin aus Melilotus officinalis. In: Arzneim Forsch 20:1626-1628. 1970.

Földi-Börcsök E, Bedall FK, Rahlfs VW, Die antiphlogistische und ödemhemmende Wirkung von Cumarin aus Melilotus officinalis. In: Arzneim Forsch 21:2025-2030. 1971.

Hammouda FM, Rizk AM, Seif EL-Nazar MM, Abou-Youssef AA, Ghaleb HA, Madkour MK, Pholand AE, Wood G, Flavonoids and coumarins from elilotus. In: Fitotherapia 54(6):249-255. 1983.

Hong ND et al., (1983) Korean J Pharmacognosy 14(2):51.

Johne HO, Experimentelle und klinische Untersuchung mit dem Melilotuspräparat Esberiven. In: Ärztl Forsch 14:473-474. 1960.

Marshall M, Wüstenberg P, Klinik und Therapie der chronischen enösen Insuffizienz. In: Klinik und Therapie der chronischen venösen Insuffizienz, Braun Fachverlage, Karlsruhe 1994.

Mislin H, Die Wirkung von Cumarin aus Melilotus officinalis auf die Funktion des Lymphangioms. In: Arzneim Forsch 21:852-853. 1971.

Plouvier V, (1963) Compt Rend 257:4061.

Wüstenberg, P, Baumann G, Verdacht der Toxizität von Cumarin nicht bestätigt. In: PZ 139(13):1058. 1994.

Further information in:

Kern W, List PH, Hörhammer L (Hrsg.), Hagers Handbuch der Pharmazeutischen Praxis, 4. Aufl., Bde 1-8, Springer Verlag Berlin, Heidelberg, New York, 1969.

Madaus G, Lehrbuch der Biologischen Arzneimittel, Bde 1-3, Nachdruck, Georg Olms Verlag Hildesheim 1979.

Roth L, Daunderer M, Kormann K: Giftpflanzen, Pflanzengifte, 4. Aufl., Ecomed Fachverlag Landsberg Lech 1993.

Steinegger E, Hänsel R, Pharmakognosie, 5. Aufl., Springer Verlag Heidelberg 1992.

Teuscher E, Lindequist U, Biogene Gifte - Biologie, Chemie, Pharmakologie, 2. Aufl., Fischer Verlag Stuttgart 1994.

Teuscher E, Biogene Arzneimittel, 5. Aufl., Wiss. Verlagsges. Stuttgart 1997.

Wagner H, Wiesenauer M, Phytotherapie. Phytopharmaka und pflanzliche Homöopathika, Fischer-Verlag, Stuttgart, Jena, New York 1995.

Wichtl M (Hrsg.), Teedrogen, 4. Aufl., Wiss. Verlagsges. Stuttgart 1997.

Melissa Officinalis

Lemon Balm

DESCRIPTION

Medicinal Parts: The medicinal parts are the oil extracted by distillation, the dried leaves, the fresh leaves, and the whole plant.

Flower and Fruit: The small white bilabiate flowers are in 6 one-sided false whorls in the axils of the upper leaves. The calyx is campanulate, bilabiate, and has a shortly dentate upper lip. The corolla tube is curved upwards. The upper lip is slightly domed and divided in two parts, the lower lip is 3-lobed with an extended middle lobe. The flower has 4 stamens. The fruit is an oblong-ovate, 1.5 to 2 mm long, and chestnut brown nutlet.

Leaves, Stem and Root: The plant is an up to 90 cm high perennial with an erect, quadrangular, branched, and sparsely haired to glabrous stem. The leaves are petiolate and have an ovate to rhomboid, 2 to 6 cm long and 1.5 to 5 cm wide crenate leaf blade, which is shortly pointed at the end, and stunted or wedge-shaped at the base. It is usually only pubescent above or completely glabrous.

Characteristics: Before flowering, the taste and smell is lemon-like, later becoming astringent to balm-like and warming.

Habitat: The plant is indigenous to the east Mediterranean region and west Asia and is cultivated in central Europe or established in the wild.

Production: The leaves are collected before flowering or before there is too much branching. Leaves and stem are separated and comminuted and dried quickly at temperatures between 30 to 40°C.

Not To Be Confused With: Nepeta cataria. var. citriodora (lemon cat mint).

Other Names: Sweet Mary, Honey Plant, Cure-all, Dropsy Plant, Melissa

ACTIONS AND PHARMACOLOGY

COMPOUNDS

Volatile oil (0.02-0.8%): chief components geranial (citral a), neral (citral b), citronellal (together 40-75% of the volatile oil, aroma-carrier), furthermore, linalool, geraniol, geranylactetate, methyl citronellate, trans-β-ocimene, 1-Octen-3-ol, 6-methyl-5-heptene-2-on. beta-caryophyllene, caryophyllebepoxide, germacren D, eugenol

Glycosides: of the alcoholic or phenolic components of the volatile oil, for example eugenol glucoside

Caffeic acid derivatives: rosmaric acid (up to 4.7%)

Flavonoids: including among others cynaroside, cosmosiin, rhamnocitrin, isoquercitrin

Triterpene acids: including, among others, ursolic acid. Only the very fresh drug (maximum 6 months old) is usable as a sedative, because of the low volatile oil content and its high volatility; the requirements of the German-language medication texts do not take this into consideration (no minimum content requirement given).

EFFECTS

The drug has mild sedative and carminative (spasmolytic, antibacterial, antiviral) effects.

INDICATIONS AND USAGE

■ Nervousness and insomnia

The drug is used for nervous agitation, sleeping problems, and functional gastrointestinal complaints with meteorism.

In folk medicine, the drug is utilized for decoctions of the flowering shoots for nervous complaints, lower abdominal disorders, nervous gastric complaints, hysteria and melancholia, chronic bronchial catarrh, nervous palpitations, vomiting, migraine, nervous debility, and high blood pressure.

PRECAUTIONS AND ADVERSE REACTIONS

No health hazards or side effects are known in conjunction with the proper administration of designated therapeutic dosages.

DOSAGE

Mode of Administration: Comminuted herb, herb powder, liquid extracts or dry extracts for teas and other galenic preparations; liquid and solid forms for internal and external use; combinations with other sedative and/or carminative herbs may be beneficial.

Preparation: To prepare an infusion pour one cup of hot water over 1.5 to 4.5 gm of the drug and strain after 10 minutes.

Daily Dosage: The average daily dose is 8 to 10 gm of the drug.

Storage: Store in well-sealed, non-plastic containers, protected from light and moisture for up to 1 year.

LITERATURE

Auf'mkolk M, (1985) Endocrinology 116(5):1687.

Auf'mkolk M et al., (1984) Endocrinology 115(2):527.

Auf'mkolk M et al., (1984) Horm Metab Res 16(4):183.

Brieskorn CH, Krause W, (1974) Arch Pharm 307(8):603.

Buechner KH et al., (1974) Med Klein. 69(23):1032.

Chlabicz J et al., (1984) Pharmazie 39(11):770.

Cohen RA, Kucera LS, Herrmann EC Jr, Antiviral activity of Melissa officinalis (Limon Balm) extract. In: Proc Soc Exp Biol Med 117:431-434. 1964.

Czygan FC, Melisse - Objekt der Grundlagenforschung. In: DAZ 132(12):599. 1992.

De Jong CAG, (1978) Ned Tijdschr Geneeskd 112(3):82.

Enjalbert F et al., (1983) Fitoterapia 2:59.

Forster HB et al., (1980) Planta Med 40(4):309.

Hermann EC Jr., Kucera LS, Antiviral substances in plants of the mint family (Labiatae): II. Nontanninia polyphenols of Melissa officinalis. In: Proc soc Exp Bio Med 124:869. 1967.

Koch-Heitzmann I, Schultze W, 2000 Jahre Melissa officinalis. Von der Bienenpflanze zum Virustatikum. In: ZPT 9(3):77. 1988.

Kümel G, Stoll L, Brendel M, Herpes simplex. Therapie mit rezeptfreien Topika. In: DAZ 131(30):1609. 1991.

Kucera LS, Hermann EC Jr, (1967) Proc Soc Exp Biol Med 124:865 et 874.

Mohrig A, Melissenextrakt bei Herpes simplex - die Alternative zu Nucleosid-Analoga. In: DAZ 136(50):4575-4580. 1996.

Orth-Wagner S, Ressin WJ, Friedrich I, Phytosedativum gegen Schlafstörungen. In: ZPT 16(3):147-156. 1995.

Ozarowski A, (1982) Wiad 4:7.

Pertz H, Naturally occuring clavines: Antagonism/partial agonism at 5-HT2alpha receptors and antogonism at alpha1-adrenoceptors in blood vessel. In: PM 62(5)387-392. 1996.

Richter T, Melissa officinalis - Ein Leitmotiv für 1000 Jahre Medizingeschichte. In: DAZ 133(41):3723. 1993.

Sarer E, Kokdil G, Constitutents of the essential oil from Melissa officinalis. In: PM 57:89. 1991.

Schultze W, König WA, Hilker A, Richter R, Melissenöle. In: DAZ 135(7):557-577. 1995.

Thieme H, Kithe C, (1973) Pharmazie 28(1):69.

Uehleke B, Phytobalneologie. In: ZPT 17(1):26-43. 1996.

Vogt HJ, Tausch I, Wöbling RH, Kaiser PM (1991) Melissenextrakt bei Herpes simplex. Allgemeinarzt 14:832-841.

Wagner H, Sprinkmeyer L, (1973) Dtsch Apoth Z 113:1159.

Walz A, Melisse hilft heilen. In: DAZ 136(2):26. 1996.

Wolbling RH, Milbradt R, (1984) Therapiewoche 34(9):1193.

Zitiert nach: Koch- Heitzmann I, Schültze W, (1984) Melissa officinalis. Eine alte Arzneipflanze mit neue therapeutischen Wirkungen. Dtsch Apoth Z 124:2137-2145.

Further information in:

Hänsel R, Keller K, Rimpler H, Schneider G (Hrsg.), Hagers Handbuch der Pharmazeutischen Praxis, 5. Aufl., Bde 4-6 (Drogen), Springer Verlag Berlin, Heidelberg, New York, 1992-1994.

Leung AY, Encyclopedia of Common Natural Ingredients Used in Food Drugs and Cosmetics, John Wiley & Sons Inc., New York 1980.

Madaus G, Lehrbuch der Biologischen Arzneimittel, Bde 1-3, Nachdruck, Georg Olms Verlag Hildesheim 1979.

Schulz R, Hänsel R, Rationale Phytotherapie, Springer Verlag Heidelberg 1996.

Steinegger E, Hänsel R, Pharmakognosie, 5. Aufl., Springer Verlag Heidelberg 1992.

Teuscher E, Biogene Arzneimittel, 5. Aufl., Wiss. Verlagsges. Stuttgart 1997.

Wagner H, Wiesenauer M, Phytotherapie. Phytopharmaka und pflanzliche Homöopathika, Fischer-Verlag, Stuttgart, Jena, New York 1995.

Wichtl M (Hrsg.), Teedrogen, 4. Aufl., Wiss. Verlagsges. Stuttgart 1997.

Mentha Aquatica

Wild Mint

DESCRIPTION

Medicinal Parts: The medicinal part is the dried leaf.

Flower and Fruit: The flowers are in 2 to 3 dense false axillary whorls with inconspicuous bracts. The upper ones are fused into a terminal, globular or ovate capitulum. The calyx is tubular, with 13 ribs and glabrous inside. The tips are awl-shaped to triangular. The pedicles are pubescent. The corolla is violet with a ring of hair in the tube. The fruit is hard with an ovoid, light brown nutlet.

Leaves, Stem and Root: Wild Mint is a perennial, 20 to 80 cm high plant with a branched underground rhizome and an erect stem with alternate sessile curly leaves. The stem is branched in the upper half and terminates in spikes of blue flowers. The leaves are ovate and serrated.

Characteristics: The whole plant smells of caraway. The plant is a result of many cross-breedings in gardens and fields.

Habitat: The plant grows in Europe, northern Africa, and western Asia. In has been introduced to America, Australia, and Madiera.

Production: Wild Mint is the aerial part of Mentha aquatica. The drug is derived from the dried leaves.

Other Names: Water Mint, Marsh Mint, Hairy Mint

ACTIONS AND PHARMACOLOGY

COMPOUNDS

Volatile oil: chief components - menthofurane, beta-caryophyllene, 1,8-cineole, germacren D, limonene, viridiflorol, a chemotype contains isopinocamphone as chief constituent (according to older references, also linalool, linalyl acetate, cineole, menthone)

Tannins

EFFECTS

The drug is an astringent and a stimulant.

INDICATIONS AND USAGE

Water Mint is used for diarrhea and dysmenorrhea.

PRECAUTIONS AND ADVERSE REACTIONS

No health hazards or side effects are known in conjunction with the proper administration of designated therapeutic dosages.

DOSAGE

Mode of Administration: Ground drug is used as an infusion.

Preparation: Add approximately 30 gm of the drug to 500 ml of water.

Daily Dosage: As a daily dose, drink a wineglassful during the course of the day.

LITERATURE

Hänsel R, Keller K, Rimpler H, Schneider G (Hrsg.), Hagers Handbuch der Pharmazeutischen Praxis, 5. Aufl., Bde 4-6 (Drogen), Springer Verlag Berlin, Heidelberg, New York, 1992-1994.

Mentha Arvensis Var Piperascens

Japanese Mint

DESCRIPTION

Medicinal Parts: The medicinal parts are the essential oil, which has been extracted by steam distillation, and the ensuing separation of the menthol and the dried aerial parts of the plant.

Flower and Fruit: The flowers are in dense globular, sessile, 8 to 12 blossomed false whorls with small linear-lanceolate bracts. The inflorescence is leafy at the apex. The bracts are like the leaves, smaller above. The tepals are 1.5 by 2.5 mm, broadly campanulate and hairy. The corolla is lilac, white or rarely pink. The nutlets are pale brown.

Leaves, Stem and Root: Japanese Mint is a pubescent, fragrant perennial or occasionally annual up to 60 cm. The stems are ascending or erect. The leaves 15 to 70 by 10 to 40 mm, are elliptic-lanceolate to broadly ovate, usually elliptical with the base narrowing to a petiole and shallowly dentate.

Habitat: The plant is found in Europe as far the 65th latitude, in Asia (in particular Siberia), the Caucasus, the Himalayas, China, Mongolia, Korea, Japan. It was probably introduced to North America.

Production: Mint oil consists of essential oil recovered from Mentha arvensis var. piperascens. The oil its obtained by steam distillation of the fresh, flowering herb, followed by partial removal of menthol and rectification.

Menthol is obtained from various species of Mentha, chiefly M. arvensis var. piperascens (from Japan), M. arvensis var. glabrata (from China) and M. piperata (from America). Menthol is distilled from Peppermint oil, and the product produced by the first two is inferior to the latter, but contains a higher proportion of Menthol.

ACTIONS AND PHARMACOLOGY

COMPOUNDS

Chief components: menthol (25-40%), menthone (15-30%), isomenthone (7-12%), limonene (7-12%), neomenthol (2-4%), menthyl acetate (1-5%), beta- caryophyllene (2-5%), piperitone (0.5-4%), alpha-and beta-pinene (2-4% each) The composition does not reflect the relationship of the components to one another in the plant. The volatile oil gained through steam distillation was freed of 30-50% of the menthol through winterisation and rectified.

EFFECTS

Japanese Mint has carminative, cholagogue, and antibacterial properties. It also has a secretolytic effect and is cooling on the bronchial mucosa.

INDICATIONS AND USAGE

- Common cold
- Cough/bronchitis
- Fevers and colds
- Inflammation of the mouth and pharynx
- Liver and gallbladder complaints
- Pain
- Tendency to infection

Internally, the herb is used for flatulence, functional gastrointestinal and gallbladder disorders, and catarrhs of the upper respiratory tract. Externally, it is used for myalgia and neuralgic ailments.

In folk medicine, it is used internally for functional cardiac complaints, sensitivity to weather changes, and breathing difficulties. Externally, Mint is used for functional cardiac complaints and headaches.

CONTRAINDICATIONS

Contraindications for the internal administration of the drug include occlusion of the biliary ducts, gallbladder inflammation and severe liver damage. Gallstone sufferers could experience colics due to the cholagogic effect.

PRECAUTIONS AND ADVERSE REACTIONS

General: No health hazards are known in conjunction with the proper administration of designated therapeutic dosages. The intake can lead to gastric complaints in susceptible patients. Volatile oils containing menthol can worsen the spasms of bronchial asthma. The volatile oil possesses a weak potential for sensitization due to its menthol content.

Pediatric Use: Preparations containing the oil should not be applied to the faces of infants or small children, particularly not in the nasal area (glottal spasm or bronchial spasm up to asthma-like attacks or even possible respiratory failure).

OVERDOSAGE

Cases of poisoning are not recorded. The minimal lethal dosage of menthol is estimated to be 2 gm, although individuals have survived higher dosages (8-9 gm).

DOSAGE

Mode of Administration: The essential oil and other galenic preparations are available for internal and external application. Varieties are commercially available as Brazilian, Chinese and Indian mint oil.

Daily Dosage: For internal use, the average daily dosage is 3 to 6 drops. When used as inhalation therapy, 3 to 4 drops are placed in hot water. To use externally, rub a few drops on the affected area.

In folk medicine, 2 drops are placed in a glass of water, tea or juice and taken once or twice a day. To make a heart poultice, 10 to 20 drops are placed on a compress, which is applied externally for 10 to 15 minutes. For headaches, 1 to 2 drops can be rubbed on the temples.

Storage: Store in air-tight containers protected from light; oils of different batches should not be mixed.

LITERATURE

Hänsel R, Keller K, Rimpler H, Schneider G (Hrsg.), Hagers Handbuch der Pharmazeutischen Praxis, 5. Aufl., Bde 4-6 (Drogen), Springer Verlag Berlin, Heidelberg, New York, 1992-1994.

Teuscher E, Biogene Arzneimittel, 5. Aufl., Wiss. Verlagsges. Stuttgart 1997.

Mentha Longifolia

English Horsemint

DESCRIPTION

Medicinal Parts: The medicinal part is the dried herb.

Flower and Fruit: The flowers are sometimes interrupted lower down by 1 cm thick, gray to white, downy, panicled, false spikes. The false spikes are arranged with linear, villous bracts, which are longer than the flowers. The calyx is fluffy and woolly pubescent with awl-shaped tips. The corolla is lilac to flesh-colored. The fruit is a finely-speckled nutlet.

Leaves, Stem and Root: The plant is a perennial. It has a sturdy rhizome with underground runners. The shoots are densely covered in 1 to more-celled tomentose hairs with few glands and a mild odor. The stem is erect, simple or branched, up to 1 m high, tough, and obtusely angular. The leaves are sessile, oblong-ovate to lanceolate, usually acuminate, with 6 to 12 pairs of curved pinnate veins. The underside of the leaves are gray to white tomentose.

Production: English Horsemint is the aerial part of Mentha lonifolia, the dried herb.

Habitat: The plant is common in all of Europe to southern Sweden.

ACTIONS AND PHARMACOLOGY

COMPOUNDS

Volatile oil: chief components piperitone (share 60-80%), furthermore beta- caryophyllene (5-15%), germacren D (5-15%), 1,8-cineole (2-7%), limonene (1-8%), with other chemotypes chief components D-carvone, piperitone, isomenthone + menthofurane, menthone, piperitol, menthol or linalool

Flavonoids: including among others diosmin, hesperidin, quercitrin, thymonin, apigenine-7-glucuronide

EFFECTS

English Horsemint has carminative and stimulant effects.

INDICATIONS AND USAGE

The drug is used for digestive disorders, particularly for flatulence. Historically, it has been used for all kinds of pain, headaches in particular.

PRECAUTIONS AND ADVERSE REACTIONS

No health hazards or side effects are known in conjunction with the proper administration of designated therapeutic dosages.

DOSAGE

Mode of Administration: The ground drug is used internally as an infusion; externally as a bath additive.

LITERATURE

Hänsel R, Keller K, Rimpler H, Schneider G (Hrsg.), Hagers Handbuch der Pharmazeutischen Praxis, 5. Aufl., Bde 4-6 (Drogen), Springer Verlag Berlin, Heidelberg, New York, 1992-1994.

Mentha Piperita

Peppermint

DESCRIPTION

Medicinal Parts: The medicinal parts are the oil extracted from the aerial parts of the flowering plant, the dried leaves and flowering branch tips, the fresh flowering plant, and the whole plant.

Flower and Fruit: The flowers are false spikes with numerous inconspicuous bracts. The calyx is tubular, with a ring of hair. The corolla is violet, glabrous inside and has an almost even margin divided into four parts.

Leaves, Stem and Root: The plant is a perennial, 50 to 90 cm high. The usually branched stems are normally glabrous, but sometimes they are gray-tomentose and are often tinged violet. The leaves are short-petioled, oblong-ovate and serrate. The plant has over- and underground runners.

Habitat: Common in Europe and the U.S., usually cultivated.

Production: Menthae piperitae folium is harvested several times a year. The maximum leaf harvest and highest oil content is shortly before the flowering season. The harvest is dried mechanically on drying belts at a temperature of 42°C. Menthae piperitae aetheroleum is harvested mechanically shortly after flowering and dried in the field.

Not To Be Confused With: Menthae piperitae aetheroleum should not be confused with the drug with rectified mint oil. Sometime adulterated by increasing the ester content with racemic menthal acetate.

Other Names: Brandy Mint, Lamb Mint

ACTIONS AND PHARMACOLOGY

COMPOUNDS: MENTHAE PIPERITAE FOLIUM

Volatile oil: chief components: menthol (35-45%), menthone (15-20%), menthyl acetate (3-5%), neomenthol (2.5-3.5%), isomenthone (2-3%), menthofurane (2-7%), additionally including, among others, limonene, pulegone, alpha- and beta-pinene, trans-sabinene hydrate

Caffeic acid: including, among others, rosmaric acid

Flavonoids: apigenine-, diosmetin- and luteolin glycosides, free lipophile methoxylized flavone including, among others, xanthomicrol, gardenine D

EFFECTS: MENTHAE PIPERITAE FOLIUM

The drug has a spasmolytic effect on the smooth muscle of the digestive tract. It also has cholagogic and carminative effects.

COMPOUNDS: MENTHAE PIPERITAE AETHEROLEUM

Chief components: menthol (35-45%), menthone (15-20%), menthyl acetate (3-5%), neomenthol (2.5-3.5%), isomenthone (2-3%), menthofurane (2-7%), additionally including among others limonene, pulegone, alpha- and beta-pinene, trans-sabinene hydrate

Labiatentannins: including, among others, rosmaric acid

Flavonoids: apigenine-, diosmetin- and luteolin glycosides, free lipophile methoxylized flavone including, among others, xanthomicrol, gardenine D

EFFECTS: MENTHAE PIPERITAE AETHEROLEUM

The drug has a spasmolytic effect on smooth muscle of the gastrointestinal tract. It is a carminative, cholagogue, antibacterial, and secretolytic agent; also has a cooling effect on the skin.

INDICATIONS AND USAGE

MENTHAE PIPERITAE FOLIUM

- Liver and gallbladder complaints
- Loss of appetite

The drug is used for convulsive complaints of the gastrointestinal tract as well as gallbladder and bile ducts.

In folk use, peppermint is utilized for nausea, vomiting, morning sickness, respiratory infections, and dysmenorrhea.

MENTHAE PIPERITAE AETHEROLEUM

- Common cold
- Cough/bronchitis
- Fevers and colds
- Inflammation of the mouth and pharynx
- Liver and gallbladder complaints
- Loss of appetite
- Tendency to infection

The drug is used internally for cramps of the upper gastrointestinal tract and bile ducts, irritable colon, catarrhs of the respiratory tract, and inflammation of the oral and pharyngeal mucosa.

Externally, it is used for myalgia and neuralgia.

CONTRAINDICATIONS

MENTHAE PIPERITAE AETHEROLEUM

Contraindications for the internal administration of the drug include occlusion of the biliary ducts, gallbladder inflammation, and severe liver damage. Gallstone carriers could experience colic due to the cholagogic effect.

PRECAUTIONS AND ADVERSE REACTIONS

MENTHAE PIPERITAE FOLIUM

No health hazards are known in conjunction with the proper administration of designated therapeutic dosages. Gallstone carriers could experience colic due to the cholagogic effect.

MENTHAE PIPERITAE AETHEROLEUM

General: No health hazards are known in conjunction with the proper administration of designated therapeutic dosages. The intake can lead to gastric complaints in susceptible persons. The volatile oil possesses a weak potential for sensitization due to its menthol content. One is advised against administration of the drug in the presence of a tendency to gastroesophageal reflux.

Pediatric Use: Preparations containing the oil should not be applied to the faces of infants or small children, particularly not in the nasal area (glottal spasm or bronchial spasm up to asthma-like attacks or even possible respiratory failure).

OVERDOSAGE

Cases of poisoning are not recorded. The minimal lethal dosage of menthol is estimated to be 2 gm, although individuals have survived higher dosages (8 to 9 gm).

DOSAGE

MENTHAE PIPERITAE FOLIUM

Mode of Administration: Comminuted herb for infusions, extracts of peppermint leaves for internal use.

Preparation: To prepare an infusion, pour 150 ml of hot water over 1 dessertspoonful of the drug, strain after 10 minutes (one study has shown that the maximum level of menthol and methon is present after this time).

Daily Dosage: The average daily dose of the drug is 3 to 6 gm. The average daily dose of the tincture (1:10) is 5 to 15 gm.

MENTHAE PIPERITAE AETHEROLEUM

Mode of Administration: The essential oil and the galenic preparations are for internal and external use.

Daily Dosage: The average daily internal dose is 6 to 12 drops; inhalation, 3 to 4 drops in hot water; for irritable colon, 0.6 ml in an enteric coated form.

Externally, a few drops rubbed into the affected skin areas. The drug is available as semi-solid and oily preparations (5 to 20%); aqueous-ethanol preparations (5 to 10%); nasal ointments with 1 to 5% essential oil.

Storage: Peppermint should be stored cool and dry and protected from light in non-plastic containers.

LITERATURE

MENTHAE PIPERITAE FOLIUM

Bowen ICH, Cubbin IJ, (1993) Mentha piperita and Mentha spicata. In: De Smet PAGM

Bromm B, Scharein E, Darsow U, Ring J, (1995) Effects of menthol and cold on histamine-induced itch and skin reactions in man. Neuroscience Lett 187:157-160.

Burrow A, Eccles R, Jones AS, (1983) The effects of camphor, eucalyptus and menthol vapor on nasal resistance to airflow and nasal sensation. Acta Otolaryng (Stockholm) 96: 157-161.

Clark M, (1981) Econ Bot 35:59.

Dew MJ, Evans BK, Rhodes J, (1984) Peppermint oil for the irritable bowel syndrome: a multicentre trial. Br J Clin Pract 38:394-395.

Eccles R, Jones AS, (1982) The effects of menthol on nasal resistance to airflow. J Laryngology Otology 97:705-709.

Eccles R, Lancashire B, Tolley NS, (1987) Experimental studies on nasal sensation of airflow. Acta Otolaryngol (Stockholm) 103:303-306.

Eccles R, Morris S, Tolley NS, (1988) The effects of nasal anaesthesia upon nasal sensation of airflow. Acta Otolaryngol (Stockholm) 106:152-155.

Fintelmann V, Möglichkeiten und Grenzen der Phytotherapie bei Magen-Darm- Krankheiten. In: ZPT 10(1):29. 1989.

Fintelmann V, Phytopharmaka in der Gastroenterologie. In: ZPT 15(3):137. 1994.

Friederich HC, Vogelsberg, H, Neiss A, (1978) Ein Beitrag zur Bewertung von intern wirksamen Venenpharmaka. Z Hautkrankheiten 53 (11):369-374.

Göbel H, Schmidt G (1995a) Effekt von Pfefferminz- und Eukalyptusölpräparationen in experimentellen Kopfschmerzmodellen. Z Phytother 16:23-33.

Göbel H, Schmidt G, Dworschak M, Stolze H, Heuss D (1995) Essential plant oils and headache mechanisms. Phytomedicine 2:93-102.

Göbel H, Schmidt G, Dworschak M, Stolze H, Heuss D (1995b) Essential plant oils and headache mechanisms. Phytomedicine 2:93-103.

Göbel H, Schmidt G, Effekt von Pfefferminz- und Eukalyptusölpräparationen in experimentellen Kopfschmerzmodellen. In: ZPT 16(1):23-33. 1995.

Göbel H, Schmidt G, Soyka D, (1994) Effect of peppermint and eucalyptus oil preparations on neurophysiological and experimental algesimetric headache parameters. Cephalalgia 14:228-234.

Gräfe AK, Besonderheiten der Arzneimitteltherapie im Säuglings- und Kindesalter. In: PZ 140(30):2659-2667. 1995.

Hamann KF, Bonkowsky V, (1987) Minzölwirkung auf die Nasenschleimhaut von Gesunden. Dtsch Apoth Z 125:429-436.

Harries N et al., (1978) J Clin Pharm 2:171.

Hawthorn M, Ferranthe J, Luchowski E, Rutledge A, Wie XY, Triggle DJ, (1988) The actions of peppermint oil and menthol on calcium channel dependent processes in intestinal, neuronal and cardiac preparations. Aliment Pharmacol Therap 2:101-118.

Hefendehl FW, Murray MJ, (1973) Planta Med 23:101.

Heinze A, (1995c) Oleum menthae piperitae: Wirkmechanismen und klinische Effektivität bei Kopfschmerz vom Spannungstyp. In: Loew D, Rietbrock N (Hrsg) Phytopharmaka in Forschung und klinischer Anwendung. Steinkopff Verlag, Darmstadt, S 177-184.

Herrmann EC Jr., Kucera LS, Antiviral substances in plants of the mint family (Labiatae). III. Peppermint (Mentha piperita) and other mint plants. In: Proc Soc Exp Biol Med 124:874-878. 1995.

Hills JM, Aaronson PI, (1991) The mechanisms of action of peppermint oil on gastrointestinal smooth muscle. Gastroenterol 101:55-65.

Kantarev N, Peicev P, (1977) Folia Med 19(1):41.

Keller K, Hänsel R, Chandler RF, (eds) Adverse Effects of Herbal Drugs 1. Springer Verlag, Berlin Heidelberg New York, S 171-178.

Kucera LS, Hermann EC Jr, (1967) Proc Soc Exp Biol Med 124:865 et 874.

Leiber B, (1967) Dieskussionsbemerkung. In: Dost FH, Leiber B (Hrsg) Menthol and menthol-containing external remedies. Thieme Stuttgart 1967, S. 22.

Leicester RJ, Hunt RH, (1982) Peppermint oil to reduce solonic spasm during endoscopy. Lancet: 989.

Nash P, Gould SR, Barnardo DE, (1986) Peppermint oil does not relieve the pain of irritable bowel syndrome. Br J Clin Pract 40:292-293.

Nöller HG, (1967) Elektronische Messungen an der Nasenschleimhaut unter Mentholwirkung. In: Menthol and menthol-containung external remedies. Thieme, Stuttgart, S 146-153, 179.

Rees WDW, Evans BK, Rhoes J, (1979) Treating irritable bowel syndrome with peppermint oil. Brit med J II:835-838.

Reuter HD, Pflanzliche Gallentherapeutika (Teil I) und (Teil II). In: ZPT 16(1):13-20 u. 77-89. 1995.

Rohmeder J, Menthol: Verum statt Racemicum. In: PZ 139(4):300. 1994.

Sommerville KW, Richmond CR, Bell GD, (1984) Delayed release peppermint oil capsules (Colpermin) for the spastic colon syndrome: a pharmacokinetic study. Br J Clin Pharmac 18:638-640.

Taylor BA, Luscombe DK, Duthie HL, (1983) Inhibitory effect of peppermint on gastrointestinal smooth muscle. Gut 24: A 992 (Abstract)

Weizel A (1980) Colon irritabile. Therapiewoche 30:3898-3900.

White DA, Thompson SP, Wilson CG, Bel JD (1987) A pharmacokinetic comparison of two delayedrelease peppermint oil preparations, Colpermin and Mintec for treatment of the irritable bowel syndrome. Int J Pharmaceutics 40:151-155.

Wildgrube HJ, (1988) Untersuchung zur Wirksamkeit von Pfefferminzöl auf Beschwerdebild und funktionelle Parameter bei Patienten mit Reizdarmsyndrom (Studie). NaturHeilpraxis 41:2-5.

Further information in:

Hänsel R, Keller K, Rimpler H, Schneider G (Hrsg.), Hagers Handbuch der Pharmazeutischen Praxis, 5. Aufl., Bde 4-6 (Drogen), Springer Verlag Berlin, Heidelberg, New York, 1992-1994.

Hausen B, Allergiepflanzen, Pflanzenallergene, ecomed Verlagsgesellsch. mbH, Landsberg 1988.

Leung AY, Encyclopedia of Common Natural Ingredients Used in Food Drugs and Cosmetics, John Wiley & Sons Inc., New York 1980.

Madaus G, Lehrbuch der Biologischen Arzneimittel, Bde 1-3, Nachdruck, Georg Olms Verlag Hildesheim 1979.

Schulz R, Hänsel R, Rationale Phytotherapie, Springer Verlag Heidelberg 1996.

Steinegger E, Hänsel R, Pharmakognosie, 5. Aufl., Springer Verlag Heidelberg 1992.

Teuscher E, Biogene Arzneimittel, 5. Aufl., Wiss. Verlagsges. Stuttgart 1997.

Wagner H, Wiesenauer M, Phytotherapie. Phytopharmaka und pflanzliche Homöopathika, Fischer-Verlag, Stuttgart, Jena, New York 1995.

Wichtl M (Hrsg.), Teedrogen, 4. Aufl., Wiss. Verlagsges. Stuttgart 1997.

MENTHAE PIPERITAE AETHEROLEUM

Bowen ICH, Cubbin IJ, (1993) Mentha piperita and Mentha spicata. In: De Smet PAGM

Bromm B, Scharein E, Darsow U, Ring J, (1995) Effects of menthol and cold on histamine-induced itch and skin reactions in man. Neuroscience Lett 187:157-160.

Burrow A, Eccles R, Jones AS, (1983) The effects of camphor, eucalyptus and menthol vapor on nasal resistance to airflow and nasal sensation. Acta Otolaryng (Stockholm) 96:157-161.

Clark M, (1981) Econ Bot 35:59.

Dew MJ, Evans BK, Rhodes J, (1984) Peppermint oil for the irritable bowel syndrome: a multicentre trial. Br J Clin Pract 38:394-395.

Eccles R, Jones AS, (1982) The effects of menthol on nasal resistance to airflow. J Laryngology Otology 97:705-709.

Eccles R, Lancashire B, Tolley NS, (1987) Experimental studies on nasal sensation of airflow. Acta Otolaryngol (Stockholm) 103:303-306.

Eccles R, Morris S, Tolley NS, (1988) The effects of nasal anaesthesia upon nasal sensation of airflow. Acta Otolaryngol (Stockholm) 106:152-155.

Fintelmann V, Möglichkeiten und Grenzen der Phytotherapie bei Magen-Darm- Krankheiten. In: ZPT 10(1):29. 1989.

Fintelmann V, Phytopharmaka in der Gastroenterologie. In: ZPT 15(3):137. 1994.

Friederich HC, Vogelsberg, H, Neiss A, (1978) Ein Beitrag zur Bewertung von intern wirksamen Venenpharmaka. Z Hautkrankheiten 53(11):369-374.

Göbel H, Schmidt G, (1995a) Effekt von Pfefferminz- und Eukalyptusölpräparationen in experimentellen Kopfschmerzmodellen. Z Phytother 16:23-33.

Göbel H, Schmidt G, Dworschak M, Stolze H, Heuss D, (1995) Essential plant oils and headache mechanisms. Phytomedicine 2:93-102.

Göbel H, Schmidt G, Dworschak M, Stolze H, Heuss D, (1995b) Essential plant oils and headache mechanisms. Phytomedicine 2:93-103.

Göbel H, Schmidt G, Effekt von Pfefferminz- und Eukalyptusölpräparationen in experimentellen Kopfschmerzmodellen. In: ZPT 16(1):23-33. 1995.

Göbel H, Schmidt G, Soyka D, (1994) Effect of peppermint and eucalyptus oil preparations on neurophysiological and experimental algesimetric headache parameters. Cephalalgia 14:228-234.

Gräfe AK, Besonderheiten der Arzneimitteltherapie im Säuglings- und Kindesalter. In: PZ 140(30):2659-2667. 1995.

Hamann KF, Bonkowsky V, (1987) Minzölwirkung auf die Nasenschleimhaut von Gesunden. Dtsch Apoth Z 125:429-436.

Harries N et al., (1978) J Clin Pharm 2:171.

Hawthorn M, Ferranthe J, Luchowski E, Rutledge A, Wie XY, Triggle DJ, (1988) The actions of peppermint oil and menthol on calcium channel dependent processes in intestinal, neuronal and cardiac preparations. Aliment Pharmacol Therap 2:101-118.

Hefendehl FW, Murray MJ, (1973) Planta Med 23:101.

Heinze A, (1995c) Oleum menthae piperitae: Wirkmechanismen und klinische Effektivität bei Kopfschmerz vom Spannungstyp. In: Loew D, Rietbrock N (Hrsg) Phytopharmaka in Forschung und klinischer Anwendung. Steinkopff Verlag, Darmstadt, S 177-184.

Herrmann EC Jr., Kucera LS, Antiviral substances in plants of the mint family (Labiatae). III. Peppermint (Mentha piperita) and other mint plants. In: Proc Soc Exp Biol Med 124:874-878. 1995.

Hills JM, Aaronson PI, (1991) The mechanisms of action of peppermint oil on gastrointestinal smooth muscle. Gastroenterol 101:55-65.

Kantarev N, Peicev P, (1977) Folia Med 19(1):41.

Keller K, Hänsel R, Chandler RF, (eds) Adverse Effects of Herbal Drugs 1. Springer Verlag, Berlin Heidelberg New York, S 171-178.

Kucera LS, Hermann EC Jr, (1967) Proc Soc Exp Biol Med 124:865 et 874.

Leiber B, (1967) Dieskussionsbemerkung. In: Dost FH, Leiber B (Hrsg) Menthol and menthol-containing external remedies. Thieme Stuttgart 1967, S. 22.

Leicester RJ, Hunt RH, (1982) Peppermint oil to reduce solonic spasm during endoscopy. Lancet:989.

Nash P, Gould SR, Barnardo DE, (1986) Peppermint oil does not relieve the pain of irritable bowel syndrome. Br J Clin Pract 40:292-293.

Nöller HG, (1967) Elektronische Messungen an der Nasenschleimhaut unter Mentholwirkung. In: Menthol and menthol-containung external remedies. Thieme, Stuttgart, S 146-153, 179.

Rees WDW, Evans BK, Rhoes J, (1979) Treating irritable bowel syndrome with peppermint oil. Brit med J II:835-838.

Reuter HD, Pflanzliche Gallentherapeutika (Teil I) und (Teil II). In: ZPT 16(1):13-20 u. 77-89. 1995.

Rohmeder J, Menthol: Verum statt Racemicum. In: PZ 139(4):300. 1994.

Sommerville KW, Richmond CR, Bell GD, (1984) Delayed release peppermint oil capsules (Colpermin) for the spastic colon syndrome: a pharmacokinetic study. Br J Clin Pharmac 18:638-640.

Taylor BA, Luscombe DK, Duthie HL, (1983) Inhibitory effect of peppermint on gastrointestinal smooth muscle. Gut 24: A 992 (Abstract).

Weizel A, (1980) Colon irritabile. Therapiewoche 30:3898-3900.

White DA, Thompson SP, Wilson CG, Bel JD, (1987) A pharmacokinetic comparison of two delayedrelease peppermint oil preparations, Colpermin and Mintec for treatment of the irritable bowel syndrome. Int J Pharmaceutics 40:151-155.

Wildgrube HJ (1988) Untersuchung zur Wirksamkeit von Pfefferminzöl auf Beschwerdebild und funktionelle Parameter bei Patienten mit Reizdarmsyndrom (Studie). NaturHeilpraxis 41:2-5.

Further information in:

Hänsel R, Keller K, Rimpler H, Schneider G (Hrsg.), Hagers Handbuch der Pharmazeutischen Praxis, 5. Aufl., Bde 4-6 (Drogen), Springer Verlag Berlin, Heidelberg, New York, 1992-1994.

Hausen B, Allergiepflanzen, Pflanzenallergene, ecomed Verlagsgesellsch. mbH, Landsberg 1988.

Leung AY, Encyclopedia of Common Natural Ingredients Used in Food Drugs and Cosmetics, John Wiley & Sons Inc., New York 1980.

Madaus G, Lehrbuch der Biologischen Arzneimittel, Bde 1-3, Nachdruck, Georg Olms Verlag Hildesheim 1979.

Schulz R, Hänsel R, Rationale Phytotherapie, Springer Verlag Heidelberg 1996.

Steinegger E, Hänsel R, Pharmakognosie, 5. Aufl., Springer Verlag Heidelberg 1992.

Teuscher E, Biogene Arzneimittel, 5. Aufl., Wiss. Verlagsges. Stuttgart 1997.

Wagner H, Wiesenauer M, Phytotherapie. Phytopharmaka und pflanzliche Homöopathika, Fischer-Verlag, Stuttgart, Jena, New York 1995.

Fenaroli's Handbook of Flavor Ingredients, Vol. 1., 2nd Ed., CRC Press Boca Raton 1975.

Mentha Pulegium

Pennyroyal

DESCRIPTION

Medicinal Parts: The medicinal parts are the essential oil extracted from the fresh plant, the dried aerial parts, and the whole plant.

Flower and Fruit: The flowers are in axillary, loose, and globular false whorls. The calyx is cylindrical-funnel-shaped, grooved and is awned in the tube. The lower tips are awl-shaped, the upper ones shorter and wider. The upper lip has 3 tips and is curved slightly upwards. The lower lip is divided in two and is straight. The corolla is violet, glabrous or downy. It has a tube, which suddenly widens in a sack-like manner and has a slightly developed ring of hair as well as lobes, which extend well beyond the calyx. The nutlets are glossy brown.

Leaves, Stem and Root: Pennyroyal is a glabrous to downy perennial, which grows from 10 to 40 cm high. The stem is ascendent or decumbent, branched, and slightly downy. The leaves are elliptical to narrow ovate-elliptical, short-petioled, entire-margined, translucently glandular punctate with 1 to 3 pairs of shallow teeth and curved pinnate ribs.

Characteristics: Strongly aromatic.

Habitat: The plant thrives in western, southern and central Europe, in Asia as far as Turkmenistan, Iran, in the Arab countries, and Ethiopia. It is naturalized in America.

Production: The plants are harvested during the flowering season and dried.

Other Names: Pulegium, Run-by-the-Ground, Lurk-in-the-Ditch, Pudding Grass, Piliolerial, Mosquito Plant, Squaw Balm, Squawmint Tickweed

ACTIONS AND PHARMACOLOGY

COMPOUNDS

Volatile oil (1-2%): chief constituents D-pulegone (60-90%), menthone (10-20%), isomenthone (2-10%), additionally including, among others, piperitone, neoisomenthylacetate

Tannins: presumably rosmaric acid

Flavonoids: including, among others, diosmin, hesperidin

EFFECTS

There is no scientific proof of the described effects.

INDICATIONS AND USAGE

The drug is used for digestive disorders, liver and gallbladder disorders, gout, colds, and increased micturation; externally, for skin diseases.

PRECAUTIONS AND ADVERSE REACTIONS

General: European pennyroyal oil is hepatotoxic in effect.

Acute poisonings are not to be feared in conjunction with the proper administration of designated therapeutic dosages of the foilage drug. Still, because of its hepatotoxicity, it is recommended that the drug not be used.

Pregnancy: In high doses, Pennyroyal has been reported to cause abortion. Use in pregnancy is not recommended.

OVERDOSAGE

Severely acute poisonings have been observed following administration of 5 gm of the volatile oil. Vomiting, blood pressure elevation, anesthetic-like paralysis and death through respiratory failure has been reported following larger dosages. Cases of death have been described following misuse of the volatile oil as an abortient.

DOSAGE

See: **PRECAUTIONS AND ADVERSE REACTIONS.**

Mode of Administration: Internally as a ground drug, an extract, and as a tea. The oil is applied topically.

Daily Dosage: The average daily internal dose of the dried drug is 1 to 4 gm, taken 3 times daily. Pennyroyal is prepared as an infusion. Drink one cupful at a time during the course of the day.

LITERATURE

Miller EC et al., (1983) Cancer Res 43: 1124.

Further information in:

Frohne D, Pfänder HJ, Giftpflanzen - Ein Handbuch für Apotheker, Toxikologen und Biologen, 4. Aufl., Wiss. Verlags-Ges. Stuttgart 1997.

Hänsel R, Keller K, Rimpler H, Schneider G (Hrsg.), Hagers Handbuch der Pharmazeutischen Praxis, 5. Aufl., Bde 4-6 (Drogen), Springer Verlag Berlin, Heidelberg, New York, 1992-1994.

Lewin L, Gifte und Vergiftungen, 6. Aufl., Nachdruck, Haug Verlag, Heidelberg 1992.

Madaus G, Lehrbuch der Biologischen Arzneimittel, Bde 1-3, Nachdruck, Georg Olms Verlag Hildesheim 1979.

Roth L, Daunderer M, Kormann K, Giftpflanzen, Pflanzengifte, 4. Aufl., Ecomed Fachverlag Landsberg Lech 1993.

Steinegger E, Hänsel R, Pharmakognosie, 5. Aufl., Springer Verlag Heidelberg 1992.

Mentha Spicata

Spearmint

DESCRIPTION

Medicinal Parts: The medicinal parts are the steamed distillation of the fresh, flowering, aerial parts, and the leaves collected during the flowering season and dried.

Flower and Fruit: The spike-like inflorescences consist of false whorls in the axils of the bracts. The 5-tipped calyx is campanulate, glabrous or pubescent and is surrounded by a 5-tipped, pale lilac, pink or white corolla, which is almost half as long again as the calyx. The nutlet is reticulate in pubescent plants and smooth in glabrous plants.

Leaves, Stem and Root: The plant is 30 to 60 cm during the flowering season. Runners grow from the buds at the base of the stem. The quadrangular stem is ascendent or erect and usually thickly pubescent. The leaves are oblong-ovate or lanceolate, decussate, smooth or wrinkled, regularly serrate, and glabrous to thickly pubescent. The upper leaves are sessile, the lower ones short petiolate.

Habitat: The plant probably originates from the Mediterranean region and is now naturalized in large parts of Europe and North America.

Production: Spearmint is the aerial part of Mentha spicata. Spearmint oil is the essential oil extracted from the plant.

Other Names: Curled Mint, Garden Mint, Mackerel Mint, Our Lady's Mint, Green Mint, Spire Mint, Sage of Bethlehem, Fish Mint, Lamb Mint

ACTIONS AND PHARMACOLOGY

COMPOUNDS: IN THE FOLIAGE DRUG

Volatile oil (0.8-2.5%)

Flavonoids: thymonin

Caffeic acid derivatives: including among others rosmaric acid in the volatile oil

Chief components: L-carvone (40-80%, aroma-carrier), (-)-limonene (5-15%), additionally including among others beta-bourbonene, cis- and transcarvylacetate, caryophyllene, 1,8-cineole, dihydrocarveol, trans-sabinene hydrate

EFFECTS

The oil produced contains a high proportion of carvon, which produces the spearmint smell. It has antispasmodic, carminative, and stimulant effects.

INDICATIONS AND USAGE

Spearmint is used for digestive disorders, as a remedy for flatulence.

The essential oil is used as an aromatic preparation. Spearmint leaves are used as carminative.

PRECAUTIONS AND ADVERSE REACTIONS

No health hazards or side effects are known in conjunction with the proper administration of designated therapeutic dosages. The volatile oil possesses a weak potential for sensitization due to its menthol and L-carvone content.

DOSAGE

Mode of Administration: Spearmint is mainly used internally in the form of an oil or concentrate.

LITERATURE

Hefendehl FW, Murray MJ, (1973) Planta Med 23:101.

Murray MJ et al., (1972) Crop Sci 12:723.

Subramanian SS, Nair AGR, (1972) Phytochemistry 11:452.

Further information in:

Hänsel R, Keller K, Rimpler H, Schneider G (Hrsg.), Hagers Handbuch der Pharmazeutischen Praxis, 5. Aufl., Bde 4-6 (Drogen), Springer Verlag Berlin, Heidelberg, New York, 1992-1994.

Hausen B, Allergiepflanzen, Pflanzenallergene, ecomed Verlagsgesellsch. mbH, Landsberg 1988.

Leung AY, Encyclopedia of Common Natural Ingredients Used in Food Drugs and Cosmetics, John Wiley & Sons Inc., New York 1980.

Steinegger E, Hänsel R, Pharmakognosie, 5. Aufl., Springer Verlag Heidelberg 1992.

Teuscher E, Biogene Arzneimittel, 5. Aufl., Wiss. Verlagsges. Stuttgart 1997.

Wichtl M (Hrsg.), Teedrogen, 4. Aufl., Wiss. Verlagsges. Stuttgart 1997.

Menyanthes Trifoliata

Buck Bean

DESCRIPTION

Medicinal Parts: The medicinal part is the dried herb.

Flower and Fruit: The flowers are white or reddish-white, medium-sized and many blossomed racemes on long, leafless peduncles. There are 5 sepals. The corolla is fused with 5 tips and is pubescent inside. There are 5 reddish stamens and 1 superior ovary. The fruit is an ovate capsule.

Leaves, Stem and Root: Menyanthes trifoliata is a perennial 15 to 30 cm high green, glabrous aquatic plant. The herb has a small, finger-thick, creeping rhizome. The decumbent stem varies in length according to conditions. The plant is surrounded by leaf sheaths. The leaves are on long, fleshy, grooved petioles. They are trifoliate, 5 cm long and 2.5 cm wide, with obovate leaflets.

Characteristics: The herb has a strong bitter taste.

Habitat: The plant is indigenous to Europe, Asia, and America.

Other Names: Bog Bean, Bog Myrtle, Brook Bean, Marsh Clover, Moonflower, Trefoil, Water Shamrock

ACTIONS AND PHARMACOLOGY

COMPOUNDS

Iridoide monoterpenes (bitter principles): chief components 7′,8′-dihydrofoliamenthin, additionally including among others sweroside, loganin, menthiafolin, foliamenthin

Monoterpene alkaloids: including among others gentianin

Flavonoids: including among others rutin, hyperoside

Triterpene glycosides

EFFECTS

The drug stimulates saliva and gastric juice secretion.

INDICATIONS AND USAGE

- Dyspeptic complaints
- Loss of appetite

The drug is used for loss of appetite and peptic discomfort. As a bitter, it promotes gastric secretion.

CONTRAINDICATIONS

The drug is contraindicated in diarrhea, dysentery, and colitis.

PRECAUTIONS AND ADVERSE REACTIONS

No health hazards or side effects are known in conjunction with the proper administration of designated therapeutic dosages.

OVERDOSAGE

Vomiting should be induced following overdosage of the drug.

DOSAGE

Mode of Administration: Comminuted herb for teas and other bitter-tasting preparations for internal use.

Preparation: 0.5 to 1 gm finely cut drug in boiling water, or in cold water that is rapidly heated, steep for 5 to 10 minutes, then strain.

The drug is a component of standardized preparations of various tonics.

Daily Dosage: The average daily dose is 1.5 to 3.0 gm of the drug. The dosage for the infusion is 1/2 cup, unsweetened, before each meal (1 teaspoonful = 0.9 gm of the drug).

LITERATURE

Battersby AR et al., (1967) J Chem Soc Chem Commun. 1277.

Ciaceri G, (1972) Fitoterapia 43:134.

Janeczko Z et al., A triterpenoid glycoside from Menyanthes trifoliata. In: PH 29(12):3885-3887. 1990.

Junior P, Weitere Untersuchungen zur Verteilung und Straktur der Bitterstoffe von Menyanthes trifoliata. In: PM 32(12):112. 1989.

Phillipson JD, Anderson LA, (1984) Pharm J 233:80 et 111.

Swaitek L et al., (1986) Planta Med 6:60P.

Tumón H et al., The effect of Menyanthes trifolita L. on acute renal failure might due to PAF-inhibition. In: Phytomedicine 1:39-45. 1994.

Further information in:

Kern W, List PH, Hörhammer L (Hrsg.), Hagers Handbuch der Pharmazeutischen Praxis, 4. Aufl., Bde. 1-8, Springer Verlag Berlin, Heidelberg, New York, 1969.

Madaus G, Lehrbuch der Biologischen Arzneimittel, Bde 1-3, Nachdruck, Georg Olms Verlag Hildesheim 1979.

Roth L, Daunderer M, Kormann K, Giftpflanzen, Pflanzengifte, 4. Aufl., Ecomed Fachverlag Landsberg Lech 1993.

Steinegger E, Hänsel R, Pharmakognosie, 5. Aufl., Springer Verlag Heidelberg 1992.

Teuscher E, Biogene Arzneimittel, 5. Aufl., Wiss. Verlagsges. Stuttgart 1997.

Wichtl M (Hrsg.), Teedrogen, 4. Aufl., Wiss. Verlagsges. Stuttgart 1997.

Fenaroli's Handbook of Flavor Ingredients, Vol. 1., 2nd Ed., CRC Press Boca Raton 1975.

Mercurialis Annua

Mercury Herb

DESCRIPTION

Medicinal Parts: The drug is the flowering plant.

Flower and Fruit: The plant has yellow-green flowers. The male flowers are in tightly packed, interrupted ears, on thin, hair-like pedicles. They have 12 stamens. The female flowers are short-petioled in twos or threes in the leaf axils. The style is short or non-existent. There are 2 stigmas. The fruit is a 2-headed capsule.

Leaves, Stem and Root: The plant is an annual 20 to 50 cm high plant. The stem is erect, crossed-opposite branched, obtuse, quadrangular, glabrous and segmented. The leaves are opposite, petiolate, ovate to lanceolate, light green and have a ciliate margin.

Characteristics: The plant has an unpleasant smell when rubbed, the whole plant has no latex.

Habitat: The plant grows in Europe and is naturalized in the eastern U.S.

Production: Mercury Herb is the flowering herb of Mercurialis annua.

ACTIONS AND PHARMACOLOGY

COMPOUNDS

Cyanogenic glycosides (small amounts)

Pyridone derivatives (that color the urine red): including, among others, hermidin

Saponins

Amines: including, among others, methyl amine (mercurialine)

Flavonoids: including, among others, rutin, narcissin, isorhamnetin. Nothing is known regarding the type of the toxins. The cyanogenic glycosides can hardly be responsible for the toxicity.

EFFECTS

The drug is slightly poisonous, however it can lead to diarrhea and an overactive bladder. The root and stock act as strong laxatives.

INDICATIONS AND USAGE

The drug is used for suppurating inflammation, as a laxative and diuretic, and as an adjuvant in the treatment of gastrointestinal and urinary tract diseases.

PRECAUTIONS AND ADVERSE REACTIONS

The fresh plant, in particular the root and the rhizome, are considered poisonous. Symptoms of poisonings include diarrhea, nerve paralysis and liver and kidney damage. Poisonings, including fatal ones, are only known among animals. There are no reports available on the toxicity of the drug. The intake of small doses would likely lead to no more than diarrhea.

DOSAGE

Mode of Administration: The drug is administered ground, as an extract, in juice, and in homeopathic dilutions.

LITERATURE

Frohne D, Pfänder HJ, Giftpflanzen - Ein Handbuch für Apotheker, Toxikologen und Biologen, 4. Aufl., Wiss. Verlags-Ges. Stuttgart 1997.

Kern W, List PH, Hörhammer L (Hrsg.), Hagers Handbuch der Pharmazeutischen Praxis, 4. Aufl., Bde. 1-8, Springer Verlag Berlin, Heidelberg, New York, 1969.

Lewin L, Gifte und Vergiftungen, 6. Aufl., Nachdruck, Haug Verlag, Heidelberg 1992.

Madaus G, Lehrbuch der Biologischen Arzneimittel, Bde 1-3, Nachdruck, Georg Olms Verlag Hildesheim 1979.

Roth L, Daunderer M, Kormann K, Giftpflanzen, Pflanzengifte, 4. Aufl., Ecomed Fachverlag Landsberg Lech 1993.

Teuscher E, Lindequist U, Biogene Gifte - Biologie, Chemie, Pharmakologie, 2. Aufl., Fischer Verlag Stuttgart 1994.

Mercury Herb

See Mercurialis Annua

Mezereon

See Daphne Mezereum

Milk Thistle

See Silybum Marianum

Mistletoe

See Viscum Album

Monarda Didyma

Oswego Tea

DESCRIPTION

Medicinal Parts: The medicinal part is the herb.

Flower and Fruit: The flowers are in 1 to 3 terminal richly blossomed false whorls supported by bracts whose leaflets are pale green with a reddish tinge. The calyx tips are awl-shaped. The corolla is scarlet and 3.5 to 6 cm in length. The plant is propagated by root cuttings.

Leaves, Stem and Root: The plant is a bristly-haired to glabrous 50 to 90 cm high herbaceous perennial with runners. The stems are erect, acutely quadrangular, grooved, and hard. The leaves are in pairs, ovate-lanceolate, clearly petiolate, crenate, and often rough on both sides.

Habitat: The plant is indigenous to the U.S. in swampy regions from Georgia and Michigan to Ontario, Canada.

Other Names: Scarlet Monarda, Bee Balm, Blue Balm, High Balm, Low Balm, Mountain Balm, Mountain Mint, Bergamot

ACTIONS AND PHARMACOLOGY

COMPOUNDS

Volatile oil (0.1-0.3%): including among others carvacrol, thymol, p-cymene, linalool, linalyl acetate, limonene, ocimene, alpha-pinene, camphene, Delta3-carene

Flavonoids: including among others linarin, didymin, genkwanin

Anthocyans: monardein (triacyliertes pelargonidine-3,5-diglucoside, 2 malonyl- and 1 p-cumaroyl- residue)

EFFECTS

The drug has antispasmodic, digestive, carminative, and diuretic effects; it is also used to regulate menstruation.

INDICATIONS AND USAGE

The drug is used for flatulence and other digestive disorders and menstrual complaints (PMS).

In Europe, the herb is in rare use as an aromatic, carminative, and antipryreticum.

PRECAUTIONS AND ADVERSE REACTIONS

No health hazards or side effects are known in conjunction with the proper administration of designated therapeutic dosages.

DOSAGE

Mode of Administration: Ground drug (powder) as an infusion.

LITERATURE

Hegnauer R, Chemotaxonomie der Pflanzen, Bde 1-11, Birkhäuser Verlag Basel, Boston, Berlin 1962-1997.

Kern W, List PH, Hörhammer L (Hrsg.), Hagers Handbuch der Pharmazeutischen Praxis, 4. Aufl., Bde. 1-8, Springer Verlag Berlin, Heidelberg, New York, 1969.

Monarda Punctata

Horsemint

DESCRIPTION

Medicinal Parts: The medicinal part is the herb.

Flower and Fruit: The flowers occur in axillary whorls. They are bilabiate. The corolla is yellow with red spots and two stamens. The 2 stamens and the sessile bracts are yellow and purple.

Leaves, Stem and Root: The plant is a perennial and grows up to 90 cm with a branched, round stem. The leaves are opposite, lanceolate, and downy.

Characteristics: The taste is pungent and bitter and the odor is reminiscent of thyme.

Habitat: The plant is indigenous to the eastern and central U.S.

Other Names: Spotted Monarda, Monarda Lutea, Wild Bergamot

ACTIONS AND PHARMACOLOGY

COMPOUNDS

Volatile oil: including among others thymol (20%), thymol methyl ether, thymol hydroquinone, in Monarda punctata var. maritima including among others also gamma-terpinene, geranylformiat, nerylformiat

EFFECTS

The drug has carminative, stimulant, and emmenagogic effects.

INDICATIONS AND USAGE

The drug is used for digestive disorders, flatulence, and dysmenorrhea.

PRECAUTIONS AND ADVERSE REACTIONS

No health hazards or side effects are known in conjunction with the proper administration of designated therapeutic dosages.

DOSAGE

Mode of Administration: Ground drug is used as an infusion.

LITERATURE

Kern W, List PH, Hörhammer L (Hrsg.), Hagers Handbuch der Pharmazeutischen Praxis, 4. Aufl., Bde. 1-8, Springer Verlag Berlin, Heidelberg, New York, 1969.

Moneywort

See Lysimachia Nummularia

Monkshood

See Aconitum Napellus

Morus Nigra

Black Mulberry

DESCRIPTION

Medicinal Parts: The medicinal parts are the ripe berries and the root bark.

Flower and Fruit: The plant is monoecious or dioecious. The greenish flowers are in catkin-like inflorescences. The male ones are ovate to cylindrical, the female ones are ovate or globular. The flowers have a 4-bract involucre, which enlarges and becomes fleshy in the female flowers. The female flowers have 2 stigmas, the male ones have 4 stamens. All the fruit from the catkins develop into blackberry-like false berries (which are really a series of fleshy drupes). They are edible and pleasant-tasting.

Leaves, Stem and Root: The tree grows from 6 to 12 m. The bark is gray brown. The leaves are alternate with flat-grooved, somewhat hairy petioles. They are cordate or ovate, unevenly lobed, and serrate with short rough hairs above.

Habitat: The plant is cultivated worldwide in temperate regions.

Other Names: Purple Mulberry, White Mulberry

ACTIONS AND PHARMACOLOGY

COMPOUNDS: IN THE FRUIT

Fruit acids (1.9%): including among others malic acid, citric acid

Saccharose (10%)

Pectins

Ascorbic acid (0.17%)

Flavonoids: including, among others, rutin

COMPOUNDS: IN THE LEAVES

Flavonoids: including among others rutin (2-6%)

The constituents of the rhizome rind are not known.

EFFECTS

The active agents are sugar, acids, pectin, and rutin.

INDICATIONS AND USAGE

The drug is used as a mild laxative and in the treatment of respiratory catarrh.

PRECAUTIONS AND ADVERSE REACTIONS

No health hazards or side effects are known in conjunction with the proper administration of designated therapeutic dosages.

DOSAGE

Mode of Administration: The drug is used internally.

Daily Dosage: The average daily dose is 2 to 4 ml of syrup.

LITERATURE

Deshpande VH, (1968) Tetrahedron Lett 1715.

Kimura Y et al., (1986) J Nat Prod 94(4):639.

Nomura T et al., (1983) Planta Med 47:151.

Further information in:

Kern W, List PH, Hörhammer L (Hrsg.), Hagers Handbuch der Pharmazeutischen Praxis, 4. Aufl., Bde 1-8, Springer Verlag Berlin, Heidelberg, New York, 1969.

Madaus G, Lehrbuch der Biologischen Arzneimittel, Bde 1-3, Nachdruck, Georg Olms Verlag Hildesheim 1979.

Oliver-Bever B (Ed.), Medicinal Plants of Tropical West Africa, Cambridge University Press, Cambridge 1986.

Motherwort

See Leonurus Cardiaca

Mountain Ash Berry

See Sorbus Aucuparia

Mountain Flax

See Linum Catharticum

Mountain Grape

See Mahonia Aquifolium

Mountain Laurel

See Kalmia Latifolia

Mouse Ear

See Pilosella Officinarum

Mucuna Pruriens

Cowhage

DESCRIPTION

Medicinal Parts: The medicinal parts are the hairs on the pod and the seeds.

Flower and Fruit: The flowers grow in racemes in twos and threes. They are large and white and have a bluish-purple, papilionaceous corolla. The pod is pubescent, thick and leathery and has an average length of about 10 cm. They are in the shape of the sound openings of a violin. The pod is dark brown and covered with 0.25 cm long stiff hairs. They contain 4 to 6 seeds and consist of conical, sharply acuminate cells less than 1 mm in diameter, and barbed at the apex. They are extremely irritating to the skin and must be handled with caution.

Leaves, Stem and Root: The plant is a climbing legume with long, thin branches and opposite, lanceolate leaves 15 to 30 cm in length. The petioles are pubescent.

Habitat: The plant is indigenous to tropical regions especially India, and the West Indies.

Production: Cowhage bean pods are the bean pods of Mucuna pruriens. The drug is derived from the hair of the pods.

Other Names: Cowitch, Couhage, Kiwach

ACTIONS AND PHARMACOLOGY

COMPOUNDS

Serotonin: 5-methyl-N,N-dimethyl-tryptamine

EFFECTS

Externally, Cowhage is a cutaneous stimulant and rubefacient. Internally, the drug has an anthelmintic effect. Carminative, hypotensive, hypoglycemic and cholesterol reducing effects have also been described.

Experiments carried out on frogs demonstrated that prurieninin slowed down the heart rate, lowered blood pressure, and stimulated intestinal peristalisis. The reduction in blood pressure was caused by the release of histamines, and the spasmolysis of smooth muscle was caused by indole bases.

INDICATIONS AND USAGE

The drug is used externally for rheumatic disorders and muscular pain, and internally for the treatment of worm infestation.

PRECAUTIONS AND ADVERSE REACTIONS

Once in contact with the skin, the stinging hairs lead to extremely aggressive itching and burning, accompanied by long-lasting inflammation, caused by the injection of serotonin and proteins (mucunain, proteolytic enzyme). The intake of the hairs for the purpose of fighting intestinal worms should be avoided. Internal administration of the drug in the form of extracts may well be harmless, due to the difficult absorbability of the active ingredients.

DOSAGE

Mode of Administration: The drug is available in powder form.

LITERATURE

Bell EA, Jansen DH, (1971) Nature 229:136.

Ghosal S et al., (1971) Planta Med 24:434.

Further information in:

Hegnauer R, Chemotaxonomie der Pflanzen, Bde 1-11, Birkhäuser Verlag Basel, Boston, Berlin 1962-1997.

Kern W, List PH, Hörhammer L (Hrsg.), Hagers Handbuch der Pharmazeutischen Praxis, 4. Aufl., Bde. 1-8, Springer Verlag Berlin, Heidelberg, New York, 1969.

Madaus G, Lehrbuch der Biologischen Arzneimittel, Bde 1-3, Nachdruck, Georg Olms Verlag Hildesheim 1979.

Morton JF, An Atlas of Medicinal Plants of Middle America, Charles C Thomas USA 1981.

Roth L, Daunderer M, Kormann K, Giftpflanzen, Pflanzengifte, 4. Aufl., Ecomed Fachverlag Landsberg Lech 1993.

Steinegger E, Hänsel R, Pharmakognosie, 5. Aufl., Springer Verlag Heidelberg 1992.

Teuscher E, Lindequist U, Biogene Gifte - Biologie, Chemie, Pharmakologie, 2. Aufl., Fischer Verlag Stuttgart 1994.

Teuscher E, Biogene Arzneimittel, 5. Aufl., Wiss. Verlagsges. Stuttgart 1997.

Mugwort

See Artemisia Vulgaris

Muira-Puama

See Ptychopetalum Olacoides

Mullein

See Verbascum Densiflorum

Muskmallow

See Hibiscus Abelmoschus

Mustard

See Sinapis Alba

Myosotis Arvensis

Forget-Me-Not

DESCRIPTION

Medicinal Parts: The medicinal part is the flowering plant.

Flower and Fruit: The blue flowers are in leafless racemes. The calyx is fused and leaf-like with 5 tips. The corolla is shaped like a stemmed plate, has 5 tips, and is glabrous with yellow scales in the tube. The tube is enclosed in the calyx. There are 5 stamens and a 4-valvular ovary. The fruit stems are twice as long as the caylx and stand out. The calyx is closed when the fruit ripens. The fruit is composed of 4 nutlets.

Leaves, Stem and Root: The plant is leafy and grows from 15 to 40 cm high. The stem is erect or ascendent and pubescent. The leaves are alternate. The lower leaves are petiolate and oblong-obovate, the upper ones sessile and lanceolate to lanceolate-oblong.

Habitat: The plant grows in Europe.

Production: Forget-Me-Not is the flowering plant Myosotis arvensis.

ACTIONS AND PHARMACOLOGY

COMPOUNDS

Pyrrolizidine alkaloids

Caffeic acid derivatives: rosmaric acid

The Myosotis varieties contain the active agents rosemary acid and tannins.

EFFECTS

No information is available.

INDICATIONS AND USAGE

Forget-Me-Not is used in the treatment of respiratory disorders and nose bleeds.

PRECAUTIONS AND ADVERSE REACTIONS

Hepatotoxicity and carcinogenicity are to be expected consequences when taken internally, due to the presumed presence of pyrrolizidine alkaloids with 1,2-unsaturated necic parent substances. Therefore, the drug should not be taken internally.

DOSAGE

Mode of Administration: It is administered ground and as an extract for external use.

LITERATURE

Kern W, List PH, Hörhammer L (Hrsg.), Hagers Handbuch der Pharmazeutischen Praxis, 4. Aufl., Bde. 1-8, Springer Verlag Berlin, Heidelberg, New York, 1969.

Madaus G. Lehrbuch der Biologischen Arzneimittel, Bde 1-3, Nachdruck, Georg Olms Verlag Hildesheim 1979.

Myrica Cerifera

Wax Myrtle

DESCRIPTION

Medicinal Parts: The medicinal parts are the dried root bark and the wax from the berries.

Flower and Fruit: The flowers are unisexual and have no calyx or corolla. They are small and yellowish in scaly catkins. The fruit is small groups of round, gray-white berries. These contain numerous black seeds, which have a crust of usable greenish white wax. The wax helps keep the berries in a suitable state for germination for a period of 2 to 3 years.

Leaves, Stem and Root: The evergreen shrub or small tree grows up to 10 m high. The bark has a white peeling outer layer, which covers a red-brown inner layer. The leaves are lanceolate to oblong-lanceolate, glossy or resinous, and punctate on both sides.

Characteristic: The taste is astringent and bitter and the odor is slightly aromatic.

Habitat: The plant is found in the eastern regions of the U.S. and around Lake Erie.

Other Names: Bayberry, Candleberry, Tallow Shrub, Vegetable Tallow, Waxberry,

Myrica

ACTIONS AND PHARMACOLOGY

COMPOUNDS

Volatile oil (traces)

Tannins

Resins

The constituents of the drug have not been extensively investigated.

EFFECTS

The active compounds have diaphoretic, stimulant, and astringent effects.

INDICATIONS AND USAGE

The drug is used internally for coughs and colds, and externally for skin diseases and ulcers.

PRECAUTIONS AND ADVERSE REACTIONS

No health hazards or side effects are known in conjunction with the proper administration of designated therapeutic dosages.

DOSAGE

Mode of Administration: The drug is available as a liquid extract for internal use, and in powder form.

LITERATURE

Paul BD et al., (1974) J Pharm Sci 63:958.

Yoshizawa S et al., (1987) Phytother Res 1(1):44.

Further information in:

Kern W, List PH, Hörhammer L (Hrsg.), Hagers Handbuch der Pharmazeutischen Praxis, 4. Aufl., Bde. 1-8, Springer Verlag Berlin, Heidelberg, New York, 1969.

Leung AY, Encyclopedia of Common Natural Ingredients Used in Food Drugs and Cosmetics, John Wiley & Sons Inc., New York 1980.

Madaus G, Lehrbuch der Biologischen Arzneimittel, Bde 1-3, Nachdruck, Georg Olms Verlag Hildesheim 1979.

Myrica Gale

Sweet Gale

DESCRIPTION

Medicinal Parts: The medicinal parts are the leaves and branches as well as the wax extracted from the catkins.

Flower and Fruit: There are male and female plants. The male plants produce groups of stemless catkins on the leafless branches of the previous year's growth. The fruit catkins are about the same size but thicker and are close, resinous nutlets. They are dry and compressed.

Leaves, Stem and Root: The plant is usually dioecious, but plants may change sex from year to year. Sweet Gale is a deciduous shrub up to 2.5 m high. The branches have scattered yellowish glands. The leaves are 2 to 6 cm long almost lanceolate, cuneate at the base, more or less serrate near the apex. They are pubescent beneath and have shiny yellow fragrant glands on both surfaces.

Habitat: Sweet Gale is indigenous to the higher latitudes of the Northern Hemisphere.

Production: Sweet Gale is the aerial part of Myrica gale.

Other Names: Bog Myrtle, Dutch Myrtle, Bayberry

ACTIONS AND PHARMACOLOGY

COMPOUNDS

Volatile oil (0.4-0.7%): including among others alpha-pinene, delta-cadinene, gamma-cadinene, limonene, beta-myrcene, beta-phellandrene, beta-phellandrene, 1,8-cineole

Flavonoids: including among others myricitrin

EFFECTS

Astringent and aromatic.

INDICATIONS AND USAGE

Sweet Gale has been used in digestive disorders. A strong brew of dried bark is also used in Sweden as a vermifuge and to cure itching.

PRECAUTIONS AND ADVERSE REACTIONS

The volatile oil of the drug is considered toxic. The mixing of the plant with beer, as practiced in the Middle Ages, is said to have led to manic episodes.

DOSAGE

Mode of Administration: The drug is ground. Information on preparations is not available.

LITERATURE

Malteru KE, Faegri A, (1982) Acta Pharm Suec 19: 43

Von Schantz, M, Kapétanidis I, Qualitative und qunatitative Untersuchung des ätherischen Öls von Myrica gale L. (Myricaceae). In: Pharm Acta Helv 46(10/11):649. 1071.

Further information in:

Hegnauer R, Chemotaxonomie der Pflanzen, Bde 1-11, Birkhäuser Verlag Basel, Boston, Berlin 1962-1997.

Kern W, List PH, Hörhammer L (Hrsg.), Hagers Handbuch der Pharmazeutischen Praxis, 4. Aufl., Bde. 1-8, Springer Verlag Berlin, Heidelberg, New York, 1969.

Roth L, Daunderer M, Kormann K, Giftpflanzen, Pflanzengifte, 4. Aufl., Ecomed Fachverlag Landsberg Lech 1993.

Myristica Fragrans

Nutmeg

DESCRIPTION

Medicinal Parts: The medicinal parts are the essential oil of the nutmeg, the compressed, dried aril of the nutmeg seed, the mixture of fat, oil and color pigment pressed seeds, the dried seed kernels freed from the aril and shell of the nut, calcified seed kernels and the dried seed kernels.

Flower and Fruit: Myristica fragans is either male or female, although there are male trees with female flowers and fruit. The flowers are unisexual. The male flowers are in few-flowered inflorescence; the female ones are solitary and inconspicuous. The flowers have a simple 3-lobed involucre and the filaments are fused to a tube. The fruit ripens 7 to 10 months after flowering. The fruit is fleshy, almost round, acuminate at the stem end, 3 to 6 cm long and 2.5 to 5 cm thick. The fruit is light yellow and about the size of a peach. The fruit flesh bursts open when ripe and exposes the bright red seeds aril which surrounds the dark brown seed. Within the aril the seed kernel is covered in a hard brown testis which shows the marks of the aril.

Leaves, Stem and Root: Nutmeg is an evergreen tree up to 15 m in height. The bark is smooth grayish brown, the young branches green. The alternate leaves are dark green, entire-margined, sharp edged, short-petioled, ovate-elliptical and up to 8 cm long.

Habitat: Indigenous to the Molucca Islands and New Guinea, grown in Indonesia and the West Indies.

Production: Nutmeg are the seeds of Myristica fragrans.

Other Names: Mace

ACTIONS AND PHARMACOLOGY

COMPOUNDS

Volatile oil (7-16%): In the volatile oil the chief components are monoterpene hydrocarbons (80%): including among others sabinene, alpha- pinene, beta-pinene, monoterpene alcohols (5%): including among others 1,8-cineole, phenylpropane derivatives (10-18%) including among others myristicin, elemicin

Fatty oil (30-40%): fatty acids including among others lauric, myristic, pentadecanoic, palmitic, heptadecanoic, stearic, oleic acid

Saponins

Sterols: including among others beta-sitosterol, campesterol

EFFECTS

Cutaneous stimulant, stomachic.

INDICATIONS AND USAGE

Nutmeg is used for stomach complaints.

PRECAUTIONS AND ADVERSE REACTIONS

No health hazards or side effects are known in conjunction with the proper administration of designated therapeutic dosages. The drug can trigger allergic contact dermatitis.

OVERDOSAGE

Ingestion of 1 to 3 nuts produces, through bioconversion of the phenylpropane derivatives in the human body, amphetamine derivatives. Eventually, this leads to feelings of thirst, nausea, reddening and swelling of the face, urgency, and from mild alterations of consciousness to intensive hallucinations. The stupor can last from 2 to 3 days. Following gastrointestinal emptying (inducement of vomiting, gastric lavage with burgundy-colored potassium permanganate solution, sodium sulfate), and installation of activated charcoal, the therapy for poisonings consists of treating spasms with diazepam (i.v.), treating colic with atropine; electrolyte substitution and treating possible cases of acidosis with sodium bicarbonate infusions. In case of shock, plasma volume expanders should be infused. Monitoring of kidney function is essential. Intubation and oxygen respiration may also be necessary.

DOSAGE

Mode of Administration: As an extract or essential oil. Nutmeg butter is a mixture of fatty and essential oil extracted from the seeds through pressing

Preparation: This plant yields Mace, the lacy, fleshy covering of the nut, which is scarlet when fresh and dark orange when dried, and the Nutmeg. After being separated, both parts are dried slowly. Nutmeg butter is made by macerating the nuts and steaming them. Several other nuts are often given the name nutmeg.

LITERATURE

Baldry J et al., (1976) Int Flav Food Add 7:28.

Bennett A et al., New Eng J Med 290:110.

Effertz B et al., (1979) Z Pflanzenphysiol 92:319.

Forrest JE et al., (1974) J Chem Soc Perkin Trans 1(2):205.

Forrest JE, Heacock RA, (1972) Lloydia 35:440.

Forrest TP et al., (1973) Naturwissenschaften 60:257.

Gottlieb OR, (1979) J Ethnopharmacol 1:309.

Isogai A et al., (1973) Agric Biol Chem 37:198 et 1479.

Kim et al., (1978) Biochim. Biophys Acta 537:22.

Miller EC et al., (1983) Cancer Res 43:1124.

Misra V et al., (1978) Ind J Med Res 67:482.

Pecevski J et al., (1980) Toxicol Lett 7:739.

Rasheed A et al., (1984) Planta Med 50(2):222.

Sanford KJ, Heinz DE, (1971) Pharm Acta Helv 59(9/10):242.

Sanford KJ, Heinz DE, (1971) Phytochemistry 10:1245.

Sarath-Kumara SJ et al., (1985) J Sci Food Agric 36(2):93.

Shafkan I et al., (1977) New Eng J Med 296:694.

Further information in:

Frohne D, Pfänder HJ, Giftpflanzen - Ein Handbuch für Apotheker, Toxikologen und Biologen, 4. Aufl., Wiss. Verlags-Ges. Stuttgart 1997.

Hänsel R, Keller K, Rimpler H, Schneider G (Hrsg.), Hagers Handbuch der Pharmazeutischen Praxis, 5. Aufl., Bde 4-6 (Drogen), Springer Verlag Berlin, Heidelberg, New York, 1992-1994.

Leung AY, Encyclopedia of Common Natural Ingredients Used in Food Drugs and Cosmetics, John Wiley & Sons Inc., New York 1980.

Lewin L, Gifte und Vergiftungen, 6. Aufl., Nachdruck, Haug Verlag, Heidelberg 1992.

Roth L, Daunderer M, Kormann K, Giftpflanzen, Pflanzengifte, 4. Aufl., Ecomed Fachverlag Landsberg Lech 1993.

Steinegger E, Hänsel R, Pharmakognosie, 5. Aufl., Springer Verlag Heidelberg 1992.

Teuscher E, Lindequist U, Biogene Gifte - Biologie, Chemie, Pharmakologie, 2. Aufl., Fischer Verlag Stuttgart 1994.

Teuscher E, Biogene Arzneimittel, 5. Aufl., Wiss. Verlagsges. Stuttgart 1997.

Myroxylon Balsamum

Peruvian Balsam

DESCRIPTION

Medicinal Parts: The medicinal parts are the balsam from the sweltered trunks, the resin balsam which has been extracted from damaged trunks and softened and purified through a process of melting and sweltering.

Flower and Fruit: The androgynous flowers are on 12 cm-long pedicles on simple richly blossomed racemes. The calyx is inferior, broadly tubular or oblong-campanulate, dark green and has short, rough hairs. The 5 petals are white and stemmed. The standard is almost circular. The stamens are bright red. The ovary is on a long stem and has 1 valve. The fruit is a 1-seeded, indehiscent, winged pod with brown-red, reniform. The seeds are distinctly curved.

Leaves, Stem and Root: Myroxylon balsamum is a tree up to 25 m tall with a round, spreading crown which only starts to branch at a height of 13 to 19 m. The bark is smooth, yellowish gray or brown with numerous lenticles. The leaves are usually odd-pinnate and have 4 to 7 obovate, acuminate, coreacious, short-petioled leaflets. The upper surface is dark green and the lower surface pale green.

Habitat: Indigenous to South and Central America.

Production: Peruvian balsam consists of the balsam generated from scorched tree stems of Myroxylon balsamum. Tolu balsam consists of the balsam generated from the incised tree trunks of Myroxylon balsamum. The balsam is purified by melting, straining, and solidifying.

Other Names: Balsam Tree, Balsam of Peru, Balsam of Tolu

ACTIONS AND PHARMACOLOGY

COMPOUNDS: BALSAMUM PERUVIANUM

Ester mixture, so-called cinnamein (50-70%): made up of benzyl benzoate and benzyl cinnamoate

Resins (20-30%): chief constituent cinnamic acid ester of the so-called peruresitannols (polymer)

EFFECTS: BALSAMUM PERUVIANUM

Antibacterial/antiseptic, promotion of granulation process, antiparasitic (especially for scabies)

COMPOUNDS: BALSAMUM TOLUTANUM

Ester mixture (10-20%): made up of benzyl benzoate and benzyl cinnamoate

Free benzoic acid/free cinnamic acid (10 to 30%)

Resins (up to 80%)

Volatile oil

EFFECTS: BALSAMUM TOLUTANUM

Expectorant.

INDICATIONS AND USAGE

BALSAMUM PERUVIANUM

- Fevers and colds
- Hemorrhoids
- Cough
- Bronchitis
- Tendency to infection
- Inflammation of the mouth and pharynx
- Common cold
- Wounds and burns

External Use: for infected and poorly healing wounds, for burns, decubitus ulcers, frostbite, ulcus cruris, bruises caused by prostheses, hemorrhoids.

BALSAMUM TOLUTANUM

- Cough
- Bronchitis

Catarrh of the respiratory tract.

PRECAUTIONS AND ADVERSE REACTIONS

BALSAMUM PERUVIANUM

Peruvian balsam often causes contact allergies. Urticaria, recurring aphthoid oral ulcers, Quincke's disease, and diffuse purpura can all occur, among other ailments (possibly also following internal administration, as for example in foods containing peruvian balsam). Photodermatoses and phototoxic reactions are possible. Kidney damage has been observed following internal as well as external consumption of large dosages (albuminuria, pyelitis, necroses of the canaliculus epithelia).

BALSAMUM TOLUTANUM

No health hazards or side effects are known in conjunction with the proper administration of designated therapeutic dosages. However, just as is the case with Balsamum peruvianum, allergic reactions are possible.

DOSAGE

BALSAMUM PERUVIANUM

Mode of Administration: Galenic preparations for external use.

Preparation: The resin, which before drying smells strongly of vanilla or benzoin, is collected from incisions in the bark. It is an ingredient in the preparation known as Friar's Balsam.

Daily Dosage: Galenic preparations containing 5 to 20% Peruvian balsam, for extensive surface application not more than 10% Peruvian balsam.

Duration of Application: No longer than 1 week

BALSAMUM TOLUTANUM

Mode of Administration: Preparations of Tolu balsam for internal use.

Daily Dosage: Average daily dosage is 0.5 gm of drug.

LITERATURE

BALSAMUM PERUVIANUM

Friedel HD, Dissertation Marburg. 1986.

Gharbo SA, Hussein FT, Nassra AA, UAR J Pharm Sci 11:170-173. 1970.

Glasl H, Wagner H, DAZ 114:45-47. 1974.

Lund K, Rimpler H, (1985) Dtsch Apoth Ztg 125(3):105.

Rudski E, Grzywaz Z, (1977) Dermatologia 155(2):115.

Further information in:

Hänsel R, Keller K, Rimpler H, Schneider G (Hrsg.), Hagers Handbuch der Pharmazeutischen Praxis, 5. Aufl., Bde 4-6 (Drogen), Springer Verlag Berlin, Heidelberg, New York, 1992-1994.

Leung AY, Encyclopedia of Common Natural Ingredients Used in Food Drugs and Cosmetics, John Wiley & Sons Inc., New York 1980.

Lewin L, Gifte und Vergiftungen, 6. Aufl., Nachdruck, Haug Verlag, Heidelberg 1992.

Madaus G, Lehrbuch der Biologischen Arzneimittel, Bde 1-3, Nachdruck, Georg Olms Verlag Hildesheim 1979.

Morton JF, An Atlas of Medicinal Plants of Middle America, Charles C. Thomas, USA 1981.

Roth L, Daunderer M, Kormann K, Giftpflanzen, Pflanzengifte, 4. Aufl., Ecomed Fachverlag Landsberg Lech 1993.

Steinegger E, Hänsel R, Pharmakognosie, 5. Aufl., Springer Verlag Heidelberg 1992.

Teuscher E, Biogene Arzneimittel, 5. Aufl., Wiss. Verlagsges. Stuttgart 1997.

Wagner H, Wiesenauer M, Phytotherapie. Phytopharmaka und pflanzliche Homöopathika, Fischer-Verlag, Stuttgart, Jena, New York 1995.

BALSAMUM TOLUTANUM

Harkiss KJ, Linley PA, PM 35:61-65. 1979.

Lund K, Rimpler H, (1985) Dtsch Apoth Ztg 125(3):105.

Morton JF, An Atlas of Medicinal Plants of Middle America, Charles C. Thomas, USA 1981.

Rudski E, Grzywaz Z, (1977) Dermatologia 155(2):115.

Wahlberg I, Enzell CR, Acta Chem Scand 25:352-354. 1971.

Further information in:

Hänsel R, Keller K, Rimpler H, Schneider G (Hrsg.), Hagers Handbuch der Pharmazeutischen Praxis, 5. Aufl., Bde 4-6 (Drogen), Springer Verlag Berlin, Heidelberg, New York, 1992-1994.

Leung AY, Encyclopedia of Common Natural Ingredients Used in Food Drugs and Cosmetics, John Wiley & Sons Inc., New York 1980.

Madaus G, Lehrbuch der Biologischen Arzneimittel, Bde 1-3, Nachdruck, Georg Olms Verlag Hildesheim 1979.

Steinegger E, Hänsel R, Pharmakognosie, 5. Aufl., Springer Verlag Heidelberg 1992.

Teuscher E, Biogene Arzneimittel, 5. Aufl., Wiss. Verlagsges. Stuttgart 1997.

Myrrh

See Commiphora Molmol

Myrrhis Odorata

Sweet Cicely

DESCRIPTION

Medicinal Parts: The medicinal part of the plant is whole herb.

Flower and Fruit: The white flowers appear in early summer in complex umbels. The umbels are flattened on top, many-rayed and more cyme-like at the end of the branches. The rays of the androgynous flowers are covered in thick down. The pedicles of the male flowers are hollow. In the flowering season the umbels are erect and closed. The fruit is elongate-pyramid-shaped, 2 to 2.5 cm long, compressed at the sides and brown to glossy black.

Leaves, Stem and Root: The plant is perennial and smells of anise. The rhizome is thick, gnarled, brown, branched and polycephalous. The stem is erect, 50 to 120 cm high, round, glabrous or villous, cane-like and branched higher up. The nodes are covered in long, fine hairs. The leaves are large, soft, triangular and covered underneath with short, soft bristles and are 2 to 4-pinnatisect.

Habitat: The herb is found in mountainous regions from the Pyrenees to the Caucasus and is cultivated elsewhere.

Production: Sweet Cicely root and herb are the whole plant of Myrrhis odorata.

Other Names: Sweet Chervil, Sweet Bracken, Sweet-fern, Sweet-Cus, Sweet-Humlock, Sweets, The Roman Plant, Shepherd's Needle, British Myrrh

ACTIONS AND PHARMACOLOGY

COMPOUNDS

Volatile oil: chief components are anethole, additionally anisaldehyde, limonene, chavicolmethyl ether, alpha-pinene

Flavonoids: apigenine-7-O-glucoside, luteolin-7-O-glucoside

EFFECTS

Carminative, digestive, and expectorant.

INDICATIONS AND USAGE

The herb is used as a blood purifier and an expectorant, as well as for breathing difficulties and asthma. The roots are used to treat chest and throat complaints and urinary complaints. The fresh herb is used externally for gout swelling and indurations.

PRECAUTIONS AND ADVERSE REACTIONS

No health hazards or side effects are known in conjunction with the proper administration of designated therapeutic dosages.

DOSAGE

Mode of Administration: Ground root as a tonic or infusion.

LITERATURE

Hegnauer R, Chemotaxonomie der Pflanzen, Bde 1-11, Birkhäuser Verlag Basel, Boston, Berlin 1962-1997.

Kern W, List PH, Hörhammer L (Hrsg.), Hagers Handbuch der Pharmazeutischen Praxis, 4. Aufl., Bde. 1-8, Springer Verlag Berlin, Heidelberg, New York, 1969.

Myrtle

See Myrtus Communis

Myrtus Communis

Myrtle

DESCRIPTION

Medicinal Parts: The medicinal parts are the leaves and the branches.

Flower and Fruit: The flowers are medium-sized and stiff. They are short, glandular-haired pedicles, which are covered in bracteoles and grow solitary in the leaf axils. The petals are white with fine glands and a somewhat tomentose margin. The anthers are yellow. The berries are pea-sized, orbicular or ovoid-ellipsoid, blue-black or white and are crowned by the calyx.

Leaves, Stem and Root: Myrtle is an evergreen, bushy shrub or a small up to 5 m high tree with opposite branches and quadrangular cane-shaped, initially glandular, downy branches. The leaves are glossy, glabrous, dark green, opposite-paired or whorled, ovate to lanceolate, entire, acuminate and 1-3 cm long.

Characteristics: The flowers have a sweet-spicy taste.

Habitat: The origin of the plant is unknown. It grows from the Mediterranean region to the northwestern Himalayas.

Production: Myrti folium are the dried leaves of Myrtus communis. Myrti aetheroleum is the essential oil of Myrtus communis. May and June are the best months for harvesting, since the plants oil content is at its most concentrated during this time; the essential oil is extracted from the leaves and branches by a process of steam distillation; the percentage extracted ranges from 0.1 to 0.5%.

Not To Be Confused With: The leaves of Bux semper-virens and Vaccinium vitisidaea, both of which it resembles.

ACTIONS AND PHARMACOLOGY

COMPOUNDS: MYRTI FOLIUM

Volatile oil (0.1-0.5%): composition see below

Tannins (gallotannins, condensed tannins)

Acylphloroglucinols: myrtocommulon A and B

COMPOUNDS: MYRTI AETHEROLEUM

Chief components: 1,8-cineol (15-45%), alpha-pinene (15-38%), myrtenol (1-5%), myrtenylacetate (4-20%), limonene (4-10%), alpha-terpineol (2-12%), geraniol (0.5-1.5%), geranylacetate (1-5%), myrtol is a myrtle oil fraction that boils between 160-180°C, chief components 1.8-cineol and alpha-pinene

EFFECTS: MYRTI FOLIUM AND AETHEROLEUM

Myrtol is the active constituent. It is the fraction of myrtenol, which separates at 160-180 C. It is absorbed in the intestine, stimulates the mucous membrane of the stomach and deodorizes the breath. The myrtol component is fungicidal, disinfectant, and antibacterial.

INDICATIONS AND USAGE

Acute and chronic infections of the respiratory tract such as bronchitis, whooping cough, tuberculosis of the lung; bladder conditions, diarrhea and worm infestation. It is sometimes used as a substitute for Buchu.

CONTRAINDICATIONS

No internal administration of the drug should take place in the presence of inflammatory illnesses of the gastrointestinal area or of the biliary ducts, or in the case of severe liver diseases.

PRECAUTIONS AND ADVERSE REACTIONS

General: No health hazards or side effects are known in conjunction with the proper administration of designated therapeutic dosages. In rare cases, the internal administration of myrtle oil as a drug leads to nausea, vomiting and diarrhea.

Pediatric Use: Preparations containing the oil should not be applied to the faces of infants or small children (glottal spasm or bronchial spasm or even asthma-like attacks are possible, as in respiratory failure).

OVERDOSAGE

Overdoses of myrtle oil (more than 10 gm) can lead to life-threatening poisonings, due to the high cineol content. Symptoms include, among others, fall in blood pressure, circulatory disorders, collapse and respiratory failure. Vomiting is not to be induced in the case of poisoning, because of the danger of aspiration. Following administration of activated charcoal, the therapy for poisonings consists of treating spasms with diazepam (i.v.), treating colic with atropine; electrolyte substitution and treating possible cases of acidosis with sodium bicarbonate infusions. Intubation and oxygen respiration may also be necessary.

DOSAGE

Mode of Administration: Myrtle is available in various medicinal/pharmaceutical preparations for internal use.

Daily Dosage: Single dose: 0.2 gm of drug to be taken internally.

Storage: Protect from light.

LITERATURE

Joseph MI et al., (1987) Pharmazie 42 (2): 142.

Lawrence BM, Perfumer Flavorist 15:65-66. 1990.

Peyron L, Plantes Méd Phytothér 4:279-285. 1970.

Further information in:

Hänsel R, Keller K, Rimpler H, Schneider G (Hrsg.), Hagers Handbuch der Pharmazeutischen Praxis, 5. Aufl., Bde 4-6 (Drogen), Springer Verlag Berlin, Heidelberg, New York, 1992-1994.

Madaus G, Lehrbuch der Biologischen Arzneimittel, Bde 1-3, Nachdruck, Georg Olms Verlag Hildesheim 1979.

Morton JF, An Atlas of Medicinal Plants of Middle America, Charles C Thomas USA 1981.

Roth L, Daunderer M, Kormann K, Giftpflanzen, Pflanzengifte, 4. Aufl., Ecomed Fachverlag Landsberg Lech 1993.

Steinegger E, Hänsel R, Pharmakognosie, 5. Aufl., Springer Verlag Heidelberg 1992.

Wagner H, Wiesenauer M, Phytotherapie. Phytopharmaka und pflanzliche Homöopathika, Fischer-Verlag, Stuttgart, Jena, New York 1995.

Narcissus Pseudonarcissus

Daffodil

DESCRIPTION

Medicinal Parts: The medicinal parts are the bulb, the leaves and the flowers, or the whole plant without the roots.

Flower and Fruit: The flowers are solitary and bending on compressed 2-edged pedicles. They are pale yellow. At the base of the flower there is a dry, membranous sheath which is split higher at the side. The perigone is 6-tipped and splayed like a plate. The secondary corolla is egg-yolk yellow and cylindrical, with an undulating-folded, unevenly crenate margin. The stamens are fused to the tube. The ovary is inferior, the style is thread-like and the stigma obtuse.

Leaves, Stem and Root: The plant grows from 15 to 30 cm high. The leaves are basal, sprouting from an ovate, brown bulb. They are erect, linear, flatly grooved, and have 2 grooves rather than a keel.

Characteristics: Daffodil has a weak unpleasant odor and is poisonous.

Habitat: The plant is found all over Europe and is cultivated elsewhere.

Production: Daffodil is the flowering plant Narcissus pseudonarcissus without the root.

Other Names: Lent Lily

ACTIONS AND PHARMACOLOGY

COMPOUNDS

Amaryllidacene alkaloids: including, among others, haemanthamin, galanthine, galanthamine, pluviin, masonine, homolycorin

Chelidonic acid

EFFECTS

No information is available.

INDICATIONS AND USAGE

Daffodil is used for irritation of the mucous membranes such as bronchial catarrh, whooping cough, colds and asthma.

PRECAUTIONS AND ADVERSE REACTIONS

No health hazards or side effects are known in conjunction with the proper administration of designated therapeutic dosages. The plant possesses a weak potential for sensitization, a condition called ''daffodil itch''.

OVERDOSAGE

Overdosage or accidental intake of the bulbs, (instead of cooking onions), can lead to poisonings. Symptoms include vomiting, salivation, diarrhea, and central nervous disorders following resorption.

DOSAGE

Mode of Administration: Daffodil is available as a powder and as an extract.

LITERATURE

Furusawa E, Suzuki N, Ramanathan S, Furusawa S, Cutting W, Effect of long-term administration of Narcissus alkaloid on Rauscher leukemia and combinations with standard drugs. In: Proc Soc Exp Biol Med 140:1034-1040. 1972.

Moraes-Cerdeira RM et al., Alkaloid content of different bulb parts of Narcissus cv. Ice follies. In: PM 63(1):93-94. 1997.

Suzuki N, Tania S, Furusawa S, Furusawa E, Therapeutic activity of narcissus alkaloids on Rauscher leukemia: Antiviral affect in vitro and rational drug combination in vivo. In: Proc Soc Expl Biol Med 145:771-777. 1974.

Tojo E, (+)-Narcidine, a new alkaloid from Narcissus pseudonarcissus. In: JNP 54: 1387. 1991.

Further information in:

Frohne D, Pfänder HJ, Giftpflanzen - Ein Handbuch für Apotheker, Toxikologen und Biologen, 4. Aufl., Wiss. Verlags-Ges. Stuttgart 1997.

Hausen B, Allergiepflanzen, Pflanzenallergene, ecomed Verlagsgesellsch. mbH, Landsberg 1988.

Kern W, List PH, Hörhammer L (Hrsg.): Hagers Handbuch der Pharmazeutischen Praxis, 4. Aufl., Bde. 1-8, Springer Verlag Berlin, Heidelberg, New York, 1969.

Lewin L, Gifte und Vergiftungen, 6. Aufl., Nachdruck, Haug Verlag, Heidelberg 1992.

Madaus G, Lehrbuch der Biologischen Arzneimittel, Bde 1-3, Nachdruck, Georg Olms Verlag Hildesheim 1979.

Roth L, Daunderer M, Kormann K, Giftpflanzen, Pflanzengifte, 4. Aufl., Ecomed Fachverlag Landsberg Lech 1993.

Teuscher E, Lindequist U, Biogene Gifte - Biologie, Chemie, Pharmakologie, 2. Aufl., Fischer Verlag Stuttgart 1994.

Nasturtium

See Tropaeolum Majus

Nasturtium Officinale

Watercress

DESCRIPTION

Medicinal Parts: The medicinal part is the aerial part collected during the flowering season.

Flower and Fruit: On the leading and side shoots there are terminal, raceme-like inflorescences, which are slightly umbelliferous and consist of small, white, solitary flowers. The 4 white sepals are 2 to 3 mm long and glabrous. The 4 white petals are 2.5 to 5 mm long and turn lilac. There are 2 to 4 stamens with yellow anthers and filaments, which also turn lilac. The fruit is 13 to 18 mm long, with a glabrous pod on an 8 to 12 cm stem. The seeds are flat, ovate, 1 mm long, 0.8 to 0.9 mm wide and roughly reticulate. There are about 25 sections on each seed surface.

Leaves, Stem and Root: The plant is a perennial, which grows from 25 to 90 cm and has creeping runners. The stem is angular, hollow, decumbent, rooting and branched. The somewhat fleshy leaves are alternate, usually odd-pinnate, lyrate and petiolate. They remain grass-green in winter. They have broad-elliptical, entire-margined or sweeping-crenate leaflets and roundish, broadly cordate terminal leaflets.

Characteristics: The plant has a radish-like taste and smells tangy when rubbed.

Habitat: The plant is found almost all over the world and is cultivated in many regions.

Production: Watercress consists of the fresh or dried aboveground parts of Nasturtium officinale as well as their preparations. The fresh herb is collected in the wild and dried in shady, well-aired conditions.

Not To Be Confused With: Berula erecta or Cardamine amara.

Other Names: Indian Cress

ACTIONS AND PHARMACOLOGY

COMPOUNDS

Glucosinolates in the fresh, unbruised plant: chief components gluconasturtiin, releasing mustard oil through destruction of cells, releasing phenylethylisothiocyanate, additionally including among others, glucotropaeolin (producing benzyl isothiocyanat)

Flavonoids

Vitamin C (80 mg/100 gm)

EFFECTS

Watercress has antibiotic and diuretic actions. The diuretic effect is probably due to the mustard oil content.

INDICATIONS AND USAGE

■ Cough/bronchitis

The plant is used for catarrh of the respiratory tract. In folk medicine, it is used as an appetite stimulant and for digestion complaints because of its bitter taste. Because of its Vitamin C content, it is used as a spring tonic. A decoction of the leaves in poultices and compresses for arthritis and rheumatoid arthritis is used in the folk medicine of northeastern Italy.

CONTRAINDICATIONS

Contraindications include stomach or intestinal ulcers and inflammatory renal diseases.

PRECAUTIONS AND ADVERSE REACTIONS

General: No health hazards or side effects are known in conjunction with the proper administration of designated therapeutic dosages. The intake of large quantities of the freshly-harvested plant, for example in salad, could lead to gastrointestinal complaints due to the mucous membrane-irritating effect of the mustard oil.

Pediatric Use: The drug should not be administered to children under 4 years old.

DOSAGE

Mode of Administration: The comminuted herb, freshly-pressed juice, as well as other galenic preparations of the plant are for internal use.

Preparation: In folk medicine, the comminuted drug can be taken directly. To make an infusion, pour 150 ml boiling water over 2 gm drug (1 to 2 teaspoonfuls), cover for 10 minutes and strain.

Daily Dosage: The daily dosage is 2 to 3 cups of the infusion before meals, 4 to 6 gm of the dried herb, 20 to 30 gm of the fresh herb, or 60 to 150 gm of freshly-pressed juice. Externally, the drug is applied as a poultice or a compress.

LITERATURE

MacLeod AJ, Islam R, J Sci Food Agric 26:1545-1550. 1975.

Spence RMM, Tucknott OG, PH 22:2521-2523. 1993.

Further information in:

Hänsel R, Keller K, Rimpler H, Schneider G (Hrsg.), Hagers Handbuch der Pharmazeutischen Praxis, 5. Aufl., Bde 4-6 (Drogen), Springer Verlag Berlin, Heidelberg, New York, 1992-1994.

Madaus G, Lehrbuch der Biologischen Arzneimittel, Bde 1-3, Nachdruck, Georg Olms Verlag Hildesheim 1979.

Wichtl M (Hrsg.), Teedrogen, 4. Aufl., Wiss. Verlagsges. Stuttgart 1997.

Nelumbo Nucifera

Lotus

DESCRIPTION

Medicinal Parts: The medicinal parts are the roots, the seeds, and the aerial parts of the flowering plant.

Flower and Fruit: The solitary flowers are 16 to 23 cm across, pink and scented. They grow above the leaves. The seeds are 1.7 by 1.3 cm and ovoid.

Leaves, Stem and Root: The rhizome is 10 to 20 cm long, stout, and branching. It bears numerous scale-like leaves as well as foliage leaves. The foliage leaves are peltate and have no sinuses. The petioles are 1 to 2 cm long, the lamina are 30 to 100 cm in diameter and are almost circular, glossy, and unwettable.

Habitat: The plant is indigenous to India.

ACTIONS AND PHARMACOLOGY

COMPOUNDS

Isoquinoline alkaloids: including, among others, roemerin, nuciferin, nornuciferin, liensinine, isoliensinine, neferine, lotusine, armepavin, liriodenine, asimilobin

Flavonoids: including, among others, hyperoside, isoquercitrin, quercetin glucuronide, camphor glucuronide

Tannins

EFFECTS

Active agents are the alkaloids ''nelumbin'' and roemerin, in the leaves. The drug is an astringent.

INDICATIONS AND USAGE

The powdered beans are used in the treatment of digestive disorders, particularly diarrhea. The flowers are used as an astringent for bleeding.

PRECAUTIONS AND ADVERSE REACTIONS

No health hazards or side effects are known in conjunction with the proper administration of designated therapeutic dosages.

DOSAGE

Mode of Administration: Preparations of the plant are available in powder and liquid extract form.

LITERATURE

Hegnauer R: Chemotaxonomie der Pflanzen, Bde 1-11, Birkhäuser Verlag Basel, Boston, Berlin 1962-1997.

Kern W, List PH, Hörhammer L (Hrsg.), Hagers Handbuch der Pharmazeutischen Praxis, 4. Aufl., Bde. 1-8, Springer Verlag Berlin, Heidelberg, New York, 1969.

Nepeta Cataria

Catnip

DESCRIPTION

Medicinal Parts: The medicinal parts are aerial parts of the plant collected during the flowering season.

Flower and Fruit: The inflorescence is spike-like and the lower verticillasters distant from each other. The small individual flowers are on short pedicles. The bracts are 1.5 to 3 mm and linear-awl-shaped. The sepals are 5 to 6.5 mm long and ovate. The tips are 1.5 to 2.5 mm long, linear-lanceolate and patent. The corolla is 7 to 10 mm long, is slightly longer than the calyx and is white with small purple spots.

Leaves, Stem and Root: The root of the plant is perennial. The stems are up to 1 m high, angular, erect and branched. They are leafy gray-pubescent to tomentose giving the whole plant a whitish gray appearance. The leaves are 2 to 8 cm, ovate, cordate at the base, crenate or serrate and gray-tomentose beneath. The petiole is 0.5 to 4 cm in length.

Characteristics: Aromatic, characteristic smell, reminiscent of Mint and Pennyroyal.

Habitat: Indigenous to Europe and naturalized in the U.S.

Production: Catnip is the aerial part of Nepeta cataria. The harvesting takes place in uncultivated regions. The drug is manually cut in dry and sunny weather conditions. The woodless parts of the plant are sorted out and the material is then left to dry in the shade.

Other Names: Catnep, Catrup, Catmint, Catswort, Field Balm

ACTIONS AND PHARMACOLOGY

COMPOUNDS

Volatile oil (0.2-0.7%): chief components are nepetalactone (share 80-95%), additionally including among others epi-nepetalactone, caryophyllene, camphor, thymol, carvacrol

EFFECTS

Active agents are bitter and tannin substances, as well as essential oil. Antipyretic, refrigerant, relieves cramps, sedative, diaphoretic. The tea has a diuretic effect and increases gallbladder activity.

INDICATIONS AND USAGE

Colds, colic, also for the treatment of nervous disorders and migraine, since preparations from the mint have a calming effect. It is also used in the treatment of gynecological disorders. Nepeta cataria has a long tradition in England and France as a kitchen and medicinal herb and was used occasionally as stimulating drink until the introduction of black tea.

PRECAUTIONS AND ADVERSE REACTIONS

No health hazards or side effects are known in conjunction with the proper administration of designated therapeutic dosages.

DOSAGE

Mode of Administration: Orally in ground and dried forms.

Preparation: To prepare an infusion (tea), add 10 teaspoons per liter of water, leave this to stand and draw for 10 minutes.

Daily Dosage: Drink 2 to 3 cups of the tea daily.

LITERATURE

Harvey JW et al., (1978) Lloydia 41:367.

Hatch RC, (1972) Amer J Vet Res 33:143.

Margolis JS, In: Complete Book of Recreational Drugs, Cliff House Books USA 1978.

Roitman JN, (1981) Lancet I:944.

Sakan T et al., (1967) Tetrahedron 23:4635.

Sastry SD et al., (1972) Phytochemistry 11:453.

Sherry CJ et al., (1981) Quart J Crude Drug Res 19(1):31.

Tagawa M, Murai F, (1983) Planta Med 47:109.

Young LA et al., In: Recreational Drugs, Berkeley Publishing Co. USA 1977.

Further information in:

Hegnauer R, Chemotaxonomie der Pflanzen, Bde 1-11, Birkhäuser Verlag Basel, Boston, Berlin 1962-1997.

Kern W, List PH, Hörhammer L (Hrsg.), Hagers Handbuch der Pharmazeutischen Praxis, 4. Aufl., Bde. 1-8, Springer Verlag Berlin, Heidelberg, New York, 1969.

Simon E, Chadwick AF, Craker LE (Eds.), Herbs. An Indexed Bibliography 1971-80 Archon Books USA 1984.

Steinegger E, Hänsel R, Pharmakognosie, 5. Aufl., Springer Verlag Heidelberg 1992.

Teuscher E, Lindequist U, Biogene Gifte - Biologie, Chemie, Pharmakologie, 2. Aufl., Fischer Verlag Stuttgart 1994.

Nerium Odoratum

Oleander leaf

DESCRIPTION

Medicinal Parts: The leaves are the medicinal part.

Flower and Fruit: The corolla is 4 to 7 mm in diameter, usually pink to red but sometimes white. The petals are thickly covered in glands. The tube is 2 cm long and the lobes are also 2 cm long, obtuse and patent. The anther appendages are long, pubescent and twisted. The follicles are 8 to 16 cm by 0.5 to 1 cm, erect and reddish-brown.

Leaves, Stem and Root: The evergreen plant can be tree or shrub-like. The trunks are up to 4 m high. The leaves are 6 to 12 by 1.2 to 2 cm, linear-lanceolate, sharped-edged, coriaceous, dark green and matte-glossy with a lighter under surface.

Habitat: Oleander leaf grows mainly in the Mediterranean region but also in parts of Asia. It is cultivated in Europe.

Other Names: Rose Laurel

ACTIONS AND PHARMACOLOGY

COMPOUNDS

Cardiac steroids (cardenolide): chief components are oleandrine, glucosyloleandrin, gentiobiosyloleandrine, odoroside A

EFFECTS

Positively inotropic, negatively chronotropic.

INDICATIONS AND USAGE

Oleander leaf is used for diseases and functional disorders of the heart, as well as for skin diseases.

PRECAUTIONS AND ADVERSE REACTIONS

General: No health hazards are known in conjunction with the proper administration of designated therapeutic dosages. Side effects could include, particularly in the case of overdose, nausea, vomiting, diarrhea, headache, stupor and cardiac arrhythmias.

Drug Interactions: The simultaneous administration of the drug with quinidine, calcium salts, saluretics, laxatives or glucocorticoids increases both efficacy and side effects. For symptoms of an acute poisoning and therapy see Digitalis folium.

The scientific literature (Lewin) contains numerous descriptions of fatalities.

DOSAGE

No information is available.

LITERATURE

Loew D, Phytotherapie bei Herzinsuffizienz. In: ZPT 18(2):92-96. 1997.

Loew DA, Loew AD, Pharmakokinctik von herzglykosidhaltigen Pflanzenextrakten. In: ZPT 15(4):197-202. 1994.

Siddiqui S et al., Isolation and structure of two cardiac glycosides from the laeves of Nerium oleander. In: PH 26(1):237-241. 1985.

Yamauchi T et al., Quantitative variations in the cardiac glycosides of oleander. In: PH 22:2211-2214. 1983.

Further information in:

Frohne D, Pfänder HJ, Giftpflanzen - Ein Handbuch für Apotheker, Toxikologen und Biologen, 4. Aufl., Wiss. Verlags-Ges. Stuttgart 1997.

Kern W, List PH, Hörhammer L (Hrsg.), Hagers Handbuch der Pharmazeutischen Praxis, 4. Aufl., Bde. 1-8, Springer Verlag Berlin, Heidelberg, New York, 1969.

Lewin L, Gifte und Vergiftungen, 6. Aufl., Nachdruck, Haug Verlag, Heidelberg 1992.

Madaus G, Lehrbuch der Biologischen Arzneimittel, Bde 1-3, Nachdruck, Georg Olms Verlag Hildesheim 1979.

Roth L, Daunderer M, Kormann K: Giftpflanzen, Pflanzengifte, 4. Aufl., Ecomed Fachverlag Landsberg Lech 1993.

Schulz R, Hänsel R, Rationale Phytotherapie, Springer Verlag Heidelberg 1996.

Steinegger E, Hänsel R, Pharmakognosie, 5. Aufl., Springer Verlag Heidelberg 1992.

Teuscher E, Lindequist U, Biogene Gifte - Biologie, Chemie, Pharmakologie, 2. Aufl., Fischer Verlag Stuttgart 1994.

Teuscher E, Biogene Arzneimittel, 5. Aufl., Wiss. Verlagsges. Stuttgart 1997.

Wagner H, Wiesenauer M, Phytotherapie. Phytopharmaka und pflanzliche Homöopathika, Fischer-Verlag, Stuttgart, Jena, New York 1995.

Nerve Root

See Cypripedium Calceolus

Nettle

See Urtica Dioica

New Jersey Tea

See Ceanothus Americanus

Niauli

See Melaleucea Viridiflora

Nicotiana Tabacum

Tobacco

DESCRIPTION

Medicinal Parts: The medicinal parts are the dried leaves.

Flower and Fruit: The numerous flowers are in many-branched panicles. The sepals are 12 to 25 mm long and tubular to tubular-campanulate. The tips are triangular, pointed and unequal. The corolla is 30 to 55 mm long, funnel-shaped, pale greenish-cream and often pinkish distally. The limb is 10 to 15 mm, with pointed lobes, which are sometimes subentire. The 4 stamens are unequal and sometimes slightly exerted. The capsule is 15 to 20 mm long, ellipsoid to globose.

Leaves, Stem and Root: Tobacco is an annual or biennial plant, 1 to 3 m in height. The plant has a long fibrous root and an upright, round, pubescent and stick stem, which is heavily branched at the top. The leaves are up to 50 cm in length. They are ovate to elliptical or lanceolate, pointed, alternate and sessile. They sometimes have a short, winged petiole.

Habitat: The plant originates from tropical America and is cultivated worldwide, in particular in the U.S., China, Turkey, Greece, Holland, France, Germany and most subtropical countries.

Production: Tobacco leaves are the cultivated, unfermented leaves of Nicotiana tabacum.

ACTIONS AND PHARMACOLOGY

COMPOUNDS

Pyridine alkaloids (0.5-8.0%, among select cultivars 1.5%): chief alkaloid nicotine ((-)- nicotine, 30-60% share of the alkaloid mixture), additionally, including among others, N-formylnornicotine, cotinine, myosmin, nicotyrin, anabasine, nicotellin

EFFECTS

In small doses, Tobacco increases blood pressure and the activity of the gastric mucous membrane. In larger doses it reduces blood pressure and lowers muscle tone of the gastrointestinal tract. Tobacco also stimulates respiratory and tremor centers.

INDICATIONS AND USAGE

Tobacco is used to help break the smoking habit.

In combination with a neuroleptic (complimentary drug), Tobacco has been used for the treatment of extrapyramidal disorders in children.

PRECAUTIONS AND ADVERSE REACTIONS

Tobacco leaves are severely poisonous. The chief toxin is nicotine, a liquid alkaloid, that can also be resorbed through the skin.

OVERDOSAGE

The lethal dosage for nicotine lies between 40 to 100 mg, although this can be considerably elevated through habituation (thus, with smoking tobacco, 2 to 7 g of the drug; one cigarette contains 10 mg nicotine, of which 1 to 2 mg are inhaled during smoking). Symptoms of an acute poisoning include dizziness, salivation, vomiting, diarrhea, trembling of the hands, and feelings of weakness in the legs; very high dosages can lead rapidly to spasms, unconsciousness, cardiac arrest and respiratory failure. Poisonings occur in particular through the ingestion of cigarettes by children, the handling of insecticides containing nicotine (thus through skin contact) and in connection with the harvesting of tobacco (also through cutaneous resorption). Nicotine plasters also represent a danger for children.

Following gastric lavage with burgundy-colored potassium permanganate solution, instillation of activated charcoal and sodium sulphate solution, the therapy for poisonings consists of treating spasms with diazepam (i.v.), chloral hydrate for children (rectal); cardiac massage and atropine for severe sympathetic excitation. Intubation and oxygen respiration may also be necessary. No centrally-effective analeptics are to be given.

DOSAGE

Mode of Administration: The nicotine alkaloid is used internally as a gum, and externally as a transdermal patch.

Preparation: Nicorette (chewing gum); also as transdermal patches.

Daily Dosage: Nicotine as a pure alkaloid in smoker's remedies. Nicotine (2 to 4mg) bound by polacrilin (8 to 16mg) (Nicorette) is an ion exchanger and therefore causes the slow release of the nicotine. The nicotine in the saliva is absorbed over and over again. Eventually, the doses are reduced as the breaking of the habit progresses.

LITERATURE

Anonym, Harvard-Studie: Herzkrank durch Passivrauchen. In: DAZ 137(22):1860. 1997.

Anonym, Passivrauchen:Risiko für vorzeitigen Herztod. In: DAZ 137(14):1097. 1997.

Anonym, Rauchen und Gesundheit. In: DAZ 131(25):1313. 1991.

Anonym, Rauchen während der Schwangerschaft - Lungenfunktion von Säuglingen gestört. In: DAZ 137(8):554. 1997.

Anonym, Raucherinnen schaden ihren Knochen. In: DAZ 137(26):2226. 1997.

Anonym, Risiken des Rauchens in der Schwangerschaft. In: DAZ 131(20):1010. 1991.

Anonym, Risikofaktoren:Primäre Prävention des Schlaganfalls. In: DAZ 136(24):1999-2003. 1996.

Anonym, Zigaretten:Raucher haben ein doppeltes Alzheimer-Risiko. In: DAZ 137(17):1423. 1997.

Bakoula C et al., Objective passive smoking indicators and respiratory morbidity in young children. In: DAZ 135(46):4330-4331 et 4334. 1995.

Bhide SV et al., Beitrag Tabakforsch Int 14:29. 1987.

Duncker S, Atemwegserkrankungen: Passivrauchen verschlimmert Bronchialasthma bei Kindern. In: DAZ 136(3):184. 1996.

Enzell CR, Wahlberg I, Aaasen AI, Fortschr Chem Org Naturstoffe 34:1. 1977.

Jungmayr P, Schlaganfall: Wie hoch ist das Risiko für Exraucher? In: DAZ 136(2):28. 1996.

Kammerer S, Nichtraucherschutz. Passivrauchen erhöht Lungenkrebsrisiko. In: DAZ 135(14):1264-1266. 1995.

Langheimer P, Rauchen und freie Radikale. In: DAZ 134(10):836. 1994.

Lippiello, Buch. In: The Biology of Nicotine. Current Research Issue. Lippiello PM, Collins AC, Gray JA, Robinson JH (Eds.). Raven Press New York. 1992.

Matsushima S, Ohsumi T, Sugawara S, Agric Biol Chem (Tokyo) 47:507. 1983.

Müller CE, Nicotin - Genuβmittel oder Arzneistoff. In: DAZ 135(36):3253-3268. 1995.

Olbrich A, Das Lungenemphysem - Neuere Apsekte zu Pathogenese und Therapie. In: DAZ 135(47):4393-4405. 1995.

Seigel R, Collings PR, Diaz JL, Econ Botany 32:16. 1977.

Wasielewski S, Neuropharmakologie:MAO-B-Hemmung:Psychoaktiver Zigarettenrauch. In: DAZ 136(30):2529-2530. 1996.

Wasielewski S, Zigarettenrauch: Wie Passivrauchen Herz und Kreislauf schädigt. In: DAZ 135(28):2605-2606, siehe auch S. 2606 rechts. 1995.

Willaman JJ, Hui-Li L, (1970) Lloydia 33 (3A): 1.

Further information in:

Frohne D, Pfänder HJ: Giftpflanzen - Ein Handbuch für Apotheker, Toxikologen und Biologen, 4. Aufl., Wiss. Verlags-Ges. Stuttgart 1997.

Kern W, List PH, Hörhammer L (Hrsg.), Hagers Handbuch der Pharmazeutischen Praxis, 4. Aufl., Bde. 1-8, Springer Verlag Berlin, Heidelberg, New York, 1969.

Lewin L, Gifte und Vergiftungen, 6. Aufl., Nachdruck, Haug Verlag, Heidelberg 1992.

Roth L, Daunderer M, Kormann K, Giftpflanzen, Pflanzengifte, 4. Aufl., Ecomed Fachverlag Landsberg Lech 1993.

Teuscher E, Lindequist U, Biogene Gifte - Biologie, Chemie, Pharmakologie, 2. Aufl., Fischer Verlag Stuttgart 1994.

Night-Blooming Cereus

See Selenicereus Grandiflorus

Nutmeg

See Myristica Fragrans

Nux Vomica

See Strychnos Nux Vomica

Nymphaea Odorata

American White Pond Lily

DESCRIPTION

Medicinal Parts: The medicinal parts are the cut and dried rhizome, the fresh rhizome and the rhizome with the roots.

Flower and Fruit: The androgynous flowers are solitary, 7 to 15 cm across, radial-symmetrical and have a sweet fragrance. They grow from the rhizome and grow above the water by means of a long stem. The sepals are almost free, oblong-ovate pale green on the outside, greenish white on the inside. The 23 to 32 petals are free, elliptical-lanceolate, and are narrower than the sepals. They are arranged on the axis like a screw and are pure white. The numerous carpels are sunk into the beaker-shaped axis in a ring and are partially fused with it. The fruit is a berry-like capsule, which ripens under water. The seeds are small, ovate, 2.5 mm long, smooth and have an aril. The flowers open as the sun rises and close a few hours later before the intense midday heat, remaining so until the next morning. The size of the plant varies according to depth of water.

Leaves, Stem and Root: The fragrant water lily is an aquatic plant with a strong horizontal rhizome, which grows under water. The leaves are swimming, alternate, long-petioled and have 4 air channels in the petiole. The lamina is oval-orbicular, large (15-30 cm long) and has a wedge-shaped deep indentation at the base. It is entire-margined, coriaceous, green above, purple-brown beneath. The petiole is greenish and is usually purple-tinged. The stipules are triangular to reniform.

Characteristics: Pleasant smell.

Habitat: The plant is indigenous to the eastern part of North America. It is found as far south as Mexico and El Salvador and is naturalized in Europe.

Production: American White Pond Lilly root is the rhizome of Nymphaea odorata and other varieties. The drug is derived from the cut and dried rhizome; the powdered drug is yellowish to gray-brown in color. The fluid extract is produced by percolation: 1:1 using ethanol 25%.

Other Names: Water Cabbage, Cow Cabbage, Water Lily, Water Nymph

ACTIONS AND PHARMACOLOGY

COMPOUNDS

Tannins (gallotannins, ellagitannins)

Only a very small amount of research work has been carried out on the drug; it contains large amounts of gallic and ellagic tannins.

EFFECTS

Astringent, antiseptic.

INDICATIONS AND USAGE

Internally, the plant is used for chronic diarrhea.

Externally, the plant has been used in the treatment of vaginal conditions, as a gargle in the treatment of diseases of the mouth and throat, and also as a poultice for burns and furuncles.

PRECAUTIONS AND ADVERSE REACTIONS

No health hazards or side effects are known in conjunction with the proper administration of designated therapeutic dosages.

OVERDOSAGE

No poisonings have yet been observed among humans. Animal experiments have been performed with fatal results, even though very high dosages were used. These results should be taken as a warning to exercise care.

DOSAGE

Mode of Administration: Externally for furuncles, as a hot poultice. For internal use it is available as a liquid extract, as well as in combination preparations.

Daily Dosage: Internally: in a single dose of 1 to 2 gm drug as an infusion; 1 to 4 ml of liquid extract.

LITERATURE

Odinstsova NV, (1960) Farmakol i Toxicol 23:132 (via CA 54:25303).

Su KL et al., (1983) Lloydia 36:72 and 80.

Further information in:

Hänsel R, Keller K, Rimpler H, Schneider G (Hrsg.), Hagers Handbuch der Pharmazeutischen Praxis, 5. Aufl., Bde 4-6 (Drogen), Springer Verlag Berlin, Heidelberg, New York, 1992-1994.

Madaus G, Lehrbuch der Biologischen Arzneimittel, Bde 1-3, Nachdruck, Georg Olms Verlag Hildesheim 1979.

Roth L, Daunderer M, Kormann K, Giftpflanzen, Pflanzengifte, 4. Aufl., Ecomed Fachverlag Landsberg Lech 1993.

Oak Bark

See Quercus Robur

Oats

See Avena Sativa

Ocimum Basilicum

Basil

DESCRIPTION

Medicinal Parts: The medicinal part is the fresh or dried herb.

Flower and Fruit: The 6 white, labiate flowers are in 6-blossomed, pedicled, almost sessile axillary false whorls. The calyx is bilabiate, and the corolla is 4-lobed. The lower lip is simple and the 4 stamens lie on it.

Leaves, Stem and Root: The plant grows from 20 to 40 cm high. The stem is erect, branched from the base up and downy. The leaves are ovate or oblong. They are long-petioled, acuminate, irregularly dentate or entire-margined.

Characteristics: Basil has a characteristic odor and sharp taste.

Habitat: Probably originated in India, cultivated worldwide.

Production: Basil herb consists of the dried, above-ground parts of Ocimum basilicum. Oil of basil is the essential oil extracted from the dried aerial parts of Ocimum basilicum by steam distillation.

Other Names: St. Josephwort

ACTIONS AND PHARMACOLOGY

COMPOUNDS: BASILICI HERBA

Volatile oil: chief constituents are linalool, chavicol methyl ether (estragole) and eugenol

Caffeic acid derivatives

Flavonoids

EFFECTS: BASILICI HERBA

In vitro, Basil is antimicrobial.

COMPOUNDS: BASILICI AETHEROLEUM

Chief constituents: estragole (chavicol methyl ether), linalool, eugenol

EFFECTS: BASILICI AETHEROLEUM

In vitro, the oil is antimicrobial.

INDICATIONS AND USAGE

BASILICI HERBA

Preparations of basil are used for supportive therapy for feelings of fullness and flatulence, for the stimulation of appetite and digestion, and as a diuretic.

The effectiveness for the claimed applications is not documented.

BASILICI AETHEROLEUM

Wounds, rheumatic complaints, colds and chills, contusions, joint pains, depression.

PRECAUTIONS AND ADVERSE REACTIONS

BASILICI HERBA

General: No health hazards or side effects are known in conjunction with the proper administration of designated therapeutic dosages.

Pregnancy: The herb contains about 0.5% essential oil with up to 85% estragole. Because of the high estragole content in the essential oil, the herb should not be taken during pregnancy or during lactation.

Pediatric Use: Basil should not be given to infants or toddlers.

BASILICI AETHEROLEUM

General: No health hazards or side effects are known in conjunction with the proper administration of designated therapeutic dosages.

Pregnancy: Because a mutagenic effect in vitro and a carcinogenic effect in animal experiments have been demonstrated for estragole, oil of basil should not be administered for longer periods during pregnancy and while nursing.

Pediatric Use: Basil oil should not be given to infants or small children.

DOSAGE

Until the final determination of the drug's carcinogenic potential, one should completely forgo its administration.

LITERATURE

BASILICI HERBA

Balambal R et al., (1985) J Assoc Phys (India) 33(8):507.

Czygan FCh, Balsilikum - Ocimum basilicum L. Portrait einer Arzneipflanze. In: ZPT 18(1):58-66. 1997.

Jain ML, Jain SR, (1972) Planta Med 22:66.

Lemberkovics É et al., Formation of essential oil and phenolic compounds during the vegetation period in Ocimum basilicum. In: PM 59(7):A700. 1993.

Miller EC et al., (1983) Cancer Res 43:1124.

Opdyke DLJ, (1973) Food Cosmet Toxicol 11:867.

Wagner H, Nörr H, Winterhoff H, Drogen mit ''Adaptogenwirkung'' zur Stärkung der Widerstandskräfte. In: ZPT 13(2):42. 1992.

Further information in:

Kern W, List PH, Hörhammer L (Hrsg.), Hagers Handbuch der Pharmazeutischen Praxis, 4. Aufl., Bde. 1-8, Springer Verlag Berlin, Heidelberg, New York, 1969.

Leung AY, Encyclopedia of Common Natural Ingredients Used in Food Drugs and Cosmetics, John Wiley & Sons Inc., New York 1980.

Madaus G, Lehrbuch der Biologischen Arzneimittel, Bde 1-3, Nachdruck, Georg Olms Verlag Hildesheim 1979.

Simon JE, Chadwick AF, Craker LE (Eds.), Herbs. An Indexed Bibliography 1971-80. Archon Books, USA 1984.

Wichtl M (Hrsg.), Teedrogen, 4. Aufl., Wiss. Verlagsges. Stuttgart 1997.

BASILICI AETHEROLEUM

Balambal R et al., (1985) J Assoc Phys (India) 33(8):507.

Czygan FCh, Balsilikum - Ocimum basilicum L. Portrait einer Arzneipflanze. In: ZPT 18(1):58-66. 1997.

Jain ML, Jain SR, (1972) Planta Med 22:66.

Lemberkovics É et al., Formation of essential oil and phenolic compounds during the vegetation period in Ocimum basilicum. In: PM 59(7):A700. 1993.

Miller EC et al., (1983) Cancer Res 43:1124.

Opdyke DLJ, (1973) Food Cosmet Toxicol 11:867.

Wagner H, Nörr H, Winterhoff H, Drogen mit ''Adaptogenwirkung'' zur Stärkung der Widerstandskräfte. In: ZPT 13(2):42. 1992.

Further information in:

Kern W, List PH, Hörhammer L (Hrsg.), Hagers Handbuch der Pharmazeutischen Praxis, 4. Aufl., Bde. 1-8, Springer Verlag Berlin, Heidelberg, New York, 1969.

Leung AY, Encyclopedia of Common Natural Ingredients Used in Food Drugs and Cosmetics, John Wiley & Sons Inc., New York 1980.

Madaus G, Lehrbuch der Biologischen Arzneimittel, Bde 1-3, Nachdruck, Georg Olms Verlag Hildesheim 1979.

Simon JE, Chadwick AF, Craker LE (Eds.), Herbs. An Indexed Bibliography 1971-80. Archon Books, USA 1984.

Wichtl M (Hrsg.), Teedrogen, 4. Aufl., Wiss. Verlagsges. Stuttgart 1997.

Oenanthe Aquatica

Water Fennel

DESCRIPTION

Medicinal Parts: The medicinal parts are the ripe seeds.

Flower and Fruit: The flowers are white and in many-rayed compound umbels opposite the leaves. They have no involucre but there is a small epicalyx. The calyx is distinct and the corolla irregular with a distinct border, it narrows at the base and has an involute tip. The style is long. The fruit is 5 mm long 1.5 mm wide and circular, with 5 broad obtuse ribs.

Leaves, Stem and Root: The plant grows from 30 to 120 cm high. The stem is angularly branched, hollow and soft. The lower end of the stem is under water, 3 cm thick and has long roots at the nodes. When it is not under water, the stem end is only 6 mm thick. The leaves are double pinnate, pinnatifid to pinnatisect with splayed leaflets, which are often turned backwards and have lanceolate, deeply indent-ed-serrate tips. The underwater leaves have a thread-like tip.

Habitat: Found near ponds and ditches in both the U.S. and Europe.

Production: Water Fennel fruit are the ripe seeds of Oenanthe aquatica.

Other Names: Water Dropwort, Horsebane

ACTIONS AND PHARMACOLOGY

COMPOUNDS

Volatile oil (1-2.5%): including among others (+)-beta-phellandrene, dillapiol, myristicin, 1-nonen-3-ol (androle), volatile polyynes

Polyynes: including among others all-trans-pentadeca-2,8,10-trien-4,6-diin-12-on

Fatty oil

EFFECTS

The active agents are the essential and fatty oil, resin, wax, galacton, mannan and rubber substances.

INDICATIONS AND USAGE

Expectorant and for the relief of coughs (bronchial catarrh, asthma and suppurating or festering inflammation of the lungs), also as a diuretic and carminative.

PRECAUTIONS AND ADVERSE REACTIONS

No health hazards or side effects are known in conjunction with the proper administration of designated therapeutic dosages.

DOSAGE

Mode of Administration: Ground, as an extract and as a tea.

Daily Dosage: 1.0 gm is considered a medium sized dose.

LITERATURE

Ram AS, Devi HM, (1983) Indian J Bot 6(1):21.

Further information in:

Hegnauer R, Chemotaxonomie der Pflanzen, Bde 1-11, Birkhäuser Verlag Basel, Boston, Berlin 1962-1997.

Kern W, List PH, Hörhammer L (Hrsg.), Hagers Handbuch der Pharmazeutischen Praxis, 4. Aufl., Bde. 1-8, Springer Verlag Berlin, Heidelberg, New York, 1969.

Madaus G, Lehrbuch der Biologischen Arzneimittel, Bde 1-3, Nachdruck, Georg Olms Verlag Hildesheim 1979.

Roth L, Daunderer M, Kormann K, Giftpflanzen, Pflanzengifte, 4. Aufl., Ecomed Fachverlag Landsberg Lech 1993.

Wagner H, Wiesenauer M, Phytotherapie. Phytopharmaka und pflanzliche Homöopathika, Fischer-Verlag, Stuttgart, Jena, New York 1995.

Oenanthe Crocata

Water Dropwort

DESCRIPTION

Medicinal Parts: The medicinal part is the rhizome.

Flower and Fruit: The flowers are in terminal umbels. The flowering shoots are longer than the 10 to 40 pedicled rays, which do not thicken in the fruiting phase. The fruit is 4 to 6 mm long and cylindrical.

Leaves, Stem and Root: The plant is a branched, stout perennial up to 150 cm high. The roots are fleshy and pale yellow. They have obovoid or ellipsoid tubers close to the point of attachment to the stem. The stems are hollow, striate and grooved. The basal leaves are 3- to 4-pinnate. The lobes of the basal leaves are ovate to suborbicular, cuneate at base. The lobed, crenate, cauline leaves are 2- to 3-pinnate. The lobes of the cauline leaves are ovate to linear and the segments are closer and sharper than the basal leaves.

Characteristics: The plant is poisonous.

Habitat: The plant grows beside ditches and ponds in the U.S., and parts of Europe, excluding Scandinavia, Holland, Germany, Russia, Turkey and Greece.

Production: Water Dropwort is the root of Oenanthe crocata.

Other Names: Hemlock, Water Dropwort, Dead Men's Fingers, Horsebane, Dead Tongue, Five-Fingered Root, Water Lovage

ACTIONS AND PHARMACOLOGY

COMPOUNDS

Polyynes: including, among others, the highly toxic oenanthotoxin, additionally including among others oenanthetol

EFFECTS

No information available.

INDICATIONS AND USAGE

Water Dropwort was formerly used in the treatment of epilepsy but this can no longer be recommended.

PRECAUTIONS AND ADVERSE REACTIONS

The drug is severely poisonous due to the highly toxic oenanthotoxin content.

OVERDOSAGE

Symptoms of poisoning include burning sensation in the mouth and nose, dizziness, weakness, chill, mild twitching, and speech disorders; with higher dosages, tonic-colonic spasms, temporarily slowed cardiac activity, unconsciousness, bloody foam at the mouth and death through respiratory failure.

Following gastrointestinal emptying (inducement of vomiting, gastric lavage with burgundy-colored potassium permanganate solution, sodium sulfate), and the administration of activated charcoal, the therapy for poisonings consists of treating spasms with thiobarbiturates (diazepam is said to be less effective), hemodialysis has been applied successfully.

DOSAGE

Mode of Administration: The drug is obsolete.

LITERATURE

Anet E, Lythgoe B, Silk MH, Tripett S, The chemistry of oenanthotoxin and cicutoxin. In: Chem Ind 31:757. 1952.

Bohlmann F, Rode KM, Polyacetylenic compounds: CXVII. Polyynes of Oenanthe crocata. In: Chem Ber 101(4):1163-1175. 1968.

Grindy HF, Howarth F, Pharmacological studies on hemlock water dropwort. In: Brit J Pharmacol 11:225-30. 1956.

Mitchell MJ, Routledge PA, Hemlock water dropwort poisoning - a review. In: Clin Toxicol 12(4):417-426. 1978.

Further information in:

Frohne D, Pfänder HJ, Giftpflanzen - Ein Handbuch für Apotheker, Toxikologen und Biologen, 4. Aufl., Wiss. Verlags-Ges. Stuttgart 1997.

Kern W, List PH, Hörhammer L (Hrsg.), Hagers Handbuch der Pharmazeutischen Praxis, 4. Aufl., Bde. 1-8, Springer Verlag Berlin, Heidelberg, New York, 1969.

Lewin L, Gifte und Vergiftungen, 6. Aufl., Nachdruck, Haug Verlag, Heidelberg 1992.

Madaus G, Lehrbuch der Biologischen Arzneimittel, Bde 1-3, Nachdruck, Georg Olms Verlag Hildesheim 1979.

Roth L, Daunderer M, Kormann K, Giftpflanzen, Pflanzengifte, 4. Aufl., Ecomed Fachverlag Landsberg Lech 1993.

Teuscher E, Lindequist U, Biogene Gifte - Biologie, Chemie, Pharmakologie, 2. Aufl., Fischer Verlag Stuttgart 1994.

Oenothera Biennis

Evening Primrose

DESCRIPTION

Medicinal Parts: The medicinal part is the oil from the seed.

Flower and Fruit: The fragrant flowers are 2 to 3 cm long and are solitary in the leaf axils. The open ones are lower than the buds. The sepals are lanceolate, acuminate, turned down, thin, more or less pale green and smooth on the outside with a few scattered hairs. The petals are obovate. The ovary is inferior. The style has a 4-sectioned stigma. The fruit is a linear-oblong up to 3 cm long, quadrangular, downy-villous capsule. The seeds are 1.5 mm long, dark gray to black with irregular sharp edges.

Leaves, Stem and Root: The biennial grows up to 1 m and has a spindle-shaped, fleshy turnip-like root, which produces leaf rosette in the first year, which is pressed close to the ground. The stem is erect, unbranched or branched higher up, angular and like the calyx. The ovary is a capsule covered in short glandular hairs and simple light hairs on purple papilla. The cauline leaves are short-petioled or sessile, often hanging, oblong-lanceolate, pointed, irregular and finely dentate.

Characteristics: The flowers open in the evening.

Habitat: Originally indigenous to North America it is now naturalized throughout most of Europe and parts of Asia.

Production: Evening Primrose oil is the fatty seed oil of Oenothera biennis. The oil is extracted by means of a cold-extraction process, which involves hexane in steel or glass-lined tanks. The extract is washed and the solvent is removed using low pressure.

Other Names: Fever Plant, King's Cureall, Night Willow-herb, Scabish, Sun Drop

ACTIONS AND PHARMACOLOGY

COMPOUNDS

Fatty oil: chief fatty acids linoleic acid (65-80%), gamma-linolenic acid (8-14%), oleic acid (6-11%), palmitic acid (7-10%)

EFFECTS

Anti-arteriosclerotic. In cases of atopic eczema, it compensates for the lack of gamma-linolenic acid.

INDICATIONS AND USAGE

Evening Primrose Oil is used for neurodermatitis, premenstrual syndrome and as a dietary aid. Capsules containing 0.5 gm of evening primrose oil have been approved for use in Germany, in the treatment of and to relieve symptoms of atopic eczema. Symptoms such as itching, flaking and inflammation may be reduced or cured. Also available as a dietary supplement. The drug is used to treat hyperactivity in children, lessen high cholesterol levels and ease premenstrual syndrome.

PRECAUTIONS AND ADVERSE REACTIONS

No health hazards or side effects are known in conjunction with the proper administration of designated therapeutic dosages.

DOSAGE

Mode of Administration: Available as a medicinal/pharmaceutical preparation (with gammon acid standardized proportion of evening primrose oil) in capsule form (0.5 gm).

Daily Dosage: Capsules, with a standardized percentage of 0.5 gamma acids. To be taken 3 times daily, in doses of 1 to 2 capsules.

Storage: Evening primrose oil is rinsed in nitrogen and stored in cooled tanks, which are encased in polyethylene.

LITERATURE

Berth-Jones J, Placebo controlled trial of essential fatty acid supplementation in atopic dermatitis. In: Lancet 341:1557-1560. 1993.

Haslett C et al., (1983) Int J Obesity 7(6):549.

Horrobin DF, (1983) J Reprod Med 28(7):465.

Ihrig M, Blume H, Nachtkerzenöl-Präparate: Ein Qualitätsvergleich. In: PZ 139(9):668. 1994.

Ippen H, Gamma-Linolensäure besser aus Nachtkerzen- oder aus Borretschöl? In: ZPT 16(3):167-170. 1995.

Midwinter RE et al., (1982) Lancet I, 339.

Pye J K et al., (1985) Lancet II, 373.

Seaman GVF et al., (1979) Lancet I:1139.

Ten Hoor F, (1980) Nutr Metab 24(Suppl. 1):162.

Willuhn G, Phytopharmaka in der Dermatologie. In: ZPT 16(6):325-342. 1995.

Wright S, Burton JL, (1982) Lancet II, 1120.

Further information in:

Hänsel R, Keller K, Rimpler H, Schneider G (Hrsg.), Hagers Handbuch der Pharmazeutischen Praxis, 5. Aufl., Bde 4-6 (Drogen), Springer Verlag Berlin, Heidelberg, New York, 1992-1994.

Madaus G, Lehrbuch der Biologischen Arzneimittel, Bde 1-3, Nachdruck, Georg Olms Verlag Hildesheim 1979.

Schulz R, Hänsel R, Rationale Phytotherapie, Springer Verlag Heidelberg 1996.

Steinegger E, Hänsel R, Pharmakognosie, 5. Aufl., Springer Verlag Heidelberg 1992.

Teuscher E, Biogene Arzneimittel, 5. Aufl., Wiss. Verlagsges. Stuttgart 1997.

Wagner H, Wiesenauer M, Phytotherapie. Phytopharmaka und pflanzliche Homöopathika, Fischer-Verlag, Stuttgart, Jena, New York 1995.

Olea Europaea

Olive

DESCRIPTION

Medicinal Parts: The medicinal parts are the dried leaves, the oil extracted from the ripe drupes and the fresh branches with leaves and clusters of flowers.

Flower and Fruit: The flowers are in small axillary clustered inflorescence. The calyx has 4 tips. The white corolla has a short tube and 4 lobes. The superior ovary is bilocular, each with 2 hanging anatropal ovules. The drupe has 1 to 2 seeds, is fleshy, plum-like or round, smooth, initially green then red and is blue-black when ripe. The very hard stone contains oblong compact seeds with plenty of endosperm.

Leaves, Stem and Root: The Olive tree or medium high shrub grows up to 10 m high and has pale bark and cane-like, quadrangular to round, initially downy, thorny or thornless branches. The leaves are opposite, entire, stiff, coriaceous, narrow elliptical to lanceolate or cordate with thorny tips. The upper surface is dark green, glabrous and the underside shimmers silver with hairs.

Habitat: The plant grows in almost all of the southern European countries, in the entire Mediterranean region as far as Iran and beyond the Caucasus. Olive trees are cultivated in many regions of the world including Mediterranean countries.

Production: Olive leaves consist of the fresh or dried leaves of Olea europaea. The leaves are harvested from cultivated trees and dried under shady conditions. Olive oil is the fatty oil extracted from the drupes of Olea europaea, using the "cold press" method.

Other Names: Olivier

ACTIONS AND PHARMACOLOGY

COMPOUNDS: OLEA FOLIUM

Iridoide monoterpenes: including, among others, chief components oleoropine (6-9%), additionally 6-O-oleoropine-saccharose, ligstroside, oleoroside, oleoside-7,11-dimethylether

Triterpenes: including oleanolic acid, maslinic acid

Flavonoids: luteolin-7-O-glucoside, apigenine-7-O-glucoside

EFFECTS: OLEA FOLIUM

In animal tests: hypotensive, antiarrhythmic, spasmolytic

COMPOUNDS: OLIVAE OLEUM

Chief fatty acids: oleic acid (56-83%), palmitic acid (8-20%), linoleic acid (4-20%)

EFFECTS: OLIVAE OLEUM

Contraction of the gallbladder due to the raising of the cholecystokinin level in the plasma.

INDICATIONS AND USAGE

OLEA FOLIUM

Used as diuretic for hypertonia.

Efficacy has not been sufficiently documented.

OLIVAE OLEUM

Used in dermatological preparations and in traditional oil remedies.

PRECAUTIONS AND ADVERSE REACTIONS

OLEA FOLIUM

No health hazards or side effects are known in conjunction with the proper administration of designated therapeutic dosages.

OLIVAE OLEUM

No health hazards or side effects are known in conjunction with the proper administration of designated therapeutic dosages. The internal administration of the drug can trigger colic among gallstone sufferers.

DOSAGE

OLEA FOLIUM

Mode of Administration: The drug is available for oral use in mono and combination tea mixture preparations.

Preparation: An infusion is prepared by pouring hot water over 2 teaspoonfuls drug, allow to draw for 30 minutes.

Daily Dosage: 7 to 8 gm of dried leaves for infusions with 150 ml of water. Drink 3 to 4 cups throughout the day.

OLIVAE OLEUM

Mode of Administration: Obsolete as a drug (oil remedy) because of the risks.

LITERATURE

OLEA FOLIUM

Bianchi G, Pozzi N, 3,4-Dihydroxyphenylglycol, a major C6-C2 phenolic in Olea europaea. In: PH 35(5):1335. 1994.

Bianco A et al., Partial synthesis of oleuropein. In: JNP 55(6):760-766. 1992.

Duarte J et al., Effects of oleuropeosid in isolated guinea-pig atria. In: PM 59(4):318. 1993.

Kuwajima H et al., A secoiridoid glucoside from Olea europaea. In: PH 27(6):1757. 1988.

Lasser B et al., (1983) Naturwissenschaften 70:95.

Further information in:

Hänsel R, Keller K, Rimpler H, Schneider G (Hrsg.), Hagers Handbuch der Pharmazeutischen Praxis, 5. Aufl., Bde 4-6 (Drogen), Springer Verlag Berlin, Heidelberg, New York, 1992-1994.

OLIVE OLEUM

Anonym, Positive Auswirkungen von Olivenöl auf den Blutdruck. In: ZPT 12(1):13. 1991.

Flemming S, Ist Olivenöl erlaubt? In: DAZ 131(29):1525. 1991.

Lasser B et al., (1983) Naturwissensch. 70:95.

Further information in:

Hänsel R, Keller K, Rimpler H, Schneider G (Hrsg.), Hagers Handbuch der Pharmazeutischen Praxis, 5. Aufl., Bde 4-6 (Drogen), Springer Verlag Berlin, Heidelberg, New York, 1992-1994.

Steinegger E, Hänsel R, Pharmakognosie, 5. Aufl., Springer Verlag Heidelberg 1992.

Teuscher E, Biogene Arzneimittel, 5. Aufl., Wiss. Verlagsges. Stuttgart 1997.

Oleander leaf

See Nerium Odoratum

Olive

See Olea Europaea

Onion

See Allium Cepa

Ononis Spinosa

Spiny Rest Harrow

DESCRIPTION

Medicinal Parts: The medicinal parts are the roots or flowering branches.

Flower and Fruit: The pink flowers are solitary or in pairs in the leaf axils. The calyx is campanulate with 5 segments. The standard is large and dark-striped. The fruit is a pod as long as or longer than the calyx. The fruit is ovoid and erect.

Leaves, Stem and Root: The plant is a low subshrub of about 30 to 60 cm with a long tap root. The branches are erect, spread, villous and more less densely covered in short shoots, which terminate in straight thorns. The leaves are trifoliate with 3 small, dentate, oblong leaflets.

Characteristics: The plant has an unpleasant smell.

Habitat: Spiny Rest Harrow is common in almost all of Europe.

Production: Spiny Rest Harrow root consists of the dried roots and rhizomes of Ononis spinosa. The plant is harvested in autumn.

Other Names: Cammock, Petty Whin, Stayplough, Rest-Harrow, Wild Liquorice, Stinking Tommy, Ground Furze, Land Whin

ACTIONS AND PHARMACOLOGY

COMPOUNDS

Isoflavonoids: glycosides, including, among others, trifolirhizin (maackiain-7-glucoside), ononin (formononetin-7-glucoside), ononin-6-malonylester, homopterocarpin-7-glucoside, free isoflavonoids, including, among others, formononetin, genistein, biochanin

Volatile oil (0.02-0.2%): chief components anethole, carvone, menthol

Triterpenes: including, among others, alpha-onocerin (alpha-onoceradiendiol)

EFFECTS

Preparations have a diuretic effect.

INDICATIONS AND USAGE

- Infections of the urinary tract
- Kidney and bladder stones

Preparations are used for flushing-out therapy for inflammatory diseases of the lower urinary tract and also for prevention and treatment of kidney gravel. Popularly used for gout and rheumatic complaints.

Ensure ample liquid intake.

CONTRAINDICATIONS

The drug should not be used in the presence of edema resulting from reduced cardiac or renal activity.

PRECAUTIONS AND ADVERSE REACTIONS

No health hazards or side effects are known in conjunction with the proper administration of designated therapeutic dosages.

DOSAGE

Mode of Administration: The drug is ground for teas and other galenic preparations for internal use.

Preparation: To prepare an infusion, pour boiling water over 2 to 2.5 gm finely cut or coarsely powdered drug and strain after 20 to 30 minutes (1 teaspoonful = 3 gm).

Daily Dosage: 6 to 12 gm of drug.

LITERATURE

Dedio I, Kozlowski J, (1977) Acta Pol Pharm 34:97.

Fujise Y et al., (1965) Chem Pharm Bull 13:93.

Haznagy A, Thot G, Tamas J, Constituents of the aqueous extracts from Ononis spinosa L. In: Arch Pharm 311(4):318-323. 1978.

Hilp K et al., (1975) Arch Pharm 308:429.

Horejsi V, Kocourek J, (1978) Biochim Biophys Acta 538.

Kartnig T et al., (1985) Pharm Acta Helv 60(9/19):253.

Kirmizigül S et al., Spinonin, a novel glycoside from Ononis spinosa subsp. leiosperma. In: JNP 60(4):378-381. 1997.

Koster J et al., (1983) Planta Med 48:131.

Further information in:

Kern W, List PH, Hörhammer L (Hrsg.), Hagers Handbuch der Pharmazeutischen Praxis, 4. Aufl., Bde 1-8, Springer Verlag Berlin, Heidelberg, New York, 1969.

Madaus G, Lehrbuch der Biologischen Arzneimittel, Bde 1-3, Nachdruck, Georg Olms Verlag Hildesheim 1979.

Steinegger E, Hänsel R, Pharmakognosie, 5. Aufl., Springer Verlag Heidelberg 1992.

Teuscher E, Biogene Arzneimittel, 5. Aufl., Wiss. Verlagsges. Stuttgart 1997.

Wagner H, Wiesenauer M, Phytotherapie. Phytopharmaka und pflanzliche Homöopathika, Fischer-Verlag, Stuttgart, Jena, New York 1995.

Wichtl M (Hrsg.), Teedrogen, 4. Aufl., Wiss. Verlagsges. Stuttgart 1997.

Onopordum Acanthium

Scotch Thistle

DESCRIPTION

Medicinal Parts: The medicinal parts are the herb and the root.

Flower and Fruit: The large, light red composite flowers are terminal on the branches. The bracts are linear-lanceolate, thorny-tipped, splayed at the bottom and like cobwebs. The plant only has tubular androgynous flowers. The bristles of the hair calyx are reddish, short pinnate and almost twice as long as the fruit. The flower heads fall after the fruit ripens and the seeds fall out.

Leaves, Stem and Root: The plant is biennial and grows from 30 to 150 cm. The stem is erect, branched, and appears to be winged because of the downward leaves which are broader than the stem. The leaves are rough, irregularly thorny, and dentate to pinnatisect. When young they appear almost white.

Habitat: The plant is indigenous to Britain and is cultivated elsewhere.

Other Names: Woolly Thistle

ACTIONS AND PHARMACOLOGY

COMPOUNDS

Sesquiterpene lactones (bitter principles): including, among others, onopordopicrin

Flavonoids: including, among others, luteolin-7-glucoside

Hydroxycoumarins: aesculin

Caffeic acid derivatives

Betaine: stachydrine

Polyynes

EFFECTS

The active agents are tannin, flavonglycoside, and small quantities of alkaloid. A cardiotonic effect is questionable.

INDICATIONS AND USAGE

The drug is used as a cardiac stimulant (anthroposophic).

PRECAUTIONS AND ADVERSE REACTIONS

No health hazards or side effects are known in conjunction with the proper administration of designated therapeutic dosages.

DOSAGE

Preparation: Cardiodoron® is available in the form of drops, ampule, or tablets.

LITERATURE

Kern W, List PH, Hörhammer L (Hrsg.), Hagers Handbuch der Pharmazeutischen Praxis, 4. Aufl., Bde 1-8, Springer Verlag Berlin, Heidelberg, New York, 1969.

Madaus G, Lehrbuch der Biologischen Arzneimittel, Bde 1-3, Nachdruck, Georg Olms Verlag Hildesheim 1979.

Ophioglossum Vulgatum

English Adder's Tongue

DESCRIPTION

Medicinal Parts: The medicinal parts are the root and leaves.

Flower and Fruit: The 12 to 40 ripe yellow sporangia on either side of the middle panicle form an acuminate spike.

Leaves, Stem and Root: Grows from 8 to 25 cm high. The stem covered in the remains of leaves, grow singly from the underground roots. The stems consist of a few sturdy, yellow fibers and are round, hollow and succulent; they bear the smooth, oblong-oval, acuminate, entire frond.

Characteristics: Though a member of the Fern family, it looks unlike other ferns. It has been long used as a wound remedy under the name of ''Green Oil of Charity''.

Habitat: The plant is indigenous to Britain.

Production: English Adder's Tongue is the aerial part of Ophiglossum vulgatum.

Not To Be Confused With: English Adder's Tongue is not related to American Adder's Tongue (Erythronium).

Other Names: Serpent's Tongue, Christ's Spear

ACTIONS AND PHARMACOLOGY

COMPOUNDS

Flavonoids: including among others quercetin-3-methyl ether-7-diglucoside-4′glucoside

The constituents of the drug have not been thoroughly investigated.

EFFECTS

See Erythronium americanum.

INDICATIONS AND USAGE

See Erythronium americanum.

PRECAUTIONS AND ADVERSE REACTIONS

No health hazards or side effects are known in conjunction with the proper administration of designated therapeutic dosages.

DOSAGE

Mode of Administration: See Erythronium americanum.

LITERATURE

Hegnauer R, Chemotaxonomie der Pflanzen, Bde 1-11, Birkhäuser Verlag Basel, Boston, Berlin 1962-1997.

Opium Antidote

See Combretum Micranthum

Orchis Species

Salep

DESCRIPTION

Medicinal Parts: The medicinal parts are the subterranean parts of Orchis morio and other varieties.

Flower and Fruit: The flowers form erect spikes. The surrounding leaves are sometimes large and longer than the flowers and are often colored. The pollen mass is enclosed in 1 to 2 sectioned anthers. The ovary is almost always twisted. The seed skins can be with or without a reticulate thickening.

Leaves, Stem and Root: The species are perennial, medium-sized, glabrous plants with a round, ovate or palmate tuber. The leaves are green, sheath-like and tapering.

Habitat: The plant comes from central and southern Europe.

Production: Salep tubers are the subterranean parts of Orchis morio and other varieties of Orchis.

Other Names: Cuckoo Flower, Levant Salep, Orchid, Sahlep, Saloop, Satyrion

ACTIONS AND PHARMACOLOGY

COMPOUNDS

Mucilage (up to 50%): glucans, glucomannans (partially acetylised)- starch (25%)- proteins (5-15%)

EFFECTS

The mucus is rich in mannose and starch. The mucous membrane is a demulcent.

INDICATIONS AND USAGE

The drug is used for unspecified diarrhea, particularly in children, and for heartburn, flatulence and indigestion.

PRECAUTIONS AND ADVERSE REACTIONS

No health hazards or side effects are known in conjunction with the proper administration of designated therapeutic dosages.

DOSAGE

Mode of Administration: As a powdered formulation in medicinal preparations.

Daily Dosage: Stir 1 teaspoon of powder into a glass of warm water and drink before or after meals.

LITERATURE

Kern W, List PH, Hörhammer L (Hrsg.), Hagers Handbuch der Pharmazeutischen Praxis, 4. Aufl., Bde 1-8: Springer Verlag Berlin, Heidelberg, New York, 1969.

Steinegger E, Hänsel R, Pharmakognosie, 5. Aufl., Springer Verlag Heidelberg 1992.

Oregano

See Origanum Vulgare

Origanum Majorana

Marjoram

DESCRIPTION

Medicinal Parts: The medicinal parts are the oil extracted through a process of steam distillation, the leaves and flowers stripped off the stem and dried, the fresh aerial parts of the flowering plant and the whole of the fresh flowering plant.

Flower and Fruit: The inconspicuous, sessile flowers barely extend above the gray tomentose bracts surrounding them. The calyx appears to have only 1 sepal because it has no tip. The 2 lower sepals are almost non-existent because the 3 upper ones are completely fused. The calyx is 2.5 cm long and looks like the bracts. The corolla is white to pale lilac or pink, 4 mm long with a few uneven, pointed tips. The 2 upper ones are fused together to form a lip. The stamens are enclosed in the corolla or extend above it. The fruit is a nutlet 0.75 to 1 mm long, smooth and light brown.

Leaves, Stem and Root: The plant is biennial in central Europe and in the Mediterranean region. The main shoot is heavily branched and 20 to 25 cm high. The shoots are gray-green to whitish and sometimes tinged with red. They are more or less downy to tomentose. The leaves are spatulate, short-petioled, 0.5 to 2 cm long and 0.5 cm wide, entire-margined, rounded, gray-tomentose on both surfaces, thick-ish and usually without distinct ribs. The false whorls are mostly covered by the 3 to 4 wide, circular, gray-green bracts, which are fused to globular, racemous or panicled capitula.

Characteristics: The plant has a distinctive tangy odor and a bitter taste.

Habitat: The plant is indigenous to the southeastern Mediterranean region and is cultivated in Germany.

Production: Marjoram herb consists of the dried leaf and flower of Origanum majorana (syn Majorana hortensis), gathered during the flowering season and stripped off the stems. Marjoram oil consists of the essential oil of Origanum majorana obtained by aqueous steam distillation of the leaves and flowers stripped from the stems and harvested during flowering season. Depending on the area of cultivation there may be 2 crops of the aerial plant parts per year. Drying must be fast to avoid blackening of the leaves. Marjoram aetheroleum is obtained from the flowering fresh or dried herb through a process of aqueous distillation.

ACTIONS AND PHARMACOLOGY

COMPOUNDS

Volatile oil (1-3%)

Flavonoids: including among others diosmetin, luteolin, apigenin and their C- and O-glycosides, which include vitexin, orientin, thymonin and others.

Arbutin (0.15- 0.45%)

Caffeic acid derivatives: rosmaric acid, chlorogenic acid

Water soluble polysaccharides in the volatile oil

Chief components cis-sabinene hydrate (share 40-50%), cis-sabinene hydrate acetate (20- 30%, which with steam distillation translocate into, among others alpha-terpinenes, gamma-terpinenes, terpinols, terpinene-4-ol, change of aroma), sabinenes, trans-sabinene hydrate and others

EFFECTS

Marjoram herba is antimicrobial in vitro. Marjoram aetheroleum is antimicrobial and insecticidal.

INDICATIONS AND USAGE

The drug is used for rhinitis and colds in infants, rhinitis in small children and gastritis. In folk medicine, Majoranae herba is used for cramps, depression, dizziness, gastrointestinal disorders, migraine, nervous headaches, neurasthenia, paralysis, paroxysmal coughs, rhinitis and as a diuretic. Its efficacy has not been sufficiently documented. In folk medicine, Marjoram aetheroleum is used for coughs, gall bladder complaints and gastrointestinal cramps.

PRECAUTIONS AND ADVERSE REACTIONS

General: No health hazards or side effects are known in conjunction with the proper administration of designated therapeutic dosages. The drug is not suitable for longer-term use because of its arbutin content.

Pediatric Use: Marjoram salve should not be administered to infants or small children.

DOSAGE

Mode of Administration: As an infusion, poultice, marjoram oil or marjoram herb.

Preparation: For internal use, pour 250 ml boiling water over 1 to 2 teaspoonfuls Marjoranae herba and strain after 5 minutes. When used externally, it is prepared as a mouthwash or poultice.

Daily Dosage: Sip 1 to 2 cups of tea throughout the day.

Storage: Dried Marjoram may be stored for up to 2 years in air-tight containers.

LITERATURE

Brosche T, Vostrowsky O, Über die Komponenten des ätherischen Öls aus Majorana hortensis Moench. In: Z Naturforsch 36C:23-29. 1981.

Herrmann K, (1962) Lebensm Unters Forsch. 116:224.

Kucera LS, Hermann Jr EC, (1967) Proc Soc Exp Biol Med 124: 865-874.

Lossner G, (1968) Planta Med 16:54.

Further information in:

Hänsel R, Keller K, Rimpler H, Schneider G (Hrsg.), Hagers Handbuch der Pharmazeutischen Praxis, 5. Aufl., Bde 4-6 (Drogen), Springer Verlag Berlin, Heidelberg, New York, 1992-1994 (unter Orignum majorana).

Leung AY, Encyclopedia of Common Natural Ingredients Used in Food Drugs and Cosmetics, John Wiley & Sons Inc., New York 1980.

Madaus G, Lehrbuch der Biologischen Arzneimittel, Bde 1-3, Nachdruck, Georg Olms Verlag Hildesheim 1979.

Steinegger E, Hänsel R, Pharmakognosie, 5. Aufl., Springer Verlag Heidelberg 1992.

Teuscher E, Biogene Arzneimittel, 5. Aufl., Wiss. Verlagsges. Stuttgart 1997.

Origanum Vulgare

Oregano

DESCRIPTION

Medicinal Parts: The medicinal parts are the oil extracted from the fresh or dried leaves through a process of steam distillation, the herb picked during the flowering season and freed from the thicker stems and dried, as well as the fresh flowering herb.

Flower and Fruit: The bright purple labiate flowers are in cyme-like panicles with elliptical, pointed and usually dark purple bracts, which are longer than the calyx. The calyx is tubular and has 5 even tips. The upper lip of the corolla is flat and the lower lip has 3 lobes, the middle one wider than the others. There are 4 stamens, the longer ones extending beyond the lower lip.

Leaves, Stem and Root: Origanum vulgare is a perennial, woody plant, which grows up to 90 cm. The upper part is branched. It has rhizome-like runners and is downy, bristly or velvet-like. The leaves are 10 to 40 cm long and 4 to 25 mm wide, ovate, entire-margined or slightly crenate, glabrous or pubescent, translucent punctate and petiolate.

Characteristics: The plant has an aromatic scent, similar to Origanum majorana.

Habitat: The plant is commonly distributed throughout Asia, Europe and northern Africa.

Production: Oregano consists of the above-ground parts of Origanum. It is harvested 5 cm above the ground during the flowering season and dried carefully on the field or under a roof.

Other Names: Mountain Mint, Origano, Wild Marjoram, Winter Marjoram, Wintersweet

ACTIONS AND PHARMACOLOGY

COMPOUNDS

Volatile oil (0.15-1.0%): chief components carvacrol (share 40-70%), gamma-terpinene (8-10%), p-cymene (5-10%), additionally alpha-pinene, myrcene, thymol. There are also strains with thymol, linalool, caryophyllene or germacren D as chief components

Flavonoids: including among others naringin

Caffeic acid derivatives: in particular rosmaric acid

EFFECTS

Oregano is antimicrobial.

INDICATIONS AND USAGE

The herb is used for respiratory disorders and complaints such as coughs and bronchial catarrh and as an expectorant. In folk medicine, it is used for dyspepsia, painful menstruation, rheumatoid arthritis, scrofulous, urinary tract disorders, and as a diaphoretic.

PRECAUTIONS AND ADVERSE REACTIONS

No health hazards or side effects are known in conjunction with the proper administration of designated therapeutic dosages.

DOSAGE

Mode of Administration: Oregano is used internally and externally.

Preparation: For internal use, pour 250 ml boiling water over 1 heaped teaspoonful and strain after 10 minutes; the tea can be sweetened with honey. The unsweetened infusion is used as gargle and a mouthwash. To use externally, pour 1 liter water over 100 gm drug and strain after 10 minutes; add to a full bath.

LITERATURE

Afshaypuor S et al., Volatile constituents of Origanum vulgare ssp. viride (syn. O. heracleoticum) from Iran. In: PM 63(2):179-180. 1997.

Afshaypuor S, Essential oil constituents of wild marjoram from Iran. In: PM 62, Abstracts of the 44th Ann Congress of GA, 133. 1996.

Further information in:

Hänsel R, Keller K, Rimpler H, Schneider G (Hrsg.), Hagers Handbuch der Pharmazeutischen Praxis, 5. Aufl., Bde 4-6 (Drogen), Springer Verlag Berlin, Heidelberg, New York, 1992-1994.

Madaus G, Lehrbuch der Biologischen Arzneimittel, Bde 1-3, Nachdruck, Georg Olms Verlag Hildesheim 1979.

Steinegger E, Hänsel R, Pharmakognosie, 5. Aufl., Springer Verlag Heidelberg 1992.

Orris Root

See Iris Species

Orthosiphon Spicatus

Java Tea

DESCRIPTION

Medicinal Parts: The medicinal parts are the leaves and stem tips collected during the flowering season.

Flower and Fruit: The flowers are arranged in a whorl of 6, occasionally 10 blooms. The calyx tube is short with an upright, curved upper lip. The corolla is blue to light violet. The corolla tube is about 2 cm long with a broad upper lip that has 3 indentations. The lower lip is narrow and ovate-lanceolate. The 4 stamens are blue and 2.5 to 3 cm long. The style is as long as the stamen and the ovary has a disk. The fruit breaks up into 4 oval-oblong nutlets with a bumpy surface.

Leaves, Stem and Root: The plant is a 40 to 80 cm high herb. The stem is quadrangular and glabrous to pubescent with crossed opposite leaves. The leaves are about 75 mm long, usually short-petioled, ovate-lanceolate with an irregular, roughly serrate to dentate, occasionally crenate margin. The upper surface is brownish green, the lower surface gray-green with strong, protruding ribs and glandular punctate markings. The plant is similar to peppermint.

Characteristics: The herb has a weak, unusual smell. The taste is salty, bitter and astringent.

Habitat: The plant is found in an area extending from tropical Asia to tropical Australia and is cultivated in these areas and elsewhere.

Production: Java tea consists of the dried leaf and stem tips of Orthosiphon harvested shortly before flowering. The leaves are dried in well ventilated conditions.

Not To Be Confused With: Other Orthosiphon varieties and Eupatorium varieties from Java

ACTIONS AND PHARMACOLOGY

COMPOUNDS

Volatile oil (0.02-0.06%): including among others beta-caryophyllene, alpha-humulene, caryophyllene-epoxide

Flavonoids: in particular more highly methoxylised examples (0.2%) including among others eupatorin, sinensetin, scutellarine tetramethyl ethers

Caffeic acid derivatives: including among others 2,3-dicoffeoyltartrate, rosmaric acid

Diterpene ester: orthosiphole A to E

Triterpene saponins

EFFECTS

Java Tea has been shown to be a mild diuretic, to have a spasmolytic effect on smooth muscle, and to have antimicrobial effects.

INDICATIONS AND USAGE

- Infections of the urinary tract
- Kidney and bladder stones
- Liver and gall bladder complaints

The herb is also used to flush the efferent urinary tract and to treat and prevent renal gravel. In folk medicine, it is used for bladder and kidney disorders, gallstones, gout and rheumatism.

CONTRAINDICATIONS

Irrigation therapy is contraindicated in the presence of edema resulting from reduced cardiac or renal activity.

PRECAUTIONS AND ADVERSE REACTIONS

No health hazards or side effects are known in conjunction with the proper administration of designated therapeutic dosages.

DOSAGE

Mode of Administration: Comminuted herb for infusions and other galenic preparations for internal use.

Preparation: To make an infusion, pour 150 ml hot water over the drug and strain after 10 minutes.

Daily Dosage: The daily dosage ranges from 6 to12 gm drug. Adequate fluid intake (at least 2 liters per day) is essential.

LITERATURE

Hiller K, Pharmazeutische Bewertung ausgewählter Teedrogen. In: DAZ 135(16):1425-1440. 1995.

Proksch P, Orthosiphon aristatus (BLUME) MIQUEL - der Katzenbart. In: ZPT 13(2):63. 1992.

Takeda Y et al., Orthosiphol D and E, minor diterpenes from Orthosiphon stamineus. In: PH 33:411. 1993.

Teuber R, Neue Naturstoffe aus Orthosiphon stamineus Bentham. In: Dissertation Unviversität Marburg. 1986.

Further information in:

Hänsel R, Keller K, Rimpler H, Schneider G (Hrsg.), Hagers Handbuch der Pharmazeutischen Praxis, 5. Aufl., Bde 4-6 (Drogen), Springer Verlag Berlin, Heidelberg, New York, 1992-1994.

Madaus G, Lehrbuch der Biologischen Arzneimittel, Bde 1-3, Nachdruck, Georg Olms Verlag Hildesheim 1979.

Steinegger E, Hänsel R, Pharmakognosie, 5. Aufl., Springer Verlag Heidelberg 1992.

Teuscher E, Biogene Arzneimittel, 5. Aufl., Wiss. Verlagsges. Stuttgart 1997.

Wichtl M (Hrsg.), Teedrogen, 4. Aufl., Wiss. Verlagsges. Stuttgart 1997.

Oryza Sativa

Rice

DESCRIPTION

Medicinal Parts: The medicinal parts are the seeds.

Flower and Fruit: The panicle is up to 30 cm long. The husk is 7 to 9 mm long with 5 clearly protruding veins. They have 8 cm long, light or dark red awns or have no awns at all. The seed is tightly covered by the layers of the husk and is compressed from the side.

Leaves, Stem and Root: Rice is an annual. The stem is hollow, leafy and erect. The leaves are clasping and sheath-like at the base and grow up to 1 m in length. The leaf surface is up to 60 cm long and 1.5 cm wide. They have bristly ciliate spikelets at the base.

Habitat: Rice is probably indigenous to China and India. Today it is cultivated widely in wet, tropical and sub-tropical areas.

Production: Rice is the seed of Oryza sativa.

Other Names: Nivara

ACTIONS AND PHARMACOLOGY

COMPOUNDS

Starch (70%)

Proteins (prolamines, glutelins, globulins, albumins)

Fatty oil (1.0-1.8%)

Trypsin inhibitors

Lectins

Vitamins of the B-group

EFFECTS

Rice has been shown to be effective for pain relief and sedation of the digestive tract.

INDICATIONS AND USAGE

Rice is used during recovery from disorders of the gastrointestinal tract and diarrhea.

PRECAUTIONS AND ADVERSE REACTIONS

No health hazards or side effects are known in conjunction with the proper administration of designated therapeutic dosages.

DOSAGE

Preparation: Seeds boiled in water.

LITERATURE

Huesing JE, Murdock LL, Shade RE, Rice and stinging nettle lectins - insecticidal activity similar to wheat germ agglutinin. In: PH 30:3565. 1991.

Swaminathan S, Rice, This member of the grass family is one of three on which the human species largely subsists. In: Scientific American 250(1):80. 1984.

Further information in:

Belitz HD, Grosch W, Lehrbuch der Lebensmittelchemie, 4. Aufl., Springer Verlag Berlin, Heidelberg, New York 1992.

Kern W, List PH, Hörhammer L (Hrsg.), Hagers Handbuch der Pharmazeutischen Praxis, 4. Aufl., Bde. 1-8, Springer Verlag Berlin, Heidelberg, New York, 1969.

Oswego Tea

See Monarda Didyma

Ox-Eye Daisy

See Chrysanthemum Leucanthemum

Oxalis Acetosella

Wood Sorrel

DESCRIPTION

Medicinal Parts: The medicinal part is the fresh flowering plant with the root.

Flower and Fruit: The flower is white or reddish-white, red-veined and solitary with yellow spots. The pedicle is longer than the leaves. There are 5 sepals and 5 petals, 10 stamens and 1 ovary with 5 styles. The fruit is an ovate capsule. It is pentangular, tearing open in long slits when ripe, thus freeing the seeds.

Leaves, Stem and Root: The plant grows from approximately 5 to 12 cm tall. The leaves are basal, tender, long-petioled and trifoliate. The leaflets are broad, obovate-cordate, downy and often tinged red underneath. The stem is leafless apart from bracts above the middle, which are fused at the base.

Characteristics: The plant has a pleasant sour odor.

Habitat: The plant is commonly found in woods and forests throughout Europe.

Production: Wood Sorrel is the fresh plant, in blossom, of Oxalis acetosella.

Other Names: Cuckoo Bread, Cuckowes Meat, Fairy Bells, Green Sauce, Hallelujah, Shamrock, Sour Trefoil, Stickwort, Stubwort, Surelle, Three-leaved Grass, Wood Sour

ACTIONS AND PHARMACOLOGY

COMPOUNDS

Oxalic acid (0.3-1.25%)

EFFECTS

The drug, including the green parts of the plant, contains clover acid, which in small amounts, effects gallbladder activity (diuretic). The fresh plant has a high Vitamin C content.

INDICATIONS AND USAGE

Wood Sorrel is used for liver and digestive disorders. In the past, the fresh leaves were also used to treat scurvy and wounds and inflammation of the gums.

PRECAUTIONS AND ADVERSE REACTIONS

No health hazards or side effects are known in conjunction with the proper administration of designated therapeutic dosages. Oxalic acid poisonings can occur only through the ingestion of very large quantities of the leaves, as for example in salad. The poisonings mentioned in older scientific literature seem dubious.

DOSAGE

Mode of Administration: Ground and as an extract. Wood Sorrel is no longer used as a remedy today.

LITERATURE

Tschesche R, Struckmeyer K, (1976) Chem Ber. 109:2901.

Further information in:

Kern W, List PH, Hörhammer L (Hrsg.), Hagers Handbuch der Pharmazeutischen Praxis, 4. Aufl., Bde. 1-8, Springer Verlag Berlin, Heidelberg, New York, 1969.

Madaus G, Lehrbuch der Biologischen Arzneimittel, Bde 1-3, Nachdruck, Georg Olms Verlag Hildesheim 1979.

Roth L, Daunderer M, Kormann K, Giftpflanzen, Pflanzengifte, 4. Aufl., Ecomed Fachverlag Landsberg Lech 1993.

Teuscher E, Lindequist U, Biogene Gifte - Biologie, Chemie, Pharmakologie, 2. Aufl., Fischer Verlag Stuttgart 1994.

Paeonia Officinalis

Peony

DESCRIPTION

Medicinal Parts: The medicinal parts are the dried ripe seeds, the fresh underground parts harvested in spring and the fresh root.

Flower and Fruit: The large flowers are solitary at the ends of the stems. The calyx consists of 5 green, partly corolla-like sepals. The wild species has 5 to 8 ovate, red petals that are 4 to 5 cm long. The cultivated forms have many more. The stamens are light-red with long yellow anthers. The 2 or 3 ovaries with red stigmas develop into tomentose follicles containing numerous, dark, glossy, pea-sized seeds.

Leaves, Stem and Root: In its winter state, the plant has a turnip-like rhizome and close, gnarled root fibers, brown on the outside and white inside. The stem is leafy, erect, lightly branched and about 50 cm high. The leaves are alternate, more or less petiolate with a dark green glossy upper surface and a light green finely pubescent undersurface.

Habitat: The plant is indigenous to the mountains of southern Europe from Portugal to Albania and Hungary as far as Asia Minor. It is widely cultivated as a garden plant.

Production: Peony flower consists of the petals of Paeonia officinal, Willdenow and/or Paeonia mascula. Peony root consists of the dried secondary roots of Paeonia officinals, Willdenow and/or Paeonia mascula. The cultivated peony roots are dug up in spring, cleaned and dried in the sun or artificially. The flowers are harvested in dry weather shortly after the end of flowering and dried quickly in the shade or in moderate sunshine.

ACTIONS AND PHARMACOLOGY

COMPOUNDS

Monoterpene ester glucosides of the pinan-type: chief components paeoniflorin the blossoms of Paeonia officinalis

Anthocyans: in particular paeonin (paeonidin-3,5-diglucoside)

Tannins (pentagalloyl glucose)

Flavonoids: in particular kaempferol glycosides

EFFECTS

Hypertonia has been reported in animal tests. No analgesic effect has been described.

INDICATIONS AND USAGE

Preparations of Peony are used for ailments of the respiratory tract, diseases of the skin and mucus membranes, fissures, anal fissures associated with hemorrhoids, gout and rheumatoid arthritis. In folk medicine, Peony root is used for neurasthenia and neurasthenia syndrome, neuralgias, migraines and allergic disorders such as excitability, epilepsy and whooping cough. Peony flowers were formerly used for epilepsy, as an emetic, as an emmenagogue and as an abortifacient.

PRECAUTIONS AND ADVERSE REACTIONS

No health hazards are known in conjunction with the proper administration of designated therapeutic dosages. Side effects that may occur, particularly in cases of overdosages, include gastroenteritis with vomiting, colic and diarrhea.

DOSAGE

Mode of Administration: Peony root is administered as a tincture. Peony flowers are used as an inactive ingredient in cough and fumigant teas and as a coloring agent in cough syrup.

Preparation: To make an infusion, use 1 gm Peony flowers per cup water.

Daily Dosage: Drink one cup of infusion per day.

LITERATURE

Caesar W, Die Pfingstrose. In: DAZ 130(23):1339. 1990.

Further information in:

Hänsel R, Keller K, Rimpler H, Schneider G (Hrsg.), Hagers Handbuch der Pharmazeutischen Praxis, 5. Aufl., Bde 4-6 (Drogen), Springer Verlag Berlin, Heidelberg, New York, 1992-1994.

Hikino H, Economic and Medicinal Plant Research, Vol I., Academic Press UK 1985.

Lewin L, Gifte und Vergiftungen, 6. Aufl., Nachdruck, Haug Verlag, Heidelberg 1992.

Madaus G, Lehrbuch der Biologischen Arzneimittel, Bde 1-3, Nachdruck, Georg Olms Verlag Hildesheim 1979.

Roth L, Daunderer M, Kormann K, Giftpflanzen, Pflanzengifte, 4. Aufl., Ecomed Fachverlag Landsberg Lech 1993.

Teuscher E, Lindequist U, Biogene Gifte - Biologie, Chemie, Pharmakologie, 2. Aufl., Fischer Verlag Stuttgart 1994.

Wichtl M (Hrsg.), Teedrogen, 4. Aufl., Wiss. Verlagsges. Stuttgart 1997.

Pagoda Tree

See Sophora Japonica

Panax Ginseng

Ginseng

DESCRIPTION

Medicinal Parts: The medicinal part is the dried root.

Flower and Fruit: The inflorescence is simple or branched with 1 to 3 umbels of 15 to 30 flowers. The flowers are androgynous and have greenish-yellow corollas. The ovary is inferior. The fruit is a pea-sized, globose to reniform, scarlet, smooth and glossy drupe, which contains 2 seeds.

Leaves, Stem and Root: The plant is perennial, erect and 30 to 80 cm high. It has a glabrous, round stem and bears terminal whorls of 3 to 5 palmate leaves. The leaflets are thin, finely serrate, gradually acuminate, 7 to 20 cm long and 2 to 5 cm wide. The plant has a fusiform rhizome, which is often palmate at the tip giving it a human-like form.

Habitat: Panax ginseng is indigenous to China. It is cultivated in China, Korea, Japan and Russia. Panax quinquefolius grows in the U.S.

Production: Ginseng root consists of the dried main and lateral root and root hairs of Panax ginseng.

Other Names: American Ginseng, Chinese Ginseng, Korean Ginseng

ACTIONS AND PHARMACOLOGY

COMPOUNDS

Triterpene saponins

Aglycone (20S)-protopanaxadiol: including ginsenoside Ra1, Ra2, Ra3, Rb1, Rb2, Rb3, notoginsenoside R4, Rs1, Rs2, malonylginsenoside Rb1, Rc, Rd

Aglycone (20S)-protopanaxytriol: including ginsenoside Re, Rf, Rg1, notoginsenoside R1

Aglycone oleanolic acid: including ginsenoside Ro, chikusetsusasaponin-V

Water-soluble polysaccharides: panaxane A to U

Polyynes: including falcarinol (panaxynol), falcarintriol (panaxytriol), examples estered with acetic acid or linolenic acid

EFFECTS

The main active agent is ginsenoside. In various stress models, (immobilization test and the coldness test), the resistance of laboratory rodents was increased.

INDICATIONS AND USAGE

■ Lack of stamina

Ginseng is also used as a tonic for invigoration and fortification in times of fatigue and debility and for declining capacity to work and concentrate. It is also used during convalescence.

PRECAUTIONS AND ADVERSE REACTIONS

Health risks or side effects following the proper administration of designated therapeutic dosages are not recorded.

OVERDOSAGE

Massive overdosages can bring about Ginseng Abuse Syndrome, which is characterized by sleeplessness, hypertonia and edema.

DOSAGE

Mode of Administration: Comminuted drug infusions, powder and galenic preparations for internal use. Various standardized preparations containing ginseng root are available.

Preparation: To make an infusion, pour boiling water over 3 gm comminuted drug and strain after 5 to10 minutes.

Daily Dosage: The average daily dosage is 1 to 2 gm root. The infusion may be taken 3 to 4 times a day over 3 to 4 weeks.

LITERATURE

Anonym, Kann Ginseng die Leistungsfähigkeit erhöhen? In: DAZ 132(12):XLVIII. 1992.

Anonym, Mythos-Tonikum-Arzneimittel. Ginsengextrakt bei Atemwegserkrankungen. In: DAZ 134(26):2461. 1994.

Avakian EV et al., (1984) Planta Med 50:151.

Baldwin CA et al., (1986) Pharm J 237:583.

Bauer R, Neues von ''immunmodulierenden Drogen'' und ''Drogen mit antiallergischer und antiinflammatorischer Wirkung''. In: ZPT 14(1):23-24. 1993.

Blasius H, Phytotherapie: Adaptogene Wirkung von Ginseng. In: DAZ 135(23):2136-2138. 1995.

Caesar W, Ginsengwurzel in Europa. Eine alte Geschichte. In: DAZ 131(19):935. 1991.

Fulder SJ, (1981) Am J Chin Med 9:112.

Hansen L, Boll PM, (1986) Phytochemistry 25(2):285.

Hirakura K, Morita M, Nakajima K, Ikeya Y, Mitsuhashi H, Polyacetylenes from them roots of Panax ginseng. In: PH 30:3327-3333. 1991.

Hyo-Won B, Il-Heok K, Sa-Sek H, Byung-Hun H, Mun-Hae H, Ze-Hun K, Nak-Du K, (1987) Roter Ginseng. Schriftenreihe des Staatlichen Ginseng-Monopolamtes der Republik Korea.

Kitigawa I, (1983) Yaligali Zasshi 103:612.

Konno C et al., (1984) Planta Med 50(5):434.

Matsuda H et al., (1986) Chem Pharm Bull 34(3):1153.

Obermeier A, (1980) Zur Analytik der Ginseng- und Eteutherococcusdroge. Dissertation Ludwig-Maximilians-Universität München.

Palmer BV, Montgomery ACV, Monteiro JCMP, (1978) Ginseng und mastalgia. Brit Med J I:284 (letter).

Petkov VD et al., Memory effect of standardized extracts of Panax ginseng(G 115), Ginkgo biloba(GK 501) and their combination Gincosan (PHL-00701). In: PM 59(2).106. 1993.

Pfister-Hotz G, Phytotherapie in der Geriatrie. In: ZPT 18(3):162-165. 1997.

Ploss E, (1988) Panax Ginseng C. A. Meyer. Wissenschaftlicher Bericht. Kooperation Phytopharmaka, Köln Bonn Frankfurt Bad Homburg.

Siegl RK, (1979) Ginseng abuse syndrome - problems with the panacea. J Amer Assoc 241:1614-1615.

Siegl RK, (1980) Ginseng and the high blood pressure. J Am Med Assoc 243:32.

Singh VK et al., (1983) Planta Med 47:234.

Singh VK et al., (1984) Planta Med 50:462.

Sonnenborn U, Proppert Y, (1990) Ginseng (Panax ginseng C.A. Meyer). Z Phytotherapie 11:35-49.

Sprecher E, Pflanzliche Geriatrika. In: ZPT 9(2):40. 1988.

Sprecher E, Phytotherapeutika als Wunderdrogen? Versuch einer Bewertung. In: ZPT 10(1):1. 1989.

Takahashi M, Yoshikura M, (1966) Yakugaku Zasshi 86:1051 and 1053.

Wichtl M, Pflanzliche Geriatrika. In: DAZ 132(30):1576. 1992.

Youn YS, (1987) Analytisch vergleichende Untersuchungen von Ginsengwurzeln verschiedener Provenienzen. Dissertation Freie Universität Berlin.

Further information in:

Chan, EH et al., (Eds) Advances in Chinese Medicinal Materials Research, World Scientific Pub. Co. Singapore 1985.

Frohne D, Pfänder HJ, Giftpflanzen - Ein Handbuch für potheker, Toxikologen und Biologen, 4. Aufl., Wiss. Verlagsges. mbH Stuttgart 1997.

Hänsel R, Keller K, Rimpler H, Schneider G (Hrsg.), Hagers Handbuch der Pharmazeutischen Praxis, 5. Aufl., Bde 4-6 (Drogen), Springer Verlag Berlin, Heidelberg, New York, 1992-1994.

Madaus G, Lehrbuch der Biologischen Arzneimittel, Bde 1-3, Nachdruck, Georg Olms Verlag Hildesheim 1979.

Roth L, Daunderer M, Kormann K, Giftpflanzen, Pflanzengifte, 4. Aufl., Ecomed Fachverlag Landsberg Lech 1993.

Schulz R, Hänsel R, Rationale Phytotherapie, Springer Verlag Heidelberg 1996.

Steinegger E, Hänsel R, Pharmakognosie, 5. Aufl., Springer Verlag Heidelberg 1992.

Tang W, Eisenbrand G, Chinese Drugs of Plant Origin, Springer Verlag Heidelberg 1992.

Teuscher E, Biogene Arzneimittel, 5. Aufl., Wiss. Verlagsges. mbH Stuttgart 1997.

Wagner H, Wiesenauer M, Phytotherapie. Phytopharmaka und pflanzliche Homöopathika, Fischer-Verlag, Stuttgart, Jena, New York 1995.

Papaver Rhoeas

Corn Poppy

DESCRIPTION

Medicinal Parts: The medicinal parts are the flowers and seeds.

Flower and Fruit: The flowers are solitary and terminal or axillary and have a diameter of 10 cm. The pedicles are bristly and irregularly curved. The two sepals are green, bristly and fall off. The 4 petals are orbicular, scarlet or crimson, rarely white or violet with a round, shiny, often white-bordered deep-black mark at the base. The fruit capsule is broad-elliptical, dark brown and reticulate-pitted.

Leaves, Stem and Root: Poppy is an annual, occasionally biennial, multiple-stemmed plant 25 to 90 cm high. The stems are erect to semi-erect, simple or branched with stiff, protruding hairs. They have basal rosette lanceolate leaves that are deeply indented cauline. The foliage leaves are oblong-lanceolate, pinnatefid to pinnatesect and very bristly.

Habitat: The plant is indigenous to Europe, northern Africa and temperate regions in Asia. It is established in North and South America.

Production: Corn Poppy flower consists of the dried petals of Papaver rhoeas as well as its preparations.

Other Names: Copperose, Corn Rose, Cup-Puppy, Headache, Headwark, Red Poppy

ACTIONS AND PHARMACOLOGY

COMPOUNDS

Isoquinoline alkaloids (0.1%): chief alkaloids rhoeadine, isorhoeadine, rhoeagenine

Anthocyans: including among others mecocyanin (cyanidin-3-isosophoroside), cyanin- mucilage

EFFECTS

No information is available.

INDICATIONS AND USAGE

Corn Poppy flower is used for diseases and disorders of the respiratory tract, for disturbed sleep, as a sedative and for the relief of pain. The effectiveness in the conditions indicated has not been established. In folk medicine, it is used in the manufacture of children's cough syrup, as a tea for insomnia, for pain relief, and as a sedative.

PRECAUTIONS AND ADVERSE REACTIONS

No health hazards or side effects are known in conjunction with the proper administration of designated therapeutic dosages. Reports exist in the scientific literature of children being poisoned by intake of the fresh foliage (with blossoms), with symptoms including vomiting and stomach pain. The drug itself is non-toxic due to the low level of alkaloid content.

DOSAGE

Mode of Administration: As a brightening agent in various tea mixtures, and as component of ''metabolic'' teas.

Preparation: To make an infusion, scald 2 teaspoonfuls drug, steep for 10 minutes and strain. (1 teaspoonful = approximately 8 gm drug)

Daily Dosage: As an expectorant for bronchial catarrh, drink 1 cup infusion 2 to 3 times a day. The infusion may be sweetened with honey.

LITERATURE

El-Masry S et al., (1981) Planta Med 41:61.

Fairbairn JW, Williamson EM, (1978) Phytochemistry 17:2087.

Gasic O et al., Hem Pregl 33:23. 1992.

Kalaw Y, Sariyar S, PM 55:488. 1989.

Willaman JJ, Hui-Li L, (1970) Lloydia 33 (3A): 1.

Further information in:

Frohne D, Pfänder HJ, Giftpflanzen - Ein Handbuch für Apotheker, Toxikologen und Biologen, 4. Aufl., Wiss. Verlags-Ges. Stuttgart 1997.

Kern W, List PH, Hörhammer L (Hrsg.), Hagers Handbuch der Pharmazeutischen Praxis, 4. Aufl., Bde 1-8: Springer Verlag Berlin, Heidelberg, New York, 1969.

Lewin L, Gifte und Vergiftungen, 6. Aufl., Nachdruck, Haug Verlag, Heidelberg 1992.

Roth L, Daunderer M, Kormann K, Giftpflanzen, Pflanzengifte, 4. Aufl., Ecomed Fachverlag Landsberg Lech 1993.

Teuscher E, Lindequist U, Biogene Gifte - Biologie, Chemie, Pharmakologie, 2. Aufl., Fischer Verlag Stuttgart 1994.

Wichtl M (Hrsg.), Teedrogen, 4. Aufl., Wiss. Verlagsges. Stuttgart 1997.

Papaver Somniferum

Poppy

DESCRIPTION

Medicinal Parts: The medicinal part is the latex extracted from the seed capsule.

Flower and Fruit: A solitary flower grows on a long, glabrous or pubescent pedicle. The flowers are erect with a diameter of 10 cm. There are 2 green, glabrous, falling sepals and 4 violet-white or red petals with a darker mark at the base. The fruit is round or ellipsoid and often has a very large capsule. The numerous seeds are reniform, pitted, black, blue or white-frosted.

Leaves, Stem and Root: The opium poppy is an annual that grows 30 to 150 cm high. It is a one-stemmed, blue-gray frosted plant. The stem is erect, straight or branched and produces, as does the whole plant, white milky latex. The leaves are entire, glabrous, serrated or crenate and clasping.

Characteristics: The cultivation of the plant and the extraction and sale of opium is banned in many countries.

Habitat: The plant originated in western Asia. It is cultivated worldwide commercially.

Production: Opium is the thickened latex of unripe poppy capsules, derived from incisions made in the fruit capsules of Papaver somniferum. The unripe poppy capsules are used in a similar way. Papaver somniferum is cultivated by growers. The unripe seed capsules, which are only suitable for the production of opium, are trimmed. Subsequent to drying, the processed latex is scraped off and formed into pieces of varying size. The obtained material or end product is referred to as Rohopium.

Other Names: Garden-Poppy, Mawseed, Opium Poppy

ACTIONS AND PHARMACOLOGY

COMPOUNDS

Isoquinoline alkaloids (20-30%): chief alkaloids morphine (3-23%), narcotine (2-10%), codeine (0.2-3.5%), papaverine (0.5-3%), thebaine (0.2-1%). The alkaloids are present as salts of meconic acid, lactic acid or fumaric acid.

Rubber (5-10%)

Resins

Mucilages

EFFECTS

Morphine is an analgesic that even in small doses, causes euphoria, then narcotic sleep. It slows down evacuation of the stomach, causing constipation and urine retention. Codeine is an antitussive. Papaverine is spasmolytic.

INDICATIONS AND USAGE

Morphine is used as an analgesic in colic, painful wounds, etc. Codeine is used to treat strong coughs. Papaverine is used to treat gallbladder colic, bronchial and urogenital spasms.

PRECAUTIONS AND ADVERSE REACTIONS

No health hazards are known in conjunction with the proper administration of designated therapeutic dosages. The following can occur as side effects: clonic twitching, constipation, dizziness, general weakness, headache, hyperthermia, itchy skin, rashes and trembling of the hands.

OVERDOSAGE

Overdosage leads to reduction of mental capacity, reactive euphoria, analgesia, miosis, bradycardia, slowed respiration, later to respiratory failure, cyanosis, tonic-clonic spasms, pylorospasm and sphincterism, intestinal atonia, nausea, vomiting, pulmonary and brain edemas. Numerous cases of death due to accidental poisoning, murder and suicide due to opium use are known. Following gastrointestinal emptying, (inducement of vomiting, gastric lavage with burgundy-colored potassium permanganate solution, sodium sulphate) and instillation of activated charcoal, the therapy for poisoning consists of electrolyte substitution, treating possible cases of acidosis with sodium bicarbonate infusions and administration of plasma volume expanders in the event of shock. Intubation and oxygen respiration may also be necessary. Naloxone (i.v.) is suitable as an antidote.

DOSAGE

Mode of Administration: Opium is obsolete as a drug. Morphine is administered as a pure substance and in combination with other active substances, although it has been extensively replaced by synthetic analgesia. Codeine is used by itself and in combination with other agents.

LITERATURE

Amann T, Zenk MH, Endogenes Morphin. In: DAZ 136(7):519-527. 1996.

Bethke T, Codein. In: DAZ 133(6):433. 1993.

Buch. In: Handbook of Experimental Pharmacology. Volume 104/I und 104/II: Opioids I und II. Springer-Verlag Berlin, Heidelberg, New York, 1993.

Buchbauer G et al., Headspace constituents of opium. In: PM 60(2):181. 1994.

Czygan FC, Hellas und Phytopharmaka. In: DAZ 135(51/52):4707-4711. 1995.

Freye E, Leopold C, Opiate und Opiatantagonisten. I. Theoretischen Grundlagen der Opioidwirkung. In: DAZ 131(29):1517. 1991.

Pfeifer S, Mohn - eine Arzneipflanze seit mehr als zweitausend Jahren, Teil 1 und 2. In: PA 17:467-479 et 536-554. 1962.

Répási J, Hosztafi S, Szabó Z, 5'-O-Demethylnarcotin: A New Alkaloide from Papaver somniferum. In: PM 59(5):477. 1993.

Znek MH, Über das Opium, das den Schmerz besiegt und die Sucht weckt. In: PZ 139(48):4185. 1994.

Further information in:

Frohne D, Pfänder HJ, Giftpflanzen - Ein Handbuch für Apotheker, Toxikologen und Biologen, 4. Aufl., Wiss. Verlags-Ges. Stuttgart 1997.

Kern W, List PH, Hörhammer L (Hrsg.), Hagers Handbuch der Pharmazeutischen Praxis, 4. Aufl., Bde. 1-8, Springer Verlag Berlin, Heidelberg, New York, 1969.

Lewin L, Gifte und Vergiftungen, 6. Aufl., Nachdruck, Haug Verlag, Heidelberg 1992.

Roth L, Daunderer M, Kormann K, Giftpflanzen, Pflanzengifte, 4. Aufl., Ecomed Fachverlag Landsberg Lech 1993.

Schulz R, Hänsel R, Rationale Phytotherapie, Springer Verlag Heidelberg 1996.

Steinegger E, Hänsel R, Pharmakognosie, 5. Aufl., Springer Verlag Heidelberg 1992.

Teuscher E, Biogene Arzneimittel, 5. Aufl., Wiss. Verlagsges. Stuttgart 1997.

Teuscher E, Lindequist U, Biogene Gifte - Biologie, Chemie, Pharmakologie, 2. Aufl., Fischer Verlag Stuttgart 1994.

Wagner H, Wiesenauer M, Phytotherapie. Phytopharmaka und pflanzliche Homöopathika, Fischer-Verlag, Stuttgart, Jena, New York 1995.

Papaya

See Carica Papaya

Pareira

See Chondrodendron Tomentosum

Parietaria Officinalis

Pellitory-Of-The-Wall

DESCRIPTION

Medicinal Parts: The medicinal part is the herb.

Flower and Fruit: The small, green, sessile flowers grow in axillary racemes and bloom the whole summer. The bracteoles are free and are shorter than the calyx. The filaments of the stamens are strangely jointed and so elastic that when they are touched before the flower has opened, they uncoil from their rolled up position and distribute the pollen. The achaenes are black.

Leaves, Stem and Root: The plant is a perennial, which is heavily branched, bushy, leafy and grows to 70 cm. It has a reddish hard stem and narrow petiolate, ovate-lanceolate or elliptical, long-acuminate leaves 2.5 to 5 cm long. The stem and the under surface of the leaf ribs are softly pubescent. The upper surface of the leaves is almost glabrous and the ribs sunken.

Habitat: The herb is indigenous to Europe.

Production: Pellitory-off-the-wall is the aerial part of Parietaria erecta.

Other Names: Lichwort

ACTIONS AND PHARMACOLOGY

COMPOUNDS

Flavonoids: including, among others, kaempferol-, quercetin- and isorhamnetin-3-glucosides, -3-sophoroside, -3-rutinosides, -3-neohesperidosides

Caffeic acid derivatives

Bitter principles

EFFECTS

The drug is a mild diuretic.

INDICATIONS AND USAGE

The herb is used to treat diseases of the urinary tract.

PRECAUTIONS AND ADVERSE REACTIONS

No health hazards or side effects are known in conjunction with the proper administration of designated therapeutic dosages.

DOSAGE

Mode of Administration: The herb is obsolete as a drug, but is occasionally used in medicinal preparations.

LITERATURE

Budzianowski J et al., (1985) J Nat Prod 48(2):336.

Geraci D et al., (1978) Immunochemistry 15:491.

Further information in:

Hegnauer R, Chemotaxonomie der Pflanzen, Bde 1-11, Birkhäuser Verlag Basel, Boston, Berlin 1962-1997.

Kern W, List PH, Hörhammer L (Hrsg.), Hagers Handbuch der Pharmazeutischen Praxis, 4. Aufl., Bde. 1-8, Springer Verlag Berlin, Heidelberg, New York, 1969.

Madaus G, Lehrbuch der Biologischen Arzneimittel, Bde 1-3, Nachdruck, Georg Olms Verlag Hildesheim 1979.

Paris Quadrifolia

Herb Paris

DESCRIPTION

Medicinal Parts: The medicinal part is the whole fresh plant when the fruit begins to ripen.

Flower and Fruit: The flowers are solitary and terminal. The sepals are lanceolate, acuminate, 3-veined and 4 times as wide as the linear-awl-shaped petals. The stamens are thread-like to awl-shaped and bear linear anthers in the middle. The ovary has 5 thread-like stigmas, both of which are purple-brown. The fruit is a blue-black globular berry like a small cherry.

Leaves, Stem and Root: The 15 to 30 cm high plant is a perennial herb with a creeping, fleshy rhizome. The stem is erect, round, unbranched and crowned by 4 acuminate leaves. The leaves are whorled, almost obovate, acute, entire-margined and glabrous. The leaves have 3 to 5 ribs. They are dark green and matte above, pale and slightly glossy beneath.

Characteristics: The plant has an unpleasant smell and is poisonous.

Habitat: The plant is indigenous to Europe and Asian Russia.

Production: Herb Paris is the fresh plant of Paris quadrifolia, when the fruit is ripe.

Not To Be Confused With: Poisoning can occur in children when they confuse the fruit of the Herb Paris plant with that of blueberries.

Other Names: One Berry

ACTIONS AND PHARMACOLOGY

COMPOUNDS

Triterpene saponins: chief components are pennogenintetra glycosides, additionally including 1-dehydrotrillenogenin, among others

EFFECTS

The active agents are the saponines, paristyphnin, paridin, citric acid and pectin. The parissaponins cause irritation to the applied areas, which increases absorption of the drug. The toxic principle is paristyphnin, which can cause miosis and paralysis of the respiratory system.

INDICATIONS AND USAGE

Herb Paris is used as a homeopathic remedy for headaches, neuralgia, nervous tension, dizziness, palpitations and migraine.

PRECAUTIONS AND ADVERSE REACTIONS

The drug is considered poisonous. Symptoms of poisoning following intake of the berries include nausea, vomiting, diarrhea, miosis and headache. However, no serious poisonings have been recorded in this century.

DOSAGE

Mode of Administration: Herb Paris is available in homeopathic dilutions.

LITERATURE

Nohara T et al., Chem Pharm Bull 30:1851. 1982.

Further information in:

Frohne D, Pfänder HJ, Giftpflanzen - Ein Handbuch für Apotheker, Toxikologen und Biologen, 4. Aufl., Wiss. Verlags-Ges. Stuttgart 1997.

Kern W, List PH, Hörhammer L (Hrsg.), Hagers Handbuch der Pharmazeutischen Praxis, 4. Aufl., Bde. 1-8, Springer Verlag Berlin, Heidelberg, New York, 1969.

Lewin L, Gifte und Vergiftungen, 6. Aufl., Nachdruck, Haug Verlag, Heidelberg 1992.

Madaus G, Lehrbuch der Biologischen Arzneimittel, Bde 1-3, Nachdruck, Georg Olms Verlag Hildesheim 1979.

Roth L, Daunderer M, Kormann K, Giftpflanzen, Pflanzengifte, 4. Aufl., Ecomed Fachverlag Landsberg Lech 1993.

Teuscher E, Lindequist U, Biogene Gifte - Biologie, Chemie, Pharmakologie, 2. Aufl., Fischer Verlag Stuttgart 1994.

Parsley

See Petroselinum Crispum

Parsley Piert

See Aphanes Arvensis

Parsnip

See Pastinaca Sativa

Parthenocissus Quinquefolia

American Ivy

DESCRIPTION

Medicinal Parts: The medicinal parts are the bark, the branch tips, the fresh leaves, the berries and the resin.

Flower and Fruit: The inflorescences are fairly small and in yellowish green racemes. They produce dark-purple dye. The berries are pea-sized and the seeds are cordate.

Leaves, Stem and Root: American Ivy is a high climbing shrub with dark green branches, which sometimes develop adventitious roots. The flowering branches turn into regular, double-rowed creepers, which diminish towards the top. The leaves are long-petioled and divided into 5 elliptical, ovate or obovate, roughly serrate or dentate leaflets with suddenly pointed and usually somewhat rounded-off teeth. The upper surface is dark green and the undersurface is whitish-green and matte.

Habitat: Parthenocissi quinquefoliae originated in North America and is cultivated worldwide.

Production: American Ivy bark is the bark of the trunk and branches of Parthenocissus quinquefolia.

Other Names: American Woodbine, Creeper, False Grapes, Five Leaves, Ivy, Virginia Creeper, Wild Woodbine, Wild Woodvine, Woody Climber

ACTIONS AND PHARMACOLOGY

COMPOUNDS

Up to 2% oxalic acid is contained in the berries, however there is no information available on the constituents of the rind.

EFFECTS

The plant is diaphoretic, astringent and tonic.

INDICATIONS AND USAGE

American Ivy is used for digestive disorders.

PRECAUTIONS AND ADVERSE REACTIONS

No health hazards or side effects are known in conjunction with the proper administration of designated therapeutic dosages. The berries are considered poisonous. Older scientific literature describes the death of a child following intake of the berries (Lewin).

DOSAGE

Mode of Administration: The drug is ground for use as an infusion.

LITERATURE

Kern W, List PH, Hörhammer L (Hrsg.), Hagers Handbuch der Pharmazeutischen Praxis, 4. Aufl., Bde 1-8, Springer Verlag Berlin, Heidelberg, New York, 1969.

Lewin L, Gifte und Vergiftungen, 6. Aufl., Nachdruck, Haug Verlag, Heidelberg 1992.

Roth L, Daunderer M, Kormann K, Giftpflanzen, Pflanzengifte, 4. Aufl., Ecomed Fachverlag Landsberg Lech 1993.

Pasque Flower

See Pulsatilla Pratensis

Passiflora Incarnata

Passion Flower

DESCRIPTION

Medicinal Parts: The medicinal parts are the whole or cut dried herb and the fresh aerial parts. The yellow pulp from the berry is edible. Several other related species also have edible fruit or healing properties.

Flower and Fruit: The axillary pedicle grows up to 8 cm and bears 1 flower. The flowers are androgynous and rayed with a diameter of 5 to 9 cm and have an involucre. The 5 sepals are green on the outside, white on the inside and are tough. The 5 petals are white to pale red. There is a secondary corolla inside the petals made up of 4 thread wreaths arranged in rays around the axis of the flower, which are white on the inside and purple on the outside. The ovary has 3 carpels and 3 style branches, which end in a thickened stigma. The 5 stamens are joined at the base and fused to the androgynophor.

Leaves, Stem and Root: The passion flower is a perennial vine on a strong, woody stem reaching up to about 10 m in length. The vine is initially angular, later gray and rounded with longitudinally striated bark. The leaves are alternate, petiolate, serrate and very finely pubescent. The under surface is hairier than the upper surface. There are bumpy extra-floral nectaries on the leaf blades. Stipules and tendrils grow from the leaf axils.

Habitat: The plant is indigenous to an area from the southeast U.S. to Agentina and Brazil. It is cultivated in Europe as a garden plant.

Production: Passion flower herb consists of the fresh or dried aerial parts of Passiflora incarnata. The flowering shoots are cut 10 to 15 cm above the ground, usually after the formation of the first apple-sized fruit. The harvest is dried in a hay drier or in the air. For a maximum flavonoid content in the flowering shoot, twice yearly harvest is recommended; opinions are not, however, unanimous.

Not To Be Confused With: Passiflora caeulea, Passiflora foetida or Passiflora edulis

Other Names: Granadilla, Maypop, Passion Vine

ACTIONS AND PHARMACOLOGY

COMPOUNDS

Flavonoids (up to 2.5%): in particular C-glycosylflavones, including among others isovitexin-2′′-glucoside, schaftoside, isoschaftoside, isoorientin, isoorientin-2′′-glucoside, vicenin-2, lucenin-2

Cyanogenic glycosides: gynocardine (less than 0.1%)

Volatile oil (trace)

The frequently postulated presence of harmaline alkaloids could not be confirmed.

EFFECTS

A motility-inhibiting effect has been observed in animal tests.

INDICATIONS AND USAGE

■ Nervousness and insomnia

Passion Flower is used for nervous agitation, mild insomnia and nervous gastrointestinal complaints. In folk medicine, it is used internally for depressive states such as hysteria, general nervous agitation and insomnia and externally for hemorrhoids.

PRECAUTIONS AND ADVERSE REACTIONS

No health hazards or side effects are known in conjunction with the proper administration of designated therapeutic dosages.

DOSAGE

Mode of Administration: As a comminuted herb for tea and other galenic preparations for internal use. It is contained in herbal sedative bath additives.

Preparation: To make an infusion, pour 150 ml of hot water over 1 teaspoon drug and strain after 10 minutes. To make a rinse for the external treatment of hemorrhoids, put 20 gm drug into 200 ml simmering water, strain and use when cooled.

Daily Dosage: The daily dosage is 4 to 8 gm of drug in infusions and other galenic preparations. The infusion can be taken 2 to 3 times throughout the day and one-half hour before bedtime.

LITERATURE

Anonym, Phytotherapeutika: Nachgewiesene Wirkung, aber wirksame Stoffe meist nicht bekannt. In: DAZ 137(15):1221-1222. 1997.

Aoyagi N et al., (1974) Chem Pharm Bull 22:1008.

Bennati E, (1968) Boll Chim Farm 110:664.

Bennati E, Fedeli E, (1968) Boll Chim Farm 107:716.

Busse WW et al., (1984) J All Clin Immunol 73:801.

Caesar W, Passionsblume Kulturhistorische Aspekte einer Arzneipflanze. In: DAZ 137(8):587-93. 1997.

Hänsel R, Pflanzliche Beruhigungsmittel Möglichkeiten und Grenzen der Selbstmedikation. In: DAZ 135(32):2935-2943. 1995.

Loehdefink J, Kating, H, (1974) Planta Med 25:101.

Lutomski J, Malek B, (1975) Planta Med 27:381.

Lutomski J, Wrocinski T, (1960) Bui Inst Ros Lec 6:176.

Maluf E, Barros HMT, Frochtengarten ML, Benti R, Leite JR (1991) Assessment of the Hypnotic/Sedative Effects and Toxicity of Passiflora edulis Aqueous Extract in Rodents and Humans. Phytother Res 5:262-266.

Meier B, Passiflora incarnata - Portrait einer Arzneipflanze. In: ZPT 16(2):115-126. 1995.

Meier B, Passiflorae herba - pharmazeutische Qualität. In: ZPT 16(2):90-99. 1995.

Middleton E, Drzewiecki G, (1984) Biochem Pharmacol 33:3333.

Poethke W et al., (1970) Planta Med 18:303.

Proliac A, Raynaud J, (1986) Pharmazie 41(9):673.

Schilcher H, (1968) Z Naturforsch 23B, 1393.

Schilcher H, Pflanzliche Psychopharmaka. Eine neue Klassifizierung nach Indikationsgruppen. In: DAZ 135(20):1811-1822. 1995.

Speroni E, Minghetti A, (1988) Neuropharmacological activity of extracts from Passiflora incarnata. Planta Med: 488-491.

Further information in:

Hänsel R, Keller K, Rimpler H, Schneider G (Hrsg.), Hagers Handbuch der Pharmazeutischen Praxis, 5. Aufl., Bde 4-6 (Drogen), Springer Verlag Berlin, Heidelberg, New York, 1992-1994.

Leung AY, Encyclopedia of Common Natural Ingredients Used in Food Drugs and Cosmetics, John Wiley & Sons Inc., New York, 1980.

Madaus G, Lehrbuch der Biologischen Arzneimittel, Bde 1-3, Nachdruck, Georg Olms Verlag Hildesheim 1979.

Roth L, Daunderer M, Kormann K, Giftpflanzen, Pflanzengifte, 4. Aufl., Ecomed Fachverlag Landsberg Lech 1993.

Schulz R, Hänsel R, Rationale Phytotherapie, Springer Verlag Heidelberg 1996.

Steinegger E, Hänsel R, Pharmakognosie, 5. Aufl., Springer Verlag Heidelberg 1992.

Teuscher E, Biogene Arzneimittel, 5. Aufl., Wiss. Verlagsges. Stuttgart 1997.

Wagner H, Wiesenauer M, Phytotherapie. Phytopharmaka und pflanzliche Homöopathika, Fischer-Verlag, Stuttgart, Jena, New York, 1995.

Wichtl M (Hrsg.), Teedrogen, 4. Aufl., Wiss. Verlagsges. Stuttgart 1997.

Passion Flower

See Passiflora Incarnata

Pastinaca Sativa

Parsnip

DESCRIPTION

Medicinal Parts: The medicinal parts are the dried fruit, the dried herb, the dried root and the fresh, 2-year-old root of cultivated plants.

Flower and Fruit: The golden yellow flowers are in 8 to 12-rayed umbels, which are quite flat and contain androgynous blooms. There is no involucre or epicalyx or they consist of 1 or 2 dropping bracts. The petals are even-sized, golden yellow, 0.5 mm long when rolled up and 1 mm wide. The fruit is broad-elliptical, compressed and very like a lentil, 5 to 7 mm long and 4 to 5.5 mm wide. It is yellow-brownish when ripe. The fruit is marked with oil marks and hollows.

Leaves, Stem and Root: The plant is a biennial, which grows from 30 to 100 cm. The root is fusiform or tuberous like a carrot or turnip. It is whitish and usually bears only 1 stem. The stem is erect, angular, grooved, short-haired to glabrous and branched above. The leaves are simple pinnate, glossy above, paler and soft-haired beneath. The cauline leaves are on a long sheath, which is rolled at the edge. The basal leaves are petiolate and the leaflets are ovate-oblong and deeply lobed at the base. The terminal leaflet is 3 lobed and roughly crenate to serrate.

Characteristics: The turnip-like root tastes like carrot.

Habitat: Parsnip grows wild in most parts of Europe and Asia Minor as far as western Siberia. It is naturalized in the U.S. It is cultivated in Europe, America, Australia, India, China and southern Africa.

Production: Parsnip root or herb are the dried parts of Pastinaca sativa.

Not To Be Confused With: With other types of root such as corium, parsley roots and the root of bear's breech (also known as hogweed).

ACTIONS AND PHARMACOLOGY

COMPOUNDS: PASTINACAE HERBA GT RADIX

Furocoumarins: in particular angelicin, bergapten, xanthotoxin, Imperatorin, psoralen

COMPOUNDS: PASTINACLAE HERBA

Furocoumarins: See above

Volatile oil: chief components cis- and trans-beta-ocimene, trans-beta-farnesene, terpineols, palmitolactone

Flavonoids: including, among others, rutin in the berries

Volatile oil (1.9-3.1%): chief components including, among others, aliphatic ester, in particular octylbutyrate (29-85%), in certain breeds also octylacetate, additionally other esters and some myristicin

Fatty oil: chief fatty acid petroselic acid (46%)

EFFECTS

No absolute knowledge or information is available on effects.

INDICATIONS AND USAGE

PASTINACAE RADIX

Parsnip is used for kidney complaints, fever, as a diuretic and an analgesic.

PASTINACAE HERBA

The herb is used in kidney and gastrointestinal complaints and problems of digestion.

PRECAUTIONS AND ADVERSE REACTIONS

No health hazards or side effects are known in conjunction with the proper administration of designated therapeutic dosages. An increase in UV-sensitivity is possible among light-skinned persons (due to phototoxic effect of the furocoumarins).

DOSAGE

PASTINACAE RADIX

Daily Dosage: Take 1 teaspoon of freshly grated root, containing 50% plant material, 3 times daily.

PASTINACAE HERBA

Mode of Administration: Available ground, as a decoction of the dried herb.

Preparation: 1 handful of parsnip herb cooked in 1 liter of water for 10 minutes.

Daily Dosage: For the first 8 days, drink one wine glass full 3 times daily, during the second week drink one water glass full. The daily intake can be increased up to 2 liters. The cure takes 4 to 6 weeks.

LITERATURE

Ivie GW, Holt DL, Ivey MC, Natural toxicants in human foods: psoralen an raw and cooked parsnip roots. In: Science 213:909. 1981.

Kubeczka KH et al., Über das ätherische Öl der Apiaceae (Umbeliiferae). II. Das ätherische Öl der oberirdischen Teile von Pastinaca sativa. In: PM 31(2):173-184. 1977.

Stahl E et al., Über das ätherische Öl der Apiaceae (Umbeliiferae). VI.Untersuchungen zum Vorkommen von Chemotypen bei Pastinaca sativa. In: PM 371(12):49-56. 1979.

Further information in:

Hänsel R, Keller K, Rimpler H, Schneider G (Hrsg.), Hagers Handbuch der Pharmazeutischen Praxis, 5. Aufl., Bde 4-6 (Drogen), Springer Verlag Berlin, Heidelberg, New York, 1992-1994.

Madaus G, Lehrbuch der Biologischen Arzneimittel, Bde 1-3, Nachdruck, Georg Olms Verlag Hildesheim 1979.

Teuscher E, Lindequist U, Biogene Gifte - Biologie, Chemie, Pharmakologie, 2. Aufl., Fischer Verlag Stuttgart 1994.

Patchouli

See Pogostemon Cablin

Paullinia Cupana

Guarana

DESCRIPTION

Medicinal Parts: The medicinal parts are the peeled, dried, roasted and pulverized seeds which, have been formed into a thick substance with water and the paste prepared from the seeds.

Flower and Fruit: The usually unisexual flowers are inconspicuous, yellow to whitish and fragrant. They are in 30 long panicles, which only produce female or male flowers at any one time. The fruit is a hazelnut-sized, deep yellow to red-orange 3-sectioned capsule, which bursts open when ripe and releases 1 purple-brown to black seed, which is in a cup-like aril.

Leaves, Stem and Root: The plant is a woody, evergreen perennial vine up to 10 m long, which climbs through the jungle. It is bushier in its cultivated form. The leaves are large, palmate, coriaceous, distinctly ribbed and roughly crenate-serrate.

Characteristics: A paste is formed from the pulverized and roasted seeds, formed into rolls or bars and dried. The taste is astringent, bitter then sweet and the odor is reminiscent of chocolate.

Habitat: The plant is indigenous to the Amazon basin and has been introduced into other rain forests. The main area of cultivation is between Maues and Manau in Brazil.

Production: Guarana seeds are the seeds of Paullinia cupana. A preparation is also made from the ground seeds. Over a period of approximately 75 days, the pollinated flower develops a ''ripe'' guarana raceme, which is harvested by hand from October to December. Seeds (up to 80 per raceme) are taken out of the capsule shells, soaked for a time in water and then finally separated from the arillus. Subsequent to being dried in the sun, the seeds are roasted for 2 to 3 hours in special clay ovens. Once they have cooled, the parchment-like shell is removed and the seeds are ground down. Following this, the resulting paste is smoked over aromatic charcoal. The final product is dark brown in color and in stick form.

Other Names: Brazilian Cocoa, Guarana Bread, Paullinia

ACTIONS AND PHARMACOLOGY

COMPOUNDS

Purine alkaloids: chief alkaloid caffeine (3.6-5.8%), in addition, small amounts of theophylline and theobromine

Tannins (12%): oligomeric proanthocyanidins, condensed tannins

Cyanolipides: including among others 2,4-dihydroxy-3-methylene-butyronitrile

Saponins

Starch (30%)

Proteins (15%)

EFFECTS

A stimulating effect, due to the presence of caffeine occurs. Caffeine is centrally arousing, has a positive inotropic and in high concentrations has a positive chronotropic cardiac effect. It relaxes the vascular muscles (with the exception of cerebral vessels which constrict) and the bronchial tube.

Caffeine works as a short-term diuretic and increases gastric secretion. Furthermore, it increases the release of catecholamines. The drug has been observed to inhibit blood platelet aggregation.

INDICATIONS AND USAGE

In folk medicine, it is used as a stimulant and a tonic.

PRECAUTIONS AND ADVERSE REACTIONS

General: No health hazards or side effects are known in conjunction with the proper administration of designated therapeutic dosages. Quantities corresponding to up to 400 mg caffeine per day (7 to 11 gm of the drug), spread out over the day, are toxicologically harmless to a healthy adult habituated to caffeine, as for example through regular consumption of coffee or black tea.

One must, however, remember that the quantities of caffeine considered harmless are calculated to include all of the foodstuffs and beverages containing the substance (including coffee, tea, cola, etc). Caution is advised for persons with sensitive cardiovascular systems, renal diseases, hyperthyroidism, increased tendency to spasms and certain psychic disorders such as panic anxiety.

Pregnancy: Pregnant women should avoid caffeine, and under no circumstances exceed a dosage of over 300 mg per day.

Nursing Mothers: Infants whose nursing mothers consume caffeine products could suffer from sleeping disorders.

OVERDOSAGE

The first symptoms of poisoning are dysuria, vomiting and abdominal spasms. For caffeine poisonings see *Coffeae carbo.*

DOSAGE

Mode of Administration: The seeds of Paullinia cupana are grated and taken directly as powder or diluted in water or juice as a drink. It is not in use as a drug. It is available in various medicinal preparations.

LITERATURE

Frohne D, Guaraná - der neue Muntermacher. In: DAZ 133(3):218. 1993.

Katzung W, Guaraná - ein Naturprodukt mit hohem Coffeingehalt. In: Med Mo Pharm 16(11):330-333. 1993.

Further information in:

Hänsel R, Keller K, Rimpler H, Schneider G (Hrsg.), Hagers Handbuch der Pharmazeutischen Praxis, 5. Aufl., Bde 4-6 (Drogen), Springer Verlag Berlin, Heidelberg, New York, 1992-1994.

Leung AY, Encyclopedia of Common Natural Ingredients Used in Food Drugs and Cosmetics, John Wiley & Sons Inc., New York, 1980.

Steinegger E, Hänsel R, Pharmakognosie, 5. Aufl., Springer Verlag Heidelberg 1992.

Teuscher E, Biogene Arzneimittel, 5. Aufl., Wiss. Verlagsges. Stuttgart 1997.

Wichtl M (Hrsg.), Teedrogen, 4. Aufl., Wiss. Verlagsges. Stuttgart 1997.

Pausinystalia Yohimbe

Yohimbe Bark

DESCRIPTION

Medicinal Parts: The medicinal part is the bark.

Flower and Fruit: The inflorescence consists of racemes of yellow blooms.

Leaves, Stem and Root: The evergreen tree grows up to 30 m. The bark is gray-brown, fissured and split. It is often spotted. The inner fracture is reddish brown and grooved. The leaves are oblong or elliptical.

Characteristics: The taste is bitter. The plant has no odor.

Habitat: The plant grows in the jungles of west Africa, Cameroon, Congo and Gabon.

Production: Yohimbe bark consists of the dried bark of the trunk and/or branches of Pausinystalia yohimbe (syn. Corynanthe yohimbi).

ACTIONS AND PHARMACOLOGY

COMPOUNDS

Indole alkaloids (2.7-5.9%): including among others yohimbine (quebrachine) and its stereoisomers (alpha-yohimbine, beta-yohimbine, allo-yohimbine), ajamalicin, dihydroyohimbine, corynanthein, dihydrocorynanthein, corynanthin (rauhimbin)

Tannins

EFFECTS

No information is available.

INDICATIONS AND USAGE

Yohimbe bark is used for sexual disorders, as an aphrodisiac, and for feebleness and exhaustion.

CONTRAINDICATIONS

Yohimbe bark is contraindicated in liver and kidney diseases.

PRECAUTIONS AND ADVERSE REACTIONS

No health hazards are known in conjunction with the proper administration of designated therapeutic dosages. Side effects that can appear include, among others, anxiety states, elevated blood pressure, exanthema, excitatory states, queasiness, sleeplessness, tachycardia, tremor, and vomiting.

OVERDOSAGE

Overdosage leads to salivation, mydriasis, evacuation, lowered blood pressure and disorders of the cardiac impulse-conducting system with negative-inotropic effect. Death occurs through cardiac failure. Poisoning treatment includes gastrointestinal emptying (inducement of vomiting, gastric lavage with burgundy-colored potassium permanganate solution, sodium sulphate), instillation of activated charcoal, treating cardiac rhythm disorders with lidocaine or orciprenaline; possibly using physostigmine for its anticholinergic effect, administering electrolyte substitution and treating possible cases of acidosis with sodium bicarbonate infusions. In case of shock, plasma volume expanders should be infused.

DOSAGE

No information available.

LITERATURE

Buffum J, (1982) J Psychoactive Drugs 17:131.

Clark JT et al., Science 225:847.

Further information in:

Kern W, List PH, Hörhammer L (Hrsg.), Hagers Handbuch der Pharmazeutischen Praxis, 4. Aufl., Bde. 1-8: Springer Verlag Berlin, Heidelberg, New York, 1969.

Lewin L, Gifte und Vergiftungen, 6. Aufl., Nachdruck, Haug Verlag, Heidelberg 1992.

Madaus G, Lehrbuch der Biologischen Arzneimittel, Bde 1-3, Nachdruck, Georg Olms Verlag Hildesheim 1979.

Roth L, Daunderer M, Kormann K, Giftpflanzen, Pflanzengifte, 4. Aufl., Ecomed Fachverlag Landsberg Lech 1993.

Steinegger E, Hänsel R, Pharmakognosie, 5. Aufl., Springer Verlag Heidelberg 1992.

Teuscher E, Biogene Arzneimittel, 5. Aufl., Wiss. Verlagsges. Stuttgart 1997.

Wagner H, Wiesenauer M, Phytotherapie. Phytopharmaka und pflanzliche Homöopathika, Fischer-Verlag, Stuttgart, Jena, New York, 1995.

Peanuts

See Arachis Hypogaea

Pear

See Pyrus Communis

Pellitory

See Anacyclus Pyrethrum

Pellitory-Of-The-Wall

See Parietaria Officinalis

Pennyroyal

See Mentha Pulegium

Peony

See Paeonia Officinalis

Peppermint

See Mentha Piperita

Periwinkle

See Vinca Minor

Persea Americana

Avocado

DESCRIPTION

Medicinal Parts: The medicinal parts are the oil extracted from the leaves, the fresh leaves and whole fruit including the seeds.

Flower and Fruit: The flowers are in compact or loose racemes. They are 5 to 8.2 mm long and greenish. The inner and outer perianth circles are 4 to 6 mm long and elliptical to oval-elliptical. The anthers are 3.5 mm long and the filaments are 2.3 mm. The ovary is oval or pear-shaped and downy. It develops into a drupe which is green and fleshy and up to 18 cm long. The drupe is smooth with thick oily flesh and a very large seed.

Leaves, Stem and Root: The avocado is a tree up to 40 m in height and with a trunk 60 cm in diameter. The leaves are 6 to 30 cm long and 3.5 to 19 cm wide. They are narrow to broadly elliptical. The leaf surface is sticky and the lower surface is downy.

Habitat: The plant originated in central and southern South America and is cultivated in all tropical and subtropical regions today.

Production: Avocado oil is the oil the fruit of Persea americana. Avocado oil is recovered from the of the pericarp of Persea americana and refined if necessary.

ACTIONS AND PHARMACOLOGY

COMPOUNDS

Fatty oil: chief fatty acids oleic acid, palmitic acid, linoleic acid, palmitoleic acid (tocopherols, vitamin E)

EFFECTS

Avocado oil is an emollient, which improves rough ichtyotic skin.

INDICATIONS AND USAGE

Avocado is a main ingredient in so-called natural cosmetics.

PRECAUTIONS AND ADVERSE REACTIONS

No health hazards or side effects are known in conjunction with the proper administration of designated therapeutic dosages.

DOSAGE

Mode of Administration: As an active or inactive ingredient in various preparations (bath oils, ointments etc.).

LITERATURE

Albert K, Pharm Ztg 131:2279. 1986.

Heller H, Asche W, Seifen Oele Fette Wachse 111:164. 1985.

Further information in:

Hänsel R, Keller K, Rimpler H, Schneider G (Hrsg.), Hagers Handbuch der Pharmazeutischen Praxis, 5. Aufl., Bde 4-6 (Drogen), Springer Verlag Berlin, Heidelberg, New York, 1992-1994.

Teuscher E, Biogene Arzneimittel, 5. Aufl., Wiss. Verlagsges. Stuttgart 1997

Peruvian Balsam

See Myroxylon Balsamum

Petasites Hybridus

Petasites

DESCRIPTION

Medicinal Parts: The medicinal parts are the dried or fresh leaves, the underground parts collected in autumn and dried, the aerial parts collected towards the end of the flowering season and the whole fresh plant.

Flower and Fruit: The reddish flowers appear before the leaves, immediately after the snow has melted. They grow on flowering shafts from the base of the plant. The shaft is erect, thick and has purplish scales. The ones bearing the male flowers are 15 to 20 cm high and the ones bearing the female flowers are 40 cm high. The capitula of the mainly male flowers are initially in ovate, compact racemes. The flowers are tubular campanulate. The female flowers have a thread-like, tight tube and a bilabiate margin. The involucre is in 1 to 2 rows and is reddish. A prismatic fruit with a yellowish-whitish pappus develops from the flower.

Leaves, Stem and Root: The short and gnarled rhizome lies vertical or somewhat slanted in the ground. It is about 4 cm thick, brownish and thickened at the nodes. The root creeps and branches under the surface. The leaves are large, basal, long-petioled and roundish with a deeply cordate base. It is gray underneath and irregularly dentate.

Characteristics: Petasite has the largest leaves of all indigenous flora and has an unpleasant smell.

Habitat: The species is found in northern Asia, Europe and some areas of North America.

Production: Petasite consists of the whole plant of Petasites species. Petasite leaf consists of the leaves of Petasites species. The leaves are harvested before the end of the flowering season and quickly dried. Only leaves that are the size of the palm of the hand are picked, as these are said to have a higher level of active principles than the larger leaves. Petasite root consists of the dried underground parts of Petasites hybridus. A distinction is made between androdynamic and gynodynamic varieties. The roots of the former are dug up in autumn and of the latter in spring. After being dug up they are washed and dried. If drugs containing petasin are to be extracted, then cultivation must be carried out under laboratory conditions.

Not To Be Confused With: Other Petasite varieties and the leaves of Adenostyles alliariae or Tussilago farfara.

Other Names: Blatterdock, Bog Rhubarb, Bogshorns, Butterbur, Butter-Dock, Butterfly Dock, Capdockin, Flapperdock, Langwort, P. Vulgaris, Umbrella Leaves

ACTIONS AND PHARMACOLOGY

COMPOUNDS: PETASITIDIS FOLIUM

Sesquiterpene alcohol esters: chief components, including among others, according to chemotype - petasitine, neopetasitine and isopetasitine, or furanopetasin and 9-hydroxyfuranoeremophilone

Pyrrolizidine alkaloids: senecionine, integerrimine, senkirkine, presumably only in traces

Volatile oil: including, among others, dodecanal (aroma-bearer)

Flavonoids: including, among others, isoquercitrin, astragaline

Mucilages

Tannins

EFFECTS: PETASITIDIS FOLIUM

A spasmolytic effect has been demonstrated in animals.

COMPOUNDS: PETASITIDIS RHIZOMA

Sesquiterpene alcohol esters: including, among others, chief components according to chemotype - petasitine, neopetasitine and isopetasitine or furanopetasine and 9-hydroxyfuranoeremophilone

Volatile oil (0.1-0.4%): including, among others, 1-nonen, eremophilone, furanoeremophilone

Pyrrolizidine alkaloids: senecionine, integerrimine

EFFECTS: PETASITIDIS RHIZOMA

An antispasmodic effect on smooth muscle has been observed. The pyrrolizidine alkaloids with 1,2 unsaturated necine structure have a hepatotoxic, mutagenic, teratogenic and carcinogenic effect.

INDICATIONS AND USAGE

PETASITIDIS FOLIUM

Petasite or Petasite leaves are used to stimulate the appetite and to treat nervous cramp-like states and states associated with pain, colic and headaches. In folk medicine, the leaves are used internally for respiratory disorders, liver, gallbladder or pancreas disorders, as a prophylaxis for agitation and to induce sleep. Externally, the leaves are used to heal wounds and as a poultice for malignant ulcers.

PETASITIDIS RHIZOMA

■ Kidney and bladder stones

Petasitidis root is used as an adjunct in the treatment of acute spastic pain in the efferent urinary tract, particularly if stones are present. It is also used for respiratory disorders, particularly for coughs, whooping cough and bronchial asthma. Other uses include gastrointestinal disorders, migraine and tension headaches.

CONTRAINDICATIONS

All forms of the drug should not be used during pregnancy or by nursing mothers.

PRECAUTIONS AND ADVERSE REACTIONS

PETASITIDIS FOLIUM

General: No health hazards or side effects are known in conjunction with the proper administration of designated therapeutic dosages. One should entirely forgo any administration of the drug, due to the presence of pyrrolizidine alkaloids with hepatotoxic and carcinogenic effects in the parts of the plant above ground, as even mere traces of the alkaloids present a danger. The industrial manufacture of extracts virtually free of pyrrolizidine alkaloids is possible. The drug should not be used without knowledge of the pyrrolizidine alkaloids content.

Note: Alkaloid-free varieties are cultivated.

Pregnancy: The administration of the drug during pregnancy is to be completely ruled out.

Nursing Mothers: The drug should not be consumed by nursing mothers.

PETASITIDIS RHIZOMA

One should unconditionally forgo any administration of the drug, due to the presence of pyrrolizidine alkaloids with hepatotoxic and carcinogenic effect. The industrial manufacture of extracts virtually free of pyrrolizidine alkaloids is possible.

DOSAGE

PETASITIDIS FOLIUM

Preparation: To make an infusion, pour boiling water over 1.2 to 2 gm comminuted drug and strain after 10 minutes.

Daily Dosage: Drink 2 to 3 cups of the infusion per day.

PETASITIDIS RHIZOMA

Mode of Administration: Extracts obtained with ethanol or lipophilic solvents and other galenic preparations for internal use.

Daily Dosage: Preparations equivalent to 4.5 to 7 gm drug may be used. The daily dosage must not exceed 1 mg of pyrrolizidine alkaloids with 1.2 unsaturated necine structure including their N-oxides. Infusions should be used.

LITERATURE

PETASITIDIS FOLIUM

Bicket D et al., Identification and characterization of inhibitors of peptide-leukotriene-synthesis from Petasites hybridus. In: PM 60(4):318. 1994.

Brune K, Analgetische Wirkung von Pestwurz. In: DAZ 133(37):3296. 1993.

Brune K, Bickel D, Peskar BA, Gastro-Protective Effects by Extracts of Petasites hybridus: The Role of Inhibition of Peptido-leukotriene Synthesis. In: PM 59(6):494. 1993.

Bucher K, (1951) Über ein antispastisches Prinzip in Petasites officinalis Moench. Arch Exp Path Pharmacol 213:69.

Carle R, Pflanzliche Antiphlogistika und Spasmolytika. In: ZPT 9(3):67. 1988.

Chizzola R, Distribution of the pyrrolizidine alkaloids senecionine and intergerrimine within the Petasites hybridus. In: PM 58(7):A693. 1992.

Dorsch W, Neues über antientzündliche Drogen. In: ZPT 14(1):26. 1993.

Hasler A et al., Trace analysis of pyrrolizidine alkaloids by GC-NPD of extracts from the roots of Petasites hybridus. In: PM 62, Abstracts of the 44th Ann Congress of GA, 147. 1996.

Mauz Ch et al., (1985) Pharm Acta Helv 60:4.

Meier B, Die Pestwurz - Stand der Forschung. In: ZPT 15(5):268-284. 1994.

Novotný L et al., (1961) Tetrahedron Lett 20:697.

Röder E, Pyrrolizidinhaltige Arzneipflanzen. In: DAZ 132(45):2427-2435. 1992.

Further information in:

Frohne D, Pfänder HJ, Giftpflanzen - Ein Handbuch für Apotheker, Toxikologen und Biologen, 4. Aufl., Wiss. Verlags-Ges. Stuttgart 1997.

Hänsel R, Keller K, Rimpler H, Schneider G (Hrsg.), Hagers Handbuch der Pharmazeutischen Praxis, 5. Aufl., Bde 4-6 (Drogen), Springer Verlag Berlin, Heidelberg, New York, 1992-1994.

Madaus G, Lehrbuch der Biologischen Arzneimittel, Bde 1-3, Nachdruck, Georg Olms Verlag Hildesheim 1979.

Roth L, Daunderer M, Kormann K, Giftpflanzen, Pflanzengifte, 4. Aufl., Ecomed Fachverlag Landsberg Lech 1993.

Teuscher E, Lindequist U, Biogene Gifte - Biologie, Chemie, Pharmakologie, 2. Aufl., Fischer Verlag Stuttgart 1994.

Wichtl M (Hrsg.), Teedrogen, 4. Aufl., Wiss. Verlagsges. Stuttgart 1997.

PETASITIDIS RHIZOMA

Bicket D et al., Identification and characterization of inhibitors of peptide-leukotriene-synthesis from Petasites hybridus. In: PM 60(4):318. 1994.

Brune K, Analgetische Wirkung von Pestwurz. In: DAZ 133(37):3296. 1993.

Brune K, Bickel D, Peskar BA, Gastro-Protective Effects by Extracts of Petasites hybridus: The Role of Inhibition of Peptido-leukotriene Synthesis. In: PM 59(6):494. 1993.

Bucher K, (1951) Über ein antispastisches Prinzip in Petasites officinalis Moench. Arch Exp Path Pharmacol 213:69.

Carle R, Pflanzliche Antiphlogistika und Spasmolytika. In: ZPT 9(3):67. 1988.

Chizzola R, Distribution of the pyrrolizidine alkaloids senecionine and intergerrimine within the Petasites hybridus. In: PM 58(7):A693. 1992.

Dorsch W, Neues über antientzündliche Drogen. In: ZPT 14(1):26. 1993.

Hasler A et al., Trace analysis of pyrrolizidine alkaloids by GC-NPD of extracts from the roots of Petasites hybridus. In: PM 62, Abstracts of the 44th Ann Congress of GA, 147. 1996.

Meier B, Die Pestwurz - Stand der Forschung. In: ZPT 15(5):268-284. 1994.

Röder E, Pyrrolizidinhaltige Arzneipflanzen. In: DAZ 132(45):2427-2435. 1992.

Further information in:

Frohne D, Pfänder HJ, Giftpflanzen - Ein Handbuch für Apotheker, Toxikologen und Biologen, 4. Aufl., Wiss. Verlags-Ges. Stuttgart 1997.

Hänsel R, Keller K, Rimpler H, Schneider G (Hrsg.), Hagers Handbuch der Pharmazeutischen Praxis, 5. Aufl., Bde 4-6 (Drogen), Springer Verlag Berlin, Heidelberg, New York, 1992-1994.

Madaus G, Lehrbuch der Biologischen Arzneimittel, Bde 1-3, Nachdruck, Georg Olms Verlag Hildesheim 1979.

Roth L, Daunderer M, Kormann K, Giftpflanzen, Pflanzengifte, 4. Aufl., Ecomed Fachverlag Landsberg Lech 1993.

Teuscher E, Lindequist U, Biogene Gifte - Biologie, Chemie, Pharmakologie, 2. Aufl., Fischer Verlag Stuttgart 1994.

Wichtl M (Hrsg.), Teedrogen, 4. Aufl., Wiss. Verlagsges. Stuttgart 1997.

Petroselinum Crispum

Parsley

DESCRIPTION

Medicinal Parts: The medicinal parts are the oil extracted from the parsley fruit, the dried, separated schizocarp, the fresh or dried aerial parts, the dried underground parts and the whole fresh plant at the beginning of the flowering season.

Flower and Fruit: The inflorescences are long pedicled, terminal, occasionally apical, 10 to 20 rayed yellowish umbels. The involucre has 1 to 2 bracts and the epicalyx has 6 to 8 leaves. The petals are splayed with a curved tip. The style thickening is very developed. The fruit is orbicular-ovate, 2.5 mm long and greenish-gray.

Leaves, Stem and Root: The plant is a biennial. It is glabrous, has a characteristic odor and grows from 60 to 100 cm high. The usually numerous stems grow from 1 root and are erect, round, finely grooved, glabrous and branched. The root is thin or thick fusiform to tuberous, vertical and almost fiberless. The leaves are ovate and tripinnate. The upper ones are shorter stemmed and less compound. The leaflets are tripinnate.

Characteristics: Parsley has a spicy smell.

Habitat: The plant originated in the Mediterranean region and is cultivated worldwide today.

Production: Parsley consists of the fresh or dried plant section of Petroselinium. Parsley root is the dried root of Petroselinium crispum. The fresh herb is harvested from cultivations. Parsley seed consists of the dried ripe fruits of Petroselinum crispum.

Not To Be Confused With: The leaves of Aethusa cynapium.

Other Names: Hamburg Parsley, Persely, Petersylinge, Rock Parsley

ACTIONS AND PHARMACOLOGY

COMPOUNDS: PETROSELINI HERBA ET RADIX

In the foilage:

Volatile oil (0.02-0.3%): chief components, according to breed, up to 90%

Apiole

Myristicin

1-allyl-2,3,4,5-tetramethoxybenzole: additionally including among others mentha-1,3,8-triene (up to 50% share, aroma-bearer). alpha- and beta-pinene, alpha- and beta-phellandrene, hybrid strains also exist

Furocoumarins: including, among others, bergapten, oxypeucedanin, isopimpinellin, psoralen, xanthotoxin, imperatorin

Flavonoids (1.9-5.6%): chief components apiin

Vitamins: in particular ascorbic acid (up to 165 mg per 100 gm)

In the rhizome:

Volatile oil (0.05-0.12%): chief components of Petroselinum crispum ssp. crispum apiole, myristicin, terpinolene, tuberosum apiole, beta-pinene, additionally including, among others, alpha- and beta-pinene, (+)-limonene, beta-bisabolene

Phthalides: including, among others, ligustilide, senkyunolide

Furocoumarins: including, among others, bergaptene, oxypeucedanin, isopimpinellin, psoralen, xanthotoxin, imperatorin

Flavonoids (0.2-1.3%): chief components apiin

Polyynes: including, among others, falcarinol, falcarindiol

EFFECTS: PETROSELINI HERBA ET RADIX

In animal tests, increased tone and induced uterine contractions were observed.

COMPOUNDS: PETROSELINI FRUCTUS

Volatile oil (2-6%): chief components, according to breed

Apiole (58-80%)

Myristicin (49-77%)

1-allyl-2,3,4,5-tetramethoxybenzole (50-60%)

Alpha- and beta-pinene, beta-phellandrene among others

Furocoumarins: including, among others, bergapten, oxypeucedanin, isopimpinellin, psoralen, xanthotoxin, imperatorin

Fatty oil: chief fatty acid petroselic acid (60-80%)

INDICATIONS AND USAGE

PETROSELINI HERBA ET RADIX

- Infections of the urinary tract
- Kidney and bladder stones

The herb is used for flushing the efferent urinary tract and for the prevention and treatment of kidney gravel. In folk medicine, it is used for gastrointestinal disorders, jaundice, kidney and bladder inflammation, as a diuretic and as an emmenagogue.

PETROSELINI FRUCTUS

Preparations from the fruit are used for ailments and complaints of the gastrointestinal tract, the kidney and lower urinary tract and as a digestive.

CONTRAINDICATIONS

PETROSELINI HERBA ET RADIX AND FRUCTUS

The herb is contraindicated in patients allergic to parsley or apiole, those with kidney inflammations, and in pregnant women. Irrigation therapy should not be carried out in the presence of edema resulting from reduced cardiac and kidney function.

PRECAUTIONS AND ADVERSE REACTIONS

PETROSELINI HERBA ET RADIX

General: No health hazards or side effects are known in conjunction with the proper administration of designated therapeutic dosages. The drug leads rarely to contact allergies; photodermatosis is also conceivable following intensive skin contact between freshly-harvested plant parts and light-skinned individuals.

Pregnancy: Therapeutic doses are contraindicated in pregnancy.

PETROSELINI FRUCTUS

General: No health hazards or side effects are known in conjunction with the proper administration of designated therapeutic dosages. The drug leads rarely to contact allergies, photodermatoses occur somewhat more frequently following skin contact.

Pregnancy: Parsley fruit preparations are contraindicated in pregnancy; an abortive effect has been observed.

OVERDOSAGE

PETROSELINI HERBA ET RADIX AND FRUCTUS

The administration of higher dosages of the volatile oil or of preparations with high concentrations of the volatile oil can lead to poisonings. Symptoms include elevated contractility of the smooth musculature, in particular of the urinary bladder, of the intestines and of the uterus. Other symptoms may include: anuria, bloody stools, emaciation, fatty liver, hemolysis, methemoglobinuria and mucous membrane bleeding.

DOSAGE

PETROSELINI HERBA ET RADIX

Mode of Administration: Comminuted drug for infusions as well as other galenic preparations with a comparably small proportion of essential oil to be taken orally. Dry extracts are used in pharmaceutical products, such as tablets.

Daily Dosage: The daily dosage is 6 gm drug. Adequate intake of liquid is essential for flushing out treatment.

PETROSELINI FRUCTUS

Mode of Administration: Preparations of the fruit are for internal use.

Preparation: To make an infusion, pour boiling water over 1gm freshly pressed drug and strain after 10 minutes.

Daily Dosage: The average single dose is 1 gm. Two to 3 cups of the infusion can be taken daily.

Storage: Protect from light and moisture.

LITERATURE

PETROSELINI HERBA ET RADIX

Ashraf M et al., (1980) Pak J Sci Ind Res 23(3/4):128.

Bjeldanes LF, Kim I, (1977) J Org Chem 42:2333.

Busse WW et al., (1984) J All Clin. Immunol. 73:801.

Chaudhary SK et al., (1986) Planta Med (6):462.

Gijbels MJM et al., (1985) Fitoterapia 61(1):17.

Harborne Jr. B, Williams CE, (1972) Phytochemistry 11:1741.

Innocenti G et al., (1976) Planta Med 29:165.

MacLeod AJ et al., (1985) Phytochemistry 24(11):2623.

MacLeod AJ, Snyder CH, Subramanian G, Volatile aroma constituents from parsley leafs. In: PH 24(11):2623-2627. 1985.

Middleton E, Drzewiecki G, (1984) Biochem Pharmacol 33:3333.

Neuhaus-Carlisle K et al., Calcium-antagonstic activity of extracts and constituents of Petroselinum crispum and other phenylpropane derivatives. In: PM 59(7):A582. 1992.

Sökeland J, Phytotherapie in der Urologie. In: ZPT 10(1):8. 1989.

Stahl E, Jork H, Chemische Rssen bei Arzneipflanzen. I. Mitt. Untersuchung der Kulturvarietäten europäischer Petersilienhrkünfte. In: Arch Pharmaz 297:273-281. 1964.

Warncke D, Petroselinum crispum - Die Gartenpetersilie. In: ZPT 15(1):50-58. 1994.

Zheng GQ, Kenney PM, Lam LKT, Myristicin - a potential cancer chemopreventive agent from parsley leaf oil. In: J Agric Food Chem 40(1):107. 1992.

Further information in:

Hänsel R, Keller K, Rimpler H, Schneider G (Hrsg.), Hagers Handbuch der Pharmazeutischen Praxis, 5. Aufl., Bde 4-6 (Drogen), Springer Verlag Berlin, Heidelberg, New York, 1992-1994.

Hausen B, Allergiepflanzen, Pflanzenallergene, ecomed Verlagsgesellsch. mbH, Landsberg 1988.

Leung AY, Encyclopedia of Common Natural Ingredients Used in Food Drugs and Cosmetics, John Wiley & Sons Inc., New York 1980.

Madaus G, Lehrbuch der Biologischen Arzneimittel, Bde 1-3, Nachdruck, Georg Olms Verlag Hildesheim 1979.

Roth L, Daunderer M, Kormann K, Giftpflanzen, Pflanzengifte, 4. Aufl., Ecomed Fachverlag Landsberg Lech 1993.

Steinegger E, Hänsel R, Pharmakognosie, 5. Aufl., Springer Verlag Heidelberg 1992.

Teuscher E, Lindequist U, Biogene Gifte - Biologie, Chemie, Pharmakologie, 2. Aufl., Fischer Verlag Stuttgart 1994.

Teuscher E, Biogene Arzneimittel, 5. Aufl., Wiss. Verlagsges. Stuttgart 1997.

Wagner H, Wiesenauer M, Phytotherapie. Phytopharmaka und pflanzliche Homöopathika, Fischer-Verlag, Stuttgart, Jena, New York, 1995.

Wichtl M (Hrsg.), Teedrogen, 4. Aufl., Wiss. Verlagsges. Stuttgart 1997.

PETROSELINI FRUCTUS

Ashraf M et al., (1980) Pak J Sci Ind Res 23(3/4):128.

Bjeldanes LF, Kim I, (1977) J Org Chem 42:2333.

Busse WW et al., (1984) J All Clin. Immunol. 73:801.

Chaudhary SK et al., (1986) Planta Med (6):462.

Gijbels MJM et al., (1985) Fitoterapia 61(1):17.

Harborne Jr. B, Williams CE, (1972) Phytochemistry 11:1741.

Innocenti G et al., (1976) Planta Med 29:165.

MacLeod AJ et al., (1985) Phytochemistry 24(11):2623.

Middleton E, Drzewiecki G, (1984) Biochem Pharmacol 33: 3333.

Neuhaus-Carlisle K et al., Calcium-antagonstic activity of extracts and constituents of Petroselinum crispum and other phenylpropane derivatives. In: PM 59(7):A582. 1992.

Sökeland J, Phytotherapie in der Urologie. In: ZPT 10(1):8. 1989.

Stahl E, Jork H, Chemische Rssen bei Arzneipflanzen. I. Mitt. Untersuchung der Kulturvarietäten europäischer Petersilienhrkünfte. In: Arch Pharmaz 297:273-281. 1964.

Warncke D, Petroselinum crispum - Die Gartenpetersilie. In: ZPT 15(1):50-58. 1994.

Zheng GQ, Kenney PM, Lam LKT, Myristicin - a potential cancer chemopreventive agent from parsley leaf oil. In: J Agric Food Chem 40(1):107. 1992.

Further information in:

Hänsel R, Keller K, Rimpler H, Schneider G (Hrsg.), Hagers Handbuch der Pharmazeutischen Praxis, 5. Aufl., Bde 4-6 (Drogen), Springer Verlag Berlin, Heidelberg, New York, 1992-1994.

Hausen B, Allergiepflanzen, Pflanzenallergene, ecomed Verlagsgesellsch. mbH, Landsberg 1988.

Leung AY, Encyclopedia of Common Natural Ingredients Used in Food Drugs and Cosmetics, John Wiley & Sons Inc., New York 1980.

Madaus G, Lehrbuch der Biologischen Arzneimittel, Bde 1-3, Nachdruck, Georg Olms Verlag Hildesheim 1979.

Roth L, Daunderer M, Kormann K, Giftpflanzen, Pflanzengifte, 4. Aufl., Ecomed Fachverlag Landsberg Lech 1993.

Steinegger E, Hänsel R, Pharmakognosie, 5. Aufl., Springer Verlag Heidelberg 1992.

Teuscher E, Lindequist U, Biogene Gifte - Biologie, Chemie, Pharmakologie, 2. Aufl., Fischer Verlag Stuttgart 1994.

Teuscher E, Biogene Arzneimittel, 5. Aufl., Wiss. Verlagsges. Stuttgart 1997.

Wagner H, Wiesenauer M, Phytotherapie. Phytopharmaka und pflanzliche Homöopathika, Fischer-Verlag, Stuttgart, Jena, New York 1995.

Wichtl M (Hrsg.), Teedrogen, 4. Aufl., Wiss. Verlagsges. Stuttgart 1997.

Peucedanum Ostruthium

Masterwort

DESCRIPTION

Medicinal Parts: The medicinal part is the dried root.

Flower and Fruit: The white flowers form many-blossomed compound umbels. There is no involucre. The epicalyx has only a few leaves. The calyx is indistinct. The petals have indented, pointed tips.

Leaves, Stem and Root: The plant grows from 50 to 100 cm high. The rhizome is gray-brown and produces runners. The stem is round, slightly grooved and glabrous. The basal leaves are doubly trifoliate. The leaflets are ovate to oblong, about 4 cm wide, roughly serrate and pale green beneath. The lateral leaflets are di-pinnate. The terminal leaflet is tripinnate. The cauline leaves are small with a bulbous, membranous sheath.

Characteristics: Masterwort has an aromatic-bitter taste.

Habitat: The plant grows in central Europe.

Production: Masterwort rootstock is the rhizome of Peucedanum ostruthium. The thickened rhizomes are harvested. These are dug up in autumn or in spring then cleaned, freed from any root or green residue, cut and dried at a temperature of 35°C.

ACTIONS AND PHARMACOLOGY

COMPOUNDS

Volatile oil: chief components alpha-pinene, (+)-phellandrene, (+)-limonene, esters of isobutyric and isovaleric acid

Furocoumarins: in particular imperatorin, oxypeucedanin, osthrutol gamma-chromones: peucenine

Phthalides

Polyynes

EFFECTS

The drug is said to be stomachic and to have a mild sedative effect. Its main action is as a diuretic.

INDICATIONS AND USAGE

Masterwort is used for meteorism, flatulence, Roemheld syndrome, digestive disorders, weak stomach, and intestinal catarrh.

PRECAUTIONS AND ADVERSE REACTIONS

No health hazards or side effects are known in conjunction with the proper administration of designated therapeutic dosages. Light-skinned individuals may experience an increase in UV-sensitivity, due to the phototoxic effect of the furocoumarins.

DOSAGE

Mode of Administration: Masterwort is obsolete as a drug in German-speaking countries. It is occasionally used as a constituent in medicinal preparations in combination with other bitters. It is administered as a powder or as an infusion.

Preparation: To prepare an infusion, use a cold extraction of 1 teaspoonful of the drug.

Daily Dosage: The infusion can be drunk throughout the day. If using the powder form, 0.5 gm to 2 gm can be taken 2 to 3 times daily.

Storage: Store in a dry place, in closed containers.

LITERATURE

Gijbels MJM et al., (1985) Fitoterapia 61(1):17.

Schimmer O et al., (1980) Planta Med 40(1):68.

Further information in:

Hegnauer R, Chemotaxonomie der Pflanzen, Bde 1-11, Birkhäuser Verlag Basel, Boston, Berlin 1962-1997.

Kern W, List PH, Hörhammer L (Hrsg.), Hagers Handbuch der Pharmazeutischen Praxis, 4. Aufl., Bde. 1-8, Springer Verlag Berlin, Heidelberg, New York, 1969.

Madaus G, Lehrbuch der Biologischen Arzneimittel, Bde 1-3, Nachdruck, Georg Olms Verlag Hildesheim 1979.

Teuscher E, Lindequist U, Biogene Gifte - Biologie, Chemie, Pharmakologie, 2. Aufl., Fischer Verlag Stuttgart 1994.

Peumus Boldo

Boldo

DESCRIPTION

Medicinal Parts: The medicinal parts are the leaves.

Flower and Fruit: The inflorescences are racemes of whitish or pinkish campanulate flowers. The berries are small, yellowish green and edible.

Leaves, Stem and Root: The plant is a strongly aromatic, heavily branched evergreen shrub 5 to 6 m tall. The leaves are sessile, opposite, oval, about 5 cm long with an entire and slightly revolute margin. They are rather thick and coriaceous with a protruding midrib and a row of small glands on the upper surface. Both surfaces are slightly pubescent.

Characteristics: Boldo has a bitter, aromatic odor and a camphoraceous, lemony taste.

Habitat: The plant is indigenous to Chile and Peru. It is naturalized in mountainous Mediterranean regions and on the western coast of the U.S.

Production: Boldo leaf consists of the dried leaves of Peumus boldus.

Other Names: Boldu, Boldus

ACTIONS AND PHARMACOLOGY

COMPOUNDS

Isoquinoline alkaloids of the aporphine type: main alkaloid boldine

Volatile oil: chief components are p-cymene, cineol, ascaridiole

EFFECTS

Boldo has been shown to be antispasmodic, choleretic and to increase gastric secretions.

INDICATIONS AND USAGE

- Liver and gallbladder complaints
- Loss of appetite

Boldo is also used for dyspepsia and mild spastic complaints of the gastrointestinal tract.

CONTRAINDICATIONS

Boldo is contraindicated in patients with bile duct obstruction and those with severe liver diseases. Patients who have gallstones should consult a doctor before using the drug.

PRECAUTIONS AND ADVERSE REACTIONS

No health hazards or side effects are known in conjunction with the proper administration of designated therapeutic dosages. The volatile oil should not be used, because it contains up to 40% of the toxin ascaridiole.

OVERDOSAGE

Signs of paralysis are reported to appear following intake of very high dosages. A case is described in the older scientific literature in which depression, color hallucinations, sound hallucinations, and partial motor aphasia occurred following the consumption of boldine over a period of months.

DOSAGE

Mode of Administration: Comminuted herb for infusions and other, virtually ascaridol-free preparations for internal application. Because of the ascaridol content, essential oil and distillates of boldo leaf should not be used.

Daily Dosage: The average daily dosage is 4.5 gm drug.

LITERATURE

Betts TJ, J Chromatogr 511:373. 1990.

Bombardelli, E et al., (1976) Fitoterapia 47:3.

Kreitmar H, (1952) Pharmazie 7:507.

Reuter HD, Pflanzliche Gallentherapeutika (Teil I) und (Teil II). In: ZPT 16(1):13-20 u. 77-89. 1995.

Urzúa A, Acuna P, (1983) Fitoterapia 4:175.

Wolters B, Arzneipflanzen und Volksmedizin Chiles. In: DAZ 134(39):3693. 1994.

Further information in:

Kern W, List PH, Hörhammer L (Hrsg.), Hagers Handbuch der Pharmazeutischen Praxis, 4. Aufl., Bde. 1-8, Springer Verlag Berlin, Heidelberg, New York, 1969.

Leung AY, Encyclopedia of Common Natural Ingredients Used in Food Drugs and Cosmetics, John Wiley & Sons Inc., New York 1980.

Madaus G, Lehrbuch der Biologischen Arzneimittel, Bde 1-3, Nachdruck, Georg Olms Verlag Hildesheim 1979.

Roth L, Daunderer M, Kormann K, Giftpflanzen, Pflanzengifte, 4. Aufl., Ecomed Fachverlag Landsberg Lech 1993.

Schulz R, Hänsel R, Rationale Phytotherapie, Springer Verlag Heidelberg 1996.

Steinegger E, Hänsel R, Pharmakognosie, 5. Aufl., Springer Verlag Heidelberg 1992.

Teuscher E, Biogene Arzneimittel, 5. Aufl., Wiss. Verlagsges. Stuttgart 1997.

Wichtl M (Hrsg.), Teedrogen, 4. Aufl., Wiss. Verlagsges. Stuttgart 1997.

Peyote

See Lophophora Williamsii

Phaseolus Vulgaris

Bean

DESCRIPTION

Medicinal Parts: The medicinal parts are the ripe, dried pods and the beans.

Flower and Fruit: The white, pink and lilac flowers are in lightly blossomed, peduncled racemes, which are shorter than their leaves. The calyx is bilabiate. The carina, stamens and style are twisted in a spiral. The fruit is a straight, smooth, hanging pod with a number of reniform seeds.

Leaves, Stem and Root: The annual plant grows from 30 to 60 cm high. It is heavily branched but not twining. The leaves are trifoliate, the leaflets are broad ovate and acuminate. The terminal leaflet is rhomboid.

Habitat: The plant probably originated in India and is found cultivated worldwide today. It is also supposed to have been found on old graves in Peru.

Production: The seed-free pods of Phaseolus vulgaris are harvested.

Other Names: Common Bean, Green Bean, Kidney Bean, Navy Bean, Pinto Bean, Snap Bean, String Bean, Wax Bean

ACTIONS AND PHARMACOLOGY

COMPOUNDS

Lectins: complex termed phytomitogen (tetrameric glycoproteins)

Saponins

L-pipecolic acid

Flavonoids

EFFECTS

A weak diuretic action has been demonstrated in animal and human experiments. Chromium salts present in the drug may cause an antidiabetic effect.

INDICATIONS AND USAGE

- Infections of the urinary tract
- Kidney and bladder stones

Bean is used as a supportive treatment for inability to urinate. In folk medicine, it is used as a diuretic and antidiabetic.

PRECAUTIONS AND ADVERSE REACTIONS

No health hazards or side effects are known in conjunction with the proper administration of designated therapeutic dosages, in the form of heated infusions.

OVERDOSAGE

Poisonings following the intake of large quantities of fresh green bean husks (or of raw green beans) are not to be entirely ruled out, due to the lectins content, which varies greatly among the individual select cultivars. Symptoms include vomiting, diarrhea and gastroenteritis. The lectins are destroyed in the process of cooking.

DOSAGE

Mode of Administration: As a comminuted herb for decoctions and other galenic preparations for internal use. The drug is a component of various kidney and bladder teas and of standardized preparations of diuretics and "antidiabetics".

Preparation: To make an infusion, pour boiling water over 2.5 gm drug and strain after 10 to 15 minutes while still covered. (1 teaspoonful = 1.5 gm drug)

Daily Dosage: The recommended daily dosage is 5 to 15 gm of herb.

LITERATURE

Pusztai A et al., Recent advances in the study of the nutrtional toxicity of kidney bean (Phaseolus vulgaris) lectins in rat. In: Toxicon 20(1): R195. 1982.

Further information in:

Kern W, List PH, Hörhammer L (Hrsg.), Hagers Handbuch der Pharmazeutischen Praxis, 4. Aufl., Bde. 1-8, Springer Verlag Berlin, Heidelberg, New York, 1969.

Madaus G, Lehrbuch der Biologischen Arzneimittel, Bde 1-3, Nachdruck, Georg Olms Verlag Hildesheim 1979.

Roth L, Daunderer M, Kormann K, Giftpflanzen, Pflanzengifte, 4. Aufl., Ecomed Fachverlag Landsberg Lech 1993.

Steinegger E, Hänsel R, Pharmakognosie, 5. Aufl., Springer Verlag Heidelberg 1992.

Teuscher E, Lindequist U, Biogene Gifte - Biologie, Chemie, Pharmakologie, 2. Aufl., Fischer Verlag Stuttgart 1994.

Wagner H, Wiesenauer M, Phytotherapie. Phytopharmaka und pflanzliche Homöopathika, Fischer-Verlag, Stuttgart, Jena, New York 1995.

Wichtl M (Hrsg.), Teedrogen, 4. Aufl., Wiss. Verlagsges. Stuttgart 1997.

Phoenix Dactylifera

Date Palm

DESCRIPTION

Medicinal Parts: The medicinal part is the fruit.

Flower and Fruit: The flowers are androgynous and are in branched, cob-like inflorescence. The 3 carpels form 1 ovary. The fruit is a 1-seeded berry about 5 cm long (the date with the characteristic seed.)

Leaves, Stem and Root: The date palm is a woody plant growing primarily in girth. The leaves form a large long-petioled tuft at the top of the trunk. The lamina are frond-like pinnatifid.

Habitat: Date Palm is found from India to the Sahara.

Production: Dates are the fruits of Phoenix dactylifera.

ACTIONS AND PHARMACOLOGY

COMPOUNDS

Sugar (50%): saccharose, inverted sugar

Leucoanthocyanidine

Piperidine derivatives: pipecolic acid, 5-hydroxy-pipecolic acid (baikiain is found in the seeds only)

Fatty oil (10%)

EFFECTS

No information is available.

INDICATIONS AND USAGE

Used in folk medicine as a treatment for chest complaints (coughs etc.).

PRECAUTIONS AND ADVERSE REACTIONS

No health hazards or side effects are known in conjunction with the proper administration of designated therapeutic dosages.

DOSAGE

Mode of Administration: Formerly, Date Palm was used as an infusion for internal administration.

Preparation: Honey made from dates is produced in Algeria using the dates full of juice, which are dried in the sun; the leftover liquid results in date honey. Date honey is used to treat chest complaints.

LITERATURE

Wylegalla R, Biblische Botanik: Pflanzen und Früchte aus dem gelobten Land. In: DAZ 137(11):867-869. 1997.

Further information in:

Kern W, List PH, Hörhammer L (Hrsg.), Hagers Handbuch der Pharmazeutischen Praxis, 4. Aufl., Bde 1-8, Springer Verlag Berlin, Heidelberg, New York, 1969.

Phragmites Communis

Reed Herb

DESCRIPTION

Medicinal Parts: The medicinal parts are the stem and the rhizome.

Flower and Fruit: The flowers in long panicles of up to 30 cm with a thick crown of hair.

Leaves, Stem and Root: The plant is a strong grass with a long creeping rhizome. It grows up to 3 m and has gray-green leaves.

Habitat: Common worldwide.

Production: Reed herb and rhizome are the stem (base) and rhizome of Phragmites communis.

Other Names: Reed

ACTIONS AND PHARMACOLOGY

COMPOUNDS

Flavonoids: including, among others, tricin, luteolin, chrysoeriol, rutin, isoquercitrin

Vitamin A (5 mg/100 gm)

Ascorbic acid (Vitamin C, 100 mg/100 gm)

Vitamins of the B-group

Sugar: in particular saccharose, inverted sugar

Triterpenes: including, among others, beta-amyrin, taraxerol

EFFECTS

The active agents in the herb include Vitamins A, C, B1 and B2. The plant has diuretic and diaphoretic effects.

INDICATIONS AND USAGE

Digestive disorders (as diuretic and diaphoretic). The juice is used to soothe insect bites.

The herb is used in oriental medicine for diabetes, Leukemia and breast cancer.

PRECAUTIONS AND ADVERSE REACTIONS

No health hazards or side effects are known in conjunction with the proper administration of designated therapeutic dosages.

DOSAGE

Mode of Administration: Preparations are used internally and externally. The fresh and dried herb are used as infusions.

LITERATURE

Hegnauer R, Chemotaxonomie der Pflanzen, Bde 1-11, Birkhäuser Verlag Basel, Boston, Berlin 1962-1997.

Kern W, List PH, Hörhammer L (Hrsg.), Hagers Handbuch der Pharmazeutischen Praxis, 4. Aufl., Bde. 1-8, Springer Verlag Berlin, Heidelberg, New York, 1969.

Physalis Alkekengi

Winter Cherry

DESCRIPTION

Medicinal Parts: The medicinal parts are the ripe fruit and the leaves.

Flower and Fruit: The whitish, long-pedicled flowers are solitary and nodding. The calyx is fused and 5-tipped. The corolla is fused with a slightly 5-tipped margin. There are 5 stamens and 1 superior ovary. The fruit is a cherry-sized, globular, scarlet berry, enclosed in the swollen, orange-red calyx. It contains numerous flat, reniform seeds.

Leaves, Stem and Root: The plant is a perennial and grows from 30 to 60 cm. The stems are erect or ascending and angular with opposite, long-petioled, entire-margined leaves.

Characteristics: Winter Cherry has a lantern-like, enlarged calyx when the fruit is ripe.

Habitat: The plant is indigenous to central and southern Europe, China and Indochina and is naturalized in the U.S.

Production: Winter Cherry fruits are the ripe fruits of Physalis alkekengi.

Other Names: Cape Gooseberry, Coqueret, Strawberry Tomato

ACTIONS AND PHARMACOLOGY

COMPOUNDS

Whitasteroids: among others physalines A-C, F, L-O

EFFECTS

No information is available.

INDICATIONS AND USAGE

Winter Cherry is used as a diuretic in kidney and bladder conditions and in the treatment of gout and rheumatism.

PRECAUTIONS AND ADVERSE REACTIONS

The ripe fruit is edible, but unripe fruit can cause poisoning in animals.

DOSAGE

Mode of Administration: The drug is administered in a ground form and as an extract.

LITERATURE

Christen P, Pharm Acta Helv 61:242. 1986.

Dornberger K, Untersuchungen über potentiell antineoplastisch wirksame Inhaltsstoffe von Physalis alkekengi L. var. franchettii MAST. In: PA 41:265. 1986.

Jana M, Raynaud J, (1971) Plant Med Phytother 5:301.

Kawai M et al., PH 26:3313. 1987.

Kawai M, Matsuura T, (1970) Tetrahedron 26:1743.

Vessal M, Mehrani HA, Omrani GH, Effects of an aqueous extract of Physalis alkekengi fruit on estrus cycle, reproduction and uterine craetive kinase BB-isoenzyme in rats. In: ETH 34(1):69-78. 1991.

Völksen W, Zur Kenntnis der Inhaltsstoffe und arzneilichen Verwendung einiger Physalisarten - Ph. alkekengi, Ph. franchettii, Ph. peruviana. In: DAZ 117(30):1199-1203. 1977.

Yamaguchi H et al., (1974) Yakugaku Zasshi 94:1115.

Further information in:

Frohne D, Pfänder HJ, Giftpflanzen - Ein Handbuch für Apotheker, Toxikologen und Biologen, 4. Aufl., Wiss. Verlags-Ges Stuttgart 1997.

Kern W, List PH, Hörhammer L (Hrsg.), Hagers Handbuch der Pharmazeutischen Praxis, 4. Aufl., Bde. 1-8, Springer Verlag Berlin, Heidelberg, New York, 1969.

Madaus G, Lehrbuch der Biologischen Arzneimittel, Bde 1-3, Nachdruck, Georg Olms Verlag Hildesheim 1979.

Teuscher E, Lindequist U, Biogene Gifte - Biologie, Chemie, Pharmakologie, 2. Aufl., Fischer Verlag Stuttgart 1994.

Physostigma Venenosum

Calabar Bean

DESCRIPTION

Medicinal Parts: The medicinal parts are the seeds.

Flower and Fruit: The inflorescences are pendulous racemes of bean-like flowers. The fruit is a dark brown pod up to 15 cm long containing two or three dark brown or blackish kidney-shaped seeds, that are about 2.5 cm long. They are rounded at the ends, uneven and somewhat polished with the hilum extending along the whole convex side. The cotyledons are whitish.

Leaves, Stem and Root: The plant is a large, perennial, twining, woody climber with large, pinnate, trifoliate leaves.

Habitat: The plant is indigenous to western Africa and is cultivated in India and parts of South America.

Production: The calabar bean is the seed of Physostigma venenosum.

Other Names: Chop Nut, Ordeal Bean

ACTIONS AND PHARMACOLOGY

COMPOUNDS

Indole alkaloide: main alkaloid physostigmine, secondary alkaloids

EFFECTS

Calabar Bean causes an increase in tone in the parasympathetic system and the striated muscles. In particular, it causes the pupils to contract, thus reducing intraocular pressure. It is a glandular stimulant and increases peristalsis of the gastrointestinal tract. It reduces heart rate and is a curare antidote.

INDICATIONS AND USAGE

The drug is frequently used in the treatment of glaucoma. It is also a poison antidote. Its use in the treatment of Alzheimer's disease to reduce memory loss and confusion is being investigated.

PRECAUTIONS AND ADVERSE REACTIONS

The drug is only used in the extraction of physostigmine. Symptoms of poisoning include: diarrhea, nausea, salivation, sweats and vomiting.

OVERDOSAGE

Lethal doses can cause muscle twitching, spasms, tachycardia and cyanosis through asphyxiation. Following gastric lavage, poisonings are treated with atropine; in the case of spasms, diazepam is also used. Forced diuresis can be useful. The lethal dose for an adult is 6 to 10 mg. Poisonings are possible through inappropriate administration of physostigmine eye drops, due to drainage into the mouth or nose.

DOSAGE

Mode of Administration: As an eye medication, in drops and ointments. It is used as an antidote in the form of an injection solution. For gastrointestinal use, it has been replaced by synthetic prostigmine.

Daily Dosage: Apply 1 to 2 eye drops 3 times daily to the conjunctival sac.

LITERATURE

Die G, 125 Jahre Physostigmin. In: ZPT 11(2):7. 1990.

Morbus A, Was gibt es Neues aus der Forschung? In: DAZ 133(23):2090. 1993.

Further information in:

Kern W, List PH, Hörhammer L (Hrsg.), Hagers Handbuch der Pharmazeutischen Praxis, 4. Aufl., Bde. 1-8, Springer Verlag Berlin, Heidelberg, New York, 1969.

Madaus G, Lehrbuch der Biologischen Arzneimittel, Bde 1-3, Nachdruck, Georg Olms Verlag Hildesheim 1979.

Roth L, Daunderer M, Kormann K, Giftpflanzen, Pflanzengifte, 4. Aufl., Ecomed Fachverlag Landsberg Lech 1993.

Steinegger E, Hänsel R, Pharmakognosie, 5. Aufl., Springer Verlag Heidelberg 1992.

Teuscher E, Lindequist U, Biogene Gifte - Biologie, Chemie, Pharmakologie, 2. Aufl., Fischer Verlag Stuttgart 1994.

Teuscher E, Biogene Arzneimittel, 5. Aufl., Wiss. Verlagsges. Stuttgart 1997.

Phytolacca Americana

Poke Root

DESCRIPTION

Medicinal Parts: The medicinal parts are the dried root and the berries.

Flower and Fruit: The racemes are about 10 cm long and more or less erect. The flowers are androgynous. There is a calyx without a corolla. The involucre segments are 2.5 cm, broadly ovate, greenish-white and turn reddish at the fruit. There are 10 stamens and 10 carpels, which are fused. The fruit are 10 mm depressed-globose, purplish-black berries which cover the stem like a raceme. They are similar to blueberries.

Leaves, Stem and Root: The plant is a glabrous, perennial herb, somewhat woody at the base. The root is long and fleshy. The stems are 1 to 3 m high, hollow, bifurcated and often marked with grooves. The leaves are alternate, entire-margined, unpleasantly scented, 12 to 25 cm by 5 to 10 cm, ovate-lanceolate and petiolate.

Habitat: The plant is indigenous to the U.S. and has also become common in Mediterranean countries.

Production: Poke Root and berries are the root and fruit of Phytolacca americana.

Other Names: American Nightshade, American Spinach, Bear's Grape, Branching Phytolacca, Cancer-root, Coakum-Chongras, Cokan, Crowberry, Inkberry, Jalap, Phytolacca Berry, Phytolacca Root, Pigeon Berry, Pocan, Poke, Poke Berry, Pokeweed, Red Weed, Red-Ink Plant, Scoke, Skoke, Virginian Poke

ACTIONS AND PHARMACOLOGY

COMPOUNDS

Triterpene saponins (mixture termed phytolaccatoxin): phytolaccoside A-G, phytolaccasaponin B, aglycones 28,30-dicarboxy-oleans, phytolaccagenin

Lectins (pokeweed-mitogens)

Ribosome: inactivating proteins (1-RIP), in the seeds

Betacyans (red pigments): including among others phytolaccanin (betanin), particularly in the fruits

Lignans: caffeic acid aldehyde-oligomerics; including among others americanine A, B and D

Histamine: gamma-aminobutyric acid (in the rhizomes)

Saccharose: cyclitols

EFFECTS

The active compounds have been shown to be anti-inflammatory, antirheumatic and to aid digestion.

INDICATIONS AND USAGE

Poke root is used as an emetic due to the saponinan content in the root. It is also used for rheumatic disorders. Research is being conducted to determine its antiviral effect in flu, HSV-1 and polio.

PRECAUTIONS AND ADVERSE REACTIONS

General: All parts of the plants are poisonous, due to the presence of mucous membrane-irritating saponins and of the toxic, perorally-effective lectins. The toxicity is reduced through cooking, since this destroys the lectins.

Pediatric Use: Emergency poison treatment procedures should be instituted in small children who consume even one berry.

OVERDOSAGE

Symptoms of poisoning include: diarrhea (sometimes bloody), dizziness, hypotension, severe thirst, somnolence, tachycardia, vomiting, and in severe cases, spasm and death through respiratory failure. Up to 10 berries are considered harmless for an adult, but could be dangerous for a small child. Adults who consume more than 10 berries and small children who consume any berries should be treated for poisoning. This includes stomach and intestinal emptying (inducement of vomiting, gastric lavage with burgundy-colored potassium permanganate solution, sodium sulphate) and instillation of activated charcoal. Electrolyte substitution and the use of sodium bicarbonate to treat possible acidosis may be necessary.

DOSAGE

Mode of Administration: Administered as a powder, liquid extract and tincture. The berries are used by the food industry to produce red food coloring.

Storage: The drug should be stored in paper or sacks made from cloth.

LITERATURE

Aron GM, Irvin JD, (1980) Antimicrob Agents Chem 17:1032.

Kang SS, Woo WS, Triterpenes from the berries of Phytolacca americana. In: JNP 43(4):510-513. 1980.

Lewis WH, (1979) J Am Med Ass 242(25):2759 cit: CA 93:217921 f. 1979.

MecPherson A, In: Toxic Plants, Ed. AD Kinghorn, Columbia Press 1979.

Shin KH et al., (1979) Soul Taehakkyo Saengyak Opjukjip 18: 90.

Sick WW, Shin KH, (1976) Yakhak Hoe Chi 20(3):149.

Sick WW et al., (1976) Soul Taehakkyo Saengyak Opjukjip 15: 103.

Tomlinson JA et al., (1974) J Gen Virol 22:225.

Ussberg MA et al., (1977) Ann N Y Acad Sci 284:431.

Woo WS, Kang SS, (1978) cit.: C A 88:4750z.

Further information in:

Kern W, List PH, Hörhammer L (Hrsg.), Hagers Handbuch der Pharmazeutischen Praxis, 4. Aufl., Bde. 1-8, Springer Verlag Berlin, Heidelberg, New York, 1969.

Lewin L, Gifte und Vergiftungen, 6. Aufl., Nachdruck, Haug Verlag, Heidelberg 1992.

Madaus G, Lehrbuch der Biologischen Arzneimittel, Bde 1-3, Nachdruck, Georg Olms Verlag Hildesheim 1979.

Roth L, Daunderer M, Kormann K, Giftpflanzen, Pflanzengifte, 4. Aufl., Ecomed Fachverlag Landsberg Lech 1993.

Steinegger E, Hänsel R, Pharmakognosie, 5. Aufl., Springer Verlag Heidelberg 1992.

Tang W, Eisenbrand G, Chinese Drugs of Plant Origin, Springer Verlag Heidelberg 1992.

Teuscher E, Lindequist U, Biogene Gifte - Biologie, Chemie, Pharmakologie, 2. Aufl., Fischer Verlag Stuttgart 1994.

Wagner H, Wiesenauer M, Phytotherapie. Phytopharmaka und pflanzliche Homöopathika, Fischer-Verlag, Stuttgart, Jena, New York 1995.

Picea Excelsa

Spruce

DESCRIPTION

Medicinal Parts: The medicinal parts are the oil extracted from the needles, branch tips or branches and the fresh fir shoots.

Flower and Fruit: The male flowers are strawberry colored, the female are crimson or green. The male flowers are in short stemmed, cylindrical catkins scattered over the crown. The female flowers are in elliptical-cylindrical cones at the top of the crown. The ripe cones are sessile, hanging, globular-clavate and covered in rhomboid scales, which are thin, undulating at the tip and dentate. The wings of the small seeds are 3 times as long as the seeds themselves.

Leaves, Stem and Root: Picea excelsa is a tree which grows from 30 to 60 m high and has a column-like trunk with brown-red bark and a girth of about 2 m. The trunk is usually branched. The branches are horizontal and flat. The young shoots are reddish-brown or orange-red. The crossed-opposite leaves are scaly and imbricate. The needles remain on the tree for a number of years. On the upper surface of the shoots they are pointed forwards, on the lower surface they are pointed towards the sides. They are 1.3 to 2.5 cm long, rigid or curved, rich green and have a blunt horn-like tip.

Habitat: The tree is found in northern and central Europe.

Production: The essential oil is obtained from the fresh needles and twig tops or branches of Picea abies, (Syn: picea excelsa), Abies alba, Abies sachalinensis, or Abies sibirica. The essential oil is recovered from the needles by a 5 to 6 hour continuous process of aqueous steam distillation on a sieve base of layered and crushed fresh twigs. Preparations from the fresh 10 to 15 cm long shoots of Picea abies and/or Abies alba (Syn.: Abies pectinata) are collected in the spring.

Other Names: Balm of Gilead Fir, Balsam Fir, Canada Balsam, Fir Tree, Hemlock Spruce, Norway Pine, Norway Spruce, Spruce Fir

ACTIONS AND PHARMACOLOGY

COMPOUNDS: PICEA AETHEROLEUM

From Picea abies:

Bornyl acetate (5-25%)

Limonene (10-30%)

Camphene (10-25%)

Alpha-pinene (10-25%): additionally, including among others, santene, beta-pinene, Delta3-carene, myrcene

From Picea mariana:

Bornyl acetate (37-49%)

Camphene (10-17%)

Alpha-pinene (10%): additionally, including among others, beta-pinene, limonene, Delta3-carene, myrcene, santene

From Abies alba:

Bornyl acetate (2-10%)

Limonene (25-55%)

Camphene (9-20%)

Alpha-pinene (6-35%): additionally, including among others, beta-pinene, beta-phellandrene, Delta-carene, myrcene, santene

EFFECTS: PICEA AETHEROLEUM

The plants are secretolytic, antibacterial and hyperaemic.

COMPOUNDS: PICEAE TURIONES RECENTES

Volatile oil: chief components limonene, alpha-pinene, borneol, bornyl acetate

Ascorbic acid (Vitamin C)

EFFECTS: PICEAE TURIONES RECENTES

The essential oil has a secretory and antibacterial effect on the bronchial mucous membranes. Used externally, it acts as a rubefacient and improves circulation.

INDICATIONS AND USAGE

PICEA AETHEROLEUM

- Common cold
- Cough/bronchitis
- Fevers and colds
- Inflammation of the mouth and pharynx
- Neuralgias
- Rheumatism
- Tendency to infection

The essential oil is used internally for catarrhal conditions of the respiratory tract. Externally, it is used for catarrhal conditions of the respiratory tract, rheumatic and neuralgic pain and tension states.

PICEAE TURIONES RECENTES

- Common cold
- Cough/bronchitis
- Fevers and colds
- Inflammation of the mouth and pharynx
- Muscular and nerve pains
- Tendency to infection

The drug is used internally as a respiratory tract catarrh and externally for muscle pains and neuralgia. In folk medicine, it is used internally for tuberculosis and externally as a bath additive for mentally ill patients.

CONTRAINDICATIONS

PICEA AETHEROLEUM AND TURIONES RECENTES

Contraindications include bronchial asthma and whooping cough. Patients with extensive skin injuries, acute skin diseases, feverish or infectious diseases, cardiac insufficiency or hypertonia should not use the drug as a bath additive.

PRECAUTIONS AND ADVERSE REACTIONS

PICEA AETHEROLEUM AND TURIONES RECENTES

No health hazards or side effects are known in conjunction with the proper administration of designated therapeutic dosages, although bronchial spasms could be worsened.

DOSAGE

PICEA AETHEROLEUM

Mode of Administration: Embrocations of alcohol solutions, ointments, gels, emulsions, and oils are available, as well as bath additives and inhalants.

Daily Dosage: For internal use, place 4 drops of oil on a lump of sugar or in a little water and take 3 times a day. To use as inhalation therapy, add 2 gm of oil to hot water and inhale several times a day. For external application, rub several drops of oil into the affected area using liquid and semi-solid preparations that contain 10% to 50% of the drug.

Storage: Store in closed containers.

PICEAE TURIONES RECENTES

Mode of Administration: In galenic preparations for internal and external application.

Preparation: For inhalation therapy, place 2 gm of oil in hot water and inhale the vapors. To make a bath additive, boil 200 to 300 gm drug with 1 liter water and draw for 5 minutes; add to a full bath. Make sure it is possible to relax after the bath.

Daily Dosage: For internal use, 5 to 6 gm of drug is administered per day. Four drops of the essential oil may be placed in a little water or on a lump of sugar and taken 3 times a day. The inhalation therapy can be used several times a day.

LITERATURE

PICEA AETHEROLEUM

Glasl H, Wagner H, DAZ 120:64-67. 1980.

Kubeczka KH, Schultze W, Flavour Fragrance J:2.137-148. 1987.

Schantz von M, Juvonen S, Acta Bot Fenn 73:5-51. 1966.

Schantz von M, Juvonen S, PM 15:337-341. 1967.

Further information in:

Hänsel R, Keller K, Rimpler H, Schneider G (Hrsg.), Hagers Handbuch der Pharmazeutischen Praxis, 5. Aufl., Bde 4-6 (Drogen), Springer Verlag Berlin, Heidelberg, New York, 1992-1994.

Madaus G, Lehrbuch der Biologischen Arzneimittel, Bde 1-3, Nachdruck, Georg Olms Verlag Hildesheim 1979.

Steinegger E, Hänsel R, Pharmakognosie, 5. Aufl., Springer Verlag Heidelberg 1992.

Teuscher E, Biogene Arzneimittel, 5. Aufl., Wiss. Verlagsges. Stuttgart 1997.

Wagner H, Wiesenauer M, Phytotherapie. Phytopharmaka und pflanzliche Homöopathika, Fischer-Verlag, Stuttgart, Jena, New York 1995.

PICEAE TURIONES RECENTES

Glasl H, Wagner H, DAZ 120:64-67. 1980.

Kubeczka KH, Schultze W, Flavour Fragrance J:2.137-148. 1987.

Schantz M von, Juvonen S, Acta Bot Fenn 73:5-51. 1966.

Schantz M von, Juvonen S, PM 15:337-341. 1967.

Further information in:

Hänsel R, Keller K, Rimpler H, Schneider G (Hrsg.), Hagers Handbuch der Pharmazeutischen Praxis, 5. Aufl., Bde 4-6 (Drogen), Springer Verlag Berlin, Heidelberg, New York, 1992-1994.

Madaus G, Lehrbuch der Biologischen Arzneimittel, Bde 1-3, Nachdruck, Georg Olms Verlag Hildesheim 1979.

Pilocarpus Microphyllus

Jaborandi

DESCRIPTION

Medicinal Parts: The medicinal parts are the dried leaves.

Flower and Fruit: The numerous flowers are in terminal or axillary racemes that are up to 30 cm long and 0.5 cm wide. The pedicles are 0.1 to 1.5 mm long and have alternate bracts. The flowers have a diameter of 4 to 5 cm and are glabrous. The 5 sepals are free, broadly triangular to orbicular and coriaceous. The petals have forward bending tips and are thinly coriaceous and somewhat translucent. The oval anthers have an oblong gland. The disc is 0.5 mm high and 1.3 to 1.5 mm in diameter. The ovary is 0.5 mm and extends past the disc with a head-like stigma. The mericarp has roundish, flattened, black-brown seeds.

Leaves, Stem and Root: The plant is a tree or shrub 3 to 7 m high with a trunk diameter of 3 to 7.5 cm. The branches are pubescent when young and glabrous when older. The leaves are alternate to opposite, odd-pinnate with 1 to 5 pairs of pinna. The pinna are sessile, elliptical, distinctly asymmetrical at the base and have an indented tip. The leaflets are dull green, up to 5 cm long and 3 cm wide, with entire, slightly recurved margins and an uneven base. The ribs are prominent on the upper surface and have visible oil cells.

Characteristics: The taste is bitter and the odor is slightly aromatic.

Habitat: The plant grows in the northeastern part of Brazil.

Production: Jaborandi leaves are the dried leaves of Pilocarpus microphyllus.

Other Names: Arruda Brava, Arruda do Mato, Jamguarandi, Juarandi

ACTIONS AND PHARMACOLOGY

COMPOUNDS

Imidazole alkaloids (0.5-1.0%): chief alkaloid is (+)-pilocarpins, through drying and under storage conditions changing over to some extent into isopilocarpin, companion alkaloids including pilocarpidin, pilosin and others

Volatile oil: chief components are limonene and undecanone

EFFECTS

The drug affects the parasympathetic system. It increases the secretion of saliva and sweat and stimulates the smooth muscle of the gastrointestinal tract.

INDICATIONS AND USAGE

Jaborandi has been used in the treatment of glaucoma. In folk medicine, it is used as a diaphoretic and for diarrhea.

PRECAUTIONS AND ADVERSE REACTIONS

No health hazards or side effects are known in conjunction with the proper administration of designated therapeutic dosages. The drug is used today as an industrial agent for the manufacture of pilocarpins, but is used medicinally only for homeopathic applications.

The incorrect administration of pilocarpine eyedrops can lead to poisonings through leakage into the nose or mouth. Symptoms include: bradycardia, bronchial spasms, colics, collapse and possible cardiac arrest, convulsions, drop in blood pressure, dyspnea, nausea, severe salivation, strong secretion of sweat and vomiting.

OVERDOSAGE

The lethal dose is approximately 60 mg, corresponding to 5 to 10 gm of the drug. Individuals with cardiac and circulatory illnesses are particularly susceptible. Following stomach and intestinal emptying (gastric lavage, sodium sulphate), the treatment for poisonings consists of the instillation of activated charcoal with atropine and the use of diazepam in the case of spasms. Forced dialysis and the administration of plasma volume expanders can also be useful.

DOSAGE

Mode of Administration: Jaborandi is obsolete by itself as a drug.

LITERATURE

Craveiro AA et al., (1979) J Nat Prod 42:169.

Tedeschi E, Kamionsky J, Fackler S, Sarel S, Isr J Chem 11:731-733. 1973.

Further information in:

Hänsel R, Keller K, Rimpler H, Schneider G (Hrsg.), Hagers Handbuch der Pharmazeutischen Praxis, 5. Aufl., Bde 4-6 (Drogen), Springer Verlag Berlin, Heidelberg, New York, 1992-1994.

Lewin L, Gifte und Vergiftungen, 6. Aufl., Nachdruck, Haug Verlag, Heidelberg 1992.

Madaus G, Lehrbuch der Biologischen Arzneimittel, Bde 1-3, Nachdruck, Georg Olms Verlag Hildesheim 1979.

Roth L, Daunderer M, Kormann K, Giftpflanzen, Pflanzengifte, 4. Aufl., Ecomed Fachverlag Landsberg Lech 1993.

Steinegger E, Hänsel R, Pharmakognosie, 5. Aufl., Springer Verlag Heidelberg 1992.

Teuscher E, Lindequist U, Biogene Gifte - Biologie, Chemie, Pharmakologie, 2. Aufl., Fischer Verlag Stuttgart 1994.

Teuscher E, Biogene Arzneimittel, 5. Aufl., Wiss. Verlagsges. Stuttgart 1997.

Wagner H, Wiesenauer M, Phytotherapie. Phytopharmaka und pflanzliche Homöopathika, Fischer-Verlag, Stuttgart, Jena, New York, 1995.

Pilosella Officinarum

Mouse Ear

DESCRIPTION

Medicinal Parts: The medicinal parts are the flowering aerial parts.

Flower and Fruit: The yellow, composite flowers are solitary at the end of long pedicles. There are bright yellow, lingual florets. The lateral ones are usually striped reddish underneath. The bracts are linear and acute, with a membranous margin and are covered in star-hairs. They have black glandular hairs at the base. The fruit is cylindrical and has a simple, brittle tuft of hair.

Leaves, Stem and Root: The plant is a perennial herb, which grows up to 30 cm. Erect, leafless stems grow from the rosette of basal leaves. The plant produces long, leafy runners. The leaves are oblong or obovate to lanceolate. They bear long bristles, which are thickened at the base and are star-haired to tomentose beneath.

Habitat: The plant grows in large areas of Europe and temperate Asia. It is also found in North America.

Production: Mouse Ear is the aerial part of Pilosella officinarum.

ACTIONS AND PHARMACOLOGY

COMPOUNDS

Flavonoids: including among others luteolin-7-glucoside, isoetin

Hydroxycoumarins: umbelliferone, skimmine

Tannins

EFFECTS

The plant has been shown to have diuretic, carminative and diaphoretic effects.

INDICATIONS AND USAGE

Mouse Ear is used internally in the treatment of asthma, bronchitis, coughs and whooping cough and externally in the treatment of wounds.

PRECAUTIONS AND ADVERSE REACTIONS

No health hazards or side effects are known in conjunction with the proper administration of designated therapeutic dosages.

DOSAGE

Mode of Administration: The drug is used internally and externally as a liquid extract.

LITERATURE

Bate-Smith EC et al., Phytochemistry 7:1165.

Duquenois P, (1965) Mem Soc Bot Franc 41.

Guerin JC, Reveillere HP, (1985) Ann Farm Franc 43(1):77.

Further information in:

Hegnauer R, Chemotaxonomie der Pflanzen, Bde 1-11, Birkhäuser Verlag Basel, Boston, Berlin 1962-1997.

Kern W, List PH, Hörhammer L (Hrsg.), Hagers Handbuch der Pharmazeutischen Praxis, 4. Aufl., Bde. 1-8, Springer Verlag Berlin, Heidelberg, New York, 1969.

Madaus G, Lehrbuch der Biologischen Arzneimittel, Bde 1-3, Nachdruck, Georg Olms Verlag Hildesheim 1979.

Pimenta Racemosa

Pimento

DESCRIPTION

Medicinal Parts: The medicinal parts are the berries and the oil extracted from them.

Flower and Fruit: The inflorescences are racemes of white or lilac flowers, which develop very quickly into the infructescence. The fruit is a brown, globular berry, which is about 0.75 cm in diameter. The fruit has a rough surface and the remains of the calyx are present as a toothed ring at the apex. It contains 2 reniform seeds.

Leaves, Stem and Root: The tree is an evergreen up to 12 m in height. The leaves are oblong and coriaceous.

Characteristics: The odor is aromatic and reminiscent of cloves.

Habitat: The plant is indigenous to the West Indies and is cultivated in South America, Central America and Jamaica.

Production: Pimento leaves are the foliage leaves of Pimenta racemosa. Pimentae fructus is obsolete as a drug.

Other Names: Allspice, Clove Pepper, Jamaica Pepper, Pimenta

ACTIONS AND PHARMACOLOGY

COMPOUNDS

Volatile oil (bay oil, 0.7-1.2%): chief components- eugenol (50-60%), chavicol (20%), additionally including among others eugenol methyl ether, methyl chavicol, myrcene, limonene, 3- octanon, 1-octen-3-ol, citral

EFFECTS

Pimento is antiseptic and analgesic and is a cutaneous stimulant.

INDICATIONS AND USAGE

The drug is used externally in rubefacient lotions or liniments.

PRECAUTIONS AND ADVERSE REACTIONS

No health hazards or side effects are known in conjunction with the proper administration of designated therapeutic dosages. Allergic reactions to eugenol occur rarely.

DOSAGE

Mode of Administration: Pimento preparations are administered externally as lotions or liniments.

LITERATURE

Hogg JW et al., (1971) Am Perf Cosmet 86:33.

Kato Y, (1975) Koryo 113:17 et 24.

Oishi K et al., (1974) Nippon Suisan Gakaishi 40:1241.

Saito Y et al., (1976) Eiyo To Shokuryo 29:505.

Further information in:

Kern W, List PH, Hörhammer L (Hrsg.), Hagers Handbuch der Pharmazeutischen Praxis, 4. Aufl., Bde. 1-8, Springer Verlag Berlin, Heidelberg, New York, 1969.

Leung AY, Encyclopedia of Common Natural Ingredients Used in Food Drugs and Cosmetics, John Wiley & Sons Inc., New York 1980.

Steinegger E, Hänsel R, Pharmakognosie, 5. Aufl., Springer Verlag Heidelberg 1992.

Pimento

See Pimenta Racemosa

Pimpinella Anisum

Anise

DESCRIPTION

Medicinal Parts: The medicinal parts are the essential oil from the ripe fruit and the dried fruit.

Flower and Fruit: The inflorescences are medium-sized umbels with about 7 to 15 scattered pubescent rays. There is usually no involucre, but sometimes there is a single bract. There are barely any sepals. The petals are white, about 15 mm long, and have a ciliate margin. They have small bristles on the outside and have a long indented tip. The fruit is downy, ovate to oblong and flattened at the sides.

Leaves, Stem and Root: The plant is an annual herb about 0.5 m high which is downy all over. The root is thin and fusiform and the stem is erect, round, grooved and branched above. The lower leaves are petiolate, orbicular-reniform, entire and coarsely dentate to lobed. The middle leaves are orbicular and 3-lobed, or 3-segmented with ovate or obovate segments. The upper leaves are short-petioled to sessile with narrow sheaths, they are pinnatisect with narrow tips.

Characteristics: The taste is sweet and the odor characteristic.

Habitat: The origin of the plant is unknown but it probably came from the Near East. Today, it is cultivated mainly in southern Europe, Turkey, central Asia, India, China, Japan, Central and South America.

Production: Anise consists of the dried fruits of Pimpinella anisum.

ACTIONS AND PHARMACOLOGY

COMPOUNDS

Volatile oil: chief constituent trans-anethole, beyond that, among others, chavicol methyl ether (estragole), anisaldehyde

Caffeic acid derivatives: including chlorogenic acid

Flavonoids

Fatty oil

Proteins

EFFECTS

The drug is an expectorant, is mildly antispasmodic, and is antibacterial.

INDICATIONS AND USAGE

- Common cold
- Cough/bronchitis
- Fevers and colds
- Inflammation of the mouth and pharynx
- Liver and gallbladder complaints
- Loss of appetite
- Tendency to infection

The drug is used internally for dyspeptic complaints. It is used both internally and externally for catarrhs of the respiratory tract.

CONTRAINDICATIONS

Anise is contraindicated in patients allergic to anise and anethole.

PRECAUTIONS AND ADVERSE REACTIONS

No health hazards or side effects are known in conjunction with the proper administration of designated therapeutic dosages. Sensitization has been observed very rarely.

DOSAGE

Mode of Administration: As a comminuted drug for infusions and other galenic preparations for internal use or for inhalation. The purpose of an external application of an anise preparation is the inhalation of essential oil.

Daily Dosage: When used internally, the average daily dosage is 3.0 gm of drug or 0.3 gm of the essential oil. Preparations containing 5 to 10% essential oil can be used externally.

LITERATURE

Albert Puleo M, (1980) J Ethnopharmacol 2(4):337.

Czygan FC, Anis (Anisi fructus DAB 10) - Pimpinella anisum. In: ZPT 13(3):101. 1992.

Drinkwater NR, Miller EC, Miller JA, Pitot HC, (1976) Hepatocarcinogenicity of estragole and 1'-hydroxyestragole in the mouse and mutagenicity of 1-acetoxystragole in bacteria. J Natl Canc Inst 57:1323-1331.

Gershbein LL, (1977) Food Cosmet Toxicol 15(3):173.

Kartnig T et al., (1975) Planta Med 27:1.

Kubeczka KH et al., (1976) Z Naturforsch 31b:283.

Kubeczka KH, Formacek V, New Constituents from the Essential Oils of Pimpinella. In: Brunke EJ (Ed.) Progress in Essential Oil Research, Walter de Gruyter & Co, Berlin 1986. 1986.

Kunzemann J, Herrmann K, (1977) Z Lebensm Unters Forsch 164:194.

Mueller-Limmroth W, Froenlich HH, (1980) Fortschr Med 98 (3):95.

Nofal MA, (1981) Ain Chams Univ Fac Agric Res Bull 1602: 1-10.

Reichling J, Merkel B, Elicitor-Induced Formation of Coumarin Derivatives of Pimpinella anisum. In: PM 59(2):187. 1993.

Truhaut R, LeBourhis B, Attia M, Glomot R, Newman J, Caldwell J, (1989) Chronic toxicity/carcinogenicity study of trans-anethole in rats. Food chem Tox 27:11-20.

Further information in:

Hänsel R, Keller K, Rimpler H, Schneider G (Hrsg.), Hagers Handbuch der Pharmazeutischen Praxis, 5. Aufl., Bde 4-6 (Drogen), Springer Verlag Berlin, Heidelberg, New York, 1992-1994.

Hausen B, Allergiepflanzen, Pflanzenallergene, ecomed Verlagsgesellsch. mbH, Landsberg 1988.

Leung AY, Encyclopedia of Common Natural Ingredients Used in Food Drugs and Cosmetics, John Wiley & Sons Inc., New York, 1980.

Madaus G, Lehrbuch der Biologischen Arzneimittel, Bde 1-3, Nachdruck, Georg Olms Verlag Hildesheim 1979.

Schulz R, Hänsel R, Rationale Phytotherapie, Springer Verlag Heidelberg 1996.

Steinegger E, Hänsel R, Pharmakognosie, 5. Aufl., Springer Verlag Heidelberg 1992.

Teuscher E, Biogene Arzneimittel, 5. Aufl., Wiss. Verlagsges. Stuttgart 1997.

Wagner H, Wiesenauer M, Phytotherapie. Phytopharmaka und pflanzliche Homöopathika, Fischer-Verlag, Stuttgart, Jena, New York, 1995.

Wichtl M (Hrsg.), Teedrogen, 4. Aufl., Wiss. Verlagsges. Stuttgart 1997.

Pimpinella Major

Burnet Saxifrage

DESCRIPTION

Medicinal Parts: The medicinal parts are the dried rhizome, the dried roots, and the fresh roots collected in May.

Flower and Fruit: The white flowers are in compound 5 to 15-rayed umbels. There is no involucre or epicalyx. The flowers are small. The petals are uneven with curved lobes. The style is longer than the ovary during the flowering season. The fruit is dark brown to black, oblong-ovate, compressed at the sides, 2 to 3.5 mm long, heavily grooved and has no beak.

Leaves, Stem and Root: The 50 to 100 cm high plant is a perennial, which during the flowering season, develops lateral rosettes of leaves for the following year. These are usually glabrous, occasionally finely downy to short-bristly. The root is fusiform or carrot-shaped. The root is 10 to 20 cm long and 1 to 1.5 cm thick, gray-yellow and somewhat ringed. The stem is erect, angular, grooved, hollow, glabrous, somewhat leafy and branched from the ground up. The leaves are simple pinnate and glossy. The leaflets of the lower leaves are petiolate. They are ovate or oblong-indented or serrate acuminate.

Characteristics: The fresh root smells rancid, suet or carrot-like and the taste is tangy at first then burning-hot.

Habitat: The plant grows all over Europe with the exception of Scandinavia and the southern Balkans. It has been introduced to North America.

Production: Burnet Saxifrage herb consists of the above-ground parts of Pimpinella saxifrage and/or Pimpinella major. Pimpinella root consists of the dried rhizomes and roots of Pimpinella saxifraga and/or Pimpinella major. The root is dug up in spring and autumn. The uncut root is dried at temperatures of 40°C to prevent loss of essential oils. The drying process is completed when the roots can be broken.

Not To Be Confused With: Pimpinellae radix should not be confused with other Apiaca roots. It is often adulterated with the roots of Heracleum sphondylium, Heracleum mantegazzianum and Pastinaca sativa.

Other Names: Pimpernell, Saxifrage

ACTIONS AND PHARMACOLOGY

COMPOUNDS: PIMPINELLAE HERBA

Flavonoids

The foliage of the plant has not been fully investigated.

EFFECTS: PIMPINELLAE HERBA

No information is available.

COMPOUNDS: PIMPINELLAE RADIX

Volatile oil (0.1-0.7%): chief components- trans-epoxy-pseudo-isoeugenol (20-57%), additionally pregeijeren, beta-bisabolene, germacren A-D, 1,4-dimethyl azulene

Furocoumarins(1.2-2.3%): including, among others, bergaptene, isopimpinellin, pimpinellin, isobergapten, sphondine

Hydroxycoumarins: umbelliferone, scopoletin

Caffeic acid esters: including, among others, chlorogenic acid

Polyynes

EFFECTS: PIMPINELLAE RADIX

The root has been shown to have secretolytic and secretomotoric effects on the bronchial mucous membrane.

INDICATIONS AND USAGE

PIMPINELLAE HERBA

Preparations of Burnet Saxifrage herb are used internally for lung ailments and to stimulate gastrointestinal activity. The herb is used externally for varicose veins.

PIMPINELLAE RADIX

■ Cough/bronchitis

Preparations of the root are also used for colds, chills and catarrh of the upper respiratory tract. In folk medicine, it is used internally for disorders of the urinary organs, inflammation of the bladder and kidney, bladder and kidney stones and edema. It is also used as flushing out therapy in bacterial inflammation of the efferent urinary tract. Externally, it is used for inflammation of the oral and pharyngeal mucous membrane and as a bath additive for poorly healing wounds.

PRECAUTIONS AND ADVERSE REACTIONS

PIMPINELLAE HERBA

No health hazards or side effects are known in conjunction with the proper administration of designated therapeutic dosages.

PIMPINELLAE RADIX

No health hazards or side effects are known in conjunction with the proper administration of designated therapeutic dosages. Photosensitivity may occur in light-skinned individuals.

DOSAGE

PIMPINELLAE RADIX

Mode of Administration: Burnet Saxifrage root is administered as a tincture (Tinctura Pimpinellae) and as a comminuted herb for teas and other galenic preparations for internal use.

Daily Dosage: The daily dosage is 6 to 12 gm of drug for infusions or 6 to 15 gm pimpinel tincture (1:5).

LITERATURE

PIMPINELLAE HERBA

Bohn IU, Pimpinella saxifraga und Pimpinella major-Kleine und Groβe Bibernelle. In: ZPT 12(3):98. 1991.

Kubeczka KH, Formacek V, New Constituents from the Essential Oils of Pimpinella. In: Brunke EJ (Ed.) Progress in Essential Oil Research, Walter de Gruyter & Co, Berlin 1986. 1986.

Martin R et al., (1985) Planta Med 51(3):198.

Reichling J, Martin R, Pseudoisoeugenole - eine Gruppe seltener Phenylpropanoide im Genus Pimpinella: Biosynthese unfd biologische Wirkung. In: PZW 136(5/6)225. 1991.

Further information in:

Hänsel R, Keller K, Rimpler H, Schneider G (Hrsg.), Hagers Handbuch der Pharmazeutischen Praxis, 5. Aufl., Bde 4-6 (Drogen), Springer Verlag Berlin, Heidelberg, New York, 1992-1994.

Madaus G, Lehrbuch der Biologischen Arzneimittel, Bde 1-3, Nachdruck, Georg Olms Verlag Hildesheim 1979.

PIMPINELLAE RADIX

Bohn IU, Pimpinella saxifraga und Pimpinella major-Kleine und Groβe Bibernelle. In: ZPT 12(3):98. 1991.

Kubeczka KH, Formacek V, New Constituents from the Essential Oils of Pimpinella. In: Brunke EJ (Ed.) Progress in Essential Oil Research, Walter de Gruyter & Co, Berlin 1986.

Martin R et al., (1985) Planta Med 51(3):198.

Reichling J, Martin R, Pseudoisoeugenole - eine Gruppe seltener Phenylpropanoide im Genus Pimpinella: Biosynthese unfd biologische Wirkung. In: PZW 136(5/6)225. 1991.

Further information in:

Hänsel R, Keller K, Rimpler H, Schneider G (Hrsg.), Hagers Handbuch der Pharmazeutischen Praxis, 5. Aufl., Bde 4-6 (Drogen), Springer Verlag Berlin, Heidelberg, New York, 1992-1994.

Madaus G, Lehrbuch der Biologischen Arzneimittel, Bde 1-3, Nachdruck, Georg Olms Verlag Hildesheim 1979.

Steinegger E, Hänsel R, Pharmakognosie, 5. Aufl., Springer Verlag Heidelberg 1992.

Teuscher E, Lindequist U, Biogene Gifte - Biologie, Chemie, Pharmakologie, 2. Aufl., Fischer Verlag Stuttgart 1994.

Teuscher E, Biogene Arzneimittel, 5. Aufl., Wiss. Verlagsges. Stuttgart 1997.

Wichtl M (Hrsg.), Teedrogen, 4. Aufl., Wiss. Verlagsges. Stuttgart 1997.

Pink Root

See Spigelia Marilandica

Pinus Bark

See Tsuga Canadensis

Pinus Sylvestris

Scotch Pine

DESCRIPTION

Medicinal Parts: The medicinal parts are the tar extracted from the trunks, branches and roots. The oil extracted form the fresh needles, branch tips or fresh twigs is also used medicinally as well as the pine tips from fresh and dried shoots. The purified oil from the resin balsam, the tar extracted from the wood, the young shoots and the flowering branches of male and female flowers with pollen are also used.

Flower and Fruit: The male flowers are sulfur-yellow in the form of ovate catkins. The female flowers are purple and long-pedicled and are in erect, 5 to 6 mm long cones which hang down after flowering. The ripe cones are ovate-clavate, matte brown and have rhomboid scales. The hilum is small, smooth and light brown. The seeds are 3 to 4 mm long, oblong with wings which are 3 times as long as the seed.

Leaves, Stem and Root: The tree is 10 to 30 m high with a straight, slim, cylindrical trunk or a gnarled twisted one. It has a girth of 1.8 to 3.6 m. The crown is umbrella-shaped. The bark of the older trees is gray-brown on the outside and rust red on the inside. Bark of older trees is deeply fissured below and peeling. The bark of the young trees is fox-red and thinly peeling. The buds are reddish, 6 to 12 mm long, oblong-oval and somewhat resinous. The needles are in pairs and remain on the trees for 3 years. They are various lengths, rigid, twisted, bluish-green with interrupted rows on the outside and are minimally dentate.

Habitat: Pinus sylvestris is found in Europe, Siberia, the Crimea, the Caucasus and Iran.

Production: Pine shoots (Pini turiones) consist of the fresh or dried, 3 to 5 cm long shoots of Pinus sylvestris. Pine shoots are collected at the beginning of spring. The essential oil (Pini aetheroleum) is obtained from fresh needles, tips of the branches or fresh branches with needles and tips of Pinus sylvestris, Pinus mugo ssp. pumilio, Pinus nigra or Pinus pinaster. The oil is recovered form the fresh needles and branch tips using steam distillation with a successful yield of 0.15-0.6%. Purified turpentine oil (Terebinthinae aetheroleum rectificatum) is the essential oil obtained from the turpentine of Pinus species, especially Pinus palustries (syn. Pinus australis), and Pinus pinaster.

Not To Be Confused With: Pine shoots should not be confused with the shoots of Picea abies and Abies alba. Pine oil should not be confused with ''pine oils'' that are synthetically produced.

Other Names: Dwarf-Pine, Pine Oils, Pix Liquida, Pumilio Pine, Scotch Fir, Stockholm Tar, Swiss Mountain Pine

ACTIONS AND PHARMACOLOGY

COMPOUNDS: PINI TURIONES

Volatile oil (0.2-0.5%): including among others bornyl acetate, cadinene, Delta3 -carene, limonene, phellandrene, alpha-pinene

Resins

Bitter principles: pinicrin

Ascorbic acid (Vitamin C)

EFFECTS: PINI TURIONES

Pine shoots have secretolytic and mildly antiseptic effects and stimulate the peripheral circulation.

COMPOUNDS: PINI AETHEROLEUM

From Pinus mugo: chief components include Delta3-carene (up to 35%), alpha- and beta-pinene (20%), beta-phellandrene (15%)

From Pinus nigra: chief components include alpha-pinene (48-65%), beta-pinene (up to 32%), germacren D (up to 19%)

From Pinus palustris: chief components include alpha-and beta-pinene (95%)

From Pinus silvestris: chief components include alpha-pinene (10-50%), Delta3-carene (up to 20%), camphene (up to 12%), beta-pinene (10-25%), limonene (up to 10%), additionally including among others myrcene, terpinolene, bornyl acetate

EFFECTS: PINI AETHEROLEUM

The essential oil is secretolytic, hyperemic and weakly antiseptic.

COMPOUNDS: TEREBINTHINAE AETHEROLEUM RECTIFICATUM

Chief components of the raw terpentine oil yielded from terpentine from Pinus silvestris include: (-)-alpha-pinene (ca. 39-87%), Delta3-carene (ca. 14-33%), (-)-beta-pinene (share up to 27%), limonene (6%), camphene (ca. 5%), from out of which and form out of the volatile oils of other pine species purified terpentine oil. Therebinthinae aetheroleum rectici-factum is realized through fractional distillation. It must contain at least 90% pinenes, but no more than 0.5 % Delta3-carene.

EFFECTS: TEREBINTHINAE AETHEROLEUM RECTIFICATUM

Purified turpentine oil is hyperemic and antiseptic and reduces bronchial secretions.

INDICATIONS AND USAGE

PINI TURIONES

- Blood pressure problems
- Common cold
- Cough/bronchitis
- Fevers and colds
- Inflammation of the mouth and pharynx
- Neuralgias
- Tendency to infection

Pine shoots are used internally for catarrhal conditions of the upper and lower respiratory tract. Externally, it is used for mild muscular pain and neuralgia. In folk medicine, it is used internally for uncomplicated coughs and acute bronchial diseases and topically for nasal congestion and hoarseness. Efficacy in these areas has not been documented.

PINI AETHEROLEUM

- Common cold
- Cough/bronchitis
- Fevers and colds
- Inflammation of the mouth and pharynx
- Neuralgias
- Rheumatism
- Tendency to infection

The essential oil is used internally and externally for catarrhal diseases of the upper and lower respiratory tract. Externally, it is used for rheumatic and neuralgic ailments.

TEREBINTHINAE AETHEROLEUM RECTIFICATUM

- Common cold
- Cough/bronchitis
- Fevers and colds
- Inflammation of the mouth and pharynx
- Rheumatism
- Tendency to infection

Purified turpentine oil is used internally and externally for chronic diseases of the bronchi with profuse secretion. It is used externally for rheumatic and neuralgic ailments.

CONTRAINDICATIONS

PINI TURIONES AND PINI AETHEROLEUM

Contraindications include bronchial asthma and whooping cough.

PRECAUTIONS AND ADVERSE REACTIONS

PINI TURIONES

No health hazards or side effects are known in conjunction with the proper administration of designated therapeutic dosages. Patients with extensive skin injuries, acute skin diseases, feverish or infectious diseases, cardiac insufficiency or hypertonia should not use the drug as a bath additive.

PINI AETHEROLEUM

No health hazards are known in conjunction with the proper administration of designated therapeutic dosages. Signs of irritation could appear on skin and mucous membranes. Bronchial spasms could worsen. Patients with extensive skin injuries, acute skin diseases, feverish or infectious diseases, cardiac insufficiency or hypertonia should not use the drug as a bath additive.

TEREBINTHINAE AETHEROLEUM RECTIFICATUM

General: No health hazards or side effects are known in conjunction with the proper external administration of designated therapeutic dosages. Resorptive poisonings, such as kidney and central nervous system damage, are however possible with large-area administration. Where large skin injuries, severe feverish or infectious diseases, cardiac insufficiency or hypertonia are present, entire-body baths with the volatile oil added should be carried out only following consultation with a doctor.

Kidney damage is conceivable with internal administration of therapeutic dosages. Inhalation should be avoided with acute inflammation of the breathing passages.

Pediatric Use: Cases of death, in particular among children, following intake of the oil are known from the scientific literature.

OVERDOSAGE

TEREBINTHINAE AETHEROLEUM RECTIFICATUM

Severe poisonings are possible with the intake of large dosages. Symptoms include albuminuria, diarrhea, dyspnea, dysuria, feelings of vertigo, hematuria, intestinal colic, queasiness, reddening of the face, salivation, skin efflorescences, sore throat, staggering walk, strangury, thirst, twitching, and vomiting. Poisonings can also occur through inhalation of the vapors or through skin contact. Fifty grams is the approximate lethal dosage for an adult. Cases of death, in particular among children, following intake of the oil are known from the scientific literature. Gastric lavage with bicarbonate of soda solution, intestinal emptying through administration of sodium sulphate, the administration of paraffin oil, activated charcoal and shock prophylaxis (suitable body position, quiet, warmth), should be instituted. Thereafter, therapy for poisonings consists of treating spasms with diazepam (i.v.), electrolyte substitution, and treating possible cases of acidosis with sodium bicarbonate infusions. In case of shock, plasma volume expanders should be infused. Monitoring of kidney function is essential. Intubation and oxygen respiration may also be necessary.

DOSAGE

PINI TURIONES

Mode of Administration: Pine shoot is available as a comminuted herb for internal use in teas, syrups and tinctures. Alcoholic solutions, oils or ointments are used externally.

Daily Dosage: When used internally, the average daily dosage is 9 gm of drug. When used externally, 100 gm of alcoholic extract can be added to bath water; liquid or semi-solid preparations of extracts of Pini turiones corresponding to 20 to 50% can also be used. In folk medicine, 500 ml of a 20% infusion can be used.

PINI AETHEROLEUM

Mode of Administration: The essential oil is administered in alcoholic solutions, ointments, gels, emulsions, oils or as an inhalant. It is used externally as bubble baths and bath salts.

Daily Dosage: For internal use, the daily dose is 5 gm drug. For inhalation therapy, place several drops into hot water and breathe in the vapors. When used externally, several drops of a liquid or semi-solid preparation containing 10 to 50% drug may be rubbed onto the affected area. To use as a bath additive, use 0.025 gm drug per liter water and bathe for 10 to 20 minutes at a temperature of 35°C to 38°C.

Storage: Keep protected from light in tightly sealed containers.

TEREBINTHINAE AETHEROLEUM RECTIFICATUM

Mode of Administration: Purified turpentine oil is administered externally in the form of ointments, gels, emulsions, oils, as a plaster and as an inhalant.

Daily Dosage: For inhalation therapy, place several drops in hot water and breathe in the vapors. When used externally, several drops of a liquid or semi-solid preparation containing 10 to 50% drug may be rubbed onto the affected area.

LITERATURE

PINI TURIONES

Glasl H et al., Gaschromatographische Untersuchung von Arzneibuchdrogen 7. Mitt.: GC-Untersuchung von Pinaceen-Ölen des Handels und Versuche zu ihrer Standardisierung. In: DAZ 120(2):64-67. 1980.

Ikeda RM, (1962) J Food Sci 27:455.

Roschin VI et al., (1985) Khim Prir Soedin 1:122.

Zinkel DF, (1975) Chemtech 5(4):235.

Further information in:

Hänsel R, Keller K, Rimpler H, Schneider G (Hrsg.), Hagers Handbuch der Pharmazeutischen Praxis, 5. Aufl., Bde 4-6 (Drogen), Springer Verlag Berlin, Heidelberg, New York, 1992-1994.

Leung AY, Encyclopedia of Common Natural Ingredients Used in Food Drugs and Cosmetics, John Wiley & Sons Inc., New York, 1980.

Madaus G, Lehrbuch der Biologischen Arzneimittel, Bde 1-3, Nachdruck, Georg Olms Verlag Hildesheim 1979.

PINI AETHEROLEUM

Glasl H et al., Gaschromatographische Untersuchung von Arzneibuchdrogen 7. Mitt.: GC-Untersuchung von Pinaceen-Ölen des Handels und Versuche zu ihrer Standardisierung. In: DAZ 120(2):64-67. 1980.

Ikeda RM, (1962) J Food Sci 27:455.

Roschin VI et al., (1985) Khim Prir Soedin 1:122.

Zinkel DF, (1975) Chemtech 5(4):235.

Further information in:

Hänsel R, Keller K, Rimpler H, Schneider G (Hrsg.), Hagers Handbuch der Pharmazeutischen Praxis, 5. Aufl., Bde 4-6 (Drogen), Springer Verlag Berlin, Heidelberg, New York, 1992-1994.

Leung AY, Encyclopedia of Common Natural Ingredients Used in Food Drugs and Cosmetics, John Wiley & Sons Inc., New York, 1980.

Madaus G, Lehrbuch der Biologischen Arzneimittel, Bde 1-3, Nachdruck, Georg Olms Verlag Hildesheim 1979.

Steinegger E, Hänsel R, Pharmakognosie, 5. Aufl., Springer Verlag Heidelberg 1992.

Teuscher E, Biogene Arzneimittel, 5. Aufl., Wiss. Verlagsges. Stuttgart 1997.

Wagner H, Wiesenauer M, Phytotherapie. Phytopharmaka und pflanzliche Homöopathika, Fischer-Verlag, Stuttgart, Jena, New York, 1995.

TEREBINTHINAE AETHEROLEUM RECTIFICATUM

Bauer L, (1973) Die Feinstruktur der menschlichen Bronchialschleimhaut nach Behandlung mit Ozothin. Klin Wochenschr 51:450-453.

Glasl H, Wagner H, DAZ 120:64-67. 1980.

Iconomou N et al., J Chromatogr 16:29. 1964.

Ikeda RM, (1962) J Food Sci 27:455.

Iravani J, (1972) Wirkung eines Broncholytikums auf die tracheobronchiale Reinigung. Arzneim Forsch (Drug Res) 22:1744-1746.

Roschin VI et al., (1985) Khim Prir Soedin 1:122.

Zänker KS, Blümel G, Probst J, Reiterer W, (1984) Theoretical, experimental evidence for the action of terpens as modulators in lung function. Prog Resp Res 18:302-304.

Zinkel DF, (1975) Chemtech 5(4):235.

Further information in:

Hänsel R, Keller K, Rimpler H, Schneider G (Hrsg.), Hagers Handbuch der Pharmazeutischen Praxis, 5. Aufl., Bde 4-6 (Drogen): Springer Verlag Berlin, Heidelberg, New York, 1992-1994.

Steinegger E, Hänsel R, Pharmakognosie, 5. Aufl., Springer Verlag Heidelberg 1992.

Teuscher E, Biogene Arzneimittel, 5. Aufl., Wiss. Verlagsges. Stuttgart 1997.

Wagner H, Wiesenauer M, Phytotherapie. Phytopharmaka und pflanzliche Homöopathika, Fischer-Verlag, Stuttgart, Jena, New York, 1995.

Piper Betle

Betel Nut

DESCRIPTION

Medicinal Parts: The main medicinal parts are the dried leaves; the roots and the fruit are also used.

Flower and Fruit: The inflorescences are compact, hanging, cylindrical and 3.5 to 5 cm long spikes of yellow-green flowers. There are 2 stamens in the male flowers. The female stamens have an ovary, which is pubescent at the top and has 3 to 5 stigmas. The fruit is globular, fleshy and about 6 mm in diameter. The fruit is yellow and becomes red when ripe. The seeds are also globular.

Leaves, Stem and Root: The plant is a dioecious or monoecious woody climber which can grow to 15 m. It has numerous small and short adventitious roots. The stem is thickened at the nodes and the younger parts are glabrous. The leaves have a 2.5 to 5 cm long petiole, are broadly cordate, 5 to 18 cm long and half as wide. The leaves are glabrous, light green and glossy on both surfaces with 5 to 7 radiating ribs.

Habitat: Piper betle is found in tropical southern Asia and has been introduced to east Africa, Madagascar and the West Indies.

Production: Betel Nut leaves are the leaves of Piper betle. When the leaves are green, they are gathered, pressed and dried.

Other Names: Betel

ACTIONS AND PHARMACOLOGY

COMPOUNDS

Volatile oil (0.8-1.8%): chief components- chavibetol (betel phenol), eugenol, additionally allylpyrocatechol (hydroxy-chavicol), allylpyrocatechol-mono and -diacetate, anethole, chavibetolacetate, chavicol, methyl eugenol, safrol

Neolignans: including crotepoxide, piperbetol, piperol, among others

EFFECTS

The active agents, (essential oil, starch, sugar, carbolic acid, tannin and cadine), have stimulant, antibiotic and carminative properties. The essential oil acts as an antioxidant and a preservative.

INDICATIONS AND USAGE

Betel Nut is used as an expectorant for coughs, for diphtheria, for stomach complaints, and for inflammation of the middle ear. It is also used to increase the secretion of saliva, as a stimulant, and for the treatment of worm infestation, although these effects have not been confirmed.

PRECAUTIONS AND ADVERSE REACTIONS

No health hazards or side effects are known in conjunction with the proper administration of designated therapeutic dosages.

DOSAGE

Mode of Administration: Today, the drug is obsolete.

LITERATURE

Das PC, Sarkar AK, (1979) Acta Physiol Pol. 30(3):389.

Rawat AKS et al., Ind Perf 31:146-149. 1987.

Sharma ML et al., Ind Perf 26:134-137. 1982.

Further information in:

Hänsel R, Keller K, Rimpler H, Schneider G (Hrsg.), Hagers Handbuch der Pharmazeutischen Praxis, 5. Aufl., Bde 4-6 (Drogen), Springer Verlag Berlin, Heidelberg, New York, 1992-1994.

Roth L, Daunderer M, Kormann K, Giftpflanzen, Pflanzengifte, 4. Aufl., Ecomed Fachverlag Landsberg Lech 1993.

Piper Cubeba

Cubeb

DESCRIPTION

Medicinal Parts: The medicinal parts are the dried, not fully ripe fruit.

Flower and Fruit: The male flowering spikes are about 4 cm long and have 2 or 3 stamens. The female spikes are made up of about 50 individual flowers, which mostly consist of the oblong ovary of 4 fused carpels with 4 sessile stigmas. The infructescence is 4 to 5 cm long. When ripe, the base of the ovary grows into a stem-like, cylindrical lower part. The upper portion of the fruit is globular and holds the seed, which contains a tiny embryo in a small cavity at the apex.

Leaves, Stem and Root: The plant is a 5 to 15 m high dioecious climbing shrub. The branches are initially pubescent, later glabrous. The leaves are glabrous, entire-margined, coriaceous, ovate to oblong-elliptical and up to 15 cm long and 6 cm wide.

Characteristics: The odor is warm and reminiscent of turpentine.

Habitat: The plant is indigenous to Indonesia and is cultivated in Sri Lanka, India and Malaysia.

Production: Cubebs are the fruit of Piper cubeba.

Other Names: Java Pepper, Tailed Cubebs, Tailed Pepper

ACTIONS AND PHARMACOLOGY

COMPOUNDS

Volatile oil: chief constituents- alpha- and beta-cubeben, copas, cubebol, delta-cadinenes, humules

Lignans: chief components (-)-cubebin

Fatty oil

EFFECTS

The drug is a urinary antiseptic, a stomachic and is mildly diuretic.

INDICATIONS AND USAGE

Cubeb has been used for urinary tract diseases and stomach complaints.

PRECAUTIONS AND ADVERSE REACTIONS

Health risks or side effects following the proper administration of designated therapeutic dosages are not recorded.

OVERDOSAGE

High dosages (over 8 gm) cause irritation of the urinary passages, kidney and bladder pains, albuminuria and urination problems. Beyond this, vomiting, diarrhea, cardiac pain and skin rashes can occur. After stomach and intestinal emptying, treatment of poisonings should proceed symptomatically.

DOSAGE

Mode of Administration: Cubeb is contained in medicinal preparations, such as bath additives.

LITERATURE

Batterbee, J E et al., (1969) J Chem Soc (c), 2470.

Ikeda, RM, (1962) J Food Sci 27:455.

Koul SK et al., Phenylpropanoids and (-)-ledol from Piper species. In: PH 32:478. 1993.

Lawrence BM, Perfum Flavor 5:28. 1980.

Ohta, Y et al., (1966) Tetrahedron Letters 52:6365.

Opdyke, DLJ, (1976) Food Cosmet Toxicol 14.

Prabhu, BR, Mulchandani, NB, (1985) Phytochemistry 24 (2), 329.

Further information in:

Hänsel R, Keller K, Rimpler H, Schneider G (Hrsg.), Hagers Handbuch der Pharmazeutischen Praxis, 5. Aufl., Bde 4-6 (Drogen), Springer Verlag Berlin, Heidelberg, New York, 1992-1994.

Leung AY, Encyclopedia of Common Natural Ingredients Used in Food Drugs and Cosmetics, John Wiley & Sons Inc., New York 1980.

Lewin L, Gifte und Vergiftungen, 6. Aufl., Nachdruck, Haug Verlag, Heidelberg 1992.

Madaus G, Lehrbuch der Biologischen Arzneimittel, Bde 1-3, Nachdruck, Georg Olms Verlag Hildesheim 1979.

Roth L, Daunderer M, Kormann K, Giftpflanzen, Pflanzengifte, 4. Aufl., Ecomed Fachverlag Landsberg Lech 1993.

Piper Methysticum

Kava-Kava

DESCRIPTION

Medicinal Parts: The medicinal parts are the peeled, dried, cut rhizome, which has normally been freed from the roots and the fresh rhizome with the roots.

Flower and Fruit: The plant has numerous small flowers in spike-like inflorescences 3 to 9 cm long. Only the inflorescences of the male plants flower.

Leaves, Stem and Root: The plant is a 2 to 3 m high, erect dioecious bush. The leaves are very large, measuring 13 to 28 cm by 10 to 22 cm . They have a deeply cordate base and 9 to 13 main ribs which are slightly downy on the under surface. The stipules are large. The plant has a massive, 2 to 10 kg branched and very juicy rhizome with many roots. They are blackish-gray on the outside and whitish on the inside. The fracture is mealy and somewhat splintery. The central portion is porous with irregularly twisted thin woody bundles, separated by broad medullary rays, forming meshes beneath the bark.

Characteristics: The taste is pungent and numbing. The odor is reminiscent of lilac.

Habitat: The plant is indigenous to the South Sea Islands and is mainly cultivated there.

Production: Kava-kava rhizome consists of the dried rhizomes of Piper methysticum.

Other Names: Ava, Ava Pepper, Intoxicating Pepper, Kawa

ACTIONS AND PHARMACOLOGY

COMPOUNDS

Kava lactones (kava pyrones, 5-12%): chief components (+)-kavain, 7,8-dihydro-(+)-kavain (marindinine), (+)-methysticin, 7,8-dihydro-(+)-methysticin, yangonine, desmethoxyyangonin

Chalcones

EFFECTS

The drug has anti-anxiety effects. In animal tests a potentiation of narcosis (sedation), anticonvulsive, antispasmodic, and central muscular relaxant effects were described.

INDICATIONS AND USAGE

■ Nervousness and insomnia

Kava-kava is used for nervous anxiety, stress, and restlessness.

CONTRAINDICATIONS

The drug is contraindicated in patients with endogenous depression because it increases the danger of suicide. It is also contraindicated during pregnancy and in nursing mothers.

PRECAUTIONS AND ADVERSE REACTIONS

General: No health hazards are known in conjunction with the proper administration of designated therapeutic dosages. In rare cases, administration of the drug leads to allergic reactions and slight yellowing of the skin. Gastrointestinal complaints, accomodation disorders, pupil dilation, and disorders of the oculomotor equilibrium have been reported. Slight morning tiredness can appear at the beginning of the therapy. Reduced visual power and reactivity while driving may occur, but this effect has not been confirmed.

The drug should not be taken for longer than three months without a doctor's supervision.

Drug Interactions: The drug may potentiate the effectiveness of substances that act on the central nervous system, such as alcohol, barbiturates and psychopharmacological agents.

Pregnancy: The drug is contraindicated during pregnancy.

Nursing Mothers: The drug is contraindicated in nursing mothers.

OVERDOSAGE

Overdosage can result in disorders of complex movement, accompanied by undisturbed consciousness, later tiredness and tendency to sleep.

DOSAGE

Mode of Administration: Comminuted rhizome and other galenic preparations for oral use.

Daily Dosage: The daily dosage for herbs and preparations is the equivalent of 60 to 120 mg kava pyrones.

LITERATURE

Backhaus C, Krieglstein J, (1992) Extract of kava and its methysticin constituents protect brain tissue against ischaemic damage in rodents. J Pharmacol 215:265-269.

Bhate H, Gerster G, Fracza E, (1989) Orale Prämedikation mit Zubereitungen aus Piper methysticum bei operativen Eingriffen in Epiduralanästhesie. Erfahrungsheilkunde 6:339-345.

Dingermann T, Phytopharmaka im Alter: Crataegus, Ginkgo, Hypericum und Kava-Kava. In: PZ 140(23):2017-2024. 1995.

Emser W, Bartylla K, (1991) Verbesserung der Schlafqualität. TW Neurol Psychiatr 5:636-642.

Geβner B, Cnota P, (1994) Untersuchung der Vigilanz nach Applikation von Kava-Kava-Extrakt, Diazepam oder Placebo. Z Phytother 15:30-37.

Gleitz J et al., Antithrombotic action of the kava pyrone (+)-kavain prepared from Piper methysticum on human platelets. In: PM 63(1):27-30. 1997.

Gleitz J et al., Kavain inhibits non-stereospecifically veratridine-activated Na+ channels. In: PM 62(6):580-581. 1996.

Hänsel R, Beiersdorff HU, (1955) Arzneim Forsch 9:581.

Hänsel R, Kava-Kava (Piper methysticum G. Forster), in der modernen Arzneimittelforschung Portarit einer Arzneipflanze. In: ZPT 17(3):180-195. 1996.

Hänsel R, Pflanzliche Sedativa. In: ZPT 11(1):14. 1990.

Hänsel R, Woelk H, (1995) Spektrum Kava-Kava. 2. Auflage. Aesopus Verlag GmbH, Basel.

Herberg KW, (1991) Fahrtüchtigkeit nach Einnahme von Kava-Spezial-Extrakt WS 1490. Z Allg Med 67:842-846.

Jamieson DD, Duffield PH, Cheng D, Duffield AM, (1989) Comparison of the Central Nervous System Activity of the Aqueous and Lipid Extrakt of Kava (Piper methysticum). Arch Int Pharmacodyn 301:66-80.

Johnson E, Frauendorf A, Stecker K, Stein U, (1991) Neurophysiologisches Wirkprofil und Verträglichkeit von Kava-Extrakt WS 1490. TW Neurol Psychiatr 5:349-354.

Kinzler E, Krömer J, Lehmann, (1991) Wirksamkeit eines Kava-Spezial-Extraktes bei Patienten mit Angst-, Spannungs- und Erregungszuständen nicht-psychotischer Genese. Arzneim Forsch/Drug Res 41:584-588.

Münte TF, Heinze HJ, Matzke M, Steitz J, (1993) Effects of oxacepam and an extract of Kava roots (Piper methysticum) on event-related potentials in a word recognition task. Neuropsychobiology 27:46-53.

Ruze P, (1990) Kava-induced dermopathy: a niacin deficiency? Lancet: 1442-1445.

Schmidt M, Kava-Kava. In: PTA 8(5):374. 1994.

Siegel RK, (1976) Herbal intoxication. Psychoactive effects from herbal cigarettes, tea and capsules. JAMA 236:473-476.

Smith RM, (1979) Tetrahedron 35(3):437.

Volz HP, (1995) Die anxiolytische Wirksamkeit von Kava-Spezialextrakt WS 1490 unter Langzeittherapie - eine randomisierte Doppelblindstudie. Z Phytother Abstractband, S 9.

Volz HP, Hänsel R, (1994) Kava-Kava und Kavain in der Psychopharmakotherapie. Psychopharmakotherapie 1:33-39.

Warnecke G, Pfaender H, Gerster G, Gracza E, (1990) Wirksamkeit von Kawa-Kawa-Extrakt beim klimakterischen Syndrom. Z Phytother 11:81-86.

Woelk H, Kapoula O, Lehrl S, Schröter K, Weinholz P, (1993) Behandlung von Angst-Patienten. Z Allg Med 69:271-277.

Further information in:

Hänsel R, Keller K, Rimpler H, Schneider G (Hrsg.), Hagers Handbuch der Pharmazeutischen Praxis, 5. Aufl., Bde 4-6 (Drogen), Springer Verlag Berlin, Heidelberg, New York, 1992-1994.

Lewin L, Gifte und Vergiftungen, 6. Aufl., Nachdruck, Haug Verlag, Heidelberg 1992.

Madaus G, Lehrbuch der Biologischen Arzneimittel, Bde 1-3, Nachdruck, Georg Olms Verlag Hildesheim 1979.

Roth L, Daunderer M, Kormann K, Giftpflanzen, Pflanzengifte, 4. Aufl., Ecomed Fachverlag Landsberg Lech 1993.

Schulz R, Hänsel R, Rationale Phytotherapie, Springer Verlag Heidelberg 1996.

Steinegger E, Hänsel R, Pharmakognosie, 5. Aufl., Springer Verlag Heidelberg 1992.

Teuscher E, Biogene Arzneimittel, 5. Aufl., Wiss. Verlagsges. Stuttgart 1997.

Wagner H, Wiesenauer M, Phytotherapie. Phytopharmaka und pflanzliche Homöopathika, Fischer-Verlag, Stuttgart, Jena, New York 1995.

Wichtl M (Hrsg.), Teedrogen, 4. Aufl., Wiss. Verlagsges. Stuttgart 1997.

Piper Nigrum

Black Pepper

DESCRIPTION

Medicinal Parts: The medicinal parts are the berries, which have been freed from the pericarp and the dried berry-like fruit, which has been collected before ripening.

Flower and Fruit: The inflorescences are pendulous, axillary spikes 5 to 15 cm long containing over 100 inconspicuous white florets. The florets have 1 large ovary with 3 stigmas, 2 stamens and a reduced perianth. Red berry-like drupes form the 30 to 50 flowers, which are fertilized.

Leaves, Stem and Root: The plant is actually a liane, which in cultivation is trained on posts or wire. It can grow to over 6 m. The stem is strong and woody and the leaves are cordate, glossy and pale green. The leaves are 5 to 10 cm wide, 8 to 18 cm long and are on 5 cm long petioles.

Habitat: The plant grows wild in southern India and is cultivated in tropical Asia and the Caribbean.

Production: Black peppers are the dried fruits of Piper nigrum, harvested before ripening. The whole ears are plucked and separated from the spindles that have been dried, or the fruit is first brushed from the spindles and then dried. Once the shell has been removed, the green stone-fruit is sun-dried or roasted, following this it blackens.

Not To Be Confused With: Foreign fruits of the Piperacae family. It is most frequently confused with peppershells, pepper spindles or stiles, i.e. by-products of the extraction of white pepper from black pepper.

Other Names: Piper, Pepper Bark

ACTIONS AND PHARMACOLOGY

COMPOUNDS

Volatile oil (1.2-2.6%): chief components- sabinene (15-25%), limonene (15-20%), caryophyllene (10-15%), beta-pinene (10-12%), alpha-pinene (8-12%)

Acid amides (pungent substances): chief components- piperine, additionally including among others piperylin, piperolein A and B, cumaperine

Fatty oil (10%)

EFFECTS

The drug stimulates the thermal receptors and increases secretion of saliva and gastric mucous. It has an antimicrobial effect. It influences liver and metabolic functions, and has an insecticidal effect.

INDICATIONS AND USAGE

Black Pepper is used for stomach disorders and digestion problems. In Indian medicine, it is used to treat bronchitis. It has been used externally for neuralgia or scabies.

PRECAUTIONS AND ADVERSE REACTIONS

No health hazards or side effects are known in conjunction with the proper administration of designated therapeutic dosages.

DOSAGE

Mode of Administration: Black Pepper is used internally for stomach disorders, and is used externally as an irritant ointment for neuralgia and scabies.

Daily Dosage: Single doses range from 0.3 to 0.6 gm. The daily dosage is 1.5 gm.

LITERATURE

Atal CK et al., (1975) Lloydia 38:256.

Freist W, Der scharfe Geschmack des Pfeffers - Ein altes Rätsel, nur teilweise gelöst. In: Chemie i.u. Zeit 23(3):135-142. 1991.

Kapil A, Piperine. A Potent Inhibitor of Leishmania donovani Promastigotes in vitro. In: PM 59(5):474. 1993.

Koul IB, Kapil A, Evaluation of the Liver Protective Potential of Piperine, an Active Principle of Black and Long Peppers. In: PM 59(5):413. 1993.

Raina ML et al., (1976) Planta Med 30:198.

Richard ML et al., (1976) J Food Sci 36:584.

Schröder, Buch. In: Schröder R: Kaffee, Tee und Kardamom, Ulmer-Verlag, Stuttgart. 1991.

Traxter JT, (1971) J Agric Food Chem 19:1135.

Further information in:

Fenaroli's Handbook of Flavor Ingredients, Vol. 1. 2nd Ed. Pub. CRC Press Boca Raton 1975.

Hänsel R, Keller K, Rimpler H, Schneider G (Hrsg.), Hagers Handbuch der Pharmazeutischen Praxis, 5. Aufl., Bde 4-6 (Drogen), Springer Verlag Berlin, Heidelberg, New York, 1992-1994.

Leung AY, Encyclopedia of Common Natural Ingredients Used in Food Drugs and Cosmetics, John Wiley & Sons Inc., New York 1980.

Steinegger E, Hänsel R, Pharmakognosie, 5. Aufl., Springer Verlag Heidelberg 1992.

Teuscher E, Biogene Arzneimittel, 5. Aufl., Wiss. Verlagsges. Stuttgart 1997.

Pipsissewa

See Chimaphila Umbellata

Piscidia Piscipula

Jamaica Dogwood

DESCRIPTION

Medicinal Parts: The medicinal part is the bark.

Flower and Fruit: The plant has blue to white flowers with white stripes out of which 4 pods with 4 longitudinal wings develop.

Leaves, Stem and Root: The plant is a tree or shrub up to 15 m high with compound leaves. The bark is 3 to 6 mm thick and dark gray-brown with thin, longitudinal and transverse ridges. It is roughish and wrinkled, and somewhat fissured. The fracture is tough, fibrous, showing blue-green or brownish-green patches.

Characteristics: The taste is bitter and acrid and the odor characteristic.

Habitat: The tree is indigenous to Central America and the northern parts of South America.

Production: Jamaica Dogwood is the root bark of Piscidia piscipula.

Other Names: Dogwood, Fish Poison Tree

ACTIONS AND PHARMACOLOGY

COMPOUNDS

Isoflavonoids: including among others jamaicine, ichthynone, the rotenoids rotenone, milleton, isomilletone

Tannins

EFFECTS

Research indicates that Jamaica Dogwood is mildly sedative and spasmolytic.

INDICATIONS AND USAGE

The drug is used for states of anxiety and fear and as a daytime sedative.

PRECAUTIONS AND ADVERSE REACTIONS

No health hazards or side effects are known in conjunction with the proper administration of designated therapeutic dosages.

DOSAGE

Mode of Administration: The drug and liquid extract are no longer in use. It has been used in some medicinal preparations.

LITERATURE

Aurousseau M et al., (1965) Ann Pharm Franc 23:251.

Heller W, Tamm C., (1975) Helv Chim Acta 58:974.

Nordal A et al., (1966) Acta Chem Scand 20:1431.

Pietta P, Zio C, (1983) J Chrom. 260:497.

Schwartz JSP et al., (1964) Tetrahedron 20:1317.

Stamm OA et al., (1958) Helv Chim Acta 41:2006.

Further information in:

Kern W, List PH, Hörhammer L (Hrsg.), Hagers Handbuch der Pharmazeutischen Praxis, 4. Aufl., Bde. 1-8, Springer Verlag Berlin, Heidelberg, New York, 1969.

Leung AY, Encyclopedia of Common Natural Ingredients Used in Food Drugs and Cosmetics, John Wiley & Sons Inc., New York 1980.

Madaus G, Lehrbuch der Biologischen Arzneimittel, Bde. 1-3, Nachdruck, Georg Olms Verlag Hildesheim 1979.

Steinegger E, Hänsel R, Pharmakognosie, 5. Aufl., Springer Verlag Heidelberg 1992.

Wagner H, Wiesenauer M, Phytotherapie. Phytopharmaka und pflanzliche Homöopathika, Fischer-Verlag, Stuttgart, Jena, New York 1995.

Pistacia Lentiscus

Mastic Tree

DESCRIPTION

Medicinal Parts: The medicinal part is the resin.

Flower and Fruit: The inflorescence is compact and spike-like. The flowers are yellowish or purplish. The drupe is approximately 4 mm, globose, apiculate and is red, but later turns black.

Leaves, Stem and Root: The plant is a small evergreen tree or shrub 1 to 8 m high. The trees are said to be exclusively male. The leaves are bipinnate. The 8 to 12 leaflets measure 1 to 5 cm by 0.5 to 1.5 cm. They are lanceolate to ovate-lanceolate, mucronate and coriaceous. The rhachis is broadly winged. The petioles are glabrous.

Habitat: The tree thrives in the Mediterranean region, Portugal, Turkey, on the Canaries and in tropical Africa.

Production: Mastic resin is the resin from the trunk of Pistacia lentiscus.

Other Names: Lentisk

ACTIONS AND PHARMACOLOGY

COMPOUNDS

Resins (90%): chief components are the triterpenes mastic acid, isomastic acid, oleanolic acid and tirucallol

Volatile oil (1-3%): chief component is alpha-pinene

EFFECTS

The essential oil (pines) and resin are astringent and aromatic.

INDICATIONS AND USAGE

Mastic Tree resin was formerly used in dentistry, as a material for fillings. The masticated resin releases substances that freshen the breath and tighten the gums.

PRECAUTIONS AND ADVERSE REACTIONS

General: No health hazards or side effects are known in conjunction with the proper administration of designated therapeutic dosages.

Pediatric Use: There is an occasional risk of diarrhea in small children.

DOSAGE

Mode of Administration: The resin is used for the production of chewing gum and is used in the food and drink industries.

LITERATURE

Al-Said MS et al., Evaluation of mastic, a crude drig obtaines from Pistacia lentiscus for gastric and duodenal anti-ulcer activity. In: ETH 15:271. 1986.

Marner FJ, Freyer A, Lex J, Triterpenoids from gum mastic, the resin of Pistacia lentiscus. In: PH 30(11):3709-3712. 1991.

Further information in:

Kern W, List PH, Hörhammer L (Hrsg.), Hagers Handbuch der Pharmazeutischen Praxis, 4. Aufl., Bde. 1-8, Springer Verlag Berlin, Heidelberg, New York, 1969.

Teuscher E, Biogene Arzneimittel, 5. Aufl., Wiss. Verlagsges. Stuttgart 1997.

Pitcher Plant

See Sarracenia Purpurea

Plantago Afra

Psyllium Seed

DESCRIPTION

Medicinal Parts: The medicinal parts are the ripe seeds.

Flower and Fruit: The inflorescence is a 12 mm long spike with glandular hairs and ovate-lanceolate bracts with a midrib and translucent lateral lamina. The corolla is disc-shaped with 4 translucent petals. The edge of the calyx has 4 acute lobes. The sepals are 3 to 4.5 cm and oblanceolate. The ovary is superior and the fruit is a 2-sectioned, membranous pyxidium. The seeds are dark brown, glossy and narrowly oblong in outline.

Leaves, Stem and Root: The plant is an annual that is erect with stems up to 60 cm high. The stems have ascending, pubescent branches with patent or ascending hairs and are more or less minutely glandular above. The leaves are 3 to 8 by 0.1 to 0.3 cm, linear or linear-lanceolate and are not fleshy. The bracts are 3.5 to 8 mm and all have a similar shape. They are ovate-lanceolate to lanceolate, sharp-edged or acuminate with a broad dry membranous margin without lateral ribs.

Habitat: The plant is indigenous to the Mediterranean region and western Asia. Psyllium Seeds are cultivated in Spain, Central Europe, Israel, Russia, India, Pakistan, Japan, Cuba and southern Brazil.

Production: Psyllium seed (blonde) consists of the dried, ripe seed of Plantago psyllium (syn. Plantago afra) and of Plantago indica (syn. Plantago arenaria), with a swell index of at least 10, and its formulations.

Not To Be Confused With: The seeds of other Plantago seeds.

Other Names: Plantain, Fleaseed, Flea Wort, Psyllion, Psyllios

ACTIONS AND PHARMACOLOGY

COMPOUNDS

Mucilages (10-12%, chiefly arabinoxylans)

Iridoide monoterpenes: aucubin

EFFECTS

Regulation of intestinal peristalsis.

Constipation: a decrease of the passage time of the bowel content through an increase in volume of the stool, effects an expansive reflex and, as a result, a stimulated intestinal peristalsis.

Diarrhea: can normalize the passage time of the bowel content through water bonding.

INDICATIONS AND USAGE

■ Diarrhea

Psyllium seed is used for chronic constipation and irritable colon.

CONTRAINDICATIONS

Psyllium seed is contraindicated in pathologic constriction of the gastrointestinal tract, the threat of or the presence of ileus, and in severely variable Diabetes mellitus.

PRECAUTIONS AND ADVERSE REACTIONS

General: No health hazards or side effects are known in conjunction with the proper administration of designated therapeutic dosages. Allergic reactions could, however, arise in isolated cases (rhinitis, conjunctivitis, asthma, urticaria). Incorrect administration procedures (with too little fluid) can lead to obstruction (blockage) of the esophagus or of the intestine, particularly with older people.

Drug Interactions: Absorption of other drugs taken simultaneously could be delayed.

DOSAGE

Mode of Administration: Whole or ground seeds and other galenic preparations for oral application.

Preparation: Available in standardized preparations from the U.S. and France.

Daily Dose: The recommended daily dose is 10 to 30 g drug. Observe ample intake of liquid. As a laxative, 10 g drug soaked in 100 ml water, to be followed by at least 200 ml of water (1 teaspoonful = 4.7 g drug).

LITERATURE

Anonym, Pharmaceutical Care: ''Den Mißbrauch von Laxanzien vermeiden helfen''. In: DAZ 135(20):1867-1868. 1995.

Curry CE, (1982) Laxative products. In: Handbook of Nonprescription Drugs, Am Pharmac Assoc, Washington, S 69-92.

Fintelmann V, Phytopharmaka in der Gastroenterologie. In: ZPT 15(3):137. 1994.

Jaspersen-Schib R, Ballaststoffe als Lipidsenker. In: DAZ 132(39):1991. 1992.

Karawya MS et al., PM 20:14-35. 1971.

Kennedy JF et al., Carbohydr Res 75:265-274. 1979.

Further information in:

Hänsel R, Keller K, Rimpler H, Schneider G (Hrsg.), Hagers Handbuch der Pharmazeutischen Praxis, 5. Aufl., Bde 4-6 (Drogen), Springer Verlag Berlin, Heidelberg, New York, 1992-1994.

Schulz R, Hänsel R, Rationale Phytotherapie, Springer Verlag Heidelberg 1996.

Steinegger E, Hänsel R, Pharmakognosie, 5. Aufl., Springer Verlag Heidelberg 1992.

Teuscher E, Biogene Arzneimittel, 5. Aufl., Wiss. Verlagsges. Stuttgart 1997.

Wagner H, Wiesenauer M, Phytotherapie. Phytopharmaka und pflanzliche Homöopathika, Fischer-Verlag, Stuttgart, Jena, New York 1995.

Wichtl M (Hrsg.), Teedrogen, 4. Aufl., Wiss. Verlagsges. Stuttgart 1997.

Plantago Isphagula

Psyllium

DESCRIPTION

Medicinal Parts: The medicinal part is the ripe seed.

Flower and Fruit: The flowers are on cylindrical, glabrous or finely pubescent scapes, which are only slightly longer than the leaves. They form 0.5 to 3.5 cm long spikes. The bracts are about 3 mm, suborbicular to ovate and sometimes shortly pubescent. The sepals are about 2.5 mm, similarly shaped, almost free, keeled at the apex with wide scarious margins. The anterior ones are usually pubescent. The corolla-tube is 1.5 to 2 mm long and glabrous. The lobes are 2.5 mm, ovate-orbicular, subobtuse to very shortly acuminate. The stamens are exserted up to 1 mm and the capsule is about 3 mm. The seeds are 2.2 to 2.5 mm and cymbiform.

Leaves, Stem and Root: The plant is an annual almost stemless, softly pubescent plant with one or several rosettes. The leaves are 2.5 to 12 cm by 0.1 to 0.8 cm, linear to linear-lanceolate, entire-margined or slightly denticulate and sparsely to densely villous-lanate.

Habitat: The plant grows in India, Afghanistan, Iran, Israel, northern Africa, Spain and the Canary Islands. It is cultivated in India and neighboring countries, Arizona and southern Brazil.

Production: Psyllium consists of the ripe seeds or epidermis of Plantago ovata (synonym: Plantago isphagula).

Other Names: Indian Plantago, Ispaghula, Sand Plantain, Spogel

ACTIONS AND PHARMACOLOGY

COMPOUNDS: PLANTAGINIS OVATAE SEMEN

Mucilages (20-30%, parent substances arabinoxylans)

Fatty oil

Iridoide monoterpenes: aucubin

EFFECTS: PLANTAGINIS OVATAE SEMEN

When used for diarrhea, psyllium increases the passage time of the bowel content through bonding of water. When used for constipation, it decreases the passage time of the bowel content through increase in the volume of the stool. It also lowers serum-cholesterol levels.

COMPOUNDS: PLANTAGINIS OVATAE TESTA

Mucilages (parent substances arabinoxylans)

EFFECTS: PLANTAGINIS OVATAE TESTA

When used for diarrhea, psyllium increases the passage time of the bowel content through bonding of water. When used for constipation, it decreases the passage time of the bowel content through increase in the volume of the stool. It also lowers serum-cholesterol levels. Psyllium also reduces postprandial blood sugar elevation.

INDICATIONS AND USAGE

PLANTAGINIS OVATAE SEMEN AND TESTA

- Constipation
- Diarrhea
- Raised levels of cholesterol

Psyllium is used for habitual constipation and disorders where easy bowel movements with a loose stool is desirable (e.g., in patients with anal fissures and hemorrhoids; following anal/rectal surgery; and during pregnancy) and as a secondary medication in the treatment of various kinds of diarrhea and in the treatment of irritable bowel.

CONTRAINDICATIONS

PLANTAGINIS OVATAE SEMEN AND TESTA

The drug is contraindicated in patients who have pathological narrowing in the gastrointestinal tract, obstruction or threatening obstruction of the bowel (ileus), or difficulties in regulating diabetes mellitus.

PRECAUTIONS AND ADVERSE REACTIONS

PLANTAGINIS OVATAE SEMEN AND TESTA

General: No health hazards or side effects are known in conjunction with the proper administration of designated therapeutic dosages. Allergic reactions could however arise in isolated cases (rhinitis, conjunctivitis, asthma, urticaria). Incorrect administration procedures (with too little fluid) can lead to obstruction of the esophagus or of the intestine, particularly with older people.

Drug Interactions: The absorption of other drugs taken simultaneously may be delayed. There is a possibility that insulin dosage adjustment (downward) will be necessary when diabetics use psyllium products.

DOSAGE

PLANTAGINIS OVATAE SEMEN

Mode of Administration: The whole or coarsely-chopped drug as well as other galenic preparations are used internally. Sufficient fluid must be taken with the drug (150 ml water per 5 gm drug). The dose should be taken one-half hour to one hour after taking other medication.

Daily Dosage: The daily dosage ranges from 12 to 40 gm of the drug. Unless otherwise prescribed, 1 to 3 teaspooonfuls (5 to 15 gm drug) should be soaked in a little water, and taken in the mornings and evenings with sufficient liquid (1 to 2 glasses).

PLANTAGINIS OVATAE TESTA

Mode of Administration: The whole drug as well as other galenic preparations are taken orally.

Daily Dosage: The daily dosage is 4 to 20 gm of the drug prepared accordingly. Ample intake of liquid should be ensured (150 ml of water per 5 gm drug).

LITERATURE

PLANTAGINIS OVATAE SEMEN

Anonym, Pharmaceutical Care: ''Den Mißbrauch von Laxanzien vermeiden helfen''. In: DAZ 135(20):1867-1868. 1995.

Curry CE, (1982) Laxative products. In: Handbook of Nonprescription Drugs, Am Pharmac Assoc, Washington, S 69-92.

Ershoff BH, (1976) J Food Sci 41:949.

Kasper H, (1985) Ernährungsmedizin und Diätetik. 5. Aufl. Urban & Schwarzenberg, München Wien. Leng-Peschlow E.

Fintelmann V, Phytopharmaka in der Gastroenterologie. In: ZPT 15(3):137. 1994.

Gelpi E et al., PH 8:2077-2081. 1969.

Jaspersen-Schib R, Ballaststoffe als Lipidsenker. In: DAZ 132(39):1991. 1992.

Kennedy JF et al., Carbohydr Res 75:265-274. 1979.

Khorana ML et al., (1958) Ind J Pharm 20:3.

Koedam A, Plantago - history and use. In: Pharm Weekbl 112(10):246-252. 1977.

Mengs U, (1990) No renal pigmentation by plantago ovata seeds or husks. Med Sci Res 18:37-38.

Miller JN, In: Industrial Gums, Ed. R. L. Whistler, Academic Press 1973.

Oshio H, Inouye H, (1982) Planta Med 44:204.

Popov S, (1978) IUPAC Int Symp Chem Nat Prod 11(2):61 (via CA 92:59170).

Sandhu JS et al., Carbohdr Res 93:247-259. 1981.

Tomoda M et al., (1987) Planta Med 53(1):8.

Further information in:

Chan EH et al. (Ed.), Advances in Chinese Medicinal Materials Research, World Scientific Pub. Co. Singapore 1985.

Hänsel R, Keller K, Rimpler H, Schneider G (Hrsg.), Hagers Handbuch der Pharmazeutischen Praxis, 5. Aufl., Bde 4-6 (Drogen): Springer Verlag Berlin, Heidelberg, New York, 1992-1994.

Leung AY, Encyclopedia of Common Natural Ingredients Used in Food Drugs and Cosmetics, John Wiley & Sons Inc., New York 1980.

Steinegger E, Hänsel R, Pharmakognosie, 5. Aufl., Springer Verlag Heidelberg 1992.

Teuscher E, Biogene Arzneimittel, 5. Aufl., Wiss. Verlagsges. Stuttgart 1997.

Wagner H, Wiesenauer M, Phytotherapie. Phytopharmaka und pflanzliche Homöopathika, Fischer-Verlag, Stuttgart, Jena, New York 1995.

Wichtl M (Hrsg.), Teedrogen, 4. Aufl., Wiss. Verlagsges. Stuttgart 1997.

PLANTAGINIS OVATAE TESTA

Anonym, Pharmaceutical Care: ''Den Mißbrauch von Laxanzien vermeiden helfen''. In: DAZ 135(20):1867-1868. 1995.

Curry CE, (1982) Laxative products. In: Handbook of Nonprescription Drugs, Am Pharmac Assoc, Washington, S 69-92.

Ershoff BH, (1976) J Food Sci 41:949.

Fintelmann V, Phytopharmaka in der Gastroenterologie. In: ZPT 15(3):137. 1994.

Gelpi E et al., PH 8:2077-2081. 1969.

Jaspersen-Schib R, Ballaststoffe als Lipidsenker. In: DAZ 132(39):1991. 1992.

Kasper H, (1985) Ernährungsmedizin und Diätetik. 5. Aufl. Urban & Schwarzenberg, München Wien. Leng-Peschlow E.

Kennedy JF et al., Carbohydr Res 75:265-274. 1979.

Khorana ML et al., (1958) Ind J Pharm 20:3.

Koedam A, Plantago - history and use. In: Pharm Weekbl 112(10):246-252. 1977.

Mengs U, (1990) No renal pigmentation by plantago ovata seeds or husks. Med Sci Res 18:37-38.

Miller JN, In: Industrial Gums, Ed. R. L. Whistler, Academic Press 1973.

Oshio H, Inouye H, (1982) Planta Med 44:204.

Popov S, (1978) IUPAC Int Symp Chem Nat Prod 11(2):61 (via CA 92:59170).

Sandhu JS et al., Carbohdr Res 93:247-259. 1981.

Tomoda M et al., (1987) Planta Med 53(1):8.

Further information in:

Chan EH et al. (Ed.), Advances in Chinese Medicinal Materials Research, World Scientific Pub. Co. Singapore 1985.

Hänsel R, Keller K, Rimpler H, Schneider G (Hrsg.), Hagers Handbuch der Pharmazeutischen Praxis, 5. Aufl., Bde 4-6 (Drogen): Springer Verlag Berlin, Heidelberg, New York, 1992-1994.

Leung AY, Encyclopedia of Common Natural Ingredients Used in Food Drugs and Cosmetics, John Wiley & Sons Inc., New York 1980.

Steinegger E, Hänsel R, Pharmakognosie, 5. Aufl., Springer Verlag Heidelberg 1992.

Teuscher E, Biogene Arzneimittel, 5. Aufl., Wiss. Verlagsges. Stuttgart 1997.

Wagner H, Wiesenauer M, Phytotherapie. Phytopharmaka und pflanzliche Homöopathika, Fischer-Verlag, Stuttgart, Jena, New York 1995.

Wichtl M (Hrsg.), Teedrogen, 4. Aufl., Wiss. Verlagsges. Stuttgart 1997.

Plantago Lanceolata

Plantain

DESCRIPTION

Medicinal Parts: The medicinal parts are the dried leaves, the dried herb and the fresh plant.

Flower and Fruit: The globular or shortly cylindrical spikes are on erect or ascending, 5-grooved, appressed pubescent peduncles. The flowers are small, almost colorless behind scarious, narrow-acuminate bracts. The scarious calyx is deeply divided into 4 parts and has a cylindrical tube and a margin with 4 ovate tips. There are 4 long stamens with yellowish-white filaments and anthers and 1 superior ovary. The fruit is a bivalvular, 3 to 4 mm long capsule. The seeds are oblong, 2 mm long and blackish.

Leaves, Stem and Root: The plant is perennial and grows from 5 to 50 cm high. It has a very fibrous root. All the leaves are in basal rosettes and are lanceolate or linear lanceolate, deeply 3 to 5 ribbed, entire-margined or short-dentate.

Habitat: The plant is widespread in the cool temperate regions of the world.

Production: Plantain herb consists of the fresh or dried above-ground parts of Plantago lanceolata, harvested at flowering season.

Not To Be Confused With: The similar Digitalis-lanata leaves.

Other Names: Buckhorn, Chimney-sweeps, Headsman, Ribgrass, Ribwort, Ripplegrass, Soldier's Herb

ACTIONS AND PHARMACOLOGY

COMPOUNDS

Iridoide monoterpenes (2-3%): chief components are aucubin (rhinantin) and catalpol

Mucilages: (2-6%, glucomannans, arabinogalactane, rhamnogalacturonane)

Flavonoids: including among other chief components apigenine-6,8-diglucoside, luteolin-7-glucuronide

Caffeic acid esters: chlorogenic acid, neochlorogenic acid, acteoside (verbascoside)

Tannins

Hydroxycoumarins: aesculetin

Saponins (traces)

Silicic acid

EFFECTS

The herb is astringent and antibacterial. The liquid extract and the pressed juice of fresh plantain herb possess proven bacteriostatic and bactericidal effects due to the tannin content.

INDICATIONS AND USAGE

- Common cold
- Cough/bronchitis
- Fevers and colds
- Inflammation of the mouth and pharynx
- Inflammation of the skin
- Tendency to infection

Plantain is used internally for catarrh of the respiratory tract and inflammatory alterations of the oral and pharyngeal mucosa. Externally, it is used for inflammatory reactions of the skin. In folk medicine, the pressed juice is used to treat wounds and inflammations and as a hemostyptic.

PRECAUTIONS AND ADVERSE REACTIONS

No health hazards or side effects are known in conjunction with the proper administration of designated therapeutic dosages.

DOSAGE

Mode of Administration: As a comminuted herb and other galenic preparations for internal and external use. It is available as macerations, liquid extracts, lozenges, syrup, and pressed juice of the fresh plant. The drug is available in many standardized preparations of antitussives and expectorants.

Preparation: To make an infusion, pour boiling water over 2 to 4 gm cut drug (or put in cold water which is brought to a boil) and strain after 10 minutes. (1 teaspoonful = approximately 0.7 gm drug)

Daily Dosage: The average daily dose is 3 to 6 gm of herb.

LITERATURE

Bräutigam M, Franz G, Schleimpolysaccharide aus Spitzwegerichblättern. In: DAZ 125:58. 1985.

Davini E, The quantitative isolation and antimicrobial activity of aglycone of aucubin. In: PH 25:2420. 1986.

Elich J, Die antibakterielle Aktivität einiger einheimischer Plantago-Arten. In: Disseration Universität Berlin. 1962.

Koedam A, Plantago - history and use. In: Pharm Weekbl 112(10):246-252. 1977.

Murai M et al., Phenylethanoids in the herb of Planatago lanceolata and inhibitory effects on arachidonic acid-induced mouse ear edema. In: PM 61(5):479-480. 1995.

Wunderer H, Zentral und peripher wirksame Antitussiva: eine kritische Übersicht. In: PZ 142(11):847-852. 1997.

Further information in:

Hänsel R, Keller K, Rimpler H, Schneider G (Hrsg.), Hagers Handbuch der Pharmazeutischen Praxis, 5. Aufl., Bde 4-6 (Drogen), Springer Verlag Berlin, Heidelberg, New York, 1992-1994.

Madaus G, Lehrbuch der Biologischen Arzneimittel, Bde. 1-3, Nachdruck, Georg Olms Verlag Hildesheim 1979.

Schulz R, Hänsel R, Rationale Phytotherapie, Springer Verlag Heidelberg 1996.

Steinegger E, Hänsel R, Pharmakognosie, 5. Aufl., Springer Verlag Heidelberg 1992.

Teuscher E, Biogene Arzneimittel, 5. Aufl., Wiss. Verlagsges. Stuttgart 1997.

Wagner H, Wiesenauer M, Phytotherapie. Phytopharmaka und pflanzliche Homöopathika, Fischer-Verlag, Stuttgart, Jena, New York 1995.

Wichtl M (Hrsg.), Teedrogen, 4. Aufl., Wiss. Verlagsges. Stuttgart 1997.

Plantain

See Plantago Lanceolata

Pleurisy Root

See Asclepias Tuberosa

Podophyllum Peltatum

Mayapple

DESCRIPTION

Medicinal Parts: The medicinal parts are the dried rhizome and the resin extracted from them.

Flower and Fruit: The solitary white flowers are located in the stem bifurcation between 2 leaves. When the flower drops, the developing fruit swells to the size and shape of a 2.5 to 5 cm long rosehip. It is yellow and fleshy.

Leaves, Stem and Root: The plant is a perennial reaching a height of 40 cm. It has a bifurcated, 45 cm high stem and deeply indented, umbrella-like, hand-sized leaves. The rhizome is reddish-brown and is 0.5 cm in diameter. Depending on the time of harvesting, the surface of the rhizome may be smooth or wrinkled. Nodes occur at intervals of 3 to 5 cm and the fracture is whitish.

Characteristics: The odor is unpleasant and acrid.

Habitat: The plant is indigenous to northeast North America.

Production: Mayapple rhizome consists of the dried rhizome and connected roots of Podophyllum peltatum. Mayapple resin consists of the resin of the dried and aged rhizome of Podophyllum peltatum.

Not To Be Confused With: Mayapple should not be confused with English Mandrake or Bryonia dioica.

Other Names: Duck's Foot, Ground Lemon, Hog Apple, Indian Apple, Mandrake, Raccoon Berry, Wild Lemon

ACTIONS AND PHARMACOLOGY

COMPOUNDS

Lignans: chief components podophyllotoxin (20%), additionally including among others alpha-peltatin (5%), beta-peltatin (10%), 4′-dimethyl podophyllotoxin, dioxypodophyllotoxin

EFFECTS

The drug is antimitotic.

INDICATIONS AND USAGE

■ Warts

Preparations of Mayapple are used externally for removal of pointed condyloma. The treated skin surface must not be larger than 25 sq. cm. Be sure to protect skin adjacent to the treated area.

CONTRAINDICATIONS

The drug is contraindicated in pregnancy.

PRECAUTIONS AND ADVERSE REACTIONS

General: The drug is severely irritating to skin and mucous membranes. External administration of the drug over large skin areas can also bring about resorptive poisonings. The drug should not be taken internally in allophathic medicine. With external use, the skin area to be treated should not exceed 25 sq. cm. The drug serves as an industrial drug for the extraction of podophyllotoxin and its semi-synthetic derivatives that are used in tumor therapy.

Use in Pregnancy: The drug is contraindicated in pregnancy.

OVERDOSAGE

In dosages over 0.2 gm, it causes severe abdominal pain, bloody-watery diarrhea, vomiting of liquid bile, dizziness, headache, coordination disorders, spasms, nephritis, later collapse and death in coma through respiratory failure.

Following gastrointestinal emptying (inducement of vomiting, gastric lavage with burgundy-colored potassium permanganate solution, sodium sulfate) and instillation of activated charcoal, the therapy for poisonings consists of treating spasms with diazepam (i.v.), electrolyte substitution and treating possible cases of acidosis with sodium bicarbonate infusions. In case of shock, plasma volume expanders should be used. Monitoring of kidney function is essential. Intubation and oxygen respiration may also be necessary.

DOSAGE

Mode of Administration: The dried rhizome is used for production of resin exclusively for external application.

Daily Dosage: The daily dosage is 1.5 to 3.0 gm root, 1.5 to 3.0 gm liquid extract, or 2.5 to 7.5 gm tincture.

LITERATURE

Anonym, Dermatologie: Gemeine Warze, Flachwarze und spitze Feigwarze. In: DAZ 134(22):2059. 1994.

Auterhoff H, May O, (1958) Planta Med 6:240.

Chatterjee R, (1952) Econ Bot 6:342.

Dewick P et al., (1982) Phytochemistry 20:2277.

Enzell CR, Wahlberg I, Aaasen AI, Fortschr Chem Org Naturstoffe 34:1. 1977.

Franz G, Biogene Cytostatica. In: DAZ 130(35):2003. 1990.

Hartwell JL, Detly WE, (1950) J Am. Chem Soc 72:246.

Jardine I, In: Anticancer Agents Based on Natural Product Models, Ed. Cassady JM, Douros JD., Academic Press 1980.

MacRae WD, Towers GHN, Biological activities of lignans. In: PH 23(6):1207-1220. 1984.

Stoll A et al., (1954) J Am Chem Soc 76:5004 et 6431.

Stoll A et al., (1955) J Am. Chem Soc 77:1710.

Wartburg A et al., (1957) Helv Chim. Acta 40:1331.

Further information in:

Frohne D, Pfänder HJ, Giftpflanzen - Ein Handbuch für Apotheker, Toxikologen und Biologen, 4. Aufl., Wiss. Verlags-Ges. Stuttgart 1997.

Lewin L, Gifte und Vergiftungen, 6. Aufl., Nachdruck, Haug Verlag, Heidelberg 1992.

Madaus G, Lehrbuch der Biologischen Arzneimittel, Bde. 1-3, Nachdruck, Georg Olms Verlag Hildesheim 1979.

Roth L, Daunderer M, Kormann K, Giftpflanzen, Pflanzengifte, 4. Aufl., Ecomed Fachverlag Landsberg Lech 1993.

Schulz R, Hänsel R, Rationale Phytotherapie, Springer Verlag Heidelberg 1996.

Steinegger E, Hänsel R, Pharmakognosie, 5. Aufl., Springer Verlag Heidelberg 1992.

Teuscher E, Lindequist U, Biogene Gifte - Biologie, Chemie, Pharmakologie, 2. Aufl., Fischer Verlag Stuttgart 1994.

Teuscher E, Biogene Arzneimittel, 5. Aufl., Wiss. Verlagsges. Stuttgart 1997.

Pogostemon Cablin

Patchouli

DESCRIPTION

Medicinal Parts: The medicinal parts are the young leaves and shoots and the oil extracted from them.

Flower and Fruit: The flowers, which are whitish and often have reddish marks, grow in terminal and axillary spikes.

Leaves, Stem and Root: The plant is a pubescent, perennial herb, which grows from 60 to 90 cm high. The stem is erect and quandrangular and the leaves are ovate, opposite and soft.

Characteristics: The ovate leaves have a strong characteristic odor when rubbed. The extracted oil is used in perfumery. The desired characteristics improve with age.

Habitat: The plant is cultivated in tropical and subtropical regions worldwide.

Production: Patchouli oil is extracted from the leaves of Pogostemon cablin.

Other Names: Putcha-pat, Patchouly

ACTIONS AND PHARMACOLOGY

COMPOUNDS

Volatile oil (1.5-4%): chief components are sesquiterpenes, including among others patchouli alcohol (35%), alpha-guaiene (20%), alpha-bulnesen (20%), beta-patchoulen (2%). Sesquiterpene pyridine alkaloids were isolated from the volatile oil, including among others, patchoulipyridin, epiguajpyridin

EFFECTS

No information is available.

INDICATIONS AND USAGE

There is no known medicinal use. The herb is used in perfumes and cosmetics.

PRECAUTIONS AND ADVERSE REACTIONS

No health hazards or side effects are known in conjunction with the proper administration of designated therapeutic dosages.

DOSAGE

Mode of Administration: It is used only in the perfume and cosmetic industry.

LITERATURE

Kern W, List PH, Hörhammer L (Hrsg.), Hagers Handbuch der Pharmazeutischen Praxis, 4. Aufl., Bde. 1-8, Springer Verlag Berlin, Heidelberg, New York, 1969.

Leung AY, Encyclopedia of Common Natural Ingredients Used in Food Drugs and Cosmetics, John Wiley & Sons Inc., New York 1980.

Poison Ivy

See Rhus Toxicodendron

Poisonous Buttercup

See Ranunculus Sceleratus

Poke Root

See Phytolacca Americana

Polemonium Coeruleum

Jacob's Ladder

DESCRIPTION

Medicinal Parts: The medicinal part is the herb.

Flower and Fruit: The numerous flowers grow in clusters at the end of the lateral branches. They are open, slightly hanging and have 5 sepals and 5 petals. The corolla is 2 to 2.5 cm, deep blue and has a short pollen tube. The stamens are enclosed in the tube and have yellow anthers.

Leaves, Stem and Root: The plant is a perennial. The plant is bright green and smooth. The upper section is covered in short glandular hairs. The rhizome is short and creeping and the stem is 45 to 90 cm high, hollow and quadrangular. The leaves with numerous pairs of leaflets are 1.25 to 2.5 cm long. These are pinnate and alternate.

Habitat: The plant is indigenous to central and northern Europe.

Production: Jacob's Ladder is the aerial part of Polemonium coeruleum.

Other Names: Charity, English Greek Valerian

ACTIONS AND PHARMACOLOGY

COMPOUNDS

Triterpene saponins

Flavonoids

EFFECTS

All parts of the plant contain saponin, which has astringent, diaphoretic and hemolytic effects.

INDICATIONS AND USAGE

Jacob's Ladder is used for febrile and inflammatory conditions.

PRECAUTIONS AND ADVERSE REACTIONS

No health hazards or side effects are known in conjunction with the proper administration of designated therapeutic dosages.

DOSAGE

Mode of Administration: The ground drug is used as an infusion.

LITERATURE

Reznicek G et al., A new ester saponine from Polemonium caeruleum. In: PM 59(7):A612. 1993.

Further information in:

Kern W, List PH, Hörhammer L (Hrsg.), Hagers Handbuch der Pharmazeutischen Praxis, 4. Aufl., Bde. 1-8, Springer Verlag Berlin, Heidelberg, New York, 1969.

Polemonium Reptans

Abscess Root

DESCRIPTION

Medicinal Parts: The medicinal part is the dried root.

Flower and Fruit: The hanging blue flowers are in loose terminal, glandular-haired panicles.

Leaves, Stem and Root: The plant grows to about 25 cm. It has creeping roots and a thin rhizome, which produces numerous stems and numerous pale, thin, glabrous and brittle roots. The glabrous stems are heavily branched and bear alternate or opposite, pinnatifid leaves with 6 or 7 pairs of leaflets.

Habitat: The plant is found in the U.S.

Production: Abscess root is the rhizome of Polemonium reptans.

Not To Be Confused With: The plant is known as False Jacob's Ladder because it has an astringent action similar to true Jacob's Ladder.

Other Names: American Greek Valerian, Blue Bells, False Jacob's Ladder, Sweatroot

ACTIONS AND PHARMACOLOGY

COMPOUNDS

Triterpene saponins

EFFECTS

Abscess root has astringent, diaphoretic, and expectorant effects. No current research is available.

INDICATIONS AND USAGE

The drug is used for febrile and inflammatory disorders.

PRECAUTIONS AND ADVERSE REACTIONS

No health hazards or side effects are known in conjunction with the proper administration of designated therapeutic dosages.

DOSAGE

Mode of Administration: It is ground as a drug for infusion.

LITERATURE

Hegnauer R, Chemotaxonomie der Pflanzen, Bde 1-11, Birkhäuser Verlag Basel, Boston, Berlin 1962-1997.

Polygala Amara

Bitter Milkwort

DESCRIPTION

Medicinal Parts: The medicinal part is the flowering plant with root.

Flower and Fruit: The blue or occasionally white or pink flowers are in many-blossomed racemes. Of the 5 sepals, the 2 lateral ones are large, petal-like, patent and 3-veined. The other 3 are smaller and the middle vein is green. The 3 petals are fused together with the stamens. These form 2 clusters in 2 green pockets on the larger, lower petal. The 2 upper petals form a kind of upper lip. The ovary is superior and bilocular with a spoon-like style. The fruit is an obcordate capsule which is compressed at the sides and enclosed in the sepals.

Leaves, Stem and Root: The plant grows from 5 to 15 cm high. The stems are branched at the base, decumbent or ascending. The basal leaves form a rosette and the cauline leaves are alternate, oblong-cuneate or obovate-lanceolate.

Habitat: The plant is indigenous to Europe.

Production: Bitter Milkwort herb, including its roots, is the complete plant of Polygala amara.

Other Names: European Bitter Polygala, European Senega Snakeroot, Evergreen Snakeroot, Flowering Wintergreen, Little Pollom

ACTIONS AND PHARMACOLOGY

COMPOUNDS

Saponins: chief components senegin

Bitter principles: polygalin (polygamarin)

Phenol glycosides: monotropitoside (methyl salicylic acid-primveroside)

Polygalit (1,5-anhydrosorbite)

EFFECTS

The active agents are saponin, bitter substances and methylestersalizylic acid. The drug is mildly expectorant.

INDICATIONS AND USAGE

Bitter Milkwort is used for conditions of the respiratory tract, cough, and bronchitis.

PRECAUTIONS AND ADVERSE REACTIONS

No health hazards or side effects are known in conjunction with the proper administration of designated therapeutic dosages.

DOSAGE

Mode of Administration: The drug is obsolete in many countries.

Preparation: The drug is contained in tea for the treatment of bronchitis.

LITERATURE

Hegnauer R, Chemotaxonomie der Pflanzen, Bde 1-11, Birkhäuser Verlag Basel, Boston, Berlin 1962-1997.

Kern W, List PH, Hörhammer L (Hrsg.), Hagers Handbuch der Pharmazeutischen Praxis, 4. Aufl., Bde. 1-8, Springer Verlag Berlin, Heidelberg, New York, 1969.

Madaus G, Lehrbuch der Biologischen Arzneimittel, Bde 1-3, Nachdruck, Georg Olms Verlag Hildesheim 1979.

Polygala Senega

Senega Snakeroot

DESCRIPTION

Medicinal Parts: The medicinal part is the dried root.

Flower and Fruit: The raceme is 8 cm long and is smaller than the bracts. The petals are pale red, the wings are yellowish white with green veins.

Leaves, Stem and Root: The plant is a perennial herb with up to 40 cm high stems, which sprout in the axils of the scale-like bracts of the previous year's growth. The leaves are 8 cm long and 3 cm wide, alternate, ovate-lanceolate to lanceolate, acuminate and denticulate. The upper surface is rich green; the under surface somewhat paler. The root varies in color from pale yellowish gray to brownish gray. It is usually twisted or almost spiral and has a thick, irregular, gnarled crown.

Habitat: Polygala senega is indigenous to the central and western U.S.

Production: Senega Snakeroot consists of the dried root with remains of aerial stems of Polygala senega and/or other closely related species or a mixture of Polygala species.

Not To Be Confused With: The roots of other Polygala species.

Other Names: Milkwort, Mountain Flax, Rattlesnake Root, Seneca, Senega, Seneka, Snake Root

ACTIONS AND PHARMACOLOGY

COMPOUNDS: POLYGALA SENEGA RHIZOME

Triterpene saponins (6-12%): chief components senegasaponine A-D, aglycone senegin

Oligosaccharide esters: senegosene A-I

Xantho derivatives

Methyl salicylate (traces) and its glucoside

EFFECTS: POLYGALA SENEGA RHIZOME

The rhizome is secretolytic and works as an expectorant.

COMPOUNDS: POLYGALA TENUIFOLIA RHIZOME

Triterpene saponins (6-12%): chief components onjisaponine aglycone senegin

Oligosaccharide esters: tenuifolosen A-P

EFFECTS: POLYGALA TENUIFOLIA RHIZOME

The rhizome is secretolytic and works as an expectorant.

INDICATIONS AND USAGE

■ Cough/bronchitis

The drug is used as a catarrh of the respiratory tract, as an expectorant in cases of bronchitis with minor sputum output, and tracheitis.

PRECAUTIONS AND ADVERSE REACTIONS

No health hazards or side effects are known in conjunction with the proper administration of designated therapeutic dosages. With prolonged use, gastrointestinal irritation can occur.

OVERDOSAGE

Overdosage leads to nausea, diarrhea, gastric complaints and queasiness.

DOSAGE

Mode of Administration: As a comminuted root for decoctions and other galenic preparations for internal use or as an extract. It is a component of various standardized antitussive preparations.

Preparation: To make an infusion, place 0.5 gm comminuted drug in cold water, heat to a simmer, and strain after 10 minutes. (1 teaspoonful = 2.5 gm drug)

Daily Dosage: The daily dosage is 1.5 to 3.0 gm root or liquid extract (1:2) or 2.5 to 7.5 gm tincture (1:10). To use the infusion as an expectorant, drink 1 cup of tea 2 to 3 times daily. In serious cases, the tea can be taken every two hours if the patient is observed for side effects.

LITERATURE

Corner JJ et al., (1962) Phytochemistry 1:73.

Kako M et al., Hypoglycemic effect of the rhizomes of Polygala senega in normal and diabetic mice and its main component, the triterpenoid glycoside senegin-II. In: PM 62(5)440-443. 1996.

Shibata S, In: Progress in Phytochemistry, Vol. 6, Ed. Reinhold et al., Pergamon Press 1980.

Shoji J et al., (1971) Yakugaku Zasshi 91:198.

Further information in:

Kern W, List PH, Hörhammer L (Hrsg.), Hagers Handbuch der Pharmazeutischen Praxis, 4. Aufl., Bde 1-8, Springer Verlag Berlin, Heidelberg, New York, 1969.

Madaus G, Lehrbuch der Biologischen Arzneimittel, Bde 1-3, Nachdruck, Georg Olms Verlag Hildesheim 1979.

Steinegger E, Hänsel R, Pharmakognosie, 5. Aufl., Springer Verlag Heidelberg 1992.

Teuscher E, Biogene Arzneimittel, 5. Aufl., Wiss. Verlagsges. Stuttgart 1997.

Wichtl M (Hrsg.), Teedrogen, 4. Aufl., Wiss. Verlagsges. Stuttgart 1997.

Polygonatum Multiflorum

Solomon's Seal

DESCRIPTION

Medicinal Parts: The medicinal parts of the plant are the dried rhizome and roots.

Flower and Fruit: The odorless, greenish white campanulate flowers are in 2 to 6 blossomed racemes, usually without an accompanying leaf. The perigone tube is tightly cylindrical, 9 to 20 mm long and 2 to 4 mm wide. It is drawn together over the ovary and opens out like a funnel at the top. The tepals at the tip are pubescent on the inside and the filaments are softly pubescent. The fruit is a blue-black, frosted berry, 8 to 9 mm in diameter with a disgusting, sweet taste.

Leaves, Stem and Root: The plant is a perennial 30 to 80 cm high herb. The stems are sturdy, round and glabrous. The leaves are ovate to elliptical, 5 to 15 cm long and 3 to 7.5 cm wide, narrowing suddenly at the base. They are glabrous, dark green above and gray-green frosted beneath.

Habitat: The plant is indigenous to Europe, the Near East, eastern Asia, the Himalayas, Siberia and North America.

Production: Solomon's seal rhizome is the rhizome of Polygonatum multiflorum. The root-stocks should be dug up during the dormant seasons, autumn and spring. Earth and roots are removed and the rhizomes are cut into pieces, which are a few centimeters in length.

Other Names: Dropberry, Lady's Seals, Sealroot, Sealwort, St. Mary's Seal

ACTIONS AND PHARMACOLOGY

COMPOUNDS

Steroid saponins: 2 unnamed saponins, aglycones diosgenin

Mucilages

Acetidin-2-carboxylic acid

EFFECTS

The plant is astringent and anti-inflammatory. It works as a tonic and relieves and soothes upset stomach.

INDICATIONS AND USAGE

The plant was formerly used in the treatment of respiratory and lung disorders. It was used externally in the treatment of bruises, furuncles, ulcers or boils on the fingers, hemorrhoids, redness of the skin, and for edema and hematoma.

PRECAUTIONS AND ADVERSE REACTIONS

No health hazards or side effects are known in conjunction with the proper administration of designated therapeutic dosages. Extended administration of the drug in therapeutic dosages can lead to gastrointestinal irritations.

OVERDOSAGE

Overdosage leads to nausea, diarrhea, gastric complaints, queasiness.

DOSAGE

Mode of Administration: The drug has been used internally as an infusion and externally as a poultice, but is now obsolete.

Storage: Store in paper and cloth sacks.

LITERATURE

Janeczko Z, (1980) Acta Polon. Pharm 37:559.

Kato A, Miura T, Hypoglycemic action of the rhizomes of Polygonatum officinale in normal and diabetic mice. In: PM 60(3):201. 1994.

Sugiyama M et al., Chem Pharm Bull 32:1365-1372. 1984.

Tomoda M et al., Chem Pharm Bull 21:2511-2516. 1973.

Further information in:

Frohne D, Pfänder HJ, Giftpflanzen - Ein Handbuch für Apotheker, Toxikologen und Biologen, 4. Aufl., Wiss. Verlags-Ges. Stuttgart 1997.

Hänsel R, Keller K, Rimpler H, Schneider G (Hrsg.), Hagers Handbuch der Pharmazeutischen Praxis, 5. Aufl., Bde 4-6 (Drogen), Springer Verlag Berlin, Heidelberg, New York, 1992-1994.

Madaus G, Lehrbuch der Biologischen Arzneimittel, Bde 1-3, Nachdruck, Georg Olms Verlag Hildesheim 1979.

Roth L, Daunderer M, Kormann K, Giftpflanzen, Pflanzengifte, 4. Aufl., Ecomed Fachverlag Landsberg Lech 1993.

Teuscher E, Lindequist U, Biogene Gifte - Biologie, Chemie, Pharmakologie, 2. Aufl., Fischer Verlag Stuttgart 1994.

Polygonum Aviculare

Knotweed

DESCRIPTION

Medicinal Parts: The medicinal parts are the herb, sometimes with the root, collected during the flowering season and dried, as well as the fresh aerial parts collected during the flowering season.

Flower and Fruit: The inflorescences are axillary cymes with 1 or a few flowers. The flowers are very small, short pedicled, inconspicuous and green or red with white margins. The epicalyx has 5 bracts and is fused at the base. There are 5 stamens and the superior ovary has 3 styles. The fruit is a nut, which is as long as the epicalyx and is matte brown with wrinkled stripes, ovate to almost elliptical and flattened on 3 sides.

Leaves, Stem and Root: The plant is a sturdy annual. The main stem is initially erect, up to 1 m high and heavily branched. It later becomes closely procumbent and spreads along the ground. The leaves are alternate, entire-margined, short-petioled with varying forms on the main and side shoots. They are broadly elliptical to linear-lanceolate, acute or obtuse. At the base of the leaves there is a scarious divided leaf sheath. The thin, fusiform, brownish roots produce a few hair-thin lateral roots.

Characteristics: The appearance depends on the location. It may also have an ascending stem.

Habitat: The plant is found in most temperate regions of the world.

Production: Knotweed herb consists of the dried herb, occasionally containing roots, of Polygonum aviculare, gathered during flowering season.

Other Names: Allseed Nine-joints, Armstrong, Beggarweed, Bird's Tongue, Birdweed, Centinode, Cow Grass, Crawlgrass, Doorweed, Hogweed, Knotgrass, Ninety-knot, Pigrush, Pigweed, Red Robin, Sparrow Tongue, Swine's Grass, Swynel Grass

ACTIONS AND PHARMACOLOGY

COMPOUNDS

Flavonoids (0.1-1%): chief components are avicularin (quercetin-3-arabinoside), hyperoside, quercitrin, quercetin-3-galactoside, additionally including among others vitexin, isovitexin, rhamnazine bisulphate

Silicic acid (1%): partially water-soluble

Tannins

Hydroxycoumarins: umbelliferone, scopoletin

Lignans: aviculin

EFFECTS

Knotweed has astringent properties and is an acetylcholinesterase inhibitor.

INDICATIONS AND USAGE

- Cough/bronchitis
- Inflammation of the mouth and pharynx

The herb is used as a mild catarrh of the respiratory tract for inflammatory changes to the oral and pharyngeal mucosa. In folk medicine it is used as a supportive treatment for pulmonary disorders, as a perspiration inhibitor in cases of tuberculosis, as a diuretic, as a hemostatic in cases of hemorrhage, and for skin disorders.

PRECAUTIONS AND ADVERSE REACTIONS

No health hazards or side effects are known in conjunction with the proper administration of designated therapeutic dosages.

DOSAGE

Mode of Administration: As a ground herb for teas and other galenic preparations for internal use and local application. The drug is a component of various pectoral and bronchial teas. The extract is found in standardized preparations of antitussives and diuretics.

Preparation: To make a tea, place 1.5 gm finely cut drug in cold water and bring to a simmer. Strain after 5 to 10 minutes. (1 teaspoonful = 1.4 gm drug)

Daily Dosage: The daily dosage is 4 to 6 gm of drug. As a supportive treatment for coughs and bronchial catarrh, drink 1 cup 3 to 5 times a day.

LITERATURE

Haverland F, PA 18:59-87. 1963.

Further information in:

Hänsel R, Keller K, Rimpler H, Schneider G (Hrsg.), Hagers Handbuch der Pharmazeutischen Praxis, 5. Aufl., Bde 4-6 (Drogen), Springer Verlag Berlin, Heidelberg, New York, 1992-1994.

Madaus G, Lehrbuch der Biologischen Arzneimittel, Bde 1-3, Nachdruck, Georg Olms Verlag Hildesheim 1979.

Steinegger E, Hänsel R, Pharmakognosie, 5. Aufl., Springer Verlag Heidelberg 1992.

Wichtl M (Hrsg.), Teedrogen, 4. Aufl., Wiss. Verlagsges. Stuttgart 1997.

Polygonum Bistorta

Bistort

DESCRIPTION

Medicinal Parts: The medicinal parts are the leaves and the rhizome.

Flower and Fruit: The flowering stem terminates in a compact, cylindrical, false spike of flesh-colored flowers without a terminal bud. The pedicle is winged. The flowers consist of 5 sepals, 8 stamens and an ovary with 2 to 3 styles. The flowers are in pairs, one of which is complete, the other only having a rudimentary ovary. Only the latter ripens. The complete flowers can be cross-pollinated by insects. The fruit is a three-seeded achene. The ripe seeds are small, brown and glossy.

Leaves, Stem and Root: The plant is a perennial, 30 cm to 1 m high herb on a thick, somewhat flattened and twisted S-shaped rhizome. The radical, oval leaves grow out of the rhizome to form basal rosette leaves with cordate bases, which are blue-green above and somewhat undulate.

Habitat: The plant is indigenous to Europe, North America and Asia.

Production: Bistort root and rhizome is the subterranean part of Polygonum bistorta. The root-stocks of the older plants are harvested, cleaned, and freed from green parts and rootlets. The stronger parts are then cut up and this material is dried in the sun.

Other Names: Adderwort, Dragonwort, Easter Giant, Easter Mangiant, Oderwort, Osterick, Patience Dock, Red Legs, Snakeweed, Sweet Dock

ACTIONS AND PHARMACOLOGY

COMPOUNDS

Tannins (15-36%): chiefly condensed tannins, small quantity of gallo tannins

Starch

EFFECTS

The active agents are the galenic tannin substance, starch, catechin and silicic acid. Higher concentrations of the root cause an increase in the formation of mucus. It is also an astringent.

INDICATIONS AND USAGE

The herb is used in the treatment of digestive disorders, particularly diarrhea. Externally, it is used as a gargle for mouth and throat infections and as an ablution or ointment for wounds.

PRECAUTIONS AND ADVERSE REACTIONS

No health hazards or side effects are known in conjunction with the proper administration of designated therapeutic dosages.

DOSAGE

Mode of Administration: Internally as a powdered drug for infusion, or externally as an extract or ointment.

LITERATURE

Gonnet JF, (1981) Biochem Syst Ecol 9(4):299.

Rao PRSP, Rao EV, (1977) Curr. Sci 48(18):640.

Further information in:

Kern W, List PH, Hörhammer L (Hrsg.), Hagers Handbuch der Pharmazeutischen Praxis, 4. Aufl., Bde. 1-8, Springer Verlag Berlin, Heidelberg, New York, 1969.

Polygonum Hydropiper

Smartweed

DESCRIPTION

Medicinal Parts: The medicinal parts are the leaves and the whole plant harvested during the flowering season.

Flower and Fruit: The greenish pink flowers are in loose, thin, hanging false ears. The 4-bract involucre is inconspicuous with a reddish tip and is glandular-punctate. The flowers are androgynous. There are 6 to 8 stamens, 2 of which have no function. The fruit has a flat and a domed side. The fruit is black, punctate, nut-like, roughly bumpy and surrounded by a remaining epicalyx.

Leaves, Stem and Root: The plant grows from 30 to 50 cm high. The branched stems, which are from 60 to 90 cm long, are first creeping and later semi-erect and often tinged red. The leaves are oblong-lanceolate, alternate, short-petioled, narrowed at both ends and glandular and ciliate on the under surface. The leaf sheaths at the base of the leaves are loose and glabrous-ciliated at the margin.

Characteristics: The plant has an extraordinarily hot pepper-like taste and long, thin curved, hanging flowering branches.

Habitat: The plant is indigenous to Europe, Asian Russia and the Arctic.

Production: Smartweed is the fresh plant, in bloom, of Polygonum hydropiper. The herb is cut and washed when in bloom. The roots are removed and the plant is dried in the shade.

Other Names: Water Pepper, Arsesmart

ACTIONS AND PHARMACOLOGY

COMPOUNDS

Sesquiterpenealdehydes (pungent substances): polygoidal (tadeonal), warburganal

Tannins

Flavonoids: including, among others, rhamnazine, rhamnazine bisulphate, persicarin (isorhamnetine sulphate) quercitrin, hyperoside

p-cumaroyl glycosides: hydropiperoside

EFFECTS

The drug stops bleeding.

INDICATIONS AND USAGE

Smartweed preparations are used for the ablution of bloody wounds, to treat bleeding of the womb, menstrual bleeding, bleeding of hemorrhoids and diarrhea. Smartweed also influences the elimination of urine and acts against rheumatic pain.

PRECAUTIONS AND ADVERSE REACTIONS

No health hazards or side effects are known in conjunction with the proper administration of designated therapeutic dosages.

DOSAGE

Mode of Administration: Internally as a tea made from either the fresh or dried plant.

Preparation: To prepare the tea, use 1 teaspoonful of the drug per cup and bring to a boil.

Daily Dosage: The tea should be taken 3 times a day. Just a trace or very small quantity of the powdered drug can be taken 3 times daily.

LITERATURE

Asakawa Y, Takemoto T, (1979) Experientia 35:1429.

Barnes CS, Loder JW, (1962) Aust J Chem 15:322.

Furuta, T. et al., (1986) Phytochemistry 25(2):517.

Fukujama Y et al., Hydropiperoside, a novel coumaroly glycoside from th root of Polygonum hydropiper. In: PH 22:549-552. 1983.

Kifakh SY, Blinova KF, (1984) Khim Prir Soedin 5:658.

Further information in:

Kern W, List PH, Hörhammer L (Hrsg.), Hagers Handbuch der Pharmazeutischen Praxis, 4. Aufl., Bde. 1-8, Springer Verlag Berlin, Heidelberg, New York, 1969.

Madaus G, Lehrbuch der Biologischen Arzneimittel, Bde. 1-3, Nachdruck, Georg Olms Verlag Hildesheim 1979.

Steinegger E, Hänsel R, Pharmakognosie, 5. Aufl., Springer Verlag Heidelberg 1992.

Teuscher E, Lindequist U, Biogene Gifte - Biologie, Chemie, Pharmakologie, 2. Aufl., Fischer Verlag Stuttgart 1994.

Wagner H, Wiesenauer M, Phytotherapie. Phytopharmaka und pflanzliche Homöopathika, Fischer-Verlag, Stuttgart, Jena, New York 1995.

Pomegranate

See Punica Granatum

Poplar bark

See Populus Species

Poppy

See Papaver Somniferum

Populus Species

Poplar bark

DESCRIPTION

Medicinal Parts: The medicinal parts are the bark and leaves.

Flower and Fruit: The plant is dioecious. The male flowers are in large, cylindrical hanging, thick catkins with carmine anthers. The female flowers are in thinner catkins with carmine stigmas. The seeds ripen in May or June, are very small and have a white lanate tuft of hair.

Leaves, Stem and Root: The tree may grow up to 30 m in height. The bark is initially yellow brown and later becomes black-gray and is fissured. The leaf buds are sticky. The leaves are almost circular with a dark green upper surface and a light gray-green under surface. They are dentate or lobed with obtuse teeth, initially silky-haired, later glabrous. The petioles are long, thin and compressed at the sides.

Habitat: The plant is indigenous to North America and is cultivated in many other temperate regions.

Production: Poplar bark consists of the fresh or dried bark of salicin-rich poplar. Poplar leaves consist of the leaves of salicin-rich Poplar varieties. Poplar buds consist of the dried, unopened leaf buds of Populus species.

Other Names: Black Poplar, Canadian Poplar, European Aspen, Quaking Aspen, Trembling Poplar, White Poplar

ACTIONS AND PHARMACOLOGY

COMPOUNDS: POPULI CORTEX ET FOLIUM

In Populus alba:

Glycosides and esters yielding salicylic acid: leaf 6%, bark 2% chief components are salicortin, tremulacin, salicin

In Populus nigra:

Glycosides and esters yielding salicylic acid: leaf 2%, bark 1.5% chief components are salicortin, salicin

In Populus tremula:

Glycosides and esters yielding salicylic acid: leaf 3%, bark 2% chief components are salicin, tremulacin, salicortin additionally, salireposide, populin, tremuloidin, among others

EFFECTS: POPULI CORTEX ET FOLIUM

The content of salicylate acid derivates and flavonoids are said to account for the antiphlogistic, analgesic, spasmolytic and antibacterial characteristics of the drug. The beneficial effect in micturition complaints following prostate hypertrophy due to the content of zinc lignans in the drug could be significant.

COMPOUNDS: POPULI GEMMA

Glycosides and esters yielding salicylic acid: including, among others, salicin, populin

Volatile oil: chief components alpha- and beta-caryophyllene

Flavonoids: including, among others, chrysin, tectochrysin, galengin, izalpinine, galangin-3-methyl ether, kaempferol-3-methyl ether, pinocembrin, pinocembrin-7-methyl ether, apigenin (in the sticky coating of the buds, also yielding propolis)

EFFECTS: POPULI GEMMA

The buds are antibacterial and are vulnerary.

INDICATIONS AND USAGE

POPULI CORTEX ET FOLIUM

Poplar bark is used for pain, rheumatism, and micturition complaints in prostata adenoma. Poplar bark is only available in combination preparations.

POPULI GEMMA

- Hemorrhoids
- Wounds and burns

Preparations from the bud are used for superficial skin injuries, external hemorrhoids, frostbite and sunburn.

CONTRAINDICATIONS

POPULI CORTEX ET FOLIUM

Poplar Bark is contraindicated in patients allergic to salicylates.

POPULI GEMMA

Preparations from the buds of Poplar are contraindicated in patients allergic to salicylates, propolis, and balsam of Peru.

PRECAUTIONS AND ADVERSE REACTIONS

POPULI CORTEX ET FOLIUM

No health hazards or side effects are known in conjunction with the proper administration of designated therapeutic dosages.

POPULI GEMMA

No health hazards are known in conjunction with the proper administration of designated therapeutic dosages. External administration of the drug occasionally leads to allergic skin reactions.

DOSAGE

POPULI CORTEX ET FOLIUM

Mode of Administration: As a ground drug and galenic preparations for internal use.

Daily Dosage: 10 gm.

POPULI GEMMA

Mode of Administration: Available as semi-solid preparations for application on the skin.

Daily Dosage: 5 gm drug or semi-solid preparations equivalent to 20% to 30% of drug.

LITERATURE

POPULI CORTEX ET FOLIUM

Anonym, Phytotherapie: Pflanzliche Antirheumatika - was bringen sie? In: DAZ 136(45):4012-4015. 1996.

Jossang A et al., Cinnamrutinoses A and B, glycosides from Populus tremula. In: PH 35(2):547. 1994.

Picard S et al., Isolation of a new phenolic compound from leaves of Populus deltoides. In: JNP 57(6):808-810. 1994.

Thieme H, Benecke R, (1969) Pharmazie 24:567.

Vonkruedener S et al., Effects of extracts from Populus tremula L., Solidago virgaurea L. and Fraxinus excelsior L. on various myeloperoxidase systems. In: Arzneim Forsch 46(8):809-814. 1996.

Further information in:

Fenaroli's Handbook of Flavor Ingredients, Vol. 1. 2nd Ed. Pub. CRC Press Boca Raton 1975.

Hegnauer R, Chemotaxonomie der Pflanzen, Bde 1-11, Birkhäuser Verlag Basel, Boston, Berlin 1962-1997.

Kern W, List PH, Hörhammer L (Hrsg.), Hagers Handbuch der Pharmazeutischen Praxis, 4. Aufl., Bde. 1-8, Springer Verlag Berlin, Heidelberg, New York, 1969.

Leung AY, Encyclopedia of Common Natural Ingredients Used in Food Drugs and Cosmetics, John Wiley & Sons Inc., New York 1980.

Madaus G, Lehrbuch der Biologischen Arzneimittel, Bde 1-3, Nachdruck, Georg Olms Verlag Hildesheim 1979.

Wagner H, Wiesenauer M, Phytotherapie. Phytopharmaka und pflanzliche Homöopathika, Fischer-Verlag, Stuttgart, Jena, New York 1995.

POPULI GEMMA

Anonym, Phytotherapie: Pflanzliche Antirheumatika - was bringen sie? In: DAZ 136(45):4012-4015. 1996.

Jossang A et al., Cinnamrutinoses A and B, glycosides from Populus tremula. In: PH 35(2):547. 1994.

Picard S et al., Isolation of a new phenolic compound from leaves of Populus deltoides. In: JNP 57(6):808-810. 1994.

Thieme H, Benecke R, (1969) Pharmazie 24:567.

Vonkruedener S et al., Effects of extracts from Populus tremula L., Solidago virgaurea L. and Fraxinus excelsior L. on various myeloperoxidase systems. In: Arzneim Forsch 46(8):809-814. 1996.

Further information in:

Fenaroli's Handbook of Flavor Ingredients, Vol. 1. 2nd Ed. Pub. CRC Press Boca Raton 1975.

Hegnauer R, Chemotaxonomie der Pflanzen, Bde 1-11, Birkhäuser Verlag Basel, Boston, Berlin 1962-1997.

Kern W, List PH, Hörhammer L (Hrsg.), Hagers Handbuch der Pharmazeutischen Praxis, 4. Aufl., Bde. 1-8, Springer Verlag Berlin, Heidelberg, New York, 1969.

Leung AY, Encyclopedia of Common Natural Ingredients Used in Food Drugs and Cosmetics, John Wiley & Sons Inc., New York 1980.

Madaus G, Lehrbuch der Biologischen Arzneimittel, Bde. 1-3, Nachdruck, Georg Olms Verlag Hildesheim 1979.

Wagner H, Wiesenauer M, Phytotherapie. Phytopharmaka und pflanzliche Homöopathika, Fischer-Verlag, Stuttgart, Jena, New York 1995.

Potentilla Anserina

Potentilla

DESCRIPTION

Medicinal Parts: The medicinal parts are the leaves and flowers, whole or macerated, collected during or shortly before the flowering season and dried, the fresh aerial parts, and the whole of the flowering plant including the root.

Flower and Fruit: The flowers are solitary on long pedicles of lateral shoots growing from the stem nodes. They are 1.5 to 3 cm wide. There are 5 epicalyx bracts, 5 sepals and 5 petals. The petals are twice as long as the sepals and are golden yellow, ovate and without a distinct margin. The 20 stamens have ovate anthers. The styles occur laterally, are thread-like and only thickened at the stigmas. The ripe fruit is glabrous, ovate to almost globular with grooves on one surface.

Leaves, Stem and Root: The plant is an axiled-herbacious perennial with a short, thick, branched rhizome and rosettes of basal leaves. The stems are 80 cm long, creeping, rooting at the nodes, softly pubescent and becoming glabrous. The leaves are unevenly paired, pinnate, glossy with silky white hairs beneath and fresh green above.

Characteristics: The herb has an almond-like fragrance and dry taste.

Habitat: The plant is found in temperate and colder regions of the Northern Hemisphere.

Production: Potentilla herb consists of the fresh or dried leaf and flowers of Potentilla anserina, harvested shortly before or during flowering.

Other Names: Cinquefoil, Crampweed, Goose Tansy, Goosegrass, Goosewort, Moor Grass, Prince's Feathers, Silverweed, Trailing Tansy, Wild Agrimony

ACTIONS AND PHARMACOLOGY

COMPOUNDS

Tannins (5-10%): chiefly ellagitannins

Flavonoids: including, among others, quercitrin

Hydroxycoumarins: umbelliferone, scopoletin

EFFECTS

The herb is astringent, depending on the tannin concentration. In animal studies, it has been shown to cause a distinct increase in tonus and contraction frequency on the isolated uterus.

INDICATIONS AND USAGE

- Diarrhea
- Inflammation of the mouth and pharynx
- Premenstrual syndrome

The drug is used for mild dysmenorrhea, as a support for the treatment of milder, nonspecific, acute diarrhea, and for light inflammation of the oral and pharyngeal mucosa.

PRECAUTIONS AND ADVERSE REACTIONS

No health hazards or side effects are known in conjunction with the proper administration of designated therapeutic dosages. The drug can exacerbate stomach distress.

DOSAGE

Mode of Administration: The drug is administered as a comminuted herb for infusions and decoctions, as a powdered herb, and as other galenic preparations for oral use. The drug is a component of various tea mixtures.

Preparation: To make an infusion, scald 2 gm finely cut drug, then strain after 10 minutes. (1 teaspoonful = 0.7 gm drug)

Daily Dosage: The daily dosage is 4 to 6 gm of drug.

LITERATURE

Eisenreichova E et al., Cesk Farm 23:82-84. 1974.

Kombal R, Glasl H, Flavan-3-ols and flavonoids from Potentilla anserina. In: PM 61(5):484-485. 1995.

Schimmer O, Lindenbaum M, Tannins with antimutagenic properties in the herb of Alchemilla species and Potentilla anserina. In: PM 61(2):141-145. 1995.

Further information in:

Hänsel R, Keller K, Rimpler H, Schneider G (Hrsg.), Hagers Handbuch der Pharmazeutischen Praxis, 5. Aufl., Bde 4-6 (Drogen), Springer Verlag Berlin, Heidelberg, New York, 1992-1994.

Madaus G, Lehrbuch der Biologischen Arzneimittel, Bde 1-3, Nachdruck, Georg Olms Verlag Hildesheim 1979.

Schulz R, Hänsel R, Rationale Phytotherapie, Springer Verlag Heidelberg 1996.

Steinegger E, Hänsel R, Pharmakognosie, 5. Aufl., Springer Verlag Heidelberg 1992.

Teuscher E, Biogene Arzneimittel, 5. Aufl., Wiss. Verlagsges. Stuttgart 1997.

Potentilla Erecta

Tormentil Root

DESCRIPTION

Medicinal Parts: The medicinal parts are the rhizome freed from the roots, the fresh underground parts collected in spring and the dried rhizome.

Flower and Fruit: The small, yellow, long-pedicled flowers grow opposite the leaves or at branching points on the stem. The 4 sepals have a 4 bract epicalyx. There are 4 free petals, which are obcordate and somewhat darker at the base. There are usually 16 stamens and numerous ovaries with thread-like styles. The receptacle is domed. The fruit is nut-like, hard, 1 seeded, ovate, grooved and almost smooth.

Leaves, Stem and Root: The plant is herbacious perennial about 30 cm high. The rhizome is 1 to 3 cm thick, irregular, gnarled to cylindrical, woody, dark-brown outside and blood red inside. The stem is erect or decumbent, never rooting, branching. The trifoliate rosette-like basal leaves wilt early and are gone before flowering. The cauline leaves are sessile, trifoliate and appear to be in fives because they have 2 stipules.

Characteristics: The plant is odorless and the taste astringent.

Habitat: The plant is found in the north as far as Scandinavia, in the south as far as northwest Africa, Italy, central Spain and the Balkans.

Production: Tormentil root consists of the dried rhizome taken from the root of Potentilla erecta (syn: Potentilla tormentilla Necker).

Not To Be Confused With: Radix bistortae and the rhizomes of Geum species.

Other Names: Biscuits, Bloodroot, Earthbank, English Sarsaparilla, Ewe Daisy, Flesh and Blood, Septfoil, Shepherd's Knapperty, Shepherd's Knot, Thormantle, Tormentilla

ACTIONS AND PHARMACOLOGY

COMPOUNDS

Tannins (17-22%)

Catechin tannins (15-20%): under storage conditions transforming into non-water soluble tanner's reds (turning into phlobaphenes)

Gallo tannins (3.5%): including, among others, agrimoniin, pedunculagin, levigatin B and F

Catechins: including, among others, (-)-gallocatechingallate, (-)-epigallocatechingallate, dimers and trimers of the catechin derivatives

Proanthocyanidins

Flavonoids: including, among others, kaempferol

Triterpenes: including, among others, Tormentoside, ursolic acid

EFFECTS

The plant is astringent due to the high tannin content.

INDICATIONS AND USAGE

- Diarrhea
- Inflammation of the mouth and pharynx

Tormentil Root is used for unspecified diarrheal disorders, mild mucous membrane inflammations of the mouth and pharynx, and for acute and subacute gastroenteritis.

PRECAUTIONS AND ADVERSE REACTIONS

No health hazards are known in conjunction with the proper administration of designated therapeutic dosages. Susceptible patients could experience gastric complaints or vomiting following intake of the drug.

DOSAGE

Mode of Administration: As a comminuted drug for boiling and infusing, as well as in other galenic preparations to be taken orally and applied locally. The drug is contained in various tea mixtures, such as emplastic tea, and in preparations of stomachics and antidiarrheal remedies.

Preparation: To make an infusion, place 2 to 3 gm finely cut or coarsely powdered drug in cold water, bring rapidly to a boil, steep for some time, then strain through a tea sieve. A cold water decoction may be used, as the effect of the tannin is reduced through boiling.

Daily Dosage: Tormentil tincture (1:10), use 10 to 20 drops in a glass of water daily as a mouth and throat rinse. The average daily dosage is 4 to 6 gm of drug. If used as an antidiarrheal agent, drink 1 cup of tea 3 to 4 times daily or mix 2 to 4 gm powdered drug with red wine. (1 teaspoonful equivalent to 4 gm drug)

LITERATURE

Bilia AR, Ctalano S, Fontana C, Morelli I, Palme E, A new saponin from Potentilla tormentilla. In: PM 58(7):A723. 1992.

Geiger C et al., Ellagitannins from Alchemilla xanthochlora and Potentilla erecta. In: PM 60(4):384. 1994.

Glasl H, DAZ 123:1979. 1983.

Lund K, Rimpler H, (1985) Dtsch Apoth Ztg 125(3):105.

Lund K, Rimpler H, (1985) Tormentillwurzel. Dtsch Apoth Z 125:105-107.

Lund K, Tormentillwurzelstock, Phytochemische Untersuchungen des Rhizoms von Potentilla erecta (L.) RÄUSCHEL. In: Dissertation Universität Freiburg. 1986.

Scholz E, Rimpler H, Österr Apoth Ztg 48:138. 1994.

Vennat B et al., J Pharm Belg 47:485. 1992.

Further information in:

Hänsel R, Keller K, Rimpler H, Schneider G (Hrsg.), Hagers Handbuch der Pharmazeutischen Praxis, 5. Aufl., Bde 4-6 (Drogen): Springer Verlag Berlin, Heidelberg, New York, 1992-1994.

Madaus G, Lehrbuch der Biologischen Arzneimittel, Bde 1-3, Nachdruck, Georg Olms Verlag Hildesheim 1979.

Schulz R, Hänsel R, Rationale Phytotherapie, Springer Verlag Heidelberg 1996.

Steinegger E, Hänsel R, Pharmakognosie, 5. Aufl., Springer Verlag Heidelberg 1992.

Teuscher E, Biogene Arzneimittel, 5. Aufl., Wiss. Verlagsges. Stuttgart 1997.

Wichtl M (Hrsg.), Teedrogen, 4. Aufl., Wiss. Verlagsges. Stuttgart 1997.

Potentilla Reptans

European Five-Finger Grass

DESCRIPTION

Medicinal Parts: The medicinal parts are the fresh flowering plant and the roots.

Flower and Fruit: The flowers are either solitary or in pairs and are opposite the leaves on long thin pedicles. The calyx has 5 segments and is 18 to 25 mm across. The golden yellow petals are obcordate and up to twice as long as the calyx. A ring-like swelling at the base of the stamens exudes a kind of honey. The small fruit is oblong-ovate and wrinkled.

Leaves, Stem and Root: The plant is a herbaceous perennial with a thin divided rhizome and rosettes of basal leaves. The leaves produce 30 cm to 100 cm long flowering stems from their axils, which root at the nodes. The stems are pubescent or almost glabrous, have no glands and are often tinged red. The cauline leaves are long-petioled and 5 to 7 digitate. The basal stipules are fused to the petiole. The leaflets are obovate, 10 to 70 mm long, dentate to serrate and pubescent or almost glabrous.

Habitat: The plant is common in Europe, western Asia, North America, Ethiopia and the Near East.

Production: European Five-Finger Grass and root is the complete plant of Potentilla reptans. The drug is a mixture of green and brown in color and has no particular smell or taste. The roots are harvested in September or October and then dried in a sunny, airy place.

Not To Be Confused With: P. canadensis is indigenous to the U.S. and Canada and is very similar.

Other Names: Cinquefoil, Five Fingers, Five-finger Blossom, Sunkfield, Synkfoyle

ACTIONS AND PHARMACOLOGY

COMPOUNDS

Tannins (6-12%)

Flavonoids: including among others quercetin-3,7-diglucuronid

EFFECTS

The active agent is tannin. It is astringent, and due to its tannin content, is a cure for wounds. It also reduces fever.

INDICATIONS AND USAGE

The drug is used internally for diarrhea and fever. Externally, it is used for inflammation of the mucous membranes of the mouth and of the gums, toothache, and heartburn.

PRECAUTIONS AND ADVERSE REACTIONS

No health hazards or side effects are known in conjunction with the proper administration of designated therapeutic dosages. The drug may cause a worsening of symptoms for those that complain of an irritable stomach.

DOSAGE

Mode of Administration: The ground drug is used as an infusion for internal and external use.

Preparation: To make a decoction for internal administration, use 3 gm of the drug per 100 ml water.

To make a decoction for external administration (gargles, mouthwashes, rinses, moist compresses), use 6 gm drug per 100 ml water.

For external use, add a handful of European Five-Finger Grass to a bathful of water.

Daily Dosage: For internal use, drink 2 to 3 cups of decoction daily. To help in treating sensitive, easily reddened and agitated skin and skin that is sensitive to changing weather conditions, use bathwater preparation.

LITERATURE

Hänsel R, Keller K, Rimpler H, Schneider G (Hrsg.), Hagers Handbuch der Pharmazeutischen Praxis, 5. Aufl., Bde 4-6 (Drogen), Springer Verlag Berlin, Heidelberg, New York, 1992-1994.

Premorse

See Scabiosa Succisa

Prickly Ash

See Zanthoxylum Americanum

Primrose

See Primula Elatior

Primula Elatior

Primrose

DESCRIPTION

Medicinal Parts: The medicinal parts are the flowers and roots.

Flower and Fruit: The flowers are in richly blossomed umbels with a short peduncle, turned to one side and grow in clusters (up to 259 from the center of the leaf rosette). The calyx is cylindrical and appressed with a green margin, the remaining parts of it are yellow and it is 12 to 15 cm long. The corolla is odorless, usually sulphur yellow, and has a tube with 5 triangular, orange spots. Five short filaments are encircled by the corolla. The ovary has a style with a headed stigma from which the many seeded-capsule emerges. The rough-surfaced seeds are 1.5-2.5 mm long, dark-brown and warty.

Leaves, Stem and Root: The 10 cm high plant is a herbaceous perennial with a short sturdy rhizome. The green plant parts are covered in 2 mm long segmented hairs. The leaves are revolute in the bud. They are wrinkled, ovate or ovate-oblong and are rounded at the base and narrow quickly to the winged stems. During the flowering season they are irregularly dentate with blunt teeth. The leaves are 3 to 6 cm long.

Habitat: The plant is indigenous to the whole of central Europe as far as the southern European mountains. There are many subspecies.

Production: Primrose flower consists of the dried, whole flowers with calyx of Primula veris and/or Primula elatior. Primrose root consists of the dried rhizome with roots of Primula veris and/or Primula elatior. The best time to harvest Primrose root is in the plant's third year.

Not To Be Confused With: Primrose flower should not be confused with flowers of Primula elatior. Primrose root should not be confused with the rhizomes of Vincetoxicum hirundinaria or Vincetoxicum officinale.

Other Names: Cowslip, Peagles, English Cowslip, Butter Rose, Herb PeterPaigle Peggle, Key Flower, Key of Heaven, Fairy Caps, Petty Mulleins, Buckles, Crewel, Palsywort, Plumrocks, Mayflower, Password, Arthritica, Our Lady's Keys

ACTIONS AND PHARMACOLOGY

COMPOUNDS: PRIMULAE FLOS

Triterpene saponins (up to 2% in the sepals)

Flavonoids (3%): including, among others, rutin, kaempferol-3-rutinoside, isorhamnetin-3-glucoside; gossypetin

Primin

EFFECTS: PRIMULAE FLOS

Secretolytic, expectorant.

COMPOUNDS: PRIMULAE RADIX

Triterpene saponins (5-10%): chief components primulic acid A (aglycone protoprimulagenin)

Phenol glycosides: primulaverin 3%, 2-hydroxy-5-methoxybenzoic acid methyl ester xyloglucoside) changing over during drying into the characteristically-smelling 5-methoxymethyl salicylate

EFFECTS: PRIMULAE RADIX

Secretolytic, expectorant.

The secretolytic effect is a result of the saponin content.

INDICATIONS AND USAGE

PRIMULAE FLOS

- Cough
- Bronchitis

Preparations from the flower are used in catarrh of the respiratory tract, as a mild secretolytic and as an expectorant for colds. In folk medicine, Primrose flowers are used as a remedy for nervous diseases, for headache, neuralgia, tremors, hydroticum, and as a ''heart tonic'', for sensations of dizziness and cardiac insufficiency.

PRIMULAE RADIX

- Cough
- Bronchitis

Preparations from the root are used in catarrh of the respiratory tract. In folk medicine, Primrose root is used for whooping cough, asthma, gout and neuralgic complaints.

CONTRAINDICATIONS

PRIMULAE FLOS AND PRIMULAE RADIX

Known allergies against primroses.

PRECAUTIONS AND ADVERSE REACTIONS

PRIMULAE FLOS

No health hazards or side effects are known in conjunction with the proper administration of designated therapeutic dosages. The above-ground organs of the Primula species possess very high potentials for sensitization. In the cases of Primula veris and P. elatior, the Primin content is quite low, but sensitizations are nevertheless possible.

PRIMULAE RADIX

No health hazards or side effects are known in conjunction with the proper administration of designated therapeutic dosages.

OVERDOSAGE

PRIMULAE FLOS

Overdose can lead to gastric complaints and nausea.

PRIMULAE RADIX

Overdoses can lead to queasiness, nausea, gastric complaints and diarrhea.

DOSAGE

PRIMULAE FLOS

Mode of Administration: Comminuted herb for teas and other galenic preparations for internal use. Extracts of the drug are contained in bronchial, ''blood cleaning'', and ''vascular and circulatory'' teas.

Preparation: To prepare a tea, use 2 to 4 gm of drug, pour over boiling water and strain after 10 minutes. (1 teaspoonful = 1.3 gm drug)

Daily Dosage: 4 gm of drug; up to 1.5 to 3 gm of tincture. Bronchial tea can be sweetened with honey and taken repeatedly throughout the day.

PRIMULAE RADIX

Mode of Administration: Comminuted drug for teas and cold macerations, as well as other galenic preparations for internal use. The drug is available in standardized preparations of antitussives and expectorants.

Preparation: To prepare an infusion, use 0.2-0.5 gm finely cut drug in cold water, bring to a simmer, steep for 5 minutes, then strain. (1 teaspoonful = 3.5 gm drug)

Daily Dosage: 0.5 to 1.5 gm of drug; up to 7.5 gm of tincture. Dosage for the infusion is 1 cup of tea, sweetened with honey, used as an expectorant every 2 to 3 hours.

LITERATURE

PRIMULAE FLOS

Büechi S, Antivirale Saponine, pharmakologische und klinische Untersuchungen. In: DAZ 136(2):89-98. 1996.

Busse WW et al., (1984) J All Clin Immunol. 73:801.

Çalis I, Yürüker A, Rüegger H, Wright AD, Sticher O, Triterpene saponins from Primula veris ssp. macrocalyx and Primula elatiro ssp. meyeri. In: JNP 55:1299-1306. 1992.

Grecu VL, Cucu V, (1975) Planta Med 25:247.

Karl C et al., (1981) Planta Med 41:96.

Middleton E, Drzewiecki G, (1984) Biochem. Pharmacol. 33:3333.

Thieme H, Winkler HJ, (1971) Pharmazie 7:434.

Further information in:

Hänsel R, Keller K, Rimpler H, Schneider G (Hrsg.), Hagers Handbuch der Pharmazeutischen Praxis, 5. Aufl., Bde 4-6 (Drogen), Springer Verlag Berlin, Heidelberg, New York, 1992-1994.

Madaus G, Lehrbuch der Biologischen Arzneimittel, Bde 1-3, Nachdruck, Georg Olms Verlag Hildesheim 1979.

Steinegger E, Hänsel R, Pharmakognosie, 5. Aufl., Springer Verlag Heidelberg 1992.

Teuscher E, Lindequist U, Biogene Gifte - Biologie, Chemie, Pharmakologie, 2. Aufl., Fischer Verlag Stuttgart 1994.

Teuscher E, Biogene Arzneimittel, 5. Aufl., Wiss. Verlagsges. Stuttgart 1997.

Wichtl M (Hrsg.), Teedrogen, 4. Aufl., Wiss. Verlagsges. Stuttgart 1997.

PRIMULAE RADIX

Büechi S, Antivirale Saponine, pharmakologische und klinische Untersuchungen. In: DAZ 136(2):89-98. 1996.

Busse WW et al., (1984) J All Clin Immunol. 73:801.

Çalis I, Yürüker A, Rüegger H, Wright AD, Sticher O, Triterpene saponins from Primula veris ssp. macrocalyx and Primula elatiro ssp. meyeri. In: JNP 55:1299-1306. 1992.

Grecu VL, Cucu V, (1975) Planta Med 25:247.

Karl C et al., (1981) Planta Med 41:96.

Middleton E, Drzewiecki G, (1984) Biochem. Pharmacol. 33:3333.

Thieme H, Winkler HJ, (1971) Pharmazie 7:434.

Wagner H et al., Radix-Primulae-Extrakte. HPLC-Analyse. In: DAZ 126:1489-1493. 1986.

Further information in:

Hänsel R, Keller K, Rimpler H, Schneider G (Hrsg.), Hagers Handbuch der Pharmazeutischen Praxis, 5. Aufl., Bde 4-6 (Drogen), Springer Verlag Berlin, Heidelberg, New York, 1992-1994.

Madaus G, Lehrbuch der Biologischen Arzneimittel, Bde 1-3, Nachdruck, Georg Olms Verlag Hildesheim 1979.

Steinegger E, Hänsel R, Pharmakognosie, 5. Aufl., Springer Verlag Heidelberg 1992.

Teuscher E, Biogene Arzneimittel, 5. Aufl., Wiss. Verlagsges. Stuttgart 1997.

Wichtl M (Hrsg.), Teedrogen, 4. Aufl., Wiss. Verlagsges. Stuttgart 1997.

Prunella Vulgaris

Self-Heal

DESCRIPTION

Medicinal Parts: The medicinal part is the whole flowering plant.

Flower and Fruit: The blue-violet or brownish-blue labiate flowers are clustered in semi-whorls at the end of stems and lateral branches. The accompanying leaves are red-brown. The upper lip of the calyx has 3 tips and the lower lip has 2 tips. The corolla is about 1 cm longer than the domed upper lip. The lower lip has 3 lobes. There are 4 stamens, the longer ones with a straight awl-shaped tip. The style is divided into two. The small fruit is flung out of the calyx.

Leaves, Stem and Root: The plant grows from 10 to 30 cm high. The stems are usually ascendant, sometimes creeping. The leaves are petiolate, ovate to lanceolate, dentate or entire-margined and crossed opposite.

Habitat: Prunella vulgaris is indigenous to Europe and Asia and practically all temperate regions of the world.

Production: Self-Heal is the complete plant in flower of Prunella vulgaris.

Other Names: Woundwort, Slough-Heal, Heart of the Earth, Blue Curls, Heal-All, Siclewort, Brownwort, Carpenter's Herb, Carpenter's Weed, Hercules Woundwort, Hock-Heal, Sicklewort

ACTIONS AND PHARMACOLOGY

COMPOUNDS

Tannins (up to 50%)

Bitter principles

Triterpene saponins

Triterpenes

Flavonoids: including among others rutin, hyperoside.

The constituents of the drug have not been studied closely.

EFFECTS

Active agents: tannin and bitter substances, essential oil, saponin and the glycoside ''Aukubin''.

INDICATIONS AND USAGE

The plant is used for inflammatory diseases, ulcers in the mouth and throat and gastroenteritis. It is also used as a remedy for diarrhea, hemorrhaging and gynecological disorders.

PRECAUTIONS AND ADVERSE REACTIONS

No health hazards or side effects are known in conjunction with the proper administration of designated therapeutic dosages.

DOSAGE

Mode of Administration: The ground drug is used to prepare infusions for oral use. The drug is also used as an extract and as a preparation for gargling.

Preparation: To prepare a tea, use 1 dessertspoonful of the drug per cup of water. This provides a 6 to 10% decoction of the drug. To prepare a mouthwash (rinse or gargle), boil for approximately 9 minutes.

LITERATURE

Kojima H. et al., (1987) Phytochemistry 26(4):1107.

Tabba HD, Chang RSh, Smith KM, Isolation, purification and partial characterization of prunellin, an anti-HIV component from aqueous extracts of Prunella vulgaris. In: Antiviral Res 11:263-274. 1989.

Further information in:

Hegnauer R, Chemotaxonomie der Pflanzen, Bde 1-11, Birkhäuser Verlag Basel, Boston, Berlin 1962-1997.

Kern W, List PH, Hörhammer L (Hrsg.), Hagers Handbuch der Pharmazeutischen Praxis, 4. Aufl., Bde. 1-8, Springer Verlag Berlin, Heidelberg, New York, 1969.

Prunus Amygdalus

Almond

DESCRIPTION

Medicinal Parts: The medicinal part is the ripe fruit.

Flower and Fruit: The flowers are very short-petioled in pairs and appear before the leaves. The petals are 19 to 20 mm long, pale pink to white, with dark veins. The fruit is oblong-ovoid, compressed, 3.5 to 4.6 cm long by 2.5 to 3 cm, gray-green and velvet-downy. The nut shell is yellow, hard, compressed, sharp-edged, punctate externally, smooth and glossy inside and thick or thin skinned. The seed is cinnamon brown, flattened and 2 cm long by 1.2 to 1.5 cm wide.

Leaves, Stem and Root: The plant is a medium high tree or shrub with mildly red-tinged thorny branches. The leaves have a 1.2 to 1.5 cm long, glandular petiole and glabrous, oblong-lanceolate-acuminate, finely dentate, glossy, dark green leaf blades.

Habitat: The tree is indigenous to western Asia and is extensively cultivated.

Production: Sweet almonds are the fruits of Prunus amygdalus dulces. Bitter almonds are the fruit of Prunus amygdalus amares.

Other Names: Greek Nuts, Jordan Almond, Sweet Almond, Bitter Almond

ACTIONS AND PHARMACOLOGY

COMPOUNDS: AMYGDALES DULCES

Non-dehydrating fatty oil

Chief fatty acids: oleic acid and linolenic acid

Mucilages

EFFECTS: AMYGDALES DULCES

As a demulcent.

COMPOUNDS: AMYGDALES AMARES

Cyanogenic glycosides: Amygdalin 0.2-8.5% (12-500 mg prussic acid per 100 gm accordingly)

Non-dehydrating fatty oil

Chief fatty acids: oleic acid and linolenic acid

Mucilages

EFFECTS: AMYGDALES AMARES

No information available.

INDICATIONS AND USAGE

AMYGDALAE DULCES

In cosmetics, as an expensive base for ointments and skin care.

AMYGDALES AMARES

In the past, bitter almond was used as a remedy for coughs, vomiting and nausea in the form of bitter almond water. It was also used as a taste corrigent.

PRECAUTIONS AND ADVERSE REACTIONS

AMYGDALAE DULCES

No health hazards or side effects are known in conjunction with the proper administration of designated therapeutic dosages.

AMYGDALES AMARES

Bitter Almonds are poisonous.

OVERDOSAGE

AMYGDALES AMARES

10 bitter almonds are said to be fatal for a child, 60 for an adult (a fatal dosage would presumably be already reached at a lower level, given disadvantageous conditions - higher cyanide level in the almonds, intensive chewing). Recommended antidotes include injection of solutions of dicobalt-EDTA or thiosulfates or else application of methemoglobin-forming substances, as for example, amyl nitrite. At the same time, vomiting should be induced or the stomach emptied. Circulatory support measures and/or artificial respiration might be required.

DOSAGE

AMYGDALAE DULCES

Mode of Administration: Fatty oil used as ointment base.

AMYGDALES AMARES

Mode of Administration: No longer in use.

LITERATURE

AMYGDALAE DULCES

Fincke H, Z Untersuch Lebensm 52:423. 1926.

Le Quesne PW et al., JNP 48:496. 1985.

Opdyke DLJ, (1976) Food Cosmet Toxicol: 14.

Salvo F et al., Riv Ital Sostanze Grasse 57:24. 1980.

Saura-Calixto F et al., Fette, Seifen, Anstrichm 87:4. 1985.

Further information in:

Kern W, List PH, Hörhammer L (Hrsg.), Hagers Handbuch der Pharmazeutischen Praxis, 4. Aufl., Bde. 1-8, Springer Verlag Berlin, Heidelberg, New York, 1969.

Madaus G, Lehrbuch der Biologischen Arzneimittel, Bde 1-3, Nachdruck, Georg Olms.

Steinegger E, Hänsel R, Pharmakognosie, 5. Aufl., Springer Verlag Heidelberg 1992.

Teuscher E, Biogene Arzneimittel, 5. Aufl., Wiss. Verlagsges. Stuttgart 1997.

AMYGDALES AMARES

Fincke H, Z Untersuch Lebensm 52:423. 1926.

Le Quesne PW et al., JNP 48:496. 1985.

Opdyke DLJ, (1976) Food Cosmet Toxicol: 14.

Rosenthaler L, Ber Pharm Ges 30:13. 1920.

Salvo F et al., Riv Ital Sostanze Grasse 57:24. 1980.

Saura-Calixto F et al., Fette, Seifen, Anstrichm 87:4. 1985.

Sommer W, Dissertation Albrechts-Universität Kiel. 1984.

Further information in:

Frohne D, Pfänder HJ, Giftpflanzen - Ein Handbuch für Apotheker, Toxikologen und Biologen, 4. Aufl., Wiss. Verlags-Ges Stuttgart 1997.

Kern W, List PH, Hörhammer L (Hrsg.), Hagers Handbuch der Pharmazeutischen Praxis, 4. Aufl., Bde. 1-8, Springer Verlag Berlin, Heidelberg, New York, 1969.

Lewin L, Gifte und Vergiftungen, 6. Aufl., Nachdruck, Haug Verlag, Heidelberg 1992.

Roth L, Daunderer M, Kormann K, Giftpflanzen, Pflanzengifte, 4. Aufl., Ecomed Fachverlag Landsberg Lech 1993.

Teuscher E, Lindequist U, Biogene Gifte - Biologie, Chemie, Pharmakologie, 2. Aufl., Fischer Verlag Stuttgart 1994.

Prunus Laurocerasus

Cherry Laurel

DESCRIPTION

Medicinal Parts: The medicinal parts are the dried leaves.

Flower and Fruit: The flowers are erect and in slender racemes 10 to 12 cm long with 3 mm pedicles. The petals are obovate, 3 mm long and white. The fruit is black and globular-ovoid. The smooth kernel within the fruit is ovoid and acute, with a long black weal.

Leaves, Stem and Root: The plant is an evergreen completely glabrous shrub or tree up to 6 m high. The bud scales drop early. The petioles are 1 cm long and glandless. The leaf blades are obovate-lanceolate and 8 to 15 cm long. They are curved, entire or with a finely serrate margin, coriaceous and bright green. The upper surface of the leaves is glossy. The lower surface has 1 to 4 protruding nectaries in the axils of the ribs.

Characteristics: Poisonous. The fruit is similar to black cherries, and smells of hydrocyanic acid.

Habitat: The plant is indigenous to parts of Asia and is cultivated in many temperate areas.

Production: Cherry Laurel leaves are the leaves of Prunus laurocerasus.

Not To Be Confused With: Other forms of Prunus.

Other Names: Cherry-Bay

ACTIONS AND PHARMACOLOGY

COMPOUNDS

Cyanogenic glycosides: prunasin (corresponding to 0.5-2.5%, 50-210 mg HCN/100 g)

EFFECTS

The active agents are prunasin, ursol acid, tannin, wax, fat and enzymes (emulsion).

Through prunase (from emulsion) glucose is formed, HCN and benzaldehyde - danger of poisoning is possible. The drug acts as a tonic for the stomach, an anti-irritant and a sedative.

INDICATIONS AND USAGE

Common cold, coughs. In homeopathy: for dry coughs, whooping cough, cyanose and spasms of various genesis.

PRECAUTIONS AND ADVERSE REACTIONS

No health hazards or side effects are known in conjunction with the proper administration of designated therapeutic dosages.

OVERDOSAGE

Overdoses of cherry laurel water prepared from the drug can lead to fatal poisonings. Ingestion of the leathery leaves and of the seeds is improbable; the fruit pulp is low in cyanogenic glycosides (yielding 5-20 mg HCN/100 gm). The recommended antidotes include the injection of solutions of Dicobalt-EDTA or thiosulfates, or the administration of methemoglobin-forming agents, for example amyl nitrite, 4-dimethylaminophenol. The inducement of vomiting or gastric lavage should be done in parallel fashion. Circulatory support and artificial respiration may also be required.

DOSAGE

Mode of Administration: The drug is available as a watery extract, as an aromatic, a breathing stimulant and antispasmodic.

LITERATURE

Sommer W, Dissertation Universität Kiel. 1984.

Further information in:

Frohne D, Pfänder HJ, Giftpflanzen - Ein Handbuch für Apotheker, Toxikologen und Biologen, 4. Aufl., Wiss. Verlags-Ges. Stuttgart 1997.

Kern W, List PH, Hörhammer L (Hrsg.), Hagers Handbuch der Pharmazeutischen Praxis, 4. Aufl., Bde. 1-8, Springer Verlag Berlin, Heidelberg, New York, 1969.

Leung AY, Encyclopedia of Common Natural Ingredients Used in Food Drugs and Cosmetics, John Wiley & Sons Inc., New York 1980.

Madaus G, Lehrbuch der Biologischen Arzneimittel, Bde 1-3, Nachdruck, Georg Olms Verlag Hildesheim 1979.

Roth L, Daunderer M, Kormann K, Giftpflanzen, Pflanzengifte, 4. Aufl., Ecomed Fachverlag Landsberg Lech 1993.

Steinegger E, Hänsel R, Pharmakognosie, 5. Aufl., Springer Verlag Heidelberg 1992.

Teuscher E, Lindequist U, Biogene Gifte - Biologie, Chemie, Pharmakologie, 2. Aufl., Fischer Verlag Stuttgart 1994.

Teuscher E, Biogene Arzneimittel, 5. Aufl., Wiss. Verlagsges. Stuttgart 1997.

Wagner H, Wiesenauer M, Phytotherapie. Phytopharmaka und pflanzliche Homöopathika, Fischer-Verlag, Stuttgart, Jena, New York 1995.

Prunus Serotina

Black Cherry

DESCRIPTION

Medicinal Parts: The medicinal part is the bark.

Flower and Fruit: The racemes are 6 to 15 cm long with about 30 flowers. The perianth remains when the fruit ripens. The 3 to 4 tepals are denticulate and creamy white. The fruit is 8 mm across, depressed-globose and purplish-black. The endocarp is smooth.

Leaves, Stem and Root: Wild Cherry is a deciduous tree up to 20 m high with aromatic bark. The leaves are obovate to elliptical-oblong, acuminate, finely serrate with flattened, forwardly directed teeth. They are dark, glossy green above, paler and slightly pubescent beneath.

Habitat: Prunus serotina originates from North America and is cultivated in Europe.

Production: Black Cherry bark is the bark of Prunus serotina.

Other Names: Wild Cherry, Virginian Prune, Black Choke, Choke Cherry, Rum Cherry

ACTIONS AND PHARMACOLOGY

COMPOUNDS

Cyanogenic glycosides: prunasin yielding 0.5-1.5%, 50-150 mg HCN/100 gm

Tannins

EFFECTS

Astringent, antitussive, sedative.

INDICATIONS AND USAGE

Black Cherry is used for coughs, bronchitis and whooping cough. It is also used in the treatment of nervous digestive disorders and diarrhea.

PRECAUTIONS AND ADVERSE REACTIONS

No health hazards or side effects are known in conjunction with the proper administration of designated therapeutic dosages.

OVERDOSAGE

Overdoses can lead to fatal poisonings. The recommended antidotes include the injection of solutions of Dikobalt-EDTA or thiosulfates, or the administration of methemoglobin-forming agents, for example amyl nitrite, 4-dimethylaminophenol. The inducement of vomiting or gastric lavage should be done in parallel fashion.

Circulatory support and artificial respiration could also be required.

DOSAGE

Mode of Administration: Black Cherry is available as a syrup and tincture.

LITERATURE

Frohne D, Pfänder HJ, Giftpflanzen - Ein Handbuch für Apotheker, Toxikologen und Biologen, 4. Aufl., Wiss. Verlags-Ges. Stuttgart 1997.

Kern W, List PH, Hörhammer L (Hrsg.), Hagers Handbuch der Pharmazeutischen Praxis, 4. Aufl., Bde. 1-8, Springer Verlag Berlin, Heidelberg, New York, 1969.

Leung AY, Encyclopedia of Common Natural Ingredients Used in Food Drugs and Cosmetics, John Wiley & Sons Inc., New York 1980.

Roth L, Daunderer M, Kormann K, Giftpflanzen, Pflanzengifte, 4. Aufl., Ecomed Fachverlag Landsberg Lech 1993.

Prunus Spinosa

Blackthorn

DESCRIPTION

Medicinal Parts: The medicinal parts are the flowers.

Flower and Fruit: The white, pedicled flowers are solitary but appear close to each other on the branches. They complete flowering before the leaves unfold. The calyx is campanulate with long tips, which are twice as long as the tips of the 5 petals. The fruit is dark blue, frosted and globular with a diameter approximately 10 mm.

Leaves, Stem and Root: Prunus spinosa is a bulky bush about 3 m high. The branches are velvet-haired when young. The numerous lateral branches are almost horizontal and end in sharp thorns. The bark is black-brown.

Characteristics: The fruit tastes exceptionally sour and is edible only after several frosts.

Habitat: The plant grows in Europe and parts of Asia.

Production: Blackthorn flower consists of the dried flowers of Prunus spinosa. Blackthorn fruit consists of the fresh or dried, ripe fruit of Prunus spinosa.

Not To Be Confused With: Leaves of Prunus padus

Other Names: Sloe, Wild Plum

ACTIONS AND PHARMACOLOGY

COMPOUNDS: PRUNI SPINOSAE FLOS

Flavonoids (2.5%): including among others quercitrin, rutin, hyperoside

Cyanogenic glycosides: amygdalin, traces, likely only in the fresh blossoms

EFFECTS: PRUNI SPINOSAE FLOS

No information available.

COMPOUNDS: PRUNI SPINOSAE FRUCTUS

Tannins

Cyanogenic glycosides: amygdalin, only in the seeds

Fruit acids

EFFECTS: PRUNI SPINOSAE FRUCTUS

Astringent effect on the mucous membranes.

INDICATIONS AND USAGE

PRUNI SPINOSAE FLOS

Preparations of Blackthorn flower are used for common colds, diseases and ailments of the respiratory tract, as a laxative, for diarrhea, for prophylaxis and treatment of gastric spasms, bloating, intestinal diseases and dyspepsia.

PRUNI SPINOSAE FRUCTUS

■ Inflammation of the mouth and pharynx

Preparations of the flower are used for mild inflammations of the oral and pharyngeal mucosa (as a gargle). In folk medicine, the juice of the fruit is used as a gargle for mouth, throat, and gum inflammation. The syrup and wine are employed as a purgative or diuretic and as marmalade for dyspepsia.

PRECAUTIONS AND ADVERSE REACTIONS

PRUNI SPINOSAE FLOS AND PRUNI SPINOSAE FRUCTUS

No health hazards or side effects are known in conjunction with the proper administration of designated therapeutic dosages.

DOSAGE

PRUNI SPINOSAE FLOS

Mode of Administration: The drug is a component of ''blood-cleansing teas'' and some expectorants and laxatives.

Preparation: To prepare an infusion, add 1 to 2 heaping teaspoonfuls with boiling water, steep and stir for 5 to 10 minutes, then strain.

Daily Dosage: Dosage of the infusion is 1 to 2 cups during the day or 2 cups in the evening. (1 teaspoonful = 1.0 gm drug)

Storage: Must be protected from light and moisture, at best not longer than 1 year.

PRUNI SPINOSAE FRUCTUS

Mode of Administration: Internally, comminuted herb for teas and other galenic preparations for mouth rinses.

Daily Dosage: For external use, the daily dose is 2 to 4 gm drug.

LITERATURE

PRUNI SPINOSAE FLOS

Irizar AC, Fernandez MF, Constituents of Prunus spinosa. In: JNP 55:450-454. 1992.

Further information in:

Kern W, List PH, Hörhammer L (Hrsg.), Hagers Handbuch der Pharmazeutischen Praxis, 4. Aufl., Bde. 1-8, Springer Verlag Berlin, Heidelberg, New York, 1969.

Madaus G, Lehrbuch der Biologischen Arzneimittel, Bde 1-3, Nachdruck, Georg Olms Verlag Hildesheim 1979.

Steinegger E, Hänsel R, Pharmakognosie, 5. Aufl., Springer Verlag Heidelberg 1992.

Teuscher E, Biogene Arzneimittel, 5. Aufl., Wiss. Verlagsges. Stuttgart 1997.

Wichtl M (Hrsg.), Teedrogen, 4. Aufl., Wiss. Verlagsges. Stuttgart 1997.

PRUNI SPINOSAE FRUCTUS

Irizar AC, Fernandez MF, Constituents of Prunus spinosa. In: JNP 55:450-454. 1992.

Further information in:

Kern W, List PH, Hörhammer L (Hrsg.), Hagers Handbuch der Pharmazeutischen Praxis, 4. Aufl., Bde. 1-8, Springer Verlag Berlin, Heidelberg, New York, 1969.

Madaus G, Lehrbuch der Biologischen Arzneimittel, Bde 1-3, Nachdruck, Georg Olms Verlag Hildesheim 1979.

Psyllium

See Plantago Isphagula

Psyllium Seed

See Plantago Afra

Ptelea Trifoliata

Wafer Ash

DESCRIPTION

Medicinal Parts: The medicinal parts are the leaves, the young bark and the root bark.

Flower and Fruit: The small, greenish-white flowers are in loose, terminal cymes and are dioecious. The 4 to 5 sepalled calyx and the 4 to 5 petals are downy on the outside. There are 4 to 5 stamens whose filaments are hairy at the base. The compressed ovary has a short style and stigma, which is divided in 2. The fruit is circular and winged with a broad, greenish-white, later ochre margin.

Leaves, Stem and Root: The plant is a bush or small tree up to 4 m high with glabrous, smooth, dark or red brown branches. The younger branches, leaves and petiols are downy. The leaves are large, 3-lobed, lanceolate and tapered at both ends. The leaves are entire, dark green above, lighter beneath and covered with numerous fine glandular spots.

Characteristics: The flowers are pleasantly perfumed and the fruit is bitter-tangy.

Habitat: The plant is indigenous to eastern North America and is cultivated in Europe as an ornamental bush.

Production: Wafer Ash is the root-bark of Ptelea trifoliata.

Other Names: Pickaway Anise, Prairie Grub, Scubby Trefoil, Stinking Prairie Bush, Swamp Dogwood, Three-leafed Hop Tree, Wingseed

ACTIONS AND PHARMACOLOGY

COMPOUNDS

Furoquinoline alkaloids: including among others kokusaginin, skimmianine (beta-fagarin), ptelein, dictamnine

Furocoumarins: including among others isopimpinellin, marmesine, phellopterin

EFFECTS

The active agent is the alkaloid pteleatinium chloride. Pteleatinium chloride acts against *mycobacterium tuberculosis* and yeast fungus.

INDICATIONS AND USAGE

Wafer Ash is used for stomach complaints, gall stones and rheumatism. Preparations from the bark of the root are used as tonics. The dried root bark can be made into a tea to encourage a sluggish appetite, and as a dressing for wounds.

PRECAUTIONS AND ADVERSE REACTIONS

No health hazards or side effects are known in conjunction with the proper administration of designated therapeutic dosages. The plant can trigger phototoxicosis through skin contact.

DOSAGE

Mode of Administration: Wafer Ash is used internally in the form of an extract.

LITERATURE

Kern W, List PH, Hörhammer L (Hrsg.), Hagers Handbuch der Pharmazeutischen Praxis, 4. Aufl., Bde. 1-8, Springer Verlag Berlin, Heidelberg, New York, 1969.

Roth L, Daunderer M, Kormann K, Giftpflanzen, Pflanzengifte, 4. Aufl., Ecomed Fachverlag Landsberg Lech 1993.

Pterocarpus Santalinus

Red Sandalwood

DESCRIPTION

Medicinal Parts: The medicinal part is the wood.

Flower and Fruit: The tree bears spikes of yellow flowers.

Leaves, Stem and Root: The plant is 6 to 8 m high tree with red bark.

Habitat: The plant grows in southern India, Sri Lanka and the Philippines.

Production: Red sandalwood consists of the heart wood of the trunk of Pterocarpus santalinus separated from the sapwood.

Other Names: Red Sanderswood, Rubywood, Red Saunders, Sappan

ACTIONS AND PHARMACOLOGY

COMPOUNDS

Benzxanthenone derivatives (red pigments): chief components santalins A and B

Volatile oil (traces): including, among others, pterocarpol, isopterocarpol, eudesmol

Isoflavonoids

Neoflavonoids

Stilbene derivatives

EFFECTS

No information is available.

INDICATIONS AND USAGE

Red sandalwood is used for ailments and complaints of the gastrointestinal tract, as a diuretic, an astringent, for blood purification and for coughs.

PRECAUTIONS AND ADVERSE REACTIONS

No health hazards or side effects are known in conjunction with the proper administration of designated therapeutic dosages.

DOSAGE

Mode of Administration: The drug is used as a brightening agent in various tea mixtures. In powder form, it is used as a coloring agent in toothpaste.

LITERATURE

Kumar N et al., PH 13:633. 1974.

Kumar N et al., PH 14:521. 1974.

Kumar N et al., PH 15:1417. 1976.

Seshadri TR, (1972) Phytochemistry 11:881.

Seshadri TR, PH 11:881. 1972.

Singh S et al., Fitoterapia 63:555. 1992.

Singh S et al., Fitoterapia 64:84. 1993.

Further information in:

Kern W, List PH, Hörhammer L (Hrsg.), Hagers Handbuch der Pharmazeutischen Praxis, 4. Aufl., Bde. 1-8: Springer Verlag Berlin, Heidelberg, New York, 1969.

Wichtl M (Hrsg.), Teedrogen, 4. Aufl., Wiss. Verlagsges. Stuttgart 1997.

Ptychopetalum Olacoides

Muira-Puama

DESCRIPTION

Medicinal Parts: The medicinal parts are the dried roots and the dried trunk with bark. The drug is extracted from the wood and trunk bark as well as from the roots of both varieties of Ptychopetalum.

Flower and Fruit: The inflorescences are racemous and appear in ones or twos per axil. They have 5 to 8 flowers and are about 2 cm long. The calyx is narrow and has 5 tips. The corolla is white, oblong and about 1.3 to 2 mm long. The outside is smooth and the inside is white pubescent. There are usually 10 stamens with long anthers. The ovary is clavate. The fruit is a long elliptical drupe which is initially green and changes to pink and finally to lilac-black when ripening. The pericarp is thin and the endocarp is crusty.

Leaves, Stem and Root: The plant is a 5 to 15 m high tree with a trunk 25 cm in diameter, which is vertically grooved. The leaves are oblong-lanceolate, very tapered and narrow towards the base. They are sometimes acute, coroeacious, smooth and gray or frosted to blue-green beneath. The dried leaves are matte with a dark green to black upper surface and a dark gray undersurface. The ribs are pinnatifid, curved, becoming distinct at the margin and protruding on the undersurface. The petioles are deeply grooved and do not thicken.

Habitat: The plant is indigenous to Guyana and the Amazon region of Brazil.

Production: Muira-Puama consists of the wood from the trunk and/or roots of Ptychopetalum olacoides and/or Ptychopetalum unicatum.

ACTIONS AND PHARMACOLOGY

COMPOUNDS

Triterpene acid esters: chief components are behenolic acid esters of lupeol

Sterols: beta-sitosterol, campesterol, lupeol

Volatile oil: chief components are alpha-pinene, alpha-humulene, beta-pinene, camphene, camphor, beta-caryophyllene

EFFECTS

No information is available.

INDICATIONS AND USAGE

Muira-Puama is used for the prevention of sexual disorders and as an aphrodisiac.

PRECAUTIONS AND ADVERSE REACTIONS

No health hazards or side effects are known in conjunction with the proper administration of designated therapeutic dosages.

DOSAGE

No information is available.

LITERATURE

Auterhoff H, Momberger B, Arch Pharm 304: 223-228. 1971.

Further information in:

Hänsel R, Keller K, Rimpler H, Schneider G (Hrsg.), Hagers Handbuch der Pharmazeutischen Praxis, 5. Aufl., Bde 4-6 (Drogen), Springer Verlag Berlin, Heidelberg, New York, 1992-1994.

Steinegger E, Hänsel R, Pharmakognosie, 5. Aufl., Springer Verlag Heidelberg 1992.

Puff Ball

See Lycoperdon Species

Pulmonaria Officinalis

Lungwort

DESCRIPTION

Medicinal Parts: The medicinal parts are the dried herb and the fresh, aerial parts of the flowering plant.

Flower and Fruit: The blue, later blue-violet flowers are in terminal curled cyme-like inflorescence on flowering branches. The calyx is fused and has 5 tips. The corolla is fused to a tube and the 5 tips are rotate. There are 5 stamens and a 4-valvular ovary that has 1 style. There are long and short-styled flowers. There are 5 tufts of hair at the entrance to the corolla tube. The fruit consists of 4 nuts, which are 3.5 to 4 mm in length, glabrous, glossy brown to black, mildly keeled with a distinct ring.

Leaves, Stem and Root: The plant grows from 15 to 30 cm high. The rhizome is quite thin and branched. First the rhizome produces flowering shoots and then the leaf rosettes. The shoots are fresh green and covered in glandular hairs. The stems are erect or ascending, slightly angular and pubescent. The rosette-like basal leaves are long petioled, cordate-ovate, acute, more long than wide with whitish spots. The cauline leaves are alternate, taper to a winged stem and are sharply pointed. Only the lower leaves have some pinnatifid ribs.

Characteristics: The taste is dry and slimy.

Habitat: The plant is common in many parts of Europe.

Production: Lungwort, consists of the dried plant section of Pulmonaria officinalis.

Not To Be Confused With: Other Pulmonaria species, particularly Pulmonaria mollis

Other Names: Dage of Jerusalem

ACTIONS AND PHARMACOLOGY

COMPOUNDS

Mucilages: (polygalacturonane, arabinogalactans, rhamno-galacturonane)

Flavonoids: in particular O-glycosides of the kaempferols and quercetins

Tannins

Silicic acid: more than 2.5% soluble silicic acid

Allantoin

Caffeic acid derivatives: chlorogenic acid, rosmaric acid

EFFECTS

No information is available.

INDICATIONS AND USAGE

Lungwort preparations are used in the treatment of illnesses and conditions of the respiratory tract, the gastrointestinal tract, the kidney and urinary tract as well as being used as an astringent and in the treatment of wounds.

In folk medicine, Lungwort is used in irritant-relieving cough medicine, and as a diuretic. It was formerly used in the treatment of lung diseases, i.e. tuberculosis.

PRECAUTIONS AND ADVERSE REACTIONS

No health hazards or side effects are known in conjunction with the proper administration of designated therapeutic dosages.

DOSAGE

Mode of Administration: Standardized preparations for oral use as a component of herbal teas or liquid antitussives.

Preparation: To prepare an infusion, finely cut 1.5 gm of drug and add to cold water; rapidly heat or scald with boiling water, then strain for 5 to 10 minutes.

Daily Dosage: Bronchial tea (folk remedy) should be taken repeatedly daily, in sips, with honey. (1 teaspoonful = 0.7 gm drug)

LITERATURE

Brantner A, Kartnig Th, Flavonoid glycosides from aerial parts of Pulmonaria officinalis. In: PM 61(6):582. 1995.

Luthy J et al., (1984) Pharm Acta Helv 59(9/10):242.

Müller BM, Franz G, Polysaccharide aus Pulmonaria officinalis - Wertgebende Bestandteile der Droge? In: PZW 135(6)243-251. 1990.

Further information in:

Hänsel R, Keller K, Rimpler H, Schneider G (Hrsg.), Hagers Handbuch der Pharmazeutischen Praxis, 5. Aufl., Bde 4-6 (Drogen), Springer Verlag Berlin, Heidelberg, New York, 1992-1994.

Madaus G, Lehrbuch der Biologischen Arzneimittel, Bde 1-3, Nachdruck, Georg Olms Verlag Hildesheim 1979.

Roth L, Daunderer M, Kormann K, Giftpflanzen, Pflanzengifte, 4. Aufl., Ecomed Fachverlag Landsberg Lech 1993.

Steinegger E, Hänsel R, Pharmakognosie, 5. Aufl., Springer Verlag Heidelberg 1992.

Teuscher E, Biogene Arzneimittel, 5. Aufl., Wiss. Verlagsges. Stuttgart 1997.

Wichtl M (Hrsg.), Teedrogen, 4. Aufl., Wiss. Verlagsges. Stuttgart 1997.

Pulsatilla Pratensis

Pasque Flower

DESCRIPTION

Medicinal Parts: The medicinal part is the whole fresh plant collected during the flowering season.

Flower and Fruit: The flowers are solitary and almost always nodding. They have 6 campanulate, close, bright violet tepals. These are usually thickly silky-haired on the outside with revolute tips and are 1.5 to 3 cm long. The stamens are yellow, numerous and the longer ones are at least two-thirds the length of the tepals. The carpels with the style are as long as the tepals. The ripe fruit is oblong and densely pubescent. The exserted style is up to 6 cm long.

Leaves, Stem and Root: The plant is a perennial 7 to 50 cm high and has a strong, dark, usually divided, rhizome. The basal leaves usually appear after the flowers and are not hardy. They are 3 to 4 pinnate with narrow linear acuminate end sections, which along with the petioles, are thickly white villous. The stems are erect and densely pubescent with 3 whorled high leaves, divided into linear, pubescent tips.

Characteristics: The plant is poisonous.

Habitat: The plant grows in central and eastern Europe.

Production: Pasque flower herb consists of the dried, above-ground parts of Pulsatilla vulgaris and/or Pulsatilla pratensis.

Other Names: Easter Flower, Meadow Anemone, Passe Flower, Pulsatilla, Wind Flower

ACTIONS AND PHARMACOLOGY

COMPOUNDS

Protoanemonine-forming agents: In the freshly-harvested plant, presumably the glycoside ranunculin, changes enzymatically when the plant is cut into small pieces, and probably also when it is dried, into the pungent, volatile protoanemonine that quickly dimerizes to anemonine. When dried, the plant is not capable of protoanemonine-formation.

Triterpene saponins

EFFECTS

No information is available.

INDICATIONS AND USAGE

Pasque flower is used for diseases and functional disorders of genital organs, inflammatory and infectious diseases of skin and mucosa, diseases and functional disorders of the gastrointestinal tract and the urinary tract, neuralgia, migraine, and general restlessness.

CONTRAINDICATIONS

The drug is contraindicated during pregnancy.

PRECAUTIONS AND ADVERSE REACTIONS

General: No health hazards or side effects are known in conjunction with the proper administration of designated therapeutic dosages of the dehydrated drug. Extended skin contact with the freshly-harvested, bruised plant can lead to blister formation and cauterizations that are difficult to heal due to the resulting protoanemonine that is severely irritating to skin and mucous membranes. If taken internally, severe irritation to the gastrointestinal tract, combined with colic and diarrhea, as well as irritation of the urinary drainage passages are possible.

Symptomatic treatment for external contact should consist of mucilaginosa, after irrigation with diluted potassium permanganate solution; in case of internal contact, activated charcoal should follow gastric lavage.

Use in Pregnancy: Administration of the drug during pregnancy is absolutely contraindicated.

OVERDOSAGE

Death by asphyxiation following the intake of large quantities of protoanemonine-forming plants has been observed in animal experiments.

DOSAGE

Mode of Administraion: The herb is currently used as a homeopathic remedy.

LITERATURE

Pourrat A et al., (1980) Planta Med 38:289.

Ruijgrok HWL, PM 11:338-347. 1963.

Siess M, Seybold G, Untersuchungen über die Wirkung von Pulsatilla pratensis, Cimicifuga racemosa und Aristolochia clematis auf den Östrus infantiler und kastrierter weiβer Mäuse. In: Arzneim Forsch 10:514. 1960.

Further information in:

Chan H, But P (Eds.), Pharmacology and Applications of Chinese Materia Medica, Vol 1, World Scientific Singapore 1986.

Frohne D, Pfänder HJ, Giftpflanzen - Ein Handbuch für Apotheker, Toxikologen und Biologen, 4. Aufl., Wiss. Verlags-Ges. Stuttgart 1997.

Hänsel R, Keller K, Rimpler H, Schneider G (Hrsg.), Hagers Handbuch der Pharmazeutischen Praxis, 5. Aufl., Bde 4-6 (Drogen), Springer Verlag Berlin, Heidelberg, New York, 1992-1994.

Madaus G, Lehrbuch der Biologischen Arzneimittel, Bde 1-3, Nachdruck, Georg Olms Verlag Hildesheim 1979.

Roth L, Daunderer M, Kormann K, Giftpflanzen, Pflanzengifte, 4. Aufl., Ecomed Fachverlag Landsberg Lech 1993.

Teuscher E, Lindequist U, Biogene Gifte - Biologie, Chemie, Pharmakologie, 2. Aufl., Fischer Verlag Stuttgart 1994.

Wagner H, Wiesenauer M, Phytotherapie. Phytopharmaka und pflanzliche Homöopathika, Fischer-Verlag, Stuttgart, Jena, New York 1995.

Pumpkin

See Cucurbita Pepo

Punica Granatum

Pomegranate

DESCRIPTION

Medicinal Parts: The medicinal parts are the flowers, stem, bark and rhizome.

Flower and Fruit: The flowers are funnel-shaped or rotate, usually solitary or in pairs at the tips of the branches. The calyx and receptacle are bright coral-red and have a tough margin. There are 5 to 8 bright-red, campanulate petals and numerous stamens. The filaments are orange-red and the anthers yellow-gold. The fruit is an apple-sized, round, 1.6 to 12 cm wide false berry whose skin goes from bright red to leather-brown. The seeds are roughly square and purple, later acquiring a soft red outer skin.

Leaves, Stem and Root: The plant is an erect, roughly branched shrub up to 1.5 m high or a small tree 3 to 5 m tall with a curved trunk and spiny-tipped branches. The branches are narrowly winged when young. The trunk later becomes fissured and twisted. The leaves are generally opposite or in clusters on the short shoots, simple, pinnate-veined, short-petioled, glabrous, hard and oval-lanceolate with a tough middle rib.

Habitat: The plant probably originated in Asia. Today it is widespread in the Mediterranean region as far the southern Tyrol, the Near East, South Africa, southern Asia, China, Australia, the U.S. and South America.

Production: Pomegranate bark is the bark of the trunk and branches of Punica granatum. Roots, trunk and older branches are collected at the beginning of autumn. The bark is peeled off and air-dried.

Other Names: Grenadier

ACTIONS AND PHARMACOLOGY

COMPOUNDS

In the fruit peel:

Tannins (25-28%; gallotannins): including among others punicalin (granatin D), punicalagin (granatin C), granatin A, granatin B

In the rinds of the stem and the rhizome:

Tannins (20-25%; gallotannins): including among others punicalagin, punicacortein C, casuarin

Piperidine alkaloids (0.4%): chief alkaloids isopelletierine, N-methylisopelletierine, pseudopelletierine

EFFECTS

The effect is similar to strychnine in heightening reflex arousal, which can escalate to tetanus.

In experiments, pig and poultry tapeworms are susceptible to a diluted solution of the concentrated pomegranate bark. In-vitro experiments point to piperidinal alkaloids as agents against tapeworm. Alkaloids are the toxic contents of pomegranate bark. Pomegranate stimulates the central nevous system.

INDICATIONS AND USAGE

Tape worm infestation and opportunistic intestinal worms. Astringent properties are used for diarrhea and dysentery. The drug has also been used as a gargling rinse in cases of sore throat and as an abortive. Used externally to treat hemorrhoids.

PRECAUTIONS AND ADVERSE REACTIONS

No health hazards are known in conjunction with the proper administration of designated therapeutic dosages. The high levels of tannin content can lead to gastric irritation.

OVERDOSAGE

Due to the alkaloid content, overdoses with the rind of the stem or the root (above 80 gm) lead to vomiting, including the vomiting of blood, later to dizziness, chills, vision disorders, collapse and possible death through respiratory failure.

Total blindness (amaurosis) can occur within a few hours or a few days, that then disappears again after the passage of several weeks. Following gastrointestinal emptying (inducement of vomiting, gastric lavage with burgundy-colored potassium permanganate solution, sodium sulfate), instillation of activated charcoal and shock prophylaxis (quiet, warmth), the therapy for poisonings consists of treating spasms with diazepam (i.v.), electrolyte substitution and treating possible cases of acidosis with sodium bicarbonate infusions. In case of shock, plasma volume expanders should be administered. Monitoring of kidney function is essential. Intubation and oxygen respiration may also be necessary.

DOSAGE

Mode of Administration: Oral preparations have been used against tapeworm, but more modern methods are used today.

Preparation: One part drug is boiled with 5 parts water.

Daily Dosage: For tapeworm: dose of 3 times 65 ml. by means of a duodenal probe in intervals of 30 minutes, with the administration of a laxative one hour later.

As pomegranate bark juice extract, the medium single dose against tapeworm is 20 gm.

Storage: In closed containers, protected from moisture.

LITERATURE

Beckham N, Phyto-oestrogens and compounds that affect oestrogen metabolism. In: Aust Herbalism 7:11-16. 1995.

Foder GB, Colasenko B, In: Alkaloids, Vol. 3'', Ed. SW. Pelletier, John Wiley 1985.

Neuhöfer H et al., The occurence of pelletierine derivatives in Punica granatum. In: 37. Annual Congr Med Plant Res Braunschweig 1989 P1-13. 1989.

Schilling G, Schick H, On the structure of punicalagin and punicalin. In: Liebigs Ann Chem (11):2240. 1985.

Tanake T et al., (1986) Chem Pharm Bull 34(2):656.

Wylegalla R, Biblische Botanik: Pflanzen und Früchte aus dem gelobten Land. In: DAZ 137(11):867-869. 1997.

Further information in:

Hänsel R, Keller K, Rimpler H, Schneider G (Hrsg.), Hagers Handbuch der Pharmazeutischen Praxis, 5. Aufl., Bde 4-6 (Drogen), Springer Verlag Berlin, Heidelberg, New York, 1992-1994.

Lewin L, Gifte und Vergiftungen, 6. Aufl., Nachdruck, Haug Verlag, Heidelberg 1992.

Madaus G, Lehrbuch der Biologischen Arzneimittel, Bde 1-3, Nachdruck, Georg Olms Verlag Hildesheim 1979.

Roth L, Daunderer M, Kormann K, Giftpflanzen, Pflanzengifte, 4. Aufl., Ecomed Fachverlag Landsberg Lech 1993.

Purple Coneflower

See Echinacea

Purple Loosestrife

See Lythrum Salicaria

Pyrethrum

See Chrysanthemum Cinerariifolium

Pyrola Rotundifolia

Wintergreen

DESCRIPTION

Medicinal Parts: The medicinal parts are the leaves.

Flower and Fruit: The white, sometimes reddish flowers are in many-blossomed, nodding racemes turning to all sides. The calyx is divided in 5 almost to the base and has lanceolate, revolute, splayed tips. The corolla has 5 petals and is flatly campanulate. The 10 stamens are curved upwards. The ovary is superior with 5 sections and a downward curving style. The fruit is a 5-sectioned capsule.

Leaves, Stem and Root: The plant grows from 15 to 30 cm high. The stem is erect, obtusely angular, glabrous, and has 2 sheath-like bracts. The leaves in the basal rosette are petiolate, orbicular and glabrous. They are grass-green, glossy, somewhat cordate at the base, shallowly crenate, coriaceous and evergreen.

Characteristics: The flowers have a slight, pleasant fragrance and the leaves are astringent.

Habitat: The plant originated in the South Sea Islands but now is naturalized in other climates.

Production: Wintergreen leaves are the leaves of Pyrola rotundifolia.

ACTIONS AND PHARMACOLOGY

COMPOUNDS

Hydroquinone derivatives (4-8%): chief components isohomoarbutin, additionally homoarbutin (arbutin)

Naphthacene derivatives (naphthoquinone): chimaphilin (2,7-dimethyl-1,4-naphthoquinone)

Tannins (up to 18%)

EFFECTS

No information is available.

INDICATIONS AND USAGE

It is used for bladder inflammation and urinary tract diseases, diseases of the prostate, and kidney disorders.

PRECAUTIONS AND ADVERSE REACTIONS

No health hazards or side effects are known in conjunction with the proper administration of designated therapeutic dosages. The drug possesses a weak sensitizing effect, due to its chimaphilin content. The drug is not suitable for long-term use, because of its hydroquinone glycoside content.

DOSAGE

Mode of Administration: The drug is administered ground and as an extract.

LITERATURE

Hegnauer R, Chemotaxonomie der Pflanzen, Bde 1-11, Birkhäuser Verlag Basel, Boston, Berlin 1962-1997.

Kern W, List PH, Hörhammer L (Hrsg.), Hagers Handbuch der Pharmazeutischen Praxis, 4. Aufl., Bde. 1-8, Springer Verlag Berlin, Heidelberg, New York, 1969 (unter Pirola rotundifolia).

Madaus G, Lehrbuch der Biologischen Arzneimittel, Bde 1-3, Nachdruck, Georg Olms Verlag Hildesheim 1979 (unter Pirola rotundifolia).

Pyrus Communis

Pear

DESCRIPTION

Medicinal Parts: The medicinal part is the fruit.

Flower and Fruit: The fruit is typically pear-shaped with a more or less tough skin. The core has a number of carpels, which are large and edible. The seeds are pointed at 1 end and rounded at the other. When ripe, they are dark brown to black, glabrous and about 0.5 cm long.

Leaves, Stem and Root: The pear is a tree, up to 20 m tall, with a long-clavate crown. The bark is dark brown to black and broken into square plates. The glabrous or slightly pubescent branches are glossy brown or thorny. The leaves are 2 to 8 cm long, ovate-round, acuminate, tough and serrate. The ribs are protruding.

Habitat: The pear tree grows mainly in the temperate regions of the Northern Hemisphere.

Production: Pears are the fruit of Pyrus communis.

ACTIONS AND PHARMACOLOGY

COMPOUNDS

Fruit acids: malic acid, additionally citric acid, quinic acid

Cyanogenic glycosides: amygdalin (only in the seeds)

Aromatic substances: including, among others, (E,Z)-2,4-deca-dien-(E)-2-octen- and -(Z)-4-decenacylethylester, acetic acid hexylester

Caffeic acid derivatives: in particular 5-coffeoyl quinic acid

Pectin

EFFECTS

Astringent, refrigerant.

INDICATIONS AND USAGE

Pear is used in the treatment of mild digestive disorders and as a diuretic and laxative (syrup).

PRECAUTIONS AND ADVERSE REACTIONS

No health hazards or side effects are known in conjunction with the proper administration of designated therapeutic dosages.

DOSAGE

Mode of Administration: Fresh fruit (as food)

LITERATURE

Belitz HD, Grosch W, Lehrbuch der Lebensmittelchemie, 4. Aufl., Springer Verlag Berlin, Heidelberg, New York 1992.

Kern W, List PH, Hörhammer L (Hrsg.), Hagers Handbuch der Pharmazeutischen Praxis, 4. Aufl., Bde 1-8, Springer Verlag Berlin, Heidelberg, New York, 1969.

Quassia Amara

Bitter Wood

DESCRIPTION

Medicinal Parts: The medicinal part is the wood of the trunk and branches.

Flower and Fruit: The flowers are small and pale yellowish green. The sepals are round to ovate, fused at the base and imbricate. There are 5 petals, 10 stamens and 5 carpels. The style is fused from top to bottom. The fruit is a pea-sized drupe, which ripens from December to January. They are black, glossy, solitary, clavate and have a thin skin.

Leaves, Stem and Root: The plant is a 15 to 30 m tall tree with a diameter of 1 m. The bark is smooth and grayish. The alternate leaves are odd-pinnate. The leaflets are opposite, oblong, acuminate and uneven at the base.

Habitat: The plant grows in Jamaica.

Production: Bitter Wood is the wood of Quassia amara or Picrasma excelsa.

Not To Be Confused With: The wood of Rhus metopium.

Other Names: Quassia Wood, Bitter Ash

ACTIONS AND PHARMACOLOGY

COMPOUNDS

Decanor-triterpenes (icrasan- derivatives, 0.05-0.2%): quassinoids: chief components quassin (nigakilactone D), neoquassin and 18-hydroxyquassin beta-carboline alkaloids

EFFECTS

Bitter Wood stimulates secretion of the gastric juices, increases appetite and aids digestion. It may have choleretic properties.

INDICATIONS AND USAGE

Used as a tonic, purgative and as anthelmintic (for ascaris and thread worms).

CONTRAINDICATIONS

Bitter Wood is contraindicated in pregnancy.

PRECAUTIONS AND ADVERSE REACTIONS

General: No health hazards or side effects are known in conjunction with the proper administration of designated therapeutic dosages.

Pregnancy: Bitter Wood is contraindicated in pregnancy.

OVERDOSAGE

Overdose can lead to mucous membrane irritation, followed by vomiting. Use over extended periods of time is said to possibly lead to weak vision and total blindness.

DOSAGE

Daily Dosage: 500 mg.

Storage: Protect from light and keep dry.

LITERATURE

Barbetti P et al., Quassinoids from Quassia amara. In: PH 32:1007. 1993.

Bray DH et al., (1987) Phytother Res 1 (1):22.

Geissmann T, (1964) Ann Rev Pharmacol 4:305.

Kupchan SM, Streelman DR, (1976) J Org Chem 41:3481.

Murae T et al., (1973) Tetrahedron 29:1515.

Murae T et al., (1975) Chem Pharm Bull 23 (9):2191.

Njar VCO et al., 2-Methoxycanthin-6-on: a new alkaloid from the stem wood of Quassia amara. In: PM 59(3):259. 1992.

Njar VCO et al., Antifertility activity of Quassia amara: Quassin inhibits the steroidgenesis in rat Leydig cells in vitro. In: PM 61(2):180-182. 1995.

Ohmoto T, Koike K. (1983) Chem Pharm Bull 31:3198.

Polonsky J, (1973) Fortschr. Chem Org Naturst 30. 101.

Wagner H et al., (1979) Planta Med 36:113.

Wagner H et al., (1980) Planta Med 38:204.

Further information in:

Kern W, List PH, Hörhammer L (Hrsg.), Hagers Handbuch der Pharmazeutischen Praxis, 4. Aufl., Bde 1-8, Springer Verlag Berlin, Heidelberg, New York, 1969 (unter Pirola rotundifolia).

Leung AY, Encyclopedia of Common Natural Ingredients Used in Food Drugs and Cosmetics, John Wiley & Sons Inc., New York 1980.

Lewin L, Gifte und Vergiftungen, 6. Aufl., Nachdruck, Haug Verlag, Heidelberg 1992.

Madaus G, Lehrbuch der Biologischen Arzneimittel, Bde 1-3, Nachdruck, Georg Olms Verlag Hildesheim 1979.

Roth L, Daunderer M, Kormann K, Giftpflanzen, Pflanzengifte, 4. Aufl., Ecomed Fachverlag Landsberg Lech 1993.

Schulz R, Hänsel R, Rationale Phytotherapie, Springer Verlag Heidelberg 1996.

Steinegger E, Hänsel R, Pharmakognosie, 5. Aufl., Springer Verlag Heidelberg 1992.

Teuscher E, Biogene Arzneimittel, 5. Aufl., Wiss. Verlagsges. Stuttgart 1997.

Wagner H, Wiesenauer M, Phytotherapie. Phytopharmaka und pflanzliche Homöopathika, Fischer-Verlag, Stuttgart, Jena, New York 1995.

Wichtl M (Hrsg.), Teedrogen, 4. Aufl., Wiss. Verlagsges. Stuttgart 1997.

Quebracho

See Aspidosperma Quebracho-Blanco

Queen's Delight

See Stillingia Sylvatica

Quercus Robur

Oak Bark

DESCRIPTION

Medicinal Parts: The medicinal parts are the dried bark of the young branches and the lateral shoots, the dried bark of the trunk and branches, the dried leaves of various oak varieties and the seeds without the skin.

Flower and Fruit: The flowers are reddish brown and monoecious. The male flowers consist of a 5-part perigone with 6 to 10 stamens and are in small groups in limp, hanging catkins. The female flowers are in a bowl-shaped involucre, which clasps the base of the fruit and are solitary or in a group of up to 5. The fruit is solitary or in a group of up to 5 on 1 glabrous or occasionally sparsely pubescent stem. The fruit is oblong-ovate, acuminate and enclosed in the cupule.

Leaves, Stem and Root: The tree is about 50 m high with a broad, irregular, heavily branched crown and a trunk, which divides into gnarled, strong, bent branches. The bark is deeply fissured, thick and gray-brown. The leaves are short-petioled almost sessile, oblong-obovate, almost lobed and usually cordate at the base.

Habitat: The tree is widespread in Europe, Asia Minor and the Caucasus region.

Production: Oak bark consists of the dried bark of young branches and saplings of Quercus robur and/or Quercus petraea harvested in the spring.

Not To Be Confused With: The thin branches (lesser tannin content) or with older bark.

Other Names: English Oak, Tanner's Bark

ACTIONS AND PHARMACOLOGY

COMPOUNDS

Tannins (12-16%)

Gallo tannins

Ellagic tannins: (including among others castalagin, pedunculagin, vesvalagin), flavano-ellagic tannins (acutissimine A and B, eugenigrandin, guajavacine B, stenophyllanin C)

Catechin tannins: oligomeric proanthocyanidins

Monomeric and dimeric catechins and leucocyanidins

EFFECTS
Astringent, antiphlogistic.

INDICATIONS AND USAGE

- Diarrhea
- Fevers and colds
- Inflammation of the skin
- Cough
- Bronchitis
- Tendency to infection
- Inflammation of the mouth and pharynx
- Common cold

External: inflammatory skin diseases, local treatment of mild inflammation of the oral cavity and pharyngeal region, as well as the genital and anal area.

Internal: nonspecific, acute diarrhea; in small doses as stomachic.

CONTRAINDICATIONS
No external application is to be carried out upon large-area skin injuries. Whole-body baths are contraindicated with large-area weeping eczemas and skin injuries, with feverish and infectious illnesses, with cardiac insufficiency in stages III and IV (NYHA) and with hypertonia in stage IV (WHO).

PRECAUTIONS AND ADVERSE REACTIONS
General: No health hazards or side effects are known in conjunction with the proper administration of designated therapeutic dosages. Internal administration can lead to digestive complaints because of the secretion-inhibiting effect.

Drug Interactions: Internal use of Oak Bark may reduce or inhibit the absorption of alkaloids and other alkaline drugs.

DOSAGE
Mode of Administration: Comminuted herb for decoctions and other galenic preparations for internal and topical use. The drug is occasionally present in tea mixtures and in standardized preparations of gastrointestinal remedies. Bark extracts for external use are available commercially.

Preparation: To prepare an infusion for internal use, add 1gm finely cut or coarse powdered drug to cold water, rapidly boil, then strain. (1 teaspoonful = 3 gm drug)

To prepare rinses, compresses and gargles, add 20 gm drug per 1 liter of water; for full and partial baths, 5 gm drug scalded with 1 liter water is added to bath water.

Daily Dosage: The daily dose for internal use is 3 gm of drug. Externally, preparations listed above can be used daily.

LITERATURE

Ahn BZ et al., Arch Pharm 304:666. 1971.

Glasl H, DAZ 123:1979. 1983.

König M et al., Ellegitannins and complex tannins from Quercus petraea bark. In: JNP 57(10):1411-1415. 1994.

Pallenbach E, Scholz E, König M, Rimpler H, Proanthocyanidins from Quercus petraea bark. In: PM 59(3):264. 1993.

Scalbert A et al., PH 27:3483. 1988.

Willuhn G, Pflanzliche Dermatika. Eine kritische Übersicht. In: DAZ 132(37):1873. 1992.

Further information in:

Hänsel R, Keller K, Rimpler H, Schneider G (Hrsg.), Hagers Handbuch der Pharmazeutischen Praxis, 5. Aufl., Bde 4-6 (Drogen): Springer Verlag Berlin, Heidelberg, New York, 1992-1994.

Madaus G, Lehrbuch der Biologischen Arzneimittel, Bde. 1-3, Nachdruck, Georg Olms Verlag Hildesheim 1979.

Roth L, Daunderer M, Kormann K, Giftpflanzen, Pflanzengifte, 4. Aufl., Ecomed Fachverlag Landsberg Lech 1993.

Schulz R, Hänsel R, Rationale Phytotherapie, Springer Verlag Heidelberg 1996.

Steinegger E, Hänsel R, Pharmakognosie, 5. Aufl., Springer Verlag Heidelberg 1992.

Teuscher E, Biogene Arzneimittel, 5. Aufl., Wiss. Verlagsges. Stuttgart 1997.

Wagner H, Wiesenauer M, Phytotherapie. Phytopharmaka und pflanzliche Homöopathika, Fischer-Verlag, Stuttgart, Jena, New York 1995.

Wichtl M (Hrsg.), Teedrogen, 4. Aufl., Wiss. Verlagsges. Stuttgart 1997.

Quillaja Saponaria

Soap Bark

DESCRIPTION
Medicinal Parts: The medicinal part is the inner bark.

Flower and Fruit: The terminal inflorescence consists of white androgynous flowers with a calyx and corolla but no epicalyx. Three to five flowers are grouped on the peduncle. The flower head is 5-lobed, splayed flat and formed into a disc on the upper surface. The many-seeded carpels spread into a star shape in the ripe fruit. The seeds are winged with little or no endosperm.

Leaves, Stem and Root: The tree is up to 18 m tall. The leaves are smooth, glossy, short petioled, and oval. The bark is thick, dark and very hard.

Characteristics: The bark is odorless, very bitter and astringent.

Habitat: The plant is indigenous to Chile, Peru and is cultivated in India and California.

Production: Soap Bark is the bark of Quillaja saponaria.

Other Names: Quillai, Quillaja Bark, Soap Tree, Panama Bark, Cullay

ACTIONS AND PHARMACOLOGY

COMPOUNDS

Triterpene saponins (8.5-17%): chief saponins quillaja saponins 17 (QS 17, QS III), 18 (QS 18), 21 (QS 21), chief saponin quillaic acid

Tannins (10-15%)

EFFECTS

Expectorant, anti-inflammatory, purifying.

INDICATIONS AND USAGE

Soap Bark is used internally for coughs, chronic bronchitis and conditions of the respiratory tract. It is used externally for dandruff.

PRECAUTIONS AND ADVERSE REACTIONS

No health hazards or side effects are known in conjunction with the proper administration of designated therapeutic dosages. The drug possesses low potential for sensitization.

OVERDOSAGE

Mucus membrane irritation can occur in the event of overdose. Results include gastroenteritis, combined with vertigo, stomach pain and diarrhea.

DOSAGE

Mode of Administration: Soap Bark is used internally and externally in the form of a liquid extract or tincture.

LITERATURE

Higuchi R et al., (1987) Phytochemistry 26 (1):229.

Higuchi R et al., PH 27:1165. 1988.

Higuchi R, Komori T, PH 26:2357. 1987.

Labriola RA, Denlofeu, V, (1969) Experientia 25:124.

Lallouette P et al., (1967) C R A S Paris D 265:582.

Topping DL et al., (1980) Proc Nutr Soc Aust 5:195.

Wolters B, Arzneipflanzen und Volksmedizin Chiles. In: DAZ 134(39):3693. 1994.

Further information in:

Kern W, List PH, Hörhammer L (Hrsg.), Hagers Handbuch der Pharmazeutischen Praxis, 4. Aufl., Bde 1-8: Springer Verlag Berlin, Heidelberg, New York, 1969.

Leung AY, Encyclopedia of Common Natural Ingredients Used in Food Drugs, Cosmetics, John Wiley & Sons Inc., New York 1980.

Madaus G, Lehrbuch der Biologischen Arzneimittel, Bde 1-3, Nachdruck, Georg Olms Verlag Hildesheim 1979.

Steinegger E, Hänsel R, Pharmakognosie, 5. Aufl., Springer Verlag Heidelberg 1992.

Teuscher E, Biogene Arzneimittel, 5. Aufl., Wiss. Verlagsges. Stuttgart 1997.

Wichtl M (Hrsg.), Teedrogen, 4. Aufl., Wiss. Verlagsges. Stuttgart 1997.

Quince

See Cydonia Oblongata

Radish

See Raphanus Sativus

Ragwort

See Senecio Jacoboea

Ranunculus Acris

Buttercup

DESCRIPTION

Medicinal Parts: The medicinal part is the herb.

Flower and Fruit: The golden yellow, medium-sized flowers are on long, round pedicles. The 5 sepals and 5 petals are close. There are numerous stamens and ovaries. The broad obovate petals are very glossy and have a broad scale on the surface. The small fruit is in an almost globular capitulum.

Leaves, Stem and Root: The leafy plant grows from 30 to 80 cm. The erect stem has few branches. The petioles and pedicles are appressed and downy. The basal leaves are long-petioled and palmate with rhomboid tips, which are divided into 2 or 3. The similar cauline leaves are shorter-petioled.

Characteristics: The fresh herb is spicy and poisonous; once dried, it is no longer poisonous.

Habitat: The plant is indigenous to northern Europe.

Production: Buttercup is the fresh herb Ranunculus acris.

Other Names: Acrid Crowfoot, Batchelor's Buttons, Blisterweed, Burrwort, Globe Amaranth, Gold Cup, Meadowbloom, Yellows, Yellowweed

ACTIONS AND PHARMACOLOGY

COMPOUNDS

The glycoside ranunculin: As protoanemonine-forming agent in the freshly-harvested plant (0.36-2.66% of the fresh weight) that changes enzymatically when the plant is cut into small pieces, and probably also when it is dried, into the pungent, volatile protoanemonine that quickly dimerizes to non-mucous-membrane-irritating anemonine. Once dried, the plant may not be capable of protoanemonine formation.

Saponins

EFFECTS

The active agents are ranunculin, protoanemonin and anemonin. Upon contact with the skin, the juice of the plant causes redness, swelling and blisters. If taken internally, it can lead to burning in the mouth, vomiting, stomachache and pains in the liver.

INDICATIONS AND USAGE

Buttercup is used for blisters, bronchitis, chronic skin complaints, neuralgia and rheumatism.

PRECAUTIONS AND ADVERSE REACTIONS

No health hazards or side effects are known in conjunction with the proper administration of designated therapeutic dosages of the dehydrated drug. Extended skin contact with the freshly-harvested, bruised plant can lead to blister formation and cauterizations, which are difficult to heal, due to the resulting protoanemonine, which is severely irritating to skin and mucous membranes. If taken internally, severe irritation to the gastrointestinal tract, combined with colic and diarrhea, and irritation of the urinary drainage passages may occur.

Symptomatic treatment for external contact should consist of mucilaginosa, after irrigation with diluted potassium permanganate solution. In case of internal contact, administration of activated charcoal should follow gastric lavage.

OVERDOSAGE

Death by asphyxiation following the intake of large quantities of protoanemonine-forming plants has been observed in animal experiments.

DOSAGE

Mode of Administration: Buttercup is available as a ground, dried herb and as an extract.

LITERATURE

Bonora A et al., PH 26:2277. 1987.

Ruijgrok HWL, PM 11:338-347. 1963.

Further information in:

Frohne D, Pfänder HJ: Giftpflanzen - Ein Handbuch für Apotheker, Toxikologen und Biologen, 4. Aufl., Wiss. Verlags-Ges. Stuttgart 1997

Hegnauer R, Chemotaxonomie der Pflanzen, Bde 1-11: Birkhäuser Verlag Basel, Boston, Berlin 1962-1997.

Kern W, List PH, Hörhammer L (Hrsg.), Hagers Handbuch der Pharmazeutischen Praxis, 4. Aufl., Bde. 1-8: Springer Verlag Berlin, Heidelberg, New York, 1969.

Roth L, Daunderer M, Kormann K, Giftpflanzen, Pflanzengifte, 4. Aufl., Ecomed Fachverlag Landsberg Lech 1993.

Teuscher E, Lindequist U: Biogene Gifte - Biologie, Chemie, Pharmakologie, 2. Aufl., Fischer Verlag Stuttgart 1994.

Ranunculus Bulbosus

Bulbous Buttercup

DESCRIPTION

Medicinal Parts: The medicinal parts are the latex and the fresh flowering herb with root.

Flower and Fruit: The large golden yellow flowers consist of 5 sepals hanging down, 5 petals on grooved stems and numerous stamens and ovaries. The small fruit has a short curved beak.

Leaves, Stem and Root: The plant grows to from 10 to 30 cm high and has a tuber on the underground part of the stem. The basal leaves are long-petioled, trifoliate with orbicular and pinnasect leaflets. The middle one has a longer petiole and is sheath-like at the base. The stems are branched and tuberously thickened at the base. The plant is appressed pubescent above and patently pubescent below.

Habitat: The plant grows in the northern parts of Europe and in the northeastern U.S.

Production: Bulbous Buttercup is the whole plant in flower of Ranunculus bulbosus with root.

Other Names: Crowfoot, Cuckoo Buds, Frogwort, King's Cup, Meadowbloom, Pilewort, St. Anthony's Turnip, Frogsfoot, Goldcup

ACTIONS AND PHARMACOLOGY

COMPOUNDS

The glycoside ranunculin: changes enzymatically when the plant is cut into small pieces, and probably also when it is dried, into the pungent, volatile protoanemonine that quickly dimerizes to non-mucous membrane irritating anemonine. When dried, the plant is not capable of protoanemonine-formation.

EFFECTS

The active agents are ranunculin, protoanemonin, anemonin and labenzym. The drug is said to cause symptoms of drowsiness and tiredness and may be linked to depressive moods.

INDICATIONS AND USAGE

In homeopathy, the herb is used for skin diseases, rheumatism, gout, neuralgia, influenza, and meningitis.

CONTRAINDICATIONS

The administration of the drug during pregnancy is absolutely contraindicated.

PRECAUTIONS AND ADVERSE REACTIONS

General: No health hazards or side effects are known in conjunction with the proper administration of designated therapeutic dosages of the dehydrated drug.

Extended skin contact with the freshly-harvested, bruised plant can lead to blister formation and cauterizations that are difficult to heal due to the resulting protoanemonine, which is severely irritating to skin and mucous membranes. If taken internally, severe irritation to the gastrointestinal tract, combined with colic and diarrhea, as well as with irritation of the urinary drainage passages are possible. Symptomatic treatment for external contact should consist of mucilage, after irrigation with diluted potassium permanganate solution; in case of internal contact, activated charcoal should follow gastric lavage.

Pregnancy: The administration of the drug during pregnancy is absolutely contraindicated.

OVERDOSAGE

Death by asphyxiation following the intake of large quantities of protoanemonine-forming plants has been observed in animal experiments.

DOSAGE

Mode of Administration: The herb is used as an extract in homeopathic dilutions.

LITERATURE

Bonora A et al., PH 26:2277. 1987.

Ruijgrok HWL, PM 11:338-347. 1963.

Further information in:

Frohne D, Pfänder HJ, Giftpflanzen - Ein Handbuch für Apotheker, Toxikologen und Biologen, 4. Aufl., Wiss. Verlags-Ges. Stuttgart 1997.

Kern W, List PH, Hörhammer L (Hrsg.), Hagers Handbuch der Pharmazeutischen Praxis, 4. Aufl., Bde. 1-8: Springer Verlag Berlin, Heidelberg, New York, 1969.

Madaus G, Lehrbuch der Biologischen Arzneimittel, Bde 1-3, Nachdruck, Georg Olms Verlag Hildesheim 1979.

Roth L, Daunderer M, Kormann K, Giftpflanzen, Pflanzengifte, 4. Aufl., Ecomed Fachverlag Landsberg Lech 1993.

Teuscher E, Lindequist U, Biogene Gifte - Biologie, Chemie, Pharmakologie, 2. Aufl., Fischer Verlag Stuttgart 1994.

Ranunculus Ficaria

Lesser Celandine

DESCRIPTION

Medicinal Parts: The medicinal part is the fresh herb.

Flower and Fruit: The golden yellow flowers have a diameter of 25 mm. The calyx usually has 3 sepals, the corolla 8 or more petals which are glossy and spread out in a star-shape. Since the petals are green underneath the flowers are inconspicuous when closed. There are numerous stamens and ovaries. The fruit is 1-seeded and indehiscent.

Leaves, Stem and Root: The plant grows from 5 to 15 cm high. The stems are decumbent and bear bulbils in the leaf axils. The leaves, like the stems, are glabrous and fleshy. The lower ones are long-petioled, alternate, orbicular-cordate. The upper ones are 5-lobed. There are fleshy, cylindrical clavate tubers between the roots.

Characteristics: The herb has a hot, unpleasant taste and is toxic.

Habitat: The plant is found all over Europe, western Asia and northern Africa.

Production: Lesser Celandine is the fresh herb of Ranunculus ficaria.

Other Names: Pilewort, Figwort, Smallwort

ACTIONS AND PHARMACOLOGY

COMPOUNDS

The glycoside ranunculin as protoanemonine-forming agent: In the freshly-harvested plant (0.06-0.35% of the fresh weight, of which only 3% of the overall content of the plant is contained in the leaves used as salad, 68% in the stalks, 25% in the blossoms) that changes enzymatically when the plant is cut into small pieces, and probably also when it is dried, into the pungent, volatile protoanemonine that quickly dimerizes to non-mucus-membrane-irritating anemonine; when dried, the plant is not capable of protoanemonine-formation.

EFFECTS

Active agents are tannin, the alkaloids chelidonin and cholerytrin, the saponin fikarin and large quantities of Vitamin C.

INDICATIONS AND USAGE

Scurvy, treatment of bleeding wounds and gums, swollen joints.

PRECAUTIONS AND ADVERSE REACTIONS

The dangers of irritation of the skin and mucus membranes are relatively low with pilewort. The consumption of small quantities of the fresh leaf sheaths (before blossoming; the stem should be discarded) as a springtime salad is unproblematic.

No health hazards or side effects are known in conjunction with the proper administration of designated therapeutic dosages of the dehydrated drug. Extended skin contact with the freshly-harvested, bruised plant can lead to blister formation and cauterizations which are difficult to heal due to the resulting protoanemonine, that is severely irritating to skin and mucus membranes.

If taken internally, severe irritation to the gastrointestinal tract, combined with colic and diarrhea, as well as irritations of the urinary drainage passages, are possible. Symptomatic treatment for external contact should consist of irrigation with diluted potassium permanganate solution; in case of internal contact, administration of activated charcoal should follow gastric lavage.

OVERDOSAGE

Death by asphyxiation following the intake of large quantities of protoanemonine-forming plants has been observed in animal experiments.

DOSAGE

Mode of Administration: Ground and as an extract. The drug extracts can be added to baths to treat hemorrhoids, warts and scratches.

LITERATURE

Bonora A et al., PH 26:2277. 1987.

Kolesnik et al., (1963) CA 59:7856.

Pourrat H, Pourrat A, (1966) Bull Soc Chim Franc 2410.

Pourrat H et al., (1979) Ann Pharm Franc 37:441.

Pourrat H et al., (1982) Ann Pharm Franc 40:373.

Ruijgrok HWL, PM 11:338-347. 1963.

Texier O et al., (1984) Phytochemistry 23(12):2903.

Further information in:

Hegnauer R, Chemotaxonomie der Pflanzen, Bde 1-11: Birkhäuser Verlag Basel, Boston, Berlin 1962-1997.

Kern W, List PH, Hörhammer L (Hrsg.), Hagers Handbuch der Pharmazeutischen Praxis, 4. Aufl., Bde 1-8: Springer Verlag Berlin, Heidelberg, New York, 1969.

Madaus G, Lehrbuch der Biologischen Arzneimittel, Bde 1-3, Nachdruck, Georg Olms Verlag Hildesheim 1979.

Roth L, Daunderer M, Kormann K, Giftpflanzen, Pflanzengifte, 4. Aufl., Ecomed Fachverlag Landsberg Lech 1993.

Teuscher E, Lindequist U, Biogene Gifte - Biologie, Chemie, Pharmakologie, 2. Aufl., Fischer Verlag Stuttgart 1994.

Ranunculus Sceleratus

Poisonous Buttercup

DESCRIPTION

Medicinal Parts: The medicinal part is the herb.

Flower and Fruit: The plant produces numerous flowers. They are small, pale yellow and 4 to 10 mm in size. The petals are as long as the calyx. The sepals are revolute, ovate and downy. There are many stamens and numerous ovaries. The fruit consists of an oblong, ear-like capitula. The calyx and corolla drop easily.

Leaves, Stem and Root: The plant grows from 20 to 60 cm high with an annual root. The plant is pale, glossy, yellowish-green, fleshy and glabrous. The upper part of the stem is occasionally pubescent. The stem is erect, tubular, glabrous and branched. The leaves are palmate, the lower ones are long-petioled with 2 to 3-lobed segments, the upper ones are sessile and usually trifoliate.

Characteristics: A bruised leaf coming into contact with the skin creates a blister that heals very slowly.

Habitat: The plant is indigenous to central and northern Europe.

Production: Poisonous Buttercup is the fresh herb of R. sceleratus, which is gathered in October.

Other Names: Celery-leaved Crowfoot, Cursed Crowfoot

ACTIONS AND PHARMACOLOGY

COMPOUNDS

The glycoside ranunculin: as protoanemonine-forming agent in the freshly-harvested plant (1.4% of the fresh weight), that changes enzymatically when the plant is cut into small pieces, and probably also when it is dried, into the pungent, volatile protoanemonine that quickly dimerizes to non-mucous-membrane-irritating anemonine. When dried, the plant may not be capable of protoanemonine-formation.

Saponins

EFFECTS

The active agents are ranunculin, protoanemonin and anemonin and flavoid in the leaves. The plant is highly toxic. The juice contains protoanemonin, which causes pain and burning sensations, increases saliva secretion, and causes severe inflammation of the tongue.

INDICATIONS AND USAGE

Poisonous Buttercup is used as a skin stimulant for skin diseases (such as scabies), and leucoderma.

PRECAUTIONS AND ADVERSE REACTIONS

No health hazards or side effects are known in conjunction with the proper administration of designated therapeutic dosages of the dehydrated drug. Extended skin contact with the freshly-harvested, bruised plant can lead to blister formation and cauterizations, which are difficult to heal due to the resulting protoanemonine, which is severely irritating to skin and mucous membranes. If taken internally, severe irritation to the gastrointestinal tract, combined with colic and diarrhea, as well as irritation of the urinary drainage passages, may occur. Symptomatic treatment for external contact consists of mucilaginosa after irrigation with diluted potassium permanganate solution. In case of internal contact, administration of activated charcoal should follow gastric lavage.

OVERDOSAGE

Death by asphyxiation following the intake of large quantities of protoanemonine-forming plants has been observed in animal experiments.

DOSAGE

Mode of Administration: The herb is available as a tincture.

LITERATURE

Bonora A et al., PH 26:2277. 1987.

Ruijgrok HWL, PM 11:338-347. 1963.

Further information in:

Frohne D, Pfänder HJ, Giftpflanzen - Ein Handbuch für Apotheker, Toxikologen und Biologen, 4. Aufl., Wiss. Verlags-Ges. Stuttgart 1997.

Hegnauer R, Chemotaxonomie der Pflanzen, Bde 1-11: Birkhäuser Verlag Basel, Boston, Berlin 1962-1997.

Kern W, List PH, Hörhammer L (Hrsg.), Hagers Handbuch der Pharmazeutischen Praxis, 4. Aufl., Bde. 1-8: Springer Verlag Berlin, Heidelberg, New York, 1969.

Madaus G, Lehrbuch der Biologischen Arzneimittel, Bde 1-3, Nachdruck, Georg Olms Verlag Hildesheim 1979.

Roth L, Daunderer M, Kormann K, Giftpflanzen, Pflanzengifte, 4. Aufl., Ecomed Fachverlag Landsberg Lech 1993.

Teuscher E, Lindequist U, Biogene Gifte - Biologie, Chemie, Pharmakologie, 2. Aufl., Fischer Verlag Stuttgart 1994.

Raphanus Raphanistrum

Wild Radish

DESCRIPTION

Medicinal Parts: The medicinal part is the fresh plant before flowering.

Flower and Fruit: The flowers are bright yellow, sometimes white with violet veins. The form of the flower corresponds to that of the Cruciferae. The calyx is erect. The pods are cylindrical with vertical grooves between which the seeds are tied (like a string of pearls). The pods fall apart at these points.

Leaves, Stem and Root: The leaves are petiolate and lyrate, the upper ones are lanceolate. The leaves and lower part of the stem are stiff-haired.

Habitat: The plant has been cultivated for a very long time and is grown in all parts of the world, especially in temperate regions.

Production: Wild Radish is the fresh plant of Raphanus raphanistrum before flowering.

Other Names: Jointed-podded Charlock

ACTIONS AND PHARMACOLOGY

COMPOUNDS

Glucosinolates in the freshly-harvested, unbruised plant: chief component glucoputranjivine, that yields isopropyl mustard oil as the cells are destroyed.

EFFECTS

No information is available.

INDICATIONS AND USAGE

Wild Radish has been used for skin conditions and stomach disorders.

PRECAUTIONS AND ADVERSE REACTIONS

No health hazards or side effects are known in conjunction with the proper administration of designated therapeutic dosages. Administration of high dosages of the freshly-harvested plant can lead to mucous membrane irritation of the gastrointestinal tract.

DOSAGE

Mode of Administration: Wild Radish is administered ground and as an alcoholic extract.

LITERATURE

Kern W, List PH, Hörhammer L (Hrsg.), Hagers Handbuch der Pharmazeutischen Praxis, 4. Aufl., Bde. 1-8: Springer Verlag Berlin, Heidelberg, New York, 1969.

Raphanus Sativus

Radish

DESCRIPTION

Medicinal Parts: The medicinal part is the fresh root.

Flower and Fruit: The raceme is loose and has about 30 flowers. The pedicles are 1 to 2 cm long and are covered in scattered bristles. The sepals are 6.5 to 10 mm long, oblong, acute, glabrous or with scattered bristles and red or green. The petals are 17 to 22 mm long, obovate, slightly margined, violet or white with dark veins. The fruit is on upright, patent stems. They are upright, cylindrical, clavate and acuminate. The upper segment is up to 9 cm long and even or slightly constricted between the seeds. The fruit is straw-like on the outside. The seeds are ovate, 4 mm long and 3 mm wide, light brown with a black hilum.

Leaves, Stem and Root: The root is annual or biennial and thin. The stem is up to 1 m high, bent, cane-like, branched, glabrous or covered with bristles and often violet, particularly in the axils of the lateral branches. The lower leaves are lyrate-pinnatisect with large sweeping crenate end segments and smaller, oblong-ovate, obtuse-dentate lateral lobes. They are light green, often red-veined and covered with scattered, appressed bristles.

Characteristics: The root is large, thick, tuberous, fleshy, and has a hot taste.

Habitat: The plant is probably indigenous to China and Japan and is cultivated in most temperate regions of the world.

Production: Radish consists of the fresh roots of Raphanus sativus.

ACTIONS AND PHARMACOLOGY

COMPOUNDS

Glucosinolates (0.05-0.1% of the fresh weight) in the fresh, unbruised rhizome: chief components 4-methylthio-3-butenyl-glucosinolate, further including, among others, glucobrassin, sinigrin, glucoraphanine

EFFECTS

Secretagogue for the upper gastrointestinal tract, motility promoting, antimicrobial.

INDICATIONS AND USAGE

- Loss of appetite
- Fevers and colds
- Cough
- Bronchitis
- Tendency to infection
- Inflammation of the mouth and pharynx
- Common cold

Radish is used for peptic disorders, especially those related to dyskinesia of the bile ducts, catarrh of the upper respiratory tract.

PRECAUTIONS AND ADVERSE REACTIONS

No health hazards or side effects are known in conjunction with the proper administration of designated therapeutic dosages. Administration of higher dosages of the fresh rhizome can lead to mucus membrane irritation of the gastrointestinal tract. Due to the cholagogic effect of the drug, biliary colic could be triggered among patients with gallstones.

DOSAGE

Mode of Administration: Pressed juice or radish-honey juice for oral use.

Preparation: The gratings of 1 radish and the resulting juice are mixed with honey, then allowed to stand for 10 hours, take by the spoonful over the whole day.

Daily Dosage: Average daily dose: 50 to 100 ml pressed juice. Take 1/2 tablespoon several times daily. For patients with whooping cough, the radish-honey juice preparation described above may be used.

LITERATURE

Hänsel R, Keller K, Rimpler H, Schneider G (Hrsg.), Hagers Handbuch der Pharmazeutischen Praxis, 5. Aufl., Bde 4-6 (Drogen): Springer Verlag Berlin, Heidelberg, New York, 1992-1994.

Teuscher E, Lindequist U, Biogene Gifte - Biologie, Chemie, Pharmakologie, 2. Aufl., Fischer Verlag Stuttgart 1994.

Raspberry

See Rubus Idaeus

Rauwolfia Serpentina

Rauwolfia

DESCRIPTION

Medicinal Parts: The medicinal part is the dried root.

Flower and Fruit: The white to pink flowers are in terminal or axillary cymes, which have a diameter of 2.5 to 5 cm and are 5 to 13 cm long. The corolla tube is 11 to 19 cm long and therefore much longer than the tips, which form a plate like margin. The fruit is a bilabiate drupe, which is purple-black when ripe.

Leaves, Stem and Root: The plant is an erect, glabrous evergreen semishrub 0.5 to 1 m in height. The trunk is pale and unbranched. The leaves are concentrated towards the top of the trunk and are entire-margined in whorls of 3 to 5 and are occasionally opposite. The leaves are 7 to 18 cm long, 2.5 to 5 cm wide, oblong-ovate or lanceolate and taper to an irregular base. The petiole is 5 to 15 cm long. The rhizome is vertical and woody. The root is gray-brown with a wrinkled surface and is 23 to 22 mm in diameter.

Characteristics: The fresh root has a very bitter and unpleasant taste.

Habitat: The plant is indigenous to India, Indochina, Borneo, Sri Lanka and Sumatra.

Production: Rauwolfia root consists of the dried root of Rauwolfia serpentina. Four-year-old plants are chosen if collected in the wild, while cultivated plants are harvested at 2 years.

Not To Be Confused With: The roots of other Rauwolfia species.

ACTIONS AND PHARMACOLOGY

COMPOUNDS

Indole alkaloids (1-3%): chief alkaloids of the- yohimbine-type: reserpine, rescinnamine (reserpinine)- heteroyohimbane-type: serpentinine, serpentine, raubasine (ajmalicine)-sarpagan-type: raupine (sarpagine)- ajmalane-type: ajmaline

Starch

EFFECTS

Reserpin and other alkaloids in the Rauwolfia root have a sympathicolytic effect by removal of noradrenaline and the prevention of noradrenaline being reabsorbed in the vesicles of the noradrenergic nerve ends; this results in a hypotensive, sedative and antiarrhythmical efffect.

INDICATIONS AND USAGE

■ Nervousness and insomnia

Borderline hypertony, in particular raised sympathicotonus with sinus-tachycardia, anxiety and tension states, psychometric disturbances. The whole extract is more easily tolerated than the isolated substance with reserpin indicating the importance of the accompanying substances (so-called co-effectors).

In folk medicine, extracts of the drug are used in India as antidotes for snake bites and the poisonous bites of other reptiles. It is also used for fever, as tonic for general debilities, for constipation, for feverish intestinal diseases, diseases of the liver, rheumatism, dropsy and as a sedative for nervous and mental disorders. It is used in Indian folk medicine for snake and insect bites, fever and diarrhea.

CONTRAINDICATIONS

Rauwolfia is contraindicated in depression, ulceration, pheochromocytoma, pregnancy and lactation.

PRECAUTIONS AND ADVERSE REACTIONS

General: No health hazards are known in conjunction with the proper administration of designated therapeutic dosages. Side effects can include, among others, the following: nasal congestion, states of depression, tiredness, potency disorders. Reactive capability can be so reduced as to hinder driving ability in traffic and the effective handling of machinery (particularly in conjunction with alcohol).

Drug Interactions: Combination with alcohol severely increases the impairment of motor reactions. There is a synergistic effect with neuroleptics and barbiturates. Severe bradycardia occurs in combination with digitalis glycosides. A reduction of the effect occurs in combination with levodopa along with an increase in the undesired extra-pyramidal-motor symptoms. In combination with sympathomimetics, (in cough or flu remedies or in appetite depressors) an initial significant increase in blood pressure can occur.

DOSAGE

Mode of Administration: Ground drug, drug powder as well as other galenic preparations for internal usage.

Daily Dosage: 600 mg drug equivalent to 6 mg total alkaloids.

LITERATURE

Beim HJ, Pharmacol Rev 8:281. 1978.

Cornett GBR, World Crops 17:33. 1965.

Lounasmaa M et al., On the structure of the indole alkaloid ajmalicidine. In: PM 60(5):480. 1994.

Nattkämper G, PA 22.281. 1967.

Further information in:

Hänsel R, Keller K, Rimpler H, Schneider G (Hrsg.), Hagers Handbuch der Pharmazeutischen Praxis, 5. Aufl., Bde 4-6 (Drogen): Springer Verlag Berlin, Heidelberg, New York, 1992-1994.

Roth L, Daunderer M, Kormann K, Giftpflanzen, Pflanzengifte, 4. Aufl., Ecomed Fachverlag Landsberg Lech 1993.

Schulz R, Hänsel R, Rationale Phytotherapie, Springer Verlag Heidelberg 1996.

Steinegger E, Hänsel R, Pharmakognosie, 5. Aufl., Springer Verlag Heidelberg 1992.

Teuscher E, Biogene Arzneimittel, 5. Aufl., Wiss. Verlagsges. Stuttgart 1997.

Wagner H, Wiesenauer M, Phytotherapie. Phytopharmaka und pflanzliche Homöopathika, Fischer-Verlag, Stuttgart, Jena, New York 1995.

Wichtl M (Hrsg.), Teedrogen, 4. Aufl., Wiss. Verlagsges. Stuttgart 1997.

Red Clover

See Trifolium Pratense

Red Maple

See Acer Rubrum

Red Sandalwood

See Pterocarpus Santalinus

Red-Spur Valerian

See Centranthus Ruber

Reed Herb

See Phragmites Communis

Rhamnus Cathartica

Buckthorn

DESCRIPTION

Medicinal Parts: The medicinal parts are the whole, ripe, dried fruit and the fresh ripe fruit.

Flower and Fruit: The small, dioecious, greenish-yellow flowers are in axillary cymes. The calyx is fused and has 4 segments. The petals are small and are on the edge of the calyx tube with the short stamens. The ovary is 4-valved with a style divided in four. The fruit is a pea-sized, black berry-like drupe. The seeds are 5 mm long and triangular with a narrow split, which separates slightly at the end and is surrounded by a thick margin.

Leaves, Stem and Root: The plant is a 3 m high bush, which takes many forms or a tree that is up to 8 m high with a bent trunk. The boughs are usually stiffly spread. The branches are more or less clearly opposite, glossy, glabrous or occasionally pubescent and end in a thorn. The leaves are clustered on the older branches, opposite on the younger ones, ovate or elliptical, finely serrate with 2 to 3 lateral ribs curved towards the midrib.

Characteristics: The flowers are fragrant, the heartwood is orange-red.

Habitat: The plant is common all over northern Africa, western Asia and Europe.

Production: Buckthorn consists of the dried ripe berries of Rhamni catharticus.

Not To Be Confused With: The fruit of Frangula alnus.

Other Names: Waythorn, Highwaythorn, Hartshorn, Ramsthorn

ACTIONS AND PHARMACOLOGY

COMPOUNDS

Anthracene derivatives (2-7%): chief components are glucofrangulin A, diacetylglucofrangulin, frangulin A

Tannins (3-4%): oligomeric proanthocyanidins

Flavonoids (1-2%): including, among others, catharticin (rhamnocitrin-3-rhamnoside), xanthorhamnine (rhamnetin-3-rhamnoside)

EFFECTS

1.8-dihydroxyanthracine derivatives have a laxative effect. This works mainly through its effect on colon motility by inhibiting the stationary and stimulating the propulsive contractions. This results in faster bowel movements and a reduction of fluid absorption due to the shortened contact time. In addition, because of the stimulation of active chloride secretions, water and electrolytes are discharged.

INDICATIONS AND USAGE

■ Constipation

Buckthorn is used for constipation, bowel movement relief in cases of anal fissures and hemorrhoids and after recto-anal surgery. It is also used in preparation for diagnostic intervention of the gastrointestinal tract and to achieve softer stool. In folk medicine it is used as a diuretic (in "blood-purifying" remedies).

CONTRAINDICATIONS

Buckthorn is contraindicated in intestinal obturation, acute inflammatory intestinal diseases, appendicitis and abdominal pain of unknown origin.

PRECAUTIONS AND ADVERSE REACTIONS

General: Spasmodic gastrointestinal complaints can occur as a side effect to the drug's purgative effect. Long-term use leads to losses of electrolytes, in particular K(+)ions, and as a result of this to hyperaldosteronism, inhibition of intestinal motility and enhancement of the effect of cardioactive steroids; in rare cases also to heart arrhythmias, nephropathies, edemas and accelerated bone deterioration.

The intake of large quantities of the fresh berries could lead to European cholera or kidney irritation. The question of the increase in probability of the appearance of colonic carcinomas following long-term administration of anthracene drugs has not yet been fully clarified; recent studies show no connections between the administration of anthracene drugs and the frequency of carcinomas in the colon.

Drug Interactions: In the case of chronic use/overuse, potassium deficiency leads to an increase in the effect of cardiac glycosides as well as effecting heartbeat-regulating drugs. Potassium deficiency can be adversely affected by using the drug in combination with thiazide diuretics, corticosteroids and licorice root.

Pregnancy: Use during pregnancy or while breast feeding only after consulting a physician.

Children: The drug is not to be administered to children under 12 years of age.

DOSAGE

Mode of Administration: For internal use, comminuted drug is used for infusions, decoctions, cold macerations or elixirs. The drug is contained in purgative, metabolic, liver, gallbladder, and gastrointestinal teas.

Preparation: To prepare an infusion, scald 4 gm comminuted drug, strain after 10 to 15 minutes or put in cold water which is boiled for 2 to 3 minutes, and strain while still warm. (1 teaspoon = 3.8 gm drug)

Daily Dosage: 20 to 30 mg hydroxyanthracine derivative per day calculated as glucofrangulin A. The individual dose is the minimum required to produce a soft stool.

Stimulating laxatives should not be taken for more than 1 or 2 weeks without consulting a doctor.

LITERATURE

Anonym, Abwehr von Arzneimittelrisiken, Stufe II. In: DAZ 136(38):3253-2354. 1996.

Anonym, Anwendungseinschränkungen für Anthranoid-haltige Abführmittel angeordnet. In: PUZ 25(6):341-342. 1996.

BGA, Arzneimittelrisiken: Anthranoide. In: DAZ 132(21):1164. 1992.

Belkin M et al., (1952) J Nat Cancer Inst 13:742.

Coskun M, Int J Pharmacogn 30:151. 1992.

Demirezer LÖ, Glucofrangulinanthrone A/B, deren Oxidationsformen und davon abgeleitete Zuckerester aus Rhamnus-Arten. In: Dissertation Universität Frankfurt/Main. 1991.

Klimpel BE et al., Anthranoidhaltige Laxantien - ein Risiko für die Entwicklung von Tumoren der ableitenden Harnwege. In: PUZ 26(1):33, Jahrestagung der DPhG, Berlin, 1996. 1997.

Rauwald HW Just, J-D, (1981) Planta Med 42:244.

Thesen R, Phytotherapeutika - nicht immer harmlos. In: ZPT 9(49):105. 1988.

Further information in:

Frohne D, Pfänder HJ, Giftpflanzen - Ein Handbuch für Apotheker, Toxikologen und Biologen, 4. Aufl., Wiss. Verlags-Ges. Stuttgart 1997.

Hänsel R, Keller K, Rimpler H, Schneider G (Hrsg.), Hagers Handbuch der Pharmazeutischen Praxis, 5. Aufl., Bde 4-6 (Drogen): Springer Verlag Berlin, Heidelberg, New York, 1992-1994.

Lewin L, Gifte und Vergiftungen, 6. Aufl., Nachdruck, Haug Verlag, Heidelberg 1992.

Madaus G, Lehrbuch der Biologischen Arzneimittel, Bde 1-3, Nachdruck, Georg Olms Verlag Hildesheim 1979.

Roth L, Daunderer M, Kormann K, Giftpflanzen, Pflanzengifte, 4. Aufl., Ecomed Fachverlag Landsberg Lech 1993.

Steinegger E, Hänsel R, Pharmakognosie, 5. Aufl., Springer Verlag Heidelberg 1992.

Thomson RH, Naturally Occuring Quinones, 2nd Ed., Academic Press New York 1971.

Teuscher E, Lindequist U, Biogene Gifte - Biologie, Chemie, Pharmakologie, 2. Aufl., Fischer Verlag Stuttgart 1994.

Teuscher E, Biogene Arzneimittel, 5. Aufl., Wiss. Verlagsges. Stuttgart 1997.

Wichtl M (Hrsg.), Teedrogen, 4. Aufl., Wiss. Verlagsges. Stuttgart 1997.

Rhamnus Frangula

Buckthorn Bark

DESCRIPTION

Medicinal Parts: The medicinal parts are the dried bark and the fresh bark of the trunk and branches.

Flower and Fruit: The flowers are in 2 to 10 axillary-blossomed cymes on pedicles 1 to 3 times as long. The flowers are initially pubescent, greenish-white, conical, 3 to 4 mm long with 5 sepals and 5 petals. The sepals are 3 mm long, oblong-triangular and acute. The petals are whitish, erect, stemmed and enclose the stamens. The stamens are somewhat shorter than the petals and have large anthers and short filaments. The fruit is a globular, initially green, later red, and when ripe, a black-purple drupe about 8 cm wide containing 3 seeds. The seeds are wide, flat triangular-lentil-shaped with a very narrow groove.

Leaves, Stem and Root: The plant is a thornless, 1 to 3 m high bush or 7 m high weedy tree. The branches are piled on the boughs and densely foliated. The bark is initially green, later gray-brown and covered in gray-white lenticles. The leaf buds are pubescent. The leaves are thin, soft when young, but later become stiffer. They are broadly elliptical to obovate and about 3.5 to 5 cm long. They are usually entire-margined, slightly undulate and pubescent on the under surface of the ribs.

Characteristics: The heartwood is bright yellow-red. The odor is somewhat foul and the taste is disgustingly bitter.

Habitat: The plant is indigenous to all of Europe, western Asia, Asia Minor and the Caucasus, it has spread to the wild in North America.

Production: Buckthorn bark consists of the dried bark of the trunks and branches of Rhamnus frangula.

Other Names: Alder Buckthorn, Frangula Bark, Black Alder, Dog Wood, Arrow Wood, Persian Berries, Alder Dogwood

ACTIONS AND PHARMACOLOGY

COMPOUNDS

Anthracene derivatives: chief components glucofrangulin A, glucofrangulin A-diacetate (estered at rhamnose remainder), additionally frangulin A, frangulin C

Naphthaquinone derivatives

Peptide alkaloids (traces): including frangulanin

EFFECTS

1,8-dihydroxy-anthracene derivatives have a laxative effect. These compounds increase the motility of the colon by inhibiting stationary and stimulating propulsive contractions. The accelerated intestinal passage caused by the shortened contraction time reduces liquid absorption through the lumen. In addition, stimulation of active chloride secretion increases the water and electrolyte content of intestinal contents.

INDICATIONS AND USAGE

■ Constipation

Constipation, to ease bowel evacuation in the case of anal fissures, hemorrhoids and after rectal-anal surgery as well as in preparation for exploratory surgery in the gastrointestinal tract.

CONTRAINDICATIONS

The drug is not to be used with intestinal obduration, acutely inflammatory intestinal diseases, or if appendicitis is suspected.

PRECAUTIONS AND ADVERSE REACTIONS

General: Vomiting and spasmodic gastrointestinal complaints can occur as side effects to the drug's purgative effect or with overdoses.

The question of the increase in probability of the appearance of carcinomas in the colon following long-term administration of anthracene drugs has not yet been fully clarified; recent studies show no sure connections between the administration of anthracene drugs and the frequency of carcinomas in the colon.

Drug Interactions: Long-term use leads to losses of electrolytes, in particular K(+)ions, and as a result of this, to hyperaldosteronism, inhibition of intestinal motility and enhancement of the effect of cardioactive steroids; in rare cases also to heart arrhythmias, nephropathies, edemas and accelerated bone deterioration.

Pregnancy: The drug is not to be administered during pregnancy nor while nursing.

Pediatric Use: The drug is not to be administered to children under 12 years of age.

DOSAGE

Mode of Administration: comminuited drug, powder or dried extracts for infusions, decoctions, cold macerations or elixirs. Liquid or solid forms of medication exclusively for oral use.

Preparation: To prepare an infusion, scald 2 gm comminuted drug with boiling water and strain after 15 minutes. A cold infusion can be prepared by letting the drug steep for 12 hours at room temperature.

Daily Dosage: 20 mg to 180 mg hydroxyanthracene derivatives.

The individually correct dosage is the smallest dosage necessary to maintain a soft stool.

Note: Stimulating laxatives must not be used over an extended period (1 to 2 weeks) without medical advice.

Storage: Protect from light and dampness.

LITERATURE

Anonym, Abwehr von Arzneimittelrisiken, Stufe II. In: DAZ 136(38):3253-2354. 1996.

Anonym, Pharmaceutical Care: "Den Miβbrauch von Laxanzien vermeiden helfen". In: DAZ 135(20):1867-1868. 1995.

Demirezer LÖ, Glucofrangulinanthrone A/B, deren Oxidationsformen und davon abgeleitete Zuckerester aus Rhamnus-Arten. In: Dissertation Universität Frankfurt/Main. 1991.

Helmholz H, Ruge A, Piasecki A, Schröder S, Westendorf J, Genotoxizität der Faulbaumrinde. In: PZ 138(43):3478. 1993.

Pailer M, Haslinger E, (1972) Monatsh. Chem 103:1399.

Sydiskis RJ, Owen DG, Lohr JL, Rosler KHA, Blosmster RN, Inactivation of enveloped viruses by anthraquinones extracted from plants. In: Antimicrob Agents Chemother 35:2463-2466. 1991.

Van Os FHL, (1976) Pharmacology 14(Suppl 1)7:18.

Wagner H et al., (1978) Planta Med 33:53.

Further information in:

Frohne D, Pfänder HJ, Giftpflanzen - Ein Handbuch für Apotheker, Toxikologen und Biologen, 4. Aufl., Wiss. Verlagsges. mbH Stuttgart 1997.

Hänsel R, Keller K, Rimpler H, Schneider G (Hrsg.), Hagers Handbuch der Pharmazeutischen Praxis, 5. Aufl., Bde 4-6

(Drogen): Springer Verlag Berlin, Heidelberg, New York, 1992-1994.

Leung AY, Encyclopedia of Common Natural Ingredients Used in Food Drugs and Cosmetics, John Wiley & Sons Inc., New York 1980.

Roth L, Daunderer M, Kormann K, Giftpflanzen, Pflanzengifte, 4. Aufl., Ecomed Fachverlag Landsberg Lech 1993.

Schulz R, Hänsel R, Rationale Phytotherapie, Springer Verlag Heidelberg 1996.

Steinegger E, Hänsel R, Pharmakognosie, 5. Aufl., Springer Verlag Heidelberg 1992.

Teuscher E, Lindequist U, Biogene Gifte - Biologie, Chemie, Pharmakologie, 2. Aufl., Fischer Verlag Stuttgart 1994.

Teuscher E, Biogene Arzneimittel, 5. Aufl., Wiss. Verlagsges. mbH Stuttgart 1997.

Wagner H, Wiesenauer M, Phytotherapie. Phytopharmaka und pflanzliche Homöopathika, Fischer-Verlag, Stuttgart, Jena, New York 1995.

Wichtl M (Hrsg.), Teedrogen, 4. Aufl., Wiss. Verlagsges. Stuttgart 1997.

Rhamnus Purshianus

Cascara Sagrada

DESCRIPTION

Medicinal Parts: The medicinal part is the dried bark.

Flower and Fruit: The flowers are in axillary richly blossomed racemes. The receptacles are green and the sepals are larger than the petals. Both are white. The ovary is longer than the style and is trilocular. The fruit is dark purple and top-shaped. The seeds are ovate, black, glossy, domed on the outside and have a distinct line on the inside.

Leaves, Stem and Root: The plant is a bush or a 6 to 18 m tall tree with branches, which are gray tomentose when young. The leaves are oblong-ovate, rounded at the base or sometimes narrowing at the petiole. On the longer shoots they are up to 17 cm long and 7.5 cm wide with an 8 to 18 mm long petiole. The margins are finely dentate and the young leaves are tomentose, later becoming dark-green but not coriaceous even in autumn.

Habitat: The plant is indigenous to the western part of North America and is cultivated on the Pacific coast of the U.S., Canada and in eastern Africa.

Production: Cascara sagrada bark consists of the dried bark of Rhamnus purshiana (syn. Frangula purshiana).

Not To Be Confused With: The bark of other Rhamnus species.

Other Names: Purshiana Bark, Sagrada Bark, Sacred Bark, Bitter Bark, Yellow Bark, Dogwood Bark, California Buckthorn, Chittem Bark

ACTIONS AND PHARMACOLOGY

COMPOUNDS

Anthracene derivatives (8-10%): chief components cascarosides A and B (stereoisomeric aloin-8-glucosides), C and D (stereoisomeric 11-deoxy-aloin-8-glucosides), E and F (C-glucosyl-emodin-anthron-8-glucosides), further including among others aloin, 11-deoxyaloin

EFFECTS

1,8-dihydroxy-anthracene derivatives have a laxative effect. This effect is primarily due to the influence of the herb on the motility of the colon, inhibiting stationary and stimulating propulsive contractions. This effect results in an accelerated intestinal passage and, because of the shortened contact time, a reduction in liquid absorption. In addition, stimulation of the active chloride secretion increases water and electrolyte content.

INDICATIONS AND USAGE

■ Constipation

Cascara Segrada is used for constipation, relief of defecation with anal fissures, hemorrhoids, as a recto-anal post-operative treatment and in preparation of diagnostic interventions of the gastrointestinal tract and to obtain a soft stool.

CONTRAINDICATIONS

The drug is contraindicated in intestinal obturation, acute inflammatory intestinal disease, appendicitis and abdominal pain of unknown origin.

PRECAUTIONS AND ADVERSE REACTIONS

General: Spasmodic gastrointestinal complaints can occur as a side effect to the drug's purgative effect. Long-term use leads to losses of electrolytes, in particular K(+)ions, and as a result of this to hyperaldosteronism, inhibition of intestinal motility and enhancement of the effect of cardioactive steroids; in rare cases also to heart arrhythmias, nephropathies, edemas and accelerated bone deterioration.

Intake of the fresh rind could lead to European cholera, intestinal colic, bloody diarrhea and kidney irritation. The question of the increase in probability of the appearance of carcinomas in the colon following long-term administration of anthracene drugs has not yet been fully clarified. Recent studies show no connections between the administration of anthracene drugs and the frequency of carcinomas in the colon.

Drug Interactions: With chronic use/abuse, loss in potassium may cause an increase in efficacy of cardiac glycosides. An effect on antiarrthythmics is possible. Potassium deficiency can be increased by simultaneous application of thiazide diuretics, corticoadrenal steroids, and liquorice root.

Pregnancy: Use during pregnancy or while nursing only after consulting a physician.

Pediatric Use: The drug is not to be administered to children under 12 years of age.

DOSAGE

Mode of Administration: Liquid or solid forms of medication are exclusively for oral use. The drug is used as comminuted drug, powder or dry extracts for infusions, decoction, and as a cold maceration or elixir.

Preparation: To prepare an infusion, add 2 gm finely cut drug to boiling water and strain after 10 minutes. (1 teaspoonful = 2.5 gm drug)

Daily Dosage: 20 to 30 mg hydroxyanthracene derivatives daily, calculated as cascaroside A.

The individually correct dosage is the smallest dosage necessary to maintain a soft stool.

Stimulating laxatives must not be used over an extended period of time (1-2 weeks) without medical advice.

LITERATURE

Anonym, Abwehr von Arzneimittelrisiken, Stufe II. In: DAZ 136(38):3253-2354. 1996.

Anonym, Anwendungseinschränkungen für Anthranoid-haltige Abführmittel angeordnet. In: PUZ 25(6):341-342. 1996.

BGA, Arzneimittelrisiken: Anthranoide. In: DAZ 132(21):1164. 1992.

Dewitte P, Cuveele J, Lemli J, Bicascarosides in fluid extracts of Cascara. In: PM 57:440. 1991.

Evans FJ et al., (1975) J Pharm Pharmacol 27:91P.

Fairbairn JW et al., (1977) J Pharm Sci 66:1300.

Fairbairn JW, Simic S, (1964) J Pharm Pharmacol 16:450.

Griffini A et al., Isolation and characterisation of pure Cascarosides A, B, C, and D. In: PM 58(Suppl.7):A593. 1992.

Helmholz H, Ruge A, Piasecki A, Schröder S, Westendorf J, Genotoxizität der Faulbaumrinde. In: PZ 138(43):3478. 1993.

Klimpel BE et al., Anthranoidhaltige Laxantien - ein Risiko für die Entwicklung von Tumoren der ableitenden Harnwege. In: PUZ 26(1):33, Jahrestagung der DPhG, Berlin, 1996. 1997.

Manitto P et al., Studies on cascara, part 2. Structure of cascarosides E and F. In: JNP 58(3):419-423. 1995.

Thesen R, Phytotherapeutika - nicht immer harmlos. In: ZPT 9(49):105. 1988.

Further information in:

Hänsel R, Keller K, Rimpler H, Schneider G (Hrsg.), Hagers Handbuch der Pharmazeutischen Praxis, 5. Aufl., Bde 4-6 (Drogen): Springer Verlag Berlin, Heidelberg, New York, 1992-1994.

Leung AY, Encyclopedia of Common Natural Ingredients Used in Food Drugs, Cosmetics, John Wiley & Sons Inc., New York 1980.

Lewin L, Gifte und Vergiftungen, 6. Aufl., Nachdruck, Haug Verlag, Heidelberg 1992.

Madaus G, Lehrbuch der Biologischen Arzneimittel, Bde 1-3, Nachdruck, Georg Olms Verlag Hildesheim 1979.

Roth L, Daunderer M, Kormann K, Giftpflanzen, Pflanzengifte, 4. Aufl., Ecomed Fachverlag Landsberg Lech 1993.

Steinegger E, Hänsel R, Pharmakognosie, 5. Aufl., Springer Verlag Heidelberg 1992.

Teuscher E, Lindequist U, Biogene Gifte - Biologie, Chemie, Pharmakologie, 2. Aufl., Fischer Verlag Stuttgart 1994.

Teuscher E, Biogene Arzneimittel, 5. Aufl., Wiss. Verlagsges. Stuttgart 1997.

Wichtl M (Hrsg.), Teedrogen, 4. Aufl., Wiss. Verlagsges. Stuttgart 1997.

Rhatany

See Krameria Triandra

Rheum Palmatum

Rhubarb

DESCRIPTION

Medicinal Parts: The medicinal parts are the dried underground parts and the underground parts freed from the stem remains, smaller roots and most of the root bark in the dried form. Garden Rhubarb is Rheum ponticum.

Flower and Fruit: The inflorescence is an erect panicle foliated to the tip. The flowers consist of narrow, red, pink or whitish yellow tepals, which are curved and located far back in the mature flowers to facilitate wind pollination. The fruit is red-brown to brown, and oval. The fruit is angular, about 10.2 mm to 7.8 mm wide and usually has scarious wings. The nutlet is 6 to 10 mm long and 7 mm in diameter.

Leaves, Stem and Root: The plant is a large, sturdy herbaceous perennial. The stem grows to over 1.5 m high. The leaves are orbicular-cordate, palmate lobed, somewhat rough on the upper surface or smooth and 3 to 5 ribbed. The lobes are oblong-ovate to lanceolate, dentate or pinnatisect. The root system consists of a tuber, which after a number of years measures 10 to 15 cm in diameter and has arm-thick lateral roots.

Habitat: The plant is indigenous to the western and northwestern provinces of China and is cultivated in many regions around the world. The main producers are China and Russia.

Production: Rhubarb consists of the dried underground parts of Rheum palmatum, Rheum officinale or of both species. Stem parts, roots and most of the bark are removed from the rhizomes.

Not To Be Confused With: Other Rheum species such as Rheum rhaponticum or Rheum rhabarbarum.

ACTIONS AND PHARMACOLOGY

COMPOUNDS

Anthracene derivatives (3-12%): chief components 1- or 8β-glucosides of the aglycones rheumemodin, aloe-emodin, rhein, chrysophanol, physcion (together 60-80%), 8,8′-diglucosides of dianthrones (10-25%), including, among others, sennosides A and B

Tannins: gallo tannins, including, among others, galloylglucose, galloylsaccharose, lindleyine, isolindleyine

Flavonoids (2-3%)

Naphthohydroquinone glycosides

EFFECTS

The main effect is laxative, primarily due to the influence of the herb on the motility of the colon, inhibiting stationary and stimulating propulsive contractions. This results in an accelerated intestinal passage and because of the active chloride secretion, increases water and electrolyte content of stool.

INDICATIONS AND USAGE

■ Constipation

Constipation, bowel movement relief with anal fissures, hemorrhoids, and after recto-anal surgery and in preparation for diagnostic interventions of the gastrointestinal tract.

CONTRAINDICATIONS

Rhubarb is contraindicated in cases of intestinal obturation, acute inflammatory intestinal disease, appendicitis and abdominal pain of unknown origin.

PRECAUTIONS AND ADVERSE REACTIONS

General: Spasmodic gastrointestinal complaints can occur as a side effect to the drug's purgative effect. Long-term use leads to losses of electrolytes, in particular K(+) ions, and as a result of this to hyperaldosteronism, inhibition of intestinal motility and enhancement of the effect of cardioactive steroids; in rare cases also to heart arrhythmias, nephropathies, edemas and accelerated bone deterioration.

The question of the increase in probability of the appearance of carcinomas in the colon following long-term administration of anthracene drugs has not yet been fully clarified. Recent studies show no connections between the administration of anthracene drugs and the frequency of carcinomas in the colon.

Drug Interactions: Potassium deficiency can cause an increase in the effect of cardiacglycosides.

Pregnancy: Use during pregnancy or while nursing only after consulting a physician.

Pediatric Use: The drug is not to be administered to children under 12 years of age.

DOSAGE

Mode of Administration: Liquid or solid forms of medication are exclusively for oral use. The drug is available as comminuted drug, powder or dry extracts for teas, decoctions, cold macerations or elixirs. Extracts of the drug are often constituents of laxatives, cholagogics and gastrointestinal remedies, and are found in ''slimming cures'', ''springtime tonics'' and ''blood purifying'' teas.

Preparation: To prepare an infusion to be used as a laxative, use 1.0-2.0 gm coarse powdered drug; for a stomachic, 0.1 to 0.2 gm powdered drug stirred with sufficient liquid (may be flavored with cinnamon, ginger, or peppermint oil) or scald and strain after 5 minutes. (1 teaspoonful = approximately 2.5 gm drug)

Daily Dosage: As a laxative, the dose is 1.0 to 2.0 gm of drug prepared according to instructions above. As an astringent and stomachic, the dose is 0.1-0.2 gm.

1.2 to 4.8 gm drug corresponds to 30 to 120 mg hydroxyanthracene derivatives/day, calculated as rhein. Stimulating laxatives must not be used over an extended period (1 to 2 weeks) without medical advice.

LITERATURE

Anonym, Abwehr von Arzneimittelrisiken, Stufe II. In: DAZ 136(38):3253-2354. 1996.

Anonym, Anwendungseinschränkungen für Anthranoid-haltige Abführmittel angeordnet. In: PUZ 25(6):341-342. 1996.

BGA, Arzneimittelrisiken: Anthranoide. In: DAZ 132(21):1164. 1992.

Fairbairn JW, (1976) Pharmacol 14(Suppl 1):48.

Foust B, In: Foust MC. Rhubarb: The Wondrous Drug. Princeton University Press, Princeton, NJ 1992.

Friedrich H, Höhle J, (1966) Arch Pharm 299:857.

Iida K et al., Potent inhibitors of tyrosinase activity and melanin biosynthesis from Rheum officinale. In: PM 61(5):425-428. 1995.

Kashiwada Y et al., (1984) Chem Pharm Bull 32(9):3461.

Klimpel BE et al., Anthranoidhaltige Laxantien - ein Risiko für die Entwicklung von Tumoren der ableitenden Harnwege. In: PUZ 26(1):33, Jahrestagung der DPhG, Berlin, 1996. 1997.

Nonaka G et al., (1977) Chem Pharm Bull 25:2300.

Oshio H et al., (1974) Chem Pharm Bull 22:823.

Sanches EF, Feritas TV, Ferreiraalves DL, Velarde DT, Diniz MR, Cordeiro MN, Agostinicotta G, Biological activities of venoms from south American snakes. In: Toxicon 30(1):95. 1992.

Tsuboi et al., (1977) Chem Pharm Bull 25:2708.

Van Os FHL, (1976) Pharmacol 14(Suppl 1):7.

Zwaving JH, (1972) Planta Med 21:254.

Zwaving JH, (1974) Pharm Weekbl 109:1169.

Further information in:

Chan EH et al., (Eds.), Advances in Chinese Medicinal Materials Research, World Scientific Pub. Co. Singapore 1985.

Hänsel R, Keller K, Rimpler H, Schneider G (Hrsg.), Hagers Handbuch der Pharmazeutischen Praxis, 5. Aufl., Bde 4-6 (Drogen): Springer Verlag Berlin, Heidelberg, New York, 1992-1994.

Leung AY, Encyclopedia of Common Natural Ingredients Used in Food Drugs, Cosmetics, John Wiley & Sons Inc., New York 1980.

Lewin L, Gifte und Vergiftungen, 6. Aufl., Nachdruck, Haug Verlag, Heidelberg 1992.

Madaus G, Lehrbuch der Biologischen Arzneimittel, Bde 1-3, Nachdruck, Georg Olms Verlag Hildesheim 1979.

Roth L, Daunderer M, Kormann K, Giftpflanzen, Pflanzengifte, 4. Aufl., Ecomed Fachverlag Landsberg Lech 1993.

Schulz R, Hänsel R, Rationale Phytotherapie, Springer Verlag Heidelberg 1996.

Steinegger E, Hänsel R, Pharmakognosie, 5. Aufl., Springer Verlag Heidelberg 1992.

Tang W, Eisenbrand G, Chinese Drugs of Plant Origin, Springer Verlag Heidelberg 1992.

Teuscher E, Lindequist U, Biogene Gifte - Biologie, Chemie, Pharmakologie, 2. Aufl., Fischer Verlag Stuttgart 1994.

Teuscher E, Biogene Arzneimittel, 5. Aufl., Wiss. Verlagsges. Stuttgart 1997.

Wichtl M (Hrsg.), Teedrogen, 4. Aufl., Wiss. Verlagsges. Stuttgart 1997.

Rhododendron Ferrugineum

Rust-Red Rhododendron

DESCRIPTION

Medicinal Parts: The medicinal parts are dried foliage leaves, the dried leafy branches, and the fresh leafy branches.

Flower and Fruit: The pink flowers are in umbel-like racemes. The calyx has 5 short ovate tips. The corolla is fused and funnel-shaped with an edge divided into 5 segments. It is covered on the outside with golden yellow resin spots. There are 10 stamens and 1 superior ovary. The fruit is a 5-valved capsule. The seeds are fusiform, about 1 mm long and light brown.

Leaves, Stem and Root: The plant is an evergreen shrub up to 1 m high and is richly branched from the base upwards. The branches are sturdy and elastic with gray-brown bark. The leaves are oblong-lanceolate, tough and glabrous. The margin is entire, involuted. The leaves are dark green above, densely scaled underneath and sometimes rust-colored.

Characteristics: The leaves are not ciliate at the edge.

Habitat: The plant grows in the alpine chain from the Pyrenees to the southern Croatian mountains but not in the Carpathians.

Production: Rust-Red Rhododendron consists of the dried leaves of Rhododendron ferrugineum.

Not To Be Confused With: The leaves of R. hirsutum. The plant product may be altered through the addition of cranberry leaves.

Other Names: Rosebay, Snow Rose

ACTIONS AND PHARMACOLOGY

COMPOUNDS: RHODODENDRON AUREUM

Diterpenes of the andromedan-type (presence questionable)

Hydroquinone glycosides: arbutin

Phenyl butane derivatives: rhododendrol and its bitter glucoside rhododendrine (betuloside)-flavonoids

COMPOUNDS: RHODODENDRON FERRUGINEUM

Diterpenes of the andromedan-type (presence questionable, but probable)

Phenyl butane derivatives: rhododendrol and its bitter glucoside rhododendrine (betuloside)-flavonoids

COMPOUNDS: RHODODENDRON PONTICUM

Diterpenes of the andromedan-type: grayanotoxin I (andromedotoxin, acetylandromedol, asebotoxin, rhodotoxin), grayanotoxin II (andromedol), grayanotoxin III (andromedenol).

Phenyl butane derivatives: rhododendrol and its bitter glucoside rhododendrine (betuloside)- flavonoids

EFFECTS

No information is available.

INDICATIONS AND USAGE

Rust-Red Rhododendron is used exclusively in combination preparations in the treatment of hypertonia and muscle and joint rheumatism. In folk medicine, it is used for calculosis, geriatric complaints, gout, high blood pressure, meteorosensitiveness, migraine, muscular pain, neuralgia and rheumatic complaints.

PRECAUTIONS AND ADVERSE REACTIONS

The rhododendron species mentioned are considered poisonous. The grayanotoxins prevent the closure of the sodium channels and thus paralyze conduction.

OVERDOSAGE

Signs of poisoning in case of overdosage could include: cardiac arrhythmias, coordination disorders, diarrhea, hypotension, cold sweats, paresthesia, salivation, severe stupor, spasm bradycardia, vomiting, and eventually death through cardiac failure or apnea. Unambiguous proof of toxicity are available only for the foliage, blossoms and sap of Rhododendron ponticum.

Following gastrointestinal emptying (inducement of vomiting, gastric lavage with burgundy-colored potassium permanganate solution, sodium sulphate), administration of activated charcoal and shock prophylaxis (quiet, warmth), therapy for poisonings consists of treating spasms with diazepam (i.v.), bradycardia with atropine, electrolyte substitution, and treating possible cases of acidosis with sodium bicarbonate infusions. In case of shock, plasma volume expanders should be infused. Opiates should not be given. Monitoring of kidney function is essential. Intubation and oxygen respiration may also be necessary.

DOSAGE

Daily Dosage: The daily dosage is 5 to 6 gm drug as an infusion.

LITERATURE

Bewuβtlos nach Verzehr eines Honigbrötchens. In: DAZ 132(27):1440. 1992.

Keller S auf dem et al., PA 25:621-625. 1970.

Further information in:

Frohne D, Pfänder HJ, Giftpflanzen - Ein Handbuch für Apotheker, Toxikologen und Biologen, 4. Aufl., Wiss. Verlags-Ges. Stuttgart 1997.

Hänsel R, Keller K, Rimpler H, Schneider G (Hrsg.), Hagers Handbuch der Pharmazeutischen Praxis, 5. Aufl., Bde 4-6 (Drogen): Springer Verlag Berlin, Heidelberg, New York, 1992-1994.

Lewin L, Gifte und Vergiftungen, 6. Aufl., Nachdruck, Haug Verlag, Heidelberg 1992.

Madaus G, Lehrbuch der Biologischen Arzneimittel, Bde 1-3, Nachdruck, Georg Olms Verlag Hildesheim 1979.

Roth L, Daunderer M, Kormann K: Giftpflanzen, Pflanzengifte, 4. Aufl., Ecomed Fachverlag Landsberg Lech 1993.

Schulz R, Hänsel R, Rationale Phytotherapie, Springer Verlag Heidelberg 1996.

Tang W, Eisenbrand G, Chinese Drugs of Plant Origin, Springer Verlag Heidelberg 1992.

Teuscher E, Lindequist U, Biogene Gifte - Biologie, Chemie, Pharmakologie, 2. Aufl., Fischer Verlag Stuttgart 1994.

Wagner H, Wiesenauer M, Phytotherapie. Phytopharmaka und pflanzliche Homöopathika, Fischer-Verlag, Stuttgart, Jena, New York 1995.

Wichtl M (Hrsg.), Teedrogen, 4. Aufl., Wiss. Verlagsges. Stuttgart 1997.

Rhubarb

See Rheum Palmatum

Rhus Aromatica

Sweet Sumach

DESCRIPTION

Medicinal Parts: The medicinal parts are the dried and fresh root bark.

Flower and Fruit: The flowers are in 1 to 1.5 cm long, false spikes. They are yellow-green and often appear before the leaves. The fruit is a globular, yellow-red, pubescent drupe.

Leaves, Stem and Root: The plant is a fragrant 1 to 2.4 m high shrub with glabrous red-brown annual growth and small to 10 cm long trifoliate leaves. The leaflets are oval. The middle leaflet is cuneate at the base. The leaflets are irregularly dentate, initially pubescent on both sides later glabrous on the upper surface and only pubescent on the ribs of the lower surface.

Habitat: The plant is indigenous to Atlantic North America.

Production: Sweet sumach root-bark is the root-bark of Rhus aromatica.

ACTIONS AND PHARMACOLOGY

COMPOUNDS

Tannins (8%)- phenolglycosides: orcinol-β-D-glucoside-volatile oil (0.01-0.07%); very complex in mixture, with, including among others delta-cadinene, camphene, Delta3-carene, beta-elemene, farnesyl acetone, alpha and beta-pinene, fatty acids

Triterpenes: including among others oleanolic aldehyde

Sterols: including among others beta-sitosterol

EFFECTS

Sweet Sumach has an effect on the smooth muscles, causing changes in muscle tone and increased frequency of contraction. The plant also has antimicrobial and antiviral effects.

INDICATIONS AND USAGE

Irritable bladder, urinary incontinence. Universal use in treating kidney and bladder ailments, hemorrhage of the womb.

Uses have not been proven through clinical studies or sufficient case documentary.

PRECAUTIONS AND ADVERSE REACTIONS

No health hazards or side effects are known in conjunction with the proper administration of designated therapeutic dosages.

DOSAGE

Mode of Administration: Fluid extract, in preparations for oral use.

Daily Dosage: The standard single dose is 1.0 gm. For bed-wetting, 5 to 20 drops depending on age, to be taken 2 to 3 times daily, over an extended period.

Storage: Store in a dry place and away from direct light.

LITERATURE

Baer H, In: Toxic Plants, Ed. AD Kinghorn, Columbia Press 1979.

Effenberger S, Schilcher H, Gewürzsumachrinde. In: ZPT 11(4):113. 1990.

Schilcher H, Boesel R, Effenberger ST Segebrecht S, Neuere Untersuchungsergebnisse mit aquaretisch, antibakteriell und prostatotrop wirksamen Arzneipflanzen. In: ZPT 10(3):77. 1989.

Further information in:

Hänsel R, Keller K, Rimpler H, Schneider G (Hrsg.), Hagers Handbuch der Pharmazeutischen Praxis, 5. Aufl., Bde 4-6 (Drogen): Springer Verlag Berlin, Heidelberg, New York, 1992-1994.

Madaus G, Lehrbuch der Biologischen Arzneimittel, Bde 1-3, Nachdruck, Georg Olms Verlag Hildesheim 1979.

Rhus Toxicodendron

Poison Ivy

DESCRIPTION

Medicinal Parts: The medicinal parts are the leaves collected after flowering and dried, the fresh young shoots, the young flowering branches and the fresh leaves.

Flower and Fruit: The pedicled flowers are in axillary, pubescent panicles. They are dioecious, sometimes androgynous. The stemmed petals are whitish-green with red hearts. The fruit is an almost globular, glabrous, yellow or yellowish-white, 10-grooved drupe. The fruit varies in size and contains a viscous latex in resin channels which turns black in the air.

Leaves, Stem and Root: The plant is a dioecious shrub up to 1 m high with ascending, procumbent or climbing rooting branches and underground runners. The branches are initially green and softly pubescent, later brown and glabrous. There are numerous lenticels on the two-year old shoots. The leaves are trifoliate with 8 to 14 cm long petioles. The leaflets are oblong, acute or obtuse, entire-margined or roughly serrate in the middle. They have a dark-green upper surface and slightly pubescent lower surface, which is a lighter green.

Habitat: The plant is indigenous to North America, it is also found in east Asia and is cultivated in Germany in botanical gardens and apothecary gardens.

Production: Poison Ivy leaves are the leaves of Rhus toxicodendron. Subsequent to the flowering period, the leaves of R. toxicodendron are gathered and then well-dried. Gloves should be worn to protect hands while gathering the leaves, as they can cause unpleasant inflammation of the skin.

Not To Be Confused With: Although it is sometimes called "Ampelopsis hoggii", Rhus toxicodendron actually has nothing in common with the Ampelopsis group of vines.

Other Names: Poison Oak, Poison Vine, Epright Sumach

ACTIONS AND PHARMACOLOGY

COMPOUNDS

Alkyl phenols: urushiol, chiefly cis,cis-3-(n-heptadeca-8′,11′-dienyl)catechol, cis,cis, cis-3-(n-heptadeca-8′,11′, 14′-trienyl)catechol, cis-3-(n-heptadec-8′-enyl)catechol

Tannins

Flavonoids

EFFECTS

"Rhus poison", even in very small amounts, causes severe irritation to the area of skin, where it has been applied. Following contact it can result in reddening, swelling and herpes simplex-like blisters. It also has a strong toxic effect if taken internally. Stimulates the immune system.

INDICATIONS AND USAGE

Formerly used as a narcotic. The drug is used most extensively in homeopathy, where it is used in cases of general low resistance to infections, especially rheumatism in the joints and muscles, overexertion (stress and strain), nosebleeds, also for diverse infectious diseases.

PRECAUTIONS AND ADVERSE REACTIONS

Contact with larger quantities of the allergen can bring about resorption and generalized erythema; in severe cases also fever and unconsciousness. Severe conjunctivitis and corneal inflammations, with possible loss of sight, may result after contact with the eyes. External application of the drug should be avoided. Skin affected by accidental contact should be intensively rinsed with a soapy solution and then cleaned with ether or ethanol. The points of inflammation should be covered with bicarbonate of soda paste (mixed with water). Internal treatment is carried out with systematically effective corticosteroids. Cooling bandages give relief in mild cases.

OVERDOSAGE

Overdoses of homeopathic preparations lead to severe mucous membrane irritation, accompanied by queasiness, vomiting, intestinal colic, diarrhea, as well as to signs of resorption; for example vertigo, stupor, kidney damage (nephritis, haematuria).

Following gastrointestinal emptying (gastric lavage with burgundy-colored potassium permanganate solution, sodium sulfate), installation of activated charcoal and shock prophylaxis (quiet, warmth), the therapy for these sorts of poisonings consists of treating spasms with diazepam (i.v.), electrolyte substitution and treating possible cases of acidosis with sodium bicarbonate infusions. In case of shock, plasma volume expanders should be infused. Monitoring of kidney function is essential. Intubation and oxygen respiration may also be necessary. Furthermore, the leaves possess a very severe potential for sensitization, due to their urushiol-content. Following sensitization (which can also occur through contact with objects d'art from the Far East, such as wooden chairs that had been treated with toxicodendron lacquers), renewed contact leads within a few hours to itching eczemas and eventual blister formation.

DOSAGE

Mode of Administration: Homeopathic dilutions of the mother tincture.

Daily Dosage: Largest single dose is 0.05 gm. The largest daily dose is 0.15 gm. The standard (medium) single dose is 0.03 gm.

Storage: In tightly sealed containers, not to be kept for more than a year.

LITERATURE

Gross M et al., PH 14:2263. 1975.

Millet S et al., PH 15:553. 1976.

Randall RC, Phillips GO, Williams PA, Food Hydrocolloids 3:65-75. 1989.

Shobha SV et al., Inhibition of soybean lipoxygenase-1 by anacardic acids, cardols, and cardanols. In: JNP 57(12):1755-1757. 1994.

Symes WF, Dawson CR, Nature 171:841. 1953.

Further information in:

Frohne D, Pfänder HJ, Giftpflanzen - Ein Handbuch für Apotheker, Toxikologen und Biologen, 4. Aufl., Wiss. Verlags-Ges. Stuttgart 1997.

Hausen B, Allergiepflanzen, Pflanzenallergene, ecomed Verlagsgesellsch. mbH, Landsberg 1988.

Lewin L, Gifte und Vergiftungen, 6. Aufl., Nachdruck, Haug Verlag, Heidelberg 1992.

Madaus G, Lehrbuch der Biologischen Arzneimittel, Bde 1-3, Nachdruck, Georg Olms Verlag Hildesheim 1979.

Roth L, Daunderer M, Kormann K: Giftpflanzen, Pflanzengifte, 4. Aufl., Ecomed Fachverlag Landsberg Lech 1993 (unter Toxicodendron).

Steinegger E, Hänsel R, Pharmakognosie, 5. Aufl., Springer Verlag Heidelberg 1992.

Teuscher E, Lindequist U, Biogene Gifte - Biologie, Chemie, Pharmakologie, 2. Aufl., Fischer Verlag Stuttgart 1994.

Wagner H, Wiesenauer M, Phytotherapie. Phytopharmaka und pflanzliche Homöopathika, Fischer-Verlag, Stuttgart, Jena, New York 1995.

Ribes Nigrum

Blackcurrant

DESCRIPTION

Medicinal Parts: The medicinal parts are the leaves collected and dried after the flowering season, the fresh ripe fruit with the tops and stems and the fresh leaves collected in summer.

Flower and Fruit: The flowers form richly blossomed racemes. Each is in the axil of a pubescent bract, which is shorter than the petiole. The bract is pinnate directly under the flower and has 2 small bracteoles. The sepals are, together with the 5 small stamens, on the campanulate flower axis. The single-valved ovary and the divided style is sunk within the axis. The hanging flowers are self-pollenating. The multi-seeded, black, glandular punctate berries develop from the ovary.

Leaves, Stem and Root: The plant is a sturdy perennial bush up to 2 m high. The branches are pale, hard and initially pubescent. The leaves are alternate, petiolate, becoming quickly glabrous on the upper surface and with numerous yellow resin glands on the undersurface. The 3 to 5-lobed leaf blade has a cordate base and doubly dentate margin.

Habitat: The plant is indigenous to Eurasian forest as far as the Himalayas, Canada and Australia and is cultivated in many regions. The main exporters are Holland, Poland, France, Hungary and former Yugoslavia.

Production: Blackcurrant leaves are the leaves of Ribes nigrum. The leaves are harvested during or shortly after flowering, air-dried in the shade or at maximum temperature of 60°C. Blackcurrant fruits are the ripe fruits of Ribes nigrum. The fruit is harvested when in bloom and used immediately or deep-frozen.

Other Names: Quinsy Berries, Squinancy Berries

ACTIONS AND PHARMACOLOGY

COMPOUNDS: RIBES NIGRI FOLIUM

Flavonoids (0.5%): including among others astragalin, isoquercitrin, rutin- oligomeric proanthocyanidins- ascorbic acid (Vitamin C, 0.1-0.27%)- volatile oil (traces)

EFFECTS: RIBES NIGRI FOLIUM

Diuretic, refrigerant, hypotensive, lowers blood pressure.

COMPOUNDS: RIBES NIGRI FRUCTUS

Fruit acids (3.5%): malic acid, citric acid, isocitric acid

Invert sugar

Pectins

Flavonoids: chief components isoquercitrin, myricetinglucoside, rutin- ascorbic acid (Vitamin C, 0.1-0.3%)- anthocyans (2%): chiefly cyanidine-3- and delphinidine-3-rutinoside or else -glucoside- coffeoyl-, p-cumaroyl-, feruloylquinnic acid and coffeoyl-, p-cumaroyl-, feruloylglucoses

In the seeds fatty oil (30%) with high gamma-linolic acid content

EFFECTS: RIBES NIGRI FRUCTUS

Bacteriostatic, anti-inflammatory, mild antispasmodic.

INDICATIONS AND USAGE

RIBES NIGRI FOLIUM

Internally, the leaves are used as a tea for arthritis, gout and rheumatism, inability to urinate, bladder stones, against diarrhea, colic, hepatitis, liver ailments, convulsions, whooping cough, inflammatory disorders, particularly of the mouth and throat. The leaves are generally considered beneficial for colds and coughs. They can be used as a cleansing infusion. The bark and even the young roots possess curative properties.

Externally, preparations from the leaf are used as a treatment of wounds and insect bites.

RIBES NIGRI FRUCTUS

Internally, the fruit is used as syrup or jelly to relieve colds, sore throat, cough and stomach ache. Dried berries are used to assuage bladder ailments. The berries are also used to treat diarrhea and as a source of Vitamin C.

CONTRAINDICATIONS

RIBES NIGRI FOLIUM

Blackcurrant leaves are contraindicated in edemas resulting from reduced cardiac and renal activity.

PRECAUTIONS AND ADVERSE REACTIONS

RIBES NIGRI FOLIUM AND FRUCTUS

No health hazards or side effects are known in conjunction with the proper administration of designated therapeutic dosages.

DOSAGE

RIBES NIGRI FOLIUM

Mode of Administration: The leaves are used internally as an infusion, externally as a compress.

Preparation: Add 1 to 2 teaspoonfuls (2 to 4 gm) of blackcurrant leaves to boiling water (150 ml), strain after 10 minutes.

Daily Dosage: Internally, 3 to 4 cups of tea to be drunk during the course of the day. Externally, freshly grated blackcurrant leaves or leaves soaked in warm water, dried and used as a compress. Freshly grated leaves can also be rubbed onto insect bites.

RIBES NIGRI FRUCTUS

Mode of Administration: Internally as a fruit juice and syrup. Externally as a gargle.

Daily Dosage: Internally, 5 to 10 ml of syrup may be taken several times daily, or eaten as a jelly. Externally, gargle with the juice and equal parts of warm water.

LITERATURE

RIBES NIGRI FOLIUM

Kyerematen G, Sandberg F, (1986) Acta Pharm Suecica 23:101.

Lietti A et al., (1976) Arzneim Forsch 26(5):829.

Senchute GV, Boruch IF, (1976) Rastit Resur 12(1):113.

Further information in:

Hänsel R, Keller K, Rimpler H, Schneider G (Hrsg.), Hagers Handbuch der Pharmazeutischen Praxis, 5. Aufl., Bde 4-6 (Drogen): Springer Verlag Berlin, Heidelberg, New York, 1992-1994.

Wichtl M (Hrsg.), Teedrogen, 4. Aufl., Wiss. Verlagsges. Stuttgart 1997.

RIBES NIGRI FRUCTUS

Kyerematen G, Sandberg F, (1986) Acta Pharm Suecica 23:101.

Lietti A et al., (1976) Arzneim Forsch 26(5):829.

Senchute GV, Boruch IF, (1976) Rastit Resur 12(1):113.

Further information in:

Hänsel R, Keller K, Rimpler H, Schneider G (Hrsg.), Hagers Handbuch der Pharmazeutischen Praxis, 5. Aufl., Bde 4-6 (Drogen): Springer Verlag Berlin, Heidelberg, New York, 1992-1994.

Rice

See Oryza Sativa

Ricinus Communis

Castor Oil Plant

DESCRIPTION

Medicinal Parts: The medicinal parts are the oil extracted from the seeds, the fat extracted from the oil, the ripe seeds and the dried seeds.

Flower and Fruit: The inflorescence is terminal and almost panicled and 15 to 50 cm long. The pedicled female flowers are in the upper section and the male flowers are clustered in the lower section of the inflorescence. The male ones have a 3 to 5 part perianth with numerous, heavily branched stamens which bear up to 1,000 separate bursting anthers. The female perianth is divided in 5. The ovary is trilocular. The style has 3 red, doubly split stigma branches. The fruit is a soft, prickly or smooth, grooved capsule, 1 to 2.5 cm in diameter. The capsule bursts open when ripe flinging out the large brightly speckled seeds, which resemble pinto beans.

Leaves, Stem and Root: The plant is an annual plant in central Europe, a bi- or tri-ennial shrub in southern Europe and a perennial tree in the tropics. There is a taproot and lateral roots near the surface. The stem has alternate, palmate, reddish, simple, long-petioled leaves arranged in a spiral. The leaf blade is peltate, 10 to 60 cm long and wide, and usually divided into palmate ovate-oblong or lanceolate lobes. The ribs are palmate and the margins are irregularly serrate.

Habitat: The plant is cultivated widely today in the tropics and subtropics and in temperate latitudes where maize thrives.

Production: Castor oil is a fatty oil from the seeds of Ricinus communis. Mechanical harvesting is necessary, as the cultures are miniatures, and their capsules fail to burst open. Varieties with bursting split fruits must be cut before flowering and then threshed, these seeds yield less oil.

Not To Be Confused With: The product is often adulterated with stones, and blackened, peeled, unripe seeds. Confusion with the poisonous seeds of other Euphorbiacean is possible.

Other Names: Castor Bean, Mexico Seed, Oil Plant, Palma Christi

ACTIONS AND PHARMACOLOGY

COMPOUNDS

Fatty oil (42-55%, see below)

Proteins (20-25%)

Lectins (0.1-0.7%): including among others ricin D (RCA-60. severely toxic), RCA-120 (less toxic)

Pyridine alkaloids

Triglycerides: chief fatty acids ricinoleic acid (12-hydroxy-oleic acid, share 85-90%)

Tocopherols (Vitamin E)

EFFECTS

The oil has a purgative action. Castor oil acids are anti-absorbative and hydragogic.

The anti-viral effect of Ricini semen has been proven in experiments.

INDICATIONS AND USAGE

Internally, the drug is used as a purgative in the treatment of acute constipation, intestinal inflammation, worms and as a form of birth control. Externally, the seeds and leaves are used in powder form as a poultice for inflammatory skin disorders, boils, carbuncles, abscesses, inflammation of the middle ear and migraine.

CONTRAINDICATIONS

Castor oil is contraindicated in intestinal obturation, acute inflammatory intestinal diseases, appendicitis, abdominal pain of unknown origin, pregnancy and while nursing.

PRECAUTIONS AND ADVERSE REACTIONS

General: No health hazards or side effects are known in conjunction with the proper administration of designated therapeutic dosages of castor oil. Castor beans are severely poisonous, due to their toxic lectins content. The ricinus lectins destroy the ribosomes and thereby prevent protein synthesis. Allergy-related skin rashes have been observed in rare cases.

Drug Interactions: Long-term use leads to losses of electrolytes, in particular K+-ions, and as a result of this to hyperaldosteronism, inhibition of intestinal motility and enhancement of the effect of cardioactive steroids.

Pediatric Use: The drug is not to be administered to children under 12 years of age.

OVERDOSAGE

Overdoses can lead to gastric irritation, accompanied by queasiness, vomiting, colic and severe diarrhea. Twelve castor beans are believed to be fatal for an adult. Symptoms include severe gastroenteritis, with bloody vomiting and bloody diarrhea, kidney inflammation, loss of fluid and electrolytes and ultimately circulatory collapse. Death is usually the result of hypovolemic shock.

Following gastrointestinal emptying, (inducement of vomiting, gastric lavage with burgundy-colored potassium permanganate solution, sodium sulfate), instillation of activated charcoal and shock prophylaxis (quiet, warmth), the therapy for castor bean poisonings consists of treating spasms with diazepam (i.v.), generous supplies of fluids, electrolyte substitution and treating possible cases of acidosis with sodium bicarbonate infusions. In case of shock, plasma volume expanders should be infused. Monitoring of kidney function and blood coagulation are essential. Papain activated with H2 S is attempted as an antidote (hydrolysis of the lectins not yet resorbed).

DOSAGE

Mode of Administration: The oil is used internally and externally; in galenic preparations, as well as in combination preparations.

Daily Dosage: Internally, for acute constipation or as a purgative against worms at least 5 (2.0 gm) or 10 (1.0 gm) capsules must be taken. Externally, a paste made of ground seeds is applied to the affected skin areas twice daily. A course of treatment takes up to 15 days.

LITERATURE

Anonym, Pharmaceutical Care: "Den Miβbrauch von Laxanzien vermeiden helfen". In: DAZ 135(20):1867-1868. 1995.

BGA, Abwehr von Arzneimittelrisiken:Poly-(oxyethylen)-35-Rizinusöl. In: DAZ 132(33):1733. 1992.

Macfarlane N, Trop Sc 17:217-228. 1975.

Scarpa A, Guerci A, Various uses of the castor oil plant (Ricinus communis L.), a review. In: ETH 5(2):117. 1982.

Further information in:

Frohne D, Pfänder HJ: Giftpflanzen - Ein Handbuch für Apotheker, Toxikologen und Biologen, 4. Aufl., Wiss. Verlags-Ges. Stuttgart 1997.

Hänsel R, Keller K, Rimpler H, Schneider G (Hrsg.), Hagers Handbuch der Pharmazeutischen Praxis, 5. Aufl., Bde 4-6 (Drogen): Springer Verlag Berlin, Heidelberg, New York, 1992-1994.

Leung AY, Encyclopedia of Common Natural Ingredients Used in Food Drugs, Cosmetics, John Wiley & Sons Inc., New York 1980.

Lewin L, Gifte und Vergiftungen, 6. Aufl., Nachdruck, Haug Verlag, Heidelberg 1992.

Madaus G, Lehrbuch der Biologischen Arzneimittel, Bde 1-3, Nachdruck, Georg Olms Verlag Hildesheim 1979.

Roth L, Daunderer M, Kormann K: Giftpflanzen, Pflanzengifte, 4. Aufl., Ecomed Fachverlag Landsberg Lech 1993.

Schulz R, Hänsel R, Rationale Phytotherapie, Springer Verlag Heidelberg 1996.

Steinegger E, Hänsel R, Pharmakognosie, 5. Aufl., Springer Verlag Heidelberg 1992.

Teuscher E, Lindequist U, Biogene Gifte - Biologie, Chemie, Pharmakologie, 2. Aufl., Fischer Verlag Stuttgart 1994.

Teuscher E, Biogene Arzneimittel, 5. Aufl., Wiss. Verlagsges. Stuttgart 1997.

Wagner H, Wiesenauer M, Phytotherapie. Phytopharmaka und pflanzliche Homöopathika, Fischer-Verlag, Stuttgart, Jena, New York 1995.

Roman Chamomile

See Chamaemelum Nobile

Rosa Canina

Rose Hip

DESCRIPTION

Medicinal Parts: The medicinal parts are the petals, the rose hips with and without seeds, and the seeds.

Flower and Fruit: The large, long pedicled, white or pale pink flowers are usually solitary or in clusters of 2 or 3. The receptacle deepens to form a cup on whose upper edge, the 5 pinnatifid sepals and petals as well as numerous stamens sit. It closes with a yellow fleshy ring. There are long white silky hairs in the receptacle between which are numerous ovaries whose styles show through the opening. The ovaries grow into stiff-haired nuts surrounded by the receptacle and become the scarlet "rosehip".

Leaves, Stem and Root: The plant is an approximately 1 to 3 m high climbing and trailing prickly shrub with erect root shoots covered in sickle-shaped prickles (not thorns). The leaves are pinnatifid with 5 to 7 leaflets, which are petiolate, elliptical to ovate, serrate, glabrous, glossy and dark green above, lighter beneath.

Characteristics: The sepals turn back at the end of the flowering period and drop when the fruit ripens.

Habitat: Rosa canina grows in Europe and northern Africa and is extensively cultivated.

Production: Rose Hip consists of the ripe, fresh or dried seed receptacle of various species of the genus Rosa separated from seeds and attached trichomes. Rose Hip seeds are the ripe, dried seed of various species of the genus Rosa. The drug is a component of various diuretics.

Other Names: Brier Hip, Hip, Dog Rose, Brier Rose, Eglantine Gall, Hogseed, Dog-berry, Sweet Brier, Witches' Brier, Hep Tree, Hip Fruit, Hop Fruit

ACTIONS AND PHARMACOLOGY

COMPOUNDS: ROSAE PSEUDOFRUCTUS

Vitamins, in particular ascorbic acid (Vitamin C, 0.2-2.0%)

Fruit acids (3%): malic acid, citric acid

Pectins (15%)

Sugars (12-15%): invert sugar, saccharose

Tannins (2%)

Carotinoids

Flavonoids

EFFECTS: ROSAE PSEUDOFRUCTUS

No information is available.

COMPOUNDS: ROSAE FRUCTUS

Fatty oil (8-10%)

Tocopherol (Vitamin E 0.6%)

Volatile oil (0.3)

Proteins (10%)

EFFECTS: ROSAE FRUCTUS

Main active agents: fatty oil, essential oil, traces of Vitamin C. The pectin and fruit acid content are responsible for the diuretic and laxative effect.

INDICATIONS AND USAGE

ROSAE PSEUDOFRUCTUS

Preparations of Rose Hips are used for the prevention and treatment of colds, chills, etc., and influenza-type infections, infectious diseases, for the prevention and treatment of Vitamin C deficiencies, to increase resistance.

ROSAE FRUCTUS

Preparations of Rose Hip seed are used for diseases and ailments of the kidney and lower urinary tract, for dropsy, as a diuretic, for arthritic conditions, rheumatism, gout, sciatica.

PRECAUTIONS AND ADVERSE REACTIONS

ROSAE PSEUDOFRUCTUS AND ROSAE FRUCTUS

No health hazards or side effects are known in conjunction with the proper administration of designated therapeutic dosages.

DOSAGE

ROSAE FRUCTUS

Preparation: To prepare an infusion, scald 1 to 2 gm powdered drug, steep 10 to 15 minutes and strain.

Daily Dosage: The infusion may be taken repeatedly throughout the day as a diurectic. (1 teaspoonful = 3.5 gm drug)

LITERATURE

ROSAE PSEUDOFRUCTUS

Czygan FC, Rosa canina L. - Die Hunds- oder Heckenrose. In: ZPT 10(5):162. 1989.

Jaretzky R, Pharm Zentralh 82:229. 1941.

Kurucu S, Coskun M, Kartal M, High pressure liquid chromatographic determination of ascorbic acid in the fruits of some Rosa species growing in Turkey. In: PM 58(7):A675. 1992.

Luckner M, Beβler O, PA 21:197. 1966.

Further information in:

Kern W, List PH, Hörhammer L (Hrsg.), Hagers Handbuch der Pharmazeutischen Praxis, 4. Aufl., Bde. 1-8: Springer Verlag Berlin, Heidelberg, New York, 1969.

Leung AY, Encyclopedia of Common Natural Ingredients Used in Food Drugs, Cosmetics, John Wiley & Sons Inc., New York 1980.

Madaus G, Lehrbuch der Biologischen Arzneimittel, Bde 1-3, Nachdruck, Georg Olms Verlag Hildesheim 1979.

Steinegger E, Hänsel R, Pharmakognosie, 5. Aufl., Springer Verlag Heidelberg 1992.

Teuscher E, Biogene Arzneimittel, 5. Aufl., Wiss. Verlagsges. Stuttgart 1997.

Wagner H, Wiesenauer M, Phytotherapie. Phytopharmaka und pflanzliche Homöopathika, Fischer-Verlag, Stuttgart, Jena, New York 1995.

Wichtl M (Hrsg.), Teedrogen, 4. Aufl., Wiss. Verlagsges. Stuttgart 1997.

ROSAE FRUCTUS

Czygan FC, Rosa canina L. - Die Hunds- oder Heckenrose. In: ZPT 10(5):162. 1989.

Jaretzky R, Pharm Zentralh 82:229. 1941.

Luckner M, Beβler O, PA 21:197. 1966.

Further information in:

Kern W, List PH, Hörhammer L (Hrsg.), Hagers Handbuch der Pharmazeutischen Praxis, 4. Aufl., Bde. 1-8: Springer Verlag Berlin, Heidelberg, New York, 1969.

Leung AY, Encyclopedia of Common Natural Ingredients Used in Food Drugs, Cosmetics, John Wiley & Sons Inc., New York 1980.

Rosa Centifolia

Rose

DESCRIPTION

Medicinal Parts: The medicinal parts are the petals and the oil extracted from them.

Flower and Fruit: The flowers are usually solitary on 2 to 3 cm long pedicles. The calyx is round to pear-shaped with stem glands and gland bristles. The velvety petals are pink to purple, 2 to 3 cm long and wide. The style and stigma form the ovary, which is surrounded by carpels enclosed in the calyx. The rust-brown false fruit is 1 to 1.5 cm long.

Leaves, Stem and Root: The plant, a descendant of R. gallica is a low shrub with extensive runners and above ground reed-like shoots which are erect and branched. They usually grow to between 0.5 to 1 m and are covered with different length thorns and stem glands. The tri-to-penfoliate leaves are glandular and have dark-green stipules at the base.

Habitat: The rose is probably indigenous to Iran and is cultivated worldwide.

Production: Rose flowers consist of the dried petals of Rosa gallica, Rosa centifolia and variations, gathered prior to fully unfolding.

Other Names: Cabbage Rose, Hundred-leaved Rose

ACTIONS AND PHARMACOLOGY

COMPOUNDS

Volatile oil (0.2% in the fresh blossoms): chief components (-)-citronellol (35-55%), geraniol (share 30-40%), nerol (5-10%), phenylethanol (1-15%), further including, among others, (-)-linalool, citral

Tannins (15%): oligomeric proanthocyanidins

EFFECTS

Astringent.

INDICATIONS AND USAGE

■ Inflammation of the mouth and pharynx

Rose is used for mild inflammations of the oral and pharyngeal mucosa.

PRECAUTIONS AND ADVERSE REACTIONS

No health hazards or side effects are known in conjunction with the proper administration of designated therapeutic dosages.

DOSAGE

Mode of Administration: Comminuted herb for teas and other galenic preparations for mouth rinses.

Daily Dosage: 1 to 2 gm of drug per 200 ml of water.

LITERATURE

Kern W, List PH, Hörhammer L (Hrsg.), Hagers Handbuch der Pharmazeutischen Praxis, 4. Aufl., Bde. 1-8: Springer Verlag Berlin, Heidelberg, New York, 1969.

Leung AY, Encyclopedia of Common Natural Ingredients Used in Food Drugs, Cosmetics, John Wiley & Sons Inc., New York 1980.

Madaus G, Lehrbuch der Biologischen Arzneimittel, Bde 1-3, Nachdruck, Georg Olms Verlag Hildesheim 1979.

Rose

See Rosa Centifolia

Rose Hip

See Rosa Canina

Rosemary

See Rosmarinus Officinalis

Rosinweed

See Silphium Laciniatum

Rosmarinus Officinalis

Rosemary

DESCRIPTION

Medicinal Parts: The medicinal parts are the leaves.

Flower and Fruit: Bluish labiate flowers grow on tometose inflorescence in the leaf axils of the upper green part of the branches. The calyx is 3 to 4 mm, green or reddish, initially slightly tomentose, later 5 to 7 mm and glabrous. The venation is conspicuous. The corolla is 10 to 12 mm long, bluish, occasionally pink or white. The nutlet is brown.

Leaves, Stem and Root: The plant is an aromatic, evergreen, branched subshrub, 0.5 to 1.50 m high with erect or occasionally decumbent brown branches somewhat pubescent when young, becoming woody. The leaves are simple, linear, opposite, tomentose beneath, 15 to 40 mm by 1.2 to 3.5 mm.

Characteristics: The plant has a very pungent aroma.

Habitat: The plant is indigenous to the Mediterranean region and Portugal and is cultivated there as well as on the Crimea, in the Transcaucasus, central Asia, India, southeast Asia, South Africa, Australia and the U.S. Most of the supply comes from Morocco, Spain, Tunisia and France.

Production: Rosemary leaves consist of the fresh or dried leaves of Rosmarinus officinalis collected during flowering.

Other Names: Polar Plant, Compass-weed, Compass Plant

ACTIONS AND PHARMACOLOGY

COMPOUNDS

Volatile oil (1.0-2.5%): chief components 1,8-cineole (20-50%), alpha-pinene (15-25%), camphor (10-25%), further including among others camphene, borneol, isobutyl acetate, beta-caryophyllene, p-cymene, limonene, linalool, myrcene, alpha-terpineol, verbenol

Diterpenes (bitter): including, among others, carnosolic acid (picrosalvin), isorosmanol, rosmadial, rosmaridiphenol, rosmariquinone

Caffeic acid derivatives: chief components rosmarinic acid

Flavonoids: including, among others, cirsimarin, diosmin, hesperidin, homoplantiginin, phegopolin

Triterpenes: chief components are oleanolic acid (10%), ursolic acid (5%)

EFFECTS

The main active agent is the essential oil. Animal tests have demonstrated spasmolytic effects on the gallbladder ducts and on the upper intestine as well as a positive inotropic effect and an increase in coronary blood flow. Oil of rosemary improves circulation when applied externally, due to a certain skin irritant.

INDICATIONS AND USAGE

- Loss of appetite
- Blood pressure problems
- Liver and gallbladder complaints
- Rheumatism

Internally: Dyspeptic disorders. The drug is a component of gastrointestinal remedies (stomachic, carminatives).

Externally: Balneotherapy, hypotonic circulatory disorders, rheumatic conditions (adjuvant). In folk medicine, the plant is used as a poultice for poorly healing wounds, for eczema.

PRECAUTIONS AND ADVERSE REACTIONS

General: No health hazards or side effects are known in conjunction with the proper administration of designated therapeutic dosages. Contact allergies have been observed on occasion.

Pregnancy: One is advised against using the drug during pregnancy.

OVERDOSAGE

Very large quantities of rosemary leaves (more likely, only of rosemary oil), have been misused for the purpose of abortion, and are said to lead to deep coma, spasm, vomiting, gastroenteritis, uterine bleeding, kidney irritation, and in severe cases, accompanied by pulmonary edema, to death in humans. No documented cases have come to light.

DOSAGE

Mode of Administration: Ground drug is used for infusions. Powdered drug, dry extract and other galenic preparations are available for internal and external use. The drug is used in combination therapy with other remedies in the treatment of dyspeptic or rheumatic disorders.

Preparation: To prepare a bath additive, add 50 gm drug to 1 liter of hot water, and add to bath water. To prepare Rosemary wine, add 20 gm drug to 1 liter of wine, let stand for 5 days, shake occasionally.

Daily Dosage: Internally, the daily dose is 4 to 6 gm drug. A 1:5 tincture is available. Externally, semisolid and liquid forms with 6 to 10% essential oil are used.

LITERATURE

Anonym, Phytotherapie:Pflanzliche Antirheumatika - was bringen sie? In: DAZ 136(45):4012-4015. 1996.

Boehlens MH, Perfum Flav 10:21-24, 26 et 28-37. 1985.

Brieskorn CH, Zweyrohn G, (1970) Pharmazie 25:488.

Brieskorn CH, Domling HJ, (1969) Z Lebensm Unters Forsch 14:10.

Brieskorn CH, Michel H, (1968) Tetrahedron Letters 30:3447.

Czygan I, Czygan FC, Rosmarin - Rosmarinus officinalis L. In: ZPZ 18(3):182-186. 1997.

Haraguchi H et al., Inhibition of lipid peroxidation and superoxide generation by diterpenoids from Rosmarinus officinalis. In: PM 61(4):333-336. 1995.

Houlihan CM et al., (1985) J Am Oil Chem Soc 62(1):96.

Koedan A, Gijbels MJM, (1978) Z Natur Forsch 33C, 144.

Kreis P, Juchelka D, Motz C, Mosandl A, Chirale Inhaltstoffe ätherischer Öle. In: DAZ 131(39):1984. 1991.

Litvinenko VI et al., (1970) Planta Med 18:243.

Mascolo N et al., (1987) Phytother Res 1(1):28.

Tattje DHE, (1970) Pharm Weekbl 105:1241.

Further information in:

Fenaroli's Handbook of Flavor Ingredients, Vol. 1, 2nd Ed., CRC Press 1975.

Hänsel R, Keller K, Rimpler H, Schneider G (Hrsg.), Hagers Handbuch der Pharmazeutischen Praxis, 5. Aufl., Bde 4-6 (Drogen): Springer Verlag Berlin, Heidelberg, New York, 1992-1994.

Leung AY, Encyclopedia of Common Natural Ingredients Used in Food Drugs, Cosmetics, John Wiley & Sons Inc., New York 1980.

Madaus G, Lehrbuch der Biologischen Arzneimittel, Bde 1-3, Nachdruck, Georg Olms Verlag Hildesheim 1979.

Roth L, Daunderer M, Kormann K, Giftpflanzen, Pflanzengifte, 4. Aufl., Ecomed Fachverlag Landsberg Lech 1993.

Steinegger E, Hänsel R, Pharmakognosie, 5. Aufl., Springer Verlag Heidelberg 1992.

Teuscher E, Biogene Arzneimittel, 5. Aufl., Wiss. Verlagsges. Stuttgart 1997.

Wagner H, Wiesenauer M, Phytotherapie. Phytopharmaka und pflanzliche Homöopathika, Fischer-Verlag, Stuttgart, Jena, New York 1995.

Wichtl M (Hrsg.), Teedrogen, 4. Aufl., Wiss. Verlagsges. Stuttgart 1997.

Rubia Tinctorum

Madder

DESCRIPTION

Medicinal Parts: The medicinal part is the dried root.

Flower and Fruit: The small yellowish-green flowers are in long-peduncled, terminal or axillary cymes. The margin of the calyx is indistinct, 4 to 5 sectioned and has a tip which is curved inwards. There are 5 stamens and an inferior ovary. The fruit is a black, pea-sized, glabrous, smooth drupe containing 2 seeds.

Leaves, Stem and Root: The perennial plant grows from 60 to 100 cm high. The pencil-thick rhizome creeps widely underground. The stem is quadrangular with backward turning prickles at the edges. The stems are at time so thin that they are more descendent than erect. The leaves are in whorls, in fours below, in sixes above. They are oblong to lanceolate with 1 rib and are protrudingly reticulate beneath.

Habitat: The plant is indigenous to southern Europe, western Asia and northern Africa and is cultivated elsewhere.

Production: Madder root consists of the dried root of Rubia tinctorum.

Other Names: Dyer's Madder, Robbia

ACTIONS AND PHARMACOLOGY

COMPOUNDS

Anthracene derivatives (2-4%): rubiadine: chief components alizarin, lucidin, pseudopurpurin (purpurin carboxylic acid), purpurin, rubiadin and the glucosides or the primeroside of these compounds

EFFECTS

Decreased calcium oxalate crystallization in the kidney.

INDICATIONS AND USAGE

Madder is used for disintegration of kidney stones. It was used medicinally in menstrual and urinary disorders.

PRECAUTIONS AND ADVERSE REACTIONS

Madder root contains lucidin. Lucidin is positive in various bacterial strains using the Ames test. The substance induces concentration-dependent gene mutations and DNA strand cleavage. Therefore, there exists a strong indication that lucidin is mutagenic and carcinogenic.

DOSAGE

No information is available.

LITERATURE

Anonym, Rubiae-tinctorum-radix-haltige Humanarzneimittel, Widerruf der Zulassung. In: DAZ 133(11):888. 1993.

BGA, Arzneimittelrisiken: Anthranoide. In: DAZ 132(21):1164. 1992.

Courchesne M, Brassard P, Identification and characterization of naturally occuring rubiadins. In: JNP 56(5):722. 1993.

Nung V N et al., (1971) Plant Med Phytother 5:177.

Schümann C, Apotheker und die Entwicklung der Färberei. In: PZ 140(39):3446-3451. 1995.

Westendorf J, Phytotherapie: Anthranoide in Arzneipflanzen. In: DAZ 133(25):2345. 1993.

Westendorf J, Poginskky B, Marquardt H, Marquardt H, The genotoxicity of Lucidin, a natural component of Rubia tinctorum L., and lucidinmethylether, a component of ethanolic Rubia extracts. In: Cell Biol Toxicol in press. 19.

Further information in:

Frohne D, Pfänder HJ, Giftpflanzen - Ein Handbuch für Apotheker, Toxikologen und Biologen, 4. Aufl., Wiss. Verlags-Ges. Stuttgart 1997.

Kern W, List PH, Hörhammer L (Hrsg.), Hagers Handbuch der Pharmazeutischen Praxis, 4. Aufl., Bde 1-8: Springer Verlag Berlin, Heidelberg, New York, 1969.

Madaus G, Lehrbuch der Biologischen Arzneimittel, Bde 1-3, Nachdruck, Georg Olms Verlag Hildesheim 1979.

Thomson RH, Naturally Occuring Quinones, 2nd Ed., Academic Press New York 1971.

Teuscher E, Lindequist U, Biogene Gifte - Biologie, Chemie, Pharmakologie, 2. Aufl., Fischer Verlag Stuttgart 1994.

Teuscher E, Biogene Arzneimittel, 5. Aufl., Wiss. Verlagsges. Stuttgart 1997.

Wagner H, Wiesenauer M, Phytotherapie. Phytopharmaka und pflanzliche Homöopathika, Fischer-Verlag, Stuttgart, Jena, New York 1995.

Rubus Fruticosus

Blackberry

DESCRIPTION

Medicinal Parts: The medicinal parts are the leaves, roots and berries. American Blackberry (or Dewberry) is R. villosus.

Flower and Fruit: The white or sometimes pale pink flowers are in cymes. The calyx has 5 sepals, the corolla, 5 petals. There are numerous stamens and ovaries. The whole of the small fruit forms a black aggregate fruit, the blackberry.

Leaves and Stem: The plant is a fast-growing, thorny bush up to 2 m high. The generally blunt stems are densely covered in tough thorns, creeping or curved backwards. The leaves are usually 5-paired pinnate, glabrous above, tomentose beneath.

Habitat: The plant is indigenous to Europe and has been naturalized in America and Australia.

Production: Blackberry leaf consists of the dried, fermented or unfermented leaf, gathered during the flowering period, of Rubus fruticosus. Blackberry root consists of the underground parts of Rubus fruticosus.

Other Names: Bramble, Dewberry, Goutberry, Thimbleberry

ACTIONS AND PHARMACOLOGY

COMPOUNDS: RUBI FRUTICOSI FOLIUM

Tannins (8-14%): gallo tannins, dimeric ellagic tannins

Fruit acids: including, among others, citric acid, isocitric acid

Flavonoids

EFFECTS: RUBI FRUTICOSI FOLIUM

Has astringent and antidiarrheal effect due to high tannin content.

COMPOUNDS: RUBI FRUTICOSI RADIX

Tannins

EFFECTS: RUBI FRUTICOSI RADIX

No information is available.

INDICATIONS AND USAGE

RUBI FRUTICOSI FOLIUM

- Nonspecific, acute diarrhea
- Mild inflammation of the mucosa of the oral cavity and throat

RUBI FRUTICOSI RADIX

Blackberry root is used as a preventative for dropsy. The claimed efficacy has not been documented.

PRECAUTIONS AND ADVERSE REACTIONS

RUBI FRUTICOSI FOLIUM AND RADIX

No health hazards or side effects are known in conjunction with the proper administration of designated therapeutic dosages.

DOSAGE

RUBI FRUTICOSI FOLIUM

Mode of Administration: Comminuted drug for infusions and other preparations for internal use, as well as for mouthwashes. The drug is a component of various tea mixtures.

Preparation: To prepare an infusion, scald 1.5 gm drug, steep for 10 to 15 minutes, then strain (1 teaspoonful is equivalent to 0.6 gm drug).

Daily Dosage: 2 to 5 gm drug.

LITERATURE

RUBI FRUTICOSI FOLIUM

Henning W, (1981) Lebensm Unters Forsch 173:180.

Gupta RK et al., J Chem Soc Perkin I:2525. 1982.

Mukherjee M et al., PH 23:2881. 1984.

Wollmann Ch et al., PA 19:456. 1964.

Further information in:

Kern W, List PH, Hörhammer L (Hrsg.), Hagers Handbuch der Pharmazeutischen Praxis, 4. Aufl., Bde. 1-8: Springer Verlag Berlin, Heidelberg, New York, 1969.

Leung AY, Encyclopedia of Common Natural Ingredients Used in Food Drugs, Cosmetics, John Wiley & Sons Inc., New York 1980.

Madaus G, Lehrbuch der Biologischen Arzneimittel, Bde 1-3, Nachdruck, Georg Olms Verlag Hildesheim 1979.

Wichtl M (Hrsg.), Teedrogen, 4. Aufl., Wiss. Verlagsges. Stuttgart 1997.

RUBI FRUTICOSI RADIX

Henning W, (1981) Lebensm Unters Forsch 173:180.

Further information in:

Kern W, List PH, Hörhammer L (Hrsg.), Hagers Handbuch der Pharmazeutischen Praxis, 4. Aufl., Bde. 1-8: Springer Verlag Berlin, Heidelberg, New York, 1969.

Leung AY, Encyclopedia of Common Natural Ingredients Used in Food Drugs, Cosmetics, John Wiley & Sons Inc., New York 1980.

Rubus Idaeus

Raspberry

DESCRIPTION

Medicinal Parts: The medicinal parts are the leaves and fruit.

Flower and Fruit: The white flowers are in cymes. The calyx has 5 sepals and the corolla is 5-petalled. There are numerous stamens and ovaries. Similar to the blackberry, the whole of the small fruit forms a red aggregate fruit, the raspberry.

Leaves, Stem and Root: The plant is an approximately 2 m high deciduous bush with erect, woody stems, which are densely covered in tough thorns. The aerial part is usually biennial while the creeping root is perennial. The leaves are pale green. There are 3 leaves atop 7 leaflets.

Habitat: The plant is indigenous to Europe and Asia and is cultivated in temperate climates.

Production: Raspberry leaf consists of the leaf of Rubus idaeus.

Not To Be Confused With: Blackberry leaves.

Other Names: Red Raspberry

ACTIONS AND PHARMACOLOGY

COMPOUNDS

Tannins: gallo tannins, ellagic tannins

Flavonoids

EFFECTS

The main active agents are tannin, flavonoids, and Vitamin C.

INDICATIONS AND USAGE

Raspberry leaf is used for disorders of the gastrointestinal tract, the respiratory tract, the cardiovascular system, and the mouth and throat.

PRECAUTIONS AND ADVERSE REACTIONS

No health hazards or side effects are known in conjunction with the proper administration of designated therapeutic dosages.

DOSAGE

Mode of Administration: As a component of purgative and ''blood purifying'' teas, and in fruit tea mixtures.

Preparation: To prepare an infusion, scald 1.5 gm finely cut drug, steep for 5 minutes and then strain. (1 teaspoonful = 0.8 gm drug)

LITERATURE

Bamford DS et al., (1970) Brit J Pharmacol 40(1):161P.

Beckett A et al., (1954) J Pharm Pharmacol 6:785.

Czygan FC, Die Himbeere - Rubus idaeus L. In: ZPT 16(6):366-74. 1995.

Henning W, (1981) Lebensm Unters Forsch 173:1.

Henning W, (1981) Lebensm Unters Forsch 173:180.

Marczal G, (1963) Herba Hung 2:343.

Further information in:

Kern W, List PH, Hörhammer L (Hrsg.), Hagers Handbuch der Pharmazeutischen Praxis, 4. Aufl., Bde. 1-8: Springer Verlag Berlin, Heidelberg, New York, 1969.

Wichtl M (Hrsg.), Teedrogen, 4. Aufl., Wiss. Verlagsges. Stuttgart 1997.

Rue

See Ruta Graveolens

Rumex Acetosa

Sorrel

DESCRIPTION

Medicinal Parts: The medicinal parts are the fresh leaves and the whole herb.

Flower and Fruit: The plant has small greenish unisexual, dioecious flowers, in narrow, loose panicles. There are 6 tepals, the 3 inner ones turn red when the fruit ripens and the outer ones close. When mature they are often red-tinged, membranous, entire-margined and have a scale-like downwardly curved welt at the base. There are 6 stamens and 3 styles with paintbrush-like stigma. The fruit is a triangular, brown-black nut enclosed in the enlarged inner tepal.

Leaves, Stem and Root: The plant can grow up to 100 cm high. The leaves alternate on the erect, grooved stems which are unbranched up to the panicles. The leaves are fleshy, grass green, hastate or spit-shaped. The lower leaves are long-petioled, the upper ones are short-petioled, sessile and clasping. There is a membranous, dentate or fringed cone at the base of the leaves.

Characteristics: The stem is red-tinged, and the herb has a sour taste. It gets its acidity from the same salt as is present in Rhubarb.

Habitat: The plant is common in Europe.

Production: Sorrel is the aerial part of Rumex acetosa.

ACTIONS AND PHARMACOLOGY

COMPOUNDS

Oxalates: oxalic acid, calcium oxalate

Tannins (7-10%)

Flavonoids

Anthracene derivatives: aglycones, physcion, chryosphanol, emodin, aloe-emodin, rhein, and their glucosides, further, including, among others, aloe-emodin acetate

EFFECTS

Diuretic, stimulates secretion, improves resistance to infections (questionable).

INDICATIONS AND USAGE

The herb is used for acute and chronic inflammation of the nasal passages and respiratory tract. It is also used as an additional measure in antibacterial therapy.

PRECAUTIONS AND ADVERSE REACTIONS

No health hazards or side effects are known in conjunction with the proper administration of designated therapeutic dosages.

OVERDOSAGE

Oxalate poisonings are conceivable only with the consumption of very large quantities of the leaves as salad.

DOSAGE

Mode of Administration: The drug itself is described as obsolete.

Daily Dosage: The dosage for adults is 2 coated tablets or 50 drops (drops with 19% Ethanol) to be taken 3 times daily.

LITERATURE

No literature available.

Rumex Aquaticus

Water Dock

DESCRIPTION

Medicinal Parts: The medicinal parts are the dried roots.

Flower and Fruit: The inflorescence is a large, dense panicle. The pedicles are filiform and up to 2.5 times as long as the capsules. The capsules are 6 to 8 mm long, ovate-triangular, more or less acute, longer than wide and entire-margined.

Leaves, Stem and Root: The herb is perennial and has an erect 100 to 200 cm high stem. The basal leaves are triangular, acute, deeply cordate at base and 1.5 to 2.5 times as long as wide. The leaves are 7.5 to 10 cm wide with curly margins. The petiole is at least as long as the leaf blade. The rhizome is blackish to dark brown on the outside and porous.

Habitat: The plant is common in Europe.

Production: The root material is sliced and dried in the shade.

ACTIONS AND PHARMACOLOGY

COMPOUNDS

Oxalates: oxalic acid, calcium oxalate

Tannins

Anthracene derivatives

EFFECTS

The active agents are quercitrin, protein, fat, starch, essential oil and tannin.

The herb has digestive properties.

INDICATIONS AND USAGE

Water Dock is used for blood purification and constipation. The powdered form is also useful for cleaning the teeth or for mouth ulcers. It is used externally for sores and scorbutic conditions.

PRECAUTIONS AND ADVERSE REACTIONS

No health hazards or side effects are known in conjunction with the proper administration of designated therapeutic dosages.

OVERDOSAGE

Oxalate poisonings are conceivable only with the consumption of very large quantities of the leaves as salad.

DOSAGE

Mode of Administration: The drug is used internally and externally as a liquid extract or as a powder.

LITERATURE

Grznar K, Rada K, Farmaceut Obzor 47:195. 1978.

Sharma M et al., Indian J Chem Sect B 15B:544. 1977.

Further information in:

Kern W, List PH, Hörhammer L (Hrsg.), Hagers Handbuch der Pharmazeutischen Praxis, 4. Aufl., Bde. 1-8: Springer Verlag Berlin, Heidelberg, New York, 1969.

Rumex Crispus

Yellow Dock

DESCRIPTION

Medicinal Parts: The medicinal parts are the fresh and dried roots.

Flower and Fruit: The green androgynous flowers are in panicles. The inner tips of the perigone are entire-margined, orbicular or ovate and when the fruit ripens they are slightly longer than wide. Otherwise the flower is the same as R.acetosa, i.e. there is a 6-tepalled perigone. The inner tepals are longer than the outer ones and close. When the fruit ripens they are usually red-tinged, membranous, entire-margined and with a downward curved, scale-like welt at the base. There are 6 stamens and 3 styles with paintbrush-like stigmas. The fruit is a triangular, brown-black nut, which is enclosed by the wing-like enlarged inner tepal.

Leaves, Stem and Root: The plant is about 100 cm high. There is a carrot-like rhizome. The roots are 20 to 30 cm long, 1.25 cm thick, fleshy and are not usually branched. The rhizome is rusty brown on the outside, whitish on the inside and has a relatively thick bark. The stems are angular, grooved and usually branched from the base up. The lower leaves are large and have flat petioles. They have a cordate base, lanceolate acute to curly, alternate. The upper leaves are smaller and narrow-lanceolate.

Habitat: The plant is indigenous to Europe and Africa but grows wild in many regions of the world.

Production: Yellow Dock root is the fresh root harvested in spring from Rumex acetosa.

Other Names: Curled Dock

ACTIONS AND PHARMACOLOGY

COMPOUNDS

Oxalates: oxalic acid, calcium oxalate

Tannins (3-6%)

Flavonoids: including, among others, quercitrin

Anthracene derivatives (0.9-2.5%): aglycones physcion, chryosphanol, emodin, aloe-emodin, rhein, their glucosides

Naphthalene derivatives: neopodin 8-glucoside, lapodin

EFFECTS

No information is available.

INDICATIONS AND USAGE

Yellow Dock is used for acute and chronic inflammation of the nasal passages and respiratory tract. It is also used as an additional measure in antibacterial therapy. The plant has traditionally been used like the Red Dock (R. aquatica) for its similar properties, in decoctions for scurvy and other skin eruptions, and as a ''blood cleanser''.

PRECAUTIONS AND ADVERSE REACTIONS

No health hazards or side effects are known in conjunction with the proper administration of designated therapeutic dosages. Mucus membrane irritation, accompanied by vomiting is possible following intake of the fresh rhizome, due to its anthrone content. The anthrones are oxidized to anthraquinones through dehydration and storage.

OVERDOSAGE

Oxalate poisonings are conceivable only with the consumption of the leaves as salad, one case of death following consumption of a soup made from the leaves of the curled Yellow Dock has been described (see Frohne).

DOSAGE

Mode of Administration: Preparations are available in ground form or as an extract.

LITERATURE

Fairbairn JW, El Muhtadi FJ, (1972) Phytochemistry 11:263.

Grznar K, Rada K, Farmaceut Obzor 47:195. 1978.

Midiwo JO, Runkunga GM, (1985) Phytochemistry 24(6):1390.

Sharma M et al., Indian J Chem Sect B 15B:544. 1977.

Further information in:

Frohne D, Pfänder HJ, Giftpflanzen - Ein Handbuch für Apotheker, Toxikologen und Biologen, 4. Aufl., Wiss. Verlags-Ges. Stuttgart 1997.

Kern W, List PH, Hörhammer L (Hrsg.), Hagers Handbuch der Pharmazeutischen Praxis, 4. Aufl., Bde. 1-8: Springer Verlag Berlin, Heidelberg, New York, 1969.

Madaus G, Lehrbuch der Biologischen Arzneimittel, Bde 1-3, Nachdruck, Georg Olms Verlag Hildesheim 1979.

Morton JF, An Atlas of Medicinal Plants of Middle America, Charles C Thomas Pub. USA 1981.

Teuscher E, Lindequist U, Biogene Gifte - Biologie, Chemie, Pharmakologie, 2. Aufl., Fischer Verlag Stuttgart 1994.

Rupturewort

See Herniaria Glabra

Ruscus Aculeatus

Butcher's Broom

DESCRIPTION

Medicinal Parts: The medicinal parts are the herb and the rhizome.

Flower and Fruit: The small greenish white flowers are solitary or in a few clusters and grow from the middle of the leaves. They are dioecious. The corolla is deeply divided into 6 segments. In one variety the stamens are fused at the base. In fertile varieties the style is surrounded by a honey gland. The fertile flowers develop into cherry-sized, scarlet berries, which ripen in September and remain on the tree all winter.

Leaves, Stem and Root: The plant is a perennial evergreen, 20 to 80 cm high subshrub. The stems are erect, woody and heavily branched. The leaves are small, brown-membranous, triangular to lanceolate and scale-like. The phylloclades (short shoots spread like leaves) are oblong, stiff, double-rowed, up to 2.5 cm long and terminate in a sharp tip.

Habitat: The plant is indigenous to all of Europe, western Asia and northern Africa.

Production: Butcher's broom consists of the dried rhizome and root of Ruscus aculeatus.

Other Names: Kneeholm, Pettigree, Sweet Broom, Knee Holly, Jew's Myrtle

ACTIONS AND PHARMACOLOGY

COMPOUNDS

Steroid saponins (4-6%): chief components: ruscine, ruscoside, aglycones neoruscogenin, ruscogenin

Benzofuranes: euparone, ruscodibenzofurane

EFFECTS

In animal tests, there was an increase in venous tone, and there was an electrolyte-like reaction on the cell wall of capillaries. Butcher's Broom is antiphlogistic and diuretic.

INDICATIONS AND USAGE

- Hemorrhoids
- Venous conditions

The herb is used as supportive therapy for discomfort of chronic venous insufficiency, such as pain and heaviness, as well as cramps in the legs, itching, and swelling. Butcher's Broom is used as supportive therapy for complaint of hemorrhoids, such as itching and burning.

PRECAUTIONS AND ADVERSE REACTIONS

No health hazards or side effects are known in conjunction with the proper administration of designated therapeutic dosages.

Stomach complaints and queasiness can occur in rare cases.

DOSAGE

Mode of Administration: Extracts and their preparations for internal use.

Daily Dosage: Raw extract, equivalent to 7 to 11 mg total ruscogenin (determined as the sum of neoruscogenin and ruscogenin obtained after fermentation or acid hydrolysis).

LITERATURE

Adamek B, Drozdzik M, Samochowiec L, Wojcicki J, Clinical effect of buckwheat herb, Ruscus extract and troxerutin on retinopathy and lipids in diabetic patients. In: Phytotherapy Res 10(8):659-662. 1996.

Bombardelli E et al., (1972) Fitoterapia 43:3.

Dunaouau CH et al., Triterpenes and sterols from Ruscus aculeatus. In: PM 62(2):189-190. 1997.

Rauwald HW, Janβen B, Desglucoruscin and Desglucoruscosid als Leitstoffe des Ruscus-aculeatus-Wurzelstock. Analytische Kennzeichnung mittel HPLC und DC. In: PZW 133(1):61-68. 1988.

Schiebel-Schlosser G, Stechender Mäusedorn, eine Venenhilfe. In: PTA 8(7):586. 1994.

Vanhoutte PM (1986) in: Advances in Medicinal Phytochemistry, Ed. D Barton, WD Ollis, Pub. John Wiley 1986.

Further information in:

Kern W, List PH, Hörhammer L (Hrsg.), Hagers Handbuch der Pharmazeutischen Praxis, 4. Aufl., Bde. 1-8: Springer Verlag Berlin, Heidelberg, New York, 1969.

Steinegger E, Hänsel R, Pharmakognosie, 5. Aufl., Springer Verlag Heidelberg 1992.

Teuscher E, Biogene Arzneimittel, 5. Aufl., Wiss. Verlagsges. Stuttgart 1997.

Wagner H, Wiesenauer M, Phytotherapie. Phytopharmaka und pflanzliche Homöopathika, Fischer-Verlag, Stuttgart, Jena, New York 1995.

Wichtl M (Hrsg.), Teedrogen, 4. Aufl., Wiss. Verlagsges. Stuttgart 1997.

Rust-Red Rhododendron

See Rhododendron Ferrugineum

Ruta Graveolens

Rue

DESCRIPTION

Medicinal Parts: The medicinal parts are oil extracted from the herb, the herbal parts of the plant harvested after flowering, the fresh aerial parts of the plant collected at the beginning of the flowering season and the whole plant.

Flower and Fruit: The yellow flowers are in cymes, which are on twining branches with entire or 3-lobed bracts. The calyx is 4 to 5 segmented. There are 4 to 5 petals which are spoon-like concave, ovate and which end suddenly in the stem. The 8 to 10 stamens are in 2 circles. There is 1 short, broadly ovate ovary with 4 to 5 grooves and covered in glands. The fruit is a globular, 4 to 5 valvular, many-seeded capsule. The seeds are angular and have a black roughly bumpy skin.

Leaves, Stem and Root: The plant is a sturdy shrub 30 to 80 cm high with a woody root and a crooked, branched rhizome. The shoots are glabrous, pale green and more or less covered in oil glands. The stems are erect, rigid, round, lightly branched and woody from below. The leaves are 4 to 11 cm long and 3 to 7 cm wide, odd-pinate, with 1 to 3 pinnatesect pinna. The terminal segments are spatulate to lanceolate. The front ones are very finely crenate or serrate, somewhat fleshy, pale yellowish or bluish green.

Characteristics: The odor is tangy and the taste is hot, somewhat bitter and can cause skin irritation.

Habitat: The plant grows in the Balkans as far as Siebengebirge, upper Italy and central Italy and is cultivated elsewhere. It is completely naturalized in the southern Alps, southern France and Spain.

Production: Rue leaves consist of the dried leaves of Ruta graveolens. Rue herb consists of the dried above-ground parts of Ruta graveolens.

Other Names: Herb-of-Grace, Herbygrass

ACTIONS AND PHARMACOLOGY

COMPOUNDS

Alkaloids (0.4-0.4%): furoquinoline alkaloids: including, among others, skimmianin, gamma-fagarine, dictamnin, kokusaginine, ptelein

Acridine alkaloids: including, among others, arborinine- 2-arylquinoline alkaloids: including, among others, graveolin

Quinazoline alkaloids: including, among others, arborine

Quinoline alkaloids

Volatile oil (0.2-0.4%): chief components are 2-nonanone, 2-undecanone, further including, among others, linalyl acetate, 1,8-cineole, menthol

Flavonoids: chief component is rutin (2-5%)

Hydroxycoumarins: umbelliferone, herniarin, gravelliferon, rutacultin

Furocoumarins: bergapten, psoralen, xanthotoxin, chalepensin, isopimpinellin, isoimperatorin, rutarin, rutaretine

Pyranocoumarins: including, among others, xanthyletine

Lignans: savinin, helioxanthine

EFFECTS

Fertility inhibitor, spasmolytic and antiexudative effect.

INDICATIONS AND USAGE

Preparations of rue herb and/or leaves are used for menstrual disorders, as an effective uterine remedy and as an abortive agent. In folk medicine, Rue is used for menstrual complaints, as a contraceptive and as an abortive agent. The herb is also used for inflammation of the skin, oral and pharyngeal cavities, ear ache, toothache, for feverish infectious diseases, for cramps, as an obstetric remedy, hepatitis, dyspepsia, diarrhea and intestinal worm infestations.

PRECAUTIONS AND ADVERSE REACTIONS

General: No health hazards are known in conjunction with the proper administration of designated therapeutic dosages. The drug can lead to photosensitization, due to its furocoumarine and furoquinoline content; photodermatoses have been observed following skin contact with the fresh leaves. A sensitization is possible following skin contact.

Pregnancy: Vomiting, epigastric pain, liver damage, kidney damage, depression, sleep disorders, feelings of vertigo, delirium, fainting, tremor, and spasm, occasionally with fatal outcome, have occurred through misuse of extracts of the plant as an abortive agent.

OVERDOSAGE

Vomiting, epigastric pain, liver damage, kidney damage, depression, sleep disorders, feelings of vertigo, delirium, fainting, tremor, and spasm, occasionally with fatal outcome, have occurred in cases of overdose.

DOSAGE

Mode of Administration: Preparations are used internally and externally.

Preparation: Tea preparation or a cold decoction is prepared by adding 1 heaping teaspoonful to 1/4 liter of water. (1 teaspoonful is equivalent to 2.8 gm drug)

Daily Dosage: Medium single dose: 0.5 gm and Maximum daily dose: 1.0 gm

For topical use, leaves are used to fill hollow teeth for toothache and juice of the leaves is used for earache as an ear drop.

LITERATURE

Amling R, Phytotherapeutika in der Neurologie. In: ZPT 12(1):9. 1991.

Becela-Deller C, Die Weinraute. Heilpflanze zwischen Magie und Wissenschaft. In: DAZ 131(51/52):2705. 1991.

Becela-Deller C, Ruta graveolens L. - Weinraute. In: ZPT 16(5):275-281. 1995.

Grundon, MF, In ''The Alkaloids Vol. 11'', Pub. Royal Soc Chem (1981).

Hellwig B, Phytochemie, Hauterkrankungen und zentrales Nervensystem, 21. Seminarkongreβ der Bundesapothekerkammer in Erfurt. In: DAZ 135(38):3492 ff. 1995.

Mascolo N et al., (1987) Phytother Res 1(1):28.

Novak I et al., (1967) Planta Med 15:132.

Opdyke DLJ, (1975) Food Cosmet Toxicol 13: Suppl 713.

Paulini H, Waibel R, Kiefer J, Schimmer O, Gravacridondiolacetat, a new dihydrofuroacridone alkaloid from Ruta graveolens. In: PM 57:82. 1991.

Reisch J et al., (1967) Pharmazie 22: 220 et (1970) 25:435.

Reisch J et al., (1976) Phytochemistry 15:240.

Robbins RC, (1967) J Atheroscler Res 7:3.

Rozsa Z et al., (1980) Planta Med 39:218.

Schimmer O, Furochinolinalkaloide als biologisch aktive Naturstoffe. In: ZPT 12(5):151. 1991.

Van Duuren BL et al., (1971) J Natl Cancer Inst 46:1039.

Varga E et al., (1976) Fitoterapia 47:107.

Further information in:

Frohne D, Pfänder HJ, Giftpflanzen - Ein Handbuch für Apotheker, Toxikologen und Biologen, 4. Aufl., Wiss. Verlags-Ges. Stuttgart 1997.

Hänsel R, Keller K, Rimpler H, Schneider G (Hrsg.), Hagers Handbuch der Pharmazeutischen Praxis, 5. Aufl., Bde 4-6 (Drogen): Springer Verlag Berlin, Heidelberg, New York, 1992-1994.

Leung AY, Encyclopedia of Common Natural Ingredients Used in Food Drugs, Cosmetics, John Wiley & Sons Inc., New York 1980.

Lewin L, Gifte und Vergiftungen, 6. Aufl., Nachdruck, Haug Verlag, Heidelberg 1992.

Madaus G, Lehrbuch der Biologischen Arzneimittel, Bde 1-3, Nachdruck, Georg Olms Verlag Hildesheim 1979.

Roth L, Daunderer M, Kormann K, Giftpflanzen, Pflanzengifte, 4. Aufl., Ecomed Fachverlag Landsberg Lech 1993.

Steinegger E, Hänsel R, Pharmakognosie, 5. Aufl., Springer Verlag Heidelberg 1992.

Teuscher E, Lindequist U, Biogene Gifte - Biologie, Chemie, Pharmakologie, 2. Aufl., Fischer Verlag Stuttgart 1994.

Teuscher E, Biogene Arzneimittel, 5. Aufl., Wiss. Verlagsges. Stuttgart 1997.

Wagner H, Wiesenauer M, Phytotherapie. Phytopharmaka und pflanzliche Homöopathika, Fischer-Verlag, Stuttgart, Jena, New York 1995.

Saccharomyces Cerevisiae

Brewer's Yeast

DESCRIPTION

Medicinal Parts: The medicinal part is the mature, low fermenting Brewer's Yeast.

Flower and Fruit: The cells may be single, in pairs, in chains or they may be aggregate. On a suitable solid fertile base the individual cell colonies have smooth margins, are slightly convex to flat and are whitish to cream-yellow. Older individual colonies are slightly raised, smooth or slightly lobed sometimes in sections or folded and are yellowish to light brown. The vegetative reproduction is via multilateral budding. Ascospores are produced from the vegetative cells. There are normally 1 to 4, occasionally more, round, smooth-walled ascospores per ascus.

Characteristics: Brewer's Yeast is found extensively in the wild and they live as saprophytic parasites or symbiotically.

Habitat: Brewer's Yeast is grown worldwide.

Production: Medicinal yeast consists of fresh or dried cells of *Saccharomyces cerevisiae* and/or of *Candida utilis.*

ACTIONS AND PHARMACOLOGY

COMPOUNDS

Vitamins of the B-group (per 100 gm): thiamin 8-15 mg, riboflavin 4-8 mg, nicotinic acid amide 45-90 mg, pantothenic acid 7-25 mg, pyridoxine 4-10 mg, biotin 20 µg, folic acid 1-5 mg, vitamin B-12 20 µg

Polysaccharides: mannans, glucans

Proteins

Amines

Sterols: ergosterol, zymosterol

EFFECTS

The yeast is antibacterial and stimulates phagocytosis.

INDICATIONS AND USAGE

- Common cold
- Cough/bronchitis
- Dyspeptic complaints
- Eczema, furuncles, acne
- Fevers and colds
- Inflammation of the mouth and pharynx
- Loss of appetite
- Tendency to infection

It is also used as a dietary supplement for chronic forms of acne and furunculosis.

PRECAUTIONS AND ADVERSE REACTIONS

General: Health risks or side effects following the proper administration of designated therapeutic dosages are not recorded. The intake of large quantities can cause gas. Allergic intolerance reactions are possible (itching, urticaria, exanthema, Quinck's disease). Migraine headaches can be triggered in susceptible patients.

Drug Interactions: The simultaneous intake of monoamine oxidase inhibitors can cause an increase in blood pressure.

DOSAGE

Mode of Administration: Medicinal yeast and galenic preparations are available for internal use.

Daily Dosage: The average daily dosage is 6 gm.

LITERATURE

Aβmann C, Mikroorganismen:Biotherapeutika bei Infektionskrankheiten. In: DAZ 136(46):4136-4137. 1996.

Anonym, Hefepräparate haben sich bewährt. In: PTA 5(9):433. 1991.

Böckeler W, Thomas G (1989): In-vitro-Studien zur destabilisierenden Wirkung lyophilisierter Saccharomyces cerevisiae Hansen CBS 5926-Zellen auf Enterobakterien. Läβt sich diese Eigenschaft biochemisch erklären? In, Müller J, Ottenjann R, Seifert J (Hrsg), Ökosystem Darm, Springer-Verlag, S 142-153.

Czerucka D, Roux 1, Rampal P, (1994) Saccharomyces boulardii inhibits sectretagogue-mediated adenosin 3″, 5″-cyclic monophosphate induction in intestinal cells. Gastroenterology 106:65-72.

Ewe K, (1983) Obstipation - Pathophysiologie, Klinik, Therapie. Int Welt 6:286-292.

Gedek B, Hagenhoff G, (1989) Orale Verabreichung von lebensfähigen Zellen des Hefestammes Saccharomyces cerevisiae Hansen CBS 5926 und deren Schicksal während der Magen-Darm-Passage. Therapiewoche 38 (Sonderheft): 33-40.

Höchter W, Chase D, Hagenhoff G (1990) Saccharomyces boulardii bei akuter Erwachsenediarrhoe. Münch Med Wschr 132: 188-192.

Hojgaard L, Arffmann S, Jorgeasen M, Krag E, (1981) Tea consumption, a cause of constipation. Br Med J 282: 864.

Jahn HU, Zeitz M, (1991) Immunmodulatorische Wirkung von Saccharomyces boulardii beim Menschen. In: Seifert J, Ottenjann R, Zeitz M, Bockemühl J (Hrsg) Ökosystem Darm III. Springer-Verlag, S 159-164.

Kollaritsch HH, Tobüren D, Scheiner O, Wiedermann G, (1988) Prophylaxe der Reisediarrhoe. Münch Med Wschr 130: 671-673.

Massot J, Desconclois M, Astoin J, (1982) Protection par Saccharomyces boulardii de la diarrhée à Escherichia coli du souriceau. Ann Pharm Fr 40: 445-449.

Plein K, Hotz J, (1993) Therapeutic effect of Saccaromyces boulardii on mild residual symptoms in a stable phase of Crohn's disease with special respect to chronic diarrhea - a pilot study. Z Gastroenterol 31: 129-134.

Schmidt Ch, (1977) Unspezifische Steigerung der Phagozytoseaktivitäten von Peritoneal-makrophagen nach oraler Gabe verschiedener Hefepräparationen. Dissertation Freie Universität Berlin.

Sinai Y, Kaplan A, Hai Y et al., (1974) Enhancement of resistance to infections disease by oral administration of brewer's yeast. Infection Immunol 9: 781-787

Surawicz Ch, Elmer GW, Speelman P, McFarland LV, Chinn J, van Belle G, (1989) Die Prophylaxe Antibiotika-assoziierter Diarrhöen mit Saccharomyces boulardii. Eine prospektive Studie. Gastroenterol 96: 981-988.

Tempé JD, Steidel AL, Blehaut H, Hasselmann M, Lutun Ph, Maurier F, (1983) Prévention par Saccharomyces boulardii des diarrhées de l'alimentation entérale à débit continu. La Semaine des Hopitaux de Paris 59: 1409-1412.

Weber R, Regio Seminar Pharma: Reisemedizinische Beratung. In: DAZ 135(25):2352-2354. 1995.

Further information in:

Hänsel R, Keller K, Rimpler H, Schneider G (Hrsg.), Hagers Handbuch der Pharmazeutischen Praxis, 5. Aufl., Bde 4-6 (Drogen), Springer Verlag Berlin, Heidelberg, New York, 1992-1994 (unter Saccharomyces).

Schulz R, Hänsel R, Rationale Phytotherapie, Springer Verlag Heidelberg 1996.

Teuscher E, Biogene Arzneimittel, 5. Aufl., Wiss. Verlagsges. mbH Stuttgart 1997.

Wagner H, Wiesenauer M, Phytotherapie. Phytopharmaka und pflanzliche Homöopathika, Fischer-Verlag, Stuttgart, Jena, New York 1995.

Safflower

See Carthamus Tinctorius

Saffron

See Crocus Sativus

Sage

See Salvia Officinalis

Salep

See Orchis Species

Salix Species

White Willow

DESCRIPTION

Medicinal Parts: The medicinal part is the bark. Salix nigra is American Willow. Usually considered to be the natural origin of the modern aspirin.

Flower and Fruit: The male flowers are yellow and the female green. They are dioecious and appear at the same time as the leaves on leafy stems in erect catkins. The male catkins are densely blossomed and cylindrical, up to 6.5 cm by 1 cm and have 2 stamens. The female catkins are cylindrical, 4.5 cm by 7 mm. The seeds have a tuft of hair.

Leaves, Stem and Root: The Silver Willow is a 6 to 18 m high tree or bush with fissured gray bark and tough, sometimes egg-yellow or red-yellow, supple branches. The leaves are short-petioled, lanceolate, acuminate becoming cuneate at the base. They are finely serrate, silky-haired tomentose underneath and blue-green matte.

Characteristics: The annual twigs are not easy to break off at the base.

Habitat: The plant is indigenous to central and southern Europe.

Production: White Willow bark consists of the bark of the young, 2 to 3 year old branches harvested during early spring of Salix alba, Salix purpurea, Salix fragilis and other comparable Salix species.

Other Names: Willow, Salicin Willow, Withe Withy, Black Willow, Cartkins Willow, Pussywillow

ACTIONS AND PHARMACOLOGY

COMPOUNDS

Glycosides and esters yielding salicylic acid (1.5-12%): salicin (0.1-2%), salicortin (0.01-11%) and salicin derivatives acylated to the glucose residue (up to 6%, including, among others, fragilin, populin)

Tannins (8-20%)

Flavonoids

EFFECTS

The efficacy of the drug is due mainly to the proportion of salicin present. After the splitting of the acyl residue, the salicin glycosides convert to salicin, the precursor of salicylic acid, which also works as an antipyretic, an antiphlogistic and as an analgesic. White willow bark is the phytotherapeutic precursor to acetylsalicylic acid (aspirin).

INDICATIONS AND USAGE

- Rheumatism
- Pain

Diseases accompanied by fever, rheumatic ailments, headaches, pain caused by inflammation.

CONTRAINDICATIONS

Hypersensitivity to salicylates.

PRECAUTIONS AND ADVERSE REACTIONS

General: No health hazards are known in conjunction with the proper administration of designated therapeutic dosages. Stomach complaints could occur as side effects due to the tannin content.

Drug Interactions: Due to the salicin component, caution should be exercised when used in combination with salicylates and other non-steroidal anti-inflammatory drugs.

DOSAGE

Mode of Administration: Liquid and solid preparations for internal use. Combinations with diaphoretic drugs could be considered. Drug extracts are contained in some standardized preparations of analgesics/antirheumatics, hypnotics/sedatives, and gastrointestinal remedies.

Preparation: To prepare an infusion, use 2 to 3 gm of finely cut or coarsely powdered drug in cold water, boil, then allow to steep for 5 minutes, then strain.

Daily Dosage: Average daily dose corresponding to 60-120 mg total salicin. The dosage for an infusion is 1 cup 3 to 5 times daily. (1 teaspoonful = 1.5 gm drug)

LITERATURE

Amling R, Phytotherapeutika in der Neurologie. In: ZPT 12(1):9. 1991.

Anonym, Phytotherapie:Pflanzliche Antirheumatika - was bringen sie? In: DAZ 136(45):4012-4015. 1996.

Kreymeier J, Rheumatherapie mit Phytopharmaka. In: DAZ 137(8):611-613. 1997.

Meier B, Pflanzliche versus synthetische Arzneimittel. In: ZPT 10(6):182. 1989.

Meier B, Liebi M, Salicinhaltige Arzneimittel. Überlegungen zu Wirksamkeit und Unbedenklichkeit. In: (2):50. 1990.

Meier B et al., DAZ 125:341. 1985.

Meier B et al., DAZ 127:2401. 1987.

Meier B et al., ZPT 11:50. 1990.

Meier R et al., A chemotaxonomic survey of phenolic compounds in swiss willow species. In: PM 58(7):A698. 1992.

Nichols-Orians CM et al., PH 31:2180. 1992.

Schmid B, Heide L, The use of Salicis cortex in rheumatic disease: phytotherapie with known mode of action? In: PM 61(Abstracts of 43rd Ann Congr):94. 1995.

Schmid B, Heide L, Wirksamkeit und Verträglichkeit von Weidenrinde bei Arthrose: Design und Durchführung einer klinischen Studie. In: PUZ 26(1):33, Jahrestagung der DPhG, Berlin, 1996. 1997.

Shao Y et al., PM 55:617. 1989.

Thieme H, PM 13:431. 1965.

Thieme H, PA 20:570. 1965.

Further information in:

Kern W, List PH, Hörhammer L (Hrsg.), Hagers Handbuch der Pharmazeutischen Praxis, 4. Aufl., Bde 1-8: Springer Verlag Berlin, Heidelberg, New York, 1969.

Madaus G, Lehrbuch der Biologischen Arzneimittel, Bde 1-3, Nachdruck, Georg Olms Verlag Hildesheim 1979.

Schulz R, Hänsel R, Rationale Phytotherapie, Springer Verlag Heidelberg 1996.

Steinegger E, Hänsel R, Pharmakognosie, 5. Aufl., Springer Verlag Heidelberg 1992.

Teuscher E, Biogene Arzneimittel, 5. Aufl., Wiss. Verlagsges. Stuttgart 1997.

Wagner H, Wiesenauer M, Phytotherapie. Phytopharmaka und pflanzliche Homöopathika, Fischer-Verlag, Stuttgart, Jena, New York 1995.

Wichtl M (Hrsg.), Teedrogen, 4. Aufl., Wiss. Verlagsges. Stuttgart 1997.

Salvia Officinalis

Sage

DESCRIPTION

Medicinal Parts: The medicinal parts are dried leaves, the oils extracted from the flowers and stems, the fresh leaves, and the fresh flowering aerial parts.

Flower and Fruit: The medium-sized, pale violet, white or pink labiate flowers are in 6 to 12 blossomed false whorls, which are arranged above each other in 4 to 8 rows. The calyx is 10 to 14 mm long, funnel-shaped-campanulate, downy, glandular punctate, and bilabiate. The upper lip has 3 awned teeth, the lower lip 2. The corolla tube has a ring of hair inside. The upper lip is almost straight and the lower lip has 3 segments. There are 2 stamens with almost semi-circular bent filaments.

Leaves, Stem and Root: The plant is a bush up to 60 cm high. The stem is erect and woody at the base with leafy, quadrangular, white-gray tomentose branches. The leaves are simple, oblong or oblong-lanceolate and narrowed at the base. They are petiolate, densely and finely crenate, ribbed-wrinkled, white-gray tomentose initially, tough, and evergreen.

Characteristics: The leaves are aromatic, tangy, and bitterly astringent.

Habitat: The plant is indigenous to the Mediterranean region and has naturalized in all of Europe. It is cultivated in North America.

Production: Sage leaf consists of the fresh or dried leaf of Salvia officinalis. Sage is collected in the wild from the former Yugoslavia, the Adriatic coast and those areas that are further from the coast but are still under Mediterranean influence. The harvest takes place at different times depending on the area, from mid-July until December. October is recommended as the most favorable time to harvest Dalmatian sage.

Cultivation: it is recommended that the harvest take place from the second vegetation year at the beginning of the flowering period in the afternoon.

Drying the drug: in direct sunlight (up to 25% oil loss), in shade (2-10% oil loss), in a drying chamber (low oil loss, optimal conditions, with vertical incoming air current of 0.2 m/s, are reached at 50°C with 0.9% absolute humidity).

Not To Be Confused With: The leaves of Salvia triloba; may also be confused with other Salvia or Phlomis species.

ACTIONS AND PHARMACOLOGY

COMPOUNDS

Volatile oil (1.5-3.5%): chief constituents (when from Dalmatia) thujone (20-60%, alpha-thujone and beta-thujone), 1,8-cineole (6-16%), camphor (14-37%), further including, among others, borneol, isobutyl acetate, camphene, linalool, alpha- and beta-pinene, viridiflorol, alpha- and beta-caryophyllene (humulene)

Caffeic acid derivatives (3-6%): rosmarinic acid, chlorogenic acid

Diterpenes: chief components carnosolic acid (0.2-0.4%, picrosalvin), further including, among others, rosmanol, safficinolide

Flavonoids: including, among others, apigenin- and luteolin-7-glucosides, numerous methoxylated aglycones, including among others genkwanin, genkwanin-6-methylether

Triterpenes: chief components ursolic acid (5%)

EFFECTS

Sage has antibacterial, fungistatic, virostatic, astringent, secretolytic, and perspiration-inhibiting effects. In animal experiments, it is an antihypertensive and choleretic. It acts on the CNS and is a spasmolytic agent. Proof of an antidiabetic effect found in one study has not yet been confirmed. The essential oil has bactericidal, fungistatic, and virostatic effects.

INDICATIONS AND USAGE

- Loss of appetite
- Inflammation of the mouth and pharynx
- Excessive perspiration

Sage is used externally for inflammation of the mucous membranes of nose and throat; internally for dyspeptic symptoms and as a diaphoretic.

In folk medicine, the drug is used internally for gastric disorders such as loss of appetite, bloating, diarrhea, enteritis, and excessive perspiration. Externally, it is used as a rinse and gargle for light injuries and skin inflammation, bleeding gums, stomatitis, laryngitis, pharyngitis, and for firming the gums.

CONTRAINDICATIONS

Sage preparations are contraindicated during pregnancy.

PRECAUTIONS AND ADVERSE REACTIONS

General: No health hazards or side effects are known in conjunction with the proper administration of designated therapeutic dosages.

Pregnancy: Sage preparations should not be taken during pregnancy.

OVERDOSAGE

Sense of heat, tachycardia, feelings of vertigo and epileptiform convulsions could occur following extended intake of ethanolic extracts of the drug or of the volatile oil or through overdosage (corresponding to more than 15 gm of the sage leaves).

DOSAGE

Mode of Administration: Cut herb for infusions, alcoholic extracts, and distillates for gargles, rinses, and other topical applications, as well as for internal use. Also pressed juice of fresh plants. In folk medicine, sage is used internally as an antihidrotic infusion.

Preparation: Fortified wine for nervous exhaustion is manufactured using an 8-day maceration of 100 gm of the leaves with one liter wine.

For diabetes, a wine made by boiling 100 gm of the leaves with one liter wine for 2 minutes.

For bronchial catarrh, expectorant honey is made by mixing 50 gm of the powdered drug with 80 gm of honey.

For injuries, the drug is used as a cleanser and to heal wounds, a rinse made with wine is made by heating 100 gm of the leaves with 0.5 liter white wine for 1 minute.

For tumors, the drug is worked into an ointment base or pounded into a paste together with salt and vinegar.

To prepare an antihidrotic infusion, 20 gm of thc dried leaves are scalded with 1 liter water, steep 15 minutes, strain, compress and sweeten if required.

For cardiac insufficiency, a tonic infusion is prepared by pouring 1 liter boiling water over 50 gm of the drug, strain after 15 minutes, sweeten with sugar or honey.

The formula for decoction No. 1 is: One spoonful powdered drug scalded with 1 cup of water, quickly strained, and sweetened; decoction No. 2: 15 gm of the fresh leaves with 200 ml of water heated for 3 minutes.

Daily Dosage: The average daily internal dose is 4 to 6 gm of the drug; 0.1 to 0.3 gm of the essential oil; 2.5 to 7.5 gm of the tincture; 1.5 to 3 gm of the liquid extract.

For asthma, medicinal cigarettes are used. For nervous exhaustion, fortified wine is used. The dosage for diabetes is 1 glass of the wine preparation after mealtime. Bronchial catarrh dosage is 1 spoonful of the expectorant mornings and before bedtime.

Externally for gargles and rinses, 2.5 gm of the drug or 2 to 3 drops of essential oil in 100 ml of water as infusion or 5 gm of the alcoholic extract in 1 glass of water.

Undiluted alcohol extract is applied repeatedly to inflamed mucous membranes.

The dosage for an antihidrotic infusion is 200 ml three times daily.

For cardiac insufficiency, a tonic infusion can be taken 1 glass 4 times daily. The decoction (no. 1 or no. 2) dose is 1 glass at 1 hour intervals.

For nervous complaints and excessive perspiration, before mealtimes take 0.25 gm of the powdered drug (spoonful or capsules).

For headaches, decoction after each meal.

The leaves may be chewed occasionally in cases of foul-smelling breath.

Externally for cancerous ulcers, decoction or infusion for compresses or poultices.

Storage: Sage leaves are to be protected from light and humidity in sealed containers. Storage duration of coarsely cut drug is 18 months; powder, maximum 24 hours. The tincture is stored in tightly sealed containers away from light. The liquid extract may be kept for up to 2 years.

LITERATURE

Brieskorn CH, Bichele W, (1971) Dtsch Apoth Ztg 111:141.

Brieskorn CH, Salbei - seine Inhaltstoffe und sein therapeutischer Wert. In: ZPT 12(2):91. 1991.

Ferguson G et al., (1973) J Chem Soc Chem Comm 281.

Länger R, Mechtler C, Tanzler HO, Jurenitsch J, Differences of the composition of the essential oil within an individium of Salva officinalis. In: PM 59(7):A635. 1993.

Murko D et al., (1974) Planta Med 25:295.

Paris A, Strukelj B, Renko M, Turk V, Puki M, Umek A, Korant BD, Inhibitory effect of carnosolic acid on HIV-1 protease in cell free assays. In: JNP 56(8):1426-1430. 1993.

Raic D, Novina R, Petricic J, Acta Pharm Jugosl 35:121. 1985.

Tada M et al., Antiviral diterpenes from Salvia officinalis. In: PH 35(2):539. 1994.

Telekova D et al., PA 49:299. 1994.

Further information in:

Fenaroli's Handbook of Flavor Ingredients, Vol. 1, 2nd Ed., CRC Press 1975.

Frohne D, Pfänder HJ, Giftpflanzen - Ein Handbuch für Apotheker, Toxikologen und Biologen, 4. Aufl., Wiss. Verlags-Ges. Stuttgart 1997.

Hänsel R, Keller K, Rimpler H, Schneider G (Hrsg.), Hagers Handbuch der Pharmazeutischen Praxis, 5. Aufl., Bde 4-6 (Drogen): Springer Verlag Berlin, Heidelberg, New York, 1992-1994.

Leung AY, Encyclopedia of Common Natural Ingredients Used in Food Drugs, Cosmetics, John Wiley & Sons Inc., New York 1980.

Lewin L, Gifte und Vergiftungen, 6. Aufl., Nachdruck, Haug Verlag, Heidelberg 1992.

Madaus G, Lehrbuch der Biologischen Arzneimittel, Bde 1-3, Nachdruck, Georg Olms Verlag Hildesheim 1979.

Roth L, Daunderer M, Kormann K, Giftpflanzen, Pflanzengifte, 4. Aufl., Ecomed Fachverlag Landsberg Lech 1993.

Steinegger E, Hänsel R, Pharmakognosie, 5. Aufl., Springer Verlag Heidelberg 1992.

Teuscher E, Lindequist U, Biogene Gifte - Biologie, Chemie, Pharmakologie, 2. Aufl., Fischer Verlag Stuttgart 1994.

Teuscher E, Biogene Arzneimittel, 5. Aufl., Wiss. Verlagsges. Stuttgart 1997.

Wagner H, Wiesenauer M, Phytotherapie. Phytopharmaka und pflanzliche Homöopathika, Fischer-Verlag, Stuttgart, Jena, New York 1995.

Wichtl M (Hrsg.), Teedrogen, 4. Aufl., Wiss. Verlagsges. Stuttgart 1997.

Sambucus Ebulus

Dwarf Elder

DESCRIPTION

Medicinal Parts: The medicinal parts are the dried leaves, the ripe, dried or fresh fruit, and the dried roots collected in spring or late autumn.

Flowers and Fruit: The reddish-white flowers are in a terminal, umbrella-like, richly blossomed, paniculate cyme with 3 main branches. The calyx margin is 5-tipped. The corolla has fused petals and is rotate with 5 acuminate tips. There are 5 stamens with dark red anthers and an inferior, 3-valved ovary with 3 stigmas. The fruit is a black, globular, and berry-like drupe with at least 3 to 4 ovate seeds. The fruit stems are erect when ripe, and violet or crimson.

Leaves, Stem and Root: The plant is a perennial, herb-like plant 0.5 to 2 m high with a sturdy, finger-thick, branched rhizome which creeps deeply and horizontally. The stems are leafy, erect, sturdy, branched above, and they die off in autumn. The leaves are crossed opposite, odd-pinate with 3 to 4 pairs of ovate-lanceolate leaflets and 2 large, ovate-lanceolate, and serrate stipules.

Characteristics: The fragrance is reminiscent of sunflowers or almond.

Habitat: The plant is spread from southern Sweden through central and southern Europe, northern Africa, and western Asia as far as Iran.

Production: Dwarf Elder root is the root of Sambucus ebulus.

Other Names: Danewort, Walewort, Blood Elder, Blood Hilder

ACTIONS AND PHARMACOLOGY

COMPOUNDS

Iridoide monoterpene glycosides: ebuloside, 6′-O-apiosyl-ebuloside, 7,7-O-dihydroebuloside, secoebuloside, isosweroside

Nauseant, purgative "resins with unresolved structure"

EFFECTS

The drug is supposed to be a mild diuretic.

INDICATIONS AND USAGE

Dwarf Elder is used as an ingredient in different teas, which assist in weight reduction and alleviate rheumatism.

PRECAUTIONS AND ADVERSE REACTIONS

Health risks or side effects following the proper administration of designated therapeutic dosages are not recorded.

OVERDOSAGE

Large quantities of all parts of the plant, in particular the raw berries, according to older scientific reports, will lead to vomiting, bloody diarrhea, cyanosis, dizziness, headache, and unconsciousness. Cases of death are also mentioned.

DOSAGE

Mode of Administration: Dwarf Elder is obsolete as a drug in most countries. It is found in some tea mixtures, but is not used in medicinal preparations.

LITERATURE

Gross GA, Phytochemische Untersuchungen von Inhaltsstoffen der Zwergholunderwurzel, Dissertation Zürich. 1985.

Petkov V, Markovska V, (1981) Plant Med Phytother 15(3):172.

Further information in:

Frohne D, Pfänder HJ, Giftpflanzen - Ein Handbuch für Apotheker, Toxikologen und Biologen, 4. Aufl., Wiss. Verlagsges. mbH Stuttgart 1997.

Hänsel R, Keller K, Rimpler H, Schneider G (Hrsg.), Hagers Handbuch der Pharmazeutischen Praxis, 5. Aufl., Bde 4-6 (Drogen): Springer Verlag Berlin, Heidelberg, New York, 1992-1994.

Lewin L, Gifte und Vergiftungen, 6. Aufl., Nachdruck, Haug Verlag, Heidelberg 1992.

Madaus G, Lehrbuch der Biologischen Arzneimittel, Bde 1-3, Nachdruck, Georg Olms Verlag Hildesheim 1979.

Roth L, Daunderer M, Kormann K, Giftpflanzen, Pflanzengifte, 4. Aufl., Ecomed Fachverlag Landsberg Lech 1993.

Sambuscus Nigra

Black Elder

DESCRIPTION

Medicinal Parts: The medicinal parts are the bark peeled from the branches in spring and freed from the cork, the air-dried flowers, the leaves harvested when young and dried, the fresh or dried ripe fruit, the dried roots, the fresh leaves and inflorescences in equal parts, the fresh bark of the young branches, and the fresh leaves.

Flower and Fruit: The strongly perfumed, yellowish-white flowers are in large, flat, apical, richly and densely blossomed erect cymes with 5 main branches. The edge of the calyx is small and 5-tipped. The corolla is rotate, deep, and has 5 petals. There are 5 stamens and 1 inferior ovary. The fruit is a black-violet, berry-like drupe with blood-red juice. The seeds are brownish, ovate, and domed on the outside.

Leaves, Stem and Root: The plant is a shallow-rooted, up to 7 m high tree or bush with spreading branches containing dry white latex. The bark of the trunk is fissured, light brown to gray. The bark on the young branches is green and covered with gray lenticles. The leaves are odd 3 to 7 pinnate. They are matte green above and light blue-green beneath. The leaflets are ovate or oblong acuminate and densely serrate.

Characteristics: The flowers have a strong, numbing perfume.

Habitat: Sambuscus nigra is indigenous to almost all of Europe.

Other Names: Black-berried Alder, European Alder, Boor Tree, Elder, Bountry, Ellanwood, Ellhorn

ACTIONS AND PHARMACOLOGY

COMPOUNDS

Flavonoids (up to 3%): chief components are rutin, isoquercitrin, quercitrin, hyperoside, astragalin, nicotoflorin

Volatile oil (0.03-0.14%): higher share of free fatty acids, including among others palmitic acid (share 38%)

Caffeic acid derivatives (3%): chlorogenic acids

EFFECTS

Black Elder is a diaphoretic agent, it also increases bronchial secretion.

INDICATIONS AND USAGE

■ Cough/bronchitis

The drug is used for colds and coughs. It is a sweat-producing remedy for the treatment of feverish colds.

In folk medicine, Elder flowers are used internally as a sudorific tea and for colds and other feverish conditions. Elder is also used as an infusion, as a gargle/mouthwash and for respiratory disorders such as coughs, head colds, laryngitis, flu, and shortness of breath. Elder is used occasionally by nursing mothers to increase lactation. Externally, the herbal pads are used for swelling and inflammations.

Proof of efficacy is not available.

PRECAUTIONS AND ADVERSE REACTIONS

No health hazards or side effects are known in conjunction with the proper administration of designated therapeutic dosages.

DOSAGE

Mode of Administration: Whole herb and other galenic preparations for infusions.

Preparation: To prepare an infusion, 2 teaspoonfuls (3 to 4 gm) of elder flowers are brewed with 150 ml of simmering water and strained after 5 minutes.

Daily Dosage: The average daily dose of the drug is 10 to 15 gm. The infusion should be dosed 1 to 2 cups (as hot as possible) several times daily - especially in the afternoon and evening.

LITERATURE

Bauer R et al., (1985) Helv Chim Acta 68:2355.

Czygan FC, Holunder wird wieder gesellschaftsfähig. In: ZPT 15(2):111. 1994.

Eberhardt R, Pfannhauser W, Z Lebensm Unters Forsch 181:97. 1985.

Inoue T, Sato K, (1975) Phytochemistry 14:1871.

Lawrie W et al., (1964) Phytochemistry 3:267.

Mascolo N et al., (1987) Phytother Res 1(1):28.

Paulo E, (1976) Folia Biol 24(2):213.

Petitjean-Freytet C et al., J Pharm Belg 46:241. 1991.

Richter W, Willuhn G, (1974) Dtsch Apoth Ztg 114:947.

Richter W, Willuhn G, DAZ 114:947. 1974.

Willuhn G, Richter W, PM 31:328. 1977.

Further information in:

Hänsel R, Keller K, Rimpler H, Schneider G (Hrsg.), Hagers Handbuch der Pharmazeutischen Praxis, 5. Aufl., Bde 4-6 (Drogen): Springer Verlag Berlin, Heidelberg, New York, 1992-1994.

Leung AY, Encyclopedia of Common Natural Ingredients Used in Food Drugs, Cosmetics, John Wiley & Sons Inc., New York 1980.

Madaus G, Lehrbuch der Biologischen Arzneimittel, Bde 1-3, Nachdruck, Georg Olms Verlag Hildesheim 1979.

Schulz R, Hänsel R, Rationale Phytotherapie, Springer Verlag Heidelberg 1996.

Steinegger E, Hänsel R, Pharmakognosie, 5. Aufl., Springer Verlag Heidelberg 1992.

Teuscher E, Biogene Arzneimittel, 5. Aufl., Wiss. Verlagsges. Stuttgart 1997.

Wagner H, Wiesenauer M, Phytotherapie. Phytopharmaka und pflanzliche Homöopathika, Fischer-Verlag, Stuttgart, Jena, New York 1995.

Wichtl M (Hrsg.), Teedrogen, 4. Aufl., Wiss. Verlagsges. Stuttgart 1997.

Samphire

See Crithum Maritimum

Sandalwood

See Santalum Album

Sanguinaria Canadensis

Bloodroot

DESCRIPTION

Medicinal Parts: The medicinal parts are roots and the whole plant.

Flower and Fruit: The plant bears a white flower with 8 to 12 petals on a 15 cm long scape. It is wax-like and has golden stamens. The seed is an oblong, narrow capsule approximately 2.5 cm long.

Leaves, Stem and Root: The plant is a perennial and about 15 cm high. The rhizome is thick, round, fleshy and slightly curved at the end. It is 2.5 to 10 cm long and has orange-red rootlets. There is 1 basal palmately-lobed leaf which appears when flower dies. It is clasping, grayish green and covered in soft down, 15 to 25 cm long with 5 to 9 lobes. Protruding ribs are recognizable on the under surface.

Habitat: The plant is indigenous to the northeastern U.S.

Production: Canadian Bloodroot is the root-stock (rhizome) of Sanguinaria canadensis.

Other Names: Indian Paint, Tetterwort, Red Root, Paucon, Coon Root, Snakebite, Sweet Slumber, Indian Plant, Pauson, Sanguinaria

ACTIONS AND PHARMACOLOGY

COMPOUNDS

Isoquinoline alkaloids of the benzophenanthridine type (4-7%): chief alkaloid sanguinarine, further including, among others, chelerythrine, oxysanguinarine; protoberberine-type: berberine, coptisine; protopine-type: protopine, alpha- and beta-allocryptopine

Resins

Starch

EFFECTS

The alkaloid initially acts as a narcotic, causes severe cramping which is followed by a local paralysis of the sensitive nerve endings. The plant also has an antimicrobial effect.

INDICATIONS AND USAGE

The drug was formerly used as an expectorant, as an active antiplaque agent, and as a mouthwash.

PRECAUTIONS AND ADVERSE REACTIONS

No health hazards or side effects are known in conjunction with the proper administration of designated therapeutic dosages.

OVERDOSAGE

The drug has an emetic effect in dosages above 0.03 gm (was previously used therapeutically). Higher dosages of the drug severely irritate the mucus membranes. Results include vomiting, diarrhea, intestinal colic, and possible collapse.

DOSAGE

Mode of Administration: The drug is obsolete in most countries. Bloodroot is still used in homeopathic preparations, as an ingredient in some pharmaceutical preparations, and as a component of toothpaste and mouthwashes.

LITERATURE

Anonym, Medizinische Mundpflege mit Sanguinaria-Extrakt. In: DAZ 131(16):XLII. 1991.

Collins KR, Pat. EP 25649 (1981) Europe.

Elliott JQ, Pat. US 4515779 (1985) USA.

Ladanyi P, Pat. CH 638973 (1983) Switzerland.

Maiti M et al., Febs Lett 142:280.

Further information in:

Frohne D, Pfänder HJ, Giftpflanzen - Ein Handbuch für Apotheker, Toxikologen und Biologen, 4. Aufl., Wiss. Verlags-Ges. Stuttgart 1997.

Kern W, List PH, Hörhammer L (Hrsg.), Hagers Handbuch der Pharmazeutischen Praxis, 4. Aufl., Bde 1-8: Springer Verlag Berlin, Heidelberg, New York, 1969.

Lewin L, Gifte und Vergiftungen, 6. Aufl., Nachdruck, Haug Verlag, Heidelberg 1992.

Madaus G, Lehrbuch der Biologischen Arzneimittel, Bde 1-3, Nachdruck, Georg Olms Verlag Hildesheim 1979.

Roth L, Daunderer M, Kormann K, Giftpflanzen, Pflanzengifte, 4. Aufl., Ecomed Fachverlag Landsberg Lech 1993.

Wagner H, Wiesenauer M, Phytotherapie. Phytopharmaka und pflanzliche Homöopathika, Fischer-Verlag, Stuttgart, Jena, New York 1995.

Sanguisorba Officinalis

Great Burnet

DESCRIPTION

Medicinal Parts: The flowering plant is the medicinal part.

Flower and Fruit: The composite heads are ovate-oblong, approximately 1 to 2 cm long and consist of 5 to 10 usually androgynous flowers. The calyx has 4 dark red-brown tips, 4 stamens with stiffly patent red filaments and yellow anthers. There is 1 carpel and 1 style in the smooth spike-like quadrangular and narrowly winged fruit calyx. The fruit is a nut enclosed in the perigone tube.

Leaves, Stem and Root: The plant is a semi-rosette shrub with a strong dark brown root that produces thick fibers and a short rhizome. The stems are erect, angular, glabrous, and bifurcated. The rosette leaves are 20 to 40 cm long and consist of 7 to 15 ovate leaflets, which are cordate at the base and blue-green beneath. There are only a few cauline leaves, which taper towards the top.

Characteristics: The brown-red composite head is characteristic for this plant.

Habitat: The plant is widespread in the northern, temperate regions of Europe, temperate Asia, and North America.

Production: The plant is harvested in uncultivated regions (wild) in the former Czechoslovakia.

ACTIONS AND PHARMACOLOGY

COMPOUNDS

Flavonoids: including, among others, rutin, flavonoid sulfates

Tannins

Triterpene glycosides: aglycones pomolic acid, tormentolic acid, including, among others, ziyuglycosides I and II (sanguisorbin)

Sterols: beta-sitosterol

EFFECTS

No investigation into effects has been carried out.

INDICATIONS AND USAGE

The drug is used internally for female disorders, mennorrhagia during menopause, hot flushes, dysentery, enteritis, diarrhea, bladder restraint, hemorrhoids, phlebitis, and varicose veins. Externally, Great Burnet is used in plaster for wounds and boils. This application has not been clinically proven.

PRECAUTIONS AND ADVERSE REACTIONS

No health hazards or side effects are known in conjunction with the proper administration of designated therapeutic dosages.

DOSAGE

Mode of Administration: The drug is used internally and externally. It is available in the ground form and is used as an extract, juice or tea. A plaster is used externally.

LITERATURE

Bastow KF et al., Inhibition of DNA topoisomerase by sanguiin H-6, a cytotoxic dimeric ellagitannin from Sanguisorba officinalis. In: PM 59(3):240. 1993.

Kaneta M et al., Agric Biol Chem 43:657. 1979.

Kashiwada Y, Nonaka GI, Niskioka I, Chang JJ, Lee KH, Antitumor agents, 129. Tannins and related compounds as selective cytotoxic agents. In: JNP 55:1033-1043. 1992.

Kosuga T et al., (1981) Yakugaku Zasshi 101(6):501.

Kosuga T et al., (1984) Chem Pharm Bull 32(11):448.

Nonaka GI et al., (1982) J Chem Soc Perkin Trans. 10(4):1067.

Nonaka GI et al., (1984) Chem Pharm Bull 32(2):483.

Reher G et al., PH 31:3909-3914. 1992.

Sunstar Inc. (1980) Pat. JP 80/120509 Japan.

Tanaka T et al., (1983) Phytochemistry 22(11):2575.

Tanaka T et al., (1984) Chem Pharm Bull 32(1):117.

Tanake T et al., (1985) J Chem Res (S)6:176.

Yosioka I et al., Chem Pharm Bull 19:1700. 1971.

Further information in:

Chang, EH et al. (Eds), Advances in Chinese Medicinal Materials Research, World Scientific Pub. Co. Singapore 1985.

Hänsel R, Keller K, Rimpler H, Schneider G (Hrsg.), Hagers Handbuch der Pharmazeutischen Praxis, 5. Aufl., Bde 4-6 (Drogen), Springer Verlag Berlin, Heidelberg, New York, 1992-1994.

Madaus G, Lehrbuch der Biologischen Arzneimittel, Bde 1-3, Nachdruck, Georg Olms Verlag Hildesheim 1979.

Sanicle

See Sanicula Europaea

Sanicula Europaea

Sanicle

DESCRIPTION

Medicinal Parts: The medicinal parts are the dried basal leaves collected during the flowering season, and the fresh flowering herb.

Flower and Fruit: The white or reddish inflorescences form a cyme with small head-like umbels with 4 to 6 linear bracts. The calyx is 5-tipped. There are 5 petals. The androgynous florets are in the center of the small umbel surrounded by 10 to 20 male florets. The fruit is almost globular, ribless with long styles curved downwards, and densely covered with barbed thorns. The mericarps are distinctly domed and almost flat at the narrow groove. There are numerous oil lines.

Leaves, Stem and Root: The plant is a perennial, approximately 20 to 40 cm high. The rhizome is solid, horizontal, short, multi-segmented, broken off and covered in thick fibers. The stem is usually undivided, erect, grooved, and has only 1 to 2 sessile leaves. The leaves are basal, long-petioled, and palmate with 5 lobes. The tips are 3-lobed. The lateral tips are divided in 2 and especially glossy underneath.

Characteristics: The taste is slightly salty, bitter, and dry.

Habitat: The plant is indigenous to Europe, Asia Minor, the Caucasus, western Siberia, northern Africa, and in the mountains of tropical Africa.

Production: The plant is collected in the wild.

Not To Be Confused With: In the drug market the herb may be mixed with leaves of Cardamine enneaphylos. In some areas, Astrantia major is labeled as sanicle and accordingly used as folk medicine.

Other Names: Poolroot, Self-heal

ACTIONS AND PHARMACOLOGY

COMPOUNDS

Triterpene saponins (up to 13%): including, among others, acyl-saniculosides A-D, aglycones including, among others, A1-barrigenol, R1-barrigenol, barringtogenol

Caffeic acid derivatives: rosmarinic acid, chlorogenic acid

Flavonoids: chief components rutin, isoquercitrin, astragalin

EFFECTS

The drug has a mild astringent and expectorant effect. It also reduces edema in animal experiments.

INDICATIONS AND USAGE

■ Cough/bronchitis

Sanicle is used for mild catarrh of the respiratory tract.

PRECAUTIONS AND ADVERSE REACTIONS

No health hazards or side effects are known in conjunction with the proper administration of designated therapeutic dosages.

DOSAGE

Mode of Administration: Comminuted drug for decoctions and other preparations for oral application.

Daily Dosage: The average daily dose is 4 to 6 gm of the herb.

Storage: The drug must be kept in sealed containers, protected from light sources.

LITERATURE

Engel S, Horn K, Phytodermatosen durch Dictamnus albus, Sanicula europaea und Philodendron consanguineum. In: Dermat Mschr 158(1):22-27. 1972.

Hiller K et al., PA 24:178. 1969.

Hiller K et al., PA 22:220-221. 1967.

Further information in:

Hänsel R, Keller K, Rimpler H, Schneider G (Hrsg.), Hagers Handbuch der Pharmazeutischen Praxis, 5. Aufl., Bde 4-6 (Drogen), Springer Verlag Berlin, Heidelberg, New York, 1992-1994.

Madaus G, Lehrbuch der Biologischen Arzneimittel, Bde 1-3, Nachdruck, Georg Olms Verlag Hildesheim 1979.

Santalum Album

Sandalwood

DESCRIPTION

Medicinal Parts: The medicinal parts are the oil extracted from the trunk wood, the heartwood freed from the sapwood and the bark, and the dried wood.

Flower and Fruit: The flowers are in numerous, small, short pedicled, odorless and erect, paniculate inflorescences. There is no calyx. The perianth is 4 to 5 mm long, campanulate and changes from yellow to deep red. There are 4 stamens at the mouth of the tube, which have bushels of simple hairs at their base. The semi-inferior ovary with 3 ovules is free in the bud and later enclosed in the disc. The fruit is a round, black, pea-sized drupe with a crown made up of the perianth remains.

Leaves, Stem and Root: The plant is a small evergreen tree up to 10 m high which flowers the whole year round. It has smooth bark and pendulous branches. The leaves are opposite, 4 to 6 cm long and 2 cm wide, lanceolate, entire-margined, and matte underneath. The petiole is approximately 1 cm long.

Habitat: The tree thrives in India and is cultivated there and on Timor and the Sunda Islands.

Production: Sandalwood consists of the heartwood which has been freed from the bark and sapwood of the trunk and branches of Santalum album or Pterocarpus santalinius.

Not To Be Confused With: Other sandalwoods, i.e. the heartwood of Pterocarpus santalinus. The white sapwood, which contains almost no essential oil, is occasionally marketed as Lignum santali albi. The brownish-yellow to brown-red rootwood is, in contrast, rich in essential oil, but is disallowed as a drug by the EB6.

Other Names: Sanderswood, White Saunders, Yellow Saunders

ACTIONS AND PHARMACOLOGY

COMPOUNDS

Volatile oil (3-5%): chief components santalols (50% cis-alpha-santalol, 20% cis-beta-santalol, 4% epi-beta-santalol), further including, among others, alpha-bergamotol, alpha-bergamotal

Tannins

Resins

EFFECTS

The essential oil of sandalwood has a urinary disinfecting effect. If used in higher doses and for longer periods it can be toxic to the kidneys.

INDICATIONS AND USAGE

- Common cold
- Cough/bronchitis
- Fevers and colds
- Infections of the urinary tract
- Inflammation of the mouth and pharynx
- Liver and gallbladder complaints
- Tendency to infection

Sandalwood is used for inflammatory conditions of the efferent urinary tract. It is generally used in combination with other diuretic or urinary disinfecting drugs.

In folk medicine, the drug is used internally for heat stroke, sunstroke, and resulting fever; as an infusion mixed with honey (in Kerala); with water cooked in rice (in Nepal); in the treatment of gonorrhea and as an anti-aphrodisiac in ayurvedisic medicine.

CONTRAINDICATIONS

Sandalwood is contraindicated in diseases of the kidney parenchyma.

PRECAUTIONS AND ADVERSE REACTIONS

No health hazards are known in conjunction with the proper administration of designated therapeutic dosages. Intake can occasionally lead to skin itching, queasiness, gastrointestinal complaints, and hematuria. The drug possesses minimal potential for sensitization.

DOSAGE

Mode of Administration: Sandalwood is used internally in preparations derived from comminuted drug for decoctions and the essential oil.

Preparation: Sandalwood oil should only be taken in an enteric-coated form.

Daily Dosage: The average daily dose is 10 gm of the drug; 1 to 1.5 gm of the essential oil.

LITERATURE

Adams DR et al., (1975) Phytochemistry 14:1459.

Brunke EJ, Dragoco Rep 35:102-109. 1980.

Demole DR et al., (1976) Helv Chim Acta 59:737.

Patnikar SK, Naik CG, (1975) Tetrahedron Letters 15:1293.

Further information in:

Hänsel R, Keller K, Rimpler H, Schneider G (Hrsg.), Hagers Handbuch der Pharmazeutischen Praxis, 5. Aufl., Bde 4-6 (Drogen), Springer Verlag Berlin, Heidelberg, New York, 1992-1994.

Lewin L, Gifte und Vergiftungen, 6. Aufl., Nachdruck, Haug Verlag, Heidelberg 1992.

Madaus G, Lehrbuch der Biologischen Arzneimittel, Bde 1-3, Nachdruck, Georg Olms Verlag Hildesheim 1979.

Roth L, Daunderer M, Kormann K, Giftpflanzen, Pflanzengifte, 4. Aufl., Ecomed Fachverlag Landsberg Lech 1993.

Steinegger E, Hänsel R, Pharmakognosie, 5. Aufl., Springer Verlag Heidelberg 1992.

Wagner H, Wiesenauer M, Phytotherapie. Phytopharmaka und pflanzliche Homöopathika, Fischer-Verlag, Stuttgart, Jena, New York 1995.

Santolina Chamaecyparissias

Lavender Cotton

DESCRIPTION

Medicinal Parts: The medicinal part is the herb.

Flower and Fruit: The flower heads are 1 cm wide, almost semi-globular, long-pedicled, homogamous, yellow, and there are no lingual florets. The corolla tube is compressed and somewhat winged with a one-sided appendage. The fruit is glabrous.

Leaves, Stem and Root: The plant is an evergreen, bushy, aromatic subshrub with brittle branches. There are 4 compact rows of leaves which are small, narrow, linear, 2 to 3 cm wide, fleshy, obtuse, paired-pinate, gray-tomentose, and occasionally green.

Habitat: The plant is common in the Mediterranean region.

Production: Lavender Cotton is the aerial part of Santoline chamaecyparissus.

ACTIONS AND PHARMACOLOGY

COMPOUNDS

Volatile oil (1%): chief components artemisiaketone (3,5,6-trimethyl-1,5-heptadien-4-on), further, myrcene, alpha-pinene

Alkaloids

EFFECTS

The drug has anti-inflammatory, digestive, stimulation of menstruation, and anthelmintic effects.

INDICATIONS AND USAGE

Lavender Cotton is used for digestive disorders, PMS, worm infestation, spasmoyticum, stomach complaints, and also to treat jaundice.

PRECAUTIONS AND ADVERSE REACTIONS

No health hazards or side effects are known in conjunction with the proper administration of designated therapeutic dosages.

DOSAGE

Mode of Administration: The herb is used internally as an infusion, and externally as a moth repellant due to its strong smell.

LITERATURE

Becchi M, Carrier M, (1980) Planta Med 38(3):267.

Giner R et al., (1986) Planta Med 6:83P.

Further information in:

Kern W, List PH, Hörhammer L (Hrsg.), Hagers Handbuch der Pharmazeutischen Praxis, 4. Aufl., Bde. 1-8: Springer Verlag Berlin, Heidelberg, New York, 1969.

Saponaria Officinalis

Soapwort

DESCRIPTION

Medicinal Parts: The medicinal parts are the fresh or dried roots and the leaves harvested during the flowering season.

Flower and Fruit: The flesh-colored, sometimes white flowers in racemes have a 5-tipped fused calyx. The petals have long stems. The ovary is superior and has 1 style. The fruit is a capsule with 4 teeth at the tip which bursts open when ripe. The seeds are reniform-globular and black-brown.

Leaves, Stem and Root: The plant is a perennial. It is leafy and about 100 cm high. The stems are round, erect, and finely downy. The leaves are crossed opposite, oblong to lanceolate, acute, entire-margined, 3-veined and taper to a short petiole.

Characteristics: The plant has a weak fragrance. The leaves and root contain bitter tasting saponine and form suds when rubbed under water.

Habitat: The plant is indigenous to the temperate regions of North America, Asia, and Europe.

Production: Soapwort herb consists of the dried, above ground parts of Saponaria officinalis. Soapwort root consists of the dried root, rhizome and runner of Saponaria officinalis. White Soapwort root consists of the dried, underground parts of Gypsphila species, particularly Gypsophila paniculata. The roots of Gypsophilae radix should be dried quickly under high temperatures or in direct sunlight. The roots are cut into 2 to 5 mm thick slices to avoid a separation of the sugars from the saponines.

Not To Be Confused With: Gypsophilae radix should not be confused with Saponaria officinalis, Glycyrrhiza echinata or Bryonia alba.

Other Names: Soapwood, Soap Root, Latherwort, Bouncing Bet, Fuller's Herb, Bruisewort, Crow Soap, Sweet Betty, Wild Sweet William, Dog Cloves, Old Maids' Pink

ACTIONS AND PHARMACOLOGY

COMPOUNDS: SAPONARIAE HERBA

Triterpene saponins: chief aglycone quillaic acid

Flavonoids: including, among others, saponarine (C-glycosyl-flavone)

Ribosome-inactivating proteins (in the seeds)

EFFECTS: SAPONARIAE HERBA

No information is available.

COMPOUNDS: GYPSOPHILAE RADIX

Triterpene saponins: including chief components gypsoside A (aglycone gypsogenin) or other gypsogenin- or quillaic acid glycosides

Phytosterols

EFFECTS: GYPSOPHILAE RADIX

The drug irritates mucous membranes and effects the permeability of the intestinal wall. It is also an antibiotic and insecticidal. In high dosage, the root is cytotoxic. It also has expectorant and emetic properties.

COMPOUNDS: SAPONARIAE RUBRAE RADIX

Triterpene saponins (2-5%): deemed saponosides, chief aglycone quillaic acid

EFFECTS: SAPONARIAE RUBRAE RADIX

The drug is an expectorant by irritation of the gastric mucosa. In high concentrations, it is cytotoxic.

INDICATIONS AND USAGE

SAPONARIAE HERBA

Soapwort preparations are used as an expectorant for cough and other diseases of the respiratory tract.

GYPSOPHILAE RADIX

■ Cough/bronchitis

The drug is used in upper respiratory catarrh. In folk medicine, the drug is used for coughs and externally for chronic skin disorders, particularly eczema.

SAPONARIAE RUBRAE RADIX

■ Cough/bronchitis

The drug is used for catarrh of the upper respiratory tract. In folk medicine, the drug is used occasionally for skin disorders and rheumatic complaints.

PRECAUTIONS AND ADVERSE REACTIONS

SAPONARIAE HERBA

No health hazards are known in conjunction with the proper administration of designated therapeutic dosages. Localized skin and mucus membrane irritations are possible through the administration of larger dosages.

GYPSOPHILAE RADIX

Health risks following the proper administration of designated therapeutic dosages are not recorded, gastric complaints may appear in isolated cases.

SAPONARIAE RUBRAE RADIX

No health hazards or side effects are known in conjunction with the proper administration of designated therapeutic dosages. In rare cases, intake leads to gastric irritation.

DOSAGE

GYPSOPHILAE RADIX

Mode of Administration: Comminuted drug for infusions, gypsophila saponin and other galenic preparations for internal use.

Daily Dosage: The average daily dose of the drug is 1.5 gm.

SAPONARIAE RUBRAE RADIX

Mode of Administration: Comminuted herb for teas and other galenic preparations for internal use. Drug extracts are contained in a few standardized preparations of antitussives.

Preparation: To prepare an infusion, use 0.4 gm of medium fine cut drug as a decoction. (1 teaspoonful = 2.6 gm of the drug).

Daily Dosage: The average daily dose is 30 to 150 mg of the drug corresponding to 3 to 15 mg of saponin.

LITERATURE

SAPONARIAE HERBA

Kern W, List PH, Hörhammer L (Hrsg.), Hagers Handbuch der Pharmazeutischen Praxis, 4. Aufl., Bde 1-8: Springer Verlag Berlin, Heidelberg, New York, 1969.

Madaus G, Lehrbuch der Biologischen Arzneimittel, Bde 1-3, Nachdruck, Georg Olms Verlag Hildesheim 1979.

GYPSOPHILAE RADIX

Kochetkov NK et al., Tetrahedron:477-482. 1963.

Mostad HB, Doehl J, J Chromatogr 396:157-168. 1987.

Further information in:

Hänsel R, Keller K, Rimpler H, Schneider G (Hrsg.), Hagers Handbuch der Pharmazeutischen Praxis, 5. Aufl., Bde 4-6 (Drogen), Springer Verlag Berlin, Heidelberg, New York, 1992-1994.

Madaus G, Lehrbuch der Biologischen Arzneimittel, Bde 1-3, Nachdruck, Georg Olms Verlag Hildesheim 1979.

Steinegger E, Hänsel R, Pharmakognosie, 5. Aufl., Springer Verlag Heidelberg 1992.

SAPONARIAE RUBRAE RADIX

Carzaniga R et al., Planta 194:461. 1994.

Henry M et al., Plantes Med Phytothér 15:192. 1981.

Further information in:

Kern W, List PH, Hörhammer L (Hrsg.), Hagers Handbuch der Pharmazeutischen Praxis, 4. Aufl., Bde. 1-8: Springer Verlag Berlin, Heidelberg, New York, 1969.

Lewin L, Gifte und Vergiftungen, 6. Aufl., Nachdruck, Haug Verlag, Heidelberg 1992.

Madaus G, Lehrbuch der Biologischen Arzneimittel, Bde 1-3, Nachdruck, Georg Olms Verlag Hildesheim 1979.

Roth L, Daunderer M, Kormann K: Giftpflanzen, Pflanzengifte, 4. Aufl., Ecomed Fachverlag Landsberg Lech 1993.

Teuscher E, Biogene Arzneimittel, 5. Aufl., Wiss. Verlagsges. Stuttgart 1997.

Wichtl M (Hrsg.), Teedrogen, 4. Aufl., Wiss. Verlagsges. Stuttgart 1997.

Sarracenia Purpurea

Pitcher Plant

DESCRIPTION

Medicinal Parts: The medicinal parts are the leaves and roots.

Flower and Fruit: The androgynous flowers usually have numerous stamens and a large 3- to 5-valved superior ovary. The style spreads into a wide, stemmed umbrella, which spreads over the stamens. The 5 stigma sit as small cone-like structures on the underside of the roof of the tips. There are numerous marginal ovules on individual axillary shafts. The fruit is a valved capsule. The small, membranous, thin-skinned seeds contain plenty of endosperm.

Leaves, Stem and Root: Sarracenia pupurea is a strange, perennial plant whose leaves, which are in a basal rosette, change into a tube or beaker-like formation, which bears a long wing-like strip on the side turned towards the stem. These beakers are often very colorful and fill up with rainwater and insects. During hot weather they are closed because of a concentration of fibers. The enclosed rainwater and insects form a mass, which probably acts as a fertilizer and has a strong odor.

Habitat: The plant is indigenous to the U.S.

Other Names: Eve's Cups, Fly-catcher, Fly-trap, Huntsman's Cup, Purple Side-saddle Flower, Side-saddle Plant, Water-cup, Smallpox plant

ACTIONS AND PHARMACOLOGY

COMPOUNDS

Piperidine alkaloids: coniine, gamma-conicein (particularly in the trapping fluid of the pitcher leaves)

EFFECTS

The active agents are sarracenia acid, tannin, resin, and the alkaloid sarracenin, which is similar to veratrin. The drug has stomachic, diuretic, and laxative effects.

INDICATIONS AND USAGE

Pitcher plant was formerly used for digestive disorders, particularly constipation, also for urinary tract diseases, and as a cure for smallpox.

PRECAUTIONS AND ADVERSE REACTIONS

No health hazards or side effects are known in conjunction with the proper administration of designated therapeutic dosages.

DOSAGE

Mode of Administration: Today, Radix and Folia Sarraceniae are completely obsolete.

LITERATURE

Foder GB, Colasenko B, In: Alkaloids, Vol. 3, Ed. SW Pelletier, Pub. John Wiley 1985.

Further information in:

Kern W, List PH, Hörhammer L (Hrsg.), Hagers Handbuch der Pharmazeutischen Praxis, 4. Aufl., Bde. 1-8: Springer Verlag Berlin, Heidelberg, New York, 1969.

Teuscher E, Lindequist U, Biogene Gifte - Biologie, Chemie, Pharmakologie, 2. Aufl., Fischer Verlag Stuttgart 1994.

Sarsaparilla

See Smilax Species

Sassafras Albidum

Sassafras

DESCRIPTION

Medicinal Parts: The medicinal parts are the essential oil of the root wood, the peeled and dried root bark, and the root wood.

Flower and Fruit: The flowers appear before the leaves. They are dioecious, small and yellowish, and form loose cymes. The perigone has 6 tepals. The male flower has 6 filaments and the female has 1 ovate ovary and 6 bent stamens. The fruit is a pea-sized, oval drupe which when ripe is dark blue in the beaker-shaped receptacle.

Leaves, Stem and Root: Sassafras albidum is a deciduous tree up to 30 m tall with numerous thin branches. The bark of the trunk and of the thicker branches is rough, deeply grooved, and grayish. The bark of the outer branches is green. The alternate leaves are petiolate and 7 to 12 cm long. Some are simple ovate, others deeply 2 or 3 lobed. The root bark is a bright, rust-brown color, in irregular pieces, soft, brittle and corky, in distinct layers, showing numerous oil glands. The root itself is brownish-white, showing clear concentric rings traversed by narrow medullary rays.

Characteristics: The taste is sweet and slightly astringent and the odor is pleasant and aromatic.

Habitat: The plant is common to eastern North America, Mexico, and Taiwan.

Production: Sassafras wood is the root woods of Sassafras albidium. Woody, thick roots (up to 20 cm) are dug up in autumn, then shredded, cut or sawn into cubes.

Not To Be Confused With: The wood and bark of the trunk. The wood can be recognized by its annual ring growth and marrow; the bark has calculus and primary fibers. Trunk wood and bark have little smell or taste.

Other Names: Ague Tree, Cinnamon Wood, Saxifrax, Sassafrax

ACTIONS AND PHARMACOLOGY

COMPOUNDS

Volatile oil (6-9%): chief components safrole (up to 90%), 5-methoxyeugenol (up to 30%), asarone (up to 18%), camphor (up to 5%)

Isoquinoline alkaloids: of the aporphine and reticuline type (less than 0.1%)

EFFECTS

The drug has a mild diuretic effect (uncertain). Toxic characteristics are regulated by sassafras aetheroleum.

INDICATIONS AND USAGE

Sassafras is used for disorders of the urinary tract. The drug was a former ingredient of ''blood-cleaning tea'', has also been used for skin disorders, catarrh, rheumatism, and syphilis (unproven).

PRECAUTIONS AND ADVERSE REACTIONS

Because of the carcinogenic effect of the safrole, neither the drug nor its volatile oil should be administered.

DOSAGE

Mode of Administration: The drug is a constituent of tea mixtures.

Preparation: To prepare an infusion, add 50 gm of the drug to 1 liter of water. To prepare tea, 1 teaspoon (3 gm) is added to boiling water, strain after 10 minutes.

Storage: Keep in metal containers, wood must be kept dry so as to retain smell and taste.

LITERATURE

Albert K, Sassafrasöl zum Abtanzen? In: PZ 142(11):878. 1997.

Borchet P et al., (1973) Cancer Res 33:575.

Brophy JJ, Goldsack RJ, House APN, Lassak EV, J Ess Oil Res 5:117-122. 1993.

Chowdhury BK et al., (1976) Phytochemistry 15:1803.

Kamdem DP et al., Chemical composition of essential oil from the root bark of Sassafras albidum. In: PM 61(6):574-575. 1995.

Kampen KR van, Sudan grass and sorghum poisoning of horse: a possible lathyrogenic disease. In: J Am Vet Medic Assoc 156, 629-630. 1970.

Miller EC et al., (1983) Cancer Res 43:1124.

Segelman AB et al., (1976) J Am Med Ass 236:477.

Sethi ML et al., (1976) Phytochemistry 15:1773.

Further information in:

Frohne D, Pfänder HJ, Giftpflanzen - Ein Handbuch für Apotheker, Toxikologen und Biologen, 4. Aufl., Wiss. Verlags-Ges. Stuttgart 1997.

Hänsel R, Keller K, Rimpler H, Schneider G (Hrsg.), Hagers Handbuch der Pharmazeutischen Praxis, 5. Aufl., Bde 4-6 (Drogen), Springer Verlag Berlin, Heidelberg, New York, 1992-1994.

Lewin L, Gifte und Vergiftungen, 6. Aufl., Nachdruck, Haug Verlag, Heidelberg 1992.

Madaus G, Lehrbuch der Biologischen Arzneimittel, Bde 1-3, Nachdruck, Georg Olms Verlag Hildesheim 1979.

Roth L, Daunderer M, Kormann K, Giftpflanzen, Pflanzengifte, 4. Aufl., Ecomed Fachverlag Landsberg Lech 1993.

Steinegger E, Hänsel R, Pharmakognosie, 5. Aufl., Springer Verlag Heidelberg 1992.

Teuscher E, Lindequist U, Biogene Gifte - Biologie, Chemie, Pharmakologie, 2. Aufl., Fischer Verlag Stuttgart 1994.

Wichtl M (Hrsg.), Teedrogen, 4. Aufl., Wiss. Verlagsges. Stuttgart 1997.

Satureja Hortensis

Savory

DESCRIPTION

Medicinal Parts: The medicinal part is the fresh or dried plant harvested during the flowering stage.

Flower and Fruit: The lilac or whitish labiate flowers are in axillary, 5-blossomed, false whorls. The calyx is tubular-campanulate, regular, and has 5 tips. The corolla does not have a ring of hair. The upper lip is straight and margined. The lower lip is divided in 3 and red-spotted at the mouth of the tube.

Leaves, Stem and Root: The plant is a herb, 30 to 45 cm in height with erect, heavily branched, and shortly pubescent stems. The leaves are crossed opposite, up to 3 cm long, short-petioled, lanceolate to linear-lanceolate, entire-margined, thickish, with a ciliate margin, and glandular punctate on both surfaces.

Characteristics: The smell is spicy and the taste is spicy and peppery.

Habitat: The plant is indigenous to southern Europe and northern Africa and is extensively cultivated.

Production: Savory is the aerial part of Satureja hortensis.

Other Names: Bean Herb

ACTIONS AND PHARMACOLOGY

COMPOUNDS

Volatile oil (0.2-3.0%): chief components carvacrol (30%), p-cymene (20-30%), alpha-thujene, alpha-pinene, beta-myrcene, alpha- and beta-terpinene, beta-caryophyllene, thymol

Tannins (4-8%)

EFFECTS

The tannin content of the drug provides astringent qualities. It has a mild antiseptic effect due to the presence of cymol and carvacrol in the essential oil.

INDICATIONS AND USAGE

Savory is used for acute gastrointestinal enteritis.

PRECAUTIONS AND ADVERSE REACTIONS

No health hazards or side effects are known in conjunction with the proper administration of designated therapeutic dosages.

DOSAGE

Mode of Administration: The drug is used internally as an infusion that is prepared from ground plant.

Daily Dosage: Three teaspoons of the drug in the form of a hot drink to be taken daily, do not boil but leave the tea to draw.

LITERATURE

Herisset A et al., (1974) Plant Med Phytother 8(4):306, 287.

Opdyke DLJ (1976) Food Cosmet Toxicol: 14.

Further information in:

Kern W, List PH, Hörhammer L (Hrsg.), Hagers Handbuch der Pharmazeutischen Praxis, 4. Aufl., Bde 1-8: Springer Verlag Berlin, Heidelberg, New York, 1969.

Leung AY: Encyclopedia of Common Natural Ingredients Used in Food Drugs, Cosmetics, John Wiley & Sons Inc., New York 1980.

Madaus G: Lehrbuch der Biologischen Arzneimittel, Bde 1-3, Nachdruck, Georg Olms Verlag Hildesheim 1979.

Savin Tops

See Juniperus Sabina

Savory

See Satureja Hortensis

Saw Palmetto

See Serenoa Repens

Scabiosa Succisa

Premorse

DESCRIPTION

Medicinal Parts: The medicinal part is the dried herb.

Flower and Fruit: The flowers are purple-blue, globular and long pedicled composite blooms, with a 2 to 3 rowed involucre. The florets are all the same size. The epicalyx has thorn-tipped teeth and the calyx has 5 bristles. The corolla is fused and has 4 tips. There are 4 stamens and 1 inferior ovary. The fruit is a nutlet.

Leaves, Stem and Root: The plant grows from 15 to 80 cm high. It has a short, finger-thick rhizome, which looks bitten off. In the first year of growth, the root resembles a carrot. Later it becomes woody and dies off except for the upper part, which accounts for its appearance. The remaining upper part then develops lateral roots. The stem is erect, sparsely branched, pubescent and has few leaves. The basal leaves are petiolate, oblong and obtuse. The cauline leaves are narrow and acute.

Habitat: Scabiosae succisae is indigenous to all of Europe.

Production: Premorse is the aerial part of Scabiosa succisa.

Other Names: Devil's Bit, Ofbit, Premorse Scaboius

ACTIONS AND PHARMACOLOGY

COMPOUNDS

Iridoide monoterpenes: including, among others, dipsacan, cephalaroside (structures unknown)

Saponins

Tannins

Flavonoids: including, among others, saponarine (C-glycosyl-flavone)

Triterpenes: including, among others, ursolic acid

EFFECTS

Premorse is a febrifuge and a diaphoretic.

INDICATIONS AND USAGE

The herb is used for febrile colds and coughs.

PRECAUTIONS AND ADVERSE REACTIONS

No health hazards or side effects are known in conjunction with the proper administration of designated therapeutic dosages.

DOSAGE

Mode of Administration: The herb is ground as a drug for infusion.

LITERATURE

Hegnauer R, Chemotaxonomie der Pflanzen, Bde 1-11: Birkhäuser Verlag Basel, Boston, Berlin 1962-1997.

Kern W, List PH, Hörhammer L (Hrsg.), Hagers Handbuch der Pharmazeutischen Praxis, 4. Aufl., Bde 1-8: Springer Verlag Berlin, Heidelberg, New York, 1969 (unter Succisa pratensis).

Madaus G, Lehrbuch der Biologischen Arzneimittel, Bde 1-3, Nachdruck, Georg Olms Verlag Hildesheim 1979.

Scarlet Pimpernel

See Anagallis Arvensis

Scolopendrium Vulgare

Hartstongue

DESCRIPTION

Medicinal Parts: The medicinal part is the frond.

Flower and Fruit: On the under surface of the fronds there are 2 rows of large sporangia lying almost horizontally whose long film stretches towards the margin.

Leaves, Stem and Root: The plant is an evergreen fern with long, wide, simple, short-petioled, and dark green fronds. They are arranged in clusters, broad linear-lanceolate, 2-lobed cordate at the base, acuminate higher up, and have a sinuate margin. The stem is covered in brown, almost hair-like scales. The root is bushy, short and sturdy.

Habitat: The plant is indigenous to almost all of Europe, North America, northern Africa, eastern Asia, and southwest and eastern Asia.

Production: Hartstongue is the aerial part of Scolopendrium vulgare.

Other Names: Hind's Tongue, Horse Tongue, Buttonhole, God's-hair

ACTIONS AND PHARMACOLOGY

COMPOUNDS

Tannins

Mucilage

Flavonoids: including, among others, kaempferol-7-rhamnoside-3-coffeoyl-7-diglucoside

Thiaminase (likely only in the fresh plant)

Sugars: saccharose, invert sugar

EFFECTS

Hartstongue is a diuretic and an aperient agent.

INDICATIONS AND USAGE

Hartstongue is used for digestive disorders and urinary tract diseases.

PRECAUTIONS AND ADVERSE REACTIONS

No health hazards or side effects are known in conjunction with the proper administration of designated therapeutic dosages.

DOSAGE

Mode of Administration: Hartstongue is used internally as an infusion.

LITERATURE

Hegnauer R, Chemotaxonomie der Pflanzen, Bde 1-11: Birkhäuser Verlag Basel, Boston, Berlin 1962-1997.

Kern W, List PH, Hörhammer L (Hrsg.), Hagers Handbuch der Pharmazeutischen Praxis, 4. Aufl., Bde 1-8: Springer Verlag Berlin, Heidelberg, New York, 1969 (unter Phyllitis scolopendrium).

Madaus G, Lehrbuch der Biologischen Arzneimittel, Bde 1-3, Nachdruck, Georg Olms Verlag Hildesheim 1979.

Scopolia

See Scopolia Carniolica

Scopolia Carniolica

Scopolia

DESCRIPTION

Medicinal Parts: The medicinal part is the dried rhizome.

Flower and Fruit: The nodding flowers are solitary and axillary on long bending pedicles. The calyx is campanulate with obtuse tips. The corolla is tubular-campanulate, glossy brown outside, and matte olive-green inside. The anthers are large and yellowish. The fruit is a 2-valved pixidium. The seeds are 3 to 4 mm long, brown-yellow, and bumpy.

Leaves, Stem and Root: The plant is perennial, erect, and grows from 30 to 60 cm high. The rhizome is horizontal, slightly bent and almost cylindrical. The rhizome grows up to 12 cm long and 5 cm thick, and is covered in tough, loose-skinned fibers. The color varies between yellowish brown to dark brownish gray. The stems bear scale-like stipules at the base which are bifurcated, fleshy, glabrous or with scattered hairs. The foliage leaves are petiolate, obovate, entire, dull green, and 12 cm by 4 to 9 cm.

Characteristics: The taste is initially sweetish, then bitter and biting, odorless.

Habitat: The plant is indigenous to southern Germany, Austria, Hungary, and southwest Russia.

Production: Scopola root consists of the dried rhizome of Scopolia carniolica.

Other Names: Scopola, Japanese Belladonna, Belladonna Scopola

ACTIONS AND PHARMACOLOGY

COMPOUNDS

Tropane alkaloids (0.2-0.5%): chief alkaloid (-)-hyoscyamine, under drying conditions changing over to some extent into atropine, further including among others scopolamine

Hydroxycoumarins: including among others scopoletins, scopoline

Caffeic acid derivatives: chlorogenic acids

EFFECTS

The drug acts as a parasympatholytic/anticholinergic via competitive antagonism of the neuromuscular transmitter acetylcholine. This antagonism affects more the muscarine-like effect of acetylcholine, less the nicotine-like effects at the ganglions and the neuromuscular end-plate. Scopolia root displays peripheral effects targeted on the vegetative nervous system and the smooth muscles, as well as central nervous effects. Because of its parasympatholytic properties, scopolia root relaxes the smooth muscle organs and eliminates spastic conditions, especially of the gastrointestinal tract and the bile ducts.

Conditions of muscular tremors and muscular rigidity, caused by central nervous impulses, are alleviated. The action on the heart is positively chronotropic and positively dromotropic.

INDICATIONS AND USAGE

■ Liver and gallbladder complaints

The drug is used for spasms of the gastrointestinal tract, bile ducts, and urinary tract for adults and for children over 6 years of age.

CONTRAINDICATIONS

The drug is contraindicated in angle-closure glaucoma, prostatic adenoma with residual urine, tachycardias, mechanical stenoses in the area of the gastrointestinal tract, and megacolon.

PRECAUTIONS AND ADVERSE REACTIONS

General: No health hazards are known in conjunction with the proper administration of designated therapeutic dosages. Accommodation disorders, heat build-up through decline in sweat secretion, micturition disorders, and obstipation can occur as side effects, particularly with overdosages.

Drug Interactions: Increased effectiveness of simultaneously administered tricyclic antidepressants, amantadine, and quinidine.

OVERDOSAGE

The four early warning symptoms of a poisoning are skin reddening, dryness of the mouth, and tachycardiac arrhythmias. Accommodation disorders, heat build-up through decline in mydriasis, sweat secretion, micturition disorders, and obstipation also occur with overdosage.

The intake of very high dosages leads to central excitation (restlessness, compulsive speech, hallucinations, delirium, manic episodes, followed by exhaustion and sleep). Lethal dosages include the danger of asphyxiation (for adults starting at 100 mg atropine, depending upon alkaloid content, between 20 to 50 gm of the drug, considerably less for children).

The treatment for poisonings includes gastric lavage, temperature-lowering measures with wet cloths (no antipyretics!), oxygen respiration for respiratory distress, intubation, parenteral physostigmine salts as antidote, diazepam for spasms and chlorpormazine for severe excitation.

DOSAGE

Mode of Administration: Comminuted root, powder, and other galenic preparations for oral application.

Daily Dosage: The average daily dose is equivalent to 0.25 mg of total alkaloids, calculated as hyoscyamine. The maximum single dose is equivalent to 1.0 mg of total alkaloids, calculated as hyoscyamine. The maximum daily dose is equivalent to 3.0 mg of total alkaloids, calculated as hyoscyamine.

LITERATURE

Nicolic R et al., Acta Pharm Jugosl 26:257. 1976.

Smart RG et al., J Forens Sci 32:303. 1987.

Further information in:

Frohne D, Pfänder HJ, Giftpflanzen - Ein Handbuch für Apotheker, Toxikologen und Biologen, 4. Aufl., Wiss. Verlags-Ges. Stuttgart 1997.

Kern W, List PH, Hörhammer L (Hrsg.), Hagers Handbuch der Pharmazeutischen Praxis, 4. Aufl., Bde. 1-8: Springer Verlag Berlin, Heidelberg, New York, 1969.

Lewin L, Gifte und Vergiftungen, 6. Aufl., Nachdruck, Haug Verlag, Heidelberg 1992.

Roth L, Daunderer M, Kormann K, Giftpflanzen, Pflanzengifte, 4. Aufl., Ecomed Fachverlag Landsberg Lech 1993.

Teuscher E, Lindequist U, Biogene Gifte - Biologie, Chemie, Pharmakologie, 2. Aufl., Fischer Verlag Stuttgart 1994.

Scotch Pine

See Pinus Sylvestris

Scotch Thistle

See Onopordum Acanthium

Scrophularia Nodosa

Figwort

DESCRIPTION

Medicinal Parts: The medicinal parts are the dried herb harvested before flowering, the herb with the root, and the root alone.

Flower and Fruit: The red-brown or greenish-yellow flowers are in terminal panicles. The calyx has 5 segments. The corolla is a bilabiate, swollen, almost globular tube. The upper lip is divided into 2 and the lower lip is 3-lobed with revolute lobes. There are 4 stamens and 1 superior ovary. The fruit is an ovate, many-seeded, and pointed green capsule.

Leaves, Stem and Root: The perennial plant grows from 50 to 100 cm high. The roots have tuberous nodes. The stem is erect, sharply quadrangular, often purple, glabrous, and has a row of hairs at the nodes. The leaves are crossed opposite, dark green, oblong, double serrate, and often cordate at the base.

Habitat: The plant is indigenous to Europe, central Asia, and North America.

Other Names: Throatwort, Carpenter's Square, Kernelwort, Heal-all, Scrofula Plant, Rosenoble

ACTIONS AND PHARMACOLOGY

COMPOUNDS

Iridoide monoterpenes

Flavonoids: including, among others, diosmin

Tannins

Saponins

EFFECTS

Figwort has a diuretic and mild laxative effect (no new research is available on the effects).

INDICATIONS AND USAGE

In homeopathy, the drug is used for low resistance, chronic tonsillitis, and tonsillar hypertony as well as lymph edema.

PRECAUTIONS AND ADVERSE REACTIONS

No health hazards or side effects are known in conjunction with the proper administration of designated therapeutic dosages.

DOSAGE

Preparation: In homeopathic preparations, the mother tincture is derived from the whole figwort plant in dilutions.

Daily Dosage: The average dose is 15 to 20 drops, to be taken 3 times daily. The drug may be administered by injection when long term treatment is used.

LITERATURE

Inouye H et al., (1974) Planta Med 25:285.

Jerznanowska Z, Pijewska L, (1954) Acta Polon. Pharm 11:1 (via CA 48:11000).

Kato Y, (1946) Folia Pharmacol Jap. 42:37 (via CA 47:1843)

Pauli GF, Ofterdinger-Daegel, S, Teborg D, Digitalis, Scrophularia & Co. In: DAZ 135(2):111.1995.

Pethes E et al., (1973) Herba Hung 12:101.

Swann K, Melville C, (1972) J Pharm Pharmacol 24:170P.

Weinges K, Von der Eltz H, (1978) Justus Liebigs Ann Chem 1968.

Further information in:

Hegnauer R, Chemotaxonomie der Pflanzen, Bde 1-11: Birkhäuser Verlag Basel, Boston, Berlin 1962-1997.

Kern W, List PH, Hörhammer L (Hrsg.), Hagers Handbuch der Pharmazeutischen Praxis, 4. Aufl., Bde 1-8: Springer Verlag Berlin, Heidelberg, New York, 1969.

Madaus G, Lehrbuch der Biologischen Arzneimittel, Bde 1-3, Nachdruck, Georg Olms Verlag Hildesheim 1979.

Wagner H, Wiesenauer M, Phytotherapie. Phytopharmaka und pflanzliche Homöopathika, Fischer-Verlag, Stuttgart, Jena, New York 1995.

Scullcap

See Scutellaria Lateriflora

Scurvy Grass

See Cochlearia Officinalis

Scutellaria Lateriflora

Scullcap

DESCRIPTION

Medicinal Parts: The medicinal part is the pulverized herb of the 3 to 4-year-old plant which is harvested in June.

Flower and Fruit: The pink to blue flowers are in short lateral false spikes. The calyx is fluffy, dorsiventral, flattened with 2 rounded, entire lips. The lower lip has a helmet-shaped, concave appendage. There are 4 ascending stamens with pairs of ciliated anthers. The fruit is a globular to flattened-ovoid warty nut.

Leaves, Stem and Root: The plant is a perennial herb up to 60 cm in height covered thickly with simple and glandular hairs. The stem is erect and heavily branched. The foliage leaves are usually ovate to lanceolate or linear, petioled, entire-margined or crenate.

Characteristics: The herb has a bitter, slightly astringent taste.

Habitat: The plant is indigenous to North America and is cultivated in Europe.

Production: Scullcap is the aerial part of Scutellaria lateriflora.

Other Names: Blue Pimpernel, Helmet Flower, Hoodwort, Mad-dog Weed, Madweed, Quaker Bonnet

ACTIONS AND PHARMACOLOGY

COMPOUNDS

Tridoide monoterpenes

Flavonoids: including among others scutellarin

Volatile oil

Tannins

EFFECTS

The active agents in the leaves are scutellarin, essential oil as well as fatty oil, tannin, and resin. Scullcap has sedative, antispasmodic (little research), anti-inflammatory, and also lipid peroxidation inhibitor effects.

INDICATIONS AND USAGE

The drug was formerly used for hysteria and nervous tension, epilepsy, chorea, and other nervous disorders. It has also been used as a bitter tonic and febrifuge.

PRECAUTIONS AND ADVERSE REACTIONS

No health hazards or side effects are known in conjunction with the proper administration of designated therapeutic dosages.

DOSAGE

Mode of Administration: The herb is available as a powder and liquid extract for internal use.

LITERATURE

Barberan FAT, (1986) Fitoterapia 57(2):67.

Kimura Y et al., (1984) Planta Med 50:290.

Kimura Y et al., (1985) Planta Med 51:132.

Kimura Y et al., (1987) Phytother Res 1(1):48.

Kooiman P, (1972) Acta Bot Neerl. 21(4):417.

Kubo M et al., (1984) Chem Pharm Bull 32(7):2724.

Nicollier GF et al., (1981) J Agric Food Chem 29:1179.

Takido M et al., (1979) Yakugaku Zasshi 99(4):443-444.

Yagma, MS, Benson GG, (1979) J Nat Prod 42(2):229.

Further information in:

Chang, EH et al. (Eds.), Advances in Chinese Medicinal Materials Research, World Scientific Pub. Co. Singapore 1985.

Kern W, List PH, Hörhammer L (Hrsg.), Hagers Handbuch der Pharmazeutischen Praxis, 4. Aufl., Bde 1-8: Springer Verlag Berlin, Heidelberg, New York, 1969.

Madaus G, Lehrbuch der Biologischen Arzneimittel, Bde 1-3, Nachdruck, Georg Olms Verlag Hildesheim 1979.

Sea Buckthorn

See Hippophaë Rhamnoides

Sedum Acre

Common Stonecrop

DESCRIPTION

Medicinal Parts: The medicinal parts are the fresh or dried aerial parts collected during the flowering season.

Flower and Fruit: The flowers are leafy, twining cymes on short pedicles. There are 5 ovate sepals and 5 petals which are 7 to 9 mm long, lanceolate, twice as long as the calyx and golden yellow. The fruit is a follicle, which splits after flowering, forming a 5-rayed star. They are 3 to 5 mm long and have numerous seeds.

Leaves, Stem and Root: The plant is perennial and 2 to 15 cm high. It has many heavily branched shoots, which often creep underground, forming grass. The leaves are thick, fleshy, almost round, acute, appressed, domed, rounded at the base and without any spur-like appendage.

Characteristics: The taste is slimy-hot and pepper-like.

Habitat: Sedum acre is common to all of Europe, western Siberia, the Caucasus region and North America.

Production: The flowering parts are picked when in bloom, then sun-dried, or dried using artificial heat.

Other Names: Wallpepper, Golden Moss, Wall Ginger, Bird Bread, Prick Madam, Gold Chain, Creeping Tom, Mousetail, Jach-of-the-Buttery

ACTIONS AND PHARMACOLOGY

COMPOUNDS

Piperidine alkaloids (0.3%): chief alkaloids are sedacrin, sedamin, sedinine, sedinon

Flavonoids: including, among others, glycosides of isorhamnetin, quercetin, limnocitrin

Tannins (10%)

Arbutin

EFFECTS

Investigation has shown no clinical use for Stonecrop.

INDICATIONS AND USAGE

The drug is used internally for coughs (Spain) and high blood pressure (central Europe). Externally, it is used for wounds, ulcers resulting from burns, hemorrhoids, warts, eczema, and oral ulcers.

CONTRAINDICATIONS

The drug should not to be administered in the presence of inflammatory diseases of the gastrointestinal tract and of the urinary drainage passages.

PRECAUTIONS AND ADVERSE REACTIONS

No health hazards or side effects are known in conjunction with the proper administration of designated therapeutic dosages.

OVERDOSAGE

Dosages over 10 gm of the juice or 1 to 3.5 gm of the dried foliage of the fresh plant are said to bring about queasiness, vomiting, and diarrhea. Cases of poisoning have however not been recorded in recent times.

DOSAGE

Daily Dosage: The average daily dose of the drug as a decoction (1 teaspoonful in 1 cup of water) is 3 gm (approximately 2 teaspoonfuls).

Externally for eczema and warts, the fresh plants are crushed and placed on the skin.

LITERATURE

Francis LPS, Francis GW, PM 32:268-274. 1977.

Halin F et al., Tetrahedron 41:2891. 1985.

Hootele C et al., Tetrahedron 41:5563. 1985.

Niklon B et al., Acta Pharm Jugosl 40:555. 1980.

Van der Wal R et al., PM 43:97. 1981.

Further information in:

Frohne D, Pfänder HJ, Giftpflanzen - Ein Handbuch für Apotheker, Toxikologen und Biologen, 4. Aufl., Wiss. Verlags-Ges. Stuttgart 1997.

Hänsel R, Keller K, Rimpler H, Schneider G (Hrsg.), Hagers Handbuch der Pharmazeutischen Praxis, 5. Aufl., Bde 4-6 (Drogen): Springer Verlag Berlin, Heidelberg, New York, 1992-1994.

Lewin L, Gifte und Vergiftungen, 6. Aufl., Nachdruck, Haug Verlag, Heidelberg 1992.

Madaus G, Lehrbuch der Biologischen Arzneimittel, Bde 1-3, Nachdruck, Georg Olms Verlag Hildesheim 1979.

Roth L, Daunderer M, Kormann K, Giftpflanzen, Pflanzengifte, 4. Aufl., Ecomed Fachverlag Landsberg Lech 1993.

Teuscher E, Lindequist U, Biogene Gifte - Biologie, Chemie, Pharmakologie, 2. Aufl., Fischer Verlag Stuttgart 1994.

Selenicereus Grandiflorus

Night-Blooming Cereus

DESCRIPTION

Medicinal Parts: The medicinal parts are the fresh or dried flowers and the fresh young stems and flowers and the fresh young shoots.

Flower and Fruit: The flowers are 18 to 25 cm long and have a diameter of 15 to 27 cm. They have numerous, long-acute, lanceolate tepals. The outer tepals are brown; the middle ones are light yellow and the inner ones are spatulate to acute, lanceolate and snow white. The numerous stamens are white and have yellow anthers. The styles, with the 4-rayed stigmas, become yellow towards the top. The ovary is globular and bumpy, with triangular scales and many brownish gray hairs and thorns, which are approximately 10 mm long, dark brown and bristly.

Leaves, Stem and Root: The plant has a succulent trunk. There is a snake-like, creeping or climbing branched stem, which is 4 to 8 sided or 5 to 6 sided. The stem can grow to 10 m. It is green to bluish, has no bumps and is covered in adventitious roots. The stem has white tomentose axis buds on the protruding vertical ribs with 6 to 11 needle-like, 4-6 mm-long thorns.

Characteristics: The plant has sweet-smelling flowers which only bloom for about 6 hours before wilting.

Habitat: The plant is indigenous to Central America and is cultivated mainly in Mexico.

Production: The plant is cultivated in greenhouses. The young shoots and flowers are harvested in June/July and then conserved in alcohol.

Not To Be Confused With: The flowers of Opuntia maxima, Selenicereus hamatus, and Selenicereus pteranthus. The drug is confused commercially with the flowers of Opuntia vilgaris and Opuntia ficus-indica.

Other Names: Sweet-scented Cactus

ACTIONS AND PHARMACOLOGY

COMPOUNDS

Flavonoids (1.5%): including among others, narcissin, rutin, cacticine, kaempferitine, grandiflorin, hyperoside

Amines (in the shoots): chief components are hordenine (cactine), tyramine, N-methyltyramine

Betacyans: (in the blossoms, yellow pigments)

EFFECTS
The drug has a digitalis effect, which includes cardiac stimulation, coronary and peripheral vessel dilation. The drug stimulates the motor neurons of the spinal cord. In addition, the drug may act topically as an antiphlogistic, but this is unproven.

INDICATIONS AND USAGE
Preparations of Selenicereus grandiflorus are used for nervous cardiac disorders, angina pectoris, stenocardia, and urinary ailments.

In folk medicine, the drug is used internally for hemoptysis, menorrhagia, dysmenorrhea, hemorrhage and as an infusion for cardiac complaints (Mexico). The juice of the whole plant is used for cystitis, shortness of breath and dropsy (Central America). Externally, it is used as a skin stimulant for rheumatism (Central America and Mexico).

PRECAUTIONS AND ADVERSE REACTIONS
No health hazards or side effects are known in conjunction with the proper administration of designated therapeutic dosages. The fresh juice is said to cause itching and pustules on the skin, and burning of the mouth, queasiness, vomiting and diarrhea following intake.

DOSAGE
Mode of Administration: Preparations are used internally and externally.

Preparations: Fluid extract (Extractum Cerei liquidum 1:1) and Tinctura Cerei (1:4) BPC 34.

Daily Dosage: For the folk medicine dosages, a liquid extract is used in doses up to 0.6 ml, one to 10 times daily. The tincture dosage is 0.12 to 2 ml taken 2 to 3 times daily. For tincture in sweetened water (1:10), 10 drops, 3 to 5 times daily.

LITERATURE

Willaman JJ, Schubert BG (1961) Tech. Bull 1234: USDA Washington DC.

Further information in:

Hänsel R, Keller K, Rimpler H, Schneider G (Hrsg.), Hagers Handbuch der Pharmazeutischen Praxis, 5. Aufl., Bde 4-6 (Drogen): Springer Verlag Berlin, Heidelberg, New York, 1992-1994.

Madaus G: Lehrbuch der Biologischen Arzneimittel, Bde 1-3, Nachdruck, Georg Olms Verlag Hildesheim 1979 (unter Cactus grandiflorus).

Roth L, Daunderer M, Kormann K, Giftpflanzen, Pflanzengifte, 4.Aufl., Ecomed Fachverlag Landsberg Lech 1993.

Wagner H, Wiesenauer M, Phytotherapie. Phytopharmaka und pflanzliche Homöopathika, Fischer-Verlag, Stuttgart, Jena, New York 1995.

Self-Heal

See Prunella Vulgaris

Sempervivum Tectorum

Houseleek

DESCRIPTION
Medicinal Parts: The medicinal parts are the fresh leaves before flowering and their juice.

Flower and Fruit: The pink or red flowers are in cymes on their own peduncles, which are about 22 cm high. The individual flowers are short-pedicled and splayed in a star shape. The 12 sepals and petals are twice as long as the calyx. The 24 stamens are in 2 circles. There are 24 ovaries. The small fruit is many-seeded and fused at the base.

Leaves, Stem and Root: The green succulent leaves grow directly from the perennial fibrous root and form a dense, obovate, basal rosette 5 to 10 cm in diameter. They are fleshy and juicy, flat, 2.5 to 5 cm long. The leaves are purple and sessile-oblong with a ciliate margin. They are often in carpets of tufts.

Habitat: The plant is indigenous to central and southern Europe and now grows wild in northern Europe, northern Africa, and western Asia.

Other Names: Jupiter's Eye, Jupiter's Beard, Thor's Beard, Bullock's Eye, Sengreen, Ayron, Ayegreen, Aaron's Rod, Hens and Chickens, Liveforever, Thunder Plant

ACTIONS AND PHARMACOLOGY
COMPOUNDS
Fruit acids: L(-)-malic acid, isocitric acid, succinic acid

Tannins

Mucilage

EFFECTS
The active agents are the leaves containing tannin, bitter substances, sugar, and mucous.

INDICATIONS AND USAGE
Houseleek is used internally as a decoction to relieve severe diarrhea. Externally, the drug is used for burns, ulcers, warts, and swelling caused by insect bites. It is also used for the treatment of itchy and burning skin parts. A gargle of diluted juice made from the leaves is used for stomatitis.

PRECAUTIONS AND ADVERSE REACTIONS
No health hazards or side effects are known in conjunction with the proper administration of designated therapeutic dosages.

DOSAGE

Mode of Administration: Houseleek is used internally as a decoction. The freshly pressed leaves and the juice is used externally.

LITERATURE

Kern W, List PH, Hörhammer L (Hrsg.), Hagers Handbuch der Pharmazeutischen Praxis, 4. Aufl., Bde 1-8: Springer Verlag Berlin, Heidelberg, New York, 1969.

Madaus G, Lehrbuch der Biologischen Arzneimittel, Bde 1-3, Nachdruck, Georg Olms Verlag Hildesheim 1979.

Senecio Aureus

Life Root

DESCRIPTION

Medicinal Parts: The medicinal parts are the dried herb and the fresh plant harvested during the flowering season.

Flower and Fruit: The few capitula are in a loose, many-blossomed corymb that is up to 2.5 cm wide. They are surrounded by a double involucre and consist of 8 to 12 yellow lingual, female florets. There are also numerous androgynous, tubular, ray florets, which are somewhat darker.

Leaves, Stem and Root: The plant is a perennial that grows up to 60 cm tall. The rhizome is 2 to 5 cm thick, with numerous thread-like roots. It produces an erect or ascending stem. The root bark is hard and blackish. It surrounds a ring of whitish, woody bundles and a large, dark, central pith. The stem is fluffy-haired when young, later glabrous, and bears alternate leaves. The basal leaves are up to 15 cm long. They are long-petioled, simple, round, reniform with a cordate base. The cauline leaves are shorter, incised and pinnatifid.

Characteristics: The herb has a bitter and astringent taste. The smell is slightly acrid.

Habitat: The plant is indigenous to North America.

Other Names: Squaw Weed, Golden Senecio, Golden Groundsel, Ragwort, Coughweed, Cocash Weed, Grundy Swallow

ACTIONS AND PHARMACOLOGY

COMPOUNDS

Pyrrolizidine alkaloids: chief alkaloids are floridanine, florosenine, otosenine

Sesquiterpenes of the eremophilane-type: including among others, ligularenolide, tetrahydroligularenolide, dehydrofukinone, trans-9-oxofuranoeremophilane

Flavonoids: including among others, kaempferol-3-O-glucosyl acetate, quercetin-3-O-glucosyl acetate

EFFECTS

The active agents are seneciionin (aurein), other alkaloids, and resins. The drug has menstruation stimulant, diuretic, and astringent properties.

INDICATIONS AND USAGE

Life Root is used for loss of blood (bleeding) and menopausal symptoms.

PRECAUTIONS AND ADVERSE REACTIONS

Hepatotoxicity and carcinogenicity are possible due to the pyrrolizidine alkaloids and 1,2-unsaturated necic parent substances. Life Root should not be taken internally.

DOSAGE

Daily Dosage: The average daily dose of the drug as a liquid extract is 4 gm taken 3 to 4 times daily. (See Precautions and Adverse Reactions.)

LITERATURE

Nachmann RJ, PH 22:780-782. 1983.

Resch JF et al., PM 47:255. 1983.

Röder E et al., (1983) Planta Med 49:57.

Röder E, DAZ 132:2427. 1992.

Zalkow LH et al., (1979) J Chem Soc Perkin Trans. 1: 1542.

Further information in:

Hänsel R, Keller K, Rimpler H, Schneider G (Hrsg.), Hagers Handbuch der Pharmazeutischen Praxis, 5. Aufl., Bde 4-6 (Drogen): Springer Verlag Berlin, Heidelberg, New York, 1992-1994.

Senecio Cineraria

Dusty Miller

DESCRIPTION

Medicinal Parts: The medicinal parts are the herb of the flowering plant, the fresh plant harvested before flowering, and the whole fresh, flowering plant.

Flower and Fruit: The plant has numerous yellow capitula, 12 to 15 cm in diameter, on short peduncles. The calyx only has a few sepals. There are 10 to 12 lingual florets. The fruit is striped.

Leaves, Stem and Root: Senecio cineraria is a semi-shrub up to 80 cm high. The stem is erect, heavily branched at the base, and sometimes snow-white tomentose. The leaves are densely pubescent beneath and more or less cobwebbed on the upper surface. They may have sparse greenish hairs. The lower leaves are oval to lanceolate, pinnatifid, with the outer lobes usually more long than wide.

Habitat: The plant is indigenous to the Mediterranean region, naturalized in North America and is cultivated as an ornamental plant in many countries.

Other Names: Cineraria Maritima

ACTIONS AND PHARMACOLOGY

COMPOUNDS

Pyrrolizidine alkaloids (0.9% in the blossoming foliage): including, among others, jaconine, jacobine, otosenine, retrorsine, senecionine, seneciphylline

Polyynes

EFFECTS

The active agents are the alkaloids jacobin, senecionin, and otosenin.

INDICATIONS AND USAGE

In homeopathy, the juice is used to treat eye-sight problems (for the treatment of spots before the eyes), migraine, and is used as an emmenagogue.

PRECAUTIONS AND ADVERSE REACTIONS

Hepatotoxicity and carcinogenicity are possible due to the pyrrolizidine alkaloids and the 1,2-unsaturated necic parent substances. Dusty Miller should not be taken internally for this reason.

DOSAGE

No information is available.

LITERATURE

Adams R et al., J Am Chem Soc 71:1953-1956. 1941.

Barger G et al., J Chem Soc:584. 1937.

Habib AM, PM 26:279. 1974.

Klasek A et al., Coll Czech Chem Comm 40:2524. 1975.

Nachmann RJ, PH 22:780-782. 1983.

Resch JF et al., PM 47:255. 1983.

Röder E, DAZ 132:2427. 1992.

Willaman JJ, Hui-Li L, (1970) Lloydia 33(3A):1.

Further information in:

Hänsel R, Keller K, Rimpler H, Schneider G (Hrsg.), Hagers Handbuch der Pharmazeutischen Praxis, 5. Aufl., Bde 4-6 (Drogen): Springer Verlag Berlin, Heidelberg, New York, 1992-1994 (unter Senecio bicolor).

Madaus G, Lehrbuch der Biologischen Arzneimittel, Bde 1-3, Nachdruck, Georg Olms Verlag Hildesheim 1979 (unter Cineraria maritima).

Teuscher E, Lindequist U, Biogene Gifte - Biologie, Chemie, Pharmakologie, 2. Aufl., Fischer Verlag Stuttgart 1994 (unter Senecio bicolor).

Senecio Jacoboea

Ragwort

DESCRIPTION

Medicinal Parts: The medicinal parts are the dried aerial parts of the flowering plant.

Flower and Fruit: The golden yellow composite flowers are in dense, terminal, erect, branched cymes. The linguiform ray florets are female. The disc florets are tubular and androgynous. The capitula has a diameter of 15 to 20 mm. The involucre is cylindrical. The bracts are in 1 row and are oblong-lanceolate, acuminate, black at the tip with a short 1 to 4 leaved epicalyx. The lateral fruit is glabrous and has drooping tufts of hair. The other fruit is covered in thick tufts of hair.

Leaves, Stem and Root: The plant is biennial to perennial and 30 to 90 cm high. The stem is erect, branched above and cobweb-pubescent. The basal leaves are lyrate-pinnatifid. The cauline leaves are pinnatifid with indented pinna. The lateral tips are almost at right angles and have four sectioned, slit little ears which clasp the stem.

Habitat: The plant is indigenous all over Europe, Asia Minor and northern Africa, and is naturalized in North America.

Production: Ragwort is the flowering plant of Senecio jacoboea. The plant is gathered in uncultivated regions (in the wild). The cut drug is dried away from direct sunlight.

Other Names: Ragweed, St. James Wort, Stinking Nanny, Staggerwort, Dog Standard, Cankerwort, Stammerwort

ACTIONS AND PHARMACOLOGY

COMPOUNDS

Pyrrolizidine alkaloids (0.1-0.9%): the alkaloid spectrum depends upon the chemotype. Jacobine chemotype: chief alkaloid jacobine; erucifoline chemotype: chief alkaloids erucifoline and O-acetylerucifoline

Volatile oil (traces)

EFFECTS

The principal toxins are pyrrolizidine alkaloids. Ragwort is acute and chronically poisonous in animals (proven through countless experiments).

INDICATIONS AND USAGE

The drug is used for painful menstruation, urinary tract inflammation, chronic cough, rheumatism, anemia and anemic headaches.

PRECAUTIONS AND ADVERSE REACTIONS

Hepatotoxicity and carcinogenicity are possible due to the pyrrolizidine alkaloids with 1,2-unsaturated necic parent substances in its makeup. It should not be taken internally for this reason.

DOSAGE

Mode of Administration: The drug is used externally.

Preparation: The lotion is made using 1 part of the drug and 5 parts of 10% ethanol.

Daily Dosage: The lotion is applied topically for the treatment of rheumatic arthritis.

LITERATURE

Bradbury RB, Culvenor CCJ, (1954) Austr J Chem 7. 378.

Deinzer ML et al., Science 195:497. 1977.

Schoental R, (1968) Cancer Res 28:2237.

Van Dooren, Bos R et al., (1981) Planta Med 42:385.

Van Dorren B et al., PM 42:385. 1981.

Witte L et al., PH 31:559. 1985.

Further information in:

Frohne D, Pfänder HJ: Giftpflanzen - Ein Handbuch für Apotheker, Toxikologen und Biologen, 4. Aufl., Wiss. Verlags-Ges. Stuttgart 1997.

Hänsel R, Keller K, Rimpler H, Schneider G (Hrsg.), Hagers Handbuch der Pharmazeutischen Praxis, 5. Aufl., Bde 4-6 (Drogen): Springer Verlag Berlin, Heidelberg, New York, 1992-1994.

Madaus G: Lehrbuch der Biologischen Arzneimittel, Bde 1-3, Nachdruck, Georg Olms Verlag Hildesheim 1979.

Roth L, Daunderer M, Kormann K, Giftpflanzen, Pflanzengifte, 4. Aufl., Ecomed Fachverlag Landsberg Lech 1993.

Teuscher E, Lindequist U, Biogene Gifte - Biologie, Chemie, Pharmakologie, 2. Aufl., Fischer Verlag Stuttgart 1994.

Senecio Nemorensis

Life Root

DESCRIPTION

Medicinal Parts: The medicinal part is the herb.

Flower and Fruit: The composite flower heads are in a dense, usually heavily blossomed corymb. The involucre bracts are grass or olive green, which are often tinged greenish black at the tip. The florets are yellow. The fruit is 4 mm long, long-stemmed and glabrous. During flowering, the pappus is only as long as the disc florets. By the time the fruit ripens, the pappus is 3 times as long as the fruit.

Leaves, Stem and Root: The plant is a geophytic perennial. There are runners, which are fleshy, 20 cm long and 5 cm thick. The stem is erect, 40 to 140 cm high with rounded ribs. The stem is green and red in particularly sunny locations. The stem is glabrous, to sparsely pubescent, or short-downy. The foliage leaves are lanceolate-ovate to oblong-lanceolate, acute or acuminate and serrate to double-serrate-dentate. The upper cauline leaves are usually petiolate, almost glabrous above to sparsely pubescent. The lower surface of the leaf is usually sparsely, occasionally moderately, scattered and appressed pubescent.

Habitat: The plant grows in many regions of southern and western Europe and is cultivated in some east European countries.

Other Names: Squaw Weed

ACTIONS AND PHARMACOLOGY

COMPOUNDS

Pyrrolizidine alkaloids (0.01-0.1%): including, among others, senecionine, fuchsisencionine, 7-angeloylretronecin, bulgarsenine, nemorensin, platyphyllin, sarracin

Sesquiterpenes of the eremophilane-type: including, among others, nemosenine A-D

Flavonoids: including, among others, rutin, quercitrin

Hydroxycoumarins: including, among others, aesculetin

Volatile oil (0.1%)

EFFECTS

No information is available.

INDICATIONS AND USAGE

Life Root is used for diabetes mellitus, hemorrhage, high blood pressure, spasms, and as a uterine stimulant. In folk medicine, the drug is also used in bleeding as a result of tooth extraction.

PRECAUTIONS AND ADVERSE REACTIONS

Hepatotoxicity and carcinogenicity are possible due to the presence of pyrrolizidine alkaloids and the 1,2-unsaturated necic parent substances. Life Root should not be taken internally.

DOSAGE

Preparation: One teaspoonful (1 gm) of finely cut drug is added to boiling water, steep for 5 to 10 minutes, then strain.

LITERATURE

Gottlieb R et al., DAZ 130:285. 1990.

Röder E et al., PH 16:1462. 1977.

Röder E, Pyrrolizidinhaltige Arzneipflanzen. In: DAZ 132(45):2427-2435. 1992.

Wiedenfeld H et al., Arch Pharm 315:165. 1982.

Wiedenfeld H et al., Arch Pharm 318:294. 1985.

Wiedenfeld H et al., PH 18:1083. 1979.

Wiedenfeld H et al., PM 41:124. 1981.

Wiedenfeld H et al., PM 46:426. 1986.

Wiedenfeld H et al., Sci Pharm 57:97. 1989.

Further information in:

Hänsel R, Keller K, Rimpler H, Schneider G (Hrsg.), Hagers Handbuch der Pharmazeutischen Praxis, 5. Aufl., Bde 4-6 (Drogen): Springer Verlag Berlin, Heidelberg, New York, 1992-1994.

Steinegger E, Hänsel R, Pharmakognosie, 5. Aufl., Springer Verlag Heidelberg 1992.

Teuscher E, Lindequist U, Biogene Gifte - Biologie, Chemie, Pharmakologie, 2. Aufl., Fischer Verlag Stuttgart 1994.

Wagner H, Wiesenauer M, Phytotherapie. Phytopharmaka und pflanzliche Homöopathika, Fischer-Verlag, Stuttgart, Jena, New York 1995.

Wichtl M (Hrsg.), Teedrogen, 4. Aufl., Wiss. Verlagsges. Stuttgart 1997.

Senecio Vulgaris

Groundsel

DESCRIPTION

Medicinal Parts: The medicinal part is the herb collected during the flowering season.

Flower and Fruit: The yellow composite flowers are in compact cymes. The small capitula have tubular florets but no lingual ones. The involucre and the outer bracts have black tips. The fruit is 1.2 to 2 mm long and densely downy. The pappus, which is 3 times as long as the fruit, is silky and pure white.

Leaves, Stem and Root: The plant grows from about 10 to 30 cm high. It is annual, biennial or occasionally perennial. It has a thin, fusiform, pale root, which is densely covered in lateral roots. The stem is erect, simple or branched. The leaves are glabrous or cobweb-lanate and pinnatisect. The lower leaves narrow to the petiole, the upper ones are slit at the base and clasping. The tips are oblong, obtuse, and unevenly acute dentate.

Habitat: The plant is common in all of Europe, northern and central Asia, northern Africa and has been introduced into various parts of Africa, Australia, and the Americas.

Production: Grounsel is the flowering plant of Senecio vulgaris. The herb is gathered in uncultivated regions and dried in the shade.

Other Names: Grundy Swallow, Ground Glutton, Simson

ACTIONS AND PHARMACOLOGY

COMPOUNDS

Pyrrolizidine alkaloids (up to 0.16%): chief alkaloids senecionine, seneciphylline

Flavonoids: including among others, isorhamnetin-3-O-glucosides, isorhamnetin-3-O-rutinosides, isorhamnetin-3-monosulphate

Volatile oil (traces)

EFFECTS

The toxic principle of the drug are the pyrrolizidine alkaloids.

INDICATIONS AND USAGE

Groundsel is used for the treatment of worm infestations and colic. The pressed juice is used for dysmenorrhea, epilepsy, and as a styptic in dentistry.

Efficacy has not been clinically proven. Similar to S. jacoboeae, it contains toxic and carcinogenic pyrrolizidine alkaloids.

PRECAUTIONS AND ADVERSE REACTIONS

Hepatotoxicity and carcinogenicity are possible due to the pyrrolizidine alkaloids with 1,2-unsaturated necic parent substances in its makeup. Groundsel should not be taken internally for this reason.

DOSAGE

No information is available.

LITERATURE

Bull LB et al. in: The Pyrrolizidine Alkaloids, Pub. Wiley NY 1968.

Mansour RMA, Saleh, NAM (1981) Phytochemistry 20:1180.

Qualls CW, Segall H J (1978) J Chrom. 15:202.

Toppel G, Hartmann T (1986) Planta Med 6:25P.

Van Borstel K et al., PH 28:1635-1638. 1989.

Van Dooren Bos R et al., (1981) Planta Med 42:385.

Further information in:

Hänsel R, Keller K, Rimpler H, Schneider G (Hrsg.), Hagers Handbuch der Pharmazeutischen Praxis, 5. Aufl., Bde 4-6 (Drogen): Springer Verlag Berlin, Heidelberg, New York, 1992-1994.

Madaus G, Lehrbuch der Biologischen Arzneimittel, Bde 1-3, Nachdruck, Georg Olms Verlag Hildesheim 1979.

Teuscher E, Lindequist U, Biogene Gifte - Biologie, Chemie, Pharmakologie, 2. Aufl., Fischer Verlag Stuttgart 1994.

Senega Snakeroot

See Polygala Senega

Senna

See Cassia Species

Serenoa Repens

Saw Palmetto

DESCRIPTION

Medicinal Parts: The medicinal parts are the partially dried ripe fruit, the ripe fresh fruit, and the ripe dried fruit.

Flower and Fruit: The inconspicuous cream flowers are in short, densely pubescent, paniculately branched inflorescences. The fruit is a deep purple to almost black. It is an ovate, 3 cm long, 1-seeded berry. It has a hard, but fragile pericarp that covers a pale-brown, spongy pulp. The endocarp is thin and papery. The fruit is slightly wrinkled, 1.25 to 2.5 cm long and 1.25 cm in diameter. The hard seed is pale brown, oval or globular, and has a hilum near the base. The whole panicle can weigh up to 4 kg.

Leaves, Stem and Root: The plant is a bushy palm with a maximum height of 6 m. The large, yellow-green leaves have up to 20 segments and form a crown.

Characteristics: The taste of the seeds is soapy and unpleasant.

Habitat: The plant is indigenous to the coastal regions of the southern states of the U.S., from South Carolina to Florida and southern California.

Other Names: Sabal

ACTIONS AND PHARMACOLOGY

COMPOUNDS

Sterols: beta-sitosterol, beta-sitosterol-3-O-glucosides, beta-sitosterol-3-O-diglucoside, beta-sitosterol-fatty acid esters and their glucosides, for example beta-sitosterol-3-O-myristate, beta-sitosterol-3-O-(6-O-myristyl-beta-glucosides)

Flavonoids: including, among others, isoquercitrin, kaempferol-3-glucosides, rhoifolin

Water-soluble polysaccharides: (galactoarabane with uronic acid share)

Fatty oil: free fatty acids

EFFECTS

The drug has antiandrogenic and antiexudative effects.

INDICATIONS AND USAGE

- Prostate complaints
- Irritable bladder

Saw Palmetto is used for urination problems in benign prostate hyperplasia stages I and II. This medication relieves only the difficulties associated with an enlarged prostate without reducing the enlargement.

PRECAUTIONS AND ADVERSE REACTIONS

No health hazards or side effects are known in conjunction with the proper administration of designated therapeutic dosages. Stomach complaints following intake have been observed in rare cases.

DOSAGE

Mode of Administration: Comminuted herb and other galenic preparations for oral use.

Daily dosage: The average daily dose is 1 to 2 gm of the drug or 320 mg of lipophilic ingredients extracted with lipophile solvents (hexane or ethanol 90% v/v).

LITERATURE

Anonym, Welche Bedeutung haben pflanzliche Prostatamittel. In: DAZ 133(9):720. 1993.

Aso Y, Boccon-Gibob L, Brendler CB, et al., (1993) Clinical research criteria. In: Cockett AT, Aso Y, Chatelain C, Denis L, Griffith K, Murphy G (eds) Proceedings of the second international consultation on benign prostatic hyperplasia (BPH). Paris, SCI S. 345-355.

Bach D, (1995) Medikamentöse Langheitbehandlung der BPH Ergebnisse einer prospektiven 3-Jahres-Studie mit dem Sabalextrakt IDS 89. Urologe [B]35:178-183.

Bach D, Behandlung der benignen Prostatahypertrophie. In: ZPT 17(4):209-218. 1996.

Bach D, Ebeling L, Long-term drug treatment of benign prostatic hyperplasia - Results of a prospective 3-year multicenter study using Sabal extract IDS 89. In: Phytomedicine 3(2):105-111. 1996.

Bauer R, Neues von ''immunmodulierenden Drogen'' und ''Drogen mit antiallergischer und antiinflammatorischer Wirkung''. In: ZPT 14(1):23-24. 1993.

Bazan NG, Authie D, Braquet P, Effect of Serenoa repens extract (Permixon (r)) on estradiol/testosteron-induced experimental prostate enlargement in the rat. In: Pharmacol Res 34(3/4):171-179. 1996.

Becker H, Ebeling L, (1988) Konservative Therapie der benignen Prostata-Hyperplasie (BPH) mit Cernilton (N) - Ergebnisse einer placebokontrollierten Doppelblindstudie. Urologe [B]28:301.

Becker H, Ebeling L, (1991) Phytotherapie der BPH mit Cernilton(N) - Ergebnisse einer kontrollierten Verlaufsstudie. Urologe [B]31:113.

Berges RR, Windeler J, Trampisch HJ, Senge Th, (1995) Randomised, placebo-controlled, double-blind clinical trial of β-sitosterol in patients with benign prostatic hyperplasia. Lancet 345:1529-1532.

Carraro JC et al., Comparision of phytotherapy (Permixon (R)) with finasteride in the treatment of benign prostate hyperplasia: a randomized international study of 1,098 patiens. In: Prostate 29(4):231-240. 1996.

Casarosa C, Cosci M, o di Coscio, Fratta M, (1988) Lack of effects of a lyposterolic extract of Serenoa repens on plasma levels of testosterone, follicle-stimulating hormone, luteinizing hormone. Clin Ther 10:5.

Engelmann U, Phytopharmaka und Synthetika bei der Behandlung der benignen Prostatahypertrophie. In: ZPT 18(1):13-19. 1997.

Hänsel R et al., (1964) Planta Med 12:169.

Harnischfeger G, Stolze H, (1989) Serenoa repens - Die Sägezahnpalme. Z Phytother 10:71-76.

Koch E, (1995) Pharmakologie und Wirkmechanismen von Extrakten aus Sabalfrüchten (Sabal fructus): Brennesselwurzeln (Urticae radix) und Kürbissamen (Cucurbitae peponis semen) bei der Behandlung der benignen Prostatahyperplasie. In: Loew D, Rietbrock N (Hrsg) Phytopharmaka in Forschung und klinischer Anwendung. Steinkopff Verlag, Darmstadt, S 57-79.

Mattei FM, Capone M, Acconia A, Medikamentöse Therapie der benignen Prostatahyperplasie mit einem Exktrakt der Sägepalme. In: Therapiewoche Urologie, Nephrologie 2:346-350. 1990.

Miersch WDE, Benigne Prostatahyperplasie. In: DAZ 133(29):2653. 1993.

Nahrstedt A, (1993) Pflanzliche Urologica - eine kritische Übersicht. Pharm Z 138:1439-1450.

Niederprüm HJ, Schweikert HU, Zänker KS, (1994) Testosteron 5D-reductase inhibition by free fatty acids from Sabal serrulata fruits. Phytomedicine 1:127-133.

Plosker GL, Brogden RN, Serenoa repens (Permixon (R)): A review of its pharmacological and therapeutic efficacy in benign prostatic hyperplasia. In: Drugs & Aging 9(5):379-395. 1996.

Ravenna L et al., Effects of the lipidosterolic extract of Serenoa repens (Permixon (R)) on human prostatic cell lines. In: Prostate 29(4):219-230. 1996.

Rhodes L, Primka RL, Berman CH, Vergult F, Gabriel M, Pierre-Malice M, Gibelin B, Comparision of Finasteride (Proscar(R)), a 5alpha-reductase inhibitor, and various commercial plant extracts in in vitro and in vivo 5alpha reductase inhibition. In: Prostate.

Schilcher H, (1987) Möglichkeiten und Grenzen der Phytotherapie am Beispiel pflanzlicher Urologika. Urologe [B] 27:316-319.

Schilcher H, (1987) Pflanzliche Diuretika. Urologe [B]27:215-222.

Schilcher B, In: Schilcher H: Phytotherapie in der Urologie. Hippokrates Verlag Stuttgart. 1992.

Shimada H et al., Biological active acylglycerides from the berries of saw-palmetto (Serenoa repens). In: JNP 60(4):417-418. 1997.

Wagner H, Flachsbarth H, (1981) Planta Med 41:244.

Wichtl M, Pflanzliche Geriatrika. In: DAZ 132(30):1576. 1992.

Further information in:

Hänsel R, Keller K, Rimpler H, Schneider G (Hrsg.), Hagers Handbuch der Pharmazeutischen Praxis, 5. Aufl., Bde 4-6 (Drogen): Springer Verlag Berlin, Heidelberg, New York, 1992-1994.

Madaus G, Lehrbuch der Biologischen Arzneimittel, Bde 1-3, Nachdruck, Georg Olms Verlag Hildesheim 1979.

Schulz R, Hänsel R, Rationale Phytotherapie, Springer Verlag Heidelberg 1996.

Teuscher E, Biogene Arzneimittel, 5. Aufl., Wiss. Verlagsges. Stuttgart 1997.

Wagner H, Wiesenauer M, Phytotherapie. Phytopharmaka und pflanzliche Homöopathika, Fischer-Verlag, Stuttgart, Jena, New York 1995.

Service Tree

See Sorbus Domestica

Shepherd's Purse

See Capsella Bursa Pastoris

Siberian Ginseng

See Eleutherococcus Senticosus

Silphium Laciniatum

Rosinweed

DESCRIPTION

Medicinal Parts: The medicinal part is the root.

Leaves, Stem and Root: The plant is a stately 1 to 4 m high herbaceous perennial, with an almost leafless, round shaft. The leaves are 30 to 60 cm long. They are long-petioled, simple or double pinnate leaves. The leaves are alternate, with their edges turned upwards and downwards and their surfaces facing north and south.

Characteristics: The taste of the root is bitter and then acrid. The roots are odorless.

Habitat: The plant grows in the western U.S., especially Ohio.

Other Names: Compass Weed, Polar Plant, Pilot Weed

ACTIONS AND PHARMACOLOGY

COMPOUNDS

Resins (smelling terpene-like, mastic-like)

Volatile oil

Inulin (in the rhizome)

EFFECTS

The active agents are resin, with 19% terpene and 37% of a resin acid, and inulin in the root. The drug has antispasmodic, diuretic, and diaphoretic effects.

INDICATIONS AND USAGE

In homeopathy, the drug is used for the treatment of digestive disorders.

PRECAUTIONS AND ADVERSE REACTIONS

No health hazards or side effects are known in conjunction with the proper administration of designated therapeutic dosages.

DOSAGE

Mode of Administration: Rosinweed is available as a tincture or liquid extract.

LITERATURE

Kern W, List PH, Hörhammer L (Hrsg.), Hagers Handbuch der Pharmazeutischen Praxis, 4. Aufl., Bde. 1-8: Springer Verlag Berlin, Heidelberg, New York, 1969.

Madaus G: Lehrbuch der Biologischen Arzneimittel, Bde 1-3, Nachdruck, Georg Olms Verlag Hildesheim 1979.

Silphium Perfoliatum

Cup Plant

DESCRIPTION

Medicinal Parts: The medicinal part is the root.

Flower and Fruit: The flowers are 5 to 8 cm wide, long pedicled and clustered. The sepals are overlapping and the petals are egg yolk-yellow. The disc-like flowers are androgynous with long thread-like styles. The lateral flowers are female and lingual. The double winged-fruit is compressed and has a pappus of lateral awns.

Leaves, Stem and Root: The perennial plant is a 1.25 to 2.5 m high plant with a branched rhizome. The erect, angular, smooth stem is branched higher up and foliated up to the tip. The leaves are opposite, rough, ovate, acuminate, crenate, dark green above and blue-green beneath. The lower leaves are up to 30 cm long and the upper ones are oblong-ovate, sessile and fused at the base to a cup form.

Habitat: The plant is indigenous to the western U.S., Oregon, and Texas.

Other Names: Ragged Cup, Indian Gum, Prairie Dock, Pilot Plant, Polar Plant, Rosinweed, Turpentine Weed

ACTIONS AND PHARMACOLOGY

COMPOUNDS

Saponins

Sesquiterpenes: including among others, silphinene, silphiperfolen, 8-hydroxy-presilphiperfolane

EFFECTS

The drug is a tonic and has a diaphoretic effect.

INDICATIONS AND USAGE

Cup Plant has been used for digestive disorders.

PRECAUTIONS AND ADVERSE REACTIONS

No health hazards or side effects are known in conjunction with the proper administration of designated therapeutic dosages.

DOSAGE

Mode of Administration: Cup Root is not used in modern medicine.

LITERATURE

Davidyants ES et al., (1984) Khim Prir Soedin. 5:666.

Further information in:

Hegnauer R, Chemotaxonomie der Pflanzen, Bde 1-11: Birkhäuser Verlag Basel, Boston, Berlin 1962-1997.

Silybum Marianum

Milk Thistle

DESCRIPTION

Medicinal Parts: The medicinal parts are ripe seeds.

Flower and Fruit: The inflorescences are large, solitary, purple and somewhat nodding, composite flower heads. The perigone is globular. The inner tepals are acuminate; the outer ones are tough at the base and terminate in a tip. There are only tubular florets. The fruit is brown, spotted and glossy, with a white tuft of hair.

Leaves, Stem and Root: The plant grows from 70 to 150 cm high. The stem is erect. The leaves are alternate. The lower leaves are indented-pinnatisect; the upper ones are lanceolate and clasping. There are white spots along the ribs of the leaf and yellow thorns at the margin.

Habitat: The plant is indigenous to Europe.

Other Names: Marian Thistle

ACTIONS AND PHARMACOLOGY

COMPOUNDS: CARDUI MARIAE HERBA

Flavonoids: in particular, apigenin-, luteolin- and kaempferol-glycosides

Beta-sitosterol

Polyynes: silymarin (Cardui mariae fructus) is absent; it is localized only in the seed case

EFFECTS: CARDUI MARIAE HERBA

No information is available.

COMPOUNDS: CARDUI MARIAE FRUCTUS

Silymarin (flavonal lignan mixture): chief components silybin A, silybin B (mixture known as silibinin), isosilybin A, isosilybin B, silychristin, silydianin

Flavonoids

Fatty oil

EFFECTS: CARDUI MARIAE FRUCTUS

Silymarin acts as an antagonist in many experimental liver-damage models; in particular, death cap mushroom poisoning. The therapeutic activity of silymarin is based on two sites or mechanisms. To begin with, it alters the structure of the outer cell membrane of the hepatocytes in such a way as to prevent penetration of the liver poison into the interior of the cell. Secondly, it stimulates the action of nucleolar polymerase A, resulting in an increase in ribosomal protein synthesis, and thus stimulates the regenerative ability of the liver and the formation of new hepatocytes.

The drug is also said to be a cholagogue.

INDICATIONS AND USAGE

CARDUI MARIAE HERBA

Preparations of milk thistle herb are used as a tonic, as a stimulant, for functional disorders of liver and gallbladder as well as for jaundice, gallbladder colic, and diseases of the spleen. Formerly used as a malaria treatment, emmenagogue, and for uterine complaints.

CARDUI MARIAE FRUCTUS

- Loss of appetite
- Liver and gallbladder complaints

The drug is used for dyspeptic complaints, toxic liver damage, supportive treatment in chronic inflammatory liver disease and hepatic cirrhosis. It is also used as an antidote to Death-Cap poisoning.

PRECAUTIONS AND ADVERSE REACTIONS

CARDUI MARIAE HERBA AND FRUCTUS

No health hazards or side effects are known in conjunction with the proper administration of designated therapeutic dosages.

DOSAGE

CARDUI MARIAE FRUCTUS

Mode of Administration: Comminuted drug for infusions and extracts; tinctures for liquids and solid forms.

Preparation: To prepare an infusion, add 3 gm of the drug to cold water and bring to a boil. Drain after 10 to 20 minutes.

Daily Dosage: The average daily dose is 12 to 15 gm of the drug or an equivalent of 200 to 400 mg of silymarin, calculated as silybin.

CARDUI MARIAE HERBA

Preparation: An Infusion is prepared by pouring boiling water over 1/2 teaspoonful of the drug and then straining after 5 to 10 minutes.

Daily Dosage: The average dose of the infusion is 2 to 3 cups daily.

LITERATURE

CARDUI MARIAE HERBA

Ahmed AA et al., PH 28:1751. 1989.

DAZ 25:1427. 1990.

Khafagy SM et al., Sci Pharm 49:157. 1981.

Mericli AH, PM 54:44. 1988.

Further information in:

Kern W, List PH, Hörhammer L (Hrsg.), Hagers Handbuch der Pharmazeutischen Praxis, 4. Aufl., Bde. 1-8, Springer Verlag Berlin, Heidelberg, New York, 1969.

Madaus G, Lehrbuch der Biologischen Arzneimittel, Bde 1-3, Nachdruck, Georg Olms Verlag Hildesheim 1979.

Wichtl M (Hrsg.), Teedrogen, 4. Aufl., Wiss. Verlagsges. Stuttgart 1997.

CARDUI MARIAE FRUCTUS

Baumann J, (1975) Über die Wirkung von Chelidonium, Curcuma, Absinth und Carduus marianus auf die Galle- und Pankreassekretion bei Hepatopathien. Med Mschr 29:173.

Benda I, Zenz W, (1973) Wien Med Wschr 123:512.

Desplaces A et al., (1975) Arzneim Forsch 25, 89.

Devault RL, Rosenbrook W, (1973) J Antibiotic 26:532.

Hruby K et al., (1983) Hum Toxicol 2(2):183.

Neu R, (1960) Arch Pharm 293:269.

Pelter A, Hänsel R, (1968) Tetrahedron Letters 19:2911.

Poser G, (1971) Arzneim Forsch 21:1209.

Qiu SJ et al., (1981) Chin J Cardiol 9:61.

Tuchweber B et al., (1973) J Med 4:327.

Vogel G et al., (1984) Toxicol Appl Pharmacol 51:265.

Wagner H et al., (1971) Tetrahedron Letters 22:1985.

Arnone A, Merlini L, Zanarotti A, (1979) Constituents of Silybum marianum. Structure of isosilybin and stereochemistry of isosilybin. J Chem Soc (Chem Commun):696-697.

Benda L, Dittrich H, Ferenzi P, Frank H, Wewalka F, (1980) The influence of Therapy with silymarin on the survial rate of patients with liver cirrhosis. Wien Klin Wschr 92(19):678-683.

Bode JCh, (1986) Arzneimittel für die Indikation "Lebererkrankungen". In: Dölle W, Müller-Oerlingshausen B, Schwabe U (Hrsg.), Grundlagen der Arzneimitteltherapie. Entwicklung, Beurteilung und Anwendung von Arzneimitteln. B.I.- Wissenschaftsverlag, Mannheim Wien Zürich, S 202-211.

Bode JCh, (1981) Die alkoholische Hepatitis, ein Krankheitsspektrum. Internist 220:536-545.

Dölle W, Schwabe U, (1988) Leber- und Gallenwegstherapeutika. In: Schwabe U, Paffrath D (Hrsg.), Arzneiverordnungsreport 88, Gustav Fischer, Stuttgart New York, S 242-253.

Feher J, Deak G, Muezes G, Lang I, Niederland V, Nekam K, Karteszi M, (1989) Hepatoprotective activity of silymarin legalon therapy in patients with chronic alcoholic liver disease. Orv Hetil 130(51):2723-2727.

Ferenci P, Dragosics B, Dittrich H, Frank H, Benda L, Lochs H, Meryn S, Base W, Schneider B, (1989) Randomized controlled trial of silymarin treatment in patients with cirrhosis of the liver. J Hepatol 9(1):105-113.

Fintelmann V, Albert A, (1980) Nachweis der therapeutischen Wirksamkeit von Legalon bei toxischen Lebererkrankungen im Doppelblindversuch. Therapiewoche 30(35):5589-5594.

Hahn G, Lehmann HD, Kürten M et al., (1968) Zur Pharmakologie und Toxikologie von Silymarin, des antihepatotocischen Wirkprinzips aus Silybum marianum (L.) Gaertn. Arzneim Forsch/Drug Res 18:698-704.

Hruby K, Fuhrmann M, Csomos G, Thaler H, (1983) Pharmakotherapie der Knollenblätterpilzvergiftung mit Silibinin. Wien Klein Wschr 95(7):225-231.

Koch H, (1980) Leberschutz-Therapeutika. Pharmazie in unserer Zeit 9:33-44:65-74.

Leng-Peschlow E, Strenge-Hesse A, (1991) Die Mariendistel (Silybum marianum) und Silymarin als Lebertherapeutikum. Z Phytother 12:162-174.

Lorenz D, Mennicke WH, Behrendt W, (1992) Untersuchungen zur Elimination von Silymarin bei cholecystektomierten Patienten. Planta Med 45:216-233.

Martines G, Copponi V, Cagnetta G, (1980) Aspetti del danno epatico dopo somministrazione sperimentale di alcuni farmaci. Arch Sci Med 137:367-386.

Martini GA, (1988) Hepatozelluläre Erkrankungen, Leberkrankheiten. In: Riecker G (Hrsg.), Therapie innerer Krankheiten, Springer, Berlin Heidelberg New York, S 638-652.

Marugg D, Reutter FW, (1985) Die Amanita-phalloides-Intoxikation. Moderne therapeutische Maßnahmen und klinischer Verlauf. Schweiz Rundschau Med (Praxis) 14(37):972-982.

Mennicke WH, (1975) Zur biologischen Verfügbarkeit und Verstoffwechselung von Silybin. Dtsch Apoth Ztg 115(33):1205-1206.

Peeters H (Ed.), (1976) Phosphatidylcholine. Biochemical and Clinical Aspects of Essential Phospholipids. Springer Verlag, Berlin Heidelberg New York.

Rauen HM, Schriewer H, (1971) Die antihepatotoxische Wirkung von Silymarin bei experimentellen Leberschäden der Ratte durch Tetrachlorkohlenstoff, D-Galaktosamin und Allylalkohol. Arzneim Forsch/Drug Res 21:1194-1201.

Reuter HD, (1992) Spektrum Mariendistel und andere leber- und gallewirksame Phytopharmaka. In: Bundesverband Dtschr Ärzte für Naturheilverfahren (Hrsg.) Arzneimitteltherapie heute. Aesopus Verlag, Basel.

Salmi HA, Sarna S, (1982) Effect of silymarin on chemical, functional and morphological alterations of the liver. A double-blind controlled study. Scand J Gastroenterol 17(4):517-521.

Schulz HU, Schürer M, Krumbiegel G, Wächter W, Weyhenmeyer R, Seidel G, (1995) Untersuchungen zum Freisetzungsverhalten und zur Bioäquivalenz von Silymarin-Präparaten. Arzneim Forsch/Drug Res 45:61-64.

Sonnebichler J, Zetl I, (1984) Untersuchungen zum Wirkungsmechanismus von Silibinin, Einfluβ von Silibinin auf die Synthese ribosomaler RNA, mRNA und tRNA in Rattenlebern in vivo. Hoppe-Seyler's Physiol Chem 365:555-556.

Sonnenbichler J, Zetl I, (1986) Biochemical effects of the flavonolignane silibinin in RNA, protein and DANN synthesis of rat livers. Prog Clin Biol Res 213:319-331.

Sonnenbichler J, Zetl I, (1987) Stimulating influence of a flavonolignane on proliferation, RNA synthesis and protein Synthesis in liver cells. In, Okoliczányi L, Csomós G, Crepaldi G (Eds.), Assessment and management of hepatobiliary disease. Springer, Berlin Heidelberg New York, S 265-272.

Sonnenbichler J, Zetl I, (1988) Specific binding of a flavonolignane to an estradiol receptor. In: Plant flavonoids in Biology and Medicine II, Biochemical, cellular, and medicinal properties. Alan R Liss, New York, S 369-374.

Varis K, Salmi HA, Siurala M, (1978) Die Therapie der Lebererkrankung mit Legalon; eine kontrollierte Doppelblindstudie. In: Aktuelle Hepatologie, III. Internationales Symposium Köln 15.-17. November 1978. Hanseatisches Verlagskontor. Lübeck, S 42-43.

Vogel G, (1980) The anti-amanita effect of silymarin. In: Faulstich et al., (Eds.), Amanita toxins and poisoning. Witzstrock, Baden-Baden Köln New York, S 180-187.

Wagner H, Seligmann O, Seilz M, Abraham D, Sonnenbichler J, (1976) Silydianin und Silychristin, zwei isomere Silymarine aus Silybum marianum L. Gaertn. (Mariendistel). Z Naturforsch 31b:876-884.

Further information in:

Kern W, List PH, Hörhammer L (Hrsg.), Hagers Handbuch der Pharmazeutischen Praxis, 4. Aufl., Bde 1-8, Springer Verlag Berlin, Heidelberg, New York, 1969.

Madaus G, Lehrbuch der Biologischen Arzneimittel, Bde 1-3, Nachdruck, Georg Olms Verlag Hildesheim 1979.

Roth L, Daunderer M, Kormann K, Giftpflanzen, Pflanzengifte, 4. Aufl., Ecomed Fachverlag Landsberg Lech 1993.

Schulz R, Hänsel R, Rationale Phytotherapie, Springer Verlag Heidelberg 1996.

Steinegger E, Hänsel R, Pharmakognosie, 5. Aufl., Springer Verlag Heidelberg 1992.

Teuscher E, Biogene Arzneimittel, 5. Aufl., Wiss. Verlagsges. mbH Stuttgart 1997.

Wagner H, Wiesenauer M, Phytotherapie. Phytopharmaka und pflanzliche Homöopathika, Fischer-Verlag, Stuttgart, Jena, New York 1995.

Wichtl M (Hrsg.), Teedrogen, 4. Aufl., Wiss. Verlagsges. Stuttgart 1997.

Simaruba Amara

Simaruba

DESCRIPTION

Medicinal Parts: The medicinal part is the dried root bark.

Flower and Fruit: The flowers grow in small racemes with dense matte-white petals.

Leaves, Stem and Root: Simaruba amara is a tree that grows over 18 m high. The roots are long and spread horizontally. The leaves are 22 to 27 cm long. The tree has numerous long, bent branches covered in smooth, grayish bark. The bark that is used commercially is thin and flat with a yellowish or grayish-yellow color. The bark is tough, fibrous and almost impossible to break.

Characteristics: The taste is very bitter and odorless.

Habitat: The plant grows on the Caribbean islands and the northern parts of South America.

Other Names: Dysentery Bark, Mountain Damson, Bitter Damson, Slave Wood, Stave Wood, Sumaruba

ACTIONS AND PHARMACOLOGY

COMPOUNDS

Bitter substances: quassinoids (breakdown products of triterpenes), including among others, simarubin (1%), simarubidin, simarolide, 13,18-dehydro-glaucarubinone

Tannins (20-27%)

Volatile oil (0.1-0.2%) 5-hydroxy-canthin-6-one

Alkaloids

EFFECTS

The active agents are tannin, simarubin, essential oil, and fat. Simaruba is a tonic and febrifuge.

INDICATIONS AND USAGE

Simaruba was formerly used in the treatment of febrile illnesses and dysentery. Recent research indicates that it may be effective in treating malaria. The drug is used for unspecified enteritis, diarrhea, and amarum. It possibly causes vomiting, and is also used as an abortive.

PRECAUTIONS AND ADVERSE REACTIONS

No health hazards or side effects are known in conjunction with the proper administration of designated therapeutic dosages. The drug triggers vomiting in high dosages.

DOSAGE

Mode of Administration: The drug is available as a liquid extract for internal use.

Daily Dosage: The average dose is 1 gm of the drug to be taken internally.

Storage: Protect against dampness.

LITERATURE

Bray DH et al., (1987) Phytother Res 1 (1):22.

Geissmann T, (1964) Ann Rev Pharmacol 4:305.

Kuroda K et al., (1976) Cancer Res 36:1900.

Polonsky J et al., (1978) Experientia 34 (9):1122.

Further information in:

Hegnauer R, Chemotaxonomie der Pflanzen, Bde 1-11: Birkhäuser Verlag Basel, Boston, Berlin 1962-1997.

Kern W, List PH, Hörhammer L (Hrsg.), Hagers Handbuch der Pharmazeutischen Praxis, 4. Aufl., Bde 1-8: Springer Verlag Berlin, Heidelberg, New York, 1969.

Simmondsia Chinesis

Jojoba

DESCRIPTION

Medicinal Parts: The medicinal part is the liquid Jojoba wax.

Flower and Fruit: The flowers are axillary. The male flowers are small and yellow and have no petals. The female flowers are usually solitary, inconspicuous and pale green. There may also be inflorescences in the form of panicles, umbels and cymes. Pollination is by wind. The fruit capsules contain 1 to 3 seeds although 1-seeded capsules are the most common. The seeds are approximately 2 cm long.

Leaves, Stem and Root: The plant is a heavily branched, evergreen dioecious bush. The male plants are larger, taller and less compact than the female. The desert variety develop taproots up to 3.6 m in length. The horizontal root branches reach from 60 to 90 cm in depth. The leaves are thick, coriaceous, blue-green, entire-margined and oblong. They are in pairs and depending on the dampness of the soil the leaves may remain on the bush for 2 to 3 periods of growth.

Characteristics: The oil from the fruit has a pleasant scent and taste.

Habitat: The plant is indigenous to areas extending from the Sonora dessert of the U.S. to northwest Mexico. It is cultivated particularly in India and Israel.

Production: From the cultivation (of plants) in Mexico and in South America. Liquid Jojoba wax is a clear, light yellow, oily liquid, that is extracted from the seeds of Simmondsia chilensis.

ACTIONS AND PHARMACOLOGY

COMPOUNDS

Liquid wax exters: esters in position 9-10 simple unsaturated C20- and C22-fatty acids, chiefly gadolenic acid (20:1(9), make up 70% of the fatty acids) with the corresponding alcohols, chiefly eicosanol (20:1 (9)-OH) and docosenol (22:1 (9) OH)

EFFECTS

Active agents are the simple unsaturated C20/22 - fatty acids and alcohol.

In terms of skin care, Jojoba oil, due to its robust and stable constitution, in comparison with its rancidity, is used as a carrier (substance) for oxidation sensitive substances (Vitamin A).

INDICATIONS AND USAGE

Skin care - cosmetics.

PRECAUTIONS AND ADVERSE REACTIONS

No health hazards or side effects are known in conjunction with the proper external administration of designated therapeutic dosages. Jojoba wax, taken orally, to a great extent passes through the body without being digested, but also becomes stored in intestinal cells and in the liver, and is therefore not suitable as a dietetic.

DOSAGE

Mode of Administration: In ointments and creams as a medium (or vehicle) for oxidation sensitive substances. Because the wax derived from Joboba is not affected by digestive enzymes, use in reduction diets is possible.

LITERATURE

Knoepfler NB et al., Agr Food Chem 6:118. 1958.

Miwa TK, J Am Oil Chem Soc 48:259. 1971.

Further information in:

Hänsel R, Keller K, Rimpler H, Schneider G (Hrsg.), Hagers Handbuch der Pharmazeutischen Praxis, 5. Aufl., Bde 4-6 (Drogen): Springer Verlag Berlin, Heidelberg, New York, 1992-1994.

Steinegger E, Hänsel R, Pharmakognosie, 5. Aufl., Springer Verlag Heidelberg 1992.

Teuscher E, Biogene Arzneimittel, 5. Aufl., Wiss. Verlagsges. Stuttgart 1997.

Sinapis Alba

Mustard

DESCRIPTION

Medicinal Parts: The medicinal parts are the dried seeds.

Flower and Fruit: The flowers form an umbelliferous-racemous inflorescence. The flowers are on 3 to 7 mm long, stiff-haired pedicles. When in bloom the 4 narrow, obtuse sepals lie horizontal. There are 3 green, ovate nectaries at the base of the stamens. The fruit is a 2 to 4 cm long bristly pod, divided into two chambers. Each chamber contains two to three 2.5 mm thick seeds. The chamber ends as a large curled lip. The seeds vary from brown to white and are arranged in opposite rows.

Leaves, Stem and Root: Sinapis alba is an annual plant. The lower part of the plant is covered in stiff, single hairs. The thin root is yellow to white and branched. The root produces a 30 to 60 cm high, erect, grooved and branched stem. The leaves are 4 to 10 cm long, petiolate, lyrate, pinnatifid to pinnatesect and always have 2 to 3 indented-dentate lobed pinna.

Habitat: The plant has been introduced and naturalized in all of Europe and in Siberia, east Asia, and America. The areas of cultivation are western and northern Europe and the northern U.S.

Production: White Mustard seed consists of the ripe, dried seed of Sinapis alba.

Not To Be Confused With: Other Sinapis or Brassica species. Artificial colorings such as butter yellow or turmeric may be added.

Other Names: White Mustard

ACTIONS AND PHARMACOLOGY

COMPOUNDS

Glucosinolates: chiefly sinalbin (p-hydroxybenzylglucosinolates, 2.5%), grinding the seeds into powder and then rubbing with warm water (not with hot water — enzymes would be destroyed), as well as chewing, releases the non-volatile mustard oil

P-hydroxybenzyl isothiocyanate

Fatty oil (20-35%)

Proteins (40%)

Phenyl propane derivatives: including, among others, sinapine (choline ester of sinapic acid, 1.5%)

EFFECTS

Mustard is an irritant for skin and a bacteriostatic agent.

INDICATIONS AND USAGE

- Common cold
- Cough/bronchitis
- Fevers and colds
- Inflammation of the mouth and pharynx
- Rheumatism
- Tendency to infection

Mustard flour is used to clear and brighten the voice.

Externally, mustard is used in poultices for catarrhs of the respiratory tract, for topical hyperemization of the skin as well as for segment therapy of chronic degenerative diseases affecting the joints and soft tissue. Mustard baths are used in the treatment of paralytic symptoms.

CONTRAINDICATIONS

Mustard is contraindicated in gastrointestinal ulcers and inflammatory kidney diseases. The drug should not be given to children under 6 years of age.

PRECAUTIONS AND ADVERSE REACTIONS

General: No health hazards or side effects are known in conjunction with the proper administration of designated therapeutic dosages. The danger of nerve damage exists in connection with long-term intake. Long-term external application carries the danger of skin injury. The drug possesses minimal potential for sensitization (possible cause of food allergies).

Pediatric Use: Mustard preparations should not be used in children under 6 years of age.

OVERDOSAGE

Gastrointestinal complaints could appear following the intake of large quantities, due to the mucous membrane-irritating effect of the mustard oil.

DOSAGE

Mode of Administration: The drug is used internally as well as externally. Ground or powdered seeds are used for poultices.

Preparation: To prepare an external foot bath, 20 to 30 gm of the mustard flour in 1 liter of water is used. To prepare a mustard bath, 150 gm of the mustard flour in a pouch is used in the bathwater.

Daily Dosage: The average daily dose of the drug is 60 to 240 gm. To brighten and clear the voice, Mustard flour is stirred with honey and formed into balls. One to 2 are taken orally on an empty stomach.

For external use, just prior to application, mix 50 to 70 gm of the powdered seeds with warm water to prepare a poultice. The poultice is applied for 10 to 15 minutes for adults and for 5 to 10 minutes for children, except for those with sensitive skin where the usage should be shortened. Treatment should not exceed 2 weeks.

Storage: The drug must be protected from light and moisture.

LITERATURE

Josefsson E, J Sci Food Agric 21:94. 1970.

Kerber E et al., Angew Bot 55:457. 1981.

Kjaer A, Rubinstein K, Acta Chem Scand 4:1276. 1953.

Further information in:

Frohne D, Pfänder HJ, Giftpflanzen - Ein Handbuch für Apotheker, Toxikologen und Biologen, 4. Aufl., Wiss. Verlags-Ges. Stuttgart 1997.

Hänsel R, Keller K, Rimpler H, Schneider G (Hrsg.), Hagers Handbuch der Pharmazeutischen Praxis, 5. Aufl., Bde 4-6 (Drogen): Springer Verlag Berlin, Heidelberg, New York, 1992-1994.

Steinegger E, Hänsel R, Pharmakognosie, 5. Aufl., Springer Verlag Heidelberg 1992.

Teuscher E, Lindequist U, Biogene Gifte - Biologie, Chemie, Pharmakologie, 2. Aufl., Fischer Verlag Stuttgart 1994.

Teuscher E, Biogene Arzneimittel, 5. Aufl., Wiss. Verlagsges. Stuttgart 1997.

Sisymbrium Officinale

Hedge Mustard

DESCRIPTION

Medicinal Parts: The medicinal parts are the fresh, flowering herb and the fresh aerial parts of the flowering plant.

Flower and Fruit: The inflorescences at the end of the stems and branches have no bracts and are initially umbelliferous-racemous, later stretching into spikes. The pedicles are thin and approximately 1.5 cm long, bearing the small flowers. The 4 sepals are 1.5 to 2.5 mm long, erect, pubescent, and narrowly elliptical. The petals are pale yellow and are 3 to 4 mm long. The stamens have 0.5 to 0.5 mm long anthers. The fruit is a pubescent pod appressed to the axis of the infructescence. They are 1 to 1.5 cm long and 1 to 1.5 mm thick. The seeds are about 1 mm long, ovate, compressed, unwinged with reddish, yellow-brown seed-skins, and are almost smooth.

Leaves, Stem and Root: The plant is an annual or biennial, 30 to 60 cm high, and has a thin taproot. The stem is branched, round, leafy, and covered in scattered patent hairs. The basal leaves and lower cauline leaves are petiolate-pinnatifid with 3 to 9 segments. The upper leaves are oblong-lanceolate, simple or with 2 to 4 lateral segments, and often hastate and pubescent.

Habitat: The herb is found mainly in temperate Europe but is also found as far as northern Africa and eastern Siberia.

Production: Hedge Mustard is the fresh flowering herb of Sisymbrium officinale.

Other Names: Singer's Plant, St. Barbara's Hedge Mustard, English Watercress, Erysimum, Thalictroc

ACTIONS AND PHARMACOLOGY

COMPOUNDS

Cardioactive steroid glycosides (cardenolides, 0.05% in the tips of the foliage): including among others, Corchorosid A and Helveticosid-glucosinolates: chiefly sinigrin (allylglucosinolates) and gluconapin (3-butenylglucosinolates), releasing through cell destruction the volatile mustard oil allylisothiocyanate and 3-butenylisothiocyanate

Vitamins: ascorbic acid (Vitamin C, up to 0.2 % in the fresh foliage)

EFFECTS

Hedge mustard contains cardio-effective steroids. The drug may ease cramps and pain, but this is not proven pharmacologically.

INDICATIONS AND USAGE

The drug is used for urinary tract diseases, coughs, chronic bronchitis, and inflammation of the gallbladder.

PRECAUTIONS AND ADVERSE REACTIONS

No health hazards or side effects are known in conjunction with the proper administration of designated therapeutic dosages.

OVERDOSAGE

It is conceivable that overdosage would have digitalis-like effects. Digitalis-like effects include queasiness, vomiting, diarrhea, headache, and cardiac rhythm disorders. Cases of poisonings have not, however, been recorded.

DOSAGE

Daily Dosage: The average daily internal dose of the drug is 0.5 to 1.0 gm, which would be equal to 3 to 4 cups daily of an infusion.

Externally, the infusion is used as a gargle or mouthwash, several times daily.

LITERATURE

Bachelard HS, Trikojus VM (1963) Austral. J Biol Sci 16: 147.

Ockendon JG, Buczki ST (1979) Trans Brit Mycol Soc 72:156.

Schultz OE, Gmelin R, Naturforsch Z 7b:500-506. 1952.

Further information in:

Hänsel R, Keller K, Rimpler H, Schneider G (Hrsg.), Hagers Handbuch der Pharmazeutischen Praxis, 5. Aufl., Bde 4-6 (Drogen): Springer Verlag Berlin, Heidelberg, New York, 1992-1994.

Roth L, Daunderer M, Kormann K: Giftpflanzen, Pflanzengifte, 4. Aufl., Ecomed Fachverlag Landsberg Lech 1993.

Teuscher E, Lindequist U, Biogene Gifte - Biologie, Chemie, Pharmakologie, 2. Aufl., Fischer Verlag Stuttgart 1994.

Sium Sisarum

Skirret

DESCRIPTION

Medicinal Parts: The medicinal part is the root.

Flower and Fruit: The inflorescence has 10 to 30 rayed-umbels with 1 to 5 lanceolate-narrow involucral bracts. The petals are white, about 1 mm long, broad orbicular-elliptical. The fruit is broad-ovate, about 3.5 by 2 to 2.5 mm in diameter and brownish with light ribs. The fruit segments in cross-section are obtuse pentagons with thin walls.

Leaves, Stem and Root: Sium sisarum is a perennial glabrous plant on a stubby rhizome with clustered, often tuberous roots. The stem is about 30 to 80 cm high, round and branched. The lower leaves are simple pinnate, oblong and serrate. The upper leaves are narrower and more acuminate and are usually lanceolate.

Habitat: The plant is indigenous to China and is cultivated in Europe.

Production: Skirret root is the root of Sium sisarum.

ACTIONS AND PHARMACOLOGY

COMPOUNDS

Oligosaccharides: saccharose (4-8%)

Starch (4-18%)

Mucilage

EFFECTS

No information is available.

INDICATIONS AND USAGE

In folk medicine, the drug is used for digestive disorders and loss of appetite. In the past, it was said to be good for chest complaints.

PRECAUTIONS AND ADVERSE REACTIONS

No health hazards or side effects are known in conjunction with the proper administration of designated therapeutic dosages.

DOSAGE

Mode of Administration: Skirret root is available in the powdered form for oral use.

LITERATURE

Kern W, List PH, Hörhammer L (Hrsg.), Hagers Handbuch der Pharmazeutischen Praxis, 4. Aufl., Bde. 1-8: Springer Verlag Berlin, Heidelberg, New York, 1969.

Skirret

See Sium Sisarum

Skunk Cabbage

See Symplocarpus Foetidus

Slippery Elm

See Ulmus Fulva

Smartweed

See Polygonum Hydropiper

Smilax Species

Sarsaparilla

DESCRIPTION

Medicinal Parts: The medicinal parts are the dried roots, the entire underground part, and the tuberous swellings produced by the runners.

Flower and Fruit: The flowers are white to pale green, yellow or brown. They are, dioecious, usually in axillary cymes or racemes, and contain 6-petals in 2 circles. The ovate to lanceolate tepals are curved outward. The male flowers have 6 stamens with thick filaments and anthers, which are fused at the base of the petals. The female flowers have 6, sometimes only 3, staminoids. The ovate ovary has 3 carpels, each with 1 to 2 atropic ovules and with an almost sessile, bent back, 3-lobed stigma. The fruit is a globular, red, blue or black berry with 1 to 6 seeds.

Leaves, Stem and Root: The species are evergreen shrubs or semishrubs with climbing branches and stipular tendrils. They have a short, gnarled, perennial, creeping or ascending rhizome with numerous long roots stretching over many meters. The branched, thorny, nodular stem has the thickness of an arm and is yellowish green. The leaves are in 2 rows. They are alternate, simple, and often hardy, with 3, occasionally 5 reticulately joined main ribs. The leaf sheaths are ovate and cordate, sagittate and petiolate, or often stipule-like. They turn into climbing tendrils above and break off at this point when they die.

Habitat: The species is indigenous to tropical and subtropical regions of America, eastern Asia, and India. In Europe, only the variety *S. aspera* is found in the Mediterranean region.

Production: Sarsaparilla consists of the dried root of Smilax species, such as Smilax aristolochiaefolii, Smilax regelii, and Smilax febrifuga.

ACTIONS AND PHARMACOLOGY

COMPOUNDS

Steroid saponins (0.5-3%): chief components are sarsaparilloside, along with parillin, as a breakdown product; further, including among others, desglucoparillin, desglucorhamnoparillin, aglycones sarsapogenin

EFFECTS

No information is available.

INDICATIONS AND USAGE

Preparations of Sarsaparilla root are used for skin diseases, psoriasis, rheumatic complaints, kidney diseases, and as a diuretic and diaphoretic.

PRECAUTIONS AND ADVERSE REACTIONS

No health hazards are known in conjunction with the proper administration of designated therapeutic dosages. Stomach complaints and queasiness may occur in rare cases, as could kidney irritation.

OVERDOSAGE

Overdosage could lead to European cholera, worsened diuresis and shock, among other things.

LITERATURE

Elmunajied DT et al., (1965) Phytochemistry 4(4):587.

Thurmon FM, (1942) New Eng. J Med 227(4):128.

Tschesche R et al., (1969) Chem Ber 102:1253.

Tschesche R et al., Chem Ber 102:53-61. 1969.

Tschesche R et al., Liebigs Ann Chem 699:212. 1966.

Tschesche R, In: Pharmacognosy, Phytochemistry, Ed. H Wagner, L Hörhammer, Pub. Springer-Verlag (1971).

Further information in:

Hänsel R, Keller K, Rimpler H, Schneider G (Hrsg.), Hagers Handbuch der Pharmazeutischen Praxis, 5. Aufl., Bde 4-6 (Drogen): Springer Verlag Berlin, Heidelberg, New York, 1992-1994.

Leung AY, Encyclopedia of Common Natural Ingredients Used in Food Drugs, Cosmetics, John Wiley & Sons Inc., New York 1980.

Madaus G, Lehrbuch der Biologischen Arzneimittel, Bde 1-3, Nachdruck, Georg Olmserlag Hildesheim 1979.

Roth L, Daunderer M, Kormann K, Giftpflanzen, Pflanzengifte, 4. Aufl., Ecomed Fachverlag Landsberg Lech 1993.

Teuscher E, Biogene Arzneimittel, 5. Aufl., Wiss. Verlagsges. Stuttgart 1997.

Wagner H, Wiesenauer M, Phytotherapie. Phytopharmaka und pflanzliche Homöopathika, Fischer-Verlag, Stuttgart, Jena, New York, 1995.

Sneezewort

See Achillea Ptarmica

Soap Bark

See Quillaja Saponaria

Soapwort

See Saponaria Officinalis

Solanum Dulcamara

Bittersweet Nightshade

DESCRIPTION

Medicinal Parts: The medicinal part is the stem of the plant.

Flower and Fruit: The violet flowers are arranged in 10 to 20 blossomed, long-peduncled and hanging, panicle-like forms. The calyx is fused, 5-tipped and does not drop. The corolla has a very short tube and 5 long tips, which become revolute when mature. At the base of each tip, there are 2 green spots surrounded by white. There are 5 stamens with golden yellow anthers, which lean towards each other, and 1 superior ovary. The fruit is an oblong, scarlet, and many-seeded berry.

Leaves, Stem and Root: The plant is a subshrub from 30 to 150 cm in height with a creeping, branched rhizome. The stem is twining or creeping, woody below, angular, and usually glabrous. The leaves are petiolate, the upper and lower ones are usually cordate and acute. The middle leaves are usually pinnatesect with 1 pair of lateral segments and a large terminal segment.

Habitat: The plant is common in Europe, northern Africa, eastern and western Asia, and North America.

Production: Woody Nightshade consists of the dried, 2 to 3-year-old stems of Solanum dulcamara harvested in spring prior to leafing, or late autumn after the leaves have dropped.

Other Names: Bittersweet, Dulcamara, Felonwort, Felonwood, Scarlet Berry, Violet Bloom, Blue Nightshade, Fever Twig, Nightshade, Woody, Staff Vine

ACTIONS AND PHARMACOLOGY

COMPOUNDS

Steroid alkaloid glycosides: the alkaloid spectrum varies widely with the breed

Tomatidenol variety - alpha-solamarine, beta-solamarine

Soladulcidine variety - soladulcidinetetraoside

Solasodine variety - solasonine, solamargine

Steroid saponins

Mixed varieties also occur.

EFFECTS

The drug is astringent, antimicrobial, and irritative to mucous membranes. The steroid alkaloid has an anticholinergic effect, and solasodin has an antiphlogistic effect.

INDICATIONS AND USAGE

- Eczema
- Furuncles
- Acne
- Warts

Bittersweet Nightshade is used as supportive therapy for chronic eczema.

PRECAUTIONS AND ADVERSE REACTIONS

Health risks or side effects following the proper administration of designated therapeutic dosages are not recorded. Toxic effects should not be seen in dosages under approximately 25 gm due to the low alkaloid content of the stem.

OVERDOSAGE

Poisonings among children are known through the unripe berries. More than 10 berries cause nausea, vomiting, dilated pupils, and diarrhea. Lethal dosage is estimated to be 200 berries.

DOSAGE

Mode of Administration: Comminuted herb is used in teas and other galenic preparations for internal use. The drug is also used externally in compresses and rinses.

Daily Dosage: The average daily internal dose is 1 to 3 gm of the drug. Externally, the herb is used as infusions or decoctions that have strengths equivalent to 1 to 2 gm of the drug per 250 ml of water.

LITERATURE

Frohne D, (1992) Solanum dulcamara L. - Der Bittersüße Nachtschatten. Portrait einer Arzneipflanze. Z Phytother 14: 337-342.

Hölzer I, (1992) Dulcamara-Extrakt bei Neurodermitis und chronischem Ekzem. Ergebnisse einer klinischen Prüfung. Jatros Dermatologie 6: 32-36.

JNP 56(3):430-431. 1993.

Kupchan SM et al., (1965) Science 150:1827.

Rönsch H, Schreiber K, Stubbe H, Naturwissenschaften 55:182. 1968.

Willaman JJ, Hui-Li L, (1970) Lloydia 33 (3A):1.

Willuhn G, Kothe U, (1983) Arch Pharm 316(8):678-687.

Willuhn G, Phytopharmaka in der Dermatologie. In: ZPT 16(6):325-342. 1995.

Wolters B, Antibiotische Wirkung von Solanum dulcamara. In: Naturwissenschaften 51:111. 1964.

Wolters B, Der Anteil der Steroidsaponine an der antibiotischen Wirkung von Solanum dulcamara. In: PM 13:2. 1965.

Wolters B, (1965) Planta Med 13:189.

Further information in:

Frohne D, Pfänder HJ, Giftpflanzen - Ein Handbuch für Apotheker, Toxikologen und Biologen, 4. Aufl., Wiss. Verlagsges. mbH Stuttgart 1997.

Hänsel R, Keller K, Rimpler H, Schneider G (Hrsg.), Hagers Handbuch der Pharmazeutischen Praxis, 5. Aufl., Bde 4-6 (Drogen): Springer Verlag Berlin, Heidelberg, New York, 1992-1994.

Madaus G, Lehrbuch der Biologischen Arzneimittel, Bde 1-3, Nachdruck, Georg Olms Verlag Hildesheim 1979.

Roth L, Daunderer M, Kormann K, Giftpflanzen, Pflanzengifte, 4. Aufl., Ecomed Fachverlag Landsberg Lech 1993.

Schulz R, Hänsel R, Rationale Phytotherapie, Springer Verlag Heidelberg 1996.

Steinegger E, Hänsel R, Pharmakognosie, 5. Aufl., Springer Verlag Heidelberg 1992.

Teuscher E, Biogene Arzneimittel, 5. Aufl., Wiss. Verlagsges. mbH Stuttgart 1997.

Teuscher E, Lindequist U, Biogene Gifte - Biologie, Chemie, Pharmakologie, 2. Aufl., Fischer Verlag Stuttgart 1994.

Wagner H, Wiesenauer M, Phytotherapie. Phytopharmaka und pflanzliche Homöopathika, Fischer-Verlag, Stuttgart, Jena, New York 1995.

Solanum Nigrum

Black Nightshade

DESCRIPTION

Medicinal Parts: The medicinal parts are the dried herb collected during the flowering season, the whole fresh plant collected during the flowering season and the whole fresh plant with berries.

Flower and Fruit: The small white flowers are in 6 to 10-blossomed umbel-like, nodding, axillary inflorescence. The calyx is 5-tipped and does not drop. The corolla is 5-tipped with a short tube. There are 5 stamens with clavate anthers inclining towards each other. The corolla is rotate and has 1 superior ovary. The fruit is a pea-sized black, occasionally green or yellow berry.

Leaves, Stem and Root: Solanum nigrum is an annual plant 10 to 50 cm in height. The stem is erect, leafy, angular and has outward inclined branches. The leaves are fleshy, petiolate, rhomboid or ovate. They narrow to a cuneate base, which is crenate-dentate and glabrous or sparsely pubescent.

Characteristics: The plant has a musk-like odor when wilting and is poisonous.

Habitat: The plant is found worldwide.

Production: Black Nightshade is the herb of Solanum nigrum picked in uncultivated regions (the wild) and dried in the open air.

Not To Be Confused With: Black Nightshade was often called Petty (a corruption of ''petit'') Morel, to distinguish it from the Deadly Nightshade, or Great Morel, as it is also poisonous but apparently less so.

Other Names: Garden Nightshade, Petty Morel, Poisonberry

ACTIONS AND PHARMACOLOGY

COMPOUNDS

Steroid alkaloid glycosides: (in the foliage and in unripe fruits 0-2.0%) Ripe fruits are, as a rule, free of alkaloids

Chief alkaloids: solasonine, solamargine, β-solamargine

Steroid saponins: with tigogenin as an aglycone

EFFECTS

According to folk medicine, the herb should work as an antispasmodic, pain reliever, sedative, and narcotic.

INDICATIONS AND USAGE

Internally, Black Nightshade is used for gastric irritation and cramps. Externally, the herb is used for psoriasis, hemorrhoids and abscesses. The bruised, fresh leaves can treat external inflammation, burns and ulcers.

PRECAUTIONS AND ADVERSE REACTIONS

No health hazards or side effects are known in conjunction with the proper administration of designated therapeutic dosages.

OVERDOSAGE

Overdoses resulting from the intake of large quantities of the fresh foliage with high alkaloid content, could lead to gastrointestinal signs of irritation, characterized by queasiness, vomiting, headache, in rare cases also by mydriasis.

DOSAGE

Mode of Administration: The herb is available as a ground drug and as an extract for internal and external use.

Daily Dosage: Externally, put a handful in boiling water for 10 minutes, use as a compress or as a rinse. Internally, the dose is 10 drops of extract 2 to 3 times daily.

LITERATURE

Ridout CL et al., PA 44:732. 1989.

Schreiber K, Kulturpflanze 11:451-501. 1963.

Further information in:

Frohne D, Pfänder HJ, Giftpflanzen - Ein Handbuch für Apotheker, Toxikologen und Biologen, 4. Aufl., Wiss. Verlags-Ges. Stuttgart 1997.

Hänsel R, Keller K, Rimpler H, Schneider G (Hrsg.), Hagers Handbuch der Pharmazeutischen Praxis, 5. Aufl., Bde 4-6 (Drogen): Springer Verlag Berlin, Heidelberg, New York, 1992-1994.

Lewin L, Gifte und Vergiftungen, 6. Aufl., Nachdruck, Haug Verlag, Heidelberg 1992.

Madaus G, Lehrbuch der Biologischen Arzneimittel, Bde 1-3, Nachdruck, Georg Olms Verlag Hildesheim 1979.

Roth L, Daunderer M, Kormann K, Giftpflanzen, Pflanzengifte, 4. Aufl., Ecomed Fachverlag Landsberg Lech 1993.

Teuscher E, Biogene Arzneimittel, 5. Aufl., Wiss. Verlagsges. Stuttgart 1997.

Solidago Species

Golden Rod

DESCRIPTION

Medicinal Parts: The medicinal parts are the dried aerial parts collected during the flowering season, the fresh inflorescences and the flowering twigs.

Flower and Fruit: The yellow composite flowers are in erect racemes facing all directions and are simple or compound. They are medium-sized. The involucral bracts are imbricate and arranged in numerous rows. The ray florets are narrow, lingual and female. The disc florets are funnel-shaped, 5-tipped and androgynous. The fruit is an achene, which is cylindrical with numerous ribs. It is brown, sparsely pubescent and 3.5 to 4.5 mm long with a tuft of hair.

Leaves, Stem and Root: The plant is a perennial which ranges in size from a few centimeters to over 1 m. The rhizome is cylindrical, noded, diagonally ascending and short. The stem is erect, cane-like, angularly grooved above, usually red-tinged beneath, and glabrous to loosely appressed pubescent higher up. The basal leaves are long-petioled, elliptical, acuminate and narrowing to the winged stem. The lower ones are serrate and the upper ones are entire-margined.

Habitat: The plant is indigenous to Europe, Asia, and North America.

Production: Golden Rod is the aerial part of Solidago virgaurea. It occurs in the wild in Hungary, former Yugoslavia, Bulgaria, and Poland. Golden Rod herb consists of the above-ground parts of Solidago serotina (synonym S. gigantea). It is Solidago canadensis and its hybrids, gathered during the flowering season and carefully dried.

Not To Be Confused With: Despite qualitative and quantitative differences in their effects, drugs containing Solidago gigantea or Solidago canadensis are exchanged with Solidago virgaurea on the market; confusions with Senecio species are also conceivable.

Other Names: Aaron's Rod, Woundwort

ACTIONS AND PHARMACOLOGY

COMPOUNDS: SOLIDAGINIS VIRGAUREAE HERBA

Triterpene saponins (2.4-6.2%): bisdesmoside of polygalic acid, including acyl-virgaurea-saponins 1, 2 and 3, among others

Volatile oil (0.4-0.5%): chief components gamma-cadinene

Water-soluble acidic polysaccharides

Diterpenes of the cis clerodane-type

Carotinoids (as blossom pigments)

Flavonoids (1.5%): rutin (0.8%), including, among others, hyperoside, isoquercitrin

Phenol glucosides (0.2-1.0%): leicarposide, virgaureoside A (hydroxy-benzylbenzoate-diglucoside)

Caffeic acid derivatives: including among others chlorogenic acid

EFFECTS: SOLIDAGINIS VIRGAUREAE HERBA

Golden Rod is diuretic, antiphlogistic and mildly spasmolytic.

COMPOUNDS: SOLIDAGINIS HERBA (CANADENSIS VARIETY)

Triterpene saponins (12.5%): bisdesmoside of the bayogenins, water-soluble polysaccharides, acylglycosidically-bound, bearing arabino residues: beta-1,2-fructans, acidic polysaccharides

Volatile oil (0.6%): chief components curlone, germacren D, alpha-pinene beta-sesquiphellandrene, limonene

Diterpenes of the trans-clerodane and ladanum type

Carotenoids (as blossom pigments)

Flavonoids (2.4%): rutin (1.4%), further including among others hyperoside, quercitrin, astragalin

Caffeic acid derivatives: including, among others, chlorogenic acid

COMPOUNDS: SOLIDAGIN HERBA (GIGANTEA VARIETY)

Triterpene saponins (9%): bisdesmoside of the bayogenins: GS1-GS4

Volatile oil (0.5%): chief components gamma-cadinene-diterpenes of the cis-clerodane-type, including among others 6-deoxysolidagolactone IV-18,19-olid

Carotenoids (as blossom pigments)

Flavonoids (3.8%): quercitrin (1.3%), further including, among others, hyperoside, rutin, isoquercitrin

Caffeic acid derivatives: including, among others, chlorogenic acid

EFFECTS: SOLIDAGINIS HERBA

It is diuretic, mildly antispasmodic, and antiphlogistic.

INDICATIONS AND USAGE

SOLIDAGINIS VIRGAUREAE HERBA

- Infections of the urinary tract
- Kidney and bladder stones

The herb is used for inflammatory diseases of the urinary tract and urinary stone and kidney gravel prophylaxis. In folk medicine, it is used internally for acute exacerbations of pulmonary tuberculosis, diabetes, enlargement of the liver, gout, hemorrhoids, internal bleeding, nervous bronchial asthma, prostatic hypertrophy, and rheumatism. External uses in folk medicine include inflammation of the mouth and pharyngeal cavity and the treatment of festering wounds.

SOLIDAGINIS HERBA

- Infections of the urinary tract
- Kidney and bladder stones

The herb is used as a flushing-out therapy for inflammatory diseases of the lower urinary tract, urinary calculi and kidney gravel and as a prophylaxis for urinary calculi and kidney gravel.

CONTRAINDICATIONS

SOLIDAGINIS VIRGAUREAE HERBA AND SOLIDAGINIS HERBA

Irrigation therapy is contraindicated in cases of edema resulting from reduced cardiac and/or kidney function.

PRECAUTIONS AND ADVERSE REACTIONS

SOLIDAGINIS VIRGAUREAE HERBA

No health hazards or side effects are known in conjunction with the proper administration of designated therapeutic dosages. The drug possesses a weak potential for sensitization. Care must be taken in patients with chronic renal diseases and the drug should be used in this patient population only under the supervision of a doctor.

SOLIDAGINIS HERBA

No health hazards or side effects are known in conjunction with the proper administration of designated therapeutic dosages. Care must be taken in patients with chronic renal diseases and the drug should be used in this patient population only under the supervision of a doctor.

DOSAGE

SOLIDAGINIS VIRGAUREAE HERBA

Mode of Administration: As chopped drug by itself or in combination preparations.

Preparation: To make an infusion, 1 to 2 teaspoonfuls (3 to 5 gm) of drug is scalded with simmering water (150 ml) and strained after 15 minutes.

Daily Dosage: The daily dosage is 6 to 12 gm of comminuted drug prepared as an infusion. The infusion dosage is one cupful, 2 to 4 times daily between meals. The recommended dosage for the liquid extract is 0.5 to 2 ml liquid extract (1:1) in 25% ethanol 2 to 3 times daily. A dosage of 0.5 to 1 ml tincture (1:5) in 45% ethanol, 2 to 3 times daily is commonly used. Ample fluid intake should be ensured. In folk medicine, 0.5 to 2 gm drug as an infusion is taken 3 times daily.

Storage: The drug must be protected from light and moisture.

SOLIDAGINIS HERBA

Mode of Administration: As a comminuted drug for teas and other galenic preparations for internal use.

Daily Dosage: The daily dosage is 6 to 12 gm herb. Observe ample intake of fluids of at least 2 liters per day.

LITERATURE

SOLIDAGINIS VIRGAUREAE HERBA

Bader G et al., (1987) Pharmazie 42(2):140.

Bader G, Plohmann B, Franz G, Hiller K, Saponins from Solidago virgaurea L. - Possible agent for therapy of cancer? In: PM 62, Abstracts of the 44th Ann Congress of GA, 21. 1996.

Bader G, Wray V, Hiller K, The main saponins from the arial parts and the roots of Solidago virgaurea subsp. virgaurea. In: PM 61(2);158-161. 1995.

Goswami A et al., (1984) Phytochemistry 23(4):837.

Hiller K, Pharmazeutische Bewertung ausgewählter Teedrogen. In: DAZ 135(16):1425-1440. 1995.

Hiller K, Bader G, Goldruten-Kraut Portrait einer Arzneipflanze. In: ZPT 17(2):123-130. 1996.

Inose Y, Miyase T, Ueno A, Studies on the constituents of Solidago virga-aurea L. 1. Structural elucidation of saponins in the herb. In: Chem Pharm Bull 39: 2037. 1991.

Kalemba D, Phenolic acids in four Solidago species. In: PA 47:471-472. 1992.

Lassere B et al., (1983) Naturwissenschaft 70:95.

Metzer J et al., (1984) Pharmazie 39(12):869.

Schilcher H, Boesel R, Effenberger ST Segebrecht S, Neuere Untersuchungsergebnisse mit aquaretisch, antibakteriell und prostatotrop wirksamen Arzneipflanzen. In: ZPT 10(3):77. 1989.

Sökeland J, Phytotherapie in der Urologie. In: ZPT 10(1):8. 1989.

Vonkruedener S et al., Effects of extracts from Populus tremula L., Solidago virgaurea L. and Fraxinus excelsior L. on various myeloperoxidase systems. In: Arzneim Forsch 46(8):809-814. 1996.

Further information in:

Hänsel R, Keller K, Rimpler H, Schneider G (Hrsg.), Hagers Handbuch der Pharmazeutischen Praxis, 5. Aufl., Bde 4-6 (Drogen): Springer Verlag Berlin, Heidelberg, New York, 1992-1994.

Hausen B, Allergiepflanzen, Pflanzenallergene, ecomed Verlagsgesellsch. mbH, Landsberg 1988.

Madaus G, Lehrbuch der Biologischen Arzneimittel, Bde 1-3, Nachdruck, Georg Olms Verlag Hildesheim 1979.

Roth L, Daunderer M, Kormann K, Giftpflanzen, Pflanzengifte, 4. Aufl., Ecomed Fachverlag Landsberg Lech 1993.

Steinegger E, Hänsel R, Pharmakognosie, 5. Aufl., Springer Verlag Heidelberg 1992.

Teuscher E, Biogene Arzneimittel, 5. Aufl., Wiss. Verlagsges. Stuttgart 1997.

Wagner H, Wiesenauer M, Phytotherapie. Phytopharmaka und pflanzliche Homöopathika, Fischer-Verlag, Stuttgart, Jena, New York 1995.

Wichtl M (Hrsg.), Teedrogen, 4. Aufl., Wiss. Verlagsges. Stuttgart 1997,

SOLIDAGINIS HERBA

Bader G et al., (1987) Pharmazie 42(2):140.

Goswami A et al., (1984) Phytochemistry 23(4):837.

Metzer J et al., (1984) Pharmazie 39(12):869.

Lassere B et al., (1983) Naturwissenschaft 70:95.

Reznicek G et al., PM 55:623. 1989.

Reznicek G et al., Tetrahedron Lett 30:4097. 1989.

Reznicek G, Freiler M, Schader M, Schmidt U, Determination of the content and the composition of the main saponins from Solidago gigantea AIT. Using high-perfomance liquid chromatography. In: J Chromatogr A 755(1):133-37. 1996.

Tiansheng L et al. Polyacetylenes and diterpenes from Solida canadensis. In: PH 32:1483. 1993.

Weyerstahl P, Marshall H, Christiansen C, Kalemba D, Góra J, Constituents of the essential oil of Solidago canadensis (''Goldenrod'') from Poland. In: PM 59(3):281. 1993.

Further information in:

Hänsel R, Keller K, Rimpler H, Schneider G (Hrsg.), Hagers Handbuch der Pharmazeutischen Praxis, 5. Aufl., Bde 4-6 (Drogen): Springer Verlag Berlin, Heidelberg, New York, 1992-1994.

Hausen B, Allergiepflanzen, Pflanzenallergene, ecomed Verlagsgesellsch. mbH, Landsberg 1988.

Madaus G, Lehrbuch der Biologischen Arzneimittel, Bde 1-3, Nachdruck, Georg Olms Verlag Hildesheim 1979.

Roth L, Daunderer M, Kormann K, Giftpflanzen, Pflanzengifte, 4. Aufl., Ecomed Fachverlag Landsberg Lech 1993.

Steinegger E, Hänsel R, Pharmakognosie, 5. Aufl., Springer Verlag Heidelberg 1992.

Teuscher E, Biogene Arzneimittel, 5. Aufl., Wiss. Verlagsges. Stuttgart 1997.

Wagner H, Wiesenauer M, Phytotherapie. Phytopharmaka und pflanzliche Homöopathika, Fischer-Verlag, Stuttgart, Jena, New York 1995.

Wichtl M (Hrsg.), Teedrogen, 4. Aufl., Wiss. Verlagsges. Stuttgart 1997.

Solomon's Seal

See Polygonatum Multiflorum

Sophora Japonica

Pagoda Tree

DESCRIPTION

Medicinal Parts: The medicinal parts are the ripe seeds.

Flower and Fruit: The white flowers are in large, broad, sweeping terminal panicles made up of racemes. The flowers are papilionaceous with a patent standard. The lower edge of the lateral wing petals are bent over so that one surrounds the others. The fruit is a round pod tied in around the seeds like a string of pearls.

Leaves, Stem and Trunk: The tree is reminiscent of the robinia, with a densely branched crown and is 12 to 15 m high. It has smooth, green branches. The leaves are odd-pinnate with 11 to 15 leaflets. The leaflets are ovate, acute, dark green above and glaucous beneath. The main leaf petiole is very thick at the base.

Habitat: The plant is indigenous to China and Japan and is found in Europe as an ornamental and roadside tree.

Production: Pagoda Tree seeds are the ripe seeds of Sophora japonica.

ACTIONS AND PHARMACOLOGY

COMPOUNDS

Quinolizidine alkaloids (0-0.04%): including, among others, cytisine, N-methyl cytisine, matrine, sophocarpin

Toxic lectins

Polysaccharides: galactomannans

Fatty oil

Proteins

EFFECTS

The active agent, rutin, increases the permeability of the capillaries.

INDICATIONS AND USAGE

Pagoda Tree is used in homeopathy for dysentery.

PRECAUTIONS AND ADVERSE REACTIONS

No health hazards, side effects, or cases of poisoning are known in conjunction with the proper administration of designated therapeutic dosages. Nevertheless, according to older reports, regular consumption of the seed meal can bring about facial edema and even death. Cystine poisonings are conceivable through the intake of very high dosages.

DOSAGE

Mode of Administration: As a mother tincture in homeopathic dilutions. Sophora is used by the pharmaceutical industry in the production of rutin (a substance which influences the resolution and porousness of the dilation of the capillaries). The drug is contained in medicinal preparations, which are used to stabilize blood circulation and as a cure for nervous disorders and inflammation.

LITERATURE

Izaddoost M, PH 14:203. 1975.

Further information in:

Kern W, List PH, Hörhammer L (Hrsg.), Hagers Handbuch der Pharmazeutischen Praxis, 4. Aufl., Bde. 1-8: Springer Verlag Berlin, Heidelberg, New York, 1969.

Roth L, Daunderer M, Kormann K, Giftpflanzen, Pflanzengifte, 4. Aufl., Ecomed Fachverlag Landsberg Lech 1993.

Tang W, Eisenbrand G, Chinese Drugs of Plant Origin, Springer Verlag Heidelberg 1992.

Teuscher E, Lindequist U, Biogene Gifte - Biologie, Chemie, Pharmakologie, 2. Aufl., Fischer Verlag Stuttgart 1994.

Sorbus Aucuparia

Mountain Ash Berry

DESCRIPTION

Medicinal Parts: The medicinal parts are the ripe, dried fruit or the dried and then boiled fruit.

Flower and Fruit: The inflorescence is broadly umbelliferous-racemous, erect, richly blossomed, loosely tomentose and completely or almost completely glabrous. The calyx has 5 segments. There are 5 white petals and numerous stamens. The ovary is inferior and has 2 to 4 free styles, which are pubescent in the lower portion. The false fruit is almost globular with a diameter of 9 to 10 mm and is scarlet. There are usually 3 seeds, which are narrow-oblong, acute and reddish.

Leaves, Stem and Root: The tree is usually medium-sized up to 16 m high with an open round crown. The bark is smooth and pale gray, later becoming vertically fissured and blackish. The leaves are odd-pinnate with 5 to 11 almost sessile leaflets. The leaves are oblong-lanceolate, irregularly thorny-tipped and serrate.

Characteristics: The flowers have an unpleasant smell and the berries are sharp-tasting and sour. S. moravica tastes sweet in contrast.

Habitat: The plant is indigenous almost everywhere in Europe, in western Siberia, parts of Asia and North America.

Production: Mountain Ash berry consists of the fresh or dried fruit, or fruit cooked and dried thereafter, of Sorbus aucuparia. The ripe, shiny red fruit is harvested from August to October, mainly in Poland, Hungary, in the former Soviet Union, and in the former Czechoslovakia.

Other Names: Rowan Tree, Witchen, Sorb Apple

ACTIONS AND PHARMACOLOGY

COMPOUNDS

Parasorboside (bitter): forming parasorbic acid through cell destruction (lactone of the (5S)-Hydroxyhex-2-en-acyl-1, pungent in odor, mucus-membrane-irritating, 0.1-0.3% of the fresh weight); destroyed or volatilised through drying and cooking; present only in traces (under 0.01%) in the cultivated variety containing few bitter substances.

Cyanogenic glycosides: in the seeds 0.2-0.5% amygdalin; in the fruit pulp, little prunasin

Fruit acids: malic acid (3-5%), tartaric acid

Sugar alcohols: sorbitol (10%)- mono- and oligosaccharides: saccharose, glucose, fructose, sorbose

Vitamins: ascorbic acid (Vitamin C, 0.03-0.13%)

Tannins

EFFECTS
No information is available.

INDICATIONS AND USAGE

Mountain Ash berry and its preparations are used for kidney diseases, for diabetes, rheumatism, disorders of uric acid metabolism and for dissolution of uric acid deposits. In folk medicine, Mountain Ash Berry is used for catarrh, internal inflammations, menstrual complaints, in the alkalization of the blood, to support the metabolism and for Vitamin C deficiency. A puree of the berries is used for diarrhea, and the freshly pressed juice (or juice with sugar) is used for conditions of the lungs and pleura in association with fever.

PRECAUTIONS AND ADVERSE REACTIONS

No health hazards or side effects are known in conjunction with the proper administration of designated therapeutic dosages of the dehydrated drug or with the consumption of fruit sauces, jams, jellies, juices, etc. produced through cooking.

OVERDOSAGE

Because of the resulting build-up of the mucus-membrane-irritating parasorbic acid, the intake of very large quantities of the fresh fruits leads to gastroenteritis, vomiting, queasiness, gastric pain, diarrhea, kidney damage (albuminuria, glycosuria) and to polymorphic xanthemas.

DOSAGE

Mode of Administration: Fresh berries are used in the manufacture of marmalade, jelly, stewed fruit, juice, liqueur and vinegar. Dried fruit is used in tea mixtures.

Note: Fresh mountain ash berry contains parasorbic acid, which causes local irritation. During the drying process, the compound is largely degraded. It is fully destroyed upon cooking.

LITERATURE

Fikenscher LH et al., PM 41:313. 1981.

Letzig E et al., Nahrung 7:591. 1963.

Sicher O, Salama O, PM 39:269. 1980.

Further information in:

Frohne D, Pfänder HJ, Giftpflanzen - Ein Handbuch für Apotheker, Toxikologen und Biologen, 4. Aufl., Wiss. Verlags-Ges. Stuttgart 1997.

Hänsel R, Keller K, Rimpler H, Schneider G (Hrsg.), Hagers Handbuch der Pharmazeutischen Praxis, 5. Aufl., Bde 4-6 (Drogen): Springer Verlag Berlin, Heidelberg, New York, 1992-1994.

Lewin L, Gifte und Vergiftungen, 6. Aufl., Nachdruck, Haug Verlag, Heidelberg 1992.

Madaus G, Lehrbuch der Biologischen Arzneimittel, Bde 1-3, Nachdruck, Georg Olms Verlag Hildesheim 1979.

Roth L, Daunderer M, Kormann K, Giftpflanzen, Pflanzengifte, 4. Aufl., Ecomed Fachverlag Landsberg Lech 1993.

Teuscher E, Lindequist U, Biogene Gifte - Biologie, Chemie, Pharmakologie, 2. Aufl., Fischer Verlag Stuttgart 1994.

Sorbus Domestica

Ash

DESCRIPTION

Medicinal Parts: The medicinal part is the ripe fruit.

Flower and Fruit: The inflorescence is umbelliferous-racemous and tomentose. The sepals and petals are also tomentose. The petals are white to light red and the carpels are pubescent. The dividing membranes are not split. There are 2 ovules in each ovary chamber. The fruit is false pear-shaped-globular, yellow, speckled red on the sun side. The seed is flat, brown and sharp-edged.

Leaves, Stem and Root: Sorbus domestica is a bush or tree up to 13 m high, with branches which are initially gray-tomentose, later glabrous. The winter buds are glabrous or have hairy tips and are sticky. The leaves are pinnatifid with 13 to 21 sessile, serrate and acuminate leaflets. The serrate teeth are long and finely acuminate. The lower surface is bluish green and initially villous-cobweb pubescent, later glabrous.

Habitat: The plant is cultivated in Europe and elsewhere.

Production: Ash berries are the fruit of Sorbus domestica.

Other Names: Service Tree, Cheque Tree

ACTIONS AND PHARMACOLOGY

COMPOUNDS
Sugar alcohols: sorbitol

EFFECTS
The active agents are pectin, tannin, organic acids (sorbin acid), sorbitol. The fruit has astringent, anti-inflammatory and pain relieving properties.

INDICATIONS AND USAGE
Internally, the berries act as an astringent for the intestinal tract. Externally, preparations are used for skin cleansing.

PRECAUTIONS AND ADVERSE REACTIONS
No health hazards or side effects are known in conjunction with the proper administration of designated therapeutic dosages.

DOSAGE
Mode of Administration: Externally: wash (cleanse) the affected areas of the skin with a decoction, also for the treatment of prematurely aged skin; suppressed (subsumed) under the administration of Sorbus aucuparia.

LITERATURE
None.

Sorbus Torminalis

Ash

DESCRIPTION
Medicinal Parts: The medicinal parts are the ripe fruit. It is always the fruit that is used in the various preparations.

Flower and Fruit: The flowers are in erect, loose umbelliferous panicles on loosely tomentose, later glabrous pedicles. The petals are white and the anthers light yellow. The false fruit is orbicular-oblong and 1.5 cm long. The fruit is initially reddish-yellow, later brown and speckled. The 4 seeds are oblong, deltoid, 7 mm long and dark red-brown.

Leaves, Stem and Root: The plant is at times a small, but sometimes up to 22 m tall tree with a widely-domed crown. The bark is dark brown or gray. It is cracked into scaly plates to fairly high up. The older branches are glabrous, gray-brown, glossy and angular with lighter lenticles. The younger branches are loosely tomentose, greenish, later reddish-brown. The buds are broad ovoid and glabrous with shiny green scales. The buds are brown at the edge and loosely pubescent or glabrous. The leaves have 5 cm long, thin, downy, loosely tomentose petioles, which are fresh green. The petioles turn blood-red in autumn.

Habitat: The plant is common in northern temperate zones and is cultivated in many regions.

Production: Ash berries are the fruits of Sorbus torminalis.

Other Names: Wild Sorvice

ACTIONS AND PHARMACOLOGY
COMPOUNDS
Sugar alcohols: sorbitol

The fruits do not contain parasorboside, in contrast to those of Sorbus aucuparia.

The drug has not been fully researched.

EFFECTS
See Sorbus aucuparia.

INDICATIONS AND USAGE
See Sorbus aucuparia.

PRECAUTIONS AND ADVERSE REACTIONS
No health hazards or side effects are known in conjunction with the proper administration of designated therapeutic dosages.

DOSAGE
Mode of Administration: See Sorbus aucuparia.

LITERATURE
There is no literature available.

Sorghum Vulgare

Broom Corn

DESCRIPTION
Medicinal Parts: The medicinal parts are the seeds.

Flower and Fruit: The flowers and inflorescences are large spadix-like and solitary. They may also be in pairs and terminal on long, stiff, indistinct panicles. The panicles may be bushy-branched or occasionally tangled-branched. The individual spikelets are usually ovate to round and the spelts are usually broad-lanceolate. The spelts become hard, shiny and dentated at the tip. The seeds are small, round, and white.

Leaves, Stem and Root: The plant is reed-like and similar to maize but is not as tall.

Habitat: The plant is common in Spain, Italy and southern Europe. It is widely cultivated in the U.S.

Production: Broom Corn seeds are the seeds of Sorghum vulgare.

Other Names: Darri, Durri, Guinea Corn, Sorghum

ACTIONS AND PHARMACOLOGY
COMPOUNDS
Cyanogenic glycosides: dhurrin (in the fruits, in contrast with the foliage [250-700 mg/100 gm] only in very low concentrations: 0.005-5 mg/100 gm)

Starch (70%)

Proteins (10%)

Fatty oil (3%)

Vitamins of the B group: thiamin (B1), riboflavine (B2)

EFFECTS

Broom Corn is a demulcent that is soothing to the alimentary tract.

INDICATIONS AND USAGE

Preparations of the seeds are used for digestive disorders, but it is mainly used as a cereal grain.

PRECAUTIONS AND ADVERSE REACTIONS

No health hazards or side effects are known in conjunction with the proper administration of designated therapeutic dosages.

DOSAGE

Mode of Administration: Broom Corn can be administered as an infusion, but is mostly used as a cereal grain.

LITERATURE

Erb N et al. PM 41:84. 1981.

Seigler D, Cyanogene Glykoside (Vortragsref.). In: DAZ 132(25):1365. 1992.

Further information in:

Kern W, List PH, Hörhammer L (Hrsg.), Hagers Handbuch der Pharmazeutischen Praxis, 4. Aufl., Bde. 1-8: Springer Verlag Berlin, Heidelberg, New York, 1969.

Teuscher E, Lindequist U: Biogene Gifte - Biologie, Chemie, Pharmakologie, 2. Aufl., Fischer Verlag Stuttgart 1994.

Sorrel

See Rumex Acetosa

Soybean

See Glycine Soja

Spearmint

See Mentha Spicata

Speedwell

See Veronica Officinalis

Spergularia Rubra

Arenaria Rubra

DESCRIPTION

Medicinal Parts: The medicinal part is the herb.

Flower and Fruit: The bracts of the inflorescence are almost as large as the leaves. The sepals and petals are 3 to 4 mm. The petals are usually pink, sometimes white. There are 5 to 10 stamens. The capsule is 4 to 5 mm and about equal in size to the sepals. The seeds are 0.45 to 0.55 mm, unwinged, dark brown, subtrigonal and more or less flattened.

Leaves, Stem and Root: The plant is annual to perennial with a slender to somewhat woody taproot, which is smooth and somewhat sticky. From beneath, it produces numerous, 5 to 22 cm long, diffuse, decumbent or procumbent stems. The leaves are narrow, linear and have very short, lanceolate, acute, silver, scarious stipules.

Habitat: The plant is common in Europe, Russia, Australia, North America and Asia.

Production: Arenaria Rubra is the aerial part of Spergularia rubra.

Other Names: Common Sandspurry, Sabline Rouge, Sandwort

ACTIONS AND PHARMACOLOGY

COMPOUNDS

Triterpene saponins

Resins

EFFECTS

The herb has diuretic effects.

INDICATIONS AND USAGE

Arenaria Rubra is used for conditions of the urinary tract, such as cystitis, dysuria and urinary calculus.

PRECAUTIONS AND ADVERSE EFFECTS

No health hazards or side effects are known in conjunction with the proper administration of designated therapeutic dosages.

DOSAGE

Mode of Administration: The herb is used internally as a liquid extract.

LITERATURE

Kern W, List PH, Hörhammer L (Hrsg.), Hagers Handbuch der Pharmazeutischen Praxis, 4. Aufl., Bde 1-8: Springer Verlag Berlin, Heidelberg, New York, 1969.

Spigelia Marilandica

Pink Root

DESCRIPTION

Medicinal Parts: The medicinal parts are the dried rhizomes and roots.

Fruit and Flower: The inflorescences are terminal, sometimes branched spikes inclined to one side. The flowers are erect. The high leaves are tiny or awl-shaped in fives, and they are narrow. The 5-petaled corolla is red or yellow. The fruit is a 2-valved capsule. The seeds are angular and packed tightly in the fruit.

Leaves, Stem and Root: The plant is a perennial that grows up to 45 cm high and has fibrous, twisted roots. The stem is quadrangular and glabrous. The foliage leaves are opposite, membranous, ovate to ovate-lanceolate, acuminate, rounded at the base, entire-margined and sessile. The stipules are small.

Habitat: The plant is indigenous to the U.S.

Production: Pink Root and herb are the rhizome and aerial part of Spigelia marilandica.

Other Names: American Wormgrass, Indian Pink, Maryland Pink, Pinkroot, Starbloom, Wormgrass

ACTIONS AND PHARMACOLOGY

COMPOUNDS

The drug has not been investigated in recent times. Older sources include, among others, references to the presence of acidic resins, volatile oil, tannins, waxes and a volatile base (presumably identical with isoquinoline).

EFFECTS

Pink Root has anthelmintic actions.

INDICATIONS AND USAGE

The herb is used for worm infestation.

PRECAUTIONS AND ADVERSE REACTIONS

According to older sources, the drug allegedly contains a toxin that paralyzes the spinal marrow and leads to death through asphyxiation.

DOSAGE

Mode of Administration: As a powered root or herb or as a liquid extract.

LITERATURE

Hänsel R, Keller K, Rimpler H, Schneider G (Hrsg.), Hagers Handbuch der Pharmazeutischen Praxis, 5. Aufl., Bde 4-6 (Drogen): Springer Verlag Berlin, Heidelberg, New York, 1992-1994.

Lewin L, Gifte und Vergiftungen, 6. Aufl., Nachdruck, Haug Verlag, Heidelberg 1992.

Spikenard

See Aralia Racemosa

Spinach

See Spinacia Oleracea

Spinacia Oleracea

Spinach

DESCRIPTION

Medicinal Parts: The medicinal part is the leaves.

Leaves, Stem and Root: Spinach is an annual plant, which can be planted at various times during the vegetation period to guarantee a year-round supply. The stems may grow up to 1 m or more and are erect. The leaves are ovate to deltoid-hastate, entire or dentate. When the plant ripens, the bracteoles are almost orbicular-obovate, usually wider than long. They often have a divergent spine at the apex.

Habitat: The plant probably originated in Iran and is cultivated worldwide today.

Production: Spinach consists of the fresh or dried leaf of Spinacia oleracea.

ACTIONS AND PHARMACOLOGY

COMPOUNDS

Triterpene saponins: including, among others, spinach saponins A and B- oxalic acid (in young leaves 6-8%, in older leaves up to 16%)

Histamine (up to 140 mg/100 gm fresh weight)

Flavonoids: including, among others, Patuletin, spinacetin, spinatoside

Chlorophyll (0.3-1.0%)

Vitamins: including, among others, ascorbic acid (Vitamin C, 40-155 mg/100g)

Nitrates (depending upon the fertilizer 0.3-0.6%)

EFFECTS

No information is available.

INDICATIONS AND USAGE

Spinach preparations are used for ailments and complaints of the gastrointestinal tract, as a blood-generating remedy, to stimulate growth in children, as an appetite stimulant, for fatigue, and for supporting convalescence.

PRECAUTIONS AND ADVERSE REACTIONS

General: No health hazards or side effects are known in conjunction with the proper administration of designated therapeutic dosages. The relatively high nitrate content makes it advisable to forgo both consuming spinach as a foodstuff too often, and circumstances leading to reduction (as for example leaving it standing at room temperature), in order to avoid nitrite formation.

Pediatric Use: Infants should not receive spinach as a foodstuff until after their fourth month (danger of methemoglobin formation through nitrites).

DOSAGE

No information is available.

LITERATURE

Hegnauer R, Chemotaxonomie der Pflanzen, Bde 1-11: Birkhäuser Verlag Basel, Boston, Berlin 1962-1997.

Kern W, List PH, Hörhammer L (Hrsg.), Hagers Handbuch der Pharmazeutischen Praxis, 4. Aufl., Bde. 1-8: Springer Verlag Berlin, Heidelberg, New York, 1969.

Teuscher E, Lindequist U, Biogene Gifte - Biologie, Chemie, Pharmakologie, 2. Aufl., Fischer Verlag Stuttgart 1994.

Spiny Rest Harrow

See Ononis Spinosa

Spruce

See Picea Excelsa

Squill

See Drimia Maritima

St. Benedict Thistle

See Cnicus Benedictus

St. John's Wort

See Hypericum Perforatum

Stachys Palustris

Woundwort

DESCRIPTION

Medicinal Parts: The medicinal part is the fresh and dried herb.

Flower and Fruit: The closely sessile flowers have very small bracteoles. They are arranged in false whorls of 6 florets joined in groups of 10 to 20 into a spike. The calyx is tubular-campanulate, violet-tinged with awned tips. The corolla is dull violet and the style is pink. The nutlet is globular, 2 mm long, lightly striped and glossy dark brown.

Leaves, Stem and Root: The plant is a perennial, with long runners and barrel-like white swellings between the nodes. The shoots are usually loose and have partly appressed, partly patent silky hairs. They are pubescent or almost glabrous and almost odorless. The stems are erect or ascendent from the ground, 30 to 60 cm high, simple or branched, tough, usually with pubescent edges. The internodes are 2 to 10 cm long. The leaves are sessile or very short-petioled, usually clasping, ribbed, matte green and loosely appressed pubescent on both surfaces.

Habitat: The plant is common in Europe.

Production: Woundwort is the aerial part of Stachys palustris or Stachys sylvatica.

Not To Be Confused With: S. palustris is Marsh Woundwort and S. sylvatica is Hedge Woundwort. Several other plants have the name Woundwort, among them, Prunella vulgaris and Achillea millefolium.

Other Names: Marsh Stachys

ACTIONS AND PHARMACOLOGY

COMPOUNDS

Iridoide monoterpenes

Betaines: (-)- and (+)-stachydrine flavonoids: including, among others, palustrin

EFFECTS

Woundwort is said to be a disinfectant, an antispasmodic, and a cure for wounds.

INDICATIONS AND USAGE

The herb is used externally for the treatment of wounds and internally for abdominal pain, cramps, dizziness, fever, gout, and menstrual disorders.

PRECAUTIONS AND ADVERSE REACTIONS

No health hazards or side effects are known in conjunction with the proper administration of designated therapeutic dosages.

DOSAGE

Mode of Administration: As an extract or poultice for external application.

LITERATURE

Barberan FAT, (1986) Fitoterapia 57(2):67.

Kooiman P, (1972) Acta Bot Neerl. 21(4):417.

Miller FM, Chow LM (1954) J Am Chem Soc 76:1353.

Further information in:

Hegnauer R, Chemotaxonomie der Pflanzen, Bde 1-11: Birkhäuser Verlag Basel, Boston, Berlin 1962-1997.

Kern W, List PH, Hörhammer L (Hrsg.), Hagers Handbuch der Pharmazeutischen Praxis, 4. Aufl., Bde 1-8: Springer Verlag Berlin, Heidelberg, New York, 1969.

Star Anise

See Illicium Verum

Stavesacre

See Delphinium Staphisagria

Stellaria Media

Chickweed

DESCRIPTION

Medicinal Parts: The medicinal part is the fresh flowering or dried herb.

Flower and Fruit: The solitary white flowers are in leaf or branch axils. They open at 9 am and, in good weather, remain open for 12 hours. The 5 double petals are shorter than the oblong-lanceolate sepals. There are 2 to 5 stamens and 3 stigma. The fruit is globular or ovate and covered in teeth. It opens when ripe and the seeds are shaken out through the movement of the plant.

Leaves, Stem and Root: The plant is 5 to 30 cm high. The stem is decumbent and weak, heavily branched and often grows to an impressive length. It creeps along the ground, is fleshy, pale green, and slightly thickened at the nodes. The leaves are opposite, orbicular-ovate. The lower ones are long-petioled and the upper ones are sessile. They are 1.25 cm long and 0.70 cm wide and sit in pairs on the stem.

Characteristics: The stem is pubescent on one side.

Habitat: The plant is found worldwide as a weed.

Production: Chickweed is the fresh herb in flower of Stellaria media.

Other Names: Adder's Mouth, Passerina, Satin Flower, Starweed, Starwort, Stitchwort, Tongue-grass, Winterweed

ACTIONS AND PHARMACOLOGY

COMPOUNDS

Flavonoids: including, among others, rutin

Ascorbic acid (Vitamin C, 0.1-0.15%)

Alkaloids

INDICATIONS AND USAGE

Internally, Chickweed is used for rheumatism, gout, stiffness of the joints, tuberculosis, and diseases of the blood. Externally, it is used for poorly healing wounds, hemorrhoids, inflammation of the eyes, eczema and other diverse skin diseases.

PRECAUTIONS AND ADVERSE REACTIONS

No health hazards or side effects are known in conjunction with the proper administration of designated therapeutic dosages.

DOSAGE

Mode of Administration: The herb is used as a tea or in the form of juice for poultices, and in baths for medicinal purposes.

LITERATURE

Tsotsoriya G et al., (1977) Kromatogr Met Farm 172 (via CA 90:51421).

Further information in:

Kern W, List PH, Hörhammer L (Hrsg.), Hagers Handbuch der Pharmazeutischen Praxis, 4. Aufl., Bde 1-8: Springer Verlag Berlin, Heidelberg, New York, 1969.

Madaus G, Lehrbuch der Biologischen Arzneimittel, Bde 1-3, Nachdruck, Georg Olms Verlag Hildesheim 1979.

Watt JM, Breyer-Brandwijk MG, The Medicinal, Poisonous Plants of Southern, Eastern Africa, 2nd Ed, Livingstone 1962.

Stillingia Sylvatica

Queen's Delight

DESCRIPTION

Medicinal Parts: The medicinal part is the fresh or dried root.

Flower and Fruit: The yellow flowers are in terminal spikes and are apetalous. The fruit is a 3-seeded capsule.

Leaves, Stem and Root: The plant is a perennial herb up to 100 cm tall. It has an angular, smooth stem, which contains a milky latex. The leaves are sessile, coriaceous and narrow at the base. They are variable in form and color and are 3 to 11 cm long. The root is usually reddish-white on the outside and has numerous resin glands.

Characteristics: The taste is bitter and acrid, the smell is characteristic and unpleasant.

Habitat: The plant is indigenous to the southern U.S.

Production: Queen's Delight root is the root of Stillingia sylvatica.

Other Names: Cockup Hat, Marcory, Silver Leaf, Stillingia, Yaw Root

ACTIONS AND PHARMACOLOGY

COMPOUNDS

Diterpenes: including, among others, prostatin (12-deoxyphorbolester), gnidilatidin (orthoester of the daphnane-type), factors S2-S5

Volatile oil

EFFECTS

The juice of the green root causes inflammation of the skin and swelling. The drug has laxative, tonic, and diuretic properties.

INDICATIONS AND USAGE

The herb is used as a 'blood purifier', for digestive disorders, and for the treatment of liver, gall and skin diseases.

PRECAUTIONS AND ADVERSE REACTIONS

The drug is strongly irritating to skin and mucous membranes. Taken internally, it triggers vomiting (it is used as an emetic) and diarrhea (it is used as a laxative). Skin contact leads to inflammation and swelling. The diterpenes cause inflammation and are likely to be carcinogenic and virus-activating. It should not be administered.

DOSAGE

Mode of Administration: As a liquid extract or tincture.

Storage: The drug should not be kept for longer than 2 years.

LITERATURE

Adolf A, Hecker E (1980) Tetrahedron Letters 21:2887.

Zahn P et al. Investigations of homeopathic drugs derived from Hippomane mancinella and Stillingia sylvatica: A potential iatrogenic risk of cancer? In: PM 59(7):A684. 1993.

Further information in:

British Herbal Pharmacopoeia, British Herbal Medicine Association, UK 1983.

Hegnauer R, Chemotaxonomie der Pflanzen, Bde 1-11: Birkhäuser Verlag Basel, Boston, Berlin 1962-1997.

Kern W, List PH, Hörhammer L (Hrsg.), Hagers Handbuch der Pharmazeutischen Praxis, 4. Aufl., Bde. 1-8: Springer Verlag Berlin, Heidelberg, New York, 1969.

Lewin L, Gifte und Vergiftungen, 6. Aufl., Nachdruck, Haug Verlag, Heidelberg 1992.

Madaus G, Lehrbuch der Biologischen Arzneimittel, Bde 1-3, Nachdruck, Georg Olms Verlag Hildesheim 1979.

Teuscher E, Lindequist U, Biogene Gifte - Biologie, Chemie, Pharmakologie, 2. Aufl., Fischer Verlag Stuttgart 1994.

Stone Root

See Collinsonia Canadensis

Storax

See Liquidambar Orientalis

Strawberry Leaf

See Fragaria Vesca

Strophanthus Species

Strophanthus

DESCRIPTION

Medicinal Parts: The medicinal parts are the ripe seeds, which have been freed from their appendages and dried. Most of the species are poisonous.

Flower and Fruit: The flowers are in terminal or lateral panicles with few flowers or in richly blossomed, umbelliferous panicles. Their parts are in fives. They are white or yellowish, radially symmetrical and sometimes fragrant. The calyx has 5 elliptical-lanceolate to obovate sepals and a short tube with a campanulately splayed upper part, which has 10 scales on the margin. The anthers are acute with a partly tailed middle section. The ovary is 2-valved, semi-inferior, and has numerous ovules. The fruit has 1 to 2 follicles, which are oblong, 8 to 58 cm long, splayed or horizontal on one level. The greenish-brown seeds are 8 to 25 mm long, fusiform and often flattened. The seeds have a long tuft of hair at the base which drops off and an awn-like appendage.

Leaves, Stem and Root: The plants are climbing lianes, occasionally erect shrubs, subshrubs, or trees. They contain milky latex. The leaves are opposite, ovate to elliptical, short petioled, simple, entire-margined and usually coriaceous.

Habitat: Strophanthus is indigenous to tropical parts of the Old World.

Production: Strophanthus seeds are the seeds of Strophanthus gratus. Kombe-Strophanthus seeds are the seeds of Strophanthus kombé. The plant is harvested mostly by African tribes in the wilderness or in protected areas in the vicinity of African settlements.

Not To Be Confused With: Strophanthi semen should not be confused with African Strophantus species.

Other Names: Kombé

ACTIONS AND PHARMACOLOGY

COMPOUNDS: STROPHANTHI GRATI SEMEN

Cardioactive steroid glycosides (cardenolides, 3-8%): chief glycoside strophanthin-G (ouabain, over 80%), further including acolongifloroside K, strogoside, among others

Saponins (0.2%)

Fatty oil (35%)

EFFECTS: STROPHANTHI GRATI SEMEN

The active agent, Strophanthin-G, is a heart glycoside that has actions similar to digitalis, but is milder. No clinical test results are available. The drug is poorly absorbed by the gastrointestinal tract.

COMPOUNDS: STROPHANTHI KOMBE SEMEN

Cardioactive steroid glycosides: (cardenolides, 4.0-4.5%, the mixture known as Strophanthin-K) chief glycoside K-strophanthoside (60-80%), erysimoside (15-25%), strophoside, (10-15%)

Saponins (0.2%)

Fatty oil (35%)

EFFECTS: STROPHANTHI KOMBE SEMEN

The effects are similar to Strophanthus gratus, but milder.

INDICATIONS AND USAGE

STROPHANTHI GRATI SEMEN

Strophanthus is used for arteriosclerosis, cardiac insufficiency, gastrocardial symptoms, hypertension and neurodystonia.

PRECAUTIONS AND ADVERSE REACTIONS

STROPHANTHI GRATI SEMEN AND KOMBE SEMEN

General: No health hazards are known in conjunction with the proper administration of designated therapeutic dosages. Queasiness, vomiting, headache, stupor, disturbance of color vision, and cardiac arrhythmias could occur as side effects, in particular through overdosages connected with parenteral administration of strophantin-G or glycoside mixtures.

Drug Interactions: Simultaneous administration of quinidine, calcium salts, saluretics, laxatives and glucocorticoids enhance both effects and side effects.

OVERDOSAGE

STROPHANTHI GRATI SEMEN AND KOMBE SEMEN

Queasiness, vomiting, headache, stupor, disturbance of color vision, and cardiac arrhythmias are the most likely consequence of overdosage. Overdosage is more likely to occur with parenteral administration of strophantin-G or glycoside mixtures.

For a review of symptoms of an acute poisoning and therapy, see Digitalis folium. The danger of poisoning through peroral administration is relatively low, due to the poor absorption of the glycosides.

DOSAGE

STROPHANTHI GRATI SEMEN

Mode of Administration: The drug is available as injection solutions and capsules and in combination preparations.

STROPHANTHI KOMBE SEMEN

Mode of Administration: The drug is available in monopreparations, and is rarely used in combinations.

LITERATURE

STROPHANTHI GRATI SEMEN

Brisse B, Anwendung pflanzlicher Wirkstoffe bei kardialen Erkrankungen. In: ZPT 10(4):107. 1989.

Geiger UP et al., Helv Cheim Acta 50:179. 1967.

Jäger HH et al., Helv Chim Acta 48:202. 1965.

Tittel G et al., PM 45:207. 1982.

Tittel G et al., Pharm Ind 48:822. 1986.

Further information in:

Hänsel R, Keller K, Rimpler H, Schneider G (Hrsg.), Hagers Handbuch der Pharmazeutischen Praxis, 5. Aufl., Bde 4-6 (Drogen): Springer Verlag Berlin, Heidelberg, New York, 1992-1994.

Lewin L, Gifte und Vergiftungen, 6. Aufl., Nachdruck, Haug Verlag, Heidelberg 1992.

Madaus G, Lehrbuch der Biologischen Arzneimittel, Bde 1-3, Nachdruck, Georg Olms Verlag Hildesheim 1979.

Roth L, Daunderer M, Kormann K, Giftpflanzen, Pflanzengifte, 4. Aufl., Ecomed Fachverlag Landsberg Lech 1993.

Steinegger E, Hänsel R, Pharmakognosie, 5. Aufl., Springer Verlag Heidelberg 1992.

Teuscher E, Biogene Arzneimittel, 5. Aufl., Wiss. Verlagsges. Stuttgart 1997.

Teuscher E, Lindequist U, Biogene Gifte - Biologie, Chemie, Pharmakologie, 2. Aufl., Fischer Verlag Stuttgart 1994.

Wagner H, Wiesenauer M, Phytotherapie. Phytopharmaka und pflanzliche Homöopathika, Fischer-Verlag, Stuttgart, Jena, New York 1995.

STROPHANTHI KOMBE SEMEN

Kaiser F et al., Liebigs Ann Chem 643:192. 1961.

Kaiser F et al., Naturwissenschaften 46:670. 1959.

Kartnig T et al., J Chromatogr 52:313. 1970.

Makarevich IF, Khim Prir Soedin 180. 1972.

Puchkova EI et al., Rastit Resu 11:268. 1975.

Further information in:

Hänsel R, Keller K, Rimpler H, Schneider G (Hrsg.), Hagers Handbuch der Pharmazeutischen Praxis, 5. Aufl., Bde 4-6 (Drogen): Springer Verlag Berlin, Heidelberg, New York, 1992-1994.

Lewin L, Gifte und Vergiftungen, 6. Aufl., Nachdruck, Haug Verlag, Heidelberg 1992.

Roth L, Daunderer M, Kormann K, Giftpflanzen, Pflanzengifte, 4. Aufl., Ecomed Fachverlag Landsberg Lech 1993.

Steinegger E, Hänsel R, Pharmakognosie, 5. Aufl., Springer Verlag Heidelberg 1992.

Teuscher E, Lindequist U, Biogene Gifte - Biologie, Chemie, Pharmakologie, 2. Aufl., Fischer Verlag Stuttgart 1994.

Teuscher E, Biogene Arzneimittel, 5. Aufl., Wiss. Verlagsges. Stuttgart 1997.

Strychnos Ignatii

Ignatius Beans

DESCRIPTION

Medicinal Parts: The medicinal parts are the ripe seeds and the dried root bark.

Flower and Fruit: The flowers are in dense, axillary thyrses. Their parts are arranged in fives. They are greenish-white, pubescent and have a 2-valved superior ovary. The fruit is a golden-yellow berry. The berry is up to 13 cm wide and has a hard exocarp. The fruit pulp is yellow and contains up to 40 seeds. The seeds are 2 to 3 cm long by 2 cm wide, oval or rounded-angular, obtuse and very hard.

Leaves, Stem and Root: The plant is a climbing shrub with hooked stems that are up to 20 m long. The truck is up to 10 cm thick. It is occasionally a small tree. It bears leaves that are up to 25 cm long, broad-ovate, opposite and short-petioled.

Habitat: The plant is common all over southeastern Asia and is cultivated there; especially in Vietnam and the Philippines.

Production: Ignatius beans are the seeds of *Strychnos ignatii.*

Not To Be Confused With: The seeds of S. Ianata and S. multiflora were once treated in the same manner as Ignatii seeds.

ACTIONS AND PHARMACOLOGY

COMPOUNDS

Indole alkaloids (2.5-5.6%): chief alkaloid strychnine (share 45-60%), in addition, above all, brucine, further including, among others, 12-hydroxystrychnine, alpha-colubrine, icajine, vomicine, novacine. There are also chemical strains for which brucine predominates, others in which strychnine occurs only in traces.

Fatty oil

INDICATIONS AND USAGE

Preparations made of the ignatius bean are used to treat faintness. Therapeutic use as a bitter or tonic is not recommended.

PRECAUTIONS AND ADVERSE REACTIONS

The drug is severely toxic, due to the strychnine content.

OVERDOSAGE

Symptoms of poisoning can occur after ingestion of one bean. Strychnine doses of 5 mg (30-50 mg of the drug) initially cause restlessness, feelings of anxiety, heightening of sense perception, enhanced reflexes, equilibrium disorders and painful stiffness of the neck and back musculature. Later, twitching, tonic spasms of the masseter and neck musculature, and finally, painful convulsions of the entire body are triggered by visual or tactile stimulation. Dyspnea comes following spasm of the breathing musculature. Death occurs through suffocation or exhaustion. The lethal dosage for an adult is approximately 50 mg strychnine (1-2 gm of the drug). Chronic intake of subconvulsive dosages can also lead to death under similar conditions after some weeks. Liver damage is caused by drug accumulation.

Following the administration of a watery suspension of activated charcoal, the therapy for poisoning consists of keeping external stimulation to a minimum through placement in a quiet, warm, darkened room. Convulsions should be treated with dosages of diazepam or barbital (i.v.). High-calorie glucose infusions should also be given. Intubation and oxygen respiration may also be required. Gastric lavage should be avoided, due to the danger of triggering convulsions. Analeptics or phenothiazines should not be administered. Because of the possibility of unwanted effects occurring in conjunction with the administration of therapeutic dosages, one should forgo any administration of the drug.

DOSAGE

Mode of Administration: It is used in the manufacture of strychnine and brucine.

Daily Dosage: If the drug is taken internally, the maximum single dose is 0.1 gm; the maximum daily dosage is 0.3 gm.

LITERATURE

Bisset NG, Phillipson JD, JNP 39:263. 1976.

Marini-Bettolo GB, Advances in the research of curare and Strychnos. In: Rend Accad Naz 40:1975-1976, 1-2, 61-76. 1977.

Further information in:

Hänsel R, Keller K, Rimpler H, Schneider G (Hrsg.), Hagers Handbuch der Pharmazeutischen Praxis, 5. Aufl., Bde 4-6 (Drogen): Springer Verlag Berlin, Heidelberg, New York, 1992-1994.

Lewin L, Gifte und Vergiftungen, 6. Aufl., Nachdruck, Haug Verlag, Heidelberg 1992.

Madaus G, Lehrbuch der Biologischen Arzneimittel, Bde 1-3, Nachdruck, Georg Olms Verlag Hildesheim 1979.

Roth L, Daunderer M, Kormann K, Giftpflanzen, Pflanzengifte, 4. Aufl., Ecomed Fachverlag Landsberg Lech 1993.

Teuscher E, Lindequist U, Biogene Gifte - Biologie, Chemie, Pharmakologie, 2. Aufl., Fischer Verlag Stuttgart 1994.

Wagner H, Wiesenauer M, Phytotherapie. Phytopharmaka und pflanzliche Homöopathika, Fischer-Verlag, Stuttgart, Jena, New York 1995.

Strychnos Nux Vomica

Nux Vomica

DESCRIPTION

Medicinal Parts: The medicinal parts are the ripe, dried seeds and the dried bark.

Flower and Fruit: The inflorescences are terminal and cyme-like. The flowers have a 5-tipped calyx and a white to greenish-white, plate-shaped corolla with a long tube. There are 5 almost sessile stamens in the mouth of the corolla tube. The ovary is superior, 2-valved and has a long style and a 2-lobed stigma. The fruit, when ripe, is an orange-red, globular berry with a diameter of 4 to 6 cm. The pulp is white, bitter and surrounded by a tough, brittle exocarp about 1.5 mm thick. There are usually 1 to 9 seeds in the pulp, of which 2 to 4 are erect. The seeds are disc-like, orbicular, 12 to 25 mm wide, radially striped, appressed pubescent and exceptionally bitter.

Leaves, Stem and Root: The plant is a tree up to 25 m high with a trunk circumference of up to 3 m. The branches are obtuse-quadrangular, close together, repeatedly bifurcated, glabrous and they have 1 to 2 leaf pairs. They are thickened at the nodes. The trunk bark is blackish-ash-gray and the branch bark is gray. The twigs are green and glossy. The leaves are petiolate and crossed-opposite. The leaf blade is glabrous, broadly ovate, entire-margined and has a curved main rib. The broad stipules dry later.

Habitat: The plant grows all over southeast Asia from Pakistan to Vietnam.

Production: Nux vomica consists of the seeds of Strychnos nux-vomica. The berries are picked when ripe. The hard exocarp is removed and the seeds are taken out and washed to remove any pulp residue. They are subsequently dried in the sun.

Not To Be Confused With: The seeds of Strychnos nux-blanda, Strychnos potatorum and Strychnos wallichiana. Nux vomica powder may be confused with the powder of date nuts or olive stones and with by-products of stone-nut processing.

Other Names: Poison Nut, Quaker Button's

ACTIONS AND PHARMACOLOGY

COMPOUNDS

Indole alkaloids (2.0-5.0%): chief alkaloids strychnine and brucine (approximately in a 1:1 ratio), including among others, 12-hydroxystrychnine, 15-hydroxystrychnine, alpha-colubrine, beta-colubrine, icajine

Fatty oil

Polysaccharides as insoluble reserve substances

Iridoide monoterpenes: including, among others, loganin

EFFECTS

Nux Vomica increases reflex excitability. Endogenic and exogenic stimuli reach the targeted organ without hindrance and, as a result, possess a strengthened effect that can be attributed to the alkaloid strychnine. The toxic principle strychnine deadens the inhibitory synapse of the CNS and results in overextended musculature reactions.

INDICATIONS AND USAGE

Nux vomica and its preparations are used in combinations for diseases and conditions of the gastrointestinal tract, organic and functional disorders of the heart and circulatory system, diseases of the eye, nervous conditions, depression, migraine, and climacteric complaints. In folk medicine, it is used as a tonic, an appetite stimulant, for respiratory complaints, for secondary anemia and for unspecific geriatric complaints.

PRECAUTIONS AND ADVERSE REACTIONS

The drug is severely toxic, due to the strychnine content.

OVERDOSAGE

Symptoms of poisoning can occur after ingestion of one bean. Strychnine doses of 5 mg (30-50 mg of the drug) initially cause restlessness, feelings of anxiety, heightening of sense perception, enhanced reflexes, equilibrium disorders, and painful stiffness of the neck and back musculature. Later, twitching, tonic spasms of the masseter and neck musculature, and finally painful convulsions of the entire body that are triggered by visual or tactile stimulation occur. Dyspnea comes following spasm of the breathing musculature. Death occurs through suffocation or exhaustion. The lethal dosage for an adult is approximately 50 mg strychnine (1-2 gm of the drug). Chronic intake of subconvulsive dosages can also lead to death under similar conditions after some weeks. Liver damage can result from accumulated drug.

Following the administration of a watery suspension of activated charcoal, the therapy for poisoning consists of keeping external stimulation to a minimum through placement in a quiet, warm, darkened room. Convulsions should be treated with dosages of diazepam or barbital (i.v.). High-calorie glucose infusions should also be given. Intubation and oxygen respiration may also be required. Gastric lavage should be avoided, due to the danger of triggering convulsions. Analeptics or phenothiazines should not be administered. Because of the possibility of unwanted effects occurring in conjunction with the administration of therapeutic dosages, one should forgo any administration of the drug.

DOSAGE

Mode of Administration: Nux Vomica is used almost exclusively in homeopathy. Radioactively tagged strychnine is used in medicine to detect glycinergic receptors. In industry, the drug is used as an active agent for pest control.

Daily Dosage: The average single dose is 0.02-0.05 gm; the maximum single dose is 1.0 gm; the maximum daily dosage is 2.0 gm. The drug may be used in the form of nux vomica liquid extract, nux vomica tincture, or Strychninum nitricum (maximum single dose: 0.005 gm).

LITERATURE

Bisset NG, Phillipson JD, JNP 39:263. 1976.

Galeffi C, ETH:2:129-134. 1980.

Maier W, Gröger D, Pharm Zentralhalle 107:883. 1968.

Marini-Bettolo GB, Advances in the research of curare and Strychnos. In: Rend Accad Naz 40:1975-1976, 1-2, 61-76. 1977.

Rodriguez F et al. PH 18:2065. 1980.

Further information in:

Hänsel R, Keller K, Rimpler H, Schneider G (Hrsg.), Hagers Handbuch der Pharmazeutischen Praxis, 5. Aufl., Bde 4-6 (Drogen): Springer Verlag Berlin, Heidelberg, New York, 1992-1994.

Lewin L, Gifte und Vergiftungen, 6. Aufl., Nachdruck, Haug Verlag, Heidelberg 1992.

Madaus G, Lehrbuch der Biologischen Arzneimittel, Bde 1-3, Nachdruck, Georg Olms Verlag Hildesheim 1979.

Roth L, Daunderer M, Kormann K, Giftpflanzen, Pflanzengifte, 4. Aufl., Ecomed Fachverlag Landsberg Lech 1993.

Steinegger E, Hänsel R, Pharmakognosie, 5. Aufl., Springer Verlag Heidelberg 1992.

Teuscher E, Biogene Arzneimittel, 5. Aufl., Wiss. Verlagsges. Stuttgart 1997.

Teuscher E, Lindequist U, Biogene Gifte - Biologie, Chemie, Pharmakologie, 2. Aufl., Fischer Verlag Stuttgart 1994.

Wagner H, Wiesenauer M, Phytotherapie. Phytopharmaka und pflanzliche Homöopathika, Fischer-Verlag, Stuttgart, Jena, New York 1995.

Sumbul

See Ferula Sumbul

Sundew

See Drosera Rotundifolia

Sunflower

See Helianthus Annuus

Swamp Milkweed

See Asclepias Incarnata

Sweet Cicely

See Myrrhis Odorata

Sweet Clover

See Melilotus Officinalis

Sweet Gale

See Myrica Gale

Sweet Orange

See Citrus Sinensis

Sweet Sumach

See Rhus Aromatica

Sweet Vernal Grass

See Anthoxanthum Odoratum

Swertia Chirata

Chiretta

DESCRIPTION

Medicinal Parts: The medicinal part is the herb, which is cut and dried when the seed is ripe.

Flower and Fruit: The numerous flowers are small and form a yellow panicle. The fruit is a single-valved capsule, which tastes very bitter and is odorless.

Leaves, Stem and Root: The plant is an annual and grows up to 90 cm high. The branching stem is brown or purplish, 2 to 4 mm thick, cylindrical below and becoming quadrangular towards the top. The leaves are smooth, opposite, lanceolate or ovate and entire-margined with 3 to 7 longitudinal ribs.

Habitat: The plant is indigenous to northern India and Nepal.

Production: Chiretta is the aerial part of Swertis chirata.

Other Names: Chirata, Chirayta, Indian Balmony, Indian Gentian

ACTIONS AND PHARMACOLOGY

COMPOUNDS

Iridoide monoterpenes as bitter substances (1.3%): chief components gentiopicroside and swertiamarin

Xanthone derivatives: including, among others, swerchirin

EFFECTS

Chiretta stimulates the secretion of gastric juices.

INDICATIONS AND USAGE

Chiretta is used for dyspeptic disorders, loss of appetite and problems with the production of gastric juices in the digestive system.

CONTRAINDICATIONS

The drug should not be used in patients who have gastric or duodenal ulcers due to its stimulation of gastric juice secretion.

PRECAUTIONS AND ADVERSE REACTIONS

No health hazards or side effects are known in conjunction with the proper administration of designated therapeutic dosages.

DOSAGE

Mode of Administration: The drug is a constituent part of various preparations.

Daily Dosage: The daily dosage is 15 to 20 drops, 3 times daily before meals. For nervous disorders, 10 to 15 drops is taken daily between meals.

LITERATURE

Dalal SR et al. (1953) J Ind Chem Soc 30: 455.

Ghosal S et al. (1973) J Pharm Sci 62: 926.

Goyal H et al. (1981) J Res Ayur Siddha 2 (3): 286.

Hikano H et al. (1984) Shoyakugku Zasshi 38: 359.

Komatsu M et al. (1971) Jpn Kokai 71 (27): 558.

Ray S et al. Amarogentin, a naturally occuring secoiridoid glycoside and a newly recognized inhibitor of topoisomerase I from Leishmania donovani. In: JNP 59(1):27-29. 1996.

Sharma PV (1982) Indian J Pharm Sci 44 (2): 36.

Further information in:

Kern W, List PH, Hörhammer L (Hrsg.), Hagers Handbuch der Pharmazeutischen Praxis, 4. Aufl., Bde. 1-8: Springer Verlag Berlin, Heidelberg, New York, 1969.

Leung AY, Encyclopedia of Common Natural Ingredients Used in Food Drugs, Cosmetics, John Wiley & Sons Inc., New York 1980.

Steinegger E, Hänsel R, Pharmakognosie, 5. Aufl., Springer Verlag Heidelberg 1992.

Symphytum Officinale

Comfrey

DESCRIPTION

Medicinal Parts: The medicinal parts are the fresh root and the leaves.

Flower and Fruit: The flowers are dull purple or violet. They are arranged in crowded, apical, 2-rayed, hanging cymes. The calyx is fused and has 5 tips. The corolla is also fused and is cylindrical-campanulate with a pentangular tube and 5-tipped border. The tips are revolute and there are 5 awl-shaped scales in the mouth of the tube. The scales close together in a clavate form and have a glandular tipped margin. There are 5 stamens and 1 style. The ovary is 4-valvular. The fruit are 4 smooth, glossy nutlets.

Leaves, Stem and Root: The plant grows from 30 to 120 cm in height. The root is fusiform, branched, black on the outside and white on the inside. The stem is erect and stiff-haired. The leaves are wrinkly and roughly pubescent; the lower ones and the basal ones are ovate-lanceolate and pulled together in the petiole. The upper ones are lanceolate and broad.

Characteristics: The root is slimy and horn-like when dried.

Habitat: The plant is indigenous to Europe and temperate Asia and is naturalized in U.S.

Production: Comfrey herb consists of the fresh or dried above-ground parts of Symphytum officinale, as well as their preparations in effective dosage. Comfrey leaf consists of the fresh or dried leaf of Symphytum officinale. Comfrey root consists of the fresh or dried root section of Symphytum officinale.

Other Names: Ass Ear, Black Root, Blackwort, Boneset, Bruisewort, Consound, Gum Plant, Healing Herb, Knitback, Knitbone, Salsify, Slippery Root, Wallwort

ACTIONS AND PHARMACOLOGY

COMPOUNDS: SYMPHYTI HERBA

Allantoin (0.45-1.3% in the leaves)

Mucilage

Triterpene saponins

Tannins (8-9%)

Silicic acid (4% in the leaves)

Pyrrolizidine alkaloids (0.03% in the leaves): including echinatin, lycopsamine, 7-acetyllycopsamine, echimidine, lasiocarpine, symphytine, intermedin, among others

COMPOUNDS: SYMPHYTI FOLIUM

Allantoin (0.45-1.3%)

Mucilage

Triterpene saponins

Tannins (8-9%)

Silicic acid (4%)

Pyrrolizidine alkaloids (0.03%): including echinatin, lycopsamine, 7-acetyllycopsamine, echimidine, lasiocarpine, symphytine, intermedin, among others

COMPOUNDS: SYMPHYTI RADIX

Allantoin (0.6-0.8%)

Mucilage (fructans)

Tannins (4-6%)

Triterpene saponins: including among others, symphytoxide A

Silicic acid (4%)

Pyrrolizidine alkaloids (0.04-0.6%): including echinatin, lycopsamine, 7-acetyllycopsamine, echimidine, lasiocarpine, symphytine, intermedin, symveridine, among others

EFFECTS: SYMPHYTI HERBA, FOLIUM AND RADIX

Comfrey has anti-inflammatory and antimitotic properties and promotes the formation of callus.

INDICATIONS AND USAGE

SYMPHYTI HERBA AND FOLIUM

■ Blunt injuries

Externally, it is used for bruises and sprains.

SYMPHYTI RADIX

■ Blunt injuries

Externally, Comfrey is used for bruises and sprains, to promote bone growth, and as a mouthwash and gargle for gum disease, pharyngitis, and angina. Internally, it is used for gastritis and gastrointestinal ulcers. In folk medicine, it is used for rheumatism, bronchitis, pleuritis and as an antidiarrheal agent.

CONTRAINDICATIONS

SYMPHYTI HERBA, FOLLIUM AND RADIX

Comfrey is contraindicated in pregnancy and in nursing mothers.

PRECAUTIONS AND ADVERSE REACTIONS

SYMPHYTI HERBA, FOLLIUM AND RADIX

General: No health hazards or side effects are known in conjunction with the proper administration of designated therapeutic dosages. One should entirely forgo internal administration of the drug, due to the presence, however small, of pyrrolizidine alkaloids which have hepatotoxic and carcinogenic effects. It has been determined that traces of the alkaloids present a danger. External administration where skin is intact appears to be defensible. Nevertheless, no application of daily dosages containing more than 100 mcg pyrrolizidine alkaloids with unsaturated necic structure, to include their n-oxides, should be carried out. The industrial manufacture of extracts virtually free of pyrrolizidine alkaloids is possible.

Use in Pregnancy: The drug is contraindicated during pregnancy.

Use in Nursing Mothers: Use of the drug while nursing is contraindicated.

DOSAGE

SYMPHYTI HERBA AND FOLIUM

Mode of Administration: Ointments and other preparations for external application with 5 to 20% dried drug are available, as well as equivalent preparations.

Daily Dosage: The daily applied dosage should not exceed 1 mcg of pyrrolizidine alkaloids with 1,2 unsaturated necine structure, including their N-oxides. The drug should be used for a maximum of 4 weeks.

SYMPHYTI RADIX

Mode of Administration: The crushed root, extracts, and pressed juice of the fresh plant are used for semi-solid preparations and poultices for external use. It is available as ointments and other preparations for external application with 5 to 20% dried drug and equivalent preparations. The drug is a component of standardized preparations of analgesics, antirheumatic agents, antiphlogistics, antitussives, and expectorants.

Preparation: To make an infusion, pour boiling water over 5 to 10 gm comminuted drug or powdered drug, steep 10 to 15 minutes, then strain (1 teaspoonful = 4 gm drug). For external application, a decoction of 1:10 is used, or the fresh roots are mashed.

Daily Dosage: The daily dosage should not exceed 1 mg of pyrrolizidine alkaloids with 1.2 unsaturated necine structure, including their N-oxides. The drug should be used for a maximum of 4 weeks. When using the infusion, take 1 cup 2 to 3 times daily, but not for a long duration.

LITERATURE

SYMPHYTI HERBA

Ahmad VU, Noorwala M, Mohammad FV, Sener B, A new triterpene glycoside from the roots of Symphytum officinale. In: JNP 56(3):329-334. 1993.

Bhandari P, Gray AI (1985) J Pharm Pharmacol 37:50P.

Branchlij et al., (1982) Experientia 38:1085.

Culvenor CJJ et al., (1980) Experientia 36:377.

Franz G, (1969) Planta Med 17:217.

Furuya T, Araki K, (1968) Chem Pharm Bull 16:2512.

Gracza L et al., (1985) Arch Pharm 312(12):1090.

Gray AI et al., (1983) J Pharm Pharmacol 35:13P.

Ihrig M, Pyrrolizidinalkaloidhaltige Drogen im Handverkauf? In: PZ137(40):3128. 1992.

Kozhina IS et al., (1970) Rastit Resur 6:345.

Mascolo N et al., (1987) Phytother Res 1(1):28.

Mohammad FV et al., Bisdesmosidic triterpenoidal saponins from the roots of Symphytum officinale. In: PM 61(1):94. 1995.

Mütterlein R, Arnold CG, Untersuchungen zum Pyrrolizidingehalt und Pyrrolizidinalkaloidmsuter in Symphytum officinale L. In: PZ-W 138(5/6):119. 1993.

Noorwala M et al., A bisdesmosidic triterpene glycoside from roots of Symphytum officinale. In: PH 36(2):439. 1994.

Petersen G et al., Anti-inflammatory activity of a pyrrolizidine alkaloid-free extract of roots of Symphytum officinale. In: PM 59(7):A703. 1993.

Röder E, Pyrrolizidinhaltige Arzneipflanzen. In: DAZ 132(45):2427-2435. 1992.

Schoental R et al., (1970) Cancer Res 30:2127.

Stamford IF, Tavares IA (1983) J Pharm Pharmacol 35:816.

Taylor A, Taylor NC (1963) Proc Soc Exp Biol Med 114:772.

Weston CFM et al., (1987) Brit Med J 295:183.

White RD et al., (1983) Toxicol Letters 15:25.

Further information in:

Frohne D, Pfänder HJ: Giftpflanzen - Ein Handbuch für Apotheker, Toxikologen und Biologen, 4. Aufl., Wiss. Verlags-Ges. Stuttgart 1997.

Kern W, List PH, Hörhammer L (Hrsg.): Hagers Handbuch der Pharmazeutischen Praxis, 4. Aufl., Bde 1-8: Springer Verlag Berlin, Heidelberg, New York, 1969.

Leung AY, Encyclopedia of Common Natural Ingredients Used in Food Drugs, Cosmetics, John Wiley & Sons Inc., New York, 1980.

Madaus G, Lehrbuch der Biologischen Arzneimittel, Bde 1-3, Nachdruck, Georg Olms Verlag Hildesheim 1979.

Roth L, Daunderer M, Kormann K, Giftpflanzen, Pflanzengifte, 4. Aufl., Ecomed Fachverlag Landsberg Lech 1993.

Schulz R, Hänsel R, Rationale Phytotherapie, Springer Verlag Heidelberg 1996.

Steinegger E, Hänsel R, Pharmakognosie, 5. Aufl., Springer Verlag Heidelberg 1992.

Teuscher E, Lindequist U, Biogene Gifte - Biologie, Chemie, Pharmakologie, 2. Aufl., Fischer Verlag Stuttgart 1994.

Wagner H, Wiesenauer M: Phytotherapie. Phytopharmaka und pflanzliche Homöopathika, Fischer-Verlag, Stuttgart, Jena, New York, 1995.

SYMPHYTI FOLIUM

Ahmad VU, Noorwala M, Mohammad FV, Sener B, A new triterpene glycoside from the roots of Symphytum officinale. In: JNP 56(3):329-334. 1993.

Bhandari P, Gray AI (1985) J Pharm Pharmacol 37:50P.

Branchlij et al., (1982) Experientia 38:1085.

Culvenor CJJ et al., (1980) Experientia 36:377.

Franz G (1969) Planta Med 17:217.

Furuya T, Araki K (1968) Chem Pharm Bull 16:2512.

Gracza L et al., (1985) Arch Pharm 312(12):1090.

Gray AI et al., (1983) J Pharm Pharmacol 35:13P.

Ihrig M, Pyrrolizidinalkaloidhaltige Drogen im Handverkauf? In: PZ 137(40):3128. 1992.

Kozhina IS et al., (1970) Rastit Resur 6:345.

Mascolo N et al., (1987) Phytother Res 1(1):28.

Mohammad FV et al., Bisdesmosidic triterpenoidal saponins from the roots of Symphytum officinale. In: PM 61(1):94. 1995.

Mütterlein R, Arnold CG, Untersuchungen zum Pyrrolizidingehalt und Pyrrolizidinalkaloidmsuter in Symphytum officinale L.. In: PZ-W 138(5/6):119. 1993.

Noorwala M et al., A bisdesmosidic triterpene glycoside from roots of Symphytum officinale. In: PH 36(2):439. 1994.

Petersen G et al., Anti-inflammatory activity of a pyrrolizidine alkaloid-free extract of roots of Symphytum officinale. In: PM 59(7):A703. 1993.

Röder E, Pyrrolizidinhaltige Arzneipflanzen. In: DAZ 132(45):2427-2435. 1992.

Schoental R et al., (1970) Cancer Res 30:2127.

Stamford IF, Tavares IA (1983) J Pharm Pharmacol 35:816.

Taylor A, Taylor NC (1963) Proc Soc Exp Biol Med 114:772.

Weston CFM et al., (1987) Brit Med J 295:183.

White RD et al., (1983) Toxicol Letters 15:25.

Further information in:

Frohne D, Pfänder HJ, Giftpflanzen - Ein Handbuch für Apotheker, Toxikologen und Biologen, 4. Aufl., Wiss. Verlags-Ges. Stuttgart 1997.

Kern W, List PH, Hörhammer L (Hrsg.), Hagers Handbuch der Pharmazeutischen Praxis, 4. Aufl., Bde 1-8: Springer Verlag Berlin, Heidelberg, New York, 1969.

Leung AY, Encyclopedia of Common Natural Ingredients Used in Food Drugs, Cosmetics, John Wiley & Sons Inc., New York 1980.

Madaus G, Lehrbuch der Biologischen Arzneimittel, Bde 1-3, Nachdruck, Georg Olms Verlag Hildesheim 1979.

Roth L, Daunderer M, Kormann K, Giftpflanzen, Pflanzengifte, 4. Aufl., Ecomed Fachverlag Landsberg Lech 1993.

Schulz R, Hänsel R, Rationale Phytotherapie, Springer Verlag Heidelberg 1996.

Steinegger E, Hänsel R, Pharmakognosie, 5. Aufl., Springer Verlag Heidelberg 1992.

Teuscher E, Lindequist U, Biogene Gifte - Biologie, Chemie, Pharmakologie, 2. Aufl., Fischer Verlag Stuttgart 1994.

Wagner H, Wiesenauer M, Phytotherapie. Phytopharmaka und pflanzliche Homöopathika, Fischer-Verlag, Stuttgart, Jena, New York 1995.

Wichtl M (Hrsg.), Teedrogen, 4. Aufl., Wiss. Verlagsges. Stuttgart 1997.

SYMPHYTI RADIXZ

Ahmad VU, Noorwala M, Mohammad FV, Sener B, A new triterpene glycoside from the roots of Symphytum officinale. In: JNP 56(3):329-334. 1993.

Bhandari P, Gray AI (1985) J Pharm Pharmacol 37:50P.

Branchlij et al., (1982) Experientia 38:1085.

Culvenor CJJ et al., (1980) Experientia 36:377.

Franz G (1969) Planta Med 17:217.

Furuya T, Araki K (1968) Chem Pharm Bull 16:2512.

Gracza L et al., (1985) Arch Pharm 312(12):1090.

Gray AI et al., (1983) J Pharm Pharmacol 35:13P.

Ihrig M, Pyrrolizidinalkaloidhaltige Drogen im Handverkauf? In: PZ 137(40):3128. 1992.

Kozhina IS et al., (1970) Rastit Resur 6:345.

Mascolo N et al., (1987) Phytother Res 1(1):28.

Mohammad FV et al., Bisdesmosidic triterpenoidal saponins from the roots of Symphytum officinale. In: PM 61(1):94. 1995.

Mütterlein R, Arnold CG, Untersuchungen zum Pyrrolizidingehalt und Pyrrolizidinalkaloidmsuter in Symphytum officinale L.. In: PZ-W 138(5/6):119. 1993.

Noorwala M et al., A bisdesmosidic triterpene glycoside from roots of Symphytum officinale. In: PH 36(2):439. 1994.

Petersen G et al., Anti-inflammatory activity of a pyrrolizidine alkaloid-free extract of roots of Symphytum officinale. In: PM 59(7):A703. 1993.

Röder E, Pyrrolizidinhaltige Arzneipflanzen. In: DAZ 132(45):2427-2435. 1992.

Schoental R et al., (1970) Cancer Res 30:2127.

Stamford IF, Tavares IA (1983) J Pharm Pharmacol 35:816.

Taylor A, Taylor NC (1963) Proc Soc Exp Biol Med 114:772.

Weston CFM et al., (1987) Brit Med J 295:183.

White RD et al., (1983) Toxicol Letters 15:25.

Further information in:

Frohne D, Pfänder HJ, Giftpflanzen - Ein Handbuch für Apotheker, Toxikologen und Biologen, 4. Aufl., Wiss. Verlags-Ges. Stuttgart 1997.

Kern W, List PH, Hörhammer L (Hrsg.), Hagers Handbuch der Pharmazeutischen Praxis, 4. Aufl., Bde 1-8: Springer Verlag Berlin, Heidelberg, New York, 1969.

Leung AY, Encyclopedia of Common Natural Ingredients Used in Food Drugs, Cosmetics, John Wiley & Sons Inc., New York 1980.

Madaus G, Lehrbuch der Biologischen Arzneimittel, Bde 1-3, Nachdruck, Georg Olms Verlag Hildesheim 1979.

Roth L, Daunderer M, Kormann K, Giftpflanzen, Pflanzengifte, 4. Aufl., Ecomed Fachverlag Landsberg Lech 1993.

Schulz R, Hänsel R, Rationale Phytotherapie, Springer Verlag Heidelberg 1996.

Steinegger E, Hänsel R, Pharmakognosie, 5. Aufl., Springer Verlag Heidelberg 1992.

Teuscher E, Lindequist U, Biogene Gifte - Biologie, Chemie, Pharmakologie, 2. Aufl., Fischer Verlag Stuttgart 1994.

Symplocarpus Foetidus

Skunk Cabbage

DESCRIPTION

Medicinal Parts: The medicinal parts are the seeds, the rhizome and the roots.

Flower and Fruit: The plant has numerous small purple flowers in a red-brown, oval, high, spadix-like inflorescence.

Leaves, Stem and Root: The plant is a perennial and grows up to 75 cm high. It has a thick tuberous rhizome, which is truncate at both ends, dark brown and up to about 4 cm in diameter. It is gnarled and woody and bears numerous roots and root scars. The roots are up to 8 cm long, 0.5 cm in diameter and transversely wrinkled. The leaves are like cabbage leaves and they surround the inflorescence.

Characteristics: The taste is hot and the odor is unpleasant.

Habitat: The plant is indigenous to the northern U.S.

Production: Skunk Cabbage root and rootstock are the rhizome and roots of Symplocarpus foetidus.

Other Names: Dracontium, Meadow Cabbage, Polecatweed, Skunkweed

ACTIONS AND PHARMACOLOGY

COMPOUNDS

Volatile oil (bad-smelling)

Resins

The constituents of the drug have not been fully investigated.

EFFECTS

Skunk Cabbage is an antispasmodic, a diaphoretic, an expectorant, and a sedative.

INDICATIONS AND USAGE

The plant is used for bronchitis and asthma.

PRECAUTIONS AND ADVERSE REACTIONS

No health hazards or side effects are known in conjunction with the proper administration of designated therapeutic dosages.

OVERDOSAGE

Overdosage is said to bring about queasiness and vomiting.

DOSAGE

Mode of Administration: Skunk Cabbage is administered as a liquid extract in various medicinal preparations.

LITERATURE

Adolf A, Hecker E (1980) Tetrahedron Letters 21:2887

Further information in:

Hegnauer R, Chemotaxonomie der Pflanzen, Bde 1-11: Birkhäuser Verlag Basel, Boston, Berlin 1962-1997.

Kern W, List PH, Hörhammer L (Hrsg.), Hagers Handbuch der Pharmazeutischen Praxis, 4. Aufl., Bde 1-8: Springer Verlag Berlin, Heidelberg, New York, 1969.

Syzygium Aromaticum

Clove

DESCRIPTION

Medicinal Parts: The medicinal parts are the oil extracted from the whole or macerated flower buds, the pedicles and leaves, as well as the flower buds, the dried flower buds, and the not quite ripe fruit.

Flower and Fruit: The flowers are in triply-triple-branched cymes. They are short-pedicled, whitish-pink, approximately 6 mm wide and have 2 scale-like bracteoles. The calyx tube is 1 to 1.5 cm long and cylindrical. The 4 sepals are fleshy and there are 4 petals. The fruit is 2 to 2.5 cm long, 1.3 to 1.5 cm wide and is crowned by 4 curved sepals. The fruit is 1-seeded.

Leaves, Stem and Root: The plant is a 20 m high, pyramid-shaped, evergreen tree. The diameter of the trunk is 40 cm. The branches are almost round. The leaves are 9 to 12 cm long and 3.5 cm wide. They are coriaceous, elliptical to lanceolate, short, obtusely tipped and narrowing in a cuneate form to the petiole, which is 2.5 cm long. There is 1 main rib and more than 20 lateral ones.

Characteristics: The taste and odor are characteristic.

Habitat: The plant is indigenous to the Molucca Islands and is cultivated there and in Tanzania, Madagascar, Brazil and other tropical regions.

Production: Cloves consist of the hand-picked and dried flower buds of Syzygium aromaticum (syn. Jambosa caryophyllus, Eugenia caryophyllata).

ACTIONS AND PHARMACOLOGY

COMPOUNDS

Volatile oil: chief components are eugenol, eugenyl acetate, beta-caryophyllene

Flavonoids

Tannins

Triterpenes: oleanolic acid, crataegol acid

EFFECTS

Clove is antiseptic, antibacterial, antifungal, antiviral, spasmolytic and a local anaesthetic.

INDICATIONS AND USAGE

- Common cold
- Cough/bronchitis
- Dental analgesic
- Fevers and colds
- Inflammation of the mouth and pharynx
- Tendency to infection

Clove oil is used for inflammation of the mouth and throat and mouth ulcers, and as a local analgesic and dental antiseptic.

PRECAUTIONS AND ADVERSE REACTIONS

No health hazards or side effects are known in conjunction with the proper administration of designated therapeutic dosages. Allergic reactions against eugenol occur rarely. In concentrated form, oil of cloves may be irritating to mucosa.

DOSAGE

Mode of Administration: As a powdered, ground, or whole herb for the recovery of the essential oil, and other galenic preparations for topical use.

Daily Dosage: Aqueous solutions corresponding to 1 to 5% essential oil are used externally for mouthwashes. In dentistry, the undiluted essential oil is used.

LITERATURE

Cai L, Wu ChD, Compounds from Syzygium aromaticum possesing growth inihibitory activity against oral pathogens. In: JNP 59(10):987-990. 1996.

Debelmas AM, Rochat J, (1967) Plant Med Phytother 1:23.

Deiniger R, Gewürznelken (Syzygium aromaticum) und Nelkenöl - aktuelle Phytopharmaka. In: ZPT 12(6):205. 1992.

Kato Y, (1975) Koryo 113:17 and 24.

Narayanan CS, Matthew AG (1985) Ind Perf 29(1/2):15.

Tanaka T, Orii Y, Nonaka GI, Nishioka I, Kouno I, Syziginins A and B, two ellegitannins from Syzygium aromaticum. In: PH 43(6)1345-1348. 1996.

Willuhn G, Pflanzliche Dermatika. Eine kritische Übersicht.. In: DAZ 132(37):1873. 1992.

Further information in:

Hänsel R, Keller K, Rimpler H, Schneider G (Hrsg.), Hagers Handbuch der Pharmazeutischen Praxis, 5. Aufl., Bde 4-6 (Drogen), Springer Verlag Berlin, Heidelberg, New York, 1992-1994.

Leung AY, Encyclopedia of Common Natural Ingredients Used in Food Drugs and Cosmetics, John Wiley & Sons Inc., New York 1980.

Steinegger E, Hänsel R, Pharmakognosie, 5. Aufl., Springer Verlag Heidelberg 1992.

Teuscher E, Biogene Arzneimittel, 5. Aufl., Wiss. Verlagsges. mbH Stuttgart 1997.

Wagner H, Wiesenauer M, Phytotherapie. Phytopharmaka und pflanzliche Homöopathika, Fischer-Verlag, Stuttgart, Jena, New York 1995.

Wichtl M (Hrsg.), Teedrogen, 4. Aufl., Wiss. Verlagsges. Stuttgart 1997.

Syzygium Cumini

Jambolan

DESCRIPTION

Medicinal Parts: The medicinal parts are the dried bark, the dried seed kernels, the disintegrated kernels, the dried trunk bark, and the macerated seeds.

Flower and Fruit: The flowers are in compound, triple panicles. They are sessile, whitish, fragrant, and are usually on older branches behind the leaves. The calyx tube is 4 to 6 mm long and twisted. The petals are hood-like. There are approximately 60 stamens, which are as long as the calyx tube. The drupe is initially pink, becoming black when ripe. The drupe is 1.2 to 3 cm long, globular to ovate, 1-valved, 1-seeded and edible. The seeds are subcylindrical, about 6 mm long and rather less in diameter. One end of the seed is truncated and has a central depression. Externally, they are hard, tough and blackish-brown; internally they are pinkish-brown.

Characteristics: The taste of the seeds is faintly astringent and aromatic, the odor is slight.

Habitat: The plant is indigenous to the east Indian Malayian region. It has spread as far as China and Australia and is cultivated on the Antilles.

Production: Jambolan seed consists of the dried seed of Syzygium cumini (syn. Syzygium jambolana). Because the commodity consists mostly of the dried, fallen apart cotyledons, they must be broken apart in order to produce the drug. Jambolan bark consists of the dried bark from the trunk of Syzygium cumini (syn Syzygium jambolana).

Other Names: Jambul, Jamum, Java Plum, Rose Apple

ACTIONS AND PHARMACOLOGY

COMPOUNDS: SYZYGII CUMINI SEMEN

Fatty oil (3-5%): besides oleic acid, myristic acid, palmitic acid and linoleic acid, epoxy fatty acid

Tannins (6%): including, among others, corilagin, 3,3′-Di-O-methyl ellagic acid, galloylglucose

EFFECTS: SYZYGII CUMINI SEMEN

Anti-inflammatory actions were demonstrated in animal experiments. Results of hypoglycemic and CNS experiments were not verifiable.

COMPOUNDS: SYZYGII CUMINI CORTEX

Gallic and ellagic acid derivatives: including, among others, bergenin, 3,3′-di-O-methyl ellagic acid- triterpenes and sterols: beta-sitosterol, beta-sitosterol glucoside, betuline acid, eugenine

Flavonoids: including, among others, myricetin, kaempferol, quercetin, kaempferol-3-O-glucosides

EFFECTS: SYZYGII CUMINI CORTEX

The bark has astringent effects and has been shown to be hypoglycemic in some animal experiments.

INDICATIONS AND USAGE

SYZYGII CUMINI SEMEN

Jambolan seed is used for diabetes and in combination preparations for atonic and spastic constipation, diseases of the pancreas, gastric and pancreatic complaints, nervous disorders, depression and exhaustion. It is also used as a carminative, an antispasmodic, a diuretic and an aphrodisiac. The efficacy for the claimed applications has not been documented. It is used in India for diabetes, especially for thirst symptoms associated with the disease.

SYZYGII CUMINI CORTEX

- Diarrhea
- Inflammation of the mouth and pharynx
- Inflammation of the skin

Preparations of the bark are used internally for nonspecific acute diarrhea and as a topical therapy for mild inflammation of the oral-pharyngeal mucosa. Externally, it is used for mild, superficial inflammation of the skin. In folk medicine, preparations are used internally for bronchitis, asthma and dysentery and externally for ulcers.

PRECAUTIONS AND ADVERSE REACTIONS

SYZYGII CUMINI SEMEN

No health hazards or side effects are known in conjunction with the proper administration of designated therapeutic dosages. Administration in the presence of diabetes mellitus is not recommended, due to the fact that the blood sugar-reducing effect is unproven.

SYZYGII CUMINI CORTEX

No health hazards or side effects are known in conjunction with the proper administration of designated therapeutic dosages.

DOSAGE

SYZYGII CUMINI SEMEN

Daily Dosage: In folk medicine, a single dose is made up of 30 seeds (1.9 gm) in powdered form.

SYZYGII CUMINI CORTEX

Mode of Administration: As a comminuted herb for decoctions and other galenic preparations for internal use, (gargle, infusion), and local application, (compresses).

Preparation: To make a decoction for internal and external use, place 1 to 2 teaspoonfuls of comminuted drug in about 150 ml cold water, bring to a boil, simmer for 5 to 10 minutes, and strain.

Daily Dosage: The average daily dosage is 3 to 6 gm drug.

LITERATURE

SYZYGII CUMINI SEMEN

Bhatia IS et al., PM 28:346. 1975. Saeed MT et al., J Oil Technol Assoc India 19:86-88. 1991. Bhatia IS et al., PH 10:219. 1971. Desai HK et al., Ind J Chem 13:97-98. 1975.

Jain, SR, Sharma SN, (1967) Planta Med 15(4):439.

Linde H, (1983) Arch Pharm 316(11):971.

Mukherjee SK et al., (1963) Ind Med Gaz 3:97.

Nair AGR, Subramanian S, (1962) J Sci Ind Res India 21B, 437.

Shrothi, DS et al., (1963) Ind J Med Res 51:464.

Further information in:

Hänsel R, Keller K, Rimpler H, Schneider G (Hrsg.), Hagers Handbuch der Pharmazeutischen Praxis, 5. Aufl., Bde 4-6 (Drogen): Springer Verlag Berlin, Heidelberg, New York, 1992-1994.

Hoppe HA, (1975-1987) Drogenkunde, 8. Aufl., Bde 1-3: W de Gruyter Verlag, Berlin, New York.

Oliver-Bever B (Ed.), Medicinal Plants of Tropical West Africa, Cambridge University Press, Cambridge 1986.

SYZYGII CUMINI CORTEX

Bhargava KK et al., Curr Sci 43:645-646. 1974.

Bhargava KK et al., Curr Sci 43:645. 1974.

Bhatia IS et al., PM 28:346. 1975.

Jain, SR, Sharma SN, (1967) Planta Med 15(4):439.

Kopanski L, Schnelle G, PM 54:572. 1988.

Linde H, (1983) Arch Pharm 316(11):971.

Mukherjee SK et al., (1963) Ind Med Gaz 3:97.

Nair AGR, Subramanian S, (1962) J Sci Ind Res India 21B, 437.

Sengupta D, Das PB, J Ind Chem Soc 42:255. 1965.

Shrothi DS et al., (1963) Ind J Med Res 51:464.

Further information in:

Hänsel R, Keller K, Rimpler H, Schneider G (Hrsg.), Hagers Handbuch der Pharmazeutischen Praxis, 5. Aufl., Bde 4-6 (Drogen): Springer Verlag Berlin, Heidelberg, New York, 1992-1994.

Hoppe HA, (1975-1987) Drogenkunde, 8. Aufl., Bde 1-3: W de Gruyter Verlag, Berlin, New York.

Oliver-Bever B (Ed.), Medicinal Plants of Tropical West Africa, Cambridge University Press, Cambridge 1986.

Tamarind

See Tamarindus Indica

Tamarindus Indica

Tamarind

DESCRIPTION

Medicinal Parts: The medicinal parts are the fruit pulp and the dried seeds.

Flower and Fruit: The flowers form a terminal raceme and have three, 1 cm long petals which are initially whitish, then yellowish with light-red stripes. They have a calyx with a narrow, top-shaped base and 4 thickly covering segments. The stamens are fused in a sheath, which is open at the top. The fruit is a 20 cm long and 3 cm wide, matt-brown, slightly compressed, indehiscent, bean-like pod with 3 to 12 irregular, roundish-quadrangular glossy brown, very hard, up to 14 mm long seeds in a mushy, sweet-tasting, odorless mesocarp.

Habitat: The plant is indigenous to tropical Africa and is naturalized in North and South America from Florida to Brazil. It is cultivated in subtropical China, India, Pakistan, Indochina, on the Phillippines and in Java and Spain.

Production: Tamarind paste is derived from the fruit of Tamarindus indica. The fruit is fermented for a long time in the sun. The initially red-brown fruit attains a black or black-brown hue and becomes more aromatic and sour. The paste is boiled to a glutinous mass, which is the finished product.

Other Names: Imlee

ACTIONS AND PHARMACOLOGY

COMPOUNDS

Fruit acids: tartaric acid (3-10%); including, among others, malic acid, citric acid, lactic acid

Invert sugar (25-30%)

Pectin

EFFECTS

Tamarind acts as an aperient by increasing the volume of liquid in the large intestine.

INDICATIONS AND USAGE

The drug is used for chronic or acute constipation and liver and gallbladder ailments. In India, a drink derived from the fruit is used to combat fever.

PRECAUTIONS AND ADVERSE REACTIONS

No health hazards or side effects are known in conjunction with the proper administration of designated therapeutic dosages.

DOSAGE

Mode of Administration: Usually used in combination with other laxatives, such as figs.

Daily Dosage: 10 to 50 gm of cleaned tamarind paste, pure or with other purgatives, is taken in fruit cubes.

LITERATURE

Ishola MM et al., J Sci Food Agric 51:141. 1990.

Khurana AL, Ho CT, J Liq Chromatogr 12:419-430. 1989.

Lee PL et al., (1975) J Agric Food Chem 23:1195.

Further information in:

Hänsel R, Keller K, Rimpler H, Schneider G (Hrsg.), Hagers Handbuch der Pharmazeutischen Praxis, 5. Aufl., Bde 4-6 (Drogen): Springer Verlag Berlin, Heidelberg, New York, 1992-1994.

Leung AY, Encyclopedia of Common Natural Ingredients Used in Food Drugs, Cosmetics, John Wiley & Sons Inc., New York 1980.

Madaus G, Lehrbuch der Biologischen Arzneimittel, Bde 1-3, Nachdruck, Georg Olms Verlag Hildesheim 1979.

Steinegger E, Hänsel R, Pharmakognosie, 5. Aufl., Springer Verlag Heidelberg 1992.

Teuscher E, Biogene Arzneimittel, 5. Aufl., Wiss. Verlagsges. Stuttgart 1997.

Tamus Communis

Black Bryony

DESCRIPTION

Medicinal Parts: The medicinal part is the root.

Flower and Fruit: The flowers are small greenish-white and in loose clusters. They consist of 6 petals and are found on various plants in fertile and infertile form. The fertile flowers develop into crimson berries.

Leaves, Stem and Root: Tami communis is a glabrous climber. The stem dies back in winter but the root is perennial. The leaves are cordate, smooth, acute and glossy. The root is almost cylindrical with a diameter of 2 to 3 cm. The root is 6 to 8 cm long and has scattered, thin, root fibers. Externally, the root is blackish-brown. Internally, it is whitish and produces a slimy paste when it is peeled.

Characteristics: The taste of the root is acrid and the odor is slightly earthy.

Habitat: The plant is indigenous to parts of Europe.

Production: Black Bryony root is the root of Tamus communis. The roots are gathered at the end of the vegetation period. They are dug up and the bark is peeled off and cut into slices or pieces. During this procedure, gloves should be worn to protect the hands, as the fresh roots cause serious reddening of the skin.

Other Names: Blackeye Root

ACTIONS AND PHARMACOLOGY

COMPOUNDS

Histamine-oxalate: in the form of skin- and mucous membrane-irritating needles

Mucilage

Volatile oil

Steroid saponins

EFFECTS

Black Bryony stimulates the external nerve ends. A substance similar to histamine increases blood circulation in areas of the skin to which it is applied.

INDICATIONS AND USAGE

The plant is used for agitation and redness of the skin, bruises, strains, torn muscles, gout and other rheumatic disorders, irritation of the intestine mucous membrane and as an emetic. It is also used as a tonic for hair loss, as it improves blood circulation to the scalp.

PRECAUTIONS AND ADVERSE REACTIONS

Skin contact with the fresh plant leads to the formation of rashes, swellings, pustules and wheals, due to the skin- and mucous membrane-irritating oxalate needles and histamine. Internal administration triggers signs of severe irritation in the mouth, pharyngeal space and gastrointestinal tract, combined with vomiting and intense diarrhea. Extracts from the plant are toxicologically harmless. Skin lesions are treated with cortisone foam and sterile coverings; tetanus prophylaxis might be required. If taken by mouth, following gastric lavage with burgundy-colored potassium permanganate solution and administration of activated charcoal, treat spasms with diazepam (i.v.) and colic with atropine. Monitoring of kidney function is essential. Intubation and oxygen respiration may also be necessary.

DOSAGE

Mode of Administration: The ground root is applied externally as a lotion.

LITERATURE

Aquino R et al., (1985) J Nat Prod 48(3):502.

Aquino R et al., (1985) J Nat Prod 48(5):811.

Barbakadze V, Usov AI, Isolation and characterisation of glucans from roots of Tamus communis L. In: PM 62, Abstracts of the 44th Ann Congress of GA, 127. 1996.

Ireland CR et al., (1981) Phytochemistry 20:1569.

Further information in:

Frohne D, Pfänder HJ, Giftpflanzen - Ein Handbuch für Apotheker, Toxikologen und Biologen, 4. Aufl., Wiss. Verlags-Ges. Stuttgart 1997.

Kern W, List PH, Hörhammer L (Hrsg.), Hagers Handbuch der Pharmazeutischen Praxis, 4. Aufl., Bde. 1-8: Springer Verlag Berlin, Heidelberg, New York, 1969.

Lewin L, Gifte und Vergiftungen, 6. Aufl., Nachdruck, Haug Verlag, Heidelberg 1992.

Roth L, Daunderer M, Kormann K, Giftpflanzen, Pflanzengifte, 4. Aufl., Ecomed Fachverlag Landsberg Lech 1993.

Teuscher E, Lindequist U, Biogene Gifte - Biologie, Chemie, Pharmakologie, 2. Aufl., Fischer Verlag Stuttgart 1994.

Tanacetum Parthenium

Feverfew

DESCRIPTION

Medicinal Parts: The medicinal parts are the herb of the plant.

Flower and Fruit: The 5 to 20 composite flower heads are in a dense corymb. The epicalyx has a diameter of 6 to 8 mm. The lingual florets are white and female. The ray florets are 2.5 to 7 mm. The achenes are 1.2 to 1.5 mm and 5 to 8-ribbed.

Leaves, Stem and Root: The plant is a strongly aromatic perennial. The leaves are pinnatisect to pinnatifid and yellowish-green. The basal and lower cauline leaves are more or less ovate with 3 to 7 oblong-elliptical to ovate segments, which are subpinnately divided. They are crenate or entire-margined.

Habitat: The plant originated in southeastern Europe and is now found all over Europe, Australia and North America.

Production: Feverfew leaves are the leaves of Chrysanthemum parthenium. The plant is cut before full flowering. It is dried in thin layers in the shade, at temperatures not exceeding 35°C.

Other Names: Featherfew, Featherfoil, Midsummer Daisy

ACTIONS AND PHARMACOLOGY

COMPOUNDS

Volatile oil: chief constituents are L-camphor, trans-chrysanthylacetat, including, among others, camphene, p-cymene, linalool, borneol, terpenes-4-ol

Sesquiterpene lactones

Flavonoids

Polyynes

EFFECTS

In animal experiments, Feverfew impedes or slows down platelet aggregation, prostaglandin synthesis and the release of histamines. It reduces the release of serotonin from thrombocytes and polymorphonuclear leucocytes.

INDICATIONS AND USAGE

Feverfew is used mainly for migraine, arthritis, rheumatic diseases and allergies.

In folk medicine, Feverfew is used for cramps, as a tonic, a stimulant, a digestive, and a blood purifier. Other uses in folk medicine include migraine prophylaxis, digestion problems, cramps, intestinal parasites and gynecological disorders. The herb is also used as a wash for inflammation and wounds, as a tranquilizer, an antiseptic, and following tooth extraction as a mouthwash. The infusion is used for dysmenorrhea. In post-natal care. Feverfew is used to reduce lochia. The drug is used externally as an antiseptic and insecticide.

PRECAUTIONS AND ADVERSE REACTIONS

General: No health hazards or side effects are known in conjunction with the proper administration of designated therapeutic dosages. The potential for sensitization via skin contact with the drug is high, although contact dermatitis is seen only on occasion.

Drug Interactions: Although reports are sketchy, and most involve animal subjects and *in vitro* research, there is a strong possibility that Feverfew may interact with antithrombotic medications such as aspirin and warfarin. The mechanism of action is believed to be inhibition of arachidonic acid, which is a precursor for prostaglandins that are involved in the clotting mechanism.

DOSAGE

Mode of Administration: Feverfew preparations are used both internally and externally.

Preparation: To make an infusion, use 2 teaspoonfuls of the drug per cup, allow to draw for 15 minutes. To make a strong infusion, double the amount and allow to draw for 25 minutes.

Dosage: The recommended daily dosage is 50 mg to 1.2 gm of leaf powder. In folk medicine, 3 cups of the infusion are taken per day. The stronger infusions are used for washes.

Storage: Store in sealed containers.

LITERATURE

Abad MJ, Berjemo P, Villar A, Phytother Res 9:79-92. 1995.

Anderson D, Jenkinson PC, Dewdney RS, Blower SD, Johnson ES, Kadam NP, Human Toxicol 7:145-152. 1988.

Anonym, Naturmedizin: Mutterkraut gegen Migräne. In: DAZ 137(28):2424. 1997.

Awang DVC, Dawson BA, Kindack DG, Crompton CW, Heptinstall S, JNP 54:1516-1521. 1991.

Berry MI, (1984) Pharm J 232:611.

Bohlmann F, Arndt C, Bornowski H, Kleine KM, Herbst P, Chem Ber 97:1179-1192. 1964.

Bohlmann F, Zdero C, (1982) Phytochemistry 21(10):2543.

Brown AMG et al., Inhibition of human neutrophils by aqueous and organic extracts of Tanacetum ssp. In: PM 62, Abstracts of the 44th Ann Congress of GA, 66. 1996.

Brown AMG et al., Pharmacological activity of feverfew (Tanacetum parthenium (L.) Schultz-Bip): Assessment by inhibition of human polymorphnuclear leukocyte chemiluminescence in-vitro. In: J Pharmacy Pharmacol 49(5):558-561. 1997.

Collier HOJ et al., (1980) Lancet II:922.

Deweerdt CJ, Bootsma HPR, Hendricks H, Herbal medicines in migraine prevention. In: Phytomedicine 3(3):225-230. 1996.

Govindachari TR et al., (1964) Tetrahedron 21(6):1509.

Groenewegen WA, Heptinstall S, J Pharm Pharmacol 42:553-557. 1990.

Groenewegen WA, Heptinstall S, Lancet, No 8471, 44-45. 1986.

Groenewegen WA, Knight DW, Heptinstall S, J Pharm Pharmacol 38:709-712. 1986.

Groenewegen WA, Knight DW, Heptinstall S, Progr Med Chem 29:217-238. 1992.

Guin JD, Skidmore G, Arch Derm 123:500-503. 1987.

Hayes NA, Foreman JC, J Pharm Pharmacol 39:466-470. 1987.

Heptinstall S et al., (1985) Lancet I:1071.

Heptinstall S, Awang DVC, Dawson BA, Kindack D, Knight DW, May J, J Pharm Pharmacol 44:391-395. 1992.

Heptinstall S, Groenewegen WA, Spangenberg P, Lösche W, J Pharm Pharmacol 39:459-456. 1984.

Heptinstall S, Groenewegen WA, Spangenberg P, Lösche W, J Pharm Pharmacol 39:459-465. 1987.

Heptinstall S, Groenewegen WA, Spangenberg P, Lösche W, J Pharm Pharmacol 39:459-465. 1987.

Heptinstall S, J R Soc Med 81:373. 1988.

Hylands PJ, Hylands DM, Dev Drugs Mod Med 100-104. 1986.

Johnson ES et al., (1985) Brit Med J 291:569.

Lösche W, Mazurov AV, et al. An extract of feverfew inhibits interaction of human platelets with collagen substrates. Thromb Res. 1987; 48(5):511-518.

Lösche W, Mazurov AV, Heptinstall S, Groenewegen WA, Repin VS, Till U, Throm Res 48:511-518. 1978.

Lösche W, Mazurow AV, Voyno-Yasenetskaja TA, Groenewegen WA, Heptinstall, Repin VS, Folia Haematol 115:181184. 1988.

Lösche W, Michel E, Heptinstall S, Krause S, Groenewegen WA, Pescarmona GP, Thielmann K, Plant Med 54:381-384. 1988.

Makheja AN, Bailey JM, (1981) Lancet II:1054.

Makheja AN, Bailey JM, A platelet phospholipase inhibitor from the medicinal herb feverfew (Tanacetum parthenium). Prostaglandis Leukot Med. 1982; 8(6):653-660.

Makheja AN, Bailey JM, Prostaglandins Leukot Med 8:653-660. 1982.

Mitchell JC, Geissman TA, Dupuis G, Towers GHN, Invest Dermatol 56:98-101. 1971.

Murphy JJ, Heptinstall S, Mitchell JRA, Lancet:189-192. 1989.

Romo de Viva A, Jiminez H, (1965) Tetrahedron 21(7):1742.

Voyna-Yasenetskaja TA, Lösche W, Groenewegen WA, Heptintall S, Repin VS, Till U, J Pharm Pharmacol 40:501-502. 1988.

Warren RG, Austr J Pharm 67:475. 1986.

Willuhn G, Parthenolid - Sesquiterpenlacton zur Migräneprophylaxe. In: DAZ 133(37):3292. 1993.

Further information in:

Hausen B, Allergiepflanzen, Pflanzenallergene, ecomed Verlagsgesellsch. mbH, Landsberg 1988.

Kern W, List PH, Hörhammer L (Hrsg.), Hagers Handbuch der Pharmazeutischen Praxis, 4. Aufl., Bde. 1-8, Springer Verlag Berlin, Heidelberg, New York, 1969.

Schulz R, Hänsel R, Rationale Phytotherapie, Springer Verlag Heidelberg 1996.

Teuscher E, Lindequist U, Biogene Gifte - Biologie, Chemie, Pharmakologie, 2. Aufl., Fischer Verlag Stuttgart 1994.

Wagner H, Wiesenauer M, Phytotherapie. Phytopharmaka und pflanzliche Homöopathika, Fischer-Verlag, Stuttgart, Jena, New York 1995.

Tanacetum Vulgare

Tansy

DESCRIPTION

Medicinal Parts: The medicinal part is the dried flowering herb.

Flower and Fruit: The inflorescences are flat, round and button-like composite flowers in cymes. The bright golden yellow flowers consist only of tubular flowers. The fruit has 5 ribs without tufts of hair.

Leaves, Stem and Root: The plants grows from 60 to 120 cm high. The stem is erect, glabrous, angular, red-tinged and leafy. The leaves are alternate, simple or double pinnatifid, 15 cm long and 12 cm wide and have a long emarginate tip.

Characteristics: The herb has a strong aromatic smell. The taste is bitter and camphor-like. The plant is poisonous.

Habitat: The plant is indigenous to Europe.

Production: Tansy flower consists of the inflorescence of Chrysanthemum vulgare (syn. Tanacetum vulgare). Tansy herb consists of the above-ground parts of Chrysanthemum vulgare (syn. Tanacetum vulgare). Tansy oil is the oil extracted from Tanacetum vulgare.

Other Names: Buttons, Daisy, Hindheal, Parsley Fern

ACTIONS AND PHARMACOLOGY

COMPOUNDS: TANACETI FLOS ET HERBA

Volatile oil: components vary greatly according to breed, as main components, the following could appear: (–)-thujone, (+)-isothujone, sabinenes, umbellulone, L-camphor, L-camphor + umbellulone, bornylacetate, alpha-pinenes, 1,8-cineol, borneol, trans-chrysanthenol + trans-chrysanthenylacetate

Sesquiterpene lactones: including tanacetin, reynosine, parthenolide

Polyynes

EFFECTS: TANACETI FLOS ET HERBA

No information is available.

COMPOUNDS: TANACETI AETHEROLEUM

Components vary greatly according to breed, as main components the following could appear: (–)-thujone, (+)-isothujone, sabinenes, umbellulone, L-camphor, L-camphor + umbellulone, bornylacetate, alpha-pinenes, 1,8-cineol, borneol, or trans-chrysanthenol + trans-chrysanthenylacetate.

EFFECTS: TANACETI AETHEROLEUM

The oil was formerly used as a vermifuge.

INDICATIONS AND USAGE

TANACETI FLOS ET HERBA

Tansy preparations are used as an anthelmintic, for migraine, neuralgia, rheumatism, meteorism and loss of appetite. The effectiveness for the claimed applications has not been demonstrated.

TANACETI AETHEROLEUM

Tansy oil is used in the treatment of intestinal parasitic infestation.

PRECAUTIONS AND ADVERSE REACTIONS

TANACETI FLOS ET HERBA

The administration of therapeutic dosages of drugs that have a high thujone content (see *Tanaceti aetheroleum*) can lead to poisoning. Beyond that, there is a medium potential for sensitization via skin contact with the drug. Internal administration of the drug in allopathic dosages is to be avoided.

TANACETI AETHEROLEUM

Particularly toxic are volatile oils with high thujone content. Poisonings occur above all with the misuse of the drug as an abortifacient. Administration in allopathic dosages is to be avoided.

OVERDOSAGE

TANACETI AETHEROLEUM

Symptoms of poisoning include vomiting, abdominal pain, gastroenteritis, severe reddening of the face, mydriasis, fixed pupil, tonic-clonic spasms, cardiac arrhythmias, uterine bleeding, kidney damage and liver damage. Death occurs after 1 to 3.5 hours. The lethal dosage is approximately 15-30 gm. The treatment for poisonings can only proceed symptomatically.

DOSAGE

TANACETI FLOS ET HERBA

Daily Dosage: Administration in allopathic dosages is to be avoided.

TANACETI AETHEROLEUM

Mode of Administration: The drug is found in extract form in a small number of combination preparations.

Daily Dosage: Administration in allopathic dosages is to be avoided.

LITERATURE

Banthorpe DV et al., (1973) Planta Med 23:64.

Brown AMG et al., Tissue culture, biochemistry and pharmacology of Tanacetum ssp. In: PM 62, Abstracts of the 44th Ann Congress of GA, 33. 1996.

Hendriks H, Bos R, Woerdenbag, Der Rainfarn - eine potentielle Arzneipflanze? In: ZPT 14(6):333. 1993.

Holopainen M, (1968) Planta Med (6):20P.

Nano GM et al., (1983) Fitoterapia (4):135.

Ognyanov I, Tochorova M, (1983) Planta Med 48:181.

Schearer WR, (1984) J Nat Prod 47(6):964.

TANACETI FLOS ET HERBA

Further information in:

Frohne D, Pfänder HJ, Giftpflanzen - Ein Handbuch für Apotheker, Toxikologen und Biologen, 4. Aufl., Wiss. Verlagsges. mbH Stuttgart 1997.

Hausen B, Allergiepflanzen, Pflanzenallergene, ecomed Verlagsgesellsch. mbH, Landsberg 1988.

Kern W, List PH, Hörhammer L (Hrsg.), Hagers Handbuch der Pharmazeutischen Praxis, 4. Aufl., Bde. 1-8, Springer Verlag Berlin, Heidelberg, New York, 1969.

Lewin L, Gifte und Vergiftungen, 6. Aufl., Nachdruck, Haug Verlag, Heidelberg 1992.

Madaus G, Lehrbuch der Biologischen Arzneimittel, Bde 1-3, Nachdruck, Georg Olms Verlag Hildesheim 1979.

Roth L, Daunderer M, Kormann K, Giftpflanzen, Pflanzengifte, 4. Aufl., Ecomed Fachverlag Landsberg Lech 1993.

Teuscher E, Lindequist U, Biogene Gifte - Biologie, Chemie, Pharmakologie, 2. Aufl., Fischer Verlag Stuttgart 1994.

TANACETI AETHEROLEUM

Banthorpe DV et al., (1973) Planta Med 23:64.

Brown AMG et al., Tissue culture, biochemistry and pharmacology of Tanacetum ssp. In: PM 62, Abstracts of the 44th Ann Congress of GA, 33. 1996.

Hendriks H, Bos R, Woerdenbag, Der Rainfarn - eine potentielle Arzneipflanze? In: ZPT 14(6):333. 1993.

Holopainen M, (1968) Planta Med (6):20P.

Nano GM et al., (1983) Fitoterapia (4):135.

Ognyanov I, Tochorova M, (1983) Planta Med 48:181.

Schearer WR, (1984) J Nat Prod 47(6):964.

Further information in:

Frohne D, Pfänder HJ, Giftpflanzen - Ein Handbuch für Apotheker, Toxikologen und Biologen, 4. Aufl., Wiss. Verlagsges. mbH Stuttgart 1997.

Hausen B, Allergiepflanzen, Pflanzenallergene, ecomed Verlagsgesellsch. mbH, Landsberg 1988.

Kern W, List PH, Hörhammer L (Hrsg.), Hagers Handbuch der Pharmazeutischen Praxis, 4. Aufl., Bde. 1-8, Springer Verlag Berlin, Heidelberg, New York, 1969.

Lewin L, Gifte und Vergiftungen, 6. Aufl., Nachdruck, Haug Verlag, Heidelberg 1992.

Madaus G, Lehrbuch der Biologischen Arzneimittel, Bde 1-3, Nachdruck, Georg Olms Verlag Hildesheim 1979.

Roth L, Daunderer M, Kormann K, Giftpflanzen, Pflanzengifte, 4. Aufl., Ecomed Fachverlag Landsberg Lech 1993.

Teuscher E, Lindequist U, Biogene Gifte - Biologie, Chemie, Pharmakologie, 2. Aufl., Fischer Verlag Stuttgart 1994.

Tansy

See Tanacetum Vulgare

Taraxacum Officinale

Dandelion

DESCRIPTION

Medicinal Parts: The medicinal parts are the dried leaves harvested before the flowering season, the dried root collected in autumn, the dried aerial parts with the rhizome harvested before the flowering season and the whole fresh plant.

Flower and Fruit: The flower is a golden yellow composite flower. The composite head is solitary and has a diameter of 3 to 5 cm. All the florets are lingual and androgynous. The epicalyx is oblong-campanulate. The tepals are arranged in 3 imbricate rows, 2 of which are turned back, while the inner one is long acuminate with a white margin and is erect. The receptacle has no bracts. The fruit is small, long-beaked, light gray-brown, ribbed and has a parachute-like tuft of hair.

Leaves, Stem and Root: The plant is perennial, hardy and is found in a number of forms. It grows to about 30 cm and has a short rhizome, which turns into a many-headed, 20 to 50 cm long and 2 cm thick taproot. The hollow stem is erect or ascending. The basal leaves are glabrous or villous, usually deeply notched, lanceolate and lobed like a saw. They narrow to a red-violet tinged petiole and end in a large deltoid tip.

Characteristics: The flower opens in the morning and closes in the evening remaining closed all night and in dull weather. The plant parts contain bitter latex.

Habitat: Dandelion grows in most temperate regions of Europe and Asia.

Production: Dandelion root with herb consists of the entire plant Taraxacum officinale gathered while flowering. It is air dried.

Not To Be Confused With: Cichorium intybus and the leaves of various Leontodon species.

Other Names: Blowball, Cankerwort, Lion's Tooth, Priest's Crown, Swine Snout, Wild Endive

ACTIONS AND PHARMACOLOGY

COMPOUNDS

Sesquiterpene lactones (bitter substances): including, among others, taraxinacetyl-1′-O-glucosides, 11,13-dihydro-taraxinacetyl-1′-O-glucosides, taraxacolide-1′-O-glucosides, 4alpha,15,11beta,13-tetrahydroridentin B

Triterpenes and sterols: beta-sitosterol, beta-sitosterol-glucosides, taraxasterol, psi-taraxasterol, taraxerol, taraxol

Flavonoids: including, among others, apigenin-7-O-glucosides, luteolin-7-O-glucosides

Mucilage

Inulin

EFFECTS

Dandelion acts as a cholagogue, diuretic and appetite stimulant.

INDICATIONS AND USAGE

- Dyspeptic complaints
- Infections of the urinary tract
- Kidney and bladder stones
- Liver and gallbladder complaints
- Loss of appetite

Dandelion is used for disturbances in bile flow, stimulation of diuresis, loss of appetite, and dyspepsia. In folk medicine, it is used for liver and gallbladder disorders, hemorrhoids, congestion in the portal system, gout, rheumatic disorders, eczema, and other skin disorders. The drug has a positive diuretic effect on kidney and bladder complaints and kidney stone and gravel formation. A diabetic infusion is made from the roots and leaves.

CONTRAINDICATIONS

Contraindications include closure of the biliary ducts, gallbladder empyema and ileus. Consultation with a doctor is necessary in the presence of biliary ailments.

PRECAUTIONS AND ADVERSE REACTIONS

No health hazards are known in conjunction with the proper administration of designated therapeutic dosages. Superacid gastric complaints could be triggered, due to the drug's secretion-stimulating effect. The drug possesses weak potential for sensitization reactions.

DOSAGE

Mode of Administration: As liquid and solid preparations for oral use.

Preparation: To make a decoction, use 1 to 2 teaspoonfuls finely cut drug with 150 ml rapidly boiled water. Strain after 15 minutes and drink warm. To make an infusion, use 1 tablespoon of cut drug per 1 cup water.

Daily Dosage: When using a tincture, the recommended dosage is 10 to 15 drops 3 times daily. The decoction can be taken mornings and evenings.

Storage: The drug should be protected from light and moisture.

LITERATURE

Baba K et al., (1981) Yakugaku Zasshi 101(6):538.

Böhm K, (1959) Untersuchungen über choleretische Wirkungen einiger Arzneipflanzen. Arzneim Forsch Drug Res 9:376.

Budzianowski J, Coumarins, caffeoyltartaric acids and their artifactual estres from Taraxacum officinale. In: PM 63(3):288. 1997.

Czygan FC, Taraxacum officinale WIGGERS - Der Löwenzahn. In: ZPT 11(3):99. 1990.

Hänsel R et al., (1980) Phytochemistry 19:857.

Kotobuki Seiyaku KK, (1981) Pat. JP 81/10117 Japan.

Mascolo N et al., (1987) Phytother Res 1(1):28.

Rauwald HW, Huang DT, (1985) Phytochemistry 24(7):1557.

Further information in:

Hänsel R, Keller K, Rimpler H, Schneider G (Hrsg.), Hagers Handbuch der Pharmazeutischen Praxis, 5. Aufl., Bde 4-6 (Drogen): Springer Verlag Berlin, Heidelberg, New York, 1992-1994.

Hausen B, Allergiepflanzen, Pflanzenallergene, ecomed Verlagsgesellsch. mbH, Landsberg 1988.

Leung AY, Encyclopedia of Common Natural Ingredients Used in Food Drugs, Cosmetics, John Wiley & Sons Inc., New York 1980.

Madaus G, Lehrbuch der Biologischen Arzneimittel, Bde 1-3, Nachdruck, Georg Olms Verlag Hildesheim 1979.

Roth L, Daunderer M, Kormann K, Giftpflanzen, Pflanzengifte, 4. Aufl., Ecomed Fachverlag Landsberg Lech 1993.

Steinegger E, Hänsel R, Pharmakognosie, 5. Aufl., Springer Verlag Heidelberg 1992.

Teuscher E, Lindequist U, Biogene Gifte - Biologie, Chemie, Pharmakologie, 2. Aufl., Fischer Verlag Stuttgart 1994.

Teuscher E, Biogene Arzneimittel, 5. Aufl., Wiss. Verlagsges. Stuttgart 1997.

Wagner H, Wiesenauer M, Phytotherapie. Phytopharmaka und pflanzliche Homöopathika, Fischer-Verlag, Stuttgart, Jena, New York 1995.

Wichtl M (Hrsg.), Teedrogen, 4. Aufl., Wiss. Verlagsges. Stuttgart 1997.

Tarragon

See Artemisia Dracunculus

Taumelloolch

See Lolium Temulentum

Taxus Baccata

Yew

DESCRIPTION

Medicinal Parts: The medicinal parts are the fresh leaves, the branch twig tips, and the branches.

Flower and Fruit: The flowers are inconspicuous and dioecious. The male florets appear in autumn in yellowish catkins in the axils of the annual needle. The female florets, with only 1 pistil, are on short pedicles, which have scale-like high leaves. The hard, pea-sized, dark-brown seed is surrounded by a crimson, pulpy, beaker-shaped, sweet and edible aril.

Leaves, Stem and Root: The Yew may be a bush or small tree approximately 17 m high with a trunk diameter of over 1 m. The trunk has red-brown bark. The numerous branches are crowded and evergreen. The needles are 2 to 3 cm long, arranged in double rows, soft and acute. They are glossy dark green above, have a distinct midrib, and are lighter green beneath, matte, with no resin.

Characteristics: Yew is poisonous.

Habitat: The plant is common in large areas of Europe as far as Anatolia and Sicily.

Production: Yew leaves are the needles of Taxus baccata.

Other Names: Chinwood

ACTIONS AND PHARMACOLOGY

COMPOUNDS

Diterpene esters of the taxane-type (mixture is known as taxine, 0.6-2.0%): including, among others, taxine A, taxine B, taxol

Flavonoids: including, among others, sciadopytisin, ginkgetin, sequoia flavone (biflavonoids)

EFFECTS

Yew is a mobility inhibitor and causes a negative change in cardiac metabolism.

INDICATIONS AND USAGE

In folk medicine, the cooked yew leaves are used to promote menstruation, to treat diphtheria, epilepsy, tapeworm, tonsilitis, and as an abortifacient. The plants are highly toxic and their use is not recommended.

PRECAUTIONS AND ADVERSE REACTIONS

General: The drug is severely toxic: 50-100 gm yew needles (fresh weight) are fatal for an adult.

Use in Pregnancy: In folk medicine, the drug is used as an abortifacient.

OVERDOSAGE

Symptoms of poisoning include queasiness, vomiting, severe abdominal pain, and feelings of vertigo, followed later by unconsciousness, mydriasis, reddening of the lips, tachycardia, and superficial breathing. Death results from asphyxiation and diastolic cardiac arrest. Following gastrointestinal emptying, (inducement of vomiting, gastric lavage with burgundy-colored potassium permanganate solution, sodium sulphate), and use of activated charcoal, treatment for poisonings consists of treating spasms with diazepam or barbital (i.v.). In case of shock, plasma volume expanders should be infused. The administration of lidocaine has proven its effectiveness with cardiac rhythm disorders. Monitoring of kidney function, blood coagulation and liver values is necessary. Intubation and oxygen respiration may also be necessary.

DOSAGE

Mode of Administration: Yew is used in homeopathic dilutions of the mother tincture.

Daily Dosage: In acute conditions, 5 drops or 1 tablet of the mother tincture are taken every hour.

Storage: The mother tincture should be protected from light.

LITERATURE

Hoc S, Onkologie: Taxol, ein pflanzliches Zytostatikum. In: DAZ 133(26):2400. 1993.

Hof-Mussler S, Eiben-Zytostatikum Taxol bei Ovarialkarzinom. In: DAZ 133(1):42. 1993.

Jenniskens LHD, Identification of six taxine alkaloids from Taxus baccata needles. In: JNP 59(2):117-123. 1996.

Kelsey RG, Vance NC, Taxol and cephalomannine concentrations in the foliage and bark of shade-grown and sun-exposed Taxus baccata trees. In: JNP 55:912-917. 1992.

Kingston DGI, Sorties and surprises: unexpected reactions of taxol. In: PM 62, Abstracts of the 44th Ann Congress of GA, 5. 1996.

Kongreβbericht, Taxol in der onkologischen Therapie. In: ZPT 15(2):114. 1994.

Kubitschek J, Eibenwirkstoff gegen Malaria. In: PZ 140(8):684. 1995.

Ma W et al., New bioactive taxoids from cell cultures of Taxus baccata. In: JNP 57(1):116. 1994.

Mujumdar RB et al., (1972) Ind J Chem 10:677.

Poupat Ch et al., Noveau taxoide basique isolé des feuilles D'if, Taxus baccata: La 2-désacétyltaxine A. In: JNP 57(10):1468-1469. 1994.

Schneider B, Taxol, ein Arzneistoff der Eibe. In: DAZ 134(36):3389. 1994.

Vanek T et al., Study of the influence of year season on taxanes content in Taxus baccata bark. In: PM 59(7):A699. 1993.

Vidensek N, Lim P, Campbell A, Carlson C, Taxol content in bark, wood, root, leaf, twig and seedling from several Taxus species. In: JNP 53:1609-1610. 1994.

Vohora Kumar, (1971) Planta Med 20:100.

Wasielewski S, Taxol, ein Zytostatikum aus der pazifischen Eibe. In: UPTA 7(12):914. 1993.

Further information in:

Frohne D, Pfänder HJ, Giftpflanzen - Ein Handbuch für Apotheker, Toxikologen und Biologen, 4. Aufl., Wiss. Verlags-Ges. Stuttgart 1997.

Hänsel R, Keller K, Rimpler H, Schneider G (Hrsg.), Hagers Handbuch der Pharmazeutischen Praxis, 5. Aufl., Bde 4-6 (Drogen): Springer Verlag Berlin, Heidelberg, New York, 1992-1994.

Lewin L, Gifte und Vergiftungen, 6. Aufl., Nachdruck, Haug Verlag, Heidelberg 1992.

Madaus G, Lehrbuch der Biologischen Arzneimittel, Bde 1-3, Nachdruck, Georg Olms Verlag Hildesheim 1979.

Roth L, Daunderer M, Kormann K, Giftpflanzen, Pflanzengifte, 4. Aufl., Ecomed Fachverlag Landsberg Lech 1993.

Teuscher E, Lindequist U, Biogene Gifte - Biologie, Chemie, Pharmakologie, 2. Aufl., Fischer Verlag Stuttgart 1994.

Teuscher E, Biogene Arzneimittel, 5. Aufl., Wiss. Verlagsges. Stuttgart 1997.

Teazle

See Dipsacus Silvestris

Teucrium Chamaedrys

Germander

DESCRIPTION

Medicinal Parts: The medicinal part is the herb collected during the flowering season.

Flower and Fruit: The flowers are 10 to 12 mm long and are erect on long pedicles in 1 to 6 blossomed, false racemes inclined to one side. The calyx is tubular-campanulate, often tinged with red-violet and is pubescent. The corolla is usually carmine red, occasionally white. The stamens and styles are exserted. The nutlet is ovoid, 1.5 to 2 cm long, smooth, finely reticulate and has a large, circular, attaching surface.

Leaves, Stem and Root: The plant is a subshrub with a short-lived main root from which grow long-reaching, branched, thin woody roots and a stem-producing runner. The stems are usually erect and branched. The older branches are decumbent, the younger ones erect, tough, round and lanate. The branches are occasionally covered in glandular hairs, often red-violet. The leaves are in close pairs and are always covered in teeth. They are summer-green and have distinctly protruding pinnatifid ribs.

Habitat: The plant is indigenous to the Mediterranean region as far as Anatolia and the Urals.

Production: Germander is the aerial part of Teucrium chamaedrys.

ACTIONS AND PHARMACOLOGY

COMPOUNDS

Volatile oil (0.07%): chief components beta-caryophyllene, humulene

Iridoide monoterpenes: including, among others, harpagide, acetyl harpagide

Diterpenes: including, among others, teugin, teuflin, teuflidin, dihydroteugin, teucrin A, B, E, F, G, marrubiin

Caffeic acid derivatives: including, among others, teucroside

Flavonoids: including, among others, cirsiliol, cirsimaritin, luteolin

EFFECTS

The herb is spasmolytic and is used as a weak cholagogue, although no clear information is available. The toxic principles are unknown.

INDICATIONS AND USAGE

Germander is used as an aid in the treatment of gallbladder conditions, as a digestive aid, as a rinse for gout, for fever, and as a dietary aid.

PRECAUTIONS AND ADVERSE REACTIONS

Liver cell necroses, characterized by, (among other things), jaundice and an elevated level of aminotransferase in the blood, have been observed following intake of the drug. One case of death has been recorded. The drug is, for that reason, not to be administered.

DOSAGE

Mode of Administration: Germander is occasionally used in tea mixtures and in homeopathic preparations. SEE PRECAUTIONS

LITERATURE

Chialva F et al., J High Res Chromatogr Chromatogr Commun 5:182. 1982.

Fikenscher LH, Hegnauer R, Plant Med Phytother 3(3):183.

Malakov PY et al., PH 24:301-303. 1985.

Reinbold AM, Popa PD, (1974) Khim Prir Soedin. 589.

Rodriguez MC et al., (1984) Phytochemistry 23(7):1467.

Rodriguez MC et al., PH 23:2960-2961. 1984.

Rovesti P, (1957) Ind Perf. 12:334.

Savona G et al., PH 21:721-723. 1982.

Sticher O, Lahloub MF, (1982) Planta Med 30:124.

Further information in:

Frohne D, Pfänder HJ, Giftpflanzen - Ein Handbuch für Apotheker, Toxikologen und Biologen, 4. Aufl., Wiss. Verlags-Ges. Stuttgart 1997.

Hänsel R, Keller K, Rimpler H, Schneider G (Hrsg.), Hagers Handbuch der Pharmazeutischen Praxis, 5. Aufl., Bde 4-6 (Drogen): Springer Verlag Berlin, Heidelberg, New York, 1992-1994.

Teucrium Scordium

Water Germander

DESCRIPTION

Medicinal Parts: The medicinal parts are the herb harvested during or shortly before the flowering season and the fresh flowering herb.

Flower and Fruit: The flowers are light red, 8 to 10 mm long, with short pedicles. They are in inconspicuous clusters in 1 to 4 blossomed cymes between bracts, which are longer than the flowers. The calyx has 5 tips and is campanulate-tubular with a touch violet. The tips of the deeply divided upper lip lie on the lower lip in such a way as to make it appear 5-lobed. After flowering, the head drops. There are 4 stamens. The nutlets are 1 mm long and punctate-reticulate.

Leaves, Stem and Root: The plant is a perennial, downy herb smelling of garlic. The rhizome creeps in mud and produces overground runners, which immediately turn into leaves and flower shoots. The stems are unbranched or branched, erect, round and villous with soft-hairs. The leaves are sessile, oblong-oval and crossed opposite.

Characteristics: The plant has a garlic-like odor and a bitter taste.

Habitat: The plant is indigenous to most of Europe as far as northern Africa and central Asia.

Production: Water Germander is the aerial part of Teucrium scordium. It is picked during or shortly before flowering.

ACTIONS AND PHARMACOLOGY

COMPOUNDS

Diterpenes: including, among others, 6,20-bisdeacetylteupyreinidin, 6-deacetylteupyreinidin, 2beta, 6beta-dihydroxyteuscordin, 2beta,6beta-dihydroxyteuscordin, dihydroteugin, teuflidin, teucrin E, teugin, 2-keto-19-hydroxyteuscordin

INDICATIONS AND USAGE

The herb is used for the treatment of festering and inflamed wounds, bronchial ailments, diarrhea, fever, hemorrhoids, and intestinal parasites.

PRECAUTIONS AND ADVERSE REACTIONS

No health hazards or side effects are known in conjunction with the proper administration of designated therapeutic dosages.

DOSAGE

Mode of Administration: Water Germander is used internally and externally.

Daily Dosage: 4 teaspoonfuls of the herb (7.2 gm) is taken daily as an infusion. The same preparation can be used internally or externally.

LITERATURE

Fikenscher LH, Hegnauer R, Plant Med Phytother 3(3):183.

Papanov G, Malakov PY, (1981) Z Naturforsch (B)36:112.

Papanov GY et al., PH 24:297-299. 1985.

Singh S et al., Fitoterapia 63:555. 1992.

Further information in:

Hänsel R, Keller K, Rimpler H, Schneider G (Hrsg.), Hagers Handbuch der Pharmazeutischen Praxis, 5. Aufl., Bde 4-6 (Drogen): Springer Verlag Berlin, Heidelberg, New York, 1992-1994.

Madaus G, Lehrbuch der Biologischen Arzneimittel, Bde 1-3, Nachdruck, Georg Olms Verlag Hildesheim 1979.

Teucrium Scorodonia

Wood Sage

DESCRIPTION

Medicinal Parts: The medicinal parts are the herb, the fresh aerial parts of the flowering plant and the whole flowering plant.

Flower and Fruit: The flowers are approximately 1 cm long, pale yellow or greenish-yellow. They are solitary or in pairs on short pedicles in-one-side-inclined, terminal racemes. The calyx of the labiate flower is tubular-campanulate and bilabiate with an undivided upper and a 4-tipped lower lip. The stamens are pubescent and the anthers are violet. The nutlet is round, about 2mm long, and almost smooth.

Leaves, Stem and Root: The plant is erect, 30 to 60 cm high and has far-reaching runners. The stem is erect, paniculate-branched above, quadrangular and soft-pubescent. The leaves are petiolate, opposite, wrinkled, ovate or oblong, unevenly crenate and have a shallowly cordate base.

Characteristics: The plant smells faintly of leeks when being dried.

Habitat: The plant is common to large parts of western and central Europe including the Mediterranean region. It is rarely found in eastern Europe and Scandinavia but it has naturalized there.

Production: Wood Sage is the aerial part of Teucrium scorodonia.

Other Names: Ambroise, Garlic Sage, Hind Heal, Large-leaved Germander

ACTIONS AND PHARMACOLOGY

COMPOUNDS

Volatile oil (0.3%): containing, among others, alloaromadendrene, aristolene, beta-caryophyllene, alpha-caryophyllene (humulene), spathulenone, caryophyllene epoxide

Iridoide monoterpenes: including, among others, acetyl harpagide, reptoside

Diterpenes: the spectrum varies greatly according to strain, including among others teuscorodal, teuscorodin, teuscorodol, teuscorodonin, teuflin, teuscorolide, teupolin I

Flavonoids: including, among others, cirsiliol, cirsimaritin, luteolin

EFFECTS

The herb is a spasmolytic and an expectorant.

INDICATIONS AND USAGE

Wood Sage is used for disorders of the gastrointestinal canal, the treatment of tuberculosis, chronic bronchial catarrh, inflammation of mucous membranes of the nose and throat, spasms, hypertension, healing wounds, and liver disorders.

PRECAUTIONS AND ADVERSE REACTIONS

No health hazards or side effects are known in conjunction with the proper administration of designated therapeutic dosages.

DOSAGE

Mode of Administration: Wood Sage is obsolete as a drug in most countries.

Preparation: To treat bronchitis, a tea is made using 2 teaspoons of herb per cup.

LITERATURE

Bruno M et al., (1985) Phytochemistry 24(11):2597.

Fikenscher LH, Hegnauer R, Plant Med Phytother 3(3):183.

Marco JL et al., Phytochemistry 21(10):2567.

Marco JL et al., PH 21:2567. 1982.

Marco JL et al., PH 22:727-731. 1983.

Velasco-Negueruela A et al., PH 29:1165-1169. 1990.

Further information in:

Hänsel R, Keller K, Rimpler H, Schneider G (Hrsg.), Hagers Handbuch der Pharmazeutischen Praxis, 5. Aufl., Bde 4-6 (Drogen): Springer Verlag Berlin, Heidelberg, New York, 1992-1994.

Madaus G, Lehrbuch der Biologischen Arzneimittel, Bde 1-3, Nachdruck, Georg Olms Verlag Hildesheim 1979.

Wagner H, Wiesenauer M, Phytotherapie. Phytopharmaka und pflanzliche Homöopathika, Fischer-Verlag, Stuttgart, Jena, New York 1995.

Theobroma Cacao

Cocoa

DESCRIPTION

Medicinal Parts: The medicinal parts are the seed skins that remain after making cocoa and cocoa butter; the seeds which have been partly freed from their skins and lightly roasted; and the raw, dried, unroasted seeds.

Flower and Fruit: The inflorescences are on the main trunk and thicker branches on a so-called ''flower cup.'' The cyme-like branchlets are short, noded and persistent. There are 5 sepals, which are narrow. The petals are cap-shaped and stemmed with flag-like laminas. The stamen tube, with 5 fertile stamens and 5 awl-shaped staminoids, is short. The fruit is a 15 to 25 cm long and 10 cm thick, large berry. It is oblong or obovate, thick-skinned, yellow or reddish, grooved and sometimes bumpy and cucumber-like. The 20 to 50 seeds are arranged in rows and embedded in a pink, fruity, sweetish-sour pulp. They are pressed flat, almond-shaped, reddish-brown and without endosperm.

Leaves, Stem and Root: The plant is a 4 to 6 m, occasionally up to 13 m, tall tree with an irregular knotty trunk and a broad crown. The young branches are rounded. The leaves are coriaceous or paper-like, alternate and in 2 rows on the branches. The petiole is downy, cushioned, and 1.5 to 2 cm long. The lamina is oval or elliptical, slightly asymmetrical, rounded at the base with a conspicuous tip. The upper surface is green and pale when dry. The lower surface is paler green, glabrous or has a few, tiny, simple, branched and scattered hairs.

Habitat: The plant is cultivated globally in tropical regions.

Production: Cocoa seeds consist of the seeds of Theobroma cacao, which have been removed from their shells, fermented and lightly roasted. Cocoa consists of the testae of Theobroma cacao. Cocoa butter is the hard fat obtained from the ripe cocoa seeds of Theobroma cacao. After removal of the germ-roots and the shell from the seeds, the seeds are removed from the shell and crushed. The cocoa fat is squeezed out at a temperature of 70°C to 80°C and allowed to cool.

Other Names: Cacao, Chocolate Tree

ACTIONS AND PHARMACOLOGY

COMPOUNDS: CACAO SEMEN

Purine alkaloids: main alkaloid theobromine (2.8 to 3.5%) with less caffeine (0.1-0.4%)

Fat (50%)

Proteins

Biogenic amines: including phenyl ethyl amine, tyramine, tryptamine, serotonin

Catechin tannins

Proanthocyanidins Oxaluric acid

EFFECTS: CACAO SEMEN

Cocoa seeds can cause constipation because of the tannin content. The drug contains methylxanthines, mainly theobromin, which have a diuretic, broncholytic, and vasodilatory effect. They also stimulate cardiac muscle performance and act as a muscle relaxant.

COMPOUNDS: CACAO TESTES

Purine alkaloids: main alkaloid theobromine (0.4-1.2%) with less caffeine (0.02%)

Fat (5%)

Biogenic amine: including phenyl ethyl amine, tyramine, tryptamine, serotonin

Catechin tannins

Proanthocyanidins

EFFECTS: CACAO TESTES

Cocoa can cause constipation. Cocoa contains methylxanthines, which have a diuretic, bronchyolitic, and vasodilatory effect. They also improve cardiac muscle performance and act as a muscle relaxant.

COMPOUNDS: CACAO OLEUM

Fat: triglycerides, chief fatty acids oleic acid, stearic acid, palmitic acid

Free fatty acids

Purine alkaloids (traces)

EFFECTS: CACAO OLEUM

No information is available.

INDICATIONS AND USAGE

CACAO SEMEN

The seeds are used for infectious intestinal diseases and diarrhea.

CACAO TESTES

Preparations of cacao testae are used for liver, bladder, and kidney ailments, diabetes, as a tonic and general remedy, and as an astringent for diarrhea.

CACAO OLEUM

Cocoa Butter is used by the pharmaceutical and cosmetic industries as an inactive ingredient in dermatologic preparations.

PRECAUTIONS AND ADVERSE REACTIONS

CACAO SEMEN

General: No health hazards or side effects are known in conjunction with either the proper administration of designated therapeutic dosages or the consumption of normal amounts of chocolate products. Large dosages lead to constipation due to the tannin content. Cocoa and cocoa products can bring about allergic reactions. The amines can trigger migraine attacks.

Pediatric Use: Large quantities of chocolate products can lead to overexcitability, racing pulse and sleep disorders in children because of the caffeine content, which can be as high as 0.2% in milk chocolate and 0.4% in bitter chocolate.

CACAO TESTES

No health hazards or side effects are known in conjunction with the proper administration of designated therapeutic dosages. Cocoa and cocoa products can cause allergic reactions. Large dosages lead to constipation due to the tannin content. The amines can trigger migraine attacks.

CACAO OLEUM

No health hazards or side effects are known in conjunction with the proper administration of designated therapeutic dosages.

DOSAGE

CACAO OLEUM

Mode of Administration: Cocoa Butter is used as a pharmaceutical base for suppositories and vaginal globules. It is an additive for ointments and cosmetic preparations, such as skin creams and lip balms.

Storage: Store in a cool, dark place.

LITERATURE

CACAO SEMEN

Naturw R, 49:481. 1996.

Schröder B, In: Schröder R, Kaffee, Tee und Kardamom, Ulmer-Verlag, Stuttgart. 1991.

Further information in:

Hänsel R, Keller K, Rimpler H, Schneider G (Hrsg.), Hagers Handbuch der Pharmazeutischen Praxis, 5. Aufl., Bde 4-6 (Drogen): Springer Verlag Berlin, Heidelberg, New York, 1992-1994.

Leung AY, Encyclopedia of Common Natural Ingredients Used in Food Drugs and Cosmetics, John Wiley & Sons Inc., New York 1980.

Lewin L, Gifte und Vergiftungen, 6. Aufl., Nachdruck, Haug Verlag, Heidelberg 1992.

Roth L, Daunderer M, Kormann K, Giftpflanzen, Pflanzengifte, 4. Aufl., Ecomed Fachverlag Landsberg Lech 1993.

Teuscher E, Biogene Arzneimittel, 5. Aufl., Wiss. Verlagsges. Stuttgart 1997.

Teuscher E, Lindequist U, Biogene Gifte - Biologie, Chemie, Pharmakologie, 2. Aufl., Fischer Verlag Stuttgart 1994.

CACAO TESTES

Hänsel R, Keller K, Rimpler H, Schneider G (Hrsg.), Hagers Handbuch der Pharmazeutischen Praxis, 5. Aufl., Bde 4-6 (Drogen): Springer Verlag Berlin, Heidelberg, New York, 1992-1994.

Leung AY, Encyclopedia of Common Natural Ingredients Used in Food Drugs and Cosmetics, John Wiley & Sons Inc., New York 1980.

Lewin L, Gifte und Vergiftungen, 6. Aufl., Nachdruck, Haug Verlag, Heidelberg 1992.

Roth L, Daunderer M, Kormann K, Giftpflanzen, Pflanzengifte, 4. Aufl., Ecomed Fachverlag Landsberg Lech 1993.

Teuscher E, Lindequist U, Biogene Gifte - Biologie, Chemie, Pharmakologie, 2. Aufl., Fischer Verlag Stuttgart 1994.

Teuscher E, Biogene Arzneimittel, 5. Aufl., Wiss. Verlagsges. Stuttgart 1997.

CACAO OLEUM

Hänsel R, Keller K, Rimpler H, Schneider G (Hrsg.), Hagers Handbuch der Pharmazeutischen Praxis, 5. Aufl., Bde 4-6 (Drogen): Springer Verlag Berlin, Heidelberg, New York, 1992-1994.

Leung AY, Encyclopedia of Common Natural Ingredients Used in Food Drugs and Cosmetics, John Wiley & Sons Inc., New York 1980.

Steinegger E, Hänsel R, Pharmakognosie, 5. Aufl., Springer Verlag Heidelberg 1992.

Teuscher E, Biogene Arzneimittel, 5. Aufl., Wiss. Verlagsges. Stuttgart 1997.

Thuja Occidentalis

Thuja

DESCRIPTION

Medicinal Parts: The medicinal parts are the oil extracted from the leaves and branch tips, the young dried branches, the fresh, leafy annual branches and the fresh, leafy branches collected in spring.

Flower and Fruit: The male flowers are dark brown, the female flowers are yellow-green. They are monoecious, the male in small, terminal catkins and the female almost star-shaped. The ripe cones are brown-yellow, 6 to 8 mm long, ovate and covered in coriaceous, obtuse scales. The lower ones are patent at the tips. The seeds are brown-yellow, 3 to 5 mm long and approximately 1 mm wide. They are narrowly winged the whole way around.

Leaves, Stem and Root: The plant is a narrowly clavate, 12 to 21 m high tree with short horizontally spread branches and red-brown, striped, peeling trunk. The trunk is usually branched from the base up. The leaves are scale-like, crossed opposite, imbricate, flattened on the branch side and folded at the margins. They are dark green above and matte-green beneath. The scales on the upper part of the branches have a globular glandular swelling.

Habitat: The plant originated from eastern North America and is found in Europe mainly as an ornamental plant and is partly naturalized.

Production: Thuja herb is the young branch tips and young shoots of Thuja occidentalis. The harvest should take place in spring when the content of the active agents is optimal. The herb should be dried in the shade and handled with care.

Not To Be Confused With: Other forms of Thuja.

Other Names: Arborvitae, Hackmatack, Swamp Cedar, Tree of Life, White Cedar

ACTIONS AND PHARMACOLOGY

COMPOUNDS

Water-soluble immunostimulating polysaccharides and glycoproteins

Volatile oil (1.4-4%): chief components (-)-thujone (alpha-thujone, 59%), (+)-isothujone (beta-thujone, 7-10%), fenchone (10-15%)

Flavonoids: including, among others, quercitrin, mearusitrin, the biflavonoids hinoki flavone, amentoflavone, bilobetin-procyanidins

Lignans

Tannins

EFFECTS

The essential oil causes cramping. The podophyllotoxin derivatives are antiviral.

INDICATIONS AND USAGE

Thuja is used for respiratory tract infections and in conjunction with antibiotics in the treatment of bacterial skin infections and *Herpes Simplex*. Other possible uses include the treatment of bronchitis, rheumatism, trigeminal neuralgia, and strep throat. The drug is used in external application as an ointment for treating pains in the joints, arthritis and muscle rheumatism.

PRECAUTIONS AND ADVERSE REACTIONS

General: The drug is toxic. The toxicologically harmless polysaccharide and glycoprotein fractions of the drug are usually the parts used for therapeutic purposes.

Use in Pregnancy: The drug is misused as an abortifacient.

OVERDOSAGE

Symptoms of poisoning, in particular after misuse of the drug as an abortifacient, include queasiness, vomiting, painful diarrhea, and mucous membrane hemorrhaging. Instances of death have been reported.

Following gastrointestinal emptying (inducement of vomiting, gastric lavage with burgundy-colored potassium permanganate solution, sodium sulphate), administration of activated charcoal, and shock prophylaxis (appropriate body position, quiet, warmth), the treatment for poisoning consists of treating spasms with diazepam (i.v.), colic with atropine, administering electrolytes, and treating possible cases of acidosis with sodium bicarbonate infusions. Monitoring of kidney function is essential. Intubation and oxygen respiration may also be necessary.

DOSAGE

Mode of Administration: Thuja is used only in medicinal preparations. The mother tincture is produced in accordance with the general regulation PFX. It is a mixture of brown and green in color and has an aromatic smell and resin-like taste. It consists of 65% ethanol.

LITERATURE

Anonym, Behandlung mit pflanzlichen Immunmodulatoren. In: Symbiose 5(2):9. 1993.

Anonym, Echinacea-Präparate. In: DAZ 136(22):1814-1820. 1996.

Baumann J, Flamme D, Harnischfeger G, DAZ 127:2518-2522. 1987.

Baumann J, Vergleichende pharmakognostisch-phytochemische Untersuchungen an Drogen der Familie der Cupressaceae. In: Diplomarbeit Göttingen. 1987.

Beuscher N, Kopanski L, Purification and biological characterization of antiviral substances from Thuja occidentalis. In: PM 52:555-556. 1986.

Beuscher N, Kopanski L, Reinigung und biologische Charakterisierung von antiviralen Substanzen aus Thuja occidentalis. In: PM 52(6):555-556. 1086.

Beuscher N, Über die medikamentöse Beeinflussung zellulärer Resistenzmechanismen im Tierversuch. Aktivierung von Peritonealmakrophagen der Maus durch pflanzliche Reizkörper. In: Arzneim Forsch 32(I):134-138. 1977.

Beuscher N, Über die medikamentöse Beeinflussung zellulärer Resistenzmechanismen im Tierversuch. III. Steigerung der Leukozytenmobilisation bei der Maus durch pflanzliche Reizkörper. In: Arzneim Forsch 30(I):821-825. 1977.

Gohla S, Dissertation Universität Hamburg. 1988.

Gross G, Papillomvirus-Infektionen der Haut. In: Med Welt 36:437-440. 1985.

Khurana SMP, Effect of homoeopathic drugs on plant viruses. In: PM 20:142-146. 1971.

Sait MA, Garg BR, Indian J Dermatol Vernerol Leprol 51:96-98. 1985.

Schubert W, Die Inhaltsstoffe von Thuja occidentalis. In: Dissertation Technische Universität Braunschweig. 1987.

Tachibana Y et al., Mitogenic activities in african traditional herbal medicines. In: PM 59(4):354. 1993.

Von R, (1961) Can J Chem 39:1200.

Wagner H, Antivirales Prinzip von Thuja aufgeklärt. In: Phytoformum (Medisculab) 1/93:4. 1993.

Zellner J, Arch Pharm 262:381-397. 1924.

Further information in:

Frohne D, Pfänder HJ, Giftpflanzen - Ein Handbuch für Apotheker, Toxikologen und Biologen, 4. Aufl., Wiss. Verlags-Ges. Stuttgart 1997.

Hänsel R, Keller K, Rimpler H, Schneider G (Hrsg.), Hagers Handbuch der Pharmazeutischen Praxis, 5. Aufl., Bde 4-6 (Drogen): Springer Verlag Berlin, Heidelberg, New York, 1992-1994.

Leung AY, Encyclopedia of Common Natural Ingredients Used in Food Drugs, Cosmetics, John Wiley & Sons Inc., New York 1980.

Lewin L, Gifte und Vergiftungen, 6. Aufl., Nachdruck, Haug Verlag, Heidelberg 1992.

Madaus G, Lehrbuch der Biologischen Arzneimittel, Bde 1-3, Nachdruck, Georg Olms Verlag Hildesheim 1979.

Roth L, Daunderer M, Kormann K, Giftpflanzen, Pflanzengifte, 4. Aufl., Ecomed Fachverlag Landsberg Lech 1993.

Steinegger E, Hänsel R, Pharmakognosie, 5. Aufl., Springer Verlag Heidelberg 1992.

Teuscher E, Lindequist U, Biogene Gifte - Biologie, Chemie, Pharmakologie, 2. Aufl., Fischer Verlag Stuttgart 1994.

Teuscher E, Biogene Arzneimittel, 5. Aufl., Wiss. Verlagsges. Stuttgart 1997.

Wagner H, Wiesenauer M, Phytotherapie. Phytopharmaka und pflanzliche Homöopathika, Fischer-Verlag, Stuttgart, Jena, New York 1995.

Thyme

See Thymus Vulgaris

Thymus serpyllum

Wild Thyme

DESCRIPTION

Medicinal Parts: The medicinal parts are the steamed distillation of the dried aerial parts, the aerial shoots collecting during the flowering season and dried, the fresh aerial parts of the flowering plant and the whole plant.

Flower and Fruit: The inflorescence is globular to very elongated, often interrupted in false whorls, which are separate from each other. The calyx is tubular-campanualte with 10 distinct ribs. The 3 tips of the upper lip are short and ciliate. The 2 lower tips are awl-shaped, longer than the upper tips and ciliate. The corolla is 3 to 6 cm long with a short tube. It is light to dark purple, occasionally white.

Leaves, Stem and Root: The plant is a slightly woody subshrub, 10 to 30 cm high with or without runners. The flowering stems are erect. The non-flowering stems are decumbent, round, or mildly quadrangular, pubescent all round and rooting at all points. The leaves are small, linear or elliptical and obtuse. The leaves are also flat, narrowing to the petiole, ciliate at the base, glabrous or rough-haired with protruding nerves.

Characteristics: The odor is aromatic.

Habitat: The plant is found in all temperate regions of Eurasia.

Production: Wild thyme consists of the dried, flowering, above-ground parts of Thymus serpyllum.

Not To Be Confused With: Herba Thymi (thymian)

Other Names: Mother of Thyme, Serpyllum, Shepherd's Thyme

ACTIONS AND PHARMACOLOGY

COMPOUNDS

Volatile oil (0.2-0.6%): as a collective species, Thymus serpyllum (over 20 subspecies) encompasses a large number of chemical strains with different volatile oil make-up; chief component is usually carvacrol, further containing, among others, borneol, isobutyl acetate, caryophyllene, 1,8-cineole, citral, citronellal, citronellol, p-cymene, geraniol, geranyl acetate, linalool, linalyl acetate, alpha-pinene, gamma-terpinene, alpha-terpineol, terpinyl acetate, thymol

Flavonoids: including, among others, scutellarenine-7-O-glucosides

Caffeic acid derivatives: in particular rosmarinic acid (2.3%)

EFFECTS

Wild Thyme is antimicrobial, spasmolytic and secretomotory.

INDICATIONS AND USAGE

■ Cough/bronchitis

The herb is used for catarrhs of the upper respiratory tract. In folk medicine, it is used internally as a stomachic, carminative, expectorant, aromatic and for kidney and bladder disorders. External folk medicine uses include herbal cures, baths and alcoholic extracts in embrocations for rheumatic disorders and sprains.

PRECAUTIONS AND ADVERSE REACTIONS

No health hazards or side effects are known in conjunction with the proper administration of designated therapeutic dosages.

DOSAGE

Mode of Administration: As a comminuted drug for infusions and other preparations for internal use. The drug is a component of various standardized preparations of antitussives. Alcoholic extracts are contained in cough drops.

Preparation: To make an infusion, pour boiling water over 1.5 to 2 gm finely cut drug, steep for 10 minutes, then strain (1 teaspoonful = 1.4 gm drug).

Daily Dosage: The average daily dosage is 4 to 6 gm of herb. As a stomachic, drink one cup of the infusion before meals.

LITERATURE

Adzet T et al., PM, Suppl. 1980:52. 1980.

Länger R et al., Sci Pharm 63:325. 1995.

Further information in:

Hänsel R, Keller K, Rimpler H, Schneider G (Hrsg.), Hagers Handbuch der Pharmazeutischen Praxis, 5. Aufl., Bde 4-6 (Drogen): Springer Verlag Berlin, Heidelberg, New York, 1992-1994.

Madaus G, Lehrbuch der Biologischen Arzneimittel, Bde 1-3, Nachdruck, Georg Olms Verlag Hildesheim 1979.

Steinegger E, Hänsel R, Pharmakognosie, 5. Aufl., Springer Verlag Heidelberg 1992.

Teuscher E, Biogene Arzneimittel, 5. Aufl., Wiss. Verlagsges. Stuttgart 1997.

Wichtl M (Hrsg.), Teedrogen, 4. Aufl., Wiss. Verlagsges. Stuttgart 1997.

Thymus Vulgaris

Thyme

DESCRIPTION

Medicinal Parts: The medicinal parts are the oil extracted from the fresh, flowering herb, the dried leaves, the striped and dried leaves, and the fresh aerial part of the flowering plant.

Flower and Fruit: The blue-violet to bright red labiate flowers are in 3 to 6 blossomed axillary clusters. The calyx is bilabiate with a 3-tipped upper lip and a 2-tipped lower lip. The upper lip of the corolla is straight and the lower lip is divided in 3. The stamens are splayed from the base.

Leaves, Stem and Root: The plant is a dwarf shrub up to 50 cm high with an erect, woody and very branched-bushy and downy stem, which never roots. The leaves are short-petioled, linear or oblong-round, acute, glandular-punctate with an involute margin and a tomentose under surface.

Characteristics: The odor is aromatic and the taste tangy, somewhat bitter and camphor-like.

Habitat: The plant is indigenous to the Mediterranean region and neighboring countries, northern Africa and parts of Asia. It is extensively cultivated.

Production: Thyme consists of the stripped and dried leaves and flowers of Thymus vulgaris, Thymus zygis, or both species.

ACTIONS AND PHARMACOLOGY

COMPOUNDS

Volatile oil (1.0-2.5%): chief components thymol (20-55%), p-cymene (14-45%), carvacrol (1-10%), borneol (up to 8%), linalool (up to 8%)

Caffeic acid derivatives: rosmarinic acid

Flavonoids: including, among others, luteolin, apigenin, naringenin, cirsilineol, cirsimaritin, thymonin, partially present as glycosides

Triterpenes: including, among others, ursolic acid (2%), oleanolic acid (0.6%)

EFFECTS

Thyme is a bronchial antispasmodic, an expectorant, and an antibacterial agent.

INDICATIONS AND USAGE

- Cough
- Bronchitis

The herb is used internally for symptoms of bronchitis and whooping cough. Externally, it is used for catarrh of the upper respiratory tracts and as a skin irritative rub. It is antibacterial and deodorizing. In folk medicine, thyme is used as a stomachic for its spasmolytic effect, as a carminative, a diuretic, as a urinary disinfectant and as a vermicide.

PRECAUTIONS AND ADVERSE REACTIONS

No health hazards or side effects are known in conjunction with the proper administration of designated therapeutic dosages. The drug possesses a low potential for sensitization. Where large skin injuries or acute skin illnesses, severe feverish or infectious diseases, cardiac insufficiency or hypertonia are present, entire-body baths should be carried out only following consultation with a doctor, no matter what the active agent is.

DOSAGE

Mode of Administration: Thyme is available as a comminuted drug, powder, liquid extract or dry extract for infusions and other galenic preparations. Liquid and solid medicinal forms for internal and external application are available. Combinations with other herbs, which have expectorant action, are also available. Extracts of the drug are components of standardized preparations of antitussive and cough remedy teas.

Preparation: To prepare a tea, use 1.5 to 2 gm drug with boiling water, steep for 10 minutes, then strain. (1 teaspoonful is equivalent to 1.4 gm drug.)

Daily Dosage: The recommended daily dosage is 10 gm drug with 0.03% phenol, calculated as thymol. When using a liquid extract, 1 to 2 gm is taken 1 to 3 times daily. The tea can be taken several times a day as needed. A 5% infusion can be used for compresses.

LITERATURE

Czygan FC, Hänsel R, Thymian und Quendel - Arznei und Gewürzpflanzen. In: ZPT 14(2):104. 1992.

Haraguchi H et al., Antiperoxidative components in Thymus vulgaris. In: PM 62(3):217-221. 1996.

Hiller K, Pharmazeutische Bewertung ausgewählter Teedrogen. In: DAZ 135(16):1425-1440. 1995.

Kreis P, Juchelka D, Motz C, Mosandl A, Chirale Inhaltstoffe ätherischer Öle. In: DAZ 131(39):1984. 1991.

Messerschmidt W, PM 13:56-72. 1965.

Miguel JD, (1976) J Agric Food Chem 24:833.

Montes GM et al., (1981) An Real Acad Farm 47(3):285.

Schratz E, Hörster H, PM 19:160. 1970.

Sourgens H et al., (1982) Planta Med 45:78.

Svendsen AB, Karlsen J, (1966) Planta Med 14:376.

Vampa G et al., Plantes Med Phytothér 22:195. 1988.

Van den Broucke CO et al., (1983) Pharm Weekbl 5(1):9.

Weiss B, Flück H, Pharm Acta Helv 45:169. 1970.

Further information in:

Hänsel R, Keller K, Rimpler H, Schneider G (Hrsg.), Hagers Handbuch der Pharmazeutischen Praxis, 5. Aufl., Bde 4-6 (Drogen): Springer Verlag Berlin, Heidelberg, New York, 1992-1994.

Leung AY, Encyclopedia of Common Natural Ingredients Used in Food Drugs, Cosmetics, John Wiley & Sons Inc., New York 1980.

Madaus G, Lehrbuch der Biologischen Arzneimittel, Bde 1-3, Nachdruck, Georg Olms Verlag Hildesheim 1979.

Steinegger E, Hänsel R, Pharmakognosie, 5. Aufl., Springer Verlag Heidelberg 1992.

Teuscher E, Biogene Arzneimittel, 5. Aufl., Wiss. Verlagsges. Stuttgart 1997.

Teuscher E, Lindequist U, Biogene Gifte - Biologie, Chemie, Pharmakologie, 2. Aufl., Fischer Verlag Stuttgart 1994.

Wichtl M (Hrsg.), Teedrogen, 4. Aufl., Wiss. Verlagsges. Stuttgart 1997.

Tiarella Cordifolia

Coolwort

DESCRIPTION

Medicinal Parts: The medicinal part is the herb.

Flower and Fruit: The plant has inconspicuous white flowers in racemes. The buds are pink-tinged. The few seeds are somewhat clavate. They have a light acrid taste and are odorless.

Leaves, Stem and Root: The plant is a 15 to 20 cm high herbaceous perennial, which produces runners. The simple leaves are usually slightly 5-lobed and cordate. The basal leaves are often deep red-orange. The cauline leaves have deep red spots and veins, although the latter are often lacking.

Habitat: The plant is indigenous to North America from Virginia to Canada.

Production: Coolwort is the aerial part of Tiarella cordifolia.

Other Names: Foam Flower, Mitrewort

ACTIONS AND PHARMACOLOGY

COMPOUNDS

The effective agents of the plant are unknown.

EFFECTS

The herb is a diuretic and a tonic.

INDICATIONS AND USAGE

Coolwort is used for conditions of the urinary tract and digestive disorders.

PRECAUTIONS AND ADVERSE REACTIONS

No health hazards or side effects are known in conjunction with the proper administration of designated therapeutic dosages.

DOSAGE

Mode of Administration: The drug is ground for infusions.

LITERATURE

No literature available.

Tilia Species

Linden

DESCRIPTION

Medicinal Parts: The medicinal parts are the fresh and dried flowers.

Flower and Fruit: The yellowish-white flowers are clusters of 5 to 11 in cymes. The calyx is 5-sepaled, oblong or ovate-lanceolate, acute and deep. The 5 petals are spatulate-lanceolate with crenate tips. There are numerous stamens and 1 superior ovary, which is almost globular and has silky-haired villi. The fruit is a 1-seeded, pear-shaped, indistinctly angular, thin-shelled nut. There is a tongue-shaped, parchment-like, greenish- or yellowish-white bract at the base of the flowers.

Leaves, Stem and Root: Linden is an impressive tree up to 25 m high with a large, closed crown. The bark is fissured, gray-brown or black-gray. The bark of the branches is smooth. The branchlets are olive-green, brown or brown-red with white warts. The leaves are long-petioled, uneven at the base and broadly cordate. They have a dark upper surface and are bluish-green beneath with rust-colored tufts of down in the vein axils.

Characteristics: The flowers have a strong, sweet fragrance and the fruit tastes slightly sweet, slimy and dry.

Habitat: The tree is common in northern temperate regions.

Production: Linden charcoal consists of the charcoal obtained from the wood of Tilia cordata and/or Tilia platyphyllos. Linden leaf consists of the dried leaf of Tilia cordata and/or Tilia platyphyllos. Silver Linden flower consists of the dried flowers of Tilia tomentosa (synonym Tilia argentea). Linden wood consists of the dried sapwood of Tilia cordata and/or Tilia platyphyllos. Linden flower consists of the dried flower of Tilia cordata and/or Tilia platy-phyllos.

Not To Be Confused With: Linden flower should not be confused with Tilia tometosa and Tilia x euchlora

Other Names: Lime, Linn Flowers

ACTIONS AND PHARMACOLOGY

COMPOUNDS: TILIAE CARBO

Extremely adsorbent charcoals

EFFECTS: TILIAE CARBO

No information is available.

COMPOUNDS: TILIAE FOLIUM

Flavonoids: including, among others, linarin (acacetin-7-rutinosides)

Tannins

Mucilage

EFFECTS: TILIAE FOLIUM

No information is available.

COMPOUNDS: TILIAE TORMENTOSAE FLOS

Flavonoids: including, among others, hyperoside

Hydroxycoumarins: including, among others, calycanthoside, aesculin

Caffeic acid derivatives: chlorogenic acid

Mucilage

EFFECTS: TILIAE TORMENTOSAE FLOS

No information is available.

COMPOUNDS: TILIAE LIGNUM

Mucilage

Sterols: beta-sitosterol, stigmasterol, stigmastenol and their fatty acid esters

Triterpenes: squalene

EFFECTS: TILIAE LIGNUM

No information is available.

COMPOUNDS: TILIAE FLOS

Flavonoids (1%): including, among others, rutin, hyperoside, quercitrin, isoquercitrin, astragalin, tiliroside (astragalin-6''-p-cumaroylester)

Mucilage: arabino galactans with uronic acid share

Volatile oil (0.01-0.02%): including, among others, linalool, geraniol, 1,8-cineole, 2-phenyl ethanol

Caffeic acid derivatives: chlorogenic acid

Tannins

EFFECTS: TILIAE FLOS

Tiliae flos is a diaphoretic, an expectorant, and an irritant inhibitor.

INDICATIONS AND USAGE

TILIAE CARBO

Preparations of Linden charcoal are used internally for intestinal disorders and externally for ulcus cruris.

TILIAE FOLIUM

Preparations of Linden leaf are used as a diaphoretic.

TILIAE TORMENTOSAE FLOS

Preparations of Silver Linden flower are used for catarrhs of the respiratory tract and as an antispasmodic, expectorant and diaphoretic, as well as a diuretic.

TILIAE LIGNUM

Preparations of Linden wood are used for diseases and ailments of the liver and gallbladder systems, as well as for cellulitis.

TILIAE FLOS

■ Cough/bronchitis

The flowers are used for colds and cold-related coughs and as a diaphoretic for feverish colds and infectious diseases, where a sweating cure is needed. In folk medicine, it is occasionally used as a diuretic, a stomachic, an antispasmodic and as a sedative.

PRECAUTIONS AND ADVERSE REACTIONS

TILIAE CARBO, FOLIUM, TORMENTOSAE FLOS, LIGNUM AND FLOS

No health hazards or side effects are known in conjunction with the proper administration of designated therapeutic dosages.

DOSAGE

TILIAE FLOS

Mode of Administration: As a comminuted herb for teas and other galenic preparations for internal use. The drug is a component of some standardized urologic preparations, antitussives and sedatives and in cold remedy tea mixtures.

Preparation: To make an infusion, pour boiling water over 2 gm drug or put it in cold water, which is rapidly brought to a boil. Steep 5 to 10 minutes and strain. (1 teaspoonful = 1.8 gm drug)

Daily Dosage: The recommended daily dosage is 2 to 4 gm of drug.

LITERATURE

TILIAE CARBO

No literature available.

TILIAE FOLIUM

Kern W, List PH, Hörhammer L (Hrsg.), Hagers Handbuch der Pharmazeutischen Praxis, 4. Aufl., Bde. 1-8: Springer Verlag Berlin, Heidelberg, New York, 1969.

TILIAE TORMENTOSAE FLOS

Buchbauer G, Jirovetz L, Ätherisches Lindenblütenöl - Aromastoffanalyse. In: DAZ 132(15):748. 1992.

Further information in:

Fenaroli's Handbook of Flavor Ingredients, Vol. 1, 2nd Ed., CRC Press 1975.

Hegnauer R, Chemotaxonomie der Pflanzen, Bde 1-11: Birkhäuser Verlag Basel, Boston, Berlin 1962-1997.

Roth L, Daunderer M, Kormann K, Giftpflanzen, Pflanzengifte, 4. Aufl., Ecomed Fachverlag Landsberg Lech 1993.

TILIAE LIGNUM

Kern W, List PH, Hörhammer L (Hrsg.), Hagers Handbuch der Pharmazeutischen Praxis, 4. Aufl., Bde. 1-8: Springer Verlag Berlin, Heidelberg, New York, 1969.

TILIAE FLOS

Buchbauer G, Jirovetz L, Ätherisches Lindenblütenöl-Aromastoffanalyse. In: DAZ 132(15):748. 1992.

Hildebrandt G, Engelbrecht P, Hildebrandt-Evers G, (1954) Physiologische Grundlagen für eine tageszeitliche Ordnung der Schwitzprozeduren. Z Klin Med 152:446-468.

Kram G, Franz G, PA 49:149. 1985.

Kram G, Franz G, PM 49:149. 1983.

Further information in:

Fenaroli's Handbook of Flavor Ingredients, Vol. 1, 2nd Ed., CRC Press 1975.

Kern W, List PH, Hörhammer L (Hrsg.), Hagers Handbuch der Pharmazeutischen Praxis, 4. Aufl., Bde. 1-8: Springer Verlag Berlin, Heidelberg, New York, 1969.

Madaus G, Lehrbuch der Biologischen Arzneimittel, Bde 1-3, Nachdruck, Georg Olms Verlag Hildesheim 1979.

Schulz R, Hänsel R, Rationale Phytotherapie, Springer Verlag Heidelberg 1996.

Steinegger E, Hänsel R, Pharmakognosie, 5. Aufl., Springer Verlag Heidelberg 1992.

Teuscher E, Biogene Arzneimittel, 5. Aufl., Wiss. Verlagsges. Stuttgart 1997.

Wichtl M (Hrsg.), Teedrogen, 4. Aufl., Wiss. Verlagsges. Stuttgart 1997.

Tobacco

See Nicotiana Tabacum

Tomato

See Lycopersicon Esculentum

Tonka Beans

See Dipteryx Odorata

Tormentil Root

See Potentilla Erecta

Tragacanth

See Astragalus Gummifer

Trailing Arbutus

See Epigae Repens

Traveller's Joy

See Clematis Vitalba

Tree of Heaven

See Ailanthus Altissima

Trifolium Pratense

Red Clover

DESCRIPTION

Medicinal Parts: The medicinal parts are the dried and the fresh flower heads.

Flower and Fruit: One to 4 globular, ovate flower heads form on the tip of the stem. The calyx is tubular-campanulate. The petals are light carmine to fleshy red, occasionally yellowish-white or pure white. The fruit is a pod, which is ovate, 1-seeded and thin-skinned. The seed is oblong-ovate, yellow to brownish or violet.

Leaves, Stem and Root: The plant is a perennial herb, 15 to 40 cm high with a bushy rhizome and a basal leaf rosette. An erect, angular stem grows from the rhizome. The rhizome is covered in alternate, trifoliate, elliptical or ovate leaves, which have a characteristic arrow-shaped white spot on the upper surface. The leaflets are short-petioled, almost entire-margined, appressed, softly pubescent on both surfaces or only on the upper surface.

Habitat: The plant is indigenous to Europe, central Asia, northern Africa and is naturalized in many other parts of the world.

Production: Red Clover flowers are the flowers of Trifolium pratense. The dried flower buds are used to produce the drug.

Other Names: Purple Clover, Trefoil, Wild Clover

ACTIONS AND PHARMACOLOGY

COMPOUNDS

Volatile oil: including, among others, with benzyl alcohol, 2-phenyl ethanol, their formates and acetates, methyl salicylate, methyl anthranilate (likely only in the fresh blossoms)

Isoflavonoids: including, among others, biochanin A

Coumarin derivatives

Cyanogenic glycosides: presumably lotaustralin, linamarin

EFFECTS

Red Clover has antispasmodic and expectorant effects and also promotes the skin's healing process.

INDICATIONS AND USAGE

Internally, Red Clover is used for coughs and respiratory conditions, particularly whooping cough. Externally, it is used in the treatment of chronic skin conditions such as psoriasis and eczema.

PRECAUTIONS AND ADVERSE REACTIONS

No health hazards or side effects are known in conjunction with the proper administration of designated therapeutic dosages.

DOSAGE

Mode of Administration: The drug is used internally and externally as a liquid extract and in medicinal preparations.

Preparation: Liquid extract 1:1 can be prepared in 25% ethanol.

Daily Dosage: The daily dosage is 4 gm drug, taken as an infusion, up to 3 times a day. Alternately, 1.5 to 3 ml of the liquid extract can be taken 3 times daily.

LITERATURE

Dewick P, (1977) Phytochemistry 16:93.

Guggolz J et al., (1961) Agric Food Chem 9(4):331.

Kattaev NS et al., (1972) Khim Prir Soed 6:806.

Sachse J, (1974) J Chrom 96(1):123.

Yoshihara T et al., (1977) Agric Biol Chem 41(9):1679.

Further information in:

Fenaroli's Handbook of Flavor Ingredients, Vol. 1, 2nd Ed., CRC Press 1975.

Hänsel R, Keller K, Rimpler H, Schneider G (Hrsg.), Hagers Handbuch der Pharmazeutischen Praxis, 5. Aufl., Bde 4-6 (Drogen): Springer Verlag Berlin, Heidelberg, New York, 1992-1994.

Madaus G, Lehrbuch der Biologischen Arzneimittel, Bde 1-3, Nachdruck, Georg Olms Verlag Hildesheim 1979.

Wagner H, Wiesenauer M, Phytotherapie. Phytopharmaka und pflanzliche Homöopathika, Fischer-Verlag, Stuttgart, Jena, New York 1995.

Trigonella Foenum-Graecum

Fenugreek

DESCRIPTION

Medicinal Parts: The medicinal parts are the ripe, dried seeds.

Flower and Fruit: The 0.8 to 1.8 cm long flowers are solitary or in pairs in the leaf axils. They are almost sessile. The calyx tube is membranous and usually longer than the lanceolate tips. The corolla is usually pale yellow, occasionally darker or violet and about double the length of the calyx. The wings are about half as long as the standard and the carina is very obtuse, round and barely longer than the calyx. The fruit is a 2.5 to 10 cm long and 0.5 to 1 cm wide, more or less erect, leaning, linear and appressed pubescent pod with a long lip. The 4 to 20 seeds are flattened, divided into 2 uneven halves by a deep groove, ovate to di-shaped, yellow-brown, or brown-red, and very hard when dry.

Leaves, Stem and Root: The plant is an annual, 10 to 50 cm high herb with a long vertical taproot. The stem is sturdy, round, erect or decumbent and branched. The leaves are trifoliate and the petioles are 0.5 to 2 cm long. The leaflets are 1 to 3 cm long, obovate to oblong-lanceolate, obtusely deltoid to rounded. The stipules are fairly large, membranous, ovate, acute and more or less softly pubescent.

Habitat: The species is common all over the Mediterranean region as far as India and China and southward as far as Ethiopia. The main regions of cultivation are southern France, Turkey, northern Africa, India and China.

Production: Fenugreek consists of the ripe, dried seed of Trigonella foenum-graecum.

Other Names: Greek Hay Seed, Bird's Foot

ACTIONS AND PHARMACOLOGY

COMPOUNDS

Mucilages (25-45%, mannogalactans)

Proteins (25-30%)

Proteinase inhibitors

Steroid saponins: including trigofoenosides A to G (to some extent bitter)

Steroid saponin-peptide ester: including foenugraecin

Flavonoids: including isoorientin, isovitexin, orientin, saponaretin, vicenin-1

Trigonelline (coffearin, N-methylbetaine of the nicotinic acid)

Volatile oil (traces): aroma bearer 3-Hydroxy-4,5-dimethyl-2(5H)-furanone

EFFECTS

Externally, the drug acts as an emollient. Internally, Fenugreek reduces blood sugar, increases milk and acts as a vulnerary. The effects cannot be attributed to any specific substance or pharmacodynamic action.

INDICATIONS AND USAGE

- Loss of appetite
- Dsypeptic complaints
- Inflammation of the skin

Internal uses include loss of appetite and upper respiratory catarrh. Externally, the drug is used as poultice for local inflammation, furuncles, ulcers, inflamed swellings and eczema.

PRECAUTIONS AND ADVERSE REACTIONS

Health risks or side effects following the proper administration of designated therapeutic dosages are not recorded. Sensitization is possible through repeated external administration of the drug.

DOSAGE

Mode of Administration: Comminuted seed and other galenic preparations for internal and external use. There has recently been interest expressed in the plant as raw material for steroids.

Preparation: To prepare an infusion, leave 0.5 g drug in cold water for 3 hours and then strain. The infusion may be sweetened with honey. A poultice is prepared as a thick paste made from the powdered seeds with hot water. (50 g powdered drug per 1 liter water)

Daily Dose: The daily internal dose of the drug is 6 g. Tea preparation may be taken 1 cup several times a day.

LITERATURE

Abdo MS, Al-Khafawi AA, (1969) Planta Med 17:14.

Adamska M, Lutomski J, (1971) Planta Med 20:224.

Al-Meshal IA et al., (1985) Fitoterapia 56 (4):232.

Ali L et al., Characterization of the hypoglycemic effect of Trigonella foenum graecum seed. In: PM 61(4):358-360. 1995.

Bohlmann MB et al., (1974) Phytochemistry 13:1513.

Girardon P et al., (1985) Planta Med 51 (6):533.

Girardou P et al., PM 51:533. 1985.

Gupta RK, Jain DC, Thakur RS, PH 23:2605. 1984.

Gupta RK, Jain DC, Thakur RS, PH 24:2399. 1986.

Gupta RK, Jain DC, Thakur RS, PH 25:2205. 1986.

Hardman R et al., (1980) Phytochemistry 19:698.

Ribes G et al., (1986) Ann Nutr Metab. 28:37.

Ribes G et al., (1986) Phytother Res 1(1):40.

Ribes G et al., (1986) Proc. Soc Exp Biol Med 183:159.

Sood AR et al., (1976) Phytochemistry 15:351.

Weder JK, Heußner K, Z Lebensm Untersuch Forsch 193:242 et 321. 1991.

Further information in:

Chan, EH et al., (Eds.), Advances in Chinese Medicinal Materials Research, World Scientific Pub. Co. Singapore 1985.

Hänsel R, Keller K, Rimpler H, Schneider G (Hrsg.), Hagers Handbuch der Pharmazeutischen Praxis, 5. Aufl., Bde 4-6 (Drogen), Springer Verlag Berlin, Heidelberg, New York, 1992-1994.

Leung AY, Encyclopedia of Common Natural Ingredients Used in Food Drugs and Cosmetics, John Wiley & Sons Inc., New York 1980.

Madaus G, Lehrbuch der Biologischen Arzneimittel, Bde 1-3, Nachdruck, Georg Olms Verlag Hildesheim 1979.

Steinegger E, Hänsel R, Pharmakognosie, 5. Aufl., Springer Verlag Heidelberg 1992.

Teuscher E, Biogene Arzneimittel, 5. Aufl., Wiss. Verlagsges. mbH Stuttgart 1997.

Wichtl M (Hrsg.), Teedrogen, 4. Aufl., Wiss. Verlagsges. Stuttgart 1997.

Trillium Erectum

Beth Root

DESCRIPTION

Medicinal Parts: The medicinal parts are the rhizome and the dried root and the leaves.

Flower and Fruit: The plant has solitary, terminal, hanging flowers. The 3 green, persistent sepals and the 3 large, white to red or yellow, wilting sepals are characteristic.

Leaves, Stem and Root: The plant is a perennial, smooth herb with an erect stem, which grows from 25 to 40 cm high. It bears 3 whorled, terminal leaves under the flower, which are broad, rhomboid and lightly curled. The rhizome is matte brown, subconical, more or less compressed, 3 to 5 cm long and 2 to 3 cm in diameter. It is often ringed with oblique lines and with numerous wrinkled root fibres on the upper surface.

Characteristics: The taste is sweetish then acrid and the odor is characteristic.

Habitat: The plant is indigenous to the central and western U.S.

Production: Beth Root Stock is the rhizome of Trillium erectum, Trillium pendulum and other varieties.

Other Names: Birthroot, Indian Shamrock, Lamb's Quarters, Wake-Robin, Indian Balm, Ground Lily, Coughroot, Jew's-harp Plant, Milk Ipecac, Pariswort, Rattlesnake Root, Snake-bite, Three-leaved, Nightshade

ACTIONS AND PHARMACOLOGY

COMPOUNDS

Steroid saponins: including, among others, trillin (disogenine monoglucoside), trillarin (diosgenine diglucoside), further aglycones were able to be found following hydrolysis: kryptogenin, chlorogenin, nologenin

Tannins

EFFECTS

The active agents are diosgenin, saponins Trillen and Trillarin, as well as tannin.

The drug has astringent and expectorant properties. The drug can severely irritate the area to which it has been applied; the irritation can cause vomiting.

INDICATIONS AND USAGE

Internally, Beth Root is used for long and heavy menstruation and pain relief. Externally, it is used for varicose veins and ulcers, hematoma and hemorrhoid bleeding.

PRECAUTIONS AND ADVERSE REACTIONS

No health hazards or side effects are known in conjunction with the proper administration of designated therapeutic dosages. In higher dosages, the drug is said to be nauseant, and to have the effect of promoting menstruation.

Pregnancy: In high dosages, the drug is said to have the effect of promoting labor.

DOSAGE

Mode of Administration: The ground drug and liquid extract are used for infusions and poultices.

LITERATURE

Fukuda N et al., (1981) Chem Pharm Bull 29 (2):325.

Nakano K et al., (1982) J Chem Soc Chem Commun. 789.

Nakano K et al., (1982) Yakugaku Zasshi 102(11):1031.

Nakano K et al., (1983) Phytochemistry 22 (5):1249.

Wolters B, Zierpflanzen aus Nordamerika. In: DAZ 137(26):2253-2261. 1997.

Further information in:

Hegnauer R, Chemotaxonomie der Pflanzen, Bde 1-11: Birkhäuser Verlag Basel, Boston, Berlin 1962-1997.

Kern W, List PH, Hörhammer L (Hrsg.), Hagers Handbuch der Pharmazeutischen Praxis, 4. Aufl., Bde. 1-8: Springer Verlag Berlin, Heidelberg, New York, 1969.

Madaus G, Lehrbuch der Biologischen Arzneimittel, Bde 1-3, Nachdruck, Georg Olms Verlag Hildesheim 1979.

Roth L, Daunderer M, Kormann K, Giftpflanzen, Pflanzengifte, 4. Aufl., Ecomed Fachverlag Landsberg Lech 1993.

Trollius Europaeus

Globe Flower

DESCRIPTION

Medicinal Parts: The medicinal part is the whole fresh plant.

Flower and Fruit: Every branch of the stem bears a solitary, terminal flower. They are up to 5 cm in diameter, globular and have no calyx. The flowers usually have 10 perianth segments. The petals are lemon-yellow. The outer petals are occasionally green underneath. They are bent. The stamens are approximately 12 mm long and have a 0.5 to 5 mm long appendage.

Leaves, Stem and Root: The plant is 10 to 70 cm high and glabrous. The stem is hollow, smooth and branched upwards. The basal leaves are long-petioled and 3 to 5 lobed. The lobes are cuneate and more or less deeply indented and serrate. The cauline leaves are smaller and more or less sessile.

Habitat: The plant is indigenous to northern and central Europe.

Production: Globe flowers are the flowers of Trollius europaeus.

Other Names: Globe Ranunculus, Globe Crowfoot, Globe Trollius

ACTIONS AND PHARMACOLOGY

COMPOUNDS

Ranunculin: protoanemonine-forming substance in the freshly-harvested plant that changes enzymatically when the plant is cut into small pieces. The pungent, volatile protoanemonine quickly dimerizes to the non-mucous membrane irritating anemonine. When dried, the plant is not capable of protoanemonine-formation.

Flavonoids

Ascorbic acid (Vitamin C)

EFFECTS

The active agents are xanthophyll, expoxid and neoanthin (trollixanthin).

INDICATIONS AND USAGE

Formerly, the plant was used to treat scurvy. It loses most of its active properties on drying.

PRECAUTIONS AND ADVERSE REACTIONS

No health hazards or side effects are known in conjunction with the proper administration of designated therapeutic dosages. Extended skin contact with the freshly-harvested, bruised plant can lead to blister formation and cauterizations due to the resulting protoanemonine that is severely irritating to skin and mucous membranes.

If taken internally, severe irritation to the gastrointestinal tract, combined with colic and diarrhea, as well as irritation of the urinary drainage passages, are possible. Because of the very low level of protoanemonine-forming substances in the plant, the danger of poisoning is quite low.

DOSAGE

Mode of Administration: The drug is obsolete.

LITERATURE

Kern W, List PH, Hörhammer L (Hrsg.), Hagers Handbuch der Pharmazeutischen Praxis, 4. Aufl., Bde. 1-8: Springer Verlag Berlin, Heidelberg, New York, 1969.

Roth L, Daunderer M, Kormann K, Giftpflanzen, Pflanzengifte, 4. Aufl., Ecomed Fachverlag Landsberg Lech 1993.

Tropaeolum Majus

Nasturtium

DESCRIPTION

Medicinal Parts: The medicinal parts are the fresh herb, the whole fresh flowering plant and the seeds.

Flower and Fruit: The handsome campanulate flowers are orange with flame-red to fiery red stripes. The calyx is bilabiate, colored and has a spurred upper lip. There are 5 uneven petals. The 2 upper petals are unstemmed, the 3 lower ones are stemmed and fringed at the base. There are 8 stamens and a superior ovary with a 3-stigmaed style. The fruit is a 3-valved pericarp. It is orbicular-reniform, fleshy, wrinkled when ripe and dirty yellow.

Leaves, Stem and Root: The plant is an annual, sometimes perennial and often creeping or climbing plant, 0.3 to 5 m long. The main root is thin and forms an underground runner. The stem is round, branched, fleshy and glabrous, like the whole plant. The leaves are alternate, long-petioled, hastate and almost circular. The leaves are 3 to 5 cm and deeply lobed at the petiole.

Characteristics: The flowers are fragrant and the leafy parts smell and taste like cress.

Habitat: The plant is indigenous to warmer regions of South America and is becoming naturalized in the Mediterranean region, otherwise found as a garden or ornamental plant.

Production: Garden Nasturtium consists of the aerial parts, the seeds or leaves of Tropaeolum majus.

Other Names: Indian Cress

ACTIONS AND PHARMACOLOGY

COMPOUNDS

Glucosinolates (0.1%): in the fresh, unbruised plant: chief components are glucotropaeolin, yielding after cell destruction benzyl isothiocyanate

Ascorbic acid (Vitamin C, 300 mg/100 g fresh weight)

Oxalates

Flavonoids: including, among others, isoquercetin and quercetin glycosides

Carotinoids: as blossom pigments

EFFECTS

Benzyl mustard oil extracted from Tropaeolum majus is bacteriostatic, virostatic and antimycotic in vitro; mustard oils are eliminated mainly via the breath or are collected and eliminated in the urine; used externally, Tropaeolum acts as a rubefacient.

INDICATIONS AND USAGE

- Infections of the urinary tract
- Cough
- Bronchitis

Nastertium is used for infections of the urinary tract and catarrh of the upper respiratory tract. The drug is also used for improvement of resistance to catarrh and to support of the removal of infective substances.

CONTRAINDICATIONS

Do not intake with gastrointestinal ulcers or with kidney diseases.

Do not administer to infants or small children.

PRECAUTIONS AND ADVERSE REACTIONS

General: No health hazards or side effects are known in conjunction with the proper administration of designated therapeutic dosages. Administration of higher dosages of the fresh plant or of its volatile oil can lead to mucous membrane irritation of the gastrointestinal tract. External administration involving long-term intensive contact with the fresh plant can lead to skin irritations. The plant possesses a low potential for sensitization.

Pediatric Use: Not to be administered to infants or small children.

DOSAGE

No dosage information is available.

LITERATURE

Franz G, Kapuzinerkresse (Tropaeolum majus L.) Portrait einer Arzneipflanze. In: ZPT 17(4):255-622. 1996.

Pintao AM et al., In vitro and in vivo antitumor activity of benzyl isothiocyanate: a natural product from Tropaeolum majus. In: PH 61(3):233-236. 1995.

Further information in:

Frohne D, Pfänder HJ, Giftpflanzen - Ein Handbuch für Apotheker, Toxikologen und Biologen, 4. Aufl., Wiss. Verlags-Ges. Stuttgart 1997.

Hänsel R, Keller K, Rimpler H, Schneider G (Hrsg.), Hagers Handbuch der Pharmazeutischen Praxis, 5. Aufl., Bde 4-6 (Drogen): Springer Verlag Berlin, Heidelberg, New York, 1992-1994.

Madaus G, Lehrbuch der Biologischen Arzneimittel, Bde 1-3, Nachdruck, Georg Olms Verlag Hildesheim 1979.

Roth L, Daunderer M, Kormann K, Giftpflanzen, Pflanzengifte, 4. Aufl., Ecomed Fachverlag Landsberg Lech 1993.

Steinegger E, Hänsel R, Pharmakognosie, 5. Aufl., Springer Verlag Heidelberg 1992.

Teuscher E, Lindequist U, Biogene Gifte - Biologie, Chemie, Pharmakologie, 2. Aufl., Fischer Verlag Stuttgart 1994.

Wagner H, Wiesenauer M, Phytotherapie. Phytopharmaka und pflanzliche Homöopathika, Fischer-Verlag, Stuttgart, Jena, New York 1995.

Wichtl M (Hrsg.), Teedrogen, 4. Aufl., Wiss. Verlagsges. Stuttgart 1997.

True Unicorn Root

See Aletris Farinosa

Tsuga Canadensis

Pinus Bark

DESCRIPTION

Medicinal Parts: The medicinal parts are the latex, which exudes from the plant and the essential oil.

Flower and Fruit: The pedicle of the male flower is shorter than the scale sheath. The cones are small (1.5 to 2.5 cm long) and light brown. The wood contains no resin.

Leaves, Stem and Root: The young shoots are villous, becoming pubescent. The leaves have a leaf cushion and are flat, short (1 to 1.5 cm long) and obtuse. The upper surface is dark green and the under surface has 2 blue-white long stripes.

Habitat: The plant is indigenous to North America.

Other Names: Hemlock Bark, Canada Pitch, Hemlock Gum

ACTIONS AND PHARMACOLOGY

COMPOUNDS

Tannins (10%)

Flavonoids: hemlock tannin

Stilbene derivatives: piceatannol

EFFECTS

The active agents are the tannin, hemlock tannin and piceatannol. The drug has astringent, anti-inflammatory, diaphoretic and diuretic properties.

INDICATIONS AND USAGE

Pinus Bark is used for digestive disorders, diarrhea and diseases of the mouth and throat. It was formerly used to treat scurvy.

PRECAUTIONS AND ADVERSE REACTIONS

No health hazards or side effects are known in conjunction with the proper administration of designated therapeutic dosages. Administration in allopathic medicine is not usual.

DOSAGE

Mode of Administration: The drug is available as a liquid extract, in medicinal preparations and combinations.

LITERATURE

Hoppe HA, (1975-1987) Drogenkunde, 8. Aufl., Bde 1-3: W de Gruyter Verlag, Berlin, New York.

Kern W, List PH, Hörhammer L (Hrsg.), Hagers Handbuch der Pharmazeutischen Praxis, 4. Aufl., Bde 1-8: Springer Verlag Berlin, Heidelberg, New York, 1969.

Turkey Corn

See Dicentra Cucullaria

Turmeric

See Curcuma Domestica

Turnera Diffusa

Damiana

DESCRIPTION

Medicinal Parts: The medicinal parts are the leaves harvested during the flowering season.

Flower and Fruit: The flowers are yellow, solitary and axillary. The fruit is a small, globular, many-seeded capsule, which breaks up into 3 parts. It is aromatic and resinous.

Leaves, Stem and Root: The plant is a small shrub up to 60 cm high. The leaves are 1 to 2.5 cm long and up to 6 mm wide. They are smooth and pale green on the upper surface and glabrous with a few scattered hairs on the ribs underneath. The leaves are ovate-lanceolate, short-petioled and have 2 glands at the base. They have a few serrate teeth and recurved margins.

Habitat: The plant is found mainly in the region of the Gulf of Mexico, the Caribbean and southern Africa.

Production: Damiana leaf consists of the leaf of Turnera diffusa and its variations. Damiana herb consists of the herb of Turnera diffusa and its variations.

ACTIONS AND PHARMACOLOGY

COMPOUNDS

Volatile oil (0.5-0.9%): chief components 1,8-cineole, alpha- and beta-pinene, p-cymene

Tannins (4%)

Resins (7%)

Hydroquinone glycosides: arbutin (0.2-0.7%)

Cyanogenic glycosides: tetraphylline B (barterin)

INDICATIONS AND USAGE

Damiana preparations are used as an aphrodisiac and for prophylaxis and treatment of sexual disturbances.

PRECAUTIONS AND ADVERSE REACTIONS

No health hazards or side effects are known in conjunction with the proper administration of designated therapeutic dosages.

LITERATURE

Auterhoff H, Häufel HP, (1968) Arch Pharm 301:537.

Dominguez XA, Hinojosa M, (1976) Planta Med 30:68.

Jin J, (1966) Lloydia 29(3):250.

Further information in:

Hegnauer R, Chemotaxonomie der Pflanzen, Bde 1-11: Birkhäuser Verlag Basel, Boston, Berlin 1962-1997.

Hoppe HA, (1975-1987) Drogenkunde, 8. Aufl., Bde 1-3: W de Gruyter Verlag, Berlin, New York.

Kern W, List PH, Hörhammer L (Hrsg.), Hagers Handbuch der Pharmazeutischen Praxis, 4. Aufl., Bde 1-8: Springer Verlag Berlin, Heidelberg, New York, 1969.

Madaus G, Lehrbuch der Biologischen Arzneimittel, Bde 1-3, Nachdruck, Georg Olms Verlag Hildesheim 1979.

Steinegger E, Hänsel R, Pharmakognosie, 5. Aufl., Springer Verlag Heidelberg 1992.

Wagner H, Wiesenauer M, Phytotherapie. Phytopharmaka und pflanzliche Homöopathika, Fischer-Verlag, Stuttgart, Jena, New York 1995.

Turtle Head

See Chelone Glabra

Tussilago Farfara

Colt's Foot

DESCRIPTION

Medicinal Parts: The medicinal parts are the dried inflorescences, the dried leaves and the fresh leaves.

Flower and Fruit: The yellow compound flowers are in small, solitary capitula at the end of the scapes. The lateral florets are lingual, narrow and female. The disc florets are tubular-campanulate, 5-petalled and male. The involucral bracts are almost as long, linear-lanceolate and have a scarious margin. The fruit is 3 to 11 mm long, cylindrical, brown, glabrous and stemmed. The pappus is in a number of rows and consists of long, glossy white hairs, which are much longer than the fruit.

Leaves, Stem and Root: The plant is a perennial, 10 to 30 cm high. It has a broadly branched, underground shoot and root system with a thin round, scaly base. There is also an up to 1.8 m long, far-reaching, creeping shoot. The flower stem is a scaly, round, tomentose scape covered with lanceolate, reddish scales, which is 30 cm long when the fruit ripens. The leaves, which appear after flowering, are basal, coriaceous, cordate-round, angular, irregularly dentate, long-petioled and tomentose beneath. The leaves can reach a diameter of up to 30 cm.

Characteristics: The taste and texture is slimy-sweet and the leaves have a honey-like smell when they are rubbed.

Habitat: The plant grows wild in most of Europe, central, western and northern Asia. It has spread to the mountains of northern Africa and has been introduced into North America.

Production: Colt's Foot flower consists of the fresh or dried flowers of Tussilago farfara. Colt's Foot herb consists of the fresh or dried, above-ground parts of Tussilago farfara. Colt's Foot root consists of the fresh or dried, below-ground parts of Tussilago farfara.

Not To Be Confused With: The leaves of various Petasites species, but petasine and flavonoids can be identified using thin layer chromatography.

Other Names: British Tobacco, Bullsfoot, Butterbur, Coughwort, Flower Velure, Foal's-foot, Horse-foot, Horsehoof, Hallfoot, Ass's Foot, Foalswort, Fieldhove, Donnhove

ACTIONS AND PHARMACOLOGY

COMPOUNDS: FARFARAE FLOS, HERBA ET RADIX

Mucilages (acidic polysaccharides)

Tannins

Pyrrolizidine alkaloids (traces, not from all sources): tussilagine, isotussilagine, senkirkine, senecionin

Triterpenes: including beta-amyrin, arnidiol, faradiol

Flavonoids

EFFECTS: FARFARAE FLOS, HERBA ET RADIX

The mucin contained in the drug has a sequestering effect and envelopes the mucous membrane with a layer that protects the throat from chemical and physical irritation and thereby reduces cough irritation.

COMPOUNDS: FARFARAE FOLIUM

Mucilages (acidic polysaccharides)

Tannins

Pyrrolizidine alkaloids (traces, not from all sources): tussilagine, isotussilagine, senkirkine, senecionin

Triterpenes: including alpha- and beta-amyrin

Flavonoids

Tannins

EFFECTS: FARFARAE FOLIUM

Anti-irritant, anti-inflammatory

INDICATIONS AND USAGE

FARFARAE FLOS, HERBA ET RADIX

Preparations of Colt's Foot are used for treatment and prevention of diseases and ailments of the respiratory tract, such as coughs, hoarseness, bronchial catarrh, acute and chronic bronchitis, asthma, colds, influenza, inflammation and irritation of the oral and pharyngeal mucosa, sore throat, tonsillitis and swelling of the glands.

The efficacy for the claimed uses is not documented.

FARFARAE FOLIUM

- Cough
- Bronchitis
- Inflammation of the mouth and pharynx

Colt's Foot leaf is used for acute catarrh of the respiratory tract with cough and hoarseness and acute, mild inflammation of the oral and pharyngeal mucosa.

PRECAUTIONS AND ADVERSE REACTIONS

FARFARAE FLOS, HERBA ET RADIX

Because of the possible hepatotoxic and carcinogenic pyrrolizidine alkaloid content, the administration of the blossoms should be avoided.

FARFARAE FOLIUM

Colt's Foot leaves may no longer be brought into circulation in Austria. The intake of 10 g pyrrolizidine alkaloids with 1.2-unsaturated necic parent substances in the form of tea mixtures, of 1 g in the form of extracts may not be exceeded in Germany.

Because even traces of the alkaloids present some danger, one should forgo any administration of the drug.

Pregnancy and Nursing Mothers: Administration during pregnancy and while nursing is to be unconditionally ruled out.

DOSAGE

FARFARAE FLOS, HERBA ET RADIX

Mode of Administration: The drug is used internally through the use of tea and standardized remedies.

Preparation: To prepare a tea, add 1.5 to 2.5 g cut drug to boiling water, strain after 5 to 10 minutes. The drug is a constituent of tea preparations and phytopharmaceuticals.

FARFARAE FOLIUM

Mode of Administration: Comminuted drug for teas, pressed plant juice or other galenic preparations for internal use.

Daily Dosage: Total daily dose is up to 6 g of drug. The daily dosage must not be more than 1 mg of total pyrrolizidine alkaloids and N-oxides.

LITERATURE

FARFARAE FLOS, HERBA ET RADIX

Delaveau P et al., (1980) Planta Med 40:49.

Didry N et al., (1982) Ann Pharm Franc 40(1):75.

Engalycheva EI et al., (1982) Farmatsiya 31(2):37.

Franz G, PM 17:217. 1969.

Hiller K, Pharmazeutische Bewertung ausgewählter Teedrogen. In: DAZ 135(16):1425-1440. 1995.

Hirono I et al., (1976) Gann 67(1):125.

Hirono I et al., (1979) J Natl Canc Inst 63(2):469.

Ihrig M, Pyrrolizidinalkaloidhaltige Drogen im Handverkauf? In: PZ 137(40):3128. 1992.

Kraus C et al., (1985) Planta Med 51(2):89.

Miething H, Steinbach RA, Ermittlung der Freisetzungsraten des Pyrrolizidinalkaloids Senkirkin in Huflattich-Teegetränken. In: PZW 135(4):153. 1990.

Paβreiter CM, Co-occurence of 2-pyrrolidineacetic acid with four isomeric tussilaginic acids in Arnica species and Tussilago farfara. In: PM 58(7):A694. 1992.

Röder E et al., (1981) Plant Med 43:99.

Röder E, Pyrrolizidinhaltige Arzneipflanzen. In: DAZ 132(45):2427-2435. 1992.

Wagner H, In: Economic and Medicinal Plant Research, Vol. 1, Academic Press, UK 1985.

Wunderer H, Zentral und peripher wirksame Antitussiva: eine kritische Übersicht. In: PZ 142(11):847-852. 1997.

Further information in:

Frohne D, Pfänder HJ, Giftpflanzen - Ein Handbuch für Apotheker, Toxikologen und Biologen, 4. Aufl., Wiss. Verlagsges. mbH Stuttgart 1997.

Hänsel R, Keller K, Rimpler H, Schneider G (Hrsg.), Hagers Handbuch der Pharmazeutischen Praxis, 5. Aufl., Bde 4-6 (Drogen): Springer Verlag Berlin, Heidelberg, New York, 1992-1994.

Madaus G, Lehrbuch der Biologischen Arzneimittel, Bde 1-3, Nachdruck, Georg Olms Verlag Hildesheim 1979.

Roth L, Daunderer M, Kormann K, Giftpflanzen, Pflanzengifte, 4. Aufl., Ecomed Fachverlag Landsberg Lech 1993.

Steinegger E, Hänsel R, Pharmakognosie, 5. Aufl., Springer Verlag Heidelberg 1992.

Teuscher E, Lindequist U, Biogene Gifte - Biologie, Chemie, Pharmakologie, 2. Aufl., Fischer Verlag Stuttgart 1994.

Teuscher E, Biogene Arzneimittel, 5. Aufl., Wiss. Verlagsges. mbH Stuttgart 1997.

Wichtl M (Hrsg.), Teedrogen, 4. Aufl., Wiss. Verlagsges. Stuttgart 1997.

FARFARAE FOLIUM

Delaveau P et al., (1980) Planta Med 40:49.

Didry N et al., (1982) Ann Pharm Franc 40(1):75.

Engalycheva EI et al., (1982) Farmatsiya 31(2):37.

Franz G, PM 17:217. 1969.

Hiller K, Pharmazeutische Bewertung ausgewählter Teedrogen. In: DAZ 135(16):1425-1440. 1995.

Hirono I et al., (1976) Gann 67(1):125.

Hirono I et al., (1979) J Natl Canc Inst 63(2):469.

Ihrig M, Pyrrolizidinalkaloidhaltige Drogen im Handverkauf? In: PZ 137(40):3128. 1992.

Kraus C et al., (1985) Planta Med 51(2):89.

Miething H, Steinbach RA, Ermittlung der Freisetzungsraten des Pyrrolizidinalkaloids Senkirkin in Huflattich-Teegetränken. In: PZW 135(4):153. 1990.

Paβreiter CM, Co-occurence of 2-pyrrolidineacetic acid with four isomeric tussilaginic acids in Arnica species and Tussilago farfara. In: PM 58(7):A694. 1992.

Röder E et al., (1981) Plant Med 43:99.

Röder E, Pyrrolizidinhaltige Arzneipflanzen. In: DAZ 132(45):2427-2435. 1992.

Wagner H, In: Economic and Medicinal Plant Research, Vol. 1, Academic Press, UK 1985.

Wunderer H, Zentral und peripher wirksame Antitussiva: eine kritische Übersicht. In: PZ 142(11):847-852. 1997.

Further information in:

Frohne D, Pfänder HJ, Giftpflanzen - Ein Handbuch für Apotheker, Toxikologen und Biologen, 4. Aufl., Wiss. Verlagsges. mbH Stuttgart 1997.

Hänsel R, Keller K, Rimpler H, Schneider G (Hrsg.), Hagers Handbuch der Pharmazeutischen Praxis, 5. Aufl., Bde 4-6 (Drogen): Springer Verlag Berlin, Heidelberg, New York, 1992-1994.

Madaus G, Lehrbuch der Biologischen Arzneimittel, Bde 1-3, Nachdruck, Georg Olms Verlag Hildesheim 1979.

Roth L, Daunderer M, Kormann K, Giftpflanzen, Pflanzengifte, 4. Aufl., Ecomed Fachverlag Landsberg Lech 1993.

Steinegger E, Hänsel R, Pharmakognosie, 5. Aufl., Springer Verlag Heidelberg 1992.

Teuscher E, Lindequist U, Biogene Gifte - Biologie, Chemie, Pharmakologie, 2. Aufl., Fischer Verlag Stuttgart 1994.

Teuscher E, Biogene Arzneimittel, 5. Aufl., Wiss. Verlagsges. mbH Stuttgart 1997.

Wichtl M (Hrsg.), Teedrogen, 4. Aufl., Wiss. Verlagsges. Stuttgart 1997.

Ulmus Fulva

Slippery Elm

DESCRIPTION

Medicinal Parts: The medicinal part is the dried inner rind separated from the outer bark.

Flower and Fruit: The flowers are in dense, almost sessile clusters. There are 5 to 9 tepals and the same number of stamens. The stigmas are bright red. The fruit is almost top-shaped to broad-elliptical, 1 to 2 cm long, wide and glabrous, except for the rust-red downy center. The seeds are inserted in the center.

Leaves, Stem and Root: The tree is medium-sized and grows up to 20 m tall with spread branches forming an open crown. The younger branches are red-brown or orange and more or less downy. The bark is deeply fissured. The buds are large, rust-red and downy. The leaves are obovate to oblong, 10 to 20 cm long and have a double-serrate margin. The lamina is long acuminate and sharply asymmetrical at the base. The leaves, are dark green above and very rough, densely downy beneath. They darken in autumn.

Characteristics: The texture is mucilaginous and the odor slight but characteristic. The powdered inner bark is used for its mucilaginous quality. Taken as a drink, it relieves irritation of the mucous membrane. The same water-retaining properties allow the powder to be used as an emollient poultice.

Habitat: The plant is indigenous to North America.

Production: Slippery Elm bark is the inner bark and wood of Ulmus fulva.

Other Names: Red Elm, Sweet Elm

ACTIONS AND PHARMACOLOGY

COMPOUNDS

Mucilage: pentosans, methyl pentosans and one hexosan, yielding mainly D-galactose after hydrolysis

Tannins (very little)

EFFECTS

Slippery Elm is demulcent, emollient and soothing to the alimentary canal.

INDICATIONS AND USAGE

Internally, the drug is used in the treatment of gastritis and gastric or duodenal ulcers. Externally, it is used in the treatment of wounds, burns and skin conditions.

PRECAUTIONS AND ADVERSE REACTIONS

No health hazards or side effects are known in conjunction with the proper administration of designated therapeutic dosages.

DOSAGE

Mode of Administration: Powder for infusions used internally; poultices for external use.

LITERATURE

Hänsel R, Keller K, Rimpler H, Schneider G (Hrsg.), Hagers Handbuch der Pharmazeutischen Praxis, 5. Aufl., Bde 4-6 (Drogen): Springer Verlag Berlin, Heidelberg, New York, 1992-1994.

Ulmus Minor

Elm Bark

DESCRIPTION

Medicinal Parts: The medicinal part is the inner bark of the young branches.

Flower and Fruit: The reddish brown flowers appear before the leaves. They are androgynous, short-pedicled and in globular clusters. The perigone is campanulate-top-shaped and greenish with a purple margin. There are 3 to 4 stamens with dark violet anthers. The tree is wind pollinated. The fruit is a broad-winged, almost circular, oval or elliptical and glabrous achaene. The reddish nutlet reaches to the front margin of the notch.

Leaves, Stem and Root: Ulmus minor is a 40 m high tree with black-brown, finely fissured bark. The branches, which develop long grooves, have alternate, petiolate, 6 to 10 cm long leaves with 8 to 12 lateral ribs. The leaves are ovate. The lamina is irregular and the margin double-serrate. The petioles are 8 to 15 mm longer than the buds, which develop in spring on short branches and form into clusters before flowering.

Habitat: The plant is indigenous to Europe as far as the Mediterranean.

Production: Smooth-leaved Elm bark is the bark of Ulmus minor. The bark is gathered for therapeutic or medicinal purposes. It is manually cut in circles and the bark is removed from the young (new) twigs (the diameter of the twig should not be more than 1 cm). The long grain and the upper layer of the bark must be removed, then the bark is dried.

ACTIONS AND PHARMACOLOGY

COMPOUNDS

Mucilage: yielding mainly D-galactose, L-rhamnose, D-galacturonic acid after hydrolysis

Tannins (3%)

Caffeic acid derivatives: chlorogenic acid

Sterols: including, among others, beta-sitosterol, stigmasterol

EFFECTS

The active agents are tannin and bitter substances, also mucus. The drug has diuretic and astringent properties.

INDICATIONS AND USAGE

Internally, the drug is used for digestive disorders and severe cases of diarrhea. Externally, it is used for ablution of open wounds.

PRECAUTIONS AND ADVERSE REACTIONS

No health hazards or side effects are known in conjunction with the proper administration of designated therapeutic dosages.

DOSAGE

Mode of Administration: Elm bark is used both internally and externally in various preparations.

Preparation: The ground bark is used for infusions. A decoction from the bark can be prepared using 2 teaspoons of the drug per cup of water. Externally, a 20% decoction is used, which is diluted 1:1 with water, for the ablution of festering and open wounds.

Daily Dose: The dosage of the decoction prepared from the bark is 1 cup 2 to 3 times daily. In powder form, a dose of 2 to 5 g may be taken daily.

LITERATURE

Hänsel R, Keller K, Rimpler H, Schneider G (Hrsg.), Hagers Handbuch der Pharmazeutischen Praxis, 5. Aufl., Bde 4-6 (Drogen): Springer Verlag Berlin, Heidelberg, New York, 1992-1994.

Madaus G, Lehrbuch der Biologischen Arzneimittel, Bde 1-3, Nachdruck, Georg Olms Verlag Hildesheim 1979.

Urtica Dioica

Nettle

DESCRIPTION

Medicinal Parts: The medicinal parts are the fresh and dried flowering plant and the roots.

Flower and Fruit: The flowers are greenish-white in axillary, clustered, hanging panicles. The perigone has 4 tepals. There are 4 stamens and 1 ovary with a brush-like stigma. The flowers are dioecious. The male flowers have only stamens and the female flowers only a style or a seed-producing organ. The male flower consists of a perianth of 4 segments, which enclose an even number of stamens. The stamens curve inward in the bud stage and spring back at the end of flowering for the anthers to fling out the pollen. The fruit is a small 1-seeded nutlet.

Leaves, Stem and Root: The plant grows from 60 to 150 cm high and has a winter hard rhizome. The leaves are opposite, oblong-cordate and roughly serrate. The whole plant is covered in stinging hairs.

Habitat: The plant is common in most temperate regions of the world.

Production: Stinging nettle herb consists of the fresh or dried above-ground parts of Urtica dioica, Urtica urens and/or hybrids of these species, collected during flowering season. Stinging nettle leaf consists of fresh or dried leaves of Urtica dioica, Urtica urens and/or hybrids of these species, gathered during flowering season.

Not To Be Confused With: The leaves of Laminum album.

ACTIONS AND PHARMACOLOGY

COMPOUNDS: URTICAE HERBA ET FOLIUM

In the stings of the fresh plant: histamine, serotonin, acetylcholine, formic acid

Flavonoids (0.7-1.8%): including, among others, rutin

Silicic acid (1-4%): partially water-soluble

Volatile oil: chief components are ketones, including, among others, 2-methylhept-2-en-6-on

Potassium-ions (relatively high content)

EFFECTS: URTICAE HERBA ET FOLIUM

The herb has a diuretic effect when taken in combination with sufficient fluid intake.

COMPOUNDS: URTICAE RADIX

Sterols: beta-sitosterol, stigmasterol, campesterol, glucosides of the sterols, stigmast-4-en-3-one

Lectins (0.1%): UDA (Urtica dioica Agglutinin, isolectine mixture)

Water-soluble polysaccharides with immunostimulating effect: glucans, glucogalacturonans, acidic arabino galactans

Hydroxycoumarins: scopoletin

Lignans: including, among others, olivil, secoisolaricinol

Ceramides

EFFECTS: URTICAE RADIX

Increase in the volume of urine, increase of maximum urinary flow, reduction of residual urine.

INDICATIONS AND USAGE

URTICAE HERBA ET FOLIUM

- Infections of the urinary tract
- Kidney and bladder stones

■ Rheumatism

The drug is used internally and externally as supportive therapy for rheumatic ailments. It is used internally as flushing-out therapy for inflammatory diseases of the lower urinary tract. Also used as irrigation therapy for prevention and treatment of kidney gravel.

In folk medicine, the plant is used internally as a hematogenic remedy, diuretic for arthritis, rheumatism of the joints and muscles, and as a component of diabetic teas (this indication is not recommended by doctors). Externally, the drug is used as a hair and scalp remedy against oily hair and dandruff.

URTICAE RADIX

■ Prostate complaints, irritable bladder

Preparations of the root are used for micturition disorders in prostate adenoma stages I to II. This drug only relieves the symptoms of an enlarged prostate without eliminating the enlargement itself.

CONTRAINDICATIONS

URTICAE HERBA ET FOLIUM

The drug is contraindicated when there is fluid retention resulting from reduced cardiac or renal activity.

PRECAUTIONS AND ADVERSE REACTIONS

URTICAE HERBA ET FOLIUM

No health hazards or side effects are known in conjunction with the proper administration of designated therapeutic dosages. Possible allergic reactions (skin afflictions, edemas) have been observed in rare cases following intake of the drug.

URTICAE RADIX

No health hazards are known in conjunction with the proper administration of designated therapeutic dosages. Occasional, mild gastrointestinal complaints may occur as side effects of drug intake.

DOSAGE

URTICAE HERBA ET FOLIUM

Mode of Administration: Comminuted herb for infusions and other galenic preparations for internal use; as stinging nettle spirit for external application. Drug extracts are contained in diuretic tea mixtures and in blood-purifying teas.

Preparation: To prepare an infusion, use 1.5 g finely cut herb in cold water, briefly bring to a boil and steep for 10 minutes, then strain.

Daily Dose: The average daily dose is 8 to 12 g of drug. Observe ample intake of liquid (minimum 2 liters/day). One cup several times daily as a diuretic (1 teaspoonful = 0.8 g drug). For external application, a tincture/spiritus (1:10) may be administered.

URTICAE RADIX

Mode of Administration: Comminuted drug from the root for infusions as well as other galenic preparations for oral use.

Preparation: To prepare an infusion use 1.5 g coarse powdered drug in cold water, heat to boiling point for 1 minute, then steep, covered, for 10 minutes, and strain. (1 teaspoonful = 1.3 g drug)

Daily Dose: 4 to 6 g drug.

LITERATURE

URTICAE HERBA ET FOLIUM

Anonym (1982) Vet Hum Toxicol 24:247.

Chaurasia N, Wichtl M, PM 53:432. 1987.

Hughes RE et al., (1980) J Sci Food Agric 31:1279.

Schiebel-Schlosser G, Die Brennessel. In: PTA 8(1):53. 1994.

Schilcher H, Urtica-Arten - Die Brennessel. In: ZPT 9(5):160. 1988.

Schomakers J, Bollbach FD Hagels H, Brennesselkraut - Phytochemische und anatomische Unterscheidung der Herba-Drogen von Urtica dioica und U. urens. In: DAZ 135(7):578-584. 1995.

Further information in:

Frohne D, Pfänder HJ, Giftpflanzen - Ein Handbuch für Apotheker, Toxikologen und Biologen, 4. Aufl., Wiss. Verlags-Ges. Stuttgart 1997.

Kern W, List PH, Hörhammer L (Hrsg.), Hagers Handbuch der Pharmazeutischen Praxis, 4. Aufl., Bde 1-8: Springer Verlag Berlin, Heidelberg, New York, 1969.

Lewin L, Gifte und Vergiftungen, 6. Aufl., Nachdruck, Haug Verlag, Heidelberg 1992.

Madaus G, Lehrbuch der Biologischen Arzneimittel, Bde 1-3, Nachdruck, Georg Olms Verlag Hildesheim 1979.

Roth L, Daunderer M, Kormann K, Giftpflanzen, Pflanzengifte, 4. Aufl., Ecomed Fachverlag Landsberg Lech 1993.

Steinegger E, Hänsel R, Pharmakognosie, 5. Aufl., Springer Verlag Heidelberg 1992.

Teuscher E, Lindequist U, Biogene Gifte - Biologie, Chemie, Pharmakologie, 2. Aufl., Fischer Verlag Stuttgart 1994.

Teuscher E, Biogene Arzneimittel, 5. Aufl., Wiss. Verlagsges. Stuttgart 1997.

Wagner H, Wiesenauer M, Phytotherapie. Phytopharmaka und pflanzliche Homöopathika, Fischer-Verlag, Stuttgart, Jena, New York 1995.

Wichtl M (Hrsg.), Teedrogen, 4. Aufl., Wiss. Verlagsges. Stuttgart 1997.

URTICAE RADIX

Anonym (1982) Vet Hum Toxicol 24:247.

Anonym, Extrakt aus Brennesselwurzel wirksam bei benigner Prostatahyperplasie. In: ZPT 12(5):8. 1991.

Anonym, Phytotherapie: Pflanzliche Antirheumatika - was bringen sie? In: DAZ 136(45):4012-4015. 1996.

Anonym, Welche Bedeutung haben pflanzliche Prostatamittel. In: DAZ 133(9):720. 1993.

Dathe G, Schmid H, (1987) Phytotherapie der benignen Prostatahyperplasie (BPH). Doppelblindstudie mit Extraktum Radicis Uricae (ERU). Urologe [B]27:223-226.

Fessler B, Brennesselwurzel bei Prostataadenom. In: Med Mo Pharm 16(9):287. 1993.

Ganβer D, Spiteller G, Aromatase inhibitors from Urtica dioica. In: PM 61(2):138-140. 1995.

Goetz P, Die Behandlung der benignen Prostatahyperplasie mit Brennesselwurzeln. In: ZPT 10(6):175. 1990.

Hirano T et al., Effect of stinging nettle root extract and their steroidal components on the Na+,K+-ATPase of the benign prostic hyperplasia. In: PM 60:30. 1994.

Hryb DJ, Khan MS, Romas NA, Rosner W, (1995) The Effect of Extracts of the Roots of the Stinging Nettle (Urtica dioica) on the Interaction of SHBG with ist Receptor on Human Prostatic Membranes. Planta Med 61:31-32.

Huesing JE, Murdock LL, Shade RE, Rice and stinging nettle lectins - insecticidal activity similar to wheat germ agglutinin. In: PH 30:3565. 1991.

Hughes RE et al., (1980) J Sci Food Agric 31:1279.

Koch E, (1995) Pharmakologie und Wirkmechanismen von Extrakten aus Sabalfrüchten (Sabal fructus): Brennesselwurzeln (Urticae radix) und Kürbissamen (Cucurbitae peponis semen) bei der Behandlung der benignen Prostatahyperplasie. In: Loew D, Rietbrock N (Hrsg.) Phytopharmaka in Forschung und klinischer Anwendung. Steinkopff Verlag, Darmstadt, S 57-79.

Lauel H, Extrakt aus Radix Urticae normalisiert Hormonhaushalt. In: DAZ 130(51/52):2789. 1990.

Lichius JJ et al., Inhibition of experimentally induced mouse prostatic hyperplasia by methanolic extracts of Urtica dioica roots. In: PM 61(Abstracts of 43rd Ann Congr):89. 1995.

Lichius JJ, Muth C, A new biological evaluation of Urtica dioica root-extracts. In: PM 62, Abstracts of the 44th Ann Congress of GA, 20. 1996.

Miersch WDE, Benigne Prostatahyperplasie. In: DAZ 133(29):2653. 1993.

Nahrstedt A (1993) Pflanzliche Urologica - eine kritische Übersicht. Pharm Z 138: 1439-1450.

Nöske HD (1994) Die Effektivität pflanzlicher Prostatamittel am Beispiel von Brennesselwurzelextrakt. ÄrzteZ Naturheilverfahren 35 (1):18-27.

Sabo A et al., Radix Urticae (Urtica dioica): Influence on erythrocyte deformability and enzymes. In: PM 62, Abstracts of the 44th Ann Congress of GA, 60. 1996.

Schiebel-Schlosser G, Die Brennessel. In: PTA 8(1):53. 1994.

Schilcher H (1987a) Pflanzliche Diuretika. Urologe [B]27:215-222; (1987b) Möglichkeiten und Grenzen der Phytotherapie am Beispiel pflanzlicher Urologika. Urologe [B]27:316-319.

Schilcher H, Boesel R, Effenberger ST Segebrecht S, Neuere Untersuchungsergebnisse mit aquaretisch, antibakteriell und prostatotrop wirksamen Arzneipflanzen. In: ZPT 10(3):77. 1989.

Schilcher H, Urtica-Arten - Die Brennessel. In: ZPT 9(5):160. 1988.

Schmidt K (1983) Die Wirkung eines Radix Urticae-Extrakts und einzelner Nebenextrakte auf das SHBG des Blutplasmas bei der benignen Prostatahyperplasie. Fortschr Med 101:713-716.

Schmidt K (1983) Die Wirkung eines Radix Urticae-Extrakts und einzelner Nebenextrakte auf das SHGB des Blutplasmas bei der benignen Prostatahyperplasie. Fortschr Med 101:713-716.

Sonnenschein R (1987) Untersuchung der Wirksamkeit eines prostatotropen Phytotherapeutikums (Urtica plus) bei benigner Prostatahyperplasie und Prostatitis - eine prospektive multizentrische Studie. Urologe [B]27:232-237.

Wagner H et al., Studies on the binding of Urtica dioica agglutinin (UDA) and other lectins in an in vitro epidermal growth factor receptor test. In: Phytomedicine 1:287-290. 1994.

Wagner H, Willer F, Samtleben R, Boos G (1994) Search for the antiprostatic principle of stinging nettle (Urtica dioica) roots. Phytomedicine 1:213-224.

Willer F, Wagner H, Schecklies E, Urtica-Wurzelextrakte. In: DAZ 131(24):1217. 1991.

Further information in:

Madaus G, Lehrbuch der Biologischen Arzneimittel, Bde 1-3, Nachdruck, Georg Olms Verlag Hildesheim 1979.

Schulz R, Hänsel R, Rationale Phytotherapie, Springer Verlag Heidelberg 1996.

Steinegger E, Hänsel R, Pharmakognosie, 5. Aufl., Springer Verlag Heidelberg 1992.

Teuscher E, Biogene Arzneimittel, 5. Aufl., Wiss. Verlagsges. Stuttgart 1997.

Wichtl M (Hrsg.), Teedrogen, 4. Aufl., Wiss. Verlagsges. Stuttgart 1997.

Usnea Species

Usnea

DESCRIPTION

Medicinal Parts: Research into this species is not yet complete, making it difficult to establish which lichens are used for the extraction of which drug, and which lichens have been described by earlier botanists.

Flower and Fruit: Mycelia, compare with Cetraria. Flourishes on a variety of trees (on the trunk, branches branchlets) as a whitish, reddish, or black lichen.

Habitat: Usnea is found worldwide in cool, damp places.

Production: Usnea consists of the dried thallus of Usnea species, primarily of Usnea barbata, Usnea florida, Usnea hirta and Usnea plicata.

Other Names: Tree Moss, Old Man's Beard, Beard Moss

ACTIONS AND PHARMACOLOGY

COMPOUNDS

Llichen acids (polyketides): including among others (+)-usnic acid, thamnolic acid, lobaric acid, stictinic acid, evernic acid, barbatic acid, diffractaic acid, protocetraric acid, the lichen acid spectrums of the different species vary from one another.

Mucilage

EFFECTS

Antimicrobial.

INDICATIONS AND USAGE

■ Inflammation of the mouth and pharynx

The species are used for mild inflammation of the oral and pharyngeal mucosa.

PRECAUTIONS AND ADVERSE REACTIONS

No health hazards or side effects are known in conjunction with the proper administration of designated therapeutic dosages. Following overdosage, signs of poisoning could appear. These signs have yet to be described.

DOSAGE

Mode of Administration: Preparations for lozenges and equivalent solid forms of medication.

Daily Dose: Lozenges with preparations equivalent to 100 mg herb, One lozenge 3 to 6 times daily.

LITERATURE

Okuyama E et al., Usnic acid and diffractic acid as analgesic and antipyretic components of Usnea diffracta. In: PM 61(2):113-115. 1995.

Further information in:

Kern W, List PH, Hörhammer L (Hrsg.), Hagers Handbuch der Pharmazeutischen Praxis, 4. Aufl., Bde 1-8: Springer Verlag Berlin, Heidelberg, New York, 1969.

Roth L, Daunderer M, Kormann K, Giftpflanzen, Pflanzengifte, 4. Aufl., Ecomed Fachverlag Landsberg Lech 1993.

Steinegger E, Hänsel R, Pharmakognosie, 5. Aufl., Springer Verlag Heidelberg 1992.

Utricularia Vulgaris

Bladderwort

DESCRIPTION

Medicinal Parts: The medicinal part is the whole plant.

Flower and Fruit: The vertical peduncle is 10 to 35 cm high and bears 4 to 15 flowers in a loose raceme. The petioles are short and campanulate, 13 to 20 mm long and have a bilabiate margin.

Leaves, Stem and Root: Utricularia vulgaris is water plant, which appears at flowering time. The water shoot is 60 cm long with double-rowed leaves facing all directions. The water leaves are 1 to 8 cm long and have 2 to 3 large lobes. Each lobe is pinnatifid and ends in numerous tips. There are 8 to 209 tubes per leaf.

Habitat: Europe.

Production: Bladderwort is the whole plant of Utricularia vulgaris.

ACTIONS AND PHARMACOLOGY

COMPOUNDS

Iridoide monoterpenes: including, among others, globularin, scutellarioside II- phenylpropane derivatives: 1-p-cumaroyl-glucosides

EFFECTS

The active agents are flavonoid, cumarin and zyanidine (cyanidine). The plant has diuretic, antispasmodic and anti-inflammatory effects.

INDICATIONS AND USAGE

Formerly used internally in the treatment of urinary tract disorders and externally for burns. The active substances increase the gallbladder secretions, consequently, Bladderwort is for use against skin and mucous membrane inflammation.

PRECAUTIONS AND ADVERSE REACTIONS

No health hazards or side effects are known in conjunction with the proper administration of designated therapeutic dosages.

DOSAGE

Mode of Administration: The drug is obsolete in many parts of Germany. Bladderwort is used internally and externally in other parts of the world.

Preparation: To prepare a diuretic infusion for internal use, add 2 gm of the drug per 100 ml of water. To prepare an anti-inflammatory infusion for external use, add 6 gm of the drug per 100 ml of water.

Daily Dosage: Internally, as a diuretic infusion, drink two small cups daily. Externally, the anti-inflammatory infusion is used in mouthwashes, cleansers, cosmetic and medical packs.

LITERATURE

Hegnauer R, Chemotaxonomie der Pflanzen, Bde 1-11: Birkhäuser Verlag Basel, Boston, Berlin 1962-1997.

Uva-Ursi

See Arctostaphylos Uva-Ursi

Uzara

See Xysmalobium Undulatum

Vaccinium Myrtillus

Bilberry

DESCRIPTION

Medicinal Parts: The medicinal parts are the dried leaves, the ripe, dried fruit and the ripe fresh fruit.

Flower and Fruit: The flowers are axillary and solitary. They are 4 to 7 mm long, short-pedicled, greenish and tinged with pale pink. The calyx is fused to the ovary, persistent and indistinctly 5-lobed. The corolla is globular-jug-shaped and has 5 tips. There are 8 to 10 stamens, which are enclosed and shorter than the styles. They have glabrous filaments, which widen toward the base and 2 horn-like yellow-brown anthers, whose spurred appendage is erect. The fruit is a globular, blue-black, frosted, many-seeded berry with purple pulp.

Leaves, Stem and Root: The plant is a deciduous, dwarf shrub with sharp-edged, green branches 15 to 50 cm high. The leaves are alternate, ovate or oblong-ovate, acuminate and finely serrate.

Habitat: The plant is common to central and northern Europe, Asia and North America.

Not To Be Confused With: Myrtilli folium should not be confused with the fruits of Vaccinium uliginosum.

Other Names: Whortleberry, Blueberry, Burren myrtle, Dyeberry, Huckleberry, Hurtleberry, Wineberry, Black Whortles, Hurts, Bleaberry, Airelle, Trackleberry

ACTIONS AND PHARMACOLOGY

COMPOUNDS: MYRTILLI FOLIUM

Catechin tannins (up to 20%)

Oligomeric procyanidines

Flavonoids: including, among others, avicularin, hyperoside, isoquercitrin, quercitrin, meratine, astragaline

Iridoide monoterpenes: asperuloside, monotropein

Caffeic acid derivatives: chlorogenic acid

Phenolic acids: including, among others, salicylic acid, gentisic acid

Quinolizidine alkaloids: myrtine, epimyrtine (hybrids of Vaccinium myrtillus x V. vitis-idaea contain arbutin [hydroquine glucosides]).

EFFECTS: MYRTILLI FOLIUM

The chromium content of the drug is thought to be responsible for the antidiabetic effect.

COMPOUNDS: MYRTILLI FRUCTUS

Fruit acids: including, among others, quinic acid (3-5%), malic acid, citric acid

Tannins (5-12%, chiefly catechin tannins)

Oligomeric procyanidines

Anthocyans: chief components delphinidine-3-O-arabinoside, delphinidine-3-O-galactoside, delphinidine-3-O-glucoside

Flavonoids: including, among others, hyperoside, isoquercitrin, quercitrin, astragaline

Caffeic acid derivatives: chlorogenic acid

Pectins

EFFECTS: MYRTILLI FRUCTUS

Astringent and antidiarrheal

INDICATIONS AND USAGE

MYRTILLI FOLIUM

Bilberry has been used in Diabetes Mellitus (for prevention and treatment); complaints of the gastrointestinal tract, kidney and urinary tract, arthritis, gout and dermatitis. The drug is infrequently used as an astringent in rinses and lavages.

MYRTILLI FRUCTUS

- Diarrhea
- Inflammation of the mouth and pharynx

Internally, Bilberry is used for nonspecific, acute diarrhea (particularly in light cases of enteritis). Externally the berry is used for mild inflammation of the mucous membranes of mouth and throat.

PRECAUTIONS AND ADVERSE REACTIONS

MYRTILLI FOLIUM

No health hazards or side effects are known in conjunction with the proper administration of designated therapeutic dosages. Digestive complaints due to the high tannin content are not to be ruled out.

MYRTILLI FRUCTUS

No health hazards or side effects are known in conjunction with the proper administration of designated therapeutic dosages.

OVERDOSAGE

MYRTILLI FOLIUM

The signs of poisoning observed in animal experiments (including, among others, cachexia, anemia, icterus) appeared only in conjunction with the chronic administration of high dosages and are presumably effects of the tannins, that could also be realized with any other tanning agent.

DOSAGE

MYRTILLI FOLIUM

Preparation: To prepare an infusion, pour boiling water over 1 g finely cut drug (1 teaspoonful = approximately 0.6g) and strain after 10 to 15 minutes. Not to be taken over a long duration.

MYRTILLI FRICTUS

Mode of Administration: Macerated drug for infusions, as well as other galenic preparations for internal use and local application.

Preparation: To prepare an infusion, use 5 to 10 g mashed drug in cold water which is brought to a simmer for 10 minutes, then strained (1 teaspoonful = 4 g drug). A 10% decoction is prepared for external use.

Daily Dose: 20 to 60 g.

LITERATURE

MYRTILLI FOLIUM

Bettini V et al., (1984) Fitoterapia 55(6):323.

Bettini V et al., (1985) Fitoterapia 56(1):3.

Bomser J et al., In vitro anticancer activity of fruit extracts from Vaccinium species. In: PM 62(3):212-216. 1996.

Bosio E et al., Ginkgo biloba L. and Vaccinium myrtillus L. extracts prevent photo-induced oxidation of low density lipoproteins. In: PM 62, Abstracts of the 44th Ann Congress of GA, 24. 1996.

Cignarella A, Bertozzi D, Pinna C, Puglisi L, Hypolipidemic activity of Vaccinium myrtillus leaves on an model of genetically hyperlipidemic rat. In: PM 58(Suppl. 7):A581. 1992.

Frohne D, Vaccinium myrtillus L.- Die Heidelbeere. In: ZPT 11(6):209-211. 1999.

Kyerematen G, Sandberg F, (1986) Acta Pharm Suec. 23:101.

Sticher O et al., (1979) Planta Med 35:253.

Further information in:

Hänsel R, Keller K, Rimpler H, Schneider G (Hrsg.), Hagers Handbuch der Pharmazeutischen Praxis, 5. Aufl., Bde 4-6 (Drogen): Springer Verlag Berlin, Heidelberg, New York, 1992-1994.

Madaus G, Lehrbuch der Biologischen Arzneimittel, Bde 1-3, Nachdruck, Georg Olms Verlag Hildesheim 1979.

Roth L, Daunderer M, Kormann K, Giftpflanzen, Pflanzengifte, 4. Aufl., Ecomed Fachverlag Landsberg Lech 1993.

Teuscher E, Biogene Arzneimittel, 5. Aufl., Wiss. Verlagsges. Stuttgart 1997.

Wichtl M (Hrsg.), Teedrogen, 4. Aufl., Wiss. Verlagsges. Stuttgart 1997.

MYRTILLI FRUCTUS

Bettini V et al., (1984) Fitoterapia 55(6):323.

Bettini V et al., (1985) Fitoterapia 56(1):3.

Bomser J et al., In vitro anticancer activity of fruit extracts from Vaccinium species. In: PM 62(3):212-216. 1996.

Bosio E et al., Ginkgo biloba L. and Vaccinium myrtillus L. extracts prevent photo-induced oxidation of low density lipoproteins. In: PM 62, Abstracts of the 44th Ann Congress of GA, 24. 1996.

Cignarella A, Bertozzi D, Pinna C, Puglisi L, Hypolipidemic activity of Vaccinium myrtillus leaves on an model of genetically hyperlipidemic rat. In: PM 58(Suppl. 7):A581. 1992.

Frohne D, Vaccinium myrtillus L.- Die Heidelbeere. In: ZPT 11(6):209-211. 1999.

Kyerematen G, Sandberg F, (1986) Acta Pharm Suec 23:101.

Sticher O et al., (1979) Planta Med 35:253.

Further information in:

Hänsel R, Keller K, Rimpler H, Schneider G (Hrsg.), Hagers Handbuch der Pharmazeutischen Praxis, 5. Aufl., Bde 4-6 (Drogen), Springer Verlag Berlin, Heidelberg, New York, 1992-1994.

Madaus G, Lehrbuch der Biologischen Arzneimittel, Bde 1-3, Nachdruck, Georg Olms Verlag Hildesheim 1979.

Roth L, Daunderer M, Kormann K, Giftpflanzen, Pflanzengifte, 4. Aufl., Ecomed Fachverlag Landsberg Lech 1993.

Steinegger E, Hänsel R, Pharmakognosie, 5. Aufl., Springer Verlag Heidelberg 1992.

Teuscher E, Biogene Arzneimittel, 5. Aufl., Wiss. Verlagsges. Stuttgart 1997.

Wichtl M (Hrsg.), Teedrogen, 4. Aufl., Wiss. Verlagsges. Stuttgart 1997.

Vaccinium Uliginosum

Bog Bilberry

DESCRIPTION

Medicinal Parts: The medicinal part is the dried ripe fruit.

Flower and Fruit: The flowers are arranged in axils of small leaves at the end of short lateral branches. They are hanging and white or reddish in color. The pedicle is encircled at the base with a light brown bud husk. The calyx is fused with the ovary. The fruit is a round or pear-shaped, blue-frosted, 7 to 10 cm long, multi-seeded berry. The light brown seeds are sickle-shaped, with sharp ends and have a punctate-reticulate skin.

Leaves, Stem and Root: The plant is an angular shrub up to 80 cm high with round, gray-brown, glabrous branches and a creeping rhizome. The leaves are deciduous, obovate or oblong, entire, tough and short-petioled. The under surface has a protruding, reticulate vein system and is blue-green. The upper surface of the leaves is light matte-green to almost white.

Habitat: The plant is common throughout the Northern Hemisphere.

Production: Bog Billberries and leaves are the ripe fruit and leaves of Vaccinum uliginosum. The collection or picking occurs in uncultivated regions. The drug is either air-dried in the shade or by a means of artificial warmth.

Not To Be Confused With: The Bog Bilberry has smaller flowers and berries than the Common Bilberry. (See Vaccinium myrtillus)

ACTIONS AND PHARMACOLOGY

COMPOUNDS: IN THE LEAVES

Tannins: condensed tannins

Triterpenes: alpha-amyrin, friedelin, ursolic acid

Sterols: beta-sitosterol, beta-sitosterol-glucosides

Flavonoids: including, among others, hyperoside

COMPOUNDS: IN THE FRUITS

Anthocyans: including, among others, chief components: malvidin-3-O-glucosides, delphinidine-3-O-glucosides, delphinidine-3-O-arabinoside

Organic acids: including, among others, benzoic acid

Flavonoids: including, among others, hyperoside

EFFECTS

Active agents are tannins, anthocyanoside and flavonoids.

INDICATIONS AND USAGE

For gastric and intestinal catarrh, diarrhea and bladder complaints.

PRECAUTIONS AND ADVERSE REACTIONS

No health hazards or side effects are known in conjunction with the proper administration of designated therapeutic dosages.

OVERDOSAGE

Signs of poisoning following consumption of large quantities of the fruits have arisen very rarely. Signs of poisoning include queasiness, vomiting, states of intoxication, feelings of weakness, visual disorders. Presumably these poisonings are to be traced back to the plant being infested with the lower fungus Sclerotinia megalospora.

DOSAGE

Mode of Administration: The drug is used internally as a liquid extract (tea).

Preparation: To prepare a tea, 2 heaping teaspoons are infused with 250 ml of cold water, leave this to stand and weaken for 10 to 12 hours.

Daily Dosage: Drink 1 cup of the prepared tea, unsweetened, once or twice a day.

LITERATURE

Teuscher E, Lindequist U, Giftstoffe mikrobieller Endo- und Epiphyten. Gefahren für Mensch und Tier. In: DAZ 132(42):2231. 1992.

Further information in:

Frohne D, Pfänder HJ, Giftpflanzen - Ein Handbuch für Apotheker, Toxikologen und Biologen, 4. Aufl., Wiss. Verlags-Ges. Stuttgart 1997.

Hänsel R, Keller K, Rimpler H, Schneider G (Hrsg.), Hagers Handbuch der Pharmazeutischen Praxis, 5. Aufl., Bde 4-6 (Drogen): Springer Verlag Berlin, Heidelberg, New York, 1992-1994.

Lewin L, Gifte und Vergiftungen, 6. Aufl., Nachdruck, Haug Verlag, Heidelberg 1992.

Roth L, Daunderer M, Kormann K, Giftpflanzen, Pflanzengifte, 4. Aufl., Ecomed Fachverlag Landsberg Lech 1993.

Vaccinium Vitis-Idaea

Alpine Cranberry

DESCRIPTION

Medicinal Parts: The medicinal parts are the dried leaves and the ripe dried fruit.

Flower and Fruit: The white to reddish-tinged flowers are in cluster of various sizes. The 10 stamens are pubescent at the base and the anthers are two-tipped and have no appendage. The initially white berries turn scarlet and contain numerous rust-brown seeds that are 1.5 to 2 mm long.

Leaves, Stem and Root: The plant is a low shrub up to 30 cm high with scaly underground runners. The shoots sprout from the axillary buds of the runners. The sprouts are downy when young and later glabrous. The leaves are alternate, short-petioled, obovate and coriaceous. The upper surface is dark green and the under surface pale green and covered in glandular hairs.

Habitat: The plant is common in the Northern Hemisphere.

Production: Cranberry leaves are the foliage leaves of Vaccinium vitis-ideae. Collection takes place in uncultivated regions (Scandinavia, England). The leaves are dried in the open air.

Other Names: Cowberry, Red Bilberry, Whortleberry

ACTIONS AND PHARMACOLOGY

COMPOUNDS

Hydroquinone glycosides: arbutin (3-5%), pyroside (6′-acetyl-arbutin), hydroquinone gentiobioside, 2-O-caffeoyl arbutin

Tannins (10-20%): chiefly condensed tannins, proanthocyainidine

Flavonoids: including, among others, avicularin, hyperoside, quercitrin, isoquercitrin

Triterpenes: including, among others, beta-amyrin, oleanolic acid, ursolic acid

EFFECTS

Increase in cyclooxigenase-activity, antiviral effect, disinfection of urinary tract. Contains tannin and tannin substances from the preliminary stage.

Toxic effect is possible, the content level of arbutin and hydrochinon (mutagenic and carcinogenic effect); long term use is inadvisable.

INDICATIONS AND USAGE

Urinary tract irritation, gout, rheumatism and calculus (stone complaints).

As a substitute for bearberry leaves.

CONTRAINDICATIONS

The drug is contraindicated in pregnancy, nursing, and in children under 12 years of age.

PRECAUTIONS AND ADVERSE REACTIONS

No health hazards are known in conjunction with the proper administration of designated therapeutic dosages. Individuals with gastric sensitivity may experience queasiness and vomiting following intake of preparations made from the drug with high tannin content. Liver damage is conceivable in connection with administration of the drug over extended periods, particularly with children, due to the possible hepatotoxicity of the hydroquinones released.

Because the urine-disinfecting effect of the hydroquinones released in the urinary tract only occurs in an alkali environment, the simultaneous administration of medication and food that increases uric acid concentration in the bladder is to be avoided.

DOSAGE

Mode of Administration: As a cold maceration or tea infusion.

Daily Dose: The internal dose is 2 g as a single dose; as a decoction, the concentration is 2 g per cup.

LITERATURE

Friedrich H, Naturwissenschaften 48:304. 1961.

Sticher O et al., PM 35:253. 1979.

Thieme H et al., PA 24:236. 1969.

Thieme H, Winkler HJ, PA 21:182. 1966.

Thompson RS et al., J Chem Soc Perkin Tarns I:1387. 1972.

Further information in:

Frohne D, Pfänder HJ, Giftpflanzen - Ein Handbuch für Apotheker, Toxikologen und Biologen, 4. Aufl., Wiss. Verlags-Ges. Stuttgart 1997.

Hänsel R, Keller K, Rimpler H, Schneider G (Hrsg.), Hagers Handbuch der Pharmazeutischen Praxis, 5. Aufl., Bde 4-6 (Drogen): Springer Verlag Berlin, Heidelberg, New York, 1992-1994.

Teuscher E, Biogene Arzneimittel, 5. Aufl., Wiss. Verlagsges. Stuttgart 1997.

Valerian

See Valeriana Officinalis

Valeriana Officinalis

Valerian

DESCRIPTION

Medicinal Parts: The medicinal parts are the carefully dried underground parts and the dried roots.

Flower and Fruit: The androgynous, bright, pink-to-white flowers are in panicled cymes. The calyx consists of 10 revolute tips. The corolla is funnel-shaped with a 5-sectioned margin. The tube has a bump at the base. There are 3 stamens. The ovary is inferior and has 3 chambers. The fruit is ovate-oblong, yellow, indehiscent and has a 10-rayed tuft of white hair.

Leaves, Stem and Root: The plant is 50 to 100 cm high and has a short, cylindrical rhizome with finger-length, bushy round roots. The stem is erect and unbranched. The leaves are odd-pinnate with 11 to 23 lanceolate, indented-dentate leaflets. The lower ones are petiolate and the upper ones sessile and clasping with a white sheath.

Characteristics: The flowers are fragrant and the rhizome smells strongly when dried.

Habitat: The plant is found in Europe and in the temperate regions of Asia. It is cultivated mainly in central Europe, England, France, eastern Europe, Japan and the U.S.

Production: Valerian root, consisting of fresh underground plant parts, or parts carefully dried below 40°C of the species Valeriana officinalis. Cultivation is possible in low-lying, sandy, humus soil well supplied with lime and situated in a damp area. The root is harvested in September. The fresh roots are washed, chopped, and carefully dried in circulating air under 40°C.

Not To Be Confused With: This seldom occurs as the drug comes mostly from cultivation. The most dangerous addition to the drug are the roots of Veratrum album.

Other Names: All-heal, Amantilla, Setwall, Setewale, Capon's Tail, Heliotrope, Vandal Root

ACTIONS AND PHARMACOLOGY

COMPOUNDS

Valepotriates (valeriana-epoxy-triacylates, iridoide monoterpenes, 0.2-2.0%): chief components (50-80%) , isovaltrate (up to 46%), isovaleroxyhydroxy didrovaltrate (IVDH-valtrate, 10-20%), including, among others, didrovaltrate, acevaltrate

Volatile oil (0.2-1.0%): chief components (-)-bornyl isovalerenate and isovalerenic acid (both aroma-carriers), including, among others, (-)-bornyl acetate, isoeugenyl valerenate, isoeugenyl isovalerenate, also with some strains valerenal, valeranone, cryptofaurinol

Sesquiterpenes: valerenic acid (0.1-0.9%), 2-hydroxyvalerenic acid, 2-acetoxy-valerenic acid

Pyridine alkaloids (traces, cat pheromone): actinidine, valerianine, alpha-methylpyrrylketone

Caffeic acid derivatives: chlorogenic acid.

The subspecies within the collective species differ in their constituent substances spectra.

EFFECTS

Sedative, sleep promoting, spasmolytic, muscle relaxant.

INDICATIONS AND USAGE

■ Nervousness and insomnia

Valerian is used for restlessness, sleeping disorders based on nervous conditions, mental strain, lack of concentration, excitability, stress, headache, neurasthenia, epilepsy, hysteria, nervous cardiopathy, menstrual states of agitation, pregnancy, menopause, neuralgia, fainting, nervous stomach cramps, colic, uterine spasticity, states of angst and tonicity.

PRECAUTIONS AND ADVERSE REACTIONS

No health hazards are known in conjunction with the proper administration of designated therapeutic dosages. Gastrointestinal complaints can occur in rare cases, contact allergies in very rare ones.

With long-term administration, the following can occasionally appear: headache, restless states, sleeplessness, mydriasis, disorders of cardiac function.

Where large skin injuries or acute skin illnesses, severe feverish or infectious diseases, cardiac insufficiency or hypertonia are present, entire-body baths with the addition of the volatile oil or of extracts from the drug should be carried out only following consultation with a doctor.

DOSAGE

Mode of Administration: Valerian is used internally as expressed juice from fresh plants, tincture, extracts, and other galenic preparations. Externally, it is used as a bath additive, though efficacy is unproven for this indication.

Preparation: To prepare an infusion, use 2 to 3 g of drug per cup. A tea is prepared by adding 1 teaspoonful (3 to 5 g) of drug to 150 ml of hot water and strain after 10 to 15 minutes. For external use, 100 g of comminuted drug is mixed with 2 liters hot water; this is then added to the bath.

Daily Dose: Total internal daily dose is 15 g drug.

Infusion: One cup one to several times per day

Tea: One cup (150 ml) 2 to 3 times daily and before bedtime.

Tincture: 1/2 to 1 teaspoonful (1 to 3 ml) one to several times per day.

Tincture (1:5): several times daily 15 to 20 drops in water.

Extract: equivalent 2 to 3 g drug, one to several times per day.

Plant juice: Adults take 1 tablespoonful 3 times daily. Children take 1 teaspoonful 3 times daily.

External use: As a bath according to preparation instructions above.

Storage: Must be kept from sources of light; tinctures and extracts must be stored in tightly closed containers.

LITERATURE

Anonym, Phytotherapeutika: Nachgewiesene Wirkung, aber wirksame Stoffe meist nicht bekannt. In: DAZ 137(15):1221-1222. 1997.

Becker H et al., (1983) Planta Med 49(1):64.

Bodesheim U, Hölzl J, Isolation and receptor binding properties of alkaloids and lignans from Valeriana officinalis L. In: PA 52(5):386-391. 1997.

Bos R et al., (1983) Phytochemistry 22 (6):1505.

Bos R et al., Seasonal variation of the essential oil, valerenic acid derivatives, and valepotriates in Valeriana officinalis roots. In: PM 59(7):A698. 1993.

Bounthanh C et al., (1981) Planta Med 41:21.

Bounthanh C et al., (1983) Planta Med 49:138.

Bounthanh C, Bergmann C, Beck JP, Haag-Berrurier M, Anton R (1981) Valepotriates, a new class of cytotoxic, antitumor agents. Planta Med 41:21-28.

Braun R et al., (1982) Dtsch Apoth Ztg 122:1109.

Braun R et al., (1984) Planta Med 1.

Braun R, Dittmar W, Machut M, Weickmann S, (1982) Valepotriate mit Epoxidstruktur - beachtliche Alkylantien. Dtsch Apoth Z 122:1109-1113.

Braun R, Dittmar W, von der Hude W, Scheutwinkel-Reich M, (1985) Bacterial mutagenicity of the tranquilizing constituents of valerianaceae roots. Naunyn- Schmiedeberg's Arch Pharmacol Suppl 329:R28.

Donath F, Roots I, (1995) Untersuchung zur Erfassung der Wirkung von Baldrianextrakt (LI 156) auf das Pharmako-EEG bei 16 Probanden. Z Phytother Abstractband, S. 10.

Eickstedt KW von, (1969) Arzneim Forsch 19:995.

Eickstedt KW von, Rahmann R, (1969) Psychopharmakologische Wirkungen von Valepotriaten. Arzneim-Forsch 19:316-319.

Funk ED, Friedrich H, (1975) Planta Med 28:215.

Gross D et al., (1971) Arch Pharm 304:19.

Grusla D, (1987) Nachweis der Wirkung eines Baldrianextraktes im Rattenhirn mit der 14C-2-Desoxyglucose-Technik. Dissertation, Phillipps-Universität, Marburg.

Hänsel R, (1984) Bewertung von Baldrian-Präparaten: Differenzierung wesentlich: Dtsch Apoth Z 124:2085.

Hänsel R, Pflanzliche Beruhigungsmittel Möglichkeiten und Grenzen der Selbstmedikation. In: DAZ 135(32):2935-2943. 1995.

Hänsel R, Pflanzliche Sedativa. In: ZPT 11(1):14. 1990.

Hänsel R, Schultz J, (1982) Dtsch Apoth Ztg 122(5):215.

Hänsel R, Schulz J, (1982) Valerensäuren und Valerenal als Leitstoffe des offizinellen Baldrians. Dtsch Apoth Z 122:215-219.

Hänsel R, Schulz J, (1985) Beitrag zur Qulaitätssicherung von Baldrianextrakten. Pharm Industrie 47:531-533.

Hardy M, Kirk-Smith MD, Stretch DD (1995) Replacement of drug treatment for insomnia by ambient odour. Lancet 346:701.

Hazelhoff B, (1984) Phytochemical, Pharmacological Aspects of Valeriana compounds. Dissertation, Universität Groningen.

Hazelhoff B et al., (1979) Pharm Weekbl Sci Ed. 1:71.

Hendricks H, Bruins AB, (1980) J Chromatogr 190:321.

Hendricks R et al., (1977) Phytochemistry 16:1853.

Hendriks H et al., (1981) Planta Med 42(1):62.

Hendriks H et al., (1985) Planta Med (3):28.

Hendriks H, Bos R, Woerdenbag HJ, Koster AS, (1985) Central Nervous Depressant Activity of Valerenic Acid in the Mouse. Planta Med 51:28-31.

Hiller KO, Zetler G, (1996) Neuropharmacological Studies on Ethanol Extracts of Valeriana officinalis: Behavioural, Anticonvulsant Properties. Phytotherapy Res 10:145-151.

Hiller KO, Kato G, Anxiolytic activity of psychotropic plant extracts. I. Test of ethanolic Valeriana extract STEI Val. In: PM 62, Abstracts of the 44th Ann Congress of GA, 65. 1996.

Hiller KO, Rahlfs V, Therapeutische Äquivalenz eines hochdosierten Phytopharmakons mit Amytriptylin bei ängstlich-depressiven Versimmungen - Reanalyse einer randomisierten Studie unter besonderer Beachtung biometrischer und klinischer Aspekte. In: Forsch.

Hölzl J, Baldrian ein Mittel gegen Schlafstörungen. In: DAZ 136(10):751-759. 1996.

Jansen W, (1977) Doppelblindstudie mit Baldrisedon. Therapiewoche 27:2779-2786.

Kamm-Kohl AV, Jansen W Brockmann P, (1984) Moderne Baldriantherapie gegen nervöse Störungen im Senium. Med Welt 35:1450-1454.

Krieglstein J, Grusla D, (1988) Zentraldämpfende Inhaltsstoffe im Baldrian. Dtsch Apoth Z 128:2041-2046.

Kubitschek J, Baldrian beeinflußt die Melatoninwirkung. In: PZ 142(6):433 1997.

Leathwood PD et al., (1982) Pharmacol Biochem Behav 17:65.

Leathwood PD, Chauffard F (1983) J Psychiatr. Res 17(2):115.

Leathwood PD, Chauffard F, (1983) Quantifying the effects of mild sedatives. J Psychiat Res 17:115-122.

Leathwood PD, Chauffard F, (1984) Aqueous extract of valerian reduces latency to fall asleep in man. Planta Med 50:144-148.

Meier B, Linnenbrink N, Status und Vergleichbarkeit pflanzlicher Arzneimittel. In: DAZ 136(47):4205-4220. 1996.

Müller-Bohn T, Pflanzliche Sedativa und Antidepressiva. In: DAZ 136(24):2032-2033. 1996.

Orth-Wagner S, Ressin WJ, Friedrich I, Phytosedativum gegen Schlafstörungen. In: ZPT 16(3):147-156. 1995.

Popov S et al., (1974) Phytochemistry 13:2815.

Reidel E et al., (1982) Planta Med 46:219.

Riedel E, Hänsel R, Ehrke G, (1982) Hemmung des Gamma-Aminobuttersäureabbaus durch Valerensäurederivate. Planta Med 46:219-220.

Rücker G, Tautges J, Sieek A, Wenzel H, Frag E, (1978) Untersuchungen zur Isolierung und pharmakodynamischen Aktivität des Sesquiterpens Valeranon aus Nardostrachys jatamansi DC Arzneim-Forsch/Drug Res 28:7.

Santos MS, Ferreira F, Cunha AP et al., (1994) An Aqueous Extract of Valerian Influences the Transport of GABA in Synaptosomes. Planta Med 60:278-279.

Schilcher H, Pflanzliche Psychopharmaka. Eine neue Klassifizierung nach Indikationsgruppen. In: DAZ 135(20):1811-1822. 1995.

Schimmer O, Röder A, Valerensäuren in Fertigarzneimitteln und selbst bereiteten Auszügen aus der Wurzel von Valeriana officinalis L.s.l. In: PZW 137(1):31-36. 1992.

Schulz H, Jobert M, (1995) Die Darstellung sedierender/ Tranquilisierender Wirkungen von Phytopharmaka im quantifizierten EEG Z Phytother Abstractband, S. 10.

Schulz H, Stolz C, Müller J, (1994) The effect of a valerian extract on sleep polygraphy in poor sleepers. A pilot study. Pharmacopsychiat 27:147-151.

Schulz V, Hübner WD, Ploch M, Klinische Studien mit Psycho-Phytopharmaka. In: ZPT 18(3):141-154. 1997.

Sprecher E, Pflanzliche Geriatrika. In: ZPT 9(2):40. 1988.

Sprecher E, Über die Qualität von Phytopharmaka. In: ZPT 12(4):105. 1991.

Thies PW, Funke S, (1966) Tetrahedron Letters 11:1155.

Torii S, Fukuda H, Kanemoto H, Miyanchi R, Hamauzu Y, Kawasaki M, (1988) Contingent negative variation (CNV), the psychological effects of odour. In: Van Toller St, Dodd GH (eds) Perfumery, The psychology, biology of fragrance. Chapman, Hall, London New York, S 107-146.

Trossell K, Wahlberg K, (1966) Tetrahedron Letters 4:445.

Tyler VE, (1987) The new honest herbal. A sensible guide to herbs, related remedies. 2nd ed Stickley Co., Philadelphia, S 125-126.

Van Meer JH, Labadine RP, (1981) J Chromatogr. 205(1):206.

Veith J et al., (1986) Planta Med (3):179.

Vorbach EU, Arnold KH, (1995) Wirksamkeit und Verträglichkeit von Baldrianextrakt (LI 156) versus Placebo bei behandlungsbedürftigen Insomnien. Z Phytother Abstractband, S 11.

Werner, Arzneipflanzen in der Volksmedizin. In: DAZ 130(45):2510. 1990.

Wichtl M, Volksmedizinisch verwendete pflanzliche Arzneimittel. In: ZPT 11(3):71. 1990.

Further information in:

Hänsel R, Keller K, Rimpler H, Schneider G (Hrsg.), Hagers Handbuch der Pharmazeutischen Praxis, 5. Aufl., Bde 4-6 (Drogen): Springer Verlag Berlin, Heidelberg, New York, 1992-1994.

Leung AY, Encyclopedia of Common Natural Ingredients Used in Food Drugs, Cosmetics, John Wiley & Sons Inc., New York 1980.

Madaus G, Lehrbuch der Biologischen Arzneimittel, Bde 1-3, Nachdruck, Georg Olms Verlag Hildesheim 1979.

Roth L, Daunderer M, Kormann K, Giftpflanzen, Pflanzengifte, 4. Aufl., Ecomed Fachverlag Landsberg Lech 1993.

Schulz R, Hänsel R, Rationale Phytotherapie, Springer Verlag Heidelberg 1996.

Steinegger E, Hänsel R, Pharmakognosie, 5. Aufl., Springer Verlag Heidelberg 1992.

Teuscher E, Lindequist U, Biogene Gifte - Biologie, Chemie, Pharmakologie, 2. Aufl., Fischer Verlag Stuttgart 1994.

Teuscher E, Biogene Arzneimittel, 5. Aufl., Wiss. Verlagsges. Stuttgart 1997.

Wagner H, Wiesenauer M, Phytotherapie. Phytopharmaka und pflanzliche Homöopathika, Fischer-Verlag, Stuttgart, Jena, New York 1995.

Wichtl M (Hrsg.), Teedrogen, 4. Aufl., Wiss. Verlagsges. Stuttgart 1997.

Veratrum Album

White Hellebore

DESCRIPTION

Medicinal Parts: The medicinal parts are the rhizome and root.

Flower and Fruit: The flowers are in racemes forming a 30 to 60 cm long panicle. The pedicles are much shorter than the flowers. The yellowish-white flowers consist of 6 similar tepals, which are oblong-lanceolate, acute, denticulate and broadly splayed. There are 6 stamens, which are shorter than the perigone and 3 styles. The fruit is capsule-like.

Leaves, Stem and Root: The plant is roughly 60 to 120 cm high. The rhizome is short, cylindrical, stunted, and has numerous, long, thick and fleshy root fibers. The round, cane-like, glabrous stem is almost completely surrounded by the tight sheaths of the basal leaves. The basal leaves are whorled, broad, elliptical to linear-lanceolate and heavily ribbed.

Habitat: The plant is found from Lapland to Italy but not on the British Isles.

Production: White Hellebore root-stock is the rhizome of Veratrum album.

ACTIONS AND PHARMACOLOGY

COMPOUNDS

Steroid alkaloids (mixture is referred to as veratrin, 0.8-2.5%): including, among others, some of the- C-or-D-homo-sterane-type; including, among others, protoverine, protoveratrine A and B- solanidane-type; including, among others, isorubijervine, rubijervine

EFFECTS

The drug is a strong irritant to the sensory nerves. The steroid-alkaloids (protoveratrin A,B, gemerin, jervin), are highly-effective combinations, which through their direct influence on the heart's stimulus receptors, cause antihypertensive and cardiac frequency effects. Internally, it reduces blood pressure and heart rate. Externally, the drug causes severe irritation to the skin, including numbing and poisoning through absorption.

INDICATIONS AND USAGE

White Hellebore is used in homeopathy for the treatment of blood circulation irregularities, cold sweats, vomiting and cramps.

PRECAUTIONS AND ADVERSE REACTIONS

The drug is severely toxic and has numerous severe side effects, even in therapeutic dosages. It is no longer administered in allopathic medicine for that reason. The alkaloids are severely mucous membrane-irritating and after resorption have, by inhibiting inactivation of the sodium ions channels, a paralyzing effect upon numerous excitable cells, in particular those governing cardiac activity.

OVERDOSAGE

The first symptoms of poisoning are sneezing, lacrimation, salivation, vomiting, diarrhea, a burning sensation in the mouth and pharyngeal cavity, and inability to swallow. Then, following resorption, paresthesia, vertigo, possible blindness, paralysis of the limbs, mild convulsions, lowering of cardiac frequency, cardiac arrhythmias and hypotension occur. Death occurs either through systolic cardiac arrest or through asphyxiation. The lethal dosage is between 10 and 20 mg of the alkaloid mixture, corresponding to 1 to 2 gm of the drug. The alkaloids can be absorbed through the uninjured skin.

Treatment of poisoning consists of gastrointestinal emptying (inducement of vomiting, gastric lavage with burgundy-colored potassium permanganate solution, sodium sulphate), administration of activated charcoal and shock prophylaxis (appropriate body position, quiet, warmth). Thereafter, spasms should be treated with diazepam or barbiturates (i.v.), bradycardia should be treated with atropine, hypotension should be treated with peripherally active circulatory medications, electrolyte substitution should be employed and possible cases of acidosis should be treated with sodium bicarbonate infusions. Intubation and oxygen respiration may also be necessary

DOSAGE

Mode of Administration: The drug is used in homeopathic dilutions.

LITERATURE

Atta-Ur-Rahman, Ali RA, Choudhary MI, New steroidal alkaloids from rhizomes of Veratrum album. In: JNP 55:565-570. 1992.

Atta-Ur-Rahmann, Ali RA, Gilani A, Choudhary MI, ASftab K, Sener B, Turkz S, Isolation of antihypertensive alkaloids from rhizomes of Veratrum album. In: PM 59(6):569. 1993.

Atta-Ur-Rahman et al., Alkaloids from Veratrum album. In: PH 30(1):368. 1991.

Brossi, Buch. In: Brossi A, Cordell GA (Eds), The Alkaloids. Vol. 41. Academic Press, 1250 Sixth Avenue, San Diego, CA 92101. 1992.

Further information in:

Frohne D, Pfänder HJ, Giftpflanzen - Ein Handbuch für Apotheker, Toxikologen und Biologen, 4. Aufl., Wiss. Verlags-Ges. Stuttgart 1997.

Kern W, List PH, Hörhammer L (Hrsg.), Hagers Handbuch der Pharmazeutischen Praxis, 4. Aufl., Bde. 1-8: Springer Verlag Berlin, Heidelberg, New York, 1969.

Lewin L, Gifte und Vergiftungen, 6. Aufl., Nachdruck, Haug Verlag, Heidelberg 1992.

Madaus G, Lehrbuch der Biologischen Arzneimittel, Bde 1-3, Nachdruck, Georg Olms Verlag Hildesheim 1979.

Roth L, Daunderer M, Kormann K, Giftpflanzen, Pflanzengifte, 4. Aufl., Ecomed Fachverlag Landsberg Lech 1993.

Teuscher E, Lindequist U, Biogene Gifte - Biologie, Chemie, Pharmakologie, 2. Aufl., Fischer Verlag Stuttgart 1994.

Teuscher E, Biogene Arzneimittel, 5. Aufl., Wiss. Verlagsges. Stuttgart 1997.

Wagner H, Wiesenauer M, Phytotherapie. Phytopharmaka und pflanzliche Homöopathika, Fischer-Verlag, Stuttgart, Jena, New York 1995.

Veratrum Luteum

False Unicorn Root

DESCRIPTION

Medicinal Parts: The medicinal part is the root.

Flower and Fruit: The flowers are numerous, greenish white, without covering leaves. They are dioecious and arranged in terminal racemes of 15 cm with nod like feathers. The petals are narrow and shorter than the stamens, the filaments taper to a point. The anthers are terminal and 2-lobed. The petals of the female flowers are linear, the stamens short and the ovary ovate, deltoid and grooved. The stigmas are oblong and have 3 grooves and open upwards. The fruit is numerous and capsule-like, compressed and acute.

Leaves, Stem and Root: The plant is perennial with a strong leafy stem 30 to 90 cm high. The stem is undivided, smooth, and angular. The foliage leaves are alternate, the lower ones spatulate and the upper ones lanceolate. The basal leaves are 20 cm long, 1.25 cm wide, narrow and whorled at the base.

The rhizome is tuberous and stunted. It is approximately 1.25 cm long.

Characteristics: False Unicorn Root has a bitter taste.

Habitat: The plant grows in the Mississippi Delta region.

Other Names: Starwort, Helonias Root, Blazing Star, Fairy-wand

ACTIONS AND PHARMACOLOGY

COMPOUNDS

Steroid saponins: (mixture is referred to as chamaelirin, ca. 10%), aglycone diosgenin

EFFECTS

oxytocic, diuretic, anthelmintic

INDICATIONS AND USAGE

False Unicorn Root is used for dysmenorrhea and pregnancy complaints.

PRECAUTIONS AND ADVERSE REACTIONS

No health hazards or side effects are known in conjunction with the proper administration of designated therapeutic dosages. The appearance of gastric complaints is conceivable with the drug, due to the high saponine content, particularly in cases of overdosage.

LITERATURE

Atta-Ur-Rahman, Ali RA, Choudhary MI, New steroidal alkaloids from rhizomes of Veratrum album. In: JNP 55:565-570. 1992.

Further information in:

Hegnauer R, Chemotaxonomie der Pflanzen, Bde 1-11: Birkhäuser Verlag Basel, Boston, Berlin 1962-1997 (unter Chamaelirium luteum (L.) GRAY).

Madaus G, Lehrbuch der Biologischen Arzneimittel, Bde 1-3, Nachdruck, Georg Olms Verlag Hildesheim 1979 (unter Helionas dioica).

Wagner H, Wiesenauer M, Phytotherapie. Phytopharmaka und pflanzliche Homöopathika, Fischer-Verlag, Stuttgart, Jena, New York 1995.

Veratrum Viride

American Hellebore

DESCRIPTION

Medicinal Parts: The medicinal parts are the dried rhizome and the roots.

Flower and Fruit: The terminal inflorescence is a panicle made up of spike-like racemes. The flowers are short-pedicled, often unisexual and the perigone has 6 tepals and is almost free. The anther is reniform. The fruit is capsule-like with numerous seeds and dividing membranes. The seeds are flattened, light-brown, winged all around. The embryo is small and set in the tip of the fusiform endosperm.

Leaves, Stem and Root: The species are handsome, perennial herbs with strong leafy stems. The leaves are spiralled, broadly elliptical to linear-lanceolate, heavily ribbed and drawn together in a broad sheath. The leaves of Veratrum viride are oval to linear.

Characteristics: Characteristics of the species Veratrum viride is very similar to Veratrum album.

Habitat: The herb is indigenous to the swamps and moist ground from Canada to Georgia and westward to Minnesota.

Production: American Hellebore root is the rhizome of Veratrum viride.

Not To Be Confused With: The rhizome from Symplocarpus foetidus is thicker than that of Veratrum viride and more porous.

Other Names: Bugbane, Devil's Bite, Earth Gall, Indian Poke, Itchweed, Tickleweed

ACTIONS AND PHARMACOLOGY

COMPOUNDS

Steroid alkaloids (1%): including, among others, some of the solanidane-type, isorubijervine, rubijervine- C-nor-D-homo-sterane-type: including among others protoverine, protover-atrine A and B. In contrast with Veratrum album, the less toxic alkaloids of the solanidane-type are here in the majority.

EFFECTS

Reduces blood pressure and slows down the pulse.

INDICATIONS AND USAGE

Used as an antispasmodic, diuretic, sedative and to reduce fever.

PRECAUTIONS AND ADVERSE REACTIONS

The drug is severely toxic and has numerous severe side effects, even in therapeutic dosages. It is no longer adminis-tered in allopathic medicine for that reason. The alkaloids are severely mucous membrane-irritating and after resorption have, by inhibiting inactivation of the sodium ions channels, a paralyzing effect on numerous excitable cells, in particular those governing cardiac activity.

OVERDOSAGE

The first symptoms of poisoning are sneezing, lacrimation, salivation, vomiting, diarrhea, burning sensation in the mouth and pharyngeal space, and inability to swallow; then, following resorption: paresthesia, vertigo, possible blindness, paralysis of the limbs, also mild convulsions, lowering of cardiac frequency, cardiac arrhythmias and hypotension.

Death occurs either through systolic cardiac arrest or through asphyxiation. The alkaloids can also be absorbed through the uninjured skin.

Following gastrointestinal emptying (inducement of vomiting, gastric lavage with burgundy-colored potassium permanganate solution, sodium sulphate), installation of activated charcoal and shock prophylaxis (appropriate body position, quiet, warmth), the therapy for poisonings consists of treating spasms with diazepam or certain barbiturates (i.v.), bradycardia with atropine and hypotension with peripherally active circulatory medications. Electrolyte substitution may be necessary and possible cases of acidosis should be treated with sodium bicarbonate infusions. Intubation and oxygen respiration may also be necessary.

DOSAGE

Mode of Administration: The drug is taken orally as a tincture or as a standardized extract.

Daily Dose: 0.3 to 2ml of tincture 1:10.

Storage: Protect from light. Store in safe place. (Caution: poisonous)

LITERATURE

Brossi, B, In: Brossi A, Cordell GA (Eds), The Alkaloids. Vol. 41. Academic Press, 1250 Sixth Avenue, San Diego, CA 92101. 1992.

Kupchan, S M et al., (1961) Lloydia 24(1):17.

Further information in:

Frohne D, Pfänder HJ, Giftpflanzen - Ein Handbuch für Apotheker, Toxikologen und Biologen, 4. Aufl., Wiss. Verlags-Ges. Stuttgart 1997.

Kern W, List PH, Hörhammer L (Hrsg.), Hagers Handbuch der Pharmazeutischen Praxis, 4. Aufl., Bde 1-8: Springer Verlag Berlin, Heidelberg, New York, 1969.

Madaus G, Lehrbuch der Biologischen Arzneimittel, Bde 1-3, Nachdruck, Georg Olms Verlag Hildesheim 1979.

Roth L, Daunderer M, Kormann K, Giftpflanzen, Pflanzengifte, 4. Aufl., Ecomed Fachverlag Landsberg Lech 1993.

Teuscher E, Lindequist U, Biogene Gifte - Biologie, Chemie, Pharmakologie, 2. Aufl., Fischer Verlag Stuttgart 1994.

Verbascum Densiflorum

Mullein

DESCRIPTION

Medicinal Parts: The medicinal parts are the herb at the beginning of the flowering season, the flowers and the root.

Flower and Fruit: The large, yellow flowers with a diameter of 30 to 35 mm are in apical spike-like racemes. The calyx is divided deeply into five. The corolla is rotate, has a short tube and a 5-lobed, uneven margin. There are 5 stamens of uneven length. The 3 upper ones are lanate and have long anthers. There is 1 superior ovary. The fruit is a 2-lobed capsule.

Leaves, Stem and Root: The plant is biennial. It has petiolate basal leaves and is up to 2 m high. The stem is erect, undivided or lightly branched above. It is tomentose like the leaves and calyx. The leaves are alternate, turned downwards and finely crenate. The lower ones are lanceolate or oblong lanceolate, the upper ones, ovate.

Characteristics: The flowers have a honey-like fragrance and an almond-like taste. The leaves are slimy and bitter.

Habitat: The plant is widespread in Europe, temperate Asia and North America.

Production: Mullein flower consists of the dried petals of Verbascum densiflorum and/or of Verbascum phlomoides.

Not To Be Confused With: Other Verbascum species.

Other Names: Torch Weed, Aaron's Rod, Blanket-leaf, Candlewick Plant, Flannelflower, Feltwort, Hedge-taper, Jacob's Staff, Shepherd's Club, Velvet Plant, Shepherd's Staff, Torches, Our Lady's Flannel, Blanket Herb, Woollen, Rag Paper, Wild Ice Leaf, Clown's Lungwort, Golden Rod, Adam's Flannel, Beggar's Blanket, Clot-Bur, Cuddy's lungs, Duffle, Feltwort, Fluffweed, Hare's Beard, Hag's Taper

ACTIONS AND PHARMACOLOGY

COMPOUNDS

Mucilage (3%): including, among others, arabino galactans, xyloglucans

Triterpene saponins: chief components verbascosaponine

Iridoide monoterpenes: including, among others, aucubin, 6beta-xylosylaucubin, catalpol

Caffeic acid derivatives: verbascoside (acteoside)

Flavonoids (0.5-4.0%): including, among others, apigenin-7-O-glucosides, kaempferol-7-O-glucosides, rutin digiprolactone

Invert sugar (11%)

EFFECTS

Alleviates irritation, expectorant in cases of cold due to the active relationship between mucin (antibiotic coverage of epithelial defects) and saponins (expectorant effect).

INDICATIONS AND USAGE

■ Cough/bronchitis

Catarrh of the respiratory tract. The plant is used internally in folk medicine as a diuretic, antirheumatic agent and externally for the treatment of wounds.

PRECAUTIONS AND ADVERSE REACTIONS

No health hazards or side effects are known in conjunction with the proper administration of designated therapeutic dosages.

DOSAGE

Mode of Administration: Comminuted herb for teas and other galenic preparations for internal use. The drug is used in preparations of antitussives and in various tea mixtures.

Preparation: To prepare an infusion, pour boiling water over 1.5 to 2 g finely cut drug and strain after 10 to 15 minutes (1 teaspoonful is equivalent to 0.5 g drug).

Daily Dose: 3 to 4 g of herb.

Storage: Must be protected from light and particularly from moisture as otherwise the drug changes color to brown or dark brown due to the iridoid content.

LITERATURE

Grzybek J, Szewczyk A, Verbascum-Arten - Königskerze oder Wollblume Portrait einer Arzneipflanze. In: ZPT 17(6):389-398. 1996.

Haslinger E, Schröder H, Sci Pharm 60:202. 1992.

Klimek B, PA 48:51. 1991.

Kraus K, Franz G, DAZ 127:665. 1987.

Seifert K et al., PM 51:409. 1985.

Swiatek L et al., PM 45:153. 1982.

Swiatek L et al., Pharm Weekbl (Sci Ed) 9:246. 1987.

Further information in:

Kern W, List PH, Hörhammer L (Hrsg.), Hagers Handbuch der Pharmazeutischen Praxis, 4. Aufl., Bde. 1-8: Springer Verlag Berlin, Heidelberg, New York, 1969.

Madaus G, Lehrbuch der Biologischen Arzneimittel, Bde 1-3, Nachdruck, Georg Olms Verlag Hildesheim 1979.

Roth L, Daunderer M, Kormann K, Giftpflanzen, Pflanzengifte, 4. Aufl., Ecomed Fachverlag Landsberg Lech 1993.

Steinegger E, Hänsel R, Pharmakognosie, 5. Aufl., Springer Verlag Heidelberg 1992.

Teuscher E, Biogene Arzneimittel, 5. Aufl., Wiss. Verlagsges. Stuttgart 1997.

Wichtl M (Hrsg.), Teedrogen, 4. Aufl., Wiss. Verlagsges. Stuttgart 1997.

Verbena Officinalis

Vervain

DESCRIPTION

Medicinal Parts: The medicinal parts are the dried aerial parts collected during the flowering season, the fresh, flowering herb, the flowers and the whole fresh plant.

Flower and Fruit: The small flowers are pale lilac and arranged in thin paniculate spikes. The calyx is fused to a short, 5-tipped tube. The corolla has a 5-tipped, bent tube and a bilabiate margin. The mouth of the tube is closed by a cross of hairs. There are 4 stamens and 1 ovary which breaks up into four, 1-seeded mericarps. These are oblong-cylindrical, 1.5 to 2 mm long, warty on the inside, reticulately grooved and light brown on the outside. The seeds are grooved on the inside and have very little endosperm.

Leaves, Stem and Root: The true variety is an annual or biennial to perennial with a fusiform, branched, whitish root. The stem is erect, rigid, quadrangular and branched above. The leaves are opposite, dull green, ovate-oblong and have a short broad petiole. They are deeply divided in 3 with notched, crenate tips. They are wrinkled and roughly bristled.

Habitat: The plant is probably indigenous to the Mediterranean region. It is cultivated, however, worldwide, mainly in eastern Europe.

Production: Verbena herb consists of the above-ground parts of Verbena officinalis. The herb is predominantly cultivated in eastern Europe. It is collected in the wild and harvested in southeastern Europe. After being cut, the drug is hung in bunches to dry.

Note: Improper drying leads to hydrolytic decomposition of verbenalin.

Not To Be Confused With: Lippiae triphyllae folium.

Other Names: Enchanter's Plant, Herb of the Cross, Juno's Tears, Pigeon's Grass, Pigeonweed, Simpler's Joy, Herb of Grace

ACTIONS AND PHARMACOLOGY

COMPOUNDS

Iridoide monoterpenes (0.2-0.5%): including, among others, verbenalin, hastatoside (0.08%), further dihydroverbenalin

Flavonoids: including, among others, luteolin, scutellarin and 6-hydroxy-luteolin glycosides, artemitine, sorbifolin, pedalitin, nepetin

Caffeic acid derivatives: verbascoside, eucovoside, martynoside

EFFECTS

Experiments to demonstrate antimicrobial and antiviral activity of the drug and its effects on the immune system and on tumor cells have not been conclusively assessed.

Further animal experiments have demonstrated a rise of urinary volume, antitussive effects, secretolytic effects, and an effect on salivation and lactation. Vervain has been shown to be effective in inflammatory models.

INDICATIONS AND USAGE

Preparations of Verbena are used for diseases and ailments of the oral and pharyngeal mucosa, such as sore throats and for diseases of the respiratory tract, such as coughs, asthma and whooping cough.

In addition to the above indications, in folk medicine, the drug is used internally for pain, cramps, fatigue, nervous disorders, digestive disorders, liver and gallbladder diseases, hepatitis, kidney and urinary tract complaints, menopausal complaints, irregular menstruation, to promote lactation, for rheumatic diseases, gout, metabolic disorders, chlorosis and dropsy. The drug is used externally as a gargle for cold symptoms and for diseases of the oral and pharyngeal cavity.

Vervain is also used for antipruritic treatment of skin diseases and minor topical burns (France) and for arthritis, rheumatism, dislocations and contusions.

PRECAUTIONS AND ADVERSE REACTIONS

No health hazards or side effects are known in conjunction with the proper administration of designated therapeutic dosages.

DOSAGE

Mode of Administration: The drug has internal and external application.

Preparation: Liquid extract (1:1) in 25% ethanol. Tincture in 40% ethanol. An infusion is prepared by adding 5 to 20 g drug to 1 liter water (France).

Daily Dose: Liquid extract - take 2 to 4 ml. Tincture - take 5 to 10 ml up to 3 times per day. Folk medicine doses for the infusion is 2 to 4 g up to 3 times per day. 4.5 to 9 g of drug is the daily dose in Chinese medicine.

Storage: Vervain must be stored in a dry environment to avoid hydrolytic decomposition of verbenalin.

LITERATURE

Carnat A et al., PM 61:490. 1995.

Inouye H et al., (1974) Planta Med 25:285.

McIlroy RJ, In: The Plant Glycosides, Arnold, London 1951.

Reynaud J et al., Pharm Acta Helv 67:216. 1992.

Weber R, Dissertation Marburg. 1995.

Yip L, Pei S, Hudson JB, Towers GHN, Screening of medicinal plants from Yunnan Province in southwest China for antiviral activity. In: ETH 34:1-6. 1991.

Further information in:

Hänsel R, Keller K, Rimpler H, Schneider G (Hrsg.), Hagers Handbuch der Pharmazeutischen Praxis, 5. Aufl., Bde 4-6 (Drogen): Springer Verlag Berlin, Heidelberg, New York, 1992-1994.

Madaus G, Lehrbuch der Biologischen Arzneimittel, Bde 1-3, Nachdruck, Georg Olms Verlag Hildesheim 1979.

Wagner H, Wiesenauer M, Phytotherapie. Phytopharmaka und pflanzliche Homöopathika, Fischer-Verlag, Stuttgart, Jena, New York 1995.

Wichtl M (Hrsg.), Teedrogen, 4. Aufl., Wiss. Verlagsges. Stuttgart 1997.

Veronica Beccabunga

Brooklime

DESCRIPTION

Medicinal Parts: The medicinal parts are the fresh flowering plant freed from the root, the fresh aerial parts collected during the flowering season and the whole plant.

Flower and Fruit: The flowers are in loose, axillary, diagonal clusters. The accompanying leaves are linear, as long as or shorter than the flowers. The peduncles and pedicles are glabrous. The calyx is dorsiventral and is divided into 4. The sepals are lanceolate to spatulate and acuminate; the front ones are larger than the back ones. The corolla is rotate with a very short tube, 4 to 9 mm wide and azure blue. The ovary is green and the stigma capitual-like. The fruit is a cordate, almost globular, narrow-winged capsule. The seeds are 0.6 mm long and 0.45 mm wide. They are oval, flatly convex with a fairly smooth back and yellow.

Leaves, Stem and Root: The plant is a perennial with a creeping rhizome. The stem is ascending, up to 50 cm high, round and is filled with latex. The leaves are petiolate, ovate or broad elliptical, obtuse, narrowly serrate, glabrous and glossy.

Habitat: The plant is indigenous to almost all of Europe, western and northern Asia, northern Africa and is naturalized in eastern North America.

Production: Brooklime is the aerial part of Veronica beccabunga. The collection or picking occurs in uncultivated regions in Europe, west and north Asia, North Africa and North America.

Other Names: Beccabunga, Mouth-smart, Neckweed, Speedwell, Water Purslane, Water Pimpernel

ACTIONS AND PHARMACOLOGY

COMPOUNDS

Iridoide monoterpenes: aucubin (0.8%)

Flavonoids: including among others scutellarin glycosides. The drug has not been extensively investigated

EFFECTS

Brooklime has a diuretic effect.

INDICATIONS AND USAGE

Brooklime is used to lessen the elimination of urine. It is also used for constipation, liver complaints, dysentery and lung conditions. The drug has also been reported to be effective against bleeding of the gums.

PRECAUTIONS AND ADVERSE REACTIONS

No health hazards or side effects are known in conjunction with the proper administration of designated therapeutic dosages.

DOSAGE

Mode of Administration: In its ground form, the drug is used for infusions. It is also squeezed or pressed to make a juice.

LITERATURE

Inouye H et al., (1974) Planta Med 25:285.

Kato Y, (1946) Folia Pharmacol Jap 42:37 (via CA 47: 1843).

Swiatek L et al., Acta Pol Pharm 25:597. 1968.

Further information in:

Hänsel R, Keller K, Rimpler H, Schneider G (Hrsg.), Hagers Handbuch der Pharmazeutischen Praxis, 5. Aufl., Bde 4-6 (Drogen): Springer Verlag Berlin, Heidelberg, New York, 1992-1994.

Veronica Officinalis

Speedwell

DESCRIPTION

Medicinal Parts: The medicinal parts are the dried herb collected during the flowering season, the fresh aerial parts of the flowering plant and the dried aerial parts collected during the flowering season.

Flower and Fruit: The erect bright blue or lilac flowers are in axillary, peduncled, spike-like racemes. The flowers are small, pedicled and have 4 slightly fused sepals. The corolla has a very short tube, is flatly splayed and has 4 uneven tips. There are 2 stamens and 1 superior ovary. The fruit is a triangular capsule narrowed at the base. The fruit chambers each have 5 to 10 seeds. The seeds are about 1 mm long, oval and flat; the back of the seed is smooth.

Leaves, Stem and Root: The plant is a 10 to 20 cm high herbaceous perennial with runners that tend to form grass. The root system consists mainly of shoot-producing roots. The stem is creeping and the flower-bearing branches are erect. The whole plant is roughly pubescent. The leaves are obovate-ovate, elliptical or oblong, short-petioled and serrate.

Habitat: The plant is indigenous to almost all of Europe, parts of Asia and North America. The sources of the drug are Bulgaria, the former Yugoslavia and Hungary.

Production: Vernonica herb consists of the above-ground parts of Vernonica officinalis imported from Bulgaria, the former Yugoslavia, and Hungary. Only the flowering herb is harvested (without roots or lower parts) and subsequently dried fully in the shade before it is cut.

Not To Be Confused With: Veronica chamaedrys or Veronica allionii.

ACTIONS AND PHARMACOLOGY

COMPOUNDS

Iridoide monoterpenes (0.5-1.0%): including, among others, aucubin, catalpol, catalpol esters (including among others minecoside, verminoside, veronicoside), mussaenoside, ladroside

Flavonoids (0.7%): including, among others, luteolin-7-O-glucosides (cinaroside)

Triterpene saponins (10%)

Caffeic acid derivatives: chlorogenic acid

EFFECTS

In animal experiments, Speedwell exhibited protective effect for ulcers and acceleration of ulcer healing.

INDICATIONS AND USAGE

Veronica herb preparations are used for diseases and discomfort of the respiratory tract, gastrointestinal tract, liver, kidney and lower urinary tract, for gout, rheumatoid arthritis and rheumatic complaints.

In folk medicine, Speedwell is used internally to promote the metabolism (''blood-purifying'') and for nervous agitation. Externally, the herb is used as a gargle for inflammation of the oral and pharyngeal mucosa, promotion of wound healing, for chronic skin complaints, itching, and sweating of the feet.

PRECAUTIONS AND ADVERSE REACTIONS

No health hazards or side effects are known in conjunction with the proper administration of designated therapeutic dosages.

DOSAGE

Mode of Administration: The herb is used internally and externally.

Preparation: To prepare the infusion, pour boiling water over 1.5 g (1 g = 1 teaspoonful) finely cut drug, strain after 10 minutes. For the preparation of external lavages and compresses for ulcers, wounds and eczema, use 1 handful drug in 1 liter water and boil for 10 minutes.

Daily Dose: The average single dose of the infusion used as an expectorant is 1 cup taken 2 to 3 times daily.

Storage: Must be protected from light sources.

LITERATURE

Afifi-Yazar F, Sticher O, (1980) Helv Chim Acta 63:1905.

Afifi-Yazar FÜ et al., Helv Chim Acta 64:16. 1981.

Sticher O et al., (1982) Planta Med 45:159.

Sticher O et al., Helv Chim Acta 62:530 et 535. 1979.

Tamas M et al., Clujul Med 57:169. 1985.

Wojcik E, Acta Polon, Pharm 38:621.

Further information in:

Hänsel R, Keller K, Rimpler H, Schneider G (Hrsg.), Hagers Handbuch der Pharmazeutischen Praxis, 5. Aufl., Bde 4-6 (Drogen): Springer Verlag Berlin, Heidelberg, New York, 1992-1994.

Madaus G, Lehrbuch der Biologischen Arzneimittel, Bde 1-3, Nachdruck, Georg Olms Verlag Hildesheim 1979.

Steinegger E, Hänsel R, Pharmakognosie, 5. Aufl., Springer Verlag Heidelberg 1992.

Wichtl M (Hrsg.), Teedrogen, 4. Aufl., Wiss. Verlagsges. Stuttgart 1997.

Vervain

See Verbena Officinalis

Viburnum Prunifolium

Black Haw

DESCRIPTION

Medicinal Parts: The medicinal part is the bark of the trunk and the root.

Flower and Fruit: The flowers of the Viburnum species are white and are in richly blossomed, flat, apical cymes. The central florets are campanulate and fertile; the lateral ones are much larger, rotate and infertile. The calyx margin is small and 5-tipped. The corolla of the fertile florets is campanulate and 5-petalled. There are 5 stamens, a semi-inferior ovary and 3 sessile stigmas. The fruit of the Black Haw is a shiny black, juicy berry. The fruit of Viburnum opulus is red.

Leaves, Stem and Root: Black Haw is a deciduous tree 5 m tall. It has gray-brown bark and green, grooved branches. The leaves are opposite, petiolate, 3 to 5 lobed, roughly dentate, green on both surfaces and softly pubescent beneath.

Habitat: The plant is indigenous to the eastern and central U.S.

Production: Black Haw Bark is the bark of the trunk and branches of Viburnum prunifolium.

Other Names: Stagbush, American Sloe, European Cranberry, Cramp Bark, Guelder Rose, Snowball Tree, King's Crown, High Cranberry, Red Elder, Rose Elder, Water Elder, May Rose, Whitsun Rose, Dog Rowan Tree, Whitsun Bosses, Silver Bells, Wild Guelder Rose

ACTIONS AND PHARMACOLOGY

COMPOUNDS

Flavonoids: amentoflavon (a biflavone)

Triterpenes: including, among others, oleanolic acid, ursolic acid as well as their acetates

Hydroxycoumarins: scopoletin, aesculetin, scoplin

Caffeic acid derivatives: chlorogenic acid, isochlorogenic acid

Phenol carboxylic acids: salicylic acid, salicin

Tannins (2%)

Arbutin (traces)

EFFECTS

The drug has a spasmolytic, and to date undefined effect on the uterus.

INDICATIONS AND USAGE

Black Haw is used for complaints of dysmenorrhea.

PRECAUTIONS AND ADVERSE REACTIONS

No health hazards or side effects are known in conjunction with the proper administration of designated therapeutic dosages.

DOSAGE

Mode of Administration: Extract as a constituent of a tea mixture made from Black Haw Bark, Camomile flowers and Peppermint leaves. No medicinal preparations.

LITERATURE

Handjieva N et al., PH 27:3175. 1988.

Hörhammer L, Wagner H, Reinhardt H, Chemistry, pharmacology, and pharmaceutics of the components of

Viburnum prunifolium and V. opulus. In: Botan Mag (Tokyo) 79(Oct./Nov.): 510-525. 1966.

Jarboe CH et al., (1967) J Med Chem 10: 448.

Jarboe CH et al., (1969) J Org Chem 34: 4202.

Jensen SR et al., PH 24:487. 1985.

Further information in:

Fenaroli's Handbook of Flavor Ingredients, Vol. 1, 2nd Ed., CRC Press 1975.

Kern W, List PH, Hörhammer L (Hrsg.), Hagers Handbuch der Pharmazeutischen Praxis, 4. Aufl., Bde. 1-8: Springer Verlag Berlin, Heidelberg, New York, 1969.

Roth L, Daunderer M, Kormann K, Giftpflanzen, Pflanzengifte, 4. Aufl., Ecomed Fachverlag Landsberg Lech 1993.

Wichtl M (Hrsg.), Teedrogen, 4. Aufl., Wiss. Verlagsges. Stuttgart 1997.

Vicia Faba

Broad Bean

DESCRIPTION

Medicinal Parts: The medicinal part is the fresh flower.

Flower and Fruit: The white or bluish short-pedicled flowers have black spots on the standard. They are arranged in groups of 2 to 4 in the upper leaf axils. The calyx tips are uneven, with the upper ones shorter than the lower. The pod is leathery and velvety on the flat surface. The seeds are large, flat, ovate or oblong and brown.

Leaves, Stem and Root: The plant is 60 to 125 cm high. The stem is erect and has no climbers. The leaves are pinnate and the leaflets elliptical, fleshy, blue-green and terminate acutely. The stipules are ovate and semi-saggitate.

Habitat: The plant is indigenous to the temperate regions of the world.

Production: Broad Beans are the seeds of Vicia faba.

ACTIONS AND PHARMACOLOGY

COMPOUNDS

Pyrimidine derivatives: vicine (vicioside, 0.4-0.8%), convicine (0.1-0.6%)

Lectins: The isolectins mixture is referred to as favine- L-3,4-dihydroxyphenylalanine (L-DOPA, up to 8%)

Starch

Proteins

Tannins (2%)

EFFECTS

No information is available.

INDICATIONS AND USAGE

Formerly, Broad Bean flowers were used in the treatment of coughs, kidney and genital complaints. Externally, they are used as a poultice for skin inflammation, warts, and burns. An essence of the fresh plant after flowering is used in homeopathy.

PRECAUTIONS AND ADVERSE REACTIONS

No health hazards or side effects are known in conjunction with the proper administration of designated therapeutic dosages. Following division of the glycosides in the intestine, resorption and oxidation through dehydration of SH-groups in the erythrocyte membrane, the pyrimidine derivatives can, in high dosages, lead to hemolysis.

OVERDOSAGE

The intake of large quantities of raw or only briefly-cooked seeds can lead, in particular with individuals with genetically-caused glucose-6-phosphate-dehydrogenase-deficiency (inadequate protection of the erythrocytes through glutathione), to queasiness, vomiting, diarrhea and feelings of vertigo. In severe cases, overdosage may lead to acute hemolytic anemia with fever, icterus, hemoglobinuria, oliguria and anuria (favism). Elevations in blood pressure are also possible, because of the L-DOPA content. The treatment of the favism can be carried out through transfusion of washed erythrocytes and through administration of prednisone.

DOSAGE

Mode of Administration: Broad Bean preparations are now obsolete.

LITERATURE

Chevion M, Maer J, Glaser G, Naturally occuring food toxicant: favism-producing agents. In: CRC Handbook of Naturally Occuring Food Toxicants, CRC Press, Boca Raton, Florida. 1983.

Vered Y et al., The influence of Vicia faca (Broad bean) seedlings on urinary sodium excretion. In: PM 63(3):237-240. 1997.

Further information in:

Kern W, List PH, Hörhammer L (Hrsg.), Hagers Handbuch der Pharmazeutischen Praxis, 4. Aufl., Bde. 1-8: Springer Verlag Berlin, Heidelberg, New York, 1969.

Teuscher E, Lindequist U, Biogene Gifte - Biologie, Chemie, Pharmakologie, 2. Aufl., Fischer Verlag Stuttgart 1994.

Vinca Minor

Periwinkle

DESCRIPTION

Medicinal Parts: The medicinal parts are the dried leaves, the fresh aerial parts of the flowering plant and the whole fresh flowering plant.

Flower and Fruit: The flowers are solitary, long-pedicled, 40 to 50 mm in diameter and grow in the axils of the upper leaves. The calyx is funnel-shaped with long, narrow-linear, pointed ciliated tips. The corolla is light blue or violet with a funnel-shaped tube and 5 irregularly terminated tips. The fruit is a follicle. It is oblong, acuminate, 15 to 2 mm long and has 2 to 3 seeds.

Leaves, Stem and Root: The plant is a perennial subshrub, 10 to 60 cm high. The non-flowering shoots are prostrate root at the nodes. The flowering shoots are ascending, up to 20 cm high and woody at the base. The leaves are evergreen, ovate, tapering at the front and distinctly pinnate-ribbed. They are 5 cm by 2 cm, petiolate with finely ciliated margins, which become glabrous later.

Habitat: The plant is indigenous to northern Spain, through western France, eastwards via central and southern Europe as far as the Caucasus, and has been naturalized in many regions.

Production: Periwinkle herb consists of the above-ground parts of Vinca minor.

ACTIONS AND PHARMACOLOGY

COMPOUNDS

Indole alkaloids (0.15-1.4%): chief alkaloid vincamine (eburnamine-type, 25-65%), further, including among others, vincin, apovincamine, vincadifformin

Flavonoids

EFFECTS

No information is available.

INDICATIONS AND USAGE

Periwinkle is used for circulatory disorders, cerebral circulatory impairment and support for the metabolism of the brain.

PRECAUTIONS AND ADVERSE REACTIONS

No health hazards are known in conjunction with the proper administration of designated therapeutic dosages. Gastrointestinal complaints and skin flushing have been observed as side effects.

OVERDOSAGE

Overdosage will bring about a severe drop in blood pressure. Cases of poisonings have not yet been recorded. (Changes in blood counts were observed following the administration of extracts from the foliage in animal experiments).

Treatment of overdose or poisoning includes gastrointestinal emptying (inducement of vomiting, gastric lavage with burgundy-coloured potassium permanganate solution, sodium sulphate), instillation of activated charcoal and shock prophylaxis (appropriate body position, quiet, warmth). The therapy for poisonings consists of treating bradycardia with atropine or Alupent, cardiac arrhythmias with lidocaine or phenytoin and treating possible cases of acidosis with sodium bicarbonate infusions. In case of shock, plasma volume expanders should be infused.

DOSAGE

No information is available.

LITERATURE

Behninger C, Abel G, Schneider E, Vinca minor zeigt keine antimitotische Eigenschaften. In: ZPT 13(2):35. 1992.

Gosset-Garnier J et al., (1965) Bull Soc Chim Franc 676.

Janot MM et al., (1962) Bull Soc Chim Franc 1079.

Kaul JL, Trojanek (1966) Lloydia 29:25.

Neczypor W, PA 24:273. 1969.

Taylor, B, In: Taylor WI, Farnsworth N (Ed.): The Vinca Alkaloids, Marcel Dekker Inc., New York. 1973.

Trunzler G, Phytotherapeutische Möglichkeiten bei Herz- und arteriellen Gefäßerkrankungen. In: ZPT 10(5):147. 1989.

Vinpocetin. In: ZPT 14(1):11. 1993.

Further information in:

Hänsel R, Keller K, Rimpler H, Schneider G (Hrsg.), Hagers Handbuch der Pharmazeutischen Praxis, 5. Aufl., Bde 4-6 (Drogen): Springer Verlag Berlin, Heidelberg, New York, 1992-1994.

Madaus G, Lehrbuch der Biologischen Arzneimittel, Bde 1-3, Nachdruck, Georg Olms Verlag Hildesheim 1979.

Roth L, Daunderer M, Kormann K, Giftpflanzen, Pflanzengifte, 4. Aufl., Ecomed Fachverlag Landsberg Lech 1993.

Steinegger E, Hänsel R, Pharmakognosie, 5. Aufl., Springer Verlag Heidelberg 1992.

Teuscher E, Lindequist U, Biogene Gifte - Biologie, Chemie, Pharmakologie, 2. Aufl., Fischer Verlag Stuttgart 1994.

Teuscher E, Biogene Arzneimittel, 5. Aufl., Wiss. Verlagsges. Stuttgart 1997.

Wagner H, Wiesenauer M, Phytotherapie. Phytopharmaka und pflanzliche Homöopathika, Fischer-Verlag, Stuttgart, Jena, New York 1995.

Viola Odorata

Garden Violet

DESCRIPTION

Medicinal Parts: The medicinal parts are the essential oil from the leaves, the dried flowers, the air-dried leaves collected during the flowering season, the flowering herb, the dried rhizome, the fresh aerial parts collected during the flowering season and the whole plant.

Flower and Fruit: The dark violet flowers are solitary on 3 to 7 cm long pedicles. The flowers are 1.5 to 2 cm long and fragrant. The 5 sepals are obtuse, glabrous and have an appendage. There are 5 uneven petals which are unevenly spurred and which have a broad margin. The 5 stamens have an appendage at the tip. The flower has 3 fused ovaries. The fruit is a globular capsule, approximately 7.5 mm. It is 3 to 6 sided, clearly and densely short pubescent and often violet. It can be found pressed to the receptacle.

Leaves, Stem and Root: The violet is 5 to 10 cm high. It is a rosette plant with a short, thick but soft ground axis. The rooting runners are 10 to 20 cm long and 1.5 mm thick. They produce flowers in the second year. The shoots are a strong dark green with scattered appressed hairs or almost glabrous. The leaves are petiolate, broadly cordate, obtuse or short acuminate and crenate. The leaves, which appear first, are reniform-cordate and the younger ones are rolled up. There are lanceolate stipules at the base of the leaves.

Characteristics: The plant is strongly scented.

Habitat: The plant is indigenous to or naturalized in large parts of Europe and the Middle East as far as central Asia and is also found in North America.

Production: Sweet Violet root, consists of the dried root of Viola odorata. Sweet Violet herb is the dried plant section of Viola odorata. The rhizome is imported from the former Czechoslovakia and Rumania. The root-stock is dug up, pounded to remove any soil residue, washed and air-dried.

ACTIONS AND PHARMACOLOGY

COMPOUNDS: VIOLAE ODORATAE RHIZOMA ET HERBA

Volatile oil (0.04%): salicylic acid methyl ester (formed out of glycosidic precursors during plant drying), beta-nitropropionic acid

Saponins

Alkaloids

EFFECTS: VIOLAE ODORATAE RHIZOMA ET HERBA

The drug is said to contain saponin. Saponins can have an expectorant effect and irritate the mucus membrane when used in higher doses. There are no studies available on preparations of the drug. In animal experiments with the root, an emetic effect has been claimed. In animal experiments with the herb, antipyretic, anti-exudative and anti-expectorate effects have not been conclusively assessed.

COMPOUNDS: VIOLAE ODORATAE FLOS

Volatile oil (0.003%): aroma-carrier trans-alpha-Ionone (parmone), chief constituents (-)-zingiberene, (+)-curcumene, dihydro-beta-ionone, 2,6-nonadien-1-al, undecan-2-one, isoborneol

EFFECTS: VIOLAE ODORATAE FLOS

An antimicrobial effect may be found in an aqueous extract of the flowers, but more specific information is unavailable. Assertions of expectorant, sedative and mild diuretic effects remain experimentally undocumented.

INDICATIONS AND USAGE

VIOLAE ODORATAE RHIZOMA ET HERBA

Acute and chronic bronchitis, bronchial asthma, acute and chronic catarrh of the respiratory organs, cold symptoms of the upper respiratory tract.

The rhizome is used in folk medicine for conditions of the respiratory organs, particularly for dry catarrh and for rheumatism of the minor joints; additionally used for fever, skin diseases, inflammation of the oral mucosa, nervous strain, headache and insomnia. The herb is used internally in folk medicine for coughs, hoarseness, tuberculosis, as an expectorant for throat inflammations and bronchitis accompanied by fixed mucous, nervous strain, insomnia and hysteria. Externally, the herb is used in skin lavages for various skin diseases.

VIOLAE ODORATAE FLOS

Acute and chronic bronchitis, bronchial asthma, coughs, chest catarrh, colds and complications, spasmolytic, cough relieving. The flowers are used in folk medicine to prepare an infusion tea, which is used as an expectorant for bronchial catarrh, as an antitussive for chronic bronchitis, for whooping cough, asthma and migraine. Violet syrup is used as an expectorant and to lessen irritation for bronchial catarrh (children's remedy). The flowers are used externally in folk medicine for parasitic stomatitis and as an emollient for inflammatory diseases.

PRECAUTIONS AND ADVERSE REACTIONS

VIOLAE ODORATAE RHIZOMA, HERBA ET FLOS

No health hazards or side effects are known in conjunction with the proper administration of designated therapeutic dosages.

DOSAGE

VIOLAE ODORATAE RHIZOMA ET HERBA

Preparation: A herb infusion is prepared by adding 2 teaspoonfuls sweet violet herb with 1/4 liter water.

Daily Dose: The folk medicine average single dose of the rhizome is 1 g orally. The rhizome decoction (5%) dosage is 20 g. The dosage of the 5% rhizome infusion is 1 tablespoonful 5 to 6 times daily. The herbal infusion dosage is 1 cup 2 to 3 times daily.

VIOLAE ODORATAE FLOA

Preparation: To prepare an infusion, decoction or tea, use 1 heaping teaspoonful of drug with 1 cup of water.

Daily Dosage: The folk medicine dosage for an infusion, decoction or tea is 1 cup twice daily, or taken in sips 1 to 2 times per hour. The dosage of Violet syrup is 1 to 2 tablespoons every 2 hours.

LITERATURE

VIOLAE ODORATAE RHIZOMA ET HERBA

Farnsworth NR, (1968) Lloydia 246.

Willaman JJ, Hui-Li L, (1970) Lloydia 33 (3A):1.

Further information in:

Hänsel R, Keller K, Rimpler H, Schneider G (Hrsg.), Hagers Handbuch der Pharmazeutischen Praxis, 5. Aufl., Bde 4-6 (Drogen): Springer Verlag Berlin, Heidelberg, New York, 1992-1994.

Madaus G, Lehrbuch der Biologischen Arzneimittel, Bde 1-3, Nachdruck, Georg Olms Verlag Hildesheim 1979.

Watt JM, Breyer-Brandwijk MG, The Medicinal, Poisonous Plants of Southern, Eastern Africa, 2nd Ed, Livingstone 1962.

VIOLAE ODORATAE FLOS

Farnsworth, NR, (1968) Lloydia 246.

Roberg M, Arch Pharm 275,145. 1937.

Ruzicka L, Schinz H, Helv Chim Acta 25:760. 1942.

Uhde G et al., Helv Chim Acta 55:2621. 1972.

Willaman JJ, Hui-Li L, (1970) Lloydia 33 (3A):1.

Further information in:

Hänsel R, Keller K, Rimpler H, Schneider G (Hrsg.), Hagers Handbuch der Pharmazeutischen Praxis, 5. Aufl., Bde 4-6 (Drogen): Springer Verlag Berlin, Heidelberg, New York, 1992-1994.

Madaus G, Lehrbuch der Biologischen Arzneimittel, Bde 1-3, Nachdruck, Georg Olms Verlag Hildesheim 1979.

Watt JM, Breyer-Brandwijk MG, The Medicinal, Poisonous Plants of Southern, Eastern Africa, 2nd Ed, Livingstone 1962.

Viola Tricolor

Heartsease

DESCRIPTION

Medicinal Parts: The medicinal parts are the dried aerial parts, the fresh aerial parts of the flowering plant, and the whole plant.

Flower and Fruit: The solitary, long-pedicled flower is yellow or tricolored. It has 5 lanceolate, acute and uneven sepals with an appendage and 5 uneven petals, the largest of which is spurred. The 5 stamens also have an appendage at the tip. There are 3 fused superior ovaries. The fruit is an ellipsoid, obtusely angular capsule, which bursts open at 3 points. The seeds are pear-shaped and yellow.

Leaves, Stem and Root: Heartsease is annual to perennial and grows about 30 cm high. The shoots are usually yellowish green, glabrous or covered in scattered hairs. The stem is erect, angular, unbranched or branched, glabrous or short-haired. It has short internodes below and longer ones above. The leaves are alternate, glabrous, or short-haired. The lower leaves are cordate; the upper ones are oblong-elliptical. The stipules are lyrate-pinnatesect and have a large, crenate terminal tip.

Characteristics: The plant is odorless and the taste slimy-sweetish.

Habitat: The plant is indigenous to temperate Eurasia, from the Mediterranean to India and as far as Ireland. It is cultivated in Holland and France.

Production: Viola herb consists of the dried, above-ground parts of Viola tricolor, mainly of the subspecies vulgaris and subspecies arvensis, harvested at flowering season. The herb is cultivated predominantly in central Europe. The flowering above-ground parts are harvested in the summer months and carefully dried on a well ventilated floor or at 45°C-50°C. Two to three harvests per year are possible.

Other Names: European Wild Pansy, Johnny-jump-up, Wild Pansy

ACTIONS AND PHARMACOLOGY

COMPOUNDS

Flavonoids (0.2%): including, among others, rutin (violaquercitrin), luteolin-7-O-glucosides, scoparin, saponarine, violanthin, vicinein-2, vitexin- phenol carboxylic acid: salicylic acid (0.06-0.3%), violutoside (violutin, glucoarabinoside of the methyl salicylate)

Mucilage (10%)

Tannins (2-5%)

Hydroxycoumarins: umbelliferone

EFFECTS

The plant has antiphlogistic and anti-oxidative properties.

INDICATIONS AND USAGE

- Inflammation of the skin
- Warts

External uses include mild seborrheic skin diseases and cradle cap in children. The plant is used internally in folk medicine as a mild laxative for constipation and as an auxiliary agent to promote metabolism. Externally, the drug is used for skin affections such as wet and dry exanthema, eczema, Crusta lactea, acne, impetigo and Pruritis vulvae.

In older folk medicine the drug was used for respiratory catarrh, throat inflammation, whooping cough and for feverish colds.

PRECAUTIONS AND ADVERSE REACTIONS

No health hazards or side effects are known in conjunction with the proper administration of designated therapeutic dosages.

DOSAGE

Mode of Administration: Comminuted drug for infusions and decoctions and for other galenic preparations for external use. Heartsease is used as a source of raw material for rutin in industry.

Preparation: An external decoction is prepared using 1.5 g drug with 1 cup water. An infusion for internal use is prepared using 1.5 g drug with 1 cup water. The drug is also used as a bath additive. In folk medicine, an infusion for internal use is prepared using 5 to 10 g drug per 1 liter water.

Daily Dose: 1.5 g drug per cup of water as an infusion, 3 times daily. One-half teaspoonful of the powdered drug in hot sugar-water 3 times daily. Externally, the drug can be used as poultice.

Folk medicine usage: The dosage of the infusion is 1 tablespoonful 3 times daily. A tea is prepared by adding 1 tablespoonful of drug with 1 cup boiling water, and taking after mealtimes.

Storage: Must be kept stored away form light sources, and if possible, from moisture in well-sealed containers.

LITERATURE

Hörhammer L et al., (1965) Tetrahedron Letters 1707.

Komorowski T et al., Herba Pol 29:5. 1983.

Mánez S, Villar A, PA 44:250. 1988.

Molnár P et al., PH 25:195. 1986.

Further information in:

Fenaroli's Handbook of Flavor Ingredients, Vol. 1, 2nd Ed., CRC Press 1975

Hänsel R, Keller K, Rimpler H, Schneider G (Hrsg.), Hagers Handbuch der Pharmazeutischen Praxis, 5. Aufl., Bde 4-6 (Drogen): Springer Verlag Berlin, Heidelberg, New York, 1992-1994.

Leung AY, Encyclopedia of Common Natural Ingredients Used in Food Drugs, Cosmetics, John Wiley & Sons Inc., New York 1980.

Steinegger E, Hänsel R, Pharmakognosie, 5. Aufl., Springer Verlag Heidelberg 1992.

Teuscher E, Biogene Arzneimittel, 5. Aufl., Wiss. Verlagsges. Stuttgart 1997.

Wagner H, Wiesenauer M, Phytotherapie. Phytopharmaka und pflanzliche Homöopathika, Fischer-Verlag, Stuttgart, Jena, New York 1995.

Wichtl M (Hrsg.), Teedrogen, 4. Aufl., Wiss. Verlagsges. Stuttgart 1997.

Viscum Album

Mistletoe

DESCRIPTION

Medicinal Parts: The medicinal parts are the leaves and twigs collected before the berries form, the fresh herbs of certain host plants, the fresh leafy twigs with fruit collected in the autumn, the whole fresh plant collected from apple trees, the leaves and the berries.

Flower and Fruit: The flower is yellowish-green, dioecious and appears in insignificant, small, 3 to 5 flowered clusters. The perigone of the male flower is 4 tipped. The stamens are fused with the tips. The female flower is smaller and has 4 tepals with a thick stigma sitting on the short style. The fruit is a glossy, white, globular, pea-sized berry with thick sticky flesh. When ripe, it is white to yellowish or orange and has 1 to 2 oval or angular seeds.

Leaves, Stem and Root: The plant is a semi-parasitic, almost round bush growing on deciduous trees, which are 30 to 80 cm in diameter. The round branches are repeatedly bifurcated and thickened to knots at the joints and are the same yellowish-green as the leaves. The leaves are alternate, sessile, lanceolate or lanceolate-spatulate, coriaceous and evergreen.

Habitat: Mistletoe is found mostly in Europe and as far as Iran. It is not found in America or Australia. It is cultivated in central Europe and China.

Production: Mistletoe berries are the fresh or dried fruit of Viscum album. Mistletoe stem is the fresh or dried stem of Viscum album. Mistletoe herb consists of fresh or dried younger branches with flowers and fruits of Viscum album. The drug is collected in the wild during the spring and is air-dried or put in driers at a maximum temperature of 40°C.

Other Names: Mystyldene, All-heal, Birdlime, Devil's fuge

ACTIONS AND PHARMACOLOGY

COMPOUNDS: VISCI ALBI FRUCTUS

Mucilage (2%, referred to as Viscin): The mock berries of the mistletoe have not been fully investigated. Presumably, they lack the toxic lectins and viscotoxins.

EFFECTS: VISCI ALBI FRUCTUS

No information available.

COMPOUNDS: VISCI ALBI STIPITES

The mistletoe stems contain the same constituents as the mistletoe foliage (Visci albi herba), but because of the high percentage of support elements lacking any effective ingredients, these constituents exist only in very low concentrations.

EFFECTS: VISCI ALBI FRUCTUS

No information available.

COMPOUNDS: VISCI ALBI HERBA

Lectins (glycoproteins with 11% carbohydrate): mistletoe lectin I (ML I, VAA 1, viscumin), mistletoe lectin II (ML II), mistletoe lectin III (ML III, VAA II), the lectin fractions named are isolectin mixtures

Polypeptides (built up out of 26 amino acids, 0.05-0.1%): viscotoxins A2, A3, B, Ps 1- water-soluble polysaccharides (known as viscin, 4-5%): including, among others, galacturonans, arabino galactans

Sugar alcohols: including, among others, mannitol, quebrachitol, pinitol, viscumitol

Flavonoids: including, among others, glycosides of the quercetins, of quercetin methyl ethers, of the isorhamnetins and rhamnazins

Phenyl alyl alcohols: including, among others, syringin (syrigenin-4′-O-glucosides)

Lignans: including, among others, syringaresinol and its glycosides

Triterpenes: including, among others, alpha-amyrin (alpha-viscol), betuline acid, oleanolic acid, ursolic acid

EFFECTS: VISCI ALBI HERBA

Intracutaneous injections cause local inflammation, which can progress to necroses.

In animal tests the herb exhibits cytostatic, non-specific immune stimulation.

Note: the blood pressure-lowering effects and the therapeutic efficacy for mild forms of hypertonia (borderline hyertonia) need further investigation.

INDICATIONS AND USAGE

VISCI ALBI FRUCTUS

Regulates blood pressure, internal bleeding, epilepsy, arteriosclerosis, bleeding in the lungs, infantile convulsions, gout, hysteria, acts on the circulation, irrigating, blood purifying; major blood loss.

VISCI ALBI STIPITES

The stem of Mistletoe is used for its calming effect; in the treatment of mental and physical exhaustion; as a tranquilizer against nervous conditions such as agitation, anxiety and increased excitability.

VISCI ALBI HERBA

- Rheumatism
- Tumor therapy adjuvant

For treating degenerative inflammation of the joints by stimulating cuti-visceral reflexes following local inflammation brought about by intradermal injections. Also used as a palliative therapy for malignant tumors through non-specific stimulation. Folk medicine uses include long-term therapy for cases of mild high blood pressure and as an arteriosclerosis prophylactic.

Mistletoe tea may be used for high blood pressure, epilepsy, whooping cough, asthma, vertiginous attack, amenorrhea, diarrhea, chorea, nervous tachycardia, hysteria and nervousness.

CONTRAINDICATIONS

VISCI ALBI HERBA

Contraindications for parenteral administration of the herb include protein oversensitivity, chronic-progressive infections, as for example tuberculosis, conditions of high fever.

PRECAUTIONS AND ADVERSE REACTIONS

VISCI ALBI FRUCTUS

No health hazards or side effects are known in conjunction with the proper administration of designated therapeutic dosages. The berries are said to have emetic and evacuant effects and to have caused the death of children. Unambiguous proof for these sorts of effects does not, however, exist.

VISCI ALBI STIPITES

No health hazards or side effects are known in conjunction with the proper administration of designated therapeutic dosages.

VISCI ALBI HERBA

No health hazards are known in conjunction with the proper administration of designated therapeutic dosages. The drug is non-toxic with peroral administration. Local reactions can occur with parenteral administration of mistletoe extracts (wheal formation, possibly also necroses), chills, fever, headache, anginal complaints, orthostatic circulatory disorders and allergic reactions.

The wheal formation and the elevation of body temperature are considered signs of immune system stimulation and therefore as positive therapeutic effects.

DOSAGE

VISCI ALBI HERBA

Mode of Administration: Fresh plant, cut and powdered herb for the preparation of solutions for injections.

Preparation: A medicinal tea is prepared using 2.5 g (1 teaspoonful) finely cut drug with 1 cup cold water, steep for 12 hours at room temperature, then strain. Mistletoe wine is prepared by adding 40 g drug to 1 liter wine. The preparation is ready for use after 3 days. Other preparations are available.

Daily Dose: The recommended daily dose is 10 g drug. The dosage of medicinal tea is 1 to 2 cups daily. Mistletoe wine dosage is 3 to 4 glasses daily.

Folk medicine dosage for the treatment of hypertonia and as an arteriosclerotic prophylactic is 2 to 6 g of Mistletoe powder 3 times daily taken orally.

Storage: Mistletoe must be stored away from the light over an appropriate drying agent.

LITERATURE

VISCI ALBI FRUCTUS

Frohne D, Pfänder HJ, Giftpflanzen - Ein Handbuch für Apotheker, Toxikologen und Biologen, 4. Aufl., Wiss. Verlags-Ges. Stuttgart 1997.

Hänsel R, Keller K, Rimpler H, Schneider G (Hrsg.), Hagers Handbuch der Pharmazeutischen Praxis, 5. Aufl., Bde 4-6 (Drogen): Springer Verlag Berlin, Heidelberg, New York, 1992-1994.

Teuscher E, Lindequist U, Biogene Gifte - Biologie, Chemie, Pharmakologie, 2. Aufl., Fischer Verlág Stuttgart 1994.

VISCI ALBI HERBA AND STIPITES

Anonym, Allergie auf Mistelextrakt. In: ZPT 13(3):96. 1992.

Anonym, Die Mistel. In: DAZ 136(48):4330-4332. 1996.

Anonym, Integrative Konzepte in der Onkologie: Misteltherapie (S. 19). In: NGM Suppl. 1/94:1-36. 1994.

Anonym, Misteltherapie aus schulmedizinischer Sicht. In: DAZ 131(37):1894. 1991.

Anonym, Optimale Misteldosierung. In: PZ 140(35):3082. 1995.

Anonym, Phytotherapie: Einsatz von Mistelextrakten in der Tumortherapie. In: DAZ 135(1):73. 1995.

Anonym, Sind Mistelpräparate mehr als nur Adjuvanzien in der onkologischen Therapie? In: ZPT 15(6):353-355. 1994.

Becker H, Exner J, (1980) Z Pflanzenphysiol. 97

Berg P, Stein G, Ein Inhaltsstoff allein genügt nicht, s. auch folgenden Artikel. In: ZPT 16(5):282. 1995.

Beuth HJ, Mistel: ''In der Onkologie nur Präparate einsetzen, die auf Mistellektin standardisiert sind!'' In: ZPT 16(1):40-41. 1995.

Beuth J, Ko HL, Gabius HJ, Burrichter H, Oette K, Pulverer G, (1992) Behavior of lymphocyte subsets, expression of activation markers in response to immunotherapy with galactoside-specific lectin from mistletoe in breast cancer. Clin Invest 70:658-661

Beuth J, Ko HL, Pulverer G, Angewandte Lektinologie. In: DAZ 134(25):2331. 1994.

Beuth J, Lenartz D, Uhlenbruck G, Lektionoptimierter Mistelextrakt. In: ZPT 18(2):85-91. 1997.

Bloksma N et al., (1982) Planta Med 46:221.

Dumont S et al., Lectins from mistletoe (Viscum album L.) induce the production of cytokines by cultured human monocytes. In: PM 61(Abstracts of 43rd Ann Congr):57. 1995.

Franz G, Phytotherapie in der Tumorbehandlung. In: DAZ 130(26):1443. 1990.

Franz H, (1985) Pharmazie 40(2):97.

Franz H et al., (1981) Biochem J 195:481.

Gabius HJ, Gabius S, Die Misteltherapie auf dem naturwissenschaftlichen Prüfstand. In: PZ 139(22):1745. 1994.

Hamacher H, Mistel (Viscum album L.) - Forschung und therapeutische Anwendung. In: ZPT 18(1):34-35. 1997.

Gabius HJ, Gabius S, Joshi SS, Koch B, Schroeder M, Manzke WM, Westerhausen M, (1994) From illdefined extracts to the immunomodulatoty lectin: Will there be a reason for oncological application of mistletoe? Planta Med 60:2-7.

Gabius HJ, Gabius S, Münchner-Phytotherapietagung 1992. Neues über die Misteltherapie. In: ZPT 14(1):17. 1993.

Gabius HJ, Mythos Mistel: Anspruch und Wirklichkeit. In: PZ 140(12):1029-1030. 1995.

Hajto T, Hostanka K, Frei K, Rordorf Chr, Gabins H-J, (1990a) Increased secretion of tumor necrosis factor interleukin 1: und interleukin 6 by Heiman mononuclear cells exposed to galactoside - specific lectin from clinically applied mistletoe extract. Canc Res 50:3322.

Hajto T, Hostanka K, Gabius HI, (1989) Modulatory potency of the galactoside-specific lectin from mistletoe extract (Iscador), the host defense system in vivo in rabbits, patients. Canc Res 49:4803.

Hajto T, Hostanka K, Gabius HI, (1990) Zytokine als Lectin-induzierte Mediatoren in der Misteltherapie. Therapeutikon 4:136-145.

Hamacher H, Mistel (Viscum album L.) - Forschung und therapeutische Anwendung. In: ZPT 18(1):34-35. 1997.

Hamacher H, Scheer R, Anthroposophie/Phytotherapie: Mistel-Forschung und therapeutische Anwendung. In: DAZ 136(34):2904-2905. 1996.

Hassauer W et al., (1979) Onkologie 2(1):28.

Hauser SP, (1993) Mistel - Wunderkraut oder Medikament? Therapiewoche 43(3):76-81.

Keine H, (1989) Klinische Stdien zur Misteltherapie karzinomatöser Erkrankungen. Eine Übersicht. Therapeutikon 3:347-353.

Kleijnen J, Knopschild P, (1994) Mistletoe treatment for cancer. Review of controlled trials in humans. Phytomedicine 1:255-260.

Kwaja TA et al., (1980) Experientia 36:599.

Loew, B, In: Loew D, Rietbrock N: Phytopharmaka II: Forschung und klinische Anwendung, Steinkopff Verlag, Darmstadt, 1996.

Luther P et al., (1980) Int J Biochem 11:429.

Müller J, (1962) Ger Offen DE 1:130:112.

Olsnes S et al., (1982) J Biol Chem 257:1371.

Rentea R et al., (1981) Lab Invest. 44(1):43.

Saenz MT, Ahumada MC, Garcia MD, Extracts from Viscum and Crataegus are cytotoxic against larynx cancer cells. In: Z Naturforsch C 52(1-2):42-44. 1997.

Salzer G, Havelec L, (1978) Onkologie 1(6):264.

Salzer G, Müller H, (1978) Prax Klein Pneumol 32(11):721.

Samuellson G et al., (1981) Acta Pharm Sueca 18:179.

Schmidt S, Unkonventionelle Heilverfahren in der Tumortherapie. In: ZPT 17(2):115-117. 1996.

Schwarz T et al., Stimulation by a stable, standardised mistletoe preparation of cytokine production in an in vitro human skin bioassay. In: PM 62, Abstracts of the 44th Ann Congress of GA, 1996.

Stirpe F et al., (1982) J Biol Chem 257(22):13271.

Timoshenko AV et al., Influence of the galactoside-specific lectin from Viscum album and its subunits on cell aggregation and selected intracellular parameters of rat thymocytes. In: PM 61(2):130-133. 1995.

Uhlenbrock S, Weihnachten, Miraculix und die Anthroposophie. In: PZ 140(51/52):4602-4603. 1995.

Wagner H et al., (1986) Planta Med (2):102.

Wagner H, Die Mistel in der Tumortherapie. In: DAZ 132(20):1087/1088. 1992.

Wagner H, Jordan E, (1986) Structure, properties of polysaccarides from Viscum album (L). Oncology (Suppl 1):8-15.

Wagner H, Pflanzliche Immunstimulanzien. In: DAZ 131(4):117. 1991.

Wasielewski S, Krebserkrankungen: Streit um alternative Heilverfahren in der Onkologie. In: DAZ 135(24):2234-2235. 1995.

Woynarvski JM et al., (1980) Hoppe-Seylers Z Physiol Chem 361(10):1525 et 1535.

Further information in:

Frohne D, Pfänder HJ, Giftpflanzen - Ein Handbuch für Apotheker, Toxikologen und Biologen, 4. Aufl., Wiss. Verlags-Ges. Stuttgart 1997.

Hänsel R, Keller K, Rimpler H, Schneider G (Hrsg.), Hagers Handbuch der Pharmazeutischen Praxis, 5. Aufl., Bde 4-6 (Drogen): Springer Verlag Berlin, Heidelberg, New York, 1992-1994.

Madaus G, Lehrbuch der Biologischen Arzneimittel, Bde 1-3, Nachdruck, Georg Olms Verlag Hildesheim 1979.

Roth L, Daunderer M, Kormann K, Giftpflanzen, Pflanzengifte, 4. Aufl., Ecomed Fachverlag Landsberg Lech 1993.

Schulz R, Hänsel R, Rationale Phytotherapie, Springer Verlag Heidelberg 1996.

Steinegger E, Hänsel R, Pharmakognosie, 5. Aufl., Springer Verlag Heidelberg 1992.

Teuscher E, Lindequist U, Biogene Gifte - Biologie, Chemie, Pharmakologie, 2. Aufl., Fischer Verlag Stuttgart 1994.

Teuscher E, Biogene Arzneimittel, 5. Aufl., Wiss. Verlagsges. Stuttgart 1997.

Wagner H, Wiesenauer M, Phytotherapie. Phytopharmaka und pflanzliche Homöopathika, Fischer-Verlag, Stuttgart, Jena, New York 1995.

Wichtl M (Hrsg.), Teedrogen, 4. Aufl., Wiss. Verlagsges. Stuttgart 1997.

Vitex Agnus-Castus

Chaste Tree

DESCRIPTION

Medicinal Parts: The medicinal parts are the ripe dried fruit and the dried leaves.

Flower and Fruit: The 8 to 10 cm, blue, occasionally pink flowers form terminal, branched, spike-like inflorescences. The calyx and epicalyx of the bilabiate corolla are pubescent. The fruit is a globular to oblong, 3 to 4 mm, reddish black, 4-seeded drupe. It is surrounded up to two-thirds in cup-like fashion by the calyx. The exocarp has short-stemmed, glandular hairs.

Leaves, Stem and Root: The plant is a 1 to 6 m high bush or tree with quadrangular, gray, tomentose, young branches. The leaves are deciduous, crossed-opposite, long-petioled and palmate. They have 5 to 7 entire-margined, up to 10 cm long, lanceolate leaflets. The under surface of the leaf is white and tomentose.

Habitat: The plant is indigenous to the Mediterranean region as far as western Asia.

Production: Vitex fruits composed of the ripe, dried fruits of Vitex agnus-castus.

ACTIONS AND PHARMACOLOGY

COMPOUNDS

Iridoid glycosides: agnoside, aucubin

Flavonoids: including casticin, 3,6,7,4′-tetramethylether of 6-hydroxy-camphor oil

Volatile oil: including, among others, 1,8-cineol, limes, alpha-pinenes and beta-pinenes

Fatty oils

EFFECTS

There is evidence that aqueous-alcoholic extracts of Chaste Tree inhibit secretion of prolactin in vitro. In human pharmacology there are no data about the lowering of prolactin levels. There is no knowledge regarding pharmacokinetics. Systemic studies about toxicology are unknown.

INDICATIONS AND USAGE

■ Premenstrual syndrome (PMS)

Chaste Tree preparations are used to treat irregularities of the menstrual cycle, premenstrual complaints, and mastodynia.

CONTRAINDICATIONS

The drug is contraindicated in pregnancy and in nursing mothers.

PRECAUTIONS AND ADVERSE REACTIONS

General: Occasionally the administration of the drug leads to the formation of rashes.

Drug Interactions: Because of the dopaminergic effect of the drug, a reciprocal weakening of the effect can occur in case of ingestion of dopamine-receptor antagonists.

Pregnancy: The drug should not be administered during pregnancy

Nursing Mothers: The drug should not be used by breast-feeding mothers.

DOSAGE

Mode of Administration: Aqueous-alcoholic extracts (50 - 70% V/V) from the crushed fruits taken as liquid or dry extract.

Daily Dosage: The daily dosage of aqueous-alcoholic extracts is 30 to 40 mg of the drug.

LITERATURE

Becker H, Hemmung der Prolaktinsekretion. In: T W Gynäkologie 6:2-10. 1991.

Böhnert KJ, Hahn G, Erfahrungsheilkunde 39:494-502c. 1990.

Dittmann FW, Böhnert KJ, Peeters M, Albrecht M, Lamertz M, Schmidt U, Prämenstruelles Syndrom. Behandlung mit einem Phytopharmakon. In: TW Gynäkologie 5:60-68. 1992.

Feldmann HU, Albrecht M, Lamertz M, Böhnert KJ, Therapie bei Gelbkörperschwäche bzw. prämenstruellem Syndrom mit Vitex-agnus-castus-Tinktur. In: Gyne 11:421-425. 1990.

Jarry H, Leonhardt S, Gorkow C, Wuttke W, (1994) In vitro prolactin but not LH and FSH release is inhibited by compounds in extracts of Agnus castus, direct evidence for a dopaminergic principle by the dopamine receptor assay. Exp Clin Endocrinol 102:448-454.

Jarry H, Leonhardt S, Wuttke W, Behr B, Gorkow C, (1991) Agnus castus als dopaminerges Wirkprinzip in Mastodynon N. Z Phytother 12:77-82.

Kustrac D et al., The composition of the essential oil of Vitex agnus-castus. In: PM 58(7):A681. 1992.

Lehmann-Willenbrock E, Riedel HH, (1988) Klinische und endokrinologische Untersuchungen zur Therapie ovarieller Ausfallserscheinungen nach Hysterektromie unter Belassung der Adnexe. Zent Gynäkol 110:611-618.

Loew D, Gorkow C, Schrödter A, Reitbrock S, Merz PG, Schnieders M, Sieder C, Zur dosisabhängigen Verträglichkeit eines Agnus-castus-Spezialextraktes. In: ZPT 17(4):237-243. 1996.

Merz PG, Schrödter A, Rietbrock S, Gorkow Ch, Loew D, (1995) Prolaktinsekretion und Verträglichkeit unter der Behandlung mit einem Agnus-castus-Spezialextrakt (B1095E1). Erste Ergebnisse zum Einfluß auf die Prolaktinsekretion. In, Loew D, Rietbrock N (Hrsg) Phytopharmaka in Forschung und klinischer Anwendung. Steinkopff Verlag, Darmstadt, S 93-97.

Propping D, Böhnert KJ, Peeters M, Albrecht M, Lamertz M, Vitex´agnus-castus. Behandlung gynäkologischer Krankheitsbilder. In: Therapeutikon 5:581-585. 1991.

Reuter HD, Böhnert KJ, Schmidt U, (1995) Die Therapie des prämenstruellen Syndroms mit Vitex agnus castus. Kontrollierte Doppelblindstudie gegen Pyridoxin. Z Phytother Abstractband, S 7.

Reuter HD, Böhnert KJ, Schmidt U, Die Therapie des prämenstruellen Syndroms mit Vitex agnus castus. Kontrollierte Doppelblindstudie gegen Pyridoxin.. In: ZPT, Abstract-Band, S.7. 1995.

Röder D, Therapie von Zyklusstörungen mit Vitex agnus-castus. In: ZPT 15(3):155-159. 1994.

Wichtl M, Phytopharmaka: Agnus castus - ein Dopamin-Agonist? In: DAZ 132(8):360. 1992.

Winterhoff H, (1993) Arzneipflanzen mit endokriner Wirksamkeit. Z Phytother 14:83-94.

Winterhoff H, Gorkow C, Behr B, Die Hemmung der Laktation bei Ratten als indirekter Beweis für die Senkung von Prolaktin durch Agnus castus. In: ZPT 12(6):175-179. 1991.

Wuttke W, Gorkow Ch, Jarry J, (1995) Dopaminergic Compounds in Vitex Agnus Castus. In, Loew D, Rietbrock N (Hrsg) Phytopharmaka in Forschung und klinischer Anwendung. Steinkopff Verlag, Darmstadt, S 81-91.

Further information in:

Hänsel R, Keller K, Rimpler H, Schneider G (Hrsg.), Hagers Handbuch der Pharmazeutischen Praxis, 5. Aufl., Bde 4-6 (Drogen): Springer Verlag Berlin, Heidelberg, New York, 1992-1994.

Lewin L, Gifte und Vergiftungen, 6. Aufl., Nachdruck, Haug Verlag, Heidelberg 1992.

Madaus G, Lehrbuch der Biologischen Arzneimittel, Bde 1-3, Nachdruck, Georg Olms Verlag Hildesheim 1979.

Schulz R, Hänsel R, Rationale Phytotherapie, Springer Verlag Heidelberg 1996.

Steinegger E, Hänsel R, Pharmakognosie, 5. Aufl., Springer Verlag Heidelberg 1992.

Teuscher E, Biogene Arzneimittel, 5. Aufl., Wiss. Verlagsges. Stuttgart 1997.

Wagner H, Wiesenauer M, Phytotherapie. Phytopharmaka und pflanzliche Homöopathika, Fischer-Verlag, Stuttgart, Jena, New York 1995.

Vitis Vinifera

Grape

DESCRIPTION

Medicinal Parts: The medicinal parts are the leaves, the fruit and the juice.

Flower and Fruit: The flowers are in compound compact panicles. The petals are about 5 mm long and droop like the sepals. The fruit is oblong to globular, 6 to 22 mm long, dark blue-violet, red, green or yellow, juicy, sweet or sour. The seeds are pear-shaped, with hard skin and two long dimples on the side.

Leaves, Stem and Root: The vine is a 30 cm high climber with deep, heavily-branched roots and a woody trunk. The trunk has striped, loose bark. The brown-red to brown-yellow branches are glabrous or slightly downy and finely grooved. The leaves are orbicular, generally in 3 to 5 lobes or blades. They are deeply notched at the stem. The upper surface of the leaves is glabrous, the under surface is lanate.

Habitat: The plant is indigenous to southern Europe and western Asia and is cultivated today in all temperate regions of the world.

Production: Vine leaves are the foliage leaves of Vitis vinifera.

ACTIONS AND PHARMACOLOGY

COMPOUNDS

Flavonoids (4%): including, among others, kaempferol-3-O-glucosides, quercetin-3-O-glucosides

Tannins

Fruit acids: including, among others, tartaric acid, malic acid, succinic acid, citric acid, oxalic acid

Phenylacrylic acid derivatives: p-cumaroyl-, caffeoyl-, feruloylsuccinic acid

EFFECTS

The flavonoid in the leaves has an anti-inflammatory and ''phlebitis'' effect.

INDICATIONS AND USAGE

Grape preparations are used in venous diseases and blood circulation disorders.

PRECAUTIONS AND ADVERSE REACTIONS

No health hazards or side effects are known in conjunction with the proper administration of designated therapeutic dosages.

DOSAGE

Mode of Administration: A preparation called Antistax® (available in capsules, drops and cream) is used as an antivaricose treatment. It contains a form of flavonoid from standardized vine leaf extract and aesculin. Additionally, there are capsules, of which V. viniferae is an ingredient.

LITERATURE

Kern W, List PH, Hörhammer L (Hrsg.), Hagers Handbuch der Pharmazeutischen Praxis, 4. Aufl., Bde 1-8: Springer Verlag Berlin, Heidelberg, New York, 1969.

Wafer Ash

See Ptelea Trifoliata

Wahoo Root Bark

See Euonymus Atropurpureus

Wallflower

See Cheiranthus Cheiri

Walnut

See Juglans Regia

Water Avens

See Geum Rivale

Water Dock

See Rumex Aquaticus

Water Dropwort

See Oenanthe Crocata

Water Fennel

See Oenanthe Aquatica

Water Germander
See Teucrium Scordium

Water Plantain
See Alisma Plantago-Aquatica

Watercress
See Nasturtium Officinale

Wax Myrtle
See Myrica Cerifera

White Bryony
See Bryonia Alba

White Dead Nettle
See Lamium Album

White Hellebore
See Veratrum Album

White Horehound
See Marrubium Vulgare

White Lily
See Lilium Candidium

White Willow
See Salix Species

Wild Daisy
See Bellis Perennis

Wild Indigo
See Baptisia Tinctoria

Wild Lettuce
See Lactuca Virosa

Wild Mint
See Mentha Aquatica

Wild Radish
See Raphanus Raphanistrum

Wild Thyme
See Thymus Serpyllum

Wild Yam
See Dioscorea Villosa

Willow Herb
See Epilobium Species

Winter Cherry
See Physalis Alkekengi

Winter's Bark
See Drimys Winteri

Wintergreen

See Gaultheria Procumbens; Pyrola Rotundifolia

Witch Hazel

See Hamamelis Virginiana

Wood Anemone

See Anemone Nemorosa

Wood Betony

See Betonica Officinalis

Wood Sage

See Teucrium Scorodonia

Wood Sorrel

See Oxalis Acetosella

Woodruff

See Galium Odorata

Wormseed

See Artemisia Cina

Wormseed Oil

See Chenopodium Ambrosioides

Wormwood

See Artemisia Absinthium

Woundwort

See Anthyllis Vulneraria; Stachys Palustris

Xysmalobium Undulatum

Uzara

DESCRIPTION

Medicinal Parts: Different varieties of Pachycarpus and Xysmalobium are used for drug extraction depending on the area. The drug is therefore easier to categorize according to its definitive active substances (bitters) than to its particular varieties.

Flower and Fruit: The root has a weak and unusual odor. The taste is bitter with a burning effect after it has been chewed for a long time.

Habitat: South Africa.

Production: Uzara root consists of the dried, underground parts of 2 to 3 year old plants of Xysmalobium undulatum.

ACTIONS AND PHARMACOLOGY

COMPOUNDS

Cardioactive steroid glycosides (cardenolides, mixture referred to as uzarone or xysmalobin): including, among others, uzarin, xysmalorin, urezin, uzaroside, ascleposide

Pregnane derivatives

EFFECTS

Inhibits intestinal motility. In high dosage, Uzara has digitalis-like effects on the heart.

INDICATIONS AND USAGE

■ Diarrhea

Used traditionally in indigenous folk medicine as a treatment for diarrhea and dysentery.

CONTRAINDICATIONS

Uzara should not be administered concomitantly with other cardioactive glycosides.

PRECAUTIONS AND ADVERSE REACTIONS

No health hazards or side effects are known in conjunction with the proper administration of designated therapeutic dosages.

OVERDOSAGE

Because the glycosides are absorbed only with difficulty and because their cardiac effect is minimal, poisonings following oral intake are unlikely, although conceivable. There have been cases of fatalities following parenteral application of Uzara drugs.

DOSAGE

Mode of Administration: The drug is available as ethanol-water extracts in liquid form, or as dry extracts obtained from methanol-water extractions for internal use.

Daily Dose: Initial single dosage, preparations equivalent to 1 g herb or 75 mg total glycosides. Daily dosage equivalent from 45 to 90 mg of total glycosides, calculated as uzarin.

LITERATURE

Pauli G, Schiller H, Asymmetric key position in uzara steroids. In: PM 62, Abstracts of the 44th Ann Congress of GA, 113. 1996.

Schmidt M, Uzarawurzel. In: PTA 8(6):498. 1994.

Further information in:

Kern W, List PH, Hörhammer L (Hrsg.), Hagers Handbuch der Pharmazeutischen Praxis, 4. Aufl., Bde. 1-8: Springer Verlag Berlin, Heidelberg, New York, 1969.

Madaus G, Lehrbuch der Biologischen Arzneimittel, Bde 1-3, Nachdruck, Georg Olms Verlag Hildesheim 1979 (unter Gomphocarpus).

Roth L, Daunderer M, Kormann K, Giftpflanzen, Pflanzengifte, 4. Aufl., Ecomed Fachverlag Landsberg Lech 1993.

Steinegger E, Hänsel R, Pharmakognosie, 5. Aufl., Springer Verlag Heidelberg 1992.

Wagner H, Wiesenauer M, Phytotherapie. Phytopharmaka und pflanzliche Homöopathika, Fischer-Verlag, Stuttgart, Jena, New York 1995.

Yarrow

See Achillea Millefolium

Yellow Dock

See Rumex Crispus

Yellow Gentian

See Gentiana Lutea

Yellow Jessamine

See Gelsemium Sempervirens

Yellow Lupin

See Lupinus Luteus

Yellow Toadflax

See Linaria Vulgaris

Yerba Santa

See Eriodictyon Californicum

Yew

See Taxus Baccata

Yohimbe Bark

See Pausinystalia Yohimbe

Yucca Filamentosa

Adam's Needle

DESCRIPTION

Medicinal Parts: The medicinal parts are the leaves and the roots of non-flowering plants.

Flower and Fruit: The flowers are ivory-colored and are located in nodding, many-blossomed terminal panicles. The perigone is simple, campanulate, tinged greenish on the outside and has 6 tepals. The flower has 6 stamens and the stigma is 3-sectioned.

Leaves, Stem and Root: The plant is 120 to 240 cm in height. The leaves are in a basal rosette. They are sword-shaped and erect with a recurved tip. They are short-thorned, broadly grooved and covered on the margin with long, twisted, whitish or yellowish threads.

Habitat: The plant is indigenous to the southern states of the U.S. and is cultivated mainly as an ornamental plant in Europe.

Production: Adam's Needle leaves are the leaves of Yucca filamentosa.

ACTIONS AND PHARMACOLOGY

COMPOUNDS

Steroid saponins: aglycones including among others gitogenin, tigogenin

EFFECTS

No information is available.

INDICATIONS AND USAGE

The plant is used for liver and gallbladder disorders.

PRECAUTIONS AND ADVERSE REACTIONS

No health hazards or side effects are known in conjunction with the proper administration of designated therapeutic dosages. Intake can lead to stomach complaints because of the saponin content.

DOSAGE

Mode of Administration: Adam's Needle is available in ground form and in extracts.

LITERATURE

Kern W, List PH, Hörhammer L (Hrsg.), Hagers Handbuch der Pharmazeutischen Praxis, 4. Aufl., Bde. 1-8: Springer Verlag Berlin, Heidelberg, New York, 1969.

Madaus G, Lehrbuch der Biologischen Arzneimittel, Bde 1-3, Nachdruck, Georg Olms Verlag Hildesheim 1979.

Zanthoxylum Americanum

Prickly Ash

DESCRIPTION

Medicinal Parts: The medicinal parts are the root bark and the berries.

Flower and Fruit: The greenish-yellow flowers are in terminal umbels. The fruit is black or deep blue and enclosed in a gray shell.

Leaves, Stem and Root: The plant is an aromatic shrub or small tree up to 3 m tall. The branches are alternate and the leaves pinnatifid. The bark and the petioles are covered in sharp spines about 5 mm long. The bark is brownish gray on the outside and faintly furrowed with whitish patches and flattened spines that are about 5 mm long.

Characteristics: The leaves and berries have an aromatic lemon-like fragrance and the bark has a pungent, acrid taste.

Habitat: The plant grows in North America.

Other Names: Toothache Tree, Yellow Wood, Suterberry

ACTIONS AND PHARMACOLOGY

COMPOUNDS

Pyranocoumarins: xanthoxyletin (xanthoxyloin)

Isoquinoline alkaloids: berberine, N-methyl-isocorydin

Volatile oil

Resins

EFFECTS

Anti-inflammatory, anti-rheumatic, diaphoretic, and circulatory stimulant.

INDICATIONS AND USAGE

Prickly Ash is used for low blood pressure, rheumatic disorders, fever and inflammation.

PRECAUTIONS AND ADVERSE REACTIONS

No health hazards or side effects are known in conjunction with the proper administration of designated therapeutic dosages.

DOSAGE

Mode of Administration: Liquid extract, in preparations and in combinations.

LITERATURE

Fish F et al., (1975) Lloydia 38:268.

Fish F, Waterman PG (1973) J Pharm Pharmac. 25S, 115.

Further information in:

Kern W, List PH, Hörhammer L (Hrsg.), Hagers Handbuch der Pharmazeutischen Praxis, 4. Aufl., Bde 1-8: Springer Verlag Berlin, Heidelberg, New York, 1969.

Leung AY, Encyclopedia of Common Natural Ingredients Used in Food Drugs, Cosmetics, John Wiley & Sons Inc., New York 1980.

Madaus G, Lehrbuch der Biologischen Arzneimittel, Bde 1-3, Nachdruck, Georg Olms Verlag Hildesheim 1979.

Oliver-Bever B (Ed.), Medicinal Plants of Tropical West Africa, Cambridge University Press, Cambrigde 1986.

Roth L, Daunderer M, Kormann K, Giftpflanzen, Pflanzengifte, 4. Aufl., Ecomed Fachverlag Landsberg Lech 1993.

Zea Mays

Maize

DESCRIPTION

Medicinal Parts: The medicinal part is the seed.

Flower and Fruit: The plant is monoecious. The male flowers form terminal racemes of spikes with 2-flowered husks. The female flowers are axillary. The spikes are at varying distances from the ground and are enclosed in a number of thin leaves, the sheath-like maize husk. The spikes consist of a cylindrical substance, the cob, on which the seeds are arranged in 8 rows of 40 or more. Single whitish-green threads of a silky appearance grow from the eyes of the seeds and hang outside the husk where they catch the pollen. The maize seeds are usually yellow but can be darker to almost black.

Leaves, Stem and Root: The plant is 1 to 3 m high and sturdy with a solid stem covered in alternate, over 4 cm wide, linear leaves.

Habitat: The plant is indigenous to America and is cultivated all over the world as green fodder or as a cereal crop.

Production: Corn Silk flowers are the styles and stigmas of Zea mays. The styles of the female flowers, as they begin to grow out of the pillow-lace, are gathered for medicinal or therapeutic purposes. They are removed by hand and dried in the shade.

Other Names: Indian Corn, Corn Silk, Stigmata maydis

ACTIONS AND PHARMACOLOGY

COMPOUNDS

Volatile oil (0.2%): including among others carvacrol, alpha-terpineol, menthol, thymol

Flavonoids: including among others maysin, maysin-3′-methyl ether

Bitter substances

Saponins (2-3%)

Tannins: mainly probably proanthocyanidins

Sterols: including among others beta-sitosterol, ergosterol

Alkaloids (0.05%)

6-methoxybenzoxazolinone

Fatty oil (2%)

EFFECTS

The active agents are saponin, essential oil and tannin. Maize stimulates the cardiac muscles, increases blood pressure, acts as a diuretic and sedates the digestive tract.

INDICATIONS AND USAGE

Maize is used for disorders of the urinary tract, and is also used in Chinese medicine in the treatment of liver disorders.

PRECAUTIONS AND ADVERSE REACTIONS

No health hazards or side effects are known in conjunction with the proper administration of designated therapeutic dosages.

DOSAGE

Mode of Administration: Liquid extract, in medicinal preparations and combinations.

Preparation: Prepare an infusion using two teaspoons of the drug per cup of water. A tincture is prepared by adding 20 g of drug to 100 ml of 20% alcohol (set for 5 days).

Daily Dose: Drink 1 cup of infusion every other day. Take 2 to 3 teaspoons of tincture per day.

LITERATURE

Hahn SJ, (1973) K'at'ollick Taehak Uihak Nonmun J 25:127 (via [5]).

Further information in:

Chan H, But P, Pharmacology, Applications of Chinese Materia Medica, Vol 1, World Scientific Singapore 1986.

Hegnauer R, Chemotaxonomie der Pflanzen, Bde 1-11: Birkhäuser Verlag Basel, Boston, Berlin 1962-1997.

Kern W, List PH, Hörhammer L (Hrsg.), Hagers Handbuch der Pharmazeutischen Praxis, 4. Aufl., Bde 1-8: Springer Verlag Berlin, Heidelberg, New York, 1969.

Leung AY, Encyclopedia of Common Natural Ingredients Used in Food Drugs, Cosmetics, John Wiley & Sons Inc., New York 1980.

Madaus G, Lehrbuch der Biologischen Arzneimittel, Bde 1-3, Nachdruck, Georg Olms Verlag Hildesheim 1979.

Paris F, Schauenberg P, Guide des Plantes Medicinales, Delachaux et Niestle Switzerland 1969.

Zedoary

See Curcuma Zedoaria

Zingiber Officinale

Ginger

DESCRIPTION

Medicinal Parts: The medicinal part is the root.

Flower and Fruit: The flower scape grows directly from the root and terminates in a long, curved spike. A white or yellow flower grows from each spike.

Leaves, Stem and Root: Ginger is a creeping perennial on a thick tuberous rhizome, which spreads underground. In the first year, a green, erect, reed-like stem about 60 cm high grows from this rhizome. The plant has narrow, lanceolate to linear-lanceolate leaves 15 to 30 cm long, which die off each year.

Characteristics: The fracture is short and fibrous. The odor and taste are characteristic, aromatic and pungent.

Habitat: The plant is indigenous to southeastern Asia, and is cultivated in the U.S., India, China, West Indies and tropical regions.

Production: Ginger root consists of the peeled, finger-long, fresh or dried rhizome of Zingiber officinale.

ACTIONS AND PHARMACOLOGY

COMPOUNDS

Volatile oil (2.5-4.0%): chief components vary greatly, depending upon country of origin: (-)-zingiberene and ar-curcumene, beta-bisabolene and ar-curcumene, neral and geranial, D-camphor, beta-phellandrene, geranial, neral and linalool, (E)-alpha-farnesene, important as aroma carrier zingiberol (mixture of cis- and trans-beta-eudesmol)

Arylalkane (pungent substances)

Gingerols: chief components [6]-gingerol, [8]-gingerol, [10]-gingerol

Shogaols: chief components [6]-shogaol, [8]- shogaol, [10]-shogaol

Gingerdiols

Diarylheptanoids: including, among others, gingerenone A and B

EFFECTS

Ginger is positively inotropic. It also promotes secretion of saliva and gastric juices, and is a cholagogue. In animals it acts as an antispasmodic. In humans it increase the tone and peristalsis of the intestines. Ginger was shown to be an antiemetic in clinical trials.

INDICATIONS AND USAGE

- Loss of appetite
- Travel sickness

Ginger is also used for loss of appetite, dyspepsia, prevention of motion sickness, and as a digestive for subacidic gastritis. In folk medicine, Ginger is used as a carminative, expectorant, and astringent.

CONTRAINDICATIONS

Ginger is contraindicated in morning sickness. Because of its cholagogic effect, the drug should not be taken in the presence of gallstone conditions except after consultation with a doctor.

PRECAUTIONS AND ADVERSE REACTIONS

No health hazards or side effects are known in conjunction with the proper administration of designated therapeutic dosages.

DOSAGE

Mode of Administration: Comminuted rhizome and dry extracts for teas and other galenic preparations for internal use. The powdered drug is used in some stomach preparations.

Preparation: To prepare an infusion, pour boiling water over 0.5 to 1 g drug and strain after 5 minutes (1 teaspoonful = 3 g drug).

Daily Dose: The total daily dose of the drug is 2 to 4 g. The antiemetic dose is 2 g of the freshly powdered drug taken with some liquid.

LITERATURE

Chen CC, Ho CT, J Agric Food Chem 36:322. 1988.

Denyer CV, Jackson P, Loakes DM, Isolation of antirhinoviral sesquiterpenes from ginger (Zingiber officinale). In: JNP 57(5):658-662. 1994.

Erler J et al., Z Lebensm Unters Forsch 186:231. 1988.

Fintelmann V, Phytopharmaka in der Gastroenterologie. In: ZPT 15(3):137. 1994.

Gujral S et al., (1978) Nutr Rep Int 17:183.

Harvey DJ, J Chromatogr 212:75. 1981.

Hikino H, In: Economic, Medicinal Plant Research, Vol. 1, Acadamic Press UK 1985.

Kasahara Y, Hikino H, (1983) Shoyakugaku Zasshi 37:73.

Kawai T et al., Anti-emtic principles of Magnolia obovata bark and Zingiber officinale rhizome. In: PM 60:17. 1994.

Kikuchi F et al., (1982) Chem Pharm Bull 30. 754.

Kikuzaki H, Kobayashi M, Nakatani N, Constituents of Zingiberaceae. 4. Diarylheptanoids from Rhizomes of Zingiber officinale. In: PH 30: 3947. 1991.

Kikuzaki H, Kobayashi M, Nakatani N, Diarylheptanoids from rhizomes of Zingiber officinale. In: PH 30(11):3647-3651. 1991.

Kikuzaki H, Tsai SM, Nakatani N, Gingerdiol related compounds from the rhizomes of Zingiber officinale. In: PH 31(5):1783-1786. 1992.

Marles RJ, Kaminski J, Arnason JT, Pazos-Sanou L, Heptinstall S, Fischer NH, Crompton CW, Kindack DG, A bioassay for inhibition of serotonin release from bovine platelets. In: JNP 55:1044-1056. 1992.

Mikawa U et al., Delayed-type allergy-controlling agents containing gingerones. In: Patent Jap. 1988.

Mowrey DB, Clayson DE, (1982) Lancet II, 655.

Nagabhushan M, Amonkar AJ, Bhide SV, Mutagenicity of gingerol and shoagol and antimutagenicity in zingerone in Salmonella/microsme assay. In: Cancer-Lett (Shannon Irel) 36(2)221-233. 1987.

Narasimhan S, Govinarajan VS, (1978) J Food Tech 13:31.

Saller R, Hellenbrecht D, Zingiber officinale. In: Tägl Praxis 33(3):629. 1992.

Suekawa M et al., (1984) J Pharmacobio-Dyn 7 (11):836.

Sugaya A et al., (1975) Shoyakugaku Zasshi 29:160.

Further information in:

Chan H, But P, Pharmacology, Applications of Chinese Materia Medica, Vol 1, World Scientific Singapore 1986.

Kern W, List PH, Hörhammer L (Hrsg.), Hagers Handbuch der Pharmazeutischen Praxis, 4. Aufl., Bde 1-8: Springer Verlag Berlin, Heidelberg, New York, 1969.

Leung AY, Encyclopedia of Common Natural Ingredients Used in Food Drugs, Cosmetics, John Wiley & Sons Inc., New York 1980.

Madaus G, Lehrbuch der Biologischen Arzneimittel, Bde 1-3, Nachdruck, Georg Olms Verlag Hildesheim 1979.

Roth L, Daunderer M, Kormann K: Giftpflanzen, Pflanzengifte, 4. Aufl., Ecomed Fachverlag Landsberg Lech 1993.

Steinegger E, Hänsel R, Pharmakognosie, 5. Aufl., Springer Verlag Heidelberg 1992.

Teuscher E, Biogene Arzneimittel, 5. Aufl., Wiss. Verlagsges. Stuttgart 1997.

Wagner H, Wiesenauer M, Phytotherapie. Phytopharmaka und pflanzliche Homöopathika, Fischer-Verlag, Stuttgart, Jena, New York 1995.

Wichtl M (Hrsg.), Teedrogen, 4. Aufl., Wiss. Verlagsges. Stuttgart 1997.

Zyzyphus Jujube

Jujube

DESCRIPTION

Medicinal Parts: The medicinal part is the fruit. The Jujube berry is classed with raisins, dates and figs, and can be eaten fresh or dried.

Flower and Fruit: The flowers are small, pale yellow and solitary. The fruit is of variable size, depending on the origin, but is usually up to 3 cm long and 1.5 cm in diameter. The fruit is red, smooth and shiny when fresh, brownish-red and grooved when dried. It is pulpy and contains 1 or 2 acute, oblong seeds.

Characteristics: The taste of the fruit is sweet and mucilaginous.

Habitat: The plant grows in southern Europe, Africa, Middle East and the Far East.

Production: Jujube berries are the fruit of Zyzyphus jujube; Zyzyphus vulgaris is also used.

ACTIONS AND PHARMACOLOGY

COMPOUNDS

Triterpene saponins: zyzyphus saponins I, II and III, jujuboside-B, in the seeds jujuboside-A and -B, aglycone jujubogenine

Mucilage

Tannins (10%)

Flavonoids: including among others naringenin-6,8-di-C-glucosides, in the seeds spinosin (C-glycoflavone)

Isoquinoline alkaloids: oxonuciferin, nornuciferin

Peptide alkaloids: daechucyclopeptide, daechualkaloid-A

Triterpenes: betulinic acid, betulonic acid, maslinic acid, alphitolic acid and oleanolic acid

Hydroxycoumarins

Sugars: including, among others, saccharose, glucose, fructose, galactose

Fruit acids: including, among others, malic acid, tartaric acid

EFFECTS

Jujube is emollient, anti-allergenic, and sedative. Zyzyphus vulgaris also has a hypotensive effect.

INDICATIONS AND USAGE

Jujube is used as a nutrient to improve muscular strength and in the prophylaxis of liver disease and stress ulcers.

PRECAUTIONS AND ADVERSE REACTIONS

No health hazards or side effects are known in conjunction with the proper administration of designated therapeutic dosages.

DOSAGE

Mode of Administration: The drug is no longer in use.

LITERATURE

Ahn YS et al., (1982) Korean J Pharmacol 18 (1):17.

Cyong J et al., (1979) Proc Symp. Wakan-Yaku 12:1.

Cyong J, Hanabusa K, (1980) Phytochemistry 19:2747.

Cyong J, Takahashi, M, (1982) Chem Pharm Bull 30:1081.

Hikino H, In: Economic, Medicinal Plant Research, Vol. 1, Acadamic Press UK 1985.

Ikram M et al., (1981) J Nat Prod 44:91.

Inoue O et al., (1978) J Chem Res 144.

Okamura N et al., (1981) Chem Pharm Bull 29:676, 3507.

Shibata S et al., (1970) Phytochemistry 9:677.

Woo WS et al., (1979) Phytochemistry 18:353.

Yagi A et al., (1978) Chem Pharm Bull 26:1798.

Further information in:

Hegnauer R, Chemotaxonomie der Pflanzen, Bde 1-11: Birkhäuser Verlag Basel, Boston, Berlin 1962-1997.

Kern W, List PH, Hörhammer L (Hrsg.), Hagers Handbuch der Pharmazeutischen Praxis, 4. Aufl., Bde 1-8: Springer Verlag Berlin, Heidelberg, New York, 1969.

Wagner H, Wiesenauer M, Phytotherapie. Phytopharmaka und pflanzliche Homöopathika, Fischer-Verlag, Stuttgart, Jena, New York 1995.

Wichtl M (Hrsg.), Teedrogen, 4. Aufl., Wiss. Verlagsges. Stuttgart 1997.

Glossary

abortifacient A drug or chemical that induces abortion.

achene A small 1-seeded fruit which has a pericarp attached to the seed at only one point.

acuminate Pointed, or tapering to a slender point.

adaptogen A preparation that acts to strengthen the body and increase resistance to disease.

alterative Any drug used to favorably alter the course of an ailment and to restore health. To improve the excretion of wastes from the circulatory system.

amarum Bitters.

androgynous In botany, flowers with stamen and pistil in the same bunch.

annual A plant that completes its growth cycle in one year.

anthelmintic An agent or drug that is destructive to worms.

anther The part of the stamen that contains pollen.

antiphlogistic An agent that prevents or counteracts inflammation and fever.

antisialagogue An agent that prevents or counteracts the formation or flow of saliva.

autumnalis In botany, referring to producing, gathering, or harvesting in the autumn.

bitter An alcoholic liquid prepared by maceration or distillation of a bitter herb or herb part that is often used to improve appetite or digestion.

blood purification Removal of undesirable agents from the blood.

bracteole A small leaf arising from the floral axis.

brightening agent A substance added to the active constituents.

calculosis The condition or formation of calculi.

calyx The outer set of floral leaves consisting of fused or separate sepals.

campanulate Shaped like a bell.

capitulum A rounded or flattened cluster of sessile flowers.

capsule A closed container that contains seeds or spores.

carminative An aid to relieve gas from the alimentary canal. An agent that acts to relieve colic.

carpel A small pistil or seed vessel comprising the innermost whorl of a flower.

cataplasm A poultice or soft external application.

catarrh An inflammation of the air passages usually involving the nose, throat, or lungs.

catkin A cattail-like inflorescence bearing scaly bracts.

cauline Growing on the upper portion of a stem.

cholagogue An agent that stimulates the flow of bile from the gallbladder to the duodenum.

choleretic An agent that stimulates the production of bile by the liver.

climacteric The syndrome of physical and psychic changes that occur during the transition to menopause.

comminuted To break or crush into small pieces.

cordate A heart-shaped leaf.

coriaceous Tough, strong, and leather-like.

corolla The inner set of floral leaves that consist of separate or fused leaves.

cortex In botany, the bark of a tree or the rind of a fruit.

cotyledon A seed leaf, or the first set of leaves from the embryo in seed plants.

crenate In reference to leaf structure, having a margin cut into rounded scallops.

cyme An inflorescence where the axes always end in a single flower.

DAB Deutsches Arzneibuch (German Pharmacopoeia)

deciduous A tree that sheds its leaves at the end of the growing season.

decoction A liquid substance prepared by boiling plant parts in water or some other liquid for a period of time.

decumbent A plant, stem, or shoot that lays on the ground but terminates with an ascending apex.

dentate Tooth-like projections on the margin of a leaf.

dessertspoon A unit of measure equal to about 2½ fluidrams.

diaphoretic An agent that causes sweating or excessive perspiration.

dioecious In botany, when a plant has either a stamen or a pistil on each flower.

downy Covered with soft hairs.

dromotropic An effect on nerve fiber conduction.

dropsy An abnormal accumulation of fluid in body tissues or cavities usually related to an underlying disease.

drupe A one-seeded fruit; as in an olive or a peach.

embrocation An external medication applied as a liniment or other liquid form.

emmenagogue A substance that renews or stimulates the menstrual flow.

endosperm The albumin of the seed.

epicalyx An external accessory calyx located outside the true calyx of the flower.

eructation The act of belching.

exocarp The outer wall of a fruit covering.

extraction The portion of a plant that is removed by solvents and used in drug preparations in solid or liquid form.

febrifuge An agent that counteracts fever; an antipyretic.

floret A little flower; one of the small individual flowers that form a cluster or head.

flos Flower.

fluidextract A hydroalcoholic preparation of a botanical drug where 1 ml of the preparation contains 1 gm of the standard botanical.

folium The leaf of a plant.

fructus Fruit.

furuncle A boil or sore caused by bacterial infection of the subcutaneous tissue.

galenic preparation Medications prepared from plants as opposed to refined chemicals.

glabrous Having a smooth surface; without hair or down.

globular Spherical.

hastate Plant leaves with a triangular shape with the base coming together on each side into an acute lobe.

hilum The scar on a seed which indicates its point of attachment.

homeopathic Substances that are administered in minute amounts with the theory that substances that may cause or mimic a disease in larger amounts can be used to treat or prevent disease if given in small amounts.

imbricate Overlapping flower petals; as in the bud.

indehiscent A fruit or grain that doesn't open spontaneously when ripe.

induration The process of hardening.

inflorescence The mode of disposition of flowers or the act of flowering. The spatial arrangement of flowers along the axis.

infusion The process of steeping or soaking plant matter in a liquid to extract its medicinal properties without boiling.

involucre A ring or rosette of leaves that surround the base of a flower cluster.

labiate A lip-like part of a plant; like a calyx or corolla.

lanceolate Lance-like or spear shaped; often referring to a long, tapering leaf.

lignum Woody tissue.

maceration The softening of a solid preparation by soaking it in a liquid.

meteorism The presence of gas in the intestine or stomach.

monoecious Having stamens and pistils in separate blossoms on the same plant.

mucilage 1. A viscid substance in a plant consisting of a gum dissolved in the juice of the plant. 2. A soothing application made from plant gums.

muscarinic An effect characterized by contraction of smooth muscle, excessive salivation and perspiration, abdominal colic and excessive bronchial secretion.

nutlet The stone in a drupe.

NYHA New York Heart Association.

obstipation Persistent or intractable constipation.

panicle A loose, multiple flower cluster usually formed from numerous branches.

pedicel The stalk that supports a single flower in an inflorescence of flowers arranged upon a common peduncle.

peduncle A stalk that bears a flower or flower cluster.

percolation A liquid containing the soluble portion of a drug that has been filtered or separated from the plant matter.

perennial A plant that grows for three or more years.

perianth The external envelope of a flower which does not include the calyx and corolla if they are distinguishable.

pericarp The wall of the ripened ovary of a flower containing the germ of the fruit.

petal One of the leaves of the corolla.

petiolate The footstalk of a leaf.

pinnate Compound leaves or leaflets that have a feather-like arrangement with leaves arranged on both sides of a common axis.

pinnatisect Cleft pinnately or almost to the midrib.

pistil The seed-bearing organ of flowering plants consisting of the ovary and the stigma; usually with a style.

plaster A viscous substance that is spread on linen or cloth and applied to a part of the body for healing purposes.

poultice A soft, moist mass of plant parts that are wrapped in muslin or gauze and applied warm or hot to the skin.

pubescent In botany, having a fuzzy surface; covered with soft fine short hairs.

raceme An inflorescence where flowers are borne on stalks at an almost equal distance apart along an elongated axis that continues to grow with flowers opening in succession from below.

radix The root of a plant.

reniform When describing a leaf, kidney or bean shaped.

resin An amorphous, solid or semi-solid substance produced by plants usually as a result of terpene oxidation.

reticulate Veins, fibers, or lines crossing like a network across the surface of a leaf.

rhizome An underground stem.

roborant A tonic or substance that gives strength.

runners A plant that spreads or forms by means of runners.

scape A flower stalk or peduncle arising from the surface or from below the ground.

schizocarp A dry fruit that splits at maturity into several one-seeded carpels.

scrofulous Having an ulcerous or diseased appearance on the surface.

secretagogue An agent that promotes secretion.

secretolytic To inhibit or dry secretions.

semen A seed or seed-like fruit.

sepal One of the modified leaves comprising a calyx; usually positioned outside and surrounding the carpels.

serrate Having notched, teeth-like protrusions along the margin of a leaf that points toward the apex.

sessile Attached directly to the base of a main stem or branch without the aid of an intervening stalk.

stamen The organ of the flower that comprises the anther and filament and gives rise to the male gamete.

stipule A stalk.

stomachic An agent that promotes digestion and improves appetite.

subshrub A perennial plant which has woody stems with the exception of the terminal portion of new growth, which drops off annually.

sudorific Causing or inducing sweat.

tendril The portion of a stem, leaf, or stipule that modified into a slender, spiral-shaped, touch-sensitive specialized appendage, which acts as an anchor to aid in the plants ability to climb.

tepal Any of the modified leaves that combine to make up the perianth.

testa The hard outer coating of a seed; the exocarp.

tincture An alcoholic or hydroalcoholic mixture prepared from plant parts.

tomentose Covered with densely matted hairs.

tonic A medication used to fortify and provide increased vigor.

turiones A shoot or sprout which develops from a bud on a subterranean rootstock.

umbel Numerous flower stalks arising from the same point at the apex of the main stalk and terminating at an equal distance from the joining point.

undulate A wavy formation at the margin of a leaf, or bending in a gradual curve.

villous Having long, soft hairs.

vulnery A preparation applied externally.

wineglassful A measure equal to four fluidounces.

Poison Control Centers

Many of the centers listed below are certified by the American Association of Poison Control Centers. Certified centers are marked by an asterisk after the name. Each has to meet certain criteria. It must, for example, serve a large geographic area; it must be open 24 hours a day and provide direct-dial or toll-free access; it must be supervised by a medical director; and it must have registered pharmacists or nurses available to answer questions from the public.

The centers have a wide variety of toxicology resources, including a computerized database of some 750,000 substances maintained by MICROMEDEX, INC., an affiliate of PDR. Staff members are trained to resolve toxic situations in the home of the caller, though hospital referrals are given in some instances. The centers also offer a range of educational services to both the public and healthcare professionals. In some states, these larger centers exist side by side with smaller centers offering a more limited range of services.

Within each state, centers are listed alphabetically by city. Telephone numbers designated "TTY" are teletype lines for the hearing-impaired. "TDD" numbers reach a telecommunication device for the deaf.

ALABAMA

BIRMINGHAM

Regional Poison Control Center,
The Children's Hospital of Alabama (*)
1600 7th Ave. South
Birmingham, AL 35233-1711
Business: 205-939-9720
Emergency: 205-933-4050
205-939-9201
800-292-6678 (AL)
Fax: 205-939-9245

TUSCALOOSA

Alabama Poison Center, Tuscaloosa (*)
2503 Phoenix Dr.
Tuscaloosa, AL 35405
Business: 205-345-0600
Emergency: 205-345-0600
800-462-0800 (AL)
Fax: 205-759-7994

ALASKA

ANCHORAGE

Anchorage Poison Center,
Providence Hospital
P.O. Box 196604
3200 Providence Dr.
Anchorage, AK 99519-6604
Business: 907-562-2211
ext. 3633
Emergency: 907-261-3193
800-478-3193 (AK)
Fax: 907-261-3645

FAIRBANKS

Fairbanks Poison Control Center
1650 Cowles St.
Fairbanks, AK 99701
Business: 907-456-7182
Emergency: 907-456-7182
Fax: 907-458-5553

ARIZONA

PHOENIX

Samaritan Regional Poison Center (*)
Good Samaritan Regional Medical Center
Ancillary-1
1111 East McDowell Rd.
Phoenix, AZ 85006
Business: 602-495-4884
Emergency: 602-253-3334
800-362-0101 (AZ)
Fax: 602-256-7579

TUCSON

Arizona Poison and Drug Information Center (*)
Arizona Health Sciences Center
1501 North Campbell Ave.
Rm. #1156
Tucson, AZ 85724
Emergency: 520-626-6016
800-322-0101 (AZ)
Fax: 520-626-2720

ARKANSAS

LITTLE ROCK

Arkansas Poison and Drug Information Center,
College of Pharmacy - UAMS
4301 West Markham St.
Slot 522-2
Little Rock, AR 72205
Business: 501-661-6161
Emergency: 800-376-4766 (AR)

CALIFORNIA

FRESNO

California Poison Control System-Fresno (*)
Valley Children's Hospital
3151 North Millbrook, IN31
Fresno, CA 93703
Business: 209-241-6040
Emergency: 800-876-4766 (CA)
Fax: 209-241-6050

SACRAMENTO

California Poison Control
System-Sacramento (*)
UCDMC-HSF Room 1024
2315 Stockton Blvd.
Sacramento, CA 95817
Business: 916-734-3415
Emergency: 800-876-4766 (CA)
Fax: 916-734-7796

SAN DIEGO

California Poison Control System-San Diego (*)
UCSD Medical Center
200 West Arbor Dr.
San Diego, CA 92103-8925
Business: 619-543-3666
Emergency: 800-876-4766 (CA)
Fax: 619-692-1867

SAN FRANCISCO

San Francisco Bay Area Regional Poison Control Center,
SF General Hospital
1001 Potrero Ave.
Bldg. 80, Rm. 230
San Francisco, CA 94110
Business:
Emergency:
Fax: 415-821-8513

COLORADO

DENVER

Rocky Mountain Poison and Drug Center (*)
8802 East 9th Ave.
Denver, CO 80220-6800
Business: 303-739-1100
Emergency: 303-739-1123
800-332-3073 (CO)
Fax: 303-739-1119

CONNECTICUT

FARMINGTON

Connecticut Regional Poison Center (*)
University of Connecticut Health Center
263 Farmington Ave.
Farmington, CT 06030
Emergency: 800-343-2722 (CT)
Fax: 203-679-1623

DELAWARE

PHILADELPHIA, PA

The Poison Control Center
3600 Market St.
Suite 220
Philadelphia, PA 19104
Emergency: 800-722-7112 (PA)
215-386-2100

DISTRICT OF COLUMBIA

WASHINGTON, DC

National Capital Poison Center (*)
3201 New Mexico Ave., NW
Suite 310
Washington, DC 20016
Business: 202-362-3867
Emergency: 202-625-3333
TTY: 202-362-8563
Fax: 202-362-8377

FLORIDA

JACKSONVILLE

Florida Poison Information Center-Jacksonville (*)
University Medical Center
University of Florida Health Science Center-Jacksonville
655 W. 8th St.
Jacksonville, FL 32209
Emergency: 904-549-4480
800-282-3171 (FL)
Fax: 904-549-4063

MIAMI

Florida Poison Information Center-Miami (*)
University of Miami, School of Medicine
Department of Pediatrics
P.O. Box 016960 (R-131)
Miami, FL 33101
Emergency: 305-585-5253
800-282-3171 (FL)
Fax: 305-242-9762

TAMPA

The Florida Poison Information Center
Tampa General Hospital
P.O. Box 1289
Tampa, FL 33601
Emergency: 813-253-4444 (Tampa)
800-282-3171 (FL)
Fax: 813-253-4443

GEORGIA

ATLANTA

Georgia Poison Center (*)
Hughes Spalding Children's Hospital, Grady Health System
80 Butler St. SE
P.O. Box 26066
Atlanta, GA 30335-3801
Emergency: 404-616-9000
800-282-5846 (GA)
Fax: 404-616-6657

MACON

Regional Poison Control Center,
Medical Center of Central Georgia
777 Hemlock St.
Macon, GA 31201
Poison Ctr: 912-633-1427
Fax: 912-633-5082

IDAHO

DENVER, CO

Rocky Mountain Poison & Drug Center
8802 E. 9th Ave.
Denver, CO 80220-6800
Emergency: 800-860-0620 (ID)
303-739-1123

ILLINOIS

CHICAGO

Illinois Poison Control Center
222 South Riverside Plaza
Suite 1900
Chicago, IL 60606
Business: 312-942-7064
Emergency: 800-942-5969 (IL)
Fax: 312-803-5400

URBANA

ASPCA/National Animal Poison Control Center
1717 Philo Rd., Suite 36
Urbana, IL 61802
Business: 800-548-2423 (24-hour subscribers)
Fax: 217-337-0599

INDIANA

INDIANAPOLIS

Indiana Poison Center (*)
Methodist Hospital of Indiana
I-65 at 21st St.
Indianapolis, IN 46206-1367
Emergency: 317-929-2323
800-382-9097 (IN)
Fax: 317-929-2337

IOWA

SIOUX CITY

Iowa Poison Center
2720 Stone Park Blvd.
Sioux City, IA 51104
Business: 712-277-2222
Emergency: 800-352-2222 (IA)
Fax: 712-279-7852

KANSAS

KANSAS CITY

Mid-America Poison Control Center,
University of Kansas Medical Center
3901 Rainbow Blvd.
Room B-400
Kansas City, KS 66160-7231
Business & 913-588-6633
Emergency: 800-332-6633 (KS)
Fax: 913-588-2350

TOPEKA

Stormont-Vail Regional Medical Center Emergency Department
1500 S.W. 10th
Topeka, KS 66604-1353
Business: 913-354-6000
Emergency: 913-354-6100
Fax: 913-354-5004

KENTUCKY

LOUISVILLE

Kentucky Regional Poison Center
Medical Towers S.
Suite 572
234 E. Gray St.
Louisville, KY 40202
Business: 502-629-7264
Emergency: 502-589-8222
Fax: 502-629-7277

LOUISIANA

MONROE

Louisiana Drug and Poison Information Center (*)
Northeast Louisiana University Sugar Hall
Monroe, LA 71209-6430
Business: 318-342-1710
Emergency: 800-256-9822 (LA)
Fax: 318-342-1744

MAINE

PORTLAND

Maine Poison Center
Maine Medical Center
22 Bramhall St.
Portland, ME 04102
Business: 207-871-2950
Emergency: 800-442-6305 (ME)
Fax: 207-871-6226

MARYLAND

BALTIMORE

Maryland Poison Center (*)
20 North Pine St.
Baltimore, MD 21201
Business: 410-706-7604
Emergency: 410-706-7701
800-492-2414 (MD)
Fax: 410-706-7184

MASSACHUSETTS

BOSTON

Massachusetts Poison Control System (*)
300 Longwood Ave.
Boston, MA 02115
Emergency: 617-232-2120
800-682-9211 (MA)
Fax: 617-738-0032

MICHIGAN

DETROIT

Poison Control Center (*)
Children's Hospital of Michigan
4160 John R.,
Harper Office Bldg.
Suite 616
Detroit, MI 48201
Business: 313-745-5335
Emergency: 313-745-5711
800-764-7661 (MI)
Fax: 313-745-5493

GRAND RAPIDS

Spectrum Health Regional Poison Center (*)
1840 Wealthy SE
Grand Rapids, MI 49506-2968
Business: 616-774-5329
Emergency: 800-764-7661 (MI)
Fax: 616-774-7204

MINNESOTA

MINNEAPOLIS

Hennepin Regional Poison Center (*)
Hennepin County Medical Center
701 Park Ave.
Minneapolis, MN 55415
Business: 612-347-3144
Emergency: 800-764-7661 (MN)
612-347-3141
Fax: 612-904-4289

Minnesota Regional Poison Center (*)
8100 34th Ave. South
P.O. Box 1309
Minneapolis, MN 55440-1309
Business: 612-851-8100
Emergency: 612-221-2113
800-222-1222 (MN)
Fax: 612-851-8166

MISSISSIPPI

HATTIESBURG

Poison Center, Forrest General Hospital
400 South 28th Ave.
Hattiesburg, MS 39401
Business: 601-288-4221
Emergency: 601-288-2100

JACKSON

Mississippi Regional Poison Control, University of Mississippi Medical Center
2500 North State St.
Jackson, MS 39216
Business: 601-984-1675
Emergency: 601-354-7660
Fax: 601-984-1676

MISSOURI

KANSAS CITY

Poison Control Center, Children's Mercy Hospital
2401 Gillham Rd.
Kansas City, MO 64108
Business: 816-234-3053
Emergency: 816-234-3430
Fax: 816-234-3421

ST. LOUIS

Cardinal Glennon Children's Hospital Regional Poison Center (*)
1465 South Grand Blvd.
St. Louis, MO 63104
Emergency: 800-366-8888 (MO)
314-772-5200
Fax: 314-577-5355

MONTANA

DENVER, CO

Rocky Mountain Poison and Drug Center (*)
8802 East 9th Ave.
Denver, CO 80220-6800
Emergency: 800-525-5042 (MT)
Fax: 303-739-1119

NEBRASKA

OMAHA

The Poison Center (*)
8301 Dodge St.
Omaha, NE 68114
Emergency: 402-354-5555
(Omaha)
800-955-9119
(NE & WY)

NEVADA

DENVER, CO

Rocky Mountain Poison and Drug Center (*)
8802 East 9th Ave.
Denver, CO 80220-6800
Emergency: 800-446-6179 (NV)
303-739-1123
Fax: 303-739-1119

RENO

Poison Center, Washoe Medical Center
77 Pringle Way
Reno, NV 89520
Business: 702-328-4129
Emergency: 702-328-4129
Fax: 702-328-5555

NEW HAMPSHIRE

LEBANON

New Hampshire Poison Information Center, Dartmouth-Hitchcock Medical Center
1 Medical Center Dr.
Lebanon, NH 03756
Emergency: 603-650-5000
(ask for Poison Center)
800-562-8236 (NH)
Fax: 603-650-8986

NEW JERSEY

NEWARK

New Jersey Poison Information and Education System (*)
201 Lyons Ave.
Newark, NJ 07112
Emergency: 800-764-7661 (NJ)
Fax: 201-705-8098

PHILLIPSBURG

Warren Hospital Poison Control Center
185 Roseberry St.
Phillipsburg, NJ 08865
Business: 908-859-6768
Emergency: 908-859-6767
800-962-1253 (NJ)
Fax: 908-859-6812

NEW MEXICO

ALBUQUERQUE

New Mexico Poison and Drug Information Center (*) University of New Mexico
Health Sciences Library, Rm. 125
Albuquerque, NM 87131-1076
Emergency: 505-272-2222
800-432-6866 (NM)
Fax: 505-277-5892

NEW YORK

BUFFALO

Western New York Regional Poison Control Center Children's Hospital of Buffalo
219 Bryant St.
Buffalo, NY 14222
Business: 716-878-7657
Emergency: 716-878-7654
800-888-7655
(NY Western Regions Only)

MINEOLA

Long Island Regional Poison Control Center (*) Winthrop University Hospital
259 First St.
Mineola, NY 11501
Emergency: 516-542-2323
Fax: 516-739-2070

NEW YORK

New York City Poison Control Center (*) NYC Dept. of Health
455 First Ave., Room 123
New York, NY 10016
Business: 212-447-8154
Emergency: 212-340-4494
212-POISONS
212-447-2205
Fax: 212-447-8223

ROCHESTER

Finger Lakes Regional Poison Center (*) University of Rochester Medical Center
601 Elmwood Ave.
Box 321
Rochester, NY 14642
Business: 716-273-4155
Emergency: 716-275-3232
800-333-0542 (NY)
Fax: 716-244-1677

SLEEPY HOLLOW

Hudson Valley Regional Poison Center (*) Phelps Memorial Hospital Center
701 N. Broadway
Sleepy Hollow, NY 10590
Emergency: 914-366-3030
800-336-6997 (NY)
Fax: 914-353-1050

SYRACUSE

Central New York Poison Control Center (*) SUNY Health Science Center
750 East Adams St.
Syracuse, NY 13210
Business: 315-464-7073
Emergency: 315-476-4766
800-252-5655 (NY)
Fax: 315-464-7077

NORTH CAROLINA

ASHEVILLE

Western North Carolina Poison Control Center, Memorial Mission Hospital
509 Biltmore Ave.
Asheville, NC 28801
Emergency: 704-255-4490
800-542-4225 (NC)
Fax: 704-255-4467

CHARLOTTE

Carolinas Poison Center Carolinas Medical Center
5000 Airport Center Pkwy.
Suite B
P.O. Box 32861
Charlotte, NC 28232
Business: 704-355-3054
Emergency: 704-355-4000
800-848-6946 (NC)

NORTH DAKOTA

FARGO

North Dakota Poison Information Center, Meritcare Medical Center
720 North 4th St.
Fargo, ND 58122
Business: 701-234-6062
Emergency: 701-234-5575
800-732-2200 (ND)
Fax: 701-234-5090

OHIO

CINCINNATI

Cincinnati Drug & Poison Information Center and Regional Poison Control System (*)
2368 Victory Pkwy.
Suite 300
Cincinnati, OH 45206
Emergency: 513-558-5111
800-872-5111 (OH)
Fax: 513-558-5301

CLEVELAND

Greater Cleveland Poison Control Center
11100 Euclid Ave.
Cleveland, OH 44106
Emergency: 216-231-4455
888-231-4455
Fax: 216-844-3242

COLUMBUS

Central Ohio Poison Center (*)
700 Children's Dr.
Columbus, OH 43205-2696
Business: 614-722-2635
Emergency: 614-228-1323
800-682-7625 (OH)
Fax: 614-221-2672

Greater Dayton Area Hospital Association at Central Ohio Poison Center
700 Children's Dr.
Columbus, OH 43205
Business: 614-722-2635
Emergency: 937-222-2227
800-762-0727 (OH)

TOLEDO

Poison Information Center of NW Ohio, Medical College of Ohio Hospital
3000 Arlington Ave.
Toledo, OH 43614
Business: 419-383-3897
Emergency: 419-381-3897
800-589-3897 (OH)
Fax: 419-381-6066

OKLAHOMA

OKLAHOMA CITY

Oklahoma Poison Control Center, University of Oklahoma and Children's Hospital of Oklahoma
940 Northeast 13th St.
Oklahoma City, OK 73104
Emergency: 405-271-5454 (Bus.)
800-764-7661 (Bus.) (OK)
TDD: 405-271-1122
Fax: 405-271-1816

OREGON

PORTLAND

Oregon Poison Center (*)
Oregon Health Sciences University
3181 S.W. Sam Jackson Park Rd.
Portland, OR 97201
Emergency: 503-494-8968
800-452-7165 (OR)
Fax: 503-494-4980

PENNSYLVANIA

HERSHEY

Central Pennsylvania Poison Center (*)
University Hospital
Milton S. Hershey Medical Center
Hershey, PA 17033
Emergency: 800-521-6110 (PA)
717-531-6111
Fax: 717-531-6932

PHILADELPHIA

The Poison Control Center (*)
3600 Market St., Suite 220
Philadelphia, PA 19104-2641
Business: 215-590-2003
Emergency: 215-386-2100
800-722-7112 (PA)
Fax: 215-590-4419

PITTSBURGH

Pittsburgh Poison Center (*)
3705 Fifth Ave.
Pittsburgh, PA 15213
Business: 412-692-5600
Emergency: 412-681-6669
Fax: 412-692-7497

RHODE ISLAND

PROVIDENCE

Lifespan Poison Center
Rhode Island Hospital
593 Eddy St.
Providence, RI 02903
Emergency: 401-444-5727
Fax: 401-444-8062

SOUTH CAROLINA

COLUMBIA

Palmetto Poison Center, College of Pharmacy, University of South Carolina
Columbia, SC 29208
Business: 803-777-7909
Emergency: 803-777-1117
800-922-1117 (SC)
Fax: 803-777-6127

SOUTH DAKOTA

ABERDEEN

Poison Control Center,
St. Luke's Midland Regional Medical Center
305 South State St.
Aberdeen, SD 57401
Business: 605-622-5000
Emergency: 605-622-5100
800-592-1889 (SD, MN, ND, WY)

TENNESSEE

MEMPHIS

Southern Poison Center
875 Monroe Ave.
Suite 104
Memphis, TN 38163
Business: 901-448-6800
Emergency: 901-528-6048
800-288-9999 (TN)
Fax: 901-448-5419

NASHVILLE

Middle Tennessee Poison Center (*)
The Center for Clinical Toxicology,
Vanderbilt University Medical Center
1161 21st Ave. South
501 Oxford House
Nashville, TN 37232-4632
Business: 615-936-0760
Emergency: 615-936-2034
800-288-9999 (TN)
Fax: 615-936-2046

TEXAS

DALLAS

North Texas Poison Center (*)
5201 Harry Hines Blvd.
P.O. Box 35926
Dallas, TX 75235
Business: 214-590-6625
Emergency: 800-764-7661 (TX)
Fax: 214-590-5008

GALVESTON

Southeast Texas Poison Center (*)
The University of Texas Medical Branch
301 University Ave.
Galveston, TX 77555-1175
Emergency: 409-765-1420
800-764-7661 (TX)
Fax: 409-772-3917

TEMPLE

Central Texas Poison Center (*)
Scott & White Memorial Hospital
2401 South 31st St.
Temple, TX 76508
Business: 254-724-4636
Emergency: 800-764-7661 (TX)
254-724-7401
Fax: 254-724-1731

UTAH

SALT LAKE CITY

Utah Poison Control Center (*)
410 Chipeta Way
Suite 230
Salt Lake City, UT 84108
Emergency: 801-581-2151
800-456-7707 (UT)
Fax: 801-581-4199

VERMONT

BURLINGTON

Vermont Poison Center,
Fletcher Allen Health Care
111 Colchester Ave.
Burlington, VT 05401
Business: 802-656-2721
Emergency: 802-658-3456
Fax: 802-656-4802

VIRGINIA

CHARLOTTESVILLE

Blue Ridge Poison Center (*)
Blue Ridge University of Virginia Medical Center
Box 437
Charlottesville, VA 22908
Emergency: 804-924-5543
800-451-1428 (VA)
Fax: 804-971-8657

RICHMOND

Virginia Poison Center,
Virginia Commonwealth University
P.O. Box 980522
Richmond, VA 23298-0522
Emergency: 800-552-6337 (VA)
804-828-9123
Fax: 804-828-5291

WASHINGTON

SEATTLE

Washington Poison Center (*)
155 N.E. 100th St.
Suite 400
Seattle, WA 98125-8012
Business: 206-517-2351
Emergency: 206-526-2121
800-732-6985 (WA)
Fax: 206-526-8490

WEST VIRGINIA

CHARLESTON

West Virginia Poison Center (*)
3110 MacCorkle Ave. S.E.
Charleston, WV 25304
Business: 304-347-1212
Emergency: 304-348-4211
800-642-3625 (WV)
Fax: 304-348-9560

WISCONSIN

MADISON

Poison Control Center,
University of Wisconsin Hospital and Clinics
600 Highland Ave.
F6-133
Madison, WI 53792
Business: 608-262-7537
Emergency: 608-262-3702
800-815-8855 (WI)

MILWAUKEE

Children's Hospital Poison Center,
Children's Hospital of Wisconsin
9000 W. Wisconsin Ave.
P.O. Box 1997
Milwaukee, WI 53201
Business: 414-266-2000
Emergency: 414-266-2222
800-815-8855 (WI)
Fax: 414-266-2820

Wyoming

OMAHA, NE

The Poison Center (*)
8301 Dodge St.
Omaha, NE 68114
Emergency: 402-354-5555 (Omaha)
800-955-9119 (WY & NE)

Drug Information Centers

ALABAMA

BIRMINGHAM
Drug Information Service
University of Alabama Hospital
619 S. 20th Street
1720 Jefferson Tower
Birmingham, AL 35233-6860
Mon.-Fri. 8 AM-5 PM
Tel: 205-934-2162
Fax: 205-934-3501

Global Drug Information Center
Samford University
McWhorter School of Pharmacy
800 Lakeshore Drive
Birmingham, AL 35229-7027
Mon.-Fri. 8 AM-5 PM
Tel: 205-870-2659
Fax: 205-414-4012

HUNTSVILLE
Huntsville Hospital
Drug Information Center
101 Sivley Road
Huntsville, AL 35801
Mon.-Fri. 8 AM-5 PM
Tel: 256-517-8288
Fax: 256-517-6558

ARIZONA

TUCSON
Arizona Poison and Drug Information Center
Arizona Health Sciences Center
University Medical Center
1501 N. Campbell Ave.
Room 1156
Tucson, AZ 85724
7 days/week, 24 hours
Tel: 520-626-6016
800-362-0101 (AZ)
Fax: 520-626-2720

CALIFORNIA

LOS ANGELES
Los Angeles Regional Drug and
Poison Information Center
LAC & USC Medical Center
1200 N. State Street
Room 1107 A & B
Los Angeles, CA 90033
7 days/week, 24 hours
Tel: 213-226-2622
800-777-6476 (CA)
Fax: 213-226-4194
Poison Control Hotline:
213-222-3212

SAN DIEGO
Drug Information Analysis Service
Veterans Administration Medical Center
3350 La Jolla Village Drive
San Diego, CA 92161
Mon.-Fri. 8 AM-4:30 PM
Tel: 619-552-8585
Fax: 619-552-7582

Drug Information Center
U.S. Naval Hospital
34800 Bob Wilson Drive
San Diego, CA 92134-5000
Mon.-Fri. 8 AM-4 PM
Tel: 619-532-8414

Drug Information Service
University of California
San Diego Medical Center
135 Dickinson Street
San Diego, CA 92103-8925
Mon.-Fri. 9 AM-5 PM
Tel: 900-288-8273
619-543-6222
Fax: 619-692-1867

STANFORD
Drug Information Center
University of California
Stanford Health
Stanford Campus
300 Pasteur Drive
Room 80301
Stanford, CA 94305
Mon.-Fri. 9 AM-4 PM
Tel: 650-723-6422
Fax: 650-725-5028

COLORADO

DENVER
Rocky Mountain Drug Consultation Center
8802 E. 9th Avenue
Denver, CO 80220
Mon.-Fri. 8 AM-4:30 PM
Tel: 303-893-3784
900-370-3784
(Outside Denver
County, $1.99
per minute)

Drug Information Center
University of Colorado
Health Science Center
4200 E. 9th Avenue, Box C239
Denver, CO 80262
Mon.-Fri. 8:30 AM-4:30 PM
Tel: 303-315-8489
Fax: 303-270-3353

CONNECTICUT

FARMINGTON
Drug Information Service
University of Connecticut Health Center
263 Farmington Ave.
Farmington, CT 06030
Mon.-Fri. 8 AM-4:30 PM
Tel: 860-679-3783

HARTFORD
Drug Information Center
Hartford Hospital
P.O. Box 5037
80 Seymour Street
Hartford, CT 06102
Mon.-Fri. 8:30 AM-5 PM
Tel: 860-545-2221
860-545-2961 (main
pharmacy) after hours
Fax: 860-545-2415

NEW HAVEN
Drug Information Center
Yale-New Haven Hospital
20 York Street
New Haven, CT 06504
Mon.-Fri. 8:15 AM-4:45 PM
Tel: 203-688-2248
Fax: 203-737-4229

DISTRICT OF COLUMBIA

Drug Information Center
Washington Hospital Center
110 Irving St., NW, Room B147
Washington, DC 20010
Mon.- Fri. 7:30 AM-4 PM
Tel: 202-877-6646
Fax: 202-877-8925

Drug Information Service
Howard University Hospital
2041 Georgia Ave. NW
Washington, DC 20060
Mon.-Fri. 9 AM-5 PM
Tel: 202-865-1325
Fax: 202-745-3731

FLORIDA

GAINESVILLE
Drug Information &
Pharmacy Resource Center
Shands Hospital at
University of Florida
P.O. Box 100316
Gainesville, FL 32610-0316
Mon.-Fri. 9 AM- 5 PM
Tel: 352-395-0408
(for healthcare professionals only)
Fax: 352-338-9860

JACKSONVILLE
Drug Information Service
University Medical Center
655 W. 8th Street
Jacksonville, FL 32209
Mon.-Fri. 8 AM-5 PM
Tel: 904-549-4095
Fax: 904-549-4272

MIAMI
Drug Information Center (119)
Miami VA Medical Center
1201 NW 16th Street
Miami, FL 33125
Mon.-Fri. 7:30 AM-4:30 PM
Tel: 305-324-3237
Fax: 305-324-3394

GEORGIA

ATLANTA
Emory University Hospital Dept. of Pharmaceutical Services-Drug Information
1364 Clifton Rd. NE
Atlanta, GA 30322
Mon.-Fri. 8:30 AM-5 PM
Tel: 404-712-4640
Fax: 404-712-7577

Drug Information Service
Northside Hospital
1000 Johnson Ferry Road NE
Atlanta, GA 30342
Mon.-Fri. 9 AM-4 PM
Tel: 404-851-8676
Fax: 404-851-8682

AUGUSTA
Drug Information Center
University of Georgia
Medical College of GA
Room BIW201
1120 15th Street
Augusta, GA 30912-5600
Mon.-Fri. 8:30 AM-5 PM
Tel: 706-721-2887
Fax: 706-721-3827

IDAHO

POCATELLO
Idaho Drug Information Service
MFU 3 Box 8092
Pocatello, ID 83209
Mon.-Fri. 8 AM-5 PM
Tel: 208-236-4689
Fax: 208-236-4687

ILLINOIS

CHICAGO
Drug Information Center
Northwestern Memorial Hospital
250 E. Superior Street
Wesley 153
Chicago, IL 60611
Mon.-Fri. 8 AM-5 PM
Tel: 312-908-7573
Fax: 312-908-7956

Saint Joseph Hospital
2900 N. Lake Shore Drive
Chicago, IL 60657
8 AM-5 PM
Tel: 312-665-3140
Fax: 312-665-3462

Drug Information Services
University of Chicago
5841 S. Maryland Ave.
MC 0010
Chicago, IL 60637
Mon.-Fri. 8 AM-5 PM
Tel: 773-702-1388
Fax: 773-702-6631

Drug Information Center
University of Illinois at Chicago
Room C300, MC 883
1740 W. Taylor St.
Chicago, IL 60612
Mon.-Fri. 8 AM-4 PM
Tel: 312-996-0209
Fax: 312-413-4146

HARVEY
Drug Information Center
Ingalls Memorial Hospital
1 Ingalls Drive
Harvey, IL 60426
Mon.-Fri. 8 AM-4:30 PM
Tel: 708-333-2300
Fax: 708-210-3108

HINES
Drug Information Service
Hines Veterans Administration Hospital
Inpatient Pharmacy (119B)
P.O. Box 5000
Hines, IL 60141-5000
Mon.-Fri. 8 AM-4:30 PM
Tel: 708-343-7200

PARK RIDGE
Drug Information Center
Lutheran General Hospital
1775 Dempster St.
Park Ridge, IL 60068
Mon.-Fri. 7:30 AM-4 PM
Tel: 847-696-8128

INDIANA

INDIANAPOLIS
Drug Information Center
St. Vincent Hospital and Health Services
2001 W. 86th St.
P.O. Box 40970
Indianapolis, IN 46260
Mon.-Fri. 8 AM-4 PM
Tel: 317-338-3200
Fax: 317-338-3041

Indiana University Medical Center/Pharmacy
Dept. OH1451
550 N. University Blvd.
Indianapolis, IN 46202
Mon.-Fri. 8 AM-4:30 PM
Tel: 317-274-0353
Fax: 317-274-2327

IOWA

DES MOINES
Regional Drug Information Center
Mercy Hospital Medical Center
400 University Ave.
Des Moines, IA 50314
Mon.-Fri. 8 AM-6 PM
Tel: 515-247-3286 (answered 7 days/week, 24 hours)
Fax: 515-247-3966

IOWA CITY
Drug Information Center
University of Iowa Hospitals and Clinics
200 Hawkins Dr.
Iowa City, IA 52242
Mon.-Fri. 8 AM-5 PM
Tel: 319-356-2600
Fax: 319-356-4545

SIOUX CITY
Iowa Poison Center
2720 Stone Park Blvd.
Sioux City, IA 51104
Tel: 712-277-2222
800-352-2222 (IA)
Fax: 712-279-7852

KANSAS

KANSAS CITY
Drug Information Center
University of Kansas Medical Center
3901 Rainbow Blvd.
Kansas City, KS 66160
Mon.-Fri. 8 AM-6 PM
Tel: 913-588-2328
Fax: 913-588-2350

KENTUCKY

LEXINGTON
Drug Information Center
Chandler Medical Center
College of Pharmacy
University of Kentucky
800 Rose St., C-117
Lexington, KY 40536-0084
Mon.-Fri. 8 AM-5 PM
Tel: 606-323-5320
Fax: 606-323-2049

LOUISIANA

MONROE
Drug Information Center
St. Francis Medical Center
309 Jackson St.
Monroe, LA 71210-1901
Tel: 318-327-4250
Fax: 318-327-4125

NEW ORLEANS
Xavier University
Drug Information Center
Tulane University Hospital and Clinic
Box HC12
1415 Tulane Ave.
New Orleans, LA 70112
Mon.-Fri. 9 AM-5 PM
Tel: 504-588-5670
Fax: 504-588-5862

MARYLAND

ANDREWS AFB
Drug Information Services
89th Med Gp/SGQP
1050 W. Perimeter Rd.
Suite F1-121
Andrews AFB, MD 20331
Mon.-Fri. 7:30 AM-6 PM
Tel: 301-981-4209
Fax: 301-981-4544

ANNAPOLIS
Drug Information Services
The Anne Arundel Medical Center
Franklin & Cathedral Streets
Annapolis, MD 21401
7 days/week, 24 hours
Tel: 410-267-1130
410-267-1000
Fax: 410-267-1628

BALTIMORE
Drug Information Services
Franklin Square Hospital Center
9000 Franklin Square Dr.
Baltimore, MD 21237
7 days/week, 24 hours
Tel: 410-682-7744
Fax: 410-682-8181

Drug Information Service
Johns Hopkins Hospital
600 N. Wolfe St., Halsted 503
Baltimore, MD 21287-6180
Mon.-Fri. 8:30 AM-5 PM
Tel: 410-955-6348
Fax: 410-955-8283

Drug Information Center
University of Maryland at Baltimore
School of Pharmacy
506 W. Fayette, 3rd Floor
Baltimore, MD 21201
Mon.-Fri. 8:30 AM-5 PM
Tel: 410-706-7568
Fax: 410-706-0897

BETHESDA
Drug Information Service
National Institutes of Health
Building 10, Room 1S-259
10 Center Drive (MSC1196)
Bethesda, MD 20892-1196
Mon.-Fri. 8:30 AM-5 PM
Tel: 301-496-2407
Fax: 301-496-0210

EASTON
Drug Information Center
Memorial Hospital
219 S. Washington St.
Easton, MD 21601
7 days/week, 7 AM - Midnight
Tel: 410-822-1000
Fax: 410-820-9489

MASSACHUSETTS

BOSTON
Drug Information Services
Brigham and Women's Hospital
75 Frances St.
Boston, MA 02115
Mon.-Fri. 7 AM-3:30 PM
Tel: 617-732-7166
Fax: 617-732-7497

Drug Information Service
New England Medical Center Pharmacy
750 Washington St., Box 420
Boston, MA 02111
Mon.-Fri. 9 AM-5 PM
Tel: 617-636-8985
Fax: 617-636-5638

WORCESTER
Drug Information Center
U.M.M.C. Hospital
55 Lake Ave. North
Worcester, MA 01655
Mon.-Fri. 8:30 AM-5 PM
Tel: 508-856-3456
508-856-2775
Fax: 508-856-1850

MICHIGAN

ANN ARBOR
Drug Information Service
University of Michigan Medical Center
1500 East Medical Center Dr.
UHB2 D301 Box 0008
Ann Arbor, MI 48109
Mon.-Fri. 8 AM-5 PM
Tel: 734-936-8200
734-936-8251
Fax: 734-923-7027

DETROIT
Drug Information Services
Harper Hospital
3990 John R. St.
Detroit, MI 48201
Mon.-Fri. 8 AM-5 PM
Tel: 313-745-2006
313-745-8216
(after hours)
Fax: 313-745-1628

LANSING
Drug Information Center
Sparrow Hospital
1215 E. Michigan Ave.
Lansing, MI 48912
Mon.-Fri. 8 AM-4:30 PM
Tel: 517-483-2444
Fax: 517-483-2088

PONTIAC
Drug Information Center
St. Joseph Mercy Hospital
900 Woodward
Pontiac, MI 48341
Mon.-Fri. 8 AM-4:30 PM
Tel: 248-858-3055
Fax: 248-858-3010

ROYAL OAK
Drug Information Services
William Beaumont Hospital
3601 West 13 Mile Road
Royal Oak, MI 48073-6769
Mon.-Fri. 8 AM-4:30 PM
Tel: 248-551-4077
Fax: 248-551-4046

SOUTHFIELD
Drug Information Service
Providence Hospital
16001 West 9 Mile Rd.
P.O. Box 2043
Southfield, MI 48075
Mon.-Fri. 8 AM-4 PM
Tel: 248-424-3125
Fax: 248-424-5364

MINNESOTA

ROCHESTER
Drug Information Service
Mayo Clinic
1216 2nd St., SW
Rochester, MN 55902
Mon.-Fri. 8 AM-5 PM
Tel: 507-255-5062
507-255-5732
(after hours)
Fax: 507-255-7556

MISSISSIPPI

JACKSON
Drug Information Center
University of Mississippi Medical Center
2500 N. State St.
Jackson, MS 39216
Mon.-Fri. 8 AM-5 PM
Tel: 601-984-2060
(on call 24 hours)
Fax: 601-984-2063

MISSOURI

SPRINGFIELD
Drug Information &
Clinical Research Services
1235 E. Cherokee
Springfield, MO 65804
Mon.-Fri. 7:30 AM-4:30 PM
Tel: 417-885-3488
Fax: 417-888-7788

ST. JOSEPH
Drug Information Service
Heartland Hospital West
801 Faraon St.
St. Joseph, MO 64501
Mon.-Sat. 8 AM-8 PM
Tel: 816-271-7582
Fax: 816-271-7590

NEBRASKA

OMAHA
Drug Information Service
School of Pharmacy
Creighton University
2500 California Plaza
Omaha, NE 68178
Mon.-Fri. 8:30 AM-4:30 PM
Tel: 402-280-5101
Fax: 402-280-5149

Drug Information Center
Pharmacy Department, NHS
981090 Nebraska Medical Center
Omaha, NE 68198-1090
Mon.-Fri. 8 AM-4:30 PM
Tel: 402-559-7205
402-559-6747
Fax: 402-559-5463

NEW MEXICO

ALBUQUERQUE
New Mexico Poison &
Drug Information Center
University of New Mexico
Albuquerque, NM 87131-1076
7 days/week, 24 hours
Tel: 505-272-2222
800-432-6866 (NM)
Fax: 505-272-5892

NEW YORK

BROOKLYN
International Drug Information Center
Long Island University
Arnold & Marie Schwartz College of Pharmacy
1 University Plaza
RM-Z509
Brooklyn, NY 11201
Mon.-Fri. 9 AM-5 PM
Tel: 718-488-1064
Fax: 718-780-4056

COOPERSTOWN
Drug Information Center
The Mary Imogene Bassett Hospital
1 Atwell Rd.
Cooperstown, NY 13326
Mon.-Fri. 8:30 AM-5 PM
Tel: 607-547-3686
Fax: 607-547-3629

NEW YORK CITY
Drug Information Center
Bellevue Hospital Center
462 1st Ave.
New York, NY 10016
Mon.-Fri. 9 AM-5 PM
Tel: 212-562-6504
Fax: 212-562-6503

Drug Information Center
Memorial Sloan-Kettering Cancer Center
1275 York Ave.
RM S-702
New York, NY 10021
Mon.-Fri. 9 AM-5 PM
Tel: 212-639-7552
Fax: 212-639-2171

Drug Information Center
Mount Sinai Medical Center
1 Gustave Levy Place
New York, NY 10029
Mon.-Fri. 9 AM-5 PM
Tel: 212-241-6619
Fax: 212-348-7927

Drug Information Service
The New York Hospital
Cornell Medical Center
525 E. 68th St.
New York, NY 10021
Mon.-Fri. 9 AM-5 PM
Tel: 212-746-0741
Fax: 212-746-8506

ROCHESTER
Drug Information Service
Dept. of Pharmacy - Poison Division
University of Rochester
601 Elmwood Ave.
Rochester, NY 14642
24 HRS. 7 Days Week
Tel: 716-275-3718
716-275-2681
(after hours)
Fax: 716-473-9842

STONY BROOK
Suffolk Drug Information Center
University Hospital
S.U.N.Y. - Stony Brook
Room 3-559, Z7310
Stony Brook, NY 11794-7310
Mon.-Fri. 8 AM-3:00 PM
No Holidays
Tel: 516-444-2672
516-444-2680
(after hours)
Fax: 516-444-7935

NORTH CAROLINA

BUIES CREEK
Drug Information Center
School of Pharmacy
Campbell University
P.O. Box 1090
Buies Creek, NC 27506
Mon.-Fri. 8:30 AM - 4:30 PM
Tel: 910-893-1478
800-327-5467 (NC)
Fax: 910-893-1476

CHAPEL HILL
Drug Information Center
University of North Carolina Hospitals
101 Manning Drive
Chapel Hill, NC 27514
Mon.-Fri. 8 AM-4:30 PM
Tel: 919-966-2373
Fax: 919-966-1791

GREENSBORO
Triad Poison Center
Moses H. Cone Memorial Hospital
1200 N. Elm St.
Greensboro, NC 27401
7 days/week, 24 hours
Tel: 336-574-8105
Fax: 336-574-7198

GREENVILLE
Eastern Carolina Drug Information Center
Pitt County Memorial Hospital
Dept. of Pharmacy Service
2100 Stantonsburg Rd.
Greenville, NC 27835
Mon.-Fri. 8 AM- 5 PM
Tel: 919-816-4257
Fax: 919-816-7425

WINSTON-SALEM
Drug Information Service Center
Wake-Forest University
Baptist Medical Center
Medical Center Blvd.
Winston-Salem, NC 27157
Mon.-Fri. 8 AM-5 PM
Tel: 336-716-2037
Fax: 336-716-2186

OHIO

ADA
Drug Information Center
Raabe College of Pharmacy
Ohio Northern University
Ada, OH 45810
Mon.-Fri. 9 AM - 5 PM
Tel: 419-772-2307
Fax: 419-772-2289

CLEVELAND
Drug Information Center
Cleveland Clinic Foundation
9500 Euclid Avenue
Cleveland, OH 44195
Mon.-Fri. 8 AM - 5 PM
Tel: 216-444-6456
Fax: 216-445-6221

COLUMBUS
Central Ohio Poison Center
700 Children's Drive
Columbus, OH 43205
24 HRS. 7 Days/Week
Tel: 614-228-1323
800-682-7625 (OH)
Fax: 614-221-2672

Drug Information Center
Ohio State University Hospital
Dept. of Pharmacy
Doan Hall 368
410 W. 10th Avenue
Columbus, OH 43210-1228
Mon.-Fri. 8 AM - 4 PM
Tel: 614-293-8679
Fax: 614-293-3264

Drug Information Center
Riverside Methodist Hospital
3535 Olantangy River Road
Columbus, OH 43214
8 AM - 5 PM
Tel: 614-566-5425
Fax: 614-566-5447

OKLAHOMA

OKLAHOMA CITY

Drug Information Center
Integris Health
3300 Northwest Expressway
Oklahoma City, OK 73112
Mon.-Fri. 8 AM-4:30 PM
Tel: 405-949-3660
Fax: 405-951-8274

Drug Information Center
Presbyterian Hospital
700 NE 13th St.
Oklahoma City, OK 73104
Mon.-Fri. 7:30 AM-3:30 PM
Tel: 405-271-6226
Fax: 405-271-6281

TULSA

Drug Information Service
St. Francis Hospital
6161 S. Yale Ave.
Tulsa, OK 74136
Mon.-Fri. 9 AM-5:30 PM
Tel: 918-494-6339
Fax: 918-494-1893

PENNSYLVANIA

PHILADELPHIA

Drug Information Center
Temple University Hospital
Dept. of Pharmacy
Broad and Ontario St.
Philadelphia, PA 19140
Mon.-Fri. 8 AM-4:30 PM
Tel: 215-707-4644
Fax: 215-707-3463

Drug Information Center
Thomas Jefferson University Hospital
111 S. 11th
Philadelphia, PA 19107-5098
Mon.-Fri. 8 AM-5 PM
Tel: 215-955-8877
Fax: 215-923-3316

PITTSBURGH

The Pharmaceutical Information Center
Mylan School of Pharmacy
Duquene University
431 Mellon Hall
Pittsburgh, PA 15282
Mon.-Fri. 8 AM-4 PM
Tel: 412-396-4600
Fax: 412-396-4488

Drug Information and
Pharmacoepidemiology Center
University of Pittsburgh Medical Center
137 Victoria Hall
Pittsburgh, PA 15261
Mon.-Fri. 8:30 AM-4:30 PM
Tel: 412-624-3784
Fax: 412-624-6350

UPLAND

Drug Information Center
Crozer-Chester Medical Center
Dept. of Pharmacy
1 Medical Center Blvd.
Upland, PA 19013
Mon.-Fri. 8 AM-4:30 PM
Tel: 610-447-2851
610-447-2862 (after hours)
Fax: 215-447-2820

WILLIAMSPORT

Drug Information Center
Susquehanna Health System
Rural Avenue Campus
Williamsport, PA 17701
Mon.-Fri. 8 AM-4 PM
Tel: 717-321-3289
Fax: 717-321-3230

PUERTO RICO

SAN JUAN

Centro Information Medicamentos
Escuela de Farmacia RCM
P.O. Box 365067
San Juan, PR 00936-5067
Mon.-Fri. 8 AM-4:30 PM
Tel: 787-763-0196
Fax: 787-763-0196

RHODE ISLAND

PROVIDENCE

Drug Information Service
Dept. of Pharmacy
Rhode Island Hospital
593 Eddy Street
Providence, RI 02903
7 days/week, 24 hours
Tel: 401-444-5547
Fax: 401-444-8062

SOUTH CAROLINA

CHARLESTON

Drug Information Service
Medical University of South Carolina
171 Ashley Ave.
Room 604-SFX
Charleston, SC 29425-0810
Mon.-Fri. 8 AM-5:30 PM
Tel: 803-792-3896
800-922-5250
Fax: 803-792-5532

SPARTANBURG

Drug Information Center
Spartanburg Regional Medical Center
101 E. Wood St.
Spartanburg, SC 29303
Mon.-Fri. 8 AM-5 PM
Tel: 864-560-6910
Fax: 864-560-6017

TENNESSEE

KNOXVILLE

Drug Information Center
University of Tennessee Medical Center
1924 Alcoa Highway
Knoxville, TN 37920-6999
Mon.-Fri. 8 AM-4:30 PM
Tel: 423-544-9125

MEMPHIS

South East Regional
Drug Information Center
VA Medical Center
1030 Jefferson Ave.
Memphis, TN 38104
Mon.-Fri. 7:30 AM-4 PM
Tel: 901-523-8990

Drug Information Center
University of Tennessee
847 Monroe Avenue
Suite 238, Memphis, TN 38163
Mon.-Fri. 8:30 AM - 4:30 PM
Tel: 901-448-5555
Fax: 901-448-5419

TEXAS

GALVESTON

Drug Information Center
University of Texas Medical Branch
301 University Blvd. - G01
Galveston, TX 77555-0701
Mon.-Fri. 8 AM-5 PM
Tel: 409-772-2734
Fax: 409-747-5222

HOUSTON

Drug Information Center
Ben Taub General Hospital
Texas Southern University/HCHD
1504 Taub Loop
Houston, TX 77030
Mon.-Fri. 8 AM-5 PM
Tel: 713-793-2917
Fax: 713-793-2937

Drug Information Center
Methodist Hospital
6565 Fannin (MSDB109)
Houston, TX 77030
Mon.-Fri. 8 AM-5 PM
Tel: 713-790-4190
Fax: 713-793-1224

LACKLAND A.F.B.

Drug Information Center
Dept. of Pharmacy
Wilford Hall Medical Center
2200 Berquist Dr., Suite 1
Lackland A.F.B., TX 78236
Mon.-Fri. 7:30 AM-5 PM
Tel: 210-292-7100

LUBBOCK

Methodist Hospital Drug Information
and Consultation Service
3615 19th St.
Lubbock, TX 79410
Mon.-Fri. 8 AM-5 PM
Tel: 806-793-4012
(Attn: Pharmacy)
Fax: 806-784-5323

TEMPLE

Drug Information Center
Scott and White Memorial Hospital
2401 S. 31st St.
Temple, TX 76508
Mon.-Fri. 8 AM-6 PM
Tel: 254-724-4636
Fax: 254-724-1731

UTAH

SALT LAKE CITY

Drug Information Center
University of Utah Hospital
Dept. of Pharmacy Services
Room A-050
50 N. Medical Dr.
Salt Lake City, UT 84132
Mon.-Fri. 8:30 AM-4:30 PM
Tel: 801-581-2073
Fax: 801-585-6688

WEST VIRGINIA

MORGANTOWN

West Virginia Drug Information Center
WV University-Robert C. Byrd
Health Sciences Center
1124 HSN, P.O. Box 9550
Morgantown, WV 26506
Tel: 304-293-6640
800-352-2501 (WV)
Fax: 304-293-7672

WISCONSIN

MADISON

University of Wisconsin Hospital & Clinics
600 Highland Ave.
Madison, WI 53792
Voice mail/24 hrs. a day,
responses in 3 days
Tel: 608-262-1315
Fax: 608-263-9424

WYOMING

LARAMIE

Drug Information Center
University of Wyoming
P.O. Box 3375
Laramie, WY 82071
Mon.-Fri. 8 AM-5 PM
Tel: 307-766-6128
Fax: 307-766-2953

II. Product Development and Sourcing

Our consulting activity is done in close collaboration with the developers and manufacturers of herbal medicines. Based on our scientific and marketing knowledge we are in a position to advise intelligent and innovative product development.

Our international network of contacts in the healthcare industry provides access to the best available starting materials, the best analytical and development facilities and techniques of university and independent laboratories for pharmacological research and CROs, as well as experienced research institutions to perform human pharmacological and clinical studies.

III. R&D, Pharmacological and Clinical Research

We have performed dozens of international pharmacological and clinical trials with botanicals, including plants like Ginkgo biloba, St. John's Wort, Valerian, Garlic, Ginger, Hawthorn, Echinacea, and various others. Our activities range from the comprehensive clinical development of a research plan to the actual writing of the study protocols, supervising or actually performing the investigations.

We cooperate with a number of CROs and universities, which are experienced in various types of studies ranging from human pharmacology to placebo controlled and comparative trials and drug monitoring trials.

Our Staff:
PhytoPharm Consulting is a Berlin based company staffed with dedicated and well-trained herbal experts: physicians, botanists, pharmacists, chemists, and herbal-practitioners as well as marketing, regulatory, and PR specialists with a combined business experience.

Internet:
If you are interested in further details about our company or are looking for other subjects in the field of botanicals, please feel free to check out our web page www.phytonet.com.

The web site includes more than 500 botanical links, which may be of interest to you.

IV. Regulatory Affairs, Patents, Proprietary Technologies

1. Our 'regulatory affairs' Department is experienced in the worldwide legislation for botanicals. We are actively involved in the international botanical legislation process. Complete registration dossiers including expert reports are developed inhouse, as are IND applications, etc.

2. Patent protection and proprietary technologies for botanicals are a special expertise of ours. We work closely with experienced development companies to achieve a product-differentiation including patent protection or development of proprietary technologies.

This starts at the level of the seed material, plant specific SOPs for growth and harvesting, continues with the extraction process and refinement due to the possibilities of specific indications/use patents for botanical products.

V. Strategic Marketing and PR Support

Based on our knowledge of the market's present and future trends, critical issues, and potential technologies, we are developing strategies for companies already active in the herbal market and for those who want to enter the market.

We can supply complete marketing and PR support. Our marketing and PR activities are based on scientific principles, with the goal of differentiating the compound by quality, safety, and efficacy. We co-operate with sister companies in the field of advertisement and scientific PR and can provide our own speakers or other independent researchers from major universities internationally.

VI. International Alliances

Our strong position within the pharmaceutical and herbal industry worldwide gives us the framework to support companies developing new technologies or products, companies looking for products or collaboration as well as companies interested in mergers and acquisitions.

A special strength and top priority are our strong base in Europe and excellent contacts in the USA to support exchange of know-how of products and the establishment of co-operations, joint ventures, or the search for mergers and acquisitions.